EYE, RETINA, AND VISUAL SYSTEM OF THE MOUSE

EYE, RETINA, AND VISUAL SYSTEM OF THE MOUSE

Edited by Leo M. Chalupa and Robert W. Williams

THE MIT PRESS
CAMBRIDGE, MASSACHUSETTS
LONDON, ENGLAND

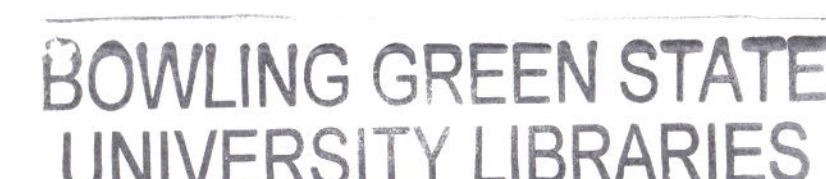

For information about special quantity discounts, please email special_sales@mitpress.mit.edu

This book was set in Baskerville by SNP Best-set Typesetter Ltd., Hong Kong.

Printed and bound in the United States of America.

Library of Congress Cataloging-in-Publication Data

Eye, retina, and visual system of the mouse / Leo M. Chalupa and Robert W. Williams, editors.
p. cm.
Includes bibliographical references and index.
ISBN 978-0-262-03381-7 (hardcover : alk. paper)
1. Mice—Sense organs. 2. Eye. 3. Visual pathways. I. Chalupa, Leo M. II. Williams, Robert W., 1952–
QL737.R6E94 2008
573.8′819353—dc22

2007047445

10 9 8 7 6 5 4 3 2 1

CONTENTS

IV DEVELOPMENT OF THE MOUSE EYE 255

V DEVELOPMENT AND PLASTICITY OF RETINAL PROJECTIONS AND VISUOTOPIC MAPS 377

VII ADVANCED GENOMIC TECHNOLOGIES: APPLICATIONS TO THE MOUSE VISUAL SYSTEM 591

PREFACE

The publication of this volume on the mouse eye and visual system seems overdue, given the burst of studies that have appeared on this topic in recent years. As the chapters in this volume illustrate, mouse models have already contributed to a wide range of scientific breakthroughs for a significant number of ocular and neurological diseases. They have also allowed us to address fundamental issues that could not be pursued using other experimental models.

As is often the case, technical rather than conceptual advances have induced or driven the move to the mouse. The major factor has been the comparatively recent ability to produce mice with precisely defined changes in gene sequence—so-called transgenic and knockout mice. As a result of this powerful technology, genes can now be turned on or off in specific cell types at specific stages of development. Of equal importance, mouse genes can now be swapped for their human equivalents. This advance should ultimately permit us to humanize cells and tissues as complex as the retina, which will allow us to test new therapies in a controlled experimental context.

Although the power of mouse models is now taken for granted, it is worth noting that until fairly recently, study of the mouse visual system was a backwater of vision research. Size matters, and the large eyes of rabbits, cats, and cows were much more tractable for biochemical, histological, and functional studies. However, a small and dedicated cadre of radiation biologists and geneticists began to exploit mice for vision research, collecting and analyzing the stream of spontaneous and induced mutations at the Jackson Laboratory, at Oak Ridge National Laboratory, at the MRC Harwell, at the German Research Center for Environmental Health (GSF, Munich), and at universities and mouse breeding and research centers. Richard Sidman, Jin Kinoshita, Matthew LaVail, Ursula Dräger, and others helped to build the mouse resource infrastructure that we now take for granted, mapping and characterizing some of the first retinal degeneration, cataract, and pigmentation mutations that disturbed visual system function.

The main activity in vision research following the catalytic studies of David Hubel and Torsten Wiesel in the 1960s and 1970s centered on fundamental problems in visual neurophysiology, development, plasticity, and pathology. Cats and macaques were the dominant species used in this program of discovery. These models are still making major contributions to our understanding of mechanisms of vision and visual system development. Because of its small size, experimental fragility, and low acuity, the mouse was generally regarded as a compromised model for this kind of systems neuroscience. Those scientists interested in development typically followed the lead of Roger Sperry and colleagues and turned to cold-blooded vertebrates, particularly fishes and frogs. The sudden introduction of transgenic and knockout technology by Rudolph Jaenisch, Mario Capecchi, Martin Evans, and Oliver Smithies radically restructured experimental possibilities. What once seemed risky or even foolish—for example, functional studies of mouse retinal ganglion cells and visual cortex—now seemed well warranted if only the experimental methods could be miniaturized to deal with an eye with an axial length of 2 mm and a brain with a total mass of 450 mg. It soon became obvious just how informative it would be to exploit this species to modify gene sequences and to test effects on development, function, plasticity, and disease progression.

This book can be considered a compendium of results from the first wave of studies. We hope that it will answer the question of just how useful mouse models can be as part of the exchange between experimental and clinical research. Study of these mouse models has already demonstrated real translational prowess. However, it is just a beginning, since large gaps in our knowledge remain to be filled, some of which, no doubt, are still blissfully outside our awareness.

We owe thanks to many colleagues. First, we are grateful to Drs. Patsy Nishina and Maureen McCall, as well as the National Eye Institute of the National Institutes of Health and the Jackson Laboratory, for having organized and supported meetings and workshops in 2004 and 2006 on the laboratory mouse in vision research. These meetings helped motivate the assembly of this book. We also thank the staff at MIT Press. For several decades, MIT Press has helped promote vision research by publishing wide-ranging texts on vision from engineering, computational, biological, psychological, and theoretical points of view. In particular, we are grateful to Barbara Murphy and Meagan Stacey for their expert assistance in bringing this project to fruition. Finally, we thank the authors whose work is included herein, for their contributions to this volume and for the sacrifices they made to meet the deadlines necessary to bring this project to a successful conclusion.

I INTRODUCTION TO THE MOUSE AS A SPECIES AND RESEARCH MODEL

1 Evolutionary History of the Genus *Mus*

PRISCILLA K. TUCKER

Knowing the evolutionary history of the house mouse is valuable not just for evolutionary and systematic biologists, who study the diversity of life, but also for biomedical researchers, who use the mouse as a research model with the assumption that certain discoveries can be generalized to humans. Understanding the biological significance of a new finding ultimately requires comparisons among populations and species in the context of their evolutionary history. For example, a newly discovered feature of the mouse may be unique to a population or to the species, it may be conserved only among species closely related to the mouse, or it may be conserved across more distantly related species such as mouse and human. Comparisons among taxa in the context of their evolutionary history also provide the researcher the ability to determine how genes, genetic or developmental pathways, physiological features, or complex traits have changed over time, and whether observed similarities between the mouse and other species are due to common ancestry or to convergence (independent evolution).

This chapter introduces the reader to the evolutionary history of species in the genus *Mus*, to which house mice and laboratory inbred strains belong. It includes an overview of species diversity in the genus and a more comprehensive account of the evolutionary history of the house mouse, the *Mus musculus* complex, from which laboratory strains are derived. It concludes with a summary of our current understanding of the evolutionary relationships among members of the genus as depicted in a phylogeny.

The house mouse is a member of the Order Rodentia, one of 29 currently recognized orders of mammals (Wilson and Reeder, 2005). The common laboratory rat (*Rattus norvegicus*) is also a member of this order. Rodentia and the Order Lagomorpha (rabbits, hares, and pikas) are considered sister taxa, each other's closest relatives, and together are thought to be closely related to a group comprising the Orders Primates, Dermoptera (flying lemurs), and Scandentia (tree shrews) (Murphy et al., 2001; Carleton and Musser, 2005; Kriegs et al., 2006). In contrast, the cat, a taxon that is also used in vision research, is a member of the Order Carnivora, a taxonomic group proposed to be more closely related to the Orders Perissodactyla (horses), Artiodactyla (even-toed ungulates), and Cetacea (whales, dolphins, and porpoises) than to either Rodentia or Primates (Murphy et al., 2001; Kriegs et al., 2006).

The genus *Mus* Linnaeus, 1758, includes a monophyletic group of 30 or more species belonging to the subfamily Murinae in the speciose rodent family Muridae (Musser and Carleton, 2005; Cucchi et al., 2006; Shimada et al., 2007). *Mus* species are found throughout the Old World from southern Africa to eastern Asia. They occupy ecologically diverse habitats such as tropical montane forests, grasslands, and deserts (Suzuki et al., 2004; Musser and Carleton, 2005; Veyrunes et al., 2005). Like many other murine rodents, most are thought to be active at night. The genus can be distinguished from other murine genera using a combination of morphological features (Marshall, 1977a, 1997b, 1978, 1981) and molecular characters (reviewed in Suzuki et al., 2004, and Veyrunes et al., 2005). Utilizing a molecular clock, a combination of mitochondrial and nuclear genes, and calibration points based on fossil dates, researchers have estimated the divergence of the genus *Mus* from other murine lineages as occurring between 11 and 8 million years ago (mya) (Chevret et al., 2005; Veyrunes et al., 2005). Fossil evidence (Flynn and Jacobs, 1983; Jacobs and Downs, 1994) and phylogeographic considerations (Suzuki et al., 2004; Veyrunes et al., 2005) place the origin of the genus in Asia.

Diversity in the genus Mus

Based on morphological characters and diploid chromosome numbers, Marshall (1977a, 1977b, 1978, 1981, 1998) recognized four subgenera: *Coelomys*, *Nannomys*, *Pyromys*, and *Mus*. Biochemical and molecular studies (Bonhomme et al., 1984; She et al., 1990; Lundrigan and Tucker, 1994; Sourrouille et al., 1995; Lundrigen et al., 2002) based on limited taxonomic sampling verified that the subgenera represent discrete evolutionary lineages (figure 1.1). The monophyly of each of these subgenera, with one exception, described subsequently, was also confirmed with morphological and molecular analyses of multiple species from each subgenus (Chevret et al., 2003, 2005), and a suite of key morphological characters to distinguish among the three Eurasian subgenera, *Pyromys*, *Coelomys*, and *Mus*, was

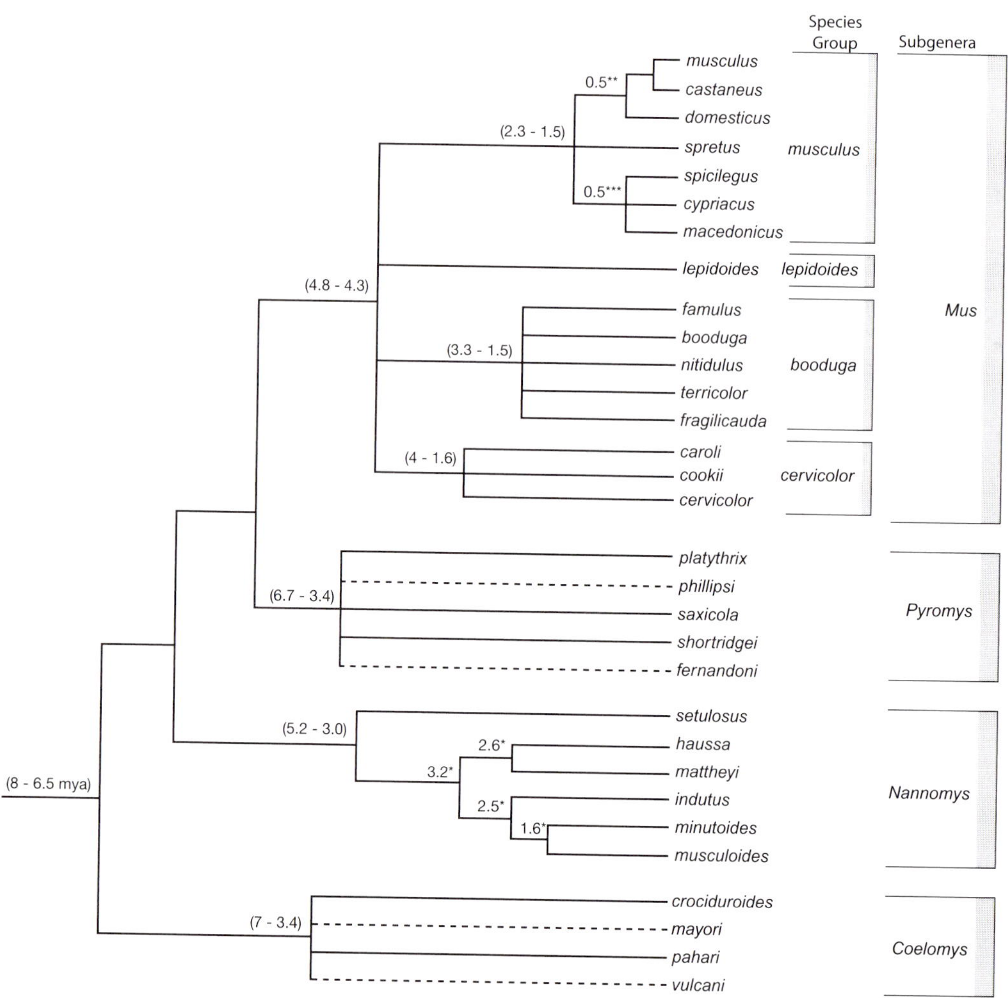

FIGURE 1.1 A synthetic phylogeny depicting evolutionary relationships among subgenera and species in the genus *Mus*. Species belonging to the four subgenera are bracketed. The phylogeny is based on recent studies using different combinations of molecular characters (Lundrigan et al., 2002; Auffray et al., 2003; Chevret et al., 2003, 2005; Suzuki et al., 2004; Tucker et al., 2005; Veyrunes et al., 2005; Cucchi et al., 2006; Shimada et al., 2007) and chromosomal characters (Veyrunes et al., 2006). Polytomies (unresolved nodes) indicate uncertainty of relationship. Estimates for divergence times (in parentheses) are ranges based on the variation in estimates calculated using DNA-DNA hybridization (She et al., 1990) or different combinations of genes, taxa, and fossil calibration dates (Suzuki et al., 2004; Chevret et al., 2005; Veyrunes et al., 2005; Cucchi et al., 2006). Where ranges are not given, divergence time estimates are from *Veyrunes et al., 2005, **Suzuki et al., 2004, and ***Cucchi et al., 2006. The recent addition of molecular data from *Mus lepidoides* to the total data (K. Aplin, pers. comm.) suggests a topology for the subgenus *Mus* in which the *M. cervicolor* group is basal and the *M. booduga* group is sister to a lineage giving rise to *M. lepidoides* and *M. musculus* species groups. *Dashed lines* indicate taxa not represented in any of the phylogenetic analyses already cited.

proposed (Chevret et al., 2003). These characters include qualitative features of the skull and dentition and the presence or absence of spinous guard hairs. Some authors (Bonhomme et al., 1984; She et al., 1990) have argued that the four subgenera should be elevated to the rank of genera based on the degree of difference in biochemical and molecular characters. Others contend that the level of genetic divergence among subgenera does not merit a change in rank (Chevret et al., 2005). Utilizing a molecular clock, different combinations of mitochondrial and nuclear genes, and different calibration points based on fossil dates, researchers have estimated the divergence of the four subgenera from 8 to 6.5 mya (Suzuki et al., 2004; Chevret et al., 2005; Veyrunes et al., 2005). For comparison, human and chimpanzee are thought to have diverged from a common ancestor approximately 6–7 mya (Brunet et al., 2002).

THE SUBGENUS *COELOMYS* THOMAS 1915: SHREW MICE Mice of this subgenus are large with a shrewlike appearance characterized by small eyes and long noses. There are four recognized species, all of which inhabit mountain forests.

They are *Mus mayori*, from Sri Lanka; *Mus pahari*, from northern India (Sikkim) to Vietnam; *Mus crociduroides*, from Sumatra; and *Mus vulcani* from Java (Marshall, 1977b). Estimates for diversification within the subgenus range from 7 to 3.4 mya (She et al., 1990; Chevret et al., 2005; Veyrunes et al., 2005).

The Subgenus *Nannomys* Peters 1876: African Pygmy Mice These are small-sized (<12 g), short-haired mice found throughout sub-Saharan Africa (Catzeflis and Denys, 1992). They are morphologically distinct from *Pyromys* and *Coelomys*. Delimitation of species within the subgenus has been difficult; the mice are morphologically similar to each other (Petter 1963, 1981; Macholan, 2001). However, they have variable diploid chromosome numbers and occupy diverse habitats, from deserts to montane forests (reviewed by Veyrunes et al., 2004). Musser and Carleton (2005) recognize 17 species, but there may be many more. Speciation within *Nannomys* is thought to have occurred between 5.2 and 3 mya (Chevret et al., 2005; Veyrunes et al., 2005).

The Subgenus *Pyromys* Thomas, 1911: Spiny Mice Five species of spiny mice are recognized. They are distinguished from each other by size, karyotype, and qualitative characteristics of the teeth and skull (Marshall, 1977a, 1977b, 1978, 1981): *Mus shortridgei*, found in grassy habitat in deciduous forests in Myanmar, Thailand, and Cambodia; *Mus saxicola*, common and widespread from Pakistan and the Himalayan foothills to southern India, with Himalayan populations lacking spiny fur; *Mus platythrix*, found in India from Bihar and Maharashtra states to the south; *Mus phillipsi*, found in India from southern Rajasthan state to the south; and *Mus fernandoni*, from Sri Lanka. Utilizing similar criteria as described for the divergence of the subgenera of *Mus*, estimates for diversification within the subgenus range from 6.7 to 3.4 mya (She et al., 1990; Chevret et al., 2005).

The Subgenus *Mus* Sensu Stricto: Field Mice, House (Commensal) Mice The 14 recognized species of subgenus *Mus* Sensu stricto are distinguished morphologically by qualitative features of the skull and dentition (Marshall, 1977a, 1997b, 1998; Auffray et al., 2003; Musser and Carleton, 2005; Cucchi et al., 2006; Shimada et al., 2007). Nine species are strictly Asian in distribution and form three phylogenetically distinct groups of taxa (Suzuki et al., 2004). These include the *Mus cervicolor* species group, the *Mus booduga* species group, and the *Mus lepidoides* species group. A fourth phylogenetically distinct group, the *Mus musculus* group, has a Palearctic distribution with the exception of one species, *Mus musculus*. Estimates for divergence of the four groups range from 4.8 to 4.3 mya or possibly later (Suzuki et al., 2004; Chevret et al., 2005).

Mus cervicolor Species Group *Mus cervicolor* is found in rice fields and in forests from Nepal and India east to Myanmar, Laos, Cambodia, Vietnam, Thailand, and Indonesia, and possibly Pakistan (reviewed in Musser and Carleton, 2005). Marshall (1977b) recognized several subspecies reflecting variation in size and/or color of fur. *Mus caroli* is typically found in rice fields and grassy habitat on the Ryuku Islands, Taiwan, and in southeastern China to Vietnam, Laos, Cambodia, Thailand, the Malay Peninsula, and the Indonesian islands of Sumatra, Java, Madura, and Flores, where it was likely introduced (reviewed in Musser and Carleton, 2005). In Thailand, populations are also known from pine savanna (Marshall, 1977b). *Mus cookii* is found primarily in mountains from India and Nepal to northern Myanmar, and in China (Yunnan Province), Thailand, Vietnam, and Laos (reviewed in Musser and Carleton, 2005). Three subspecies varying in size are recognized. Estimates of species divergence in this group range from 4 mya (Suzuki et al., 2004; Chevret et al., 2005) to 1.6 mya (She et al., 1990).

Mus booduga Species Group *Mus booduga* is known from Sri Lanka, peninsular India (north to Jammu and Kashmir), Bangladesh, southern Nepal, central Myanmar, and Pakistan (reviewed in Carleton and Musser, 2005). *Mus terricolor* is known from India, Nepal, Bangladesh, and Pakistan, and northern Sumatra, where it was likely introduced (Marshall, 1977b; reviewed in Carleton and Musser, 2005). *Mus fragilicauda* is a recently described species collected from Nahkon Ratchasima (Khorat) Province (Auffray et al., 2003) and from Laos (Suzuki et al., 2004). While similar in appearance to *Mus cervicolor*, it can be distinguished genetically, karyologically, and by subtle characteristics of the skull. All three species live in grass and cultivated rice and wheat fields. *Mus nitidulus* (Shimada et al., 2007) is a species originally identified in 1859 from south-central Myanmar. It was subsequently treated as a synonym of *M. cervicolor* (reviewed in Marshall, 1977b) until morphological and molecular analyses of recently collected specimens (Shimada et al., 2007) showed it to be a distinct lineage. Although *Mus famulus*, known only from the Nilgiri Mountains in southwestern India, was originally placed in the subfamily *Coelomys* (Marshall 1977b), based on recent molecular and morphological analyses (Chevret et al., 2003; Suzuki et al., 2004), it is now recognized as belonging to the subgenus *Mus*, and more specifically to the *Mus booduga* species group (Shimada et al., 2007). Estimates of species divergence in this group range from 3.3 mya (Suzuki et al., 2004) to 1.5 mya (Shimada et al., 2007).

Mus lepidoides Species Group This group includes a single species, *Mus lepidoides*, known only from central Myanmar and previously recognized as a subspecies of *M. booduga*

(Marshall, 1977b). Recent molecular analyses based on multiple gene sequences identify this species as a distinct lineage with no known close relatives (K. Aplin, pers. comm.). The molecular data, together with the morphological data, suggest an affinity with the *Mus musculus* species group (Shimada et al., 2008).

Mus musculus Species Group There are five species in this group, four of which have a strictly Palearctic distribution. These include *Mus macedonicus*, with a distribution from Macedonia to western Iran; *Mus spretus*, from northern Africa, the Iberian Peninsula, and southern France; *Mus spicilegus*, from southeast Austria to the Caucasus Mountains (Boursot et al., 1993); and *Mus cypriacus*, a recently described species from the island of Cyprus (Cucchi et al., 2006). The fifth species, *Mus musculus*, is found on all continents and islands except Antarctica. Its worldwide distribution is a result of its commensal association with humans. Ecological patterns for species within the *M. musculus* species group are atypical for the genus *Mus*. There are no species inhabiting forests. Rather, they are found in more open xeric habitat such as grasslands, shrublands, and temperate steppes (Suzuki et al., 2004). Estimates of the time of species divergence within this group range from 2 mya to less than 0.5 mya (She et al., 1990; Suzuki et al., 2004; Chevret et al., 2005; Cucchi et al., 2006).

Evolutionary history of the species Mus musculus

Understanding the evolutionary history of *M. musculus* is particularly important in light of the fact that most inbred strains of mice are an admixture in unequal proportions (Wade et al., 2002) of three genetically distinct yet closely related evolutionary lineages of this species, *M. musculus musculus*, *M. musculus domesticus*, and *M. musculus castaneus* (Yonegawa et al., 1980, 1982; Ferris et al., 1982, 1983b; Bishop et al., 1985; Nishioka and Lamothe, 1986; Bonhomme et al., 1987; Nishioka, 1987; Tucker et al., 1992a; Wade et al., 2002).

Mus musculus is thought to comprise three or four closely related lineages (Boursot et al., 1993, 1996; Sage et al., 1993; Moriwaki, 1994; Yonegawa et al., 1994; Din et al., 1996; Prager et al., 1996, 1998; Boissinot and Boursot, 1997; Marshall, 1998). Emphasizing evidence for distinct evolutionary histories and separate gene pools between lineages (Sage et al., 1993; Prager et al., 1996, 1998; Marshall, 1998), some authors recognize each lineage as a distinct species—*M. domesticus*, *M. musculus*, *M. castaneus*, and *M. gentilulus*. Emphasizing evidence for a continuum of gene flow across lineages, others (Boursot et al., 1993, 1996; Moriwaki, 1994; Yonegawa et al., 1994; Din et al., 1996; Boissinot and Boursot, 1997) refer to each of the lineages as subspecies: *M. musculus domesticus*, *M. m. musculus*, *M. m. castaneus*, and *M. m. gentilulus*. The "native" range for *M. m. domesticus* (*M. domesticus*) includes Western Europe, northern Africa, and the Middle East to western Iran. Populations of *M. m. domesticus* are also known from North and South America, where their occurrence is due to passive transport by Europeans to the New World. *M. m. musculus* (*M. musculus*) is found in Eastern Europe and northern Asia. *M. m. castaneus* (*M. castaneus*), as recognized by Prager et al. (1998) using mitochondrial genes, is found in Central and Southeast Asia. *M. m. gentilulus* (*M. gentilulus*) from Yemen represents a distinct mitochondrial lineage (Prager et al., 1998). Recent studies (Boursot et al., 1993, 1996; Din et al., 1996; Marshall, 1998; Prager et al., 1998) of a previously recognized subspecies, *M. m. bactrianus*, comprising mice from the Indian subcontinent, Afghanistan, and Iran, indicate that this subspecies does not constitute a cohesive genetic lineage. The subspecies *M. m. molossinus*, identified from Japan, is also not a distinct subspecies but rather a result of hybridization between *M. m. musculus* and *M. m. castaneus* (Yonegawa et al., 1986, 1988, 1994). Some populations of *M. m. molossinus* also carry *M. m. domesticus* alleles, although all but one of these populations are restricted to the Ogasawara islands and likely represent recent mixing (Bonhomme et al., 1989; Yonegawa et al., 1994). Estimates of divergence among lineages range from 350,000 to 900,000 years ago (She et al., 1990; Boursot et al., 1996; Suzuki et al., 2004).

Two hypotheses on the origin and radiation of house mice have been proposed. The first is the centrifugal model of evolution (Boursot et al., 1993, 1996; Bonhomme et al., 1994; Din et al., 1996). In this model, house mice are proposed to have originated in the northern Indian subcontinent and expanded to the west, north, and east, giving rise to *M. m. domesticus*, *M. m. musculus*, and *M. m. castaneus*, respectively (figure 1.2A). The model is based on evidence that house mice in the Indo-Pakistan region have the highest genetic (nuclear allozyme and mtDNA) variability when compared with surrounding populations (Boursot et al., 1996; Din et al., 1996). Although a subset of the nucleotide diversity from the central Indo-Pakistan populations is found in peripheral populations of *M. m castaneus*, the mtDNA lineages of *M. m. domesticus* and *M. m. musculus* are not known from the center, and the lack of evidence for intergrading populations from the center to the periphery calls into question the view of *M. musculus* as a single species (Boursot et al., 1996).

The second hypothesis is a sequential or linear model (Prager et al., 1998) and is based on additional sampling and the use of mtDNA trees to infer the relative ages of house mouse lineages. In this model, house mice originated in west-central Asia in the current range of *M. m. domesticus*, expanded to the southern Arabian Peninsula, migrated eastward and northward into south-central Asia, giving rise to

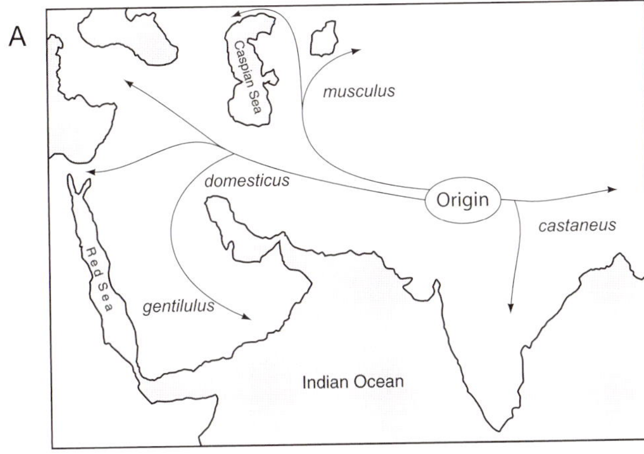

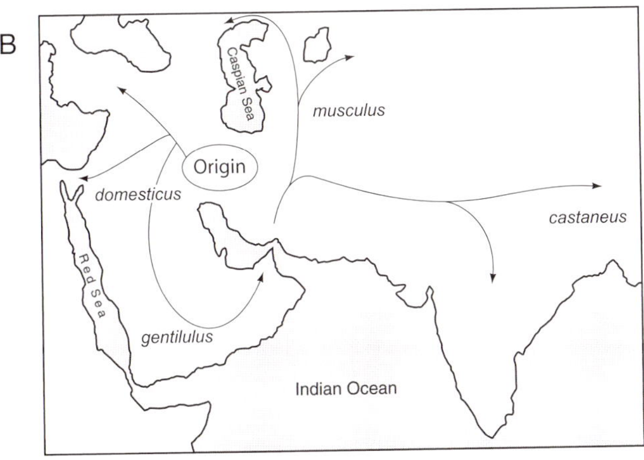

FIGURE 1.2 Maps displaying alternative hypotheses for the origin of the house mouse, *Mus musculus* (Tucker, 2007). *A*, The centrifugal model of Boursot et al. (1993, 1996), Bonhomme et al. (1994), Din et al. (1996), and Guenet and Bonhomme (2003). House mice originated in the northern Indian subcontinent and expanded to the west, north, and east, giving rise to *M. m. domesticus*, *M. m. musculus*, and *M. m. castaneus*, respectively. A fourth lineage, *M. m. gentilulus*, is recognized from the Saudi Arabian Peninsula. *B*, The sequential or linear model of Prager et al. (1998). House mice originated in west-central Asia in the current range of *M. m. domesticus*. Populations expanded west and south, into the Arabian Peninsula, giving rise to *M. m. gentilulus*. From the Arabian Peninsula, house mouse populations migrated east and north into south-central Asia, giving rise to *M. m. castaneus*, and then moved north into north-central Asia, giving rise to *M. m. musculus*.

M. m. castaneus, and then moved northward into north-central Asia, giving rise to *M. m. musculus* (figure 1.2*B*).

More recent expansions include *M. m. castaneus* into Southeast Asia, where it appears to intergrade with *M. m. musculus* in mainland China along the Yangtze River (Yonegawa et al., 1988; Frisman et al., 1990; Kawashima et al., 1995), and, as noted earlier, in Japan, where it has extensively hybridized with *M. m. musculus* (Yonegawa et al., 1986, 1988, 1994). F_2 generation laboratory crosses of both males and females of Southeast Asian *M. m. castaneus* and *M. m. musculus* from China indicate that these two subspecies are interfertile (Niwa-Kawakita, 1994). Taken together, these data suggest that there is a continuum of gene flow between *M. m. musculus* and *M. m. castaneus*.

M. m. musculus and *M. m. domesticus* are hypothesized to have independently colonized Europe via passive transport, from northwest of the Black Sea around 4000 BC and from the Mediterranean during the last millennium BC, respectively (Auffray et al., 1990; Cucchi et al., 2006; Cucchi and Vigne, 2006). These two subspecies form a narrow zone of hybridization through Central Europe that extends from the Jutland Peninsula to the Bulgarian coast of the Black Sea (Boursot et al., 1993; Sage et al., 1993). Extensive studies of the hybrid zone suggest that *M. m. musculus* and *M. m. domesticus* are partially reproductively isolated. Changes in allele frequency at diagnostic genetic markers occur over short distances, with different genomic regions introgressing differentially (Hunt and Selander, 1973; Ferris et al., 1983a; Vanlerberghe et al., 1986; Gyllensten and Wilson, 1987; Vanlerberghe et al., 1988a, 1988b; Tucker et al., 1992b; Dod et al., 1993, 2005; Sage et al., 1993; Orth et al., 1996; Munclinger et al., 2002; Payseur et al., 2004; Bozikova et al., 2005; Raufaste et al., 2005; Macholan et al., 2007). Natural hybrids also have a higher parasite load than pure *M. m. musculus* and *M. m. domesticus* (Sage et al., 1986; Moulia et al., 1993, 1995). Taken together, these data indicate hybrid breakdown between *M. m. musculus* and *M. m. domesticus*, resulting in reduced gene flow between these two subspecies.

The apparent reproductive incompatibility in nature is also found in the laboratory. Crosses between European *M. m. musculus* and some inbred strains (Forejt and Ivanyi, 1975; Forejt et al., 1991; Trachtulec et al., 1997) or between European *M. m. musculus* and European *M. m. domesticus* (Britton-Davidian et al., 2005) have resulted in sterile progeny. Furthermore, when the X chromosome from C57BL/6J, a strain that is predominantly *M. m. domesticus* in origin, is replaced by an X chromosome from a wild-derived *M. m. musculus* strain (PWD/Ph; Storchova et al., 2004) or a wild-derived *M. m. musculus* × *M. m. castaneus* strain (MSM/Ms-; Oka et al., 2004), males are sterile. These data also suggest that there is not a continuum of gene flow between *M. m. domesticus* and *M. m. musculus*.

Limited gene exchange has also been documented between *M. m. domesticus* and the more distantly related *M. spretus* where these two species overlap in their ranges (Orth et al., 2002), despite F_1 male sterility when *M. spretus* is crossed with inbred mice of mixed ancestry (i.e., *M. m. musculus* × *M. m. castaneus* × *M. m. domesticus*) in the laboratory (Bonhomme et al., 1978; Guenet et al., 1990; Pilder et al., 1991; Pilder, 1997; Elliott, 2001).

Whether house mice constitute a single species or a complex of closely related species depends on the extent of mixing among the four house mouse lineages and on one's concept of what constitutes a species. The former issue requires more studies involving greater taxonomic sampling of house mouse populations from central Asia, and the latter issue is beyond the scope of this review. However, based on studies to date, it is important to consider house mice as comprising multiple lineages, each with a distinct evolutionary history and including, for some lineages (i.e., *M. m. musculus* and *M. m. castaneus*), reticulation through hybridization, and for other lineages (i.e., *M. m. musculus* and *M. m. domesticus*), reproductive incompatibility.

When hybrid populations are identified in the wild, they should be referred to as crosses between species or subspecies; an example is Japanese house mice, *M. m. musculus* × *M. m. castaneus*. Inbred strains of mixed ancestry should also be referred to in this way. The appropriate taxonomic nomenclature for most inbred strains should be *M. m. domesticus* × *M. m. musculus* × *M. m. castaneus*, or, if one recognizes the distinct house mice lineages as species, *M. domesticus* × *M. musculus* × *M. castaneus*.

Phylogenetic relationships in the genus Mus

Comparative data from allozymes (Sage, 1981; Bonhomme et al., 1984; She et al., 1990), mtDNA restriction fragment length polymorphisms (RFLPs) (Ferris et al., 1983b; She et al., 1990), RFLPs of nuclear rDNA spacer regions (Suzuki and Kurihara, 1994), single-copy nuclear DNA (scnDNA) hybridization (She et al., 1990; Catzeflis and Denys, 1992; Chevret et al., 2003), mtDNA sequences (Fort et al., 1984; Sourrouille et al., 1995; Prager et al., 1996, 1998; Lundrigan et al., 2002; Chevret et al., 2003, 2005; Suzuki et al., 2004; Tucker et al., 2005; Veyrunes et al., 2005; Shimada et al., 2007), and nuclear sequences (Jouvin-Marche et al., 1988; Lundrigan and Tucker, 1994; Lundrigan et al., 2002, Auffray et al., 2003; Suzuki et al., 2004; Chevret et al., 2005; Tucker et al., 2005; Veyrunes et al., 2005; Shimada et al., 2007) have been used to elucidate evolutionary (phylogenetic) relationships among species of *Mus*.

Recent studies using varying combinations of molecular or chromosomal characters and species are synthesized into a single tree diagram in figure 1.1. They support monophyly for the genus *Mus*—that is, all the known species in the genus are descended from a common ancestor—as well as for each of the four recognized subgenera, *Coelomys*, *Nannomys*, *Pyromys*, and *Mus*—that is, all the known species in each of the subgenera are descended from a common ancestor (Lundrigan et al., 2002; Chevret et al., 2003, 2005; Suzuki et al., 2004; Tucker et al., 2005; Veyrunes et al., 2005, 2006). Relationships among subgenera are resolved based on chromosomal characters (Veyrunes et al., 2006). The subgenus *Coelomys* is basal, and *Nannomys* is sister to a *Pyromys-Mus* clade.

There are four well-defined monophyletic groups or clades within the subgenus *Mus*. As shown in figure 1.1, relationships among taxa within these groups are not as clearly defined. However, the recent addition of molecular data from *M. lepidoides* to the total data (K. Aplin, pers. comm.) suggests that the *M. cervicolor* group is basal and the *M. booduga* group is sister to a lineage giving rise to *M. lepidoides* and *M. musculus* species groups. In the *M. cervicolor* clade, evolutionary relationships among *M. cervicolor*, *M. cookii*, and *M. caroli* differ depending on the gene sequences used in the analysis. In combined gene analyses there is stronger support for *M. cervicolor/M. cookii* as most closely related (or sister) taxa, with *M. caroli* as more distantly related (or basal), than for *M. caroli/M. cookii* as sister taxa, with *M. cervicolor* as basal (Suzuki et al., 2004; Tucker et al., 2005). In the *M. booduga* clade, evolutionary relationships among *M. booduga*, *M. lepidoides*, *M. terricolor*, *M. fragilicauda*, *M. famulus*, and *M. nitidulus* also vary depending on the gene sequences used, and in combined gene analyses there is no resolution (Suzuki et al., 2004; Shimada et al., 2007). In the *M. musculus* clade the relationship of *M. spretus* to other species within the Palearctic clade is uncertain (Tucker et al., 2005). Comparative data from nuclear genes suggest that *M. spretus* is most closely related to an *M. spicilegus/M. macedonicus* clade, whereas the mitochondrial data place *M. spretus* as basal to both the *M. spicilegus/M. macedonicus* clade and the *M. musculus* complex. Based on mitochondrial D-loop sequence, *M. cypriacus* is most closely related to *M. macedonicus*. This relationship is not supported by sequence from a single intron from the nuclear *Abpa* (androgen-binding protein alpha) gene. Phylogenetic analyses (Tucker et al., 2005) of the *M. musculus* complex using a multigene data set places *M. m. domesticus* as basal to an *M. m. musculus/M. m. castaneus* clade. This arrangement lends support to the sequential or linear model for the evolution of house mice (Prager et al., 1998). However, this phylogeny is based on limited sampling of Asian *M. m. musculus* and *M. m. castaneus*, and thus this hypothesis needs to be more rigorously tested using a larger sample of Asian *M. m. musculus* and *M. m. castaneus*.

ACKNOWLEDGMENTS Figures were created by John Megahan, Museum of Zoology, University of Michigan. The review was supported in part by National Science Foundation grant no. DEB-9209950 and National Institutes of Health grant no. EY12994.

REFERENCES

Auffray, J.-C., Orth, A., Catalan, J., Gonzalez, J.-P., Desmarais, E., and Bonhomme, F. (2003). Phylogenetic position and description of a new species of subgenus *Mus* (Rodentia, Mammalia) from Thailand. *Zool. Scr.* 32:119–127.

AUFFRAY, J.-C., VANLERBERGHE, F., and BRITTON-DAVIDIAN, J. (1990). The house mouse progression in Eurasia: A palaeontological and archaeozoological approach. *Biol. J. Linn. Soc. Lond.* 41:13–25.

BISHOP, C. E., BOURSOT, P., BARON, B., BONHOMME, F., and HATAT, D. (1985). Most classical *Mus musculus domesticus* laboratory mouse strains carry a *Mus musculus* Y chromosome. *Nature* 325:70–72.

BOISSINOT, S., and BOURSOT, P. (1997). Discordant phylogeographic patterns between the Y chromosome and mitochondrial DNA in the house mouse: Selection on the Y chromosome? *Genetics* 146:1019–1034.

BONHOMME, F., ANAND, R., DARVICHE, D., DIN, W., and BOURSOT, P. (1994). The mouse as a ring species? In K. Moriwaki, T. Shiroishi, and H. Yonekawa (Eds.), *Genetics in wild mice: Its application to biomedical research* (pp. 13–23). Tokyo: Japan Scientific Societies Press; Basel: S. Karger.

BONHOMME, F., CATALAN, J., BRITTON-DAVIDIAN, J., CHAPMAN, V. M., MORIWAKI, K., NEVO, E., and THALER, L. (1984). Biochemical diversity and evolution in the genus *Mus*. *Biochem. Genet.* 22:275–303.

BONHOMME, F., GUENET, J.-L., DOD, B., MORIWAKI, K., and BULFIELD, G. (1987). The polyphyletic origin of laboratory inbred mice and their rate of evolution. *Biol. J. Linn. Soc. Lond.* 30:51–58.

BONHOMME, F., MARTIN S., and THALER L. (1978). Hybridation en laboratoire de *Mus musculus* et *Mus spretus Lataste*. *Experientia* 34:1140–1141.

BONHOMME, F., MIYASHITA, N., BOURSOT, P., CATALAN, J., and MORIWAKI, K. (1989). Genetical variation and polyphyletic origin in Japanese *Mus musculus*. *Heredity* 63:299–308.

BOURSOT, P., AUFFRAY, J.-C., BRITTON-DAVIDIAN, J., and BONHOMME, F. (1993). The evolution of house mice. *Annu. Rev. Ecol. Syst.* 24:119–152.

BOURSOT, P., DIN, W., ANAND, R., DARVICHE, D., DOD, B., VON DEIMLING, F., TALWAR, G. P., and BONHOMME, F. (1996). Origin and radiation of the house mouse: Mitochondrial DNA phylogeny. *J. Evol. Biol.* 9:391–415.

BOZIKOVA, E., MUNCLINGER, P., TEETER, K. C., TUCKER, P. K., MACHOLAN, M., and PIALEK, J. (2005). Mitochondrial DNA in the hybrid zone between *Mus musculus musculus* and *Mus musculus domesticus*: A comparison of two transects. *Biol. J. Linn. Soc. Lond.* 84:363–378.

BRITTON-DAVIDIAN, J., FEL-CLAIR, F., LOPEZ, J., ALIBERT, P., and BOURSOT, P. (2005). Postzygotic isolation between the two European subspecies of the house mouse: Estimates from fertility patterns in wild and laboratory-bred hybrids. *Biol. J. Linn. Soc. Lond.* 84:379–393.

BRUNET, M., GUY, F., PILBEAM, D., MACKAYE, H.T., LIKIUS, A., AHOUNTA, D., BEAUVILAIN, A., BLONDEL, C., BOCHERENS, H., et al. (2002). A new hominid from the Upper Miocene of Chad, Central Africa. *Nature* 418:145–151. Erratum in *Nature* 418:801.

CARLETON, M. D., and MUSSER, G. G. (2005). Order Rodentia. In D. E. Wilson and D. M. Reeder (Eds.), *Mammal species of the world: A taxonomic and geographic reference* (3rd ed., pp. 745–751). Baltimore: Johns Hopkins University Press.

CATZEFLIS, F. M., and DENYS, C. (1992). The African *Nannomys* (Muridae): An early offshoot from the *Mus* lineage. Evidence from scnDNA hybridization experiments and compared morphology. *Isr. J. Zool.* 38:219–231.

CHEVRET, P., JENKINS, P., and CATZEFLIS, F. (2003). Evolutionary systematics of the Indian mouse *Mus famulus* Bonhote, 1898: Molecular (DNA/DNA hybridization and 12S rRNA sequences) and morphological evidence. *Zool. J. Linn. Soc.* 137:385–401.

CHEVRET, P., VEYRUNES, F., and BRITTON-DAVIDIAN, J. (2005). Molecular phylogeny of the genus *Mus* (Rodentia: Murinae) based on mitochondrial and nuclear data. *Biol. J. Linn. Soc. Lond.* 84:417–427.

CUCCHI, T., ORTH, A., AUFFRAY, J.-C., RENAUD, S., FABRE, L., CATALAN, J., HADJISTERKOTIS, E., BONHOMME, F., and VIGNE, J. D. (2006). A new endemic species of the subgenus *Mus* (Rodentia, Mammalia) on the island of Cyprus. *Zootaxa* 1241:1–36.

CUCCHI, T., and VIGNE, J. D. (2006). Origin and diffusion of the house mouse in the Mediterranean. *Hum. Evol.* 21:95–106.

DIN, W., ANAND, R., BOURSOT, P., DARVICHE, D., DOD, B., JOUVIN-MARCHE, E., ORTH, A., TALWAR, G. P., CAZENAVE, P.-A., and BONHOMME, F. (1996). Origin and radiation of the house mouse: Clues from nuclear genes. *J. Evol. Biol.* 9:519–539.

DOD, B., JERMIN, L. S., BOURSOT, P., CHAPMAN, V. M., NIELSEN, J. T., and BONHOMME, F. (1993). Counterselection on sex chromosomes in the *Mus musculus* European hybrid zone. *J. Evol. Biol.* 6:529–546.

DOD, B., SMADJA, C., KARN, R. C., and BOURSOT, P. (2005). Testing for selection on the androgen-binding protein in the Danish hybrid zone. *Biol. J. Linn. Soc. Lond.* 84:447–459.

ELLIOTT, R. W., MILLER, D. R., PEARSHALL, R. S., HOHMAN, C., ZHANG, Y., POSLINSKI, D., TABACZYNSKI, D. A., and CHAPMAN, V. C. (2001). Genetic analysis of testis weight and fertility in an interspecies hybrid congenic strain for chromosome X. *Mamm. Genome* 12:45–51.

FERRIS, S. D., SAGE, R. D., HUANG, C.-H., NIELSEN, J. T., RITTE, U., and WILSON, A. C. (1983a). Flow of mitochondrial DNA across a species boundary. *Proc. Natl. Acad. Sci. U.S.A.* 80: 2290–2294.

FERRIS, S. D., SAGE, R. D., HUANG, C.-M., NIELSEN, J. T., RITTE, U., and WILSON, A. C. (1983b). Mitochondrial DNA evolution in mice. *Genetics* 105:681–721.

FERRIS, S. D., SAGE, R. D., and WILSON, A. C. (1982). Evidence from mtDNA sequences that common laboratory strains of inbred mice are descended from a single female. *Nature* 295:163–165.

FLYNN, L. J., and JACOBS, L. L. (1983). Effects of changing environments on Siwalik rodent fauna of northern Pakistan. *Palaeogeogr. Palaeoclimatol. Palaeoecol.* 38:129–138.

FOREJT, J., and IVANYI, P. (1975). Genetic studies on male sterility of hybrids between laboratory and wild mice (*Mus musculus* L.). *Genet. Res.* 24:189–206.

FOREJT, J., VINCEK, V., KLEIN, J., LEHRACH, H., and LOUDOVAMICKOVA, M. (1991). Genetic mapping of the t-complex region on mouse chromosome 17 including the hybrid sterility-1 gene. *Mamm. Genome* 1:84–91.

FORT P., BONHOMME, F., DARLU P., PIECHACZYK, M., JEANTEUR, P., and THALER, L. (1984). Clonal divergence of mitochondrial DNA versus population evolution of nuclear genome. *Evol. Theory* 7:81–90.

FRISMAN, L. V., KOROBITSINA, K. V., and YAKIMENKO, L. V. (1990). Genetic differentiation of U.S.S.R. house mice: Electrophoretic study of proteins. *Biol. J. Linn. Soc. Lond.* 41:65–72.

GUENET, J. L., and BONHOMME, F. (2003). Wild mice: An ever-increasing contribution to a popular mammalian model. *Trends Genet.* 19:24–31.

GUENET, J. L., NAGAMINE, C., SIMON-CHAZOTTES, D., MONTAGUTELLI, X., and BONHOMME, F. (1990). Hst-3: An X-linked hybrid sterility gene. *Genet. Res.* 56:163–165.

GYLLENSTEN, U., and WILSON, A. C. (1987). Interspecific mitochondrial DNA transfer and the colonization of Scandinavia by mice. *Genet. Res.* 49:25–29.

Hunt, W. G., and Selander, R. K. (1973). Biochemical genetics of hybridisation in European house mice. *Heredity* 31:11–33.

Jacobs, L. L., and Downs, W. R. (1994). The evolution of murine rodents in Asia. In Y. Tomida, C. Li, and T. Setoguchi (Eds.), *Rodent and lagomorph families of Asian origins and diversification* (pp. 149–156) (*National Science Museum Monographs* No. 8). *Tokyo.*

Jouvin-Marche E., Cuddihy, A., Butler, S., Hansen, J. N., Fitch, W. M., and Rudikoff, S. (1988). Modern evolution of a single-copy gene: The immunoglobulin C_k locus in wild mice. *Mol. Biol. Evol.* 5:500–511.

Kawashima, T., Miyashita, N., Tsuchiya, K., Li, H., Wang, F., Wang, C. H., Wu, X.-L., Wang, C., Jin, M.-L., et al. (1995). Geographical distribution of the *Hbb* haplotypes in the *Mus musculus* subspecies in Eastern Asia. *Jpn. J. Genet.* 70:17–23.

Kriegs, J. O., Churakov, G., Kiefmann, M., Jordan, U., Brosius, J., and Schmitz, J. (2006). Retroposed elements as archives for the evolutionary history of placental mammals. *PLoS Biol.* 4:e91.

Lundrigan, B., Jansa, S., and Tucker, P. K. (2002). Phylogenetic relationships in the genus *Mus*, based on maternally, paternally, and biparentally inherited characters. *Syst. Biol.* 53:410–431.

Lundrigan, B. L., and Tucker, P. K. (1994). Tracing paternal ancestry in mice using the Y-linked sex determining locus, *Sry*. *Mol. Biol. Evol.* 11:483–492.

Macholan, M. (2001). Multivariate analysis of morphometric variation in Asian *Mus* and sub-Saharan *Nannomys* (Rodentia: Muridae). *Zool. Anz.* 240:7–14.

Macholan, M., Munclinger, P., Sugerkova, M., Dufkova, P., Bimova, B., Bozikova, B., Zimma, J., and Pialek, J. (2007). Genetic analysis of autosomal and X-linked markers across a mouse hybrid zone. *Evolution* 61:746–771.

Marshall, J. T. (1977a). Family Muridae: Rats and mice. In B. Lekagul, and J. McNeely (Eds.), *Mammals of Thailand* (pp. 397–487). Bangkok: Association for the Conservation of Wildlife.

Marshall, J. T. (1977b). A synopsis of Asian species of *Mus* (Rodentia, Muridae). *Bull. Am. Mus. Nat. Hist.* 158:175–220.

Marshall, J. T., Jr. (1978). Classification of the genus *Mus*. In P. L. Altman, and P. D. Katz (Eds.), *Inbred and genetically defined strains of laboratory animals. Part 1. Mouse and rat* (pp. 212–220). Bethesda: Federation of the American Society of Experimental Biology.

Marshall, J. T. (1981). Taxonomy. In H. L. Foster, J. D. Small, and J. G. Fox (Eds.), *The mouse in biomedical research: Vol. 1. History, genetics, and wild mice* (pp. 17–26). New York: Academic Press.

Marshall, J. T. (1998). Identification and scientific names of Eurasian house mice and their European allies, subgenus *Mus* (Rodentia: Muridae). Unpublished manuscript.

Moriwaki, K. (1994). Introductory remarks: Wild mouse from a geneticist's viewpoint. In K. Moriwaki, T. Shiroishi, and H. Yonekawa (Eds.), *Genetics in wild mice: Its application to biomedical research* (pp. xiii–xxv). Tokyo: Japan Scientific Societies Press; Basel: S. Karger.

Moulia, C., LeBrun, N., Dallas, J., Orth, A., and Renaud, F. (1993). Experimental evidence of genetic determinism in high susceptibility to intestinal pinworm infection in mice: A hybrid zone model. *Parasitology* 106:387–393.

Moulia, C., LeBrun, N., Loubes, C., Marin, R., and Renaud, F. (1995). Hybrid vigor in parasites of interspecific crosses between two mice species. *Heredity* 74:48–52.

Munclinger, P., Bozikova, E., Sugerkova, E., Pialek, J., and Macholan, M. (2002). Genetic variation in house mice (*Mus*, Muridae, Rodentia) from the Czech and Slovak Republics. *Folia Zool. Brno.* 51:81–92.

Murphy, W. J., Eizirik, E., Johnson, W. E., Zhang, Y. P., Ryder, O. A., and O'Brien, S. J. (2001). Molecular phylogenetics and the origin of placental mammals. *Nature* 409:614–618.

Musser, G. G., and Carleton, M. D. (2005). Family Muridae. In D. E. Wilson and D. M. Reeder (Eds.), *Mammal Species of the World: A Taxonomic and Geographic Reference* (3rd ed., pp. 1247–1537). Baltimore: Johns Hopkins University Press.

Nishioka, Y. (1987). Y-chromosomal DNA polymorphism in mouse inbred strains. *Genet. Res.* 50:69–72.

Nishioka, Y., and Lamothe, E. (1986). Isolation and characterization of a Y chromosomal repetitive sequence. *Genetics* 113: 417–432.

Niwa-Kawakita, M. (1994). Reproductive depression of female mice in intersubspecific F_2 hybrids of the species *Mus musculus*. In K. Moriwaki, T. Shiroishi, and H. Yonekawa (Eds.), *Genetics in wild mice: Its application to biomedical research* (pp. 121–128). Tokyo: Japan Scientific Societies Press; Basel: S. Karger.

Oka, A., Mita, A., Sakurai-Yamatani, N., Yamamoto, H., Takagi, N., Takano-Shimizu, T., Toshimori, K., Moriwaki, K., and Shiroishi, T. (2004). Hybrid breakdown caused by substitution of the X chromosome between two mouse subspecies. *Genetics* 166:913–924.

Orth, A., Belkhir, K., Britton-Davidian, J., Boursot, P., Benazzou, T., and Bonhomme, F. (2002). Hybridation naturelle entre deux especes sympatriques de souris *Mus musculus domesticus L.* et *Mus spretus Lataste*. *C. R. Biol.* 325:89–97.

Orth, A., Lyapunova, E., Kandaurov, A., Boissinot, S., Boursot, P., Vorontsov, N., and Bonhomme, F. (1996). L'espece polytypique *Mus musculus* in Transcaucasie. *C. R. Seances Acad. Sci.*, Ser. 3, 319:435–441.

Payseur, B. A., Krenz, J. G., and Nachman, M. W. (2004). Differential patterns of introgression across the X chromosome in a hybrid zone between two species of house mice. *Evolution* 58:2064–2078.

Petter, F. (1963). Contribution a la connaissance des souris africaines. *Mammalia* 27:602–607.

Petter, F. (1981). Les souris africaines du groupe sorella (Rongeurs, Murides) *Mammalia* 45:313–320.

Pilder, S. H. (1997). Identification and linkage mapping of *Hst7*, a new *M. spretus/M. m. domesticus* chromosome 17 hybrid sterility locus. *Mamm. Genome* 8:290–291.

Pilder, S. H., Hammer, M. F., and Silver, L. M. (1991). A novel mouse chromosome 17 hybrid sterility locus: Implications for the origin of *t* haplotypes. *Genetics* 129:237–246.

Prager, E. M., Orrego C., and Sage, R. D. (1998). Genetic variation and phylogeography of central Asian and other house mice, including a major new mitochondrial lineage in Yemen. *Genetics* 150:835–861.

Prager, E. M., Tichy, H., and Sage, R. D. (1996). Mitochondrial DNA sequence variation in the Eastern house mouse, *Mus musculus*: Comparison with other house mice and report of a 75-bp tandem repeat. *Genetics* 143:427–446.

Raufaste, N., Orth, A., Belkhir, K., Senet, D., Smadja, C., Baird, S. J. E., Bonhomme, F., Dod, B., and Boursot, P. (2005). Inferences of selection and migration in the Danish house mouse hybrid zone. *Biol. J. Linn. Soc. Lond.* 84:593–616.

Sage, R. D. (1981). Wild mice. In H. L. Foster, J. D. Small, and J. G. Fox (Eds.), *The mouse in biochemical research.* (Vol. 1, pp. 39–90). New York: Academic Press.

Sage, R. D., Atchley, W. R., and Capanna, E. (1993). House mice as models in systematic biology. *Syst. Biol.* 42:523–561.

Sage, R. D., Heyneman, D., Lim, K. C., and Wilson, A. C. (1986). Wormy mice in a hybrid zone. *Nature* 324:60–63.

She, J. X., Bonhomme, F., Boursot, P., Thaler, L., and Catzeflis, F. (1990). Molecular phylogenies in the genus *Mus*: Comparative analysis of electrophoretic, scnDNA hybridization, and mtDNA RFLP data. *Biol. J. Linn. Soc. Lond.* 41:83–103.

Shimada, T., Aplin, K. P., Jenkins, P., and Suzuki, H. (2007). Rediscovery of *Mus nitidulus* Blyth (Rodentia: Muridae), an endemic murine rodent of the central basin of Myanmar. *Zootaxa* 1498:45–68.

Sourrouille, P., Hanni, C., Ruedi, M., and Catzeflis, F. M. (1995). Molecular systematics of *Mus crociduroides*, an endemic mouse of Sumatra (Muridae: Rodentia). *Mammalia* 59:91–102.

Storchova, R., Gregorova, S., Buckiova, D., Kyselova, V., Divina, P., and Forejt, J. (2004). Genetic analysis of X-linked hybrid sterility in the house mouse. *Mamm. Genome* 15:515–524.

Suzuki, H., and Kurihara, Y. (1994). Genetic variation of ribosomal RNA in the house mouse, *Mus musculus*. In K. Moriwaki, T. Shiroishi, and H. Yonekawa (Eds.), *Genetics in wild mice: Its application to biomedical research* (pp. 110–119). Tokyo: Japan Science Society Press; Basel: S. Karger.

Suzuki, H., Shimada, T., Terashima, M., Tsuchiya, K., and Aplin, K. (2004). Temporal, spatial and ecological modes of evolution of Eurasian *Mus* based on mitochondrial and nuclear genes. *Mol. Phylogenet. Evol.* 33:626–646.

Trachtulec, Z., Mnukova-Fajdelova, M., Hamvas, R. M. J., Gregorova, S., Mayer, W. E., Lehrach, H. R., Vincek, V., Forejt, J., and Klein, J. (1997). Isolation of candidate hybrid sterility 1 genes by cDNA selection in a 1.1 megabase pair region on mouse chromosome 17. *Mamm. Genome* 8:312–316.

Tucker, P. K. (2007). Systematics of the genus *Mus*. In J. Fox, S. Barthold, M. T. Davisson, C. Newcomer, F. Quimby, and A. Smith (Eds.), *The mouse in biomedical research* (Vol. 1, 2nd ed., pp. 13–23). New York: Academic Press.

Tucker, P. K., Lee, B. K., Lundrigan, B. L., and Eicher, E. M. (1992a). Geographic origin of the Y chromosomes in "old" inbred strains of mice. *Mamm. Genome* 3:254–261.

Tucker, P. K., Sage, R. D., Warner, J. H., Wilson, A. C., and Eicher, E. M. (1992b). Abrupt cline for sex chromosomes in a hybrid zone between two species of mice. *Evolution* 46:1146–1163.

Tucker, P. K., Sandstedt, S. A., and Lundrigan, B. (2005). Phylogenetic relationships in the subgenus *Mus* (genus *Mus*, family Muridae, subfamily Murinae): Examining gene trees and species trees. *Biol. J. Linn. Soc. Lond.* 84:653–662.

Vanlerberghe, F., Boursot, P., and Catalan, J. (1988a). Analyse genetique de la zone d'hybridation entre les deux sous-especes de souris *Mus musculus domesticus* et *Mus musculus musculus* en Bulgaire. *Genome* 30:427–437.

Vanlerberghe, F., Boursot, P., Nielsen, J. T., and Bonhomme, F. (1988b). A steep cline for mitochondrial DNA in Danish mice. *Genet. Res.* 52:185–193.

Vanlerberghe, F., Dod, B., Boursot, P., Bellis, M., and Bonhomme, F. (1986). Absence of Y-chromosome introgression across the hybrid zone between *Mus musculus domesticus* and *Mus musculus musculus*. *Genet. Res.* 48:191–197.

Veyrunes, F., Britton-Davidian, J., Robinson, T. J., Calvet, E., Denys, C., and Chevret, P. (2005). Molecular phylogeny of the African pygmy mice, subgenus *Nannomys* (Rodentia: Murinae, *Mus*): Implications for chromosomal evolution. *Mol. Phylogenet. Evol.* 36:358–369.

Veyrunes, F., Catalan, J., Sicard, B., Robinson, T. J., Duplantier, J.-M., Granjon, L., Dobigny, G., and Britton-Davidian, J. (2004). Autosome and sex chromosome diversity among African pygmy mice, subgenus *Nannomys* (Murinae; *Mus*). *Chromosome Res.* 12:1–14.

Veyrunes, F., Dobigny, G., Yang, F., O'Brien, P. C., Catalan, J., Robinson, T. J., and Britton-Davidian, J. (2006). Phylogenomics of the genus *Mus* (Rodentia; Muridae): Extensive genome repatterning is not restricted to the house mouse. *Proc. Biol. Soc.* 273:2925–2934.

Wade, C. M., Kulbokas III, E. J., Kirby, A. W., Zody, M. C., Mullikin, J. C., Lander, E. S., Lindblad-Toh, K., and Daly, M. J. (2002). The mosaic structure of variation in the laboratory mouse genome. *Nature* 420:574–578.

Wilson, D. E., and Reeder, D. M. (2005). Introduction. In *Mammal species of the world: A taxonomic and geographic reference* (3rd ed., pp. xxiii–xxxiv). Baltimore: Johns Hopkins University Press.

Yonegawa, H., Gotoh, O., Tagashira, Y., Matsushima, Y., Shi, L.-I., Cho, W. S., Miyashita, N., and Moriwaki, K. (1986). A hybrid origin of Japanese mice, *M. m. molossinus*. *Curr. Top. Microbiol. Immunol.* 127:62–67.

Yonegawa, H., Moriwaki, K., Gotoh, O., Miyashita, N., Matsushima, Y., Shi, L., Cho, W. S., Zhen, X.-L., and Tagashira, Y. (1988). Hybrid origin of Japanese mice "*Mus musculus molossinus*": Evidence from restriction analysis of mitochondrial DNA. *Mol. Biol. Evol.* 5:63–78.

Yonegawa, H., Moriwaki, K., Gotoh, O., Miyashita, N., Migita, S., Bonhomme, F., Hjorth, J. P., Petras, M. L., and Tagashira, Y. (1982). Origins of laboratory mice deduced from restriction patterns of mitochondrial DNA. *Differentiation* 22: 222–226.

Yonegawa, H., Moriwaki, K., Gotoh, O., Wantanabe, J., Hayashi, J.-I., Miyashita, N., Petras, M. L., and Tagashira, Y. (1980). Relationship between laboratory mice and the subspecies *Mus musculus domesticus* based on restriction endonuclease cleavage patterns of mitochondrial DNA. *Jpn. J. Gen.* 55: 289–296.

Yonegawa, H., Takahama, S., Gotoh, O., Miyashita, N., and Moriwaki, K. (1994). Genetic diversity and geographic distribution of *Mus musculus* subspecies based on the polymorphism of mitochondrial DNA. In K. Moriwaki, T. Shiroishi, and H. Yonekawa (Eds.), *Genetics in wild mice: Its application to biomedical research* (pp. 25–40). Tokyo: Japan Scientific Societies Press; Basel: S. Karger.

2 Visual and Other Sensory Abilities of Mice and Their Influence on Behavioral Measures of Cognitive Function

AIMÉE A. WONG AND RICHARD E. BROWN

Origins of inbred strains used for research

The inbred laboratory mouse has become the most widely used experimental mammal for studies of genes, brain and behavior. The power of the inbred strain is due to its isogenicity within a strain and the genetic heterogeneity among strains. Each strain possesses a distinctive phenotype that can be studied in order to determine its underlying genetic contribution to neural and behavioral phenotypes. In this way, phenotypic variations between strains and between mutants and their wild-type controls can be traced back to particular genes of interest. The advantages of using the mouse as a model organism include its small size, short generation time, large litters, the ease with which it can be handled, and its genetic comparability to humans—approximately 99% of human genes have mouse homologues (Silver, 1995; Taft et al., 2006; Tecott, 2003). Compared to other animals, the mouse genome is relatively easy to manipulate, allowing gene-gene and gene-environment interactions to be studied and thus the genetic components of human diseases to be identified. Furthermore, the mouse genome can be manipulated with innovative transgenic techniques to create a variant that, except for the mutated genes, is virtually genetically identical to its parental strain.

Inbred mice are developed by mating two unrelated strains and mating their offspring (F_1) in a series of brother-sister matings (Staats, 1968b). With each successive generation, the genetic uniformity of the strain increases, and after 20 generations of sibling matings, the resulting mice are 98.7% homozygous at all loci (Silver, 1995). The origin of inbred strains began with the DBA mouse, created by one of the founding fathers of mouse genomics, Clarence Cook Little, to study the inheritance of coat color. He bred mice carrying the recessive genes for three mutations, dilute, brown, and nonagouti, and after 20 generations of inbreeding, the first fully inbred strain (DBA) was created in 1909 (Staats, 1968a). Little's research focus shifted from inheritance of coat color to cancer susceptibility, and he built up his colony of DBA mice at the Carnegie Institute at Cold Spring Harbor to study the genetics of cancer. Little went on to develop new inbred strains, some of which were descended from fancy mice received from Miss Abbie Lathrop, a mouse supplier in Granby, Massachusetts. Little developed his line *C*, which was descended from Lathrop's stock, mating two females (number 57 and 58) to male number 52. The descendants of female 57 became the C57BL (BL for black) inbred strain, while the descendants of female 58 became the C58 inbred line. In 1920, Leonell C. Strong mated a series of DBA mice from Cold Spring Harbor with albino mice received from Halsey J. Bagg at Memorial Hospital, New York, and developed several related inbred lines of mice, including C3H, CBA, C, CHI, and C12I (Staats, 1968a). In 1921, Strong crossed an albino mouse from Little's colony in Cold Spring Harbor to Bagg's albino stock and created the A strain, which had a high incidence of mammary and lung tumors. Also at Cold Spring Harbor, Bagg's albinos were inbred by E. Carleton MacDowell and were then used exclusively by George D. Snell in work that led to his Nobel prize in 1980 for landmark immunogenetic studies on the histocompatibility locus. This research led to the production of the first genetically engineered strains of mice, so-called congenic strains, in which sections of chromosomes affecting the survival of skin grafts were transferred from one inbred line to another (http://nobelprize.org/nobel_prizes/medicine/laureates/1980/snell-lecture.pdf).

The founding of the Roscoe B. Jackson Memorial Laboratory (now the Jackson Laboratory) in Bar Harbor, Maine, in 1929 by Clarence Cook Little provided the first specialized facility for the study of the genetics of cancer and radiation biology and for the development of new inbred strains of mice and the discovery of new mutations. At present, the Jackson Laboratory (www.jax.org/about/jax_facts.html) has more than 450 inbred mouse strains available for research (Beck et al., 2000).

Transgenic and mutant mouse models

The use of inbred strains has expanded greatly in the last decade because of the availability of more advanced methods to modify the mouse genome (Peters, 2007; Tecott, 2003). These strategies fall into two general categories. The first involves introducing known mutations into the mouse genome, creating a transgenic mouse that can be examined phenotypically for consequences of the mutation. The second involves a forward genetics approach, in which inbred mice are screened for phenotypic differences and then the genetic correlates and causes of these differences are identified (Tecott, 2003; Vitaterna et al., 2006).

Although mice with spontaneously occurring mutations have been a valued resource for studying behavioral genetics, genetically engineered mice created by transgenesis, targeted mutagenesis, inducible mutagenesis, gene trapping, and chemical mutagenesis have been crucial in the search for genetic correlates of human diseases (Peters, 2007; Tecott, 2003; Vitaterna et al., 2006). With these genetic tools and the availability of the mouse genome sequence (www.ncbi.nih.gov/genome/guide/mouse/), the mouse as a model system provides a unique opportunity to study anatomical, neurochemical, and behavioral effects of aberrant gene expression and the molecular and cellular underpinnings of human neurological diseases. However, to study the genetic basis of disease, it is necessary to determine which clinical symptoms can be assessed in animal experiments. Phenotypic evaluation of each mouse model system is a prerequisite for evaluating the physiological consequences of genetic perturbations. Willott et al. (2003) suggest that a reliable and valid mouse model for a human disorder should ideally meet the following six criteria:

1. The behaviors to be studied should be readily exhibited by both mice (the primary mammalian model for genetic research) and humans (the subject of the model).
2. The behaviors should be simple enough to be accurately isolated and measured.
3. The behaviors should have relevance for everyday life or clinical conditions.
4. Assuming that genes are likely to affect behavior via neurophysiological and neurochemical mechanisms, the neural pathways and physiology of the behaviors should be reasonably well understood.
5. From a practical standpoint, quantitative measurement of the behaviors should be relatively simple, fast, and reliable, to allow testing of many mice.
6. The behaviors should vary substantially among different genetic strains of mice or mutants in order for inheritance mapping and other genetic techniques to be applied.

Meeting these criteria has become a challenge. Advances in molecular and cellular techniques for the development of new transgenic and knockout mouse strains have occurred without the development of new strategies for understanding how the manipulated genes relate to sensory systems, brain, and behavior. There are two categories of problems associated with modifying the mouse genome with respect to behavioral phenotyping strategies (Gerlai, 2001). The first problem is associated with compensatory mechanisms that could exist when a gene is knocked out. These mechanisms can cause secondary phenotypic changes that could alter developmental, physiological, or even behavioral processes. For example, "helper" genes may be able to take over the function of the targeted gene mutation, masking the functional outcome of the mutation. Or compensation for a disrupted function may lead to altered function of another mechanism, leading the investigator to falsely conclude that observed phenotypical abnormalities are due to the targeted mutation. This compensation problem is not one that can be easily solved. Gerlai (2001) suggests that gene expression changes could be measured in vitro or in vivo using quantitative reverse transcription polymerase chain reaction (RT-PCR) or gene-chip technology to assess how genes respond in concert, or transgenic studies could aim to knock out a cluster of genes that work as a functional unit, rather than a single gene.

The second problem involves the background effect of the strain that is used to maintain the genetic disruption (Gerlai, 1996). Most gene targeting is carried out in embryonic stem cells derived from the 129 inbred strain (Crawley, 2000; Gerlai, 2001; Linder, 2006). Mice receiving the targeted mutation are often mated to mice of a different strain than the genetic background of the embryonic stem cells. Resulting F_1 generation mice will have one set of chromosomes from each strain, and thus sibling matings between heterozygous F_1 generation will produce an F_2 population with mice that are wild type, homozygous and heterozygous for the null mutation. However, homozygous and heterozygous mice may be genetically different from their wild-type littermates at loci other than the targeted gene, owing to the recombination pattern of the genes of the two parental strains. Furthermore, the alleles of genes that surround the targeted locus will be of the 129 type in null mutant mice but of the other parental strain in wild-type mice. Thus, the behavioral phenotype observed in null mutant mice (and not in wild-type mice) may be due to the effect of the 129 background (Gerlai, 2001), and there are many different 129 substrains with different phenotypes (Festing et al., 1999; Simpson et al., 1997).

Many transgenic mice are maintained on a hybrid background in which one of the progenitor strains has the retinal degeneration gene *Pde6b*^{rd1} (e.g., FVB/N, C3H, Black Swiss), resulting in 25% of the offspring being homozygous for retinal degeneration. To address these problems, one can backcross the mutant hybrid multiple times to a strain

Table 2.1

Hearing and visual abilities in 14 inbred and wild-derived mouse strains from the Jackson Laboratories

Strain	Type	JAX Number	Hearing	Vision
129S1/SvImJ	Inbred	002448	Normal	Normal
A/J	Inbred	000646	Deaf < 3 mo. of age	Albino
AKR/J	Inbred	000648	Normal	Albino
BALB/cByJ	Inbred	001026	Deaf > 16 mo. of age	Albino
BALB/cJ	Inbred	000651	Normal	Albino
C3H/HeJ	Inbred	000659	Normal	*Pde66*[rd1]
C57BL/6J	Inbred	000664	Deaf > 16 mo. of age	Normal
CAST/EiJ	Wild-derived	000928	Normal	Unknown
DBA/2J	Inbred	000671	Deaf < 3 mo. of age	Glaucoma > 9 mo. of age
FVB/NJ	Inbred	001800	Normal	*Pde66*[rd1]
MOLF/EiJ	Wild-derived	000550	Normal	*Pde66*[rd1]
SJL/J	Inbred	000686	Normal	*Pde66*[rd1]
SM/J	Inbred	000687	Normal	Unknown
SPRET/EiJ	Wild-derived	001146	Normal	Unknown

Note: The Jackson Laboratory (JAX) catalogue number is given. *Pde66*[rd1] is the gene for retinal degeneration, so these mice are blind by weaning age.

without the retinal degeneration gene to create a congenic strain that carries the mutation on a desired genetic background and does not have retinal degeneration. For example, FVB/N mice are an albino strain that is commonly used for the generation of transgenic mice because of their large, strong pronuclei and high breeding performance, but they have retinal degeneration, which impairs their performance on behavioral tasks. A pigmented, sighted FVB/N strain (named FVBS/Ant) was created by repeated backcrossing of an FVB/N × 129P2/OldHsd F_1 hybrid with FVB/N mice while selecting against albinism and homozygosity of the retinal degeneration mutation (Pde6b). The FVBNS/Ant mouse is suitable for behavioral analysis as it has normal eye histology, an positive visual evoked potential response, and improved performance on visuospatial learning tasks (Errijgers et al., 2006).

Behavioral tasks used to measure sensory functions in mice

For its behavioral phenotype to be determined, a mouse must be tested in a series of behavioral tasks (Bailey et al., 2006). Performance on behavioral tasks is dependent on the sensory, motor, and cognitive abilities of the mouse. Every behavioral task depends on at least one of the sensory abilities for the mouse to correctly execute the task, but surprisingly little information is available on the sensory abilities of mice. The goal of detecting sensory deficits is to eliminate artifacts that could confound the results of tasks used to test higher cognitive function. Many commonly used strains of mice have vision or hearing deficits (table 2.1), and these sensory impairments may affect performance on behavioral tasks, as most behavioral experiments measure motor responses to sensory information. Table 2.2 shows some of the behavioral tasks most commonly used in mice and their corresponding sensory demands.

This chapter summarizes some of the behavioral tasks that are most commonly used to evaluate the sensory capabilities of mice (with an emphasis on vision), highlights strain

Table 2.2

Sensory demands of behavioral tasks used to measure higher order cognitive functions

Task	Vision	Hearing	Olfaction	Taste	Pain
Morris water maze	Yes	No	No	No	No
Cued and context conditioning	Yes	Yes	Yes	No	Yes
Passive and active avoidance	Yes	No	No	No	Yes
Conditioned taste aversion	No	No	No	Yes	No
Barnes maze	Yes	Yes	No	No	No
Olfactory tubing maze	No	Yes	Yes	No	No
Open field test	Yes	No	No	No	No
Light-dark transition test	Yes	No	No	No	No
Elevated plus maze	Yes	No	No	No	No

differences in sensory function, and discusses how strain differences in sensory ability may confound the results of learning and memory and anxiety-related behavioral tasks. The need for proper controls and for developing tasks that exploit the natural abilities of the mouse is also discussed.

Vision

Mice are not usually considered visual animals because they are nocturnal and rely principally on olfactory, auditory, and tactile information to sense predators, food, and conspecifics in their environment. Although the laboratory setting provides an unnatural environment for the mouse (food and water are provided ad libitum, constant temperature is maintained, and physical activity is greatly reduced), the eye of the laboratory mouse remains anatomically adapted for natural conditions. For example, Shupe et al. (2006) found no significant differences in outer nuclear layer thickness, linear density of the ganglion cell layer, and cone opsin expression in the eyes of wild *M. musculus*, three inbred strains (C57BL/6J, NZB/BINJ, and DBA/1J), and wild and outbred laboratory-domesticated stock of the deer mouse, *Peromyscus maniculatus*. Therefore, the laboratory mouse's visual system remains adapted to natural conditions, and use of the mouse as a model system to investigate properties of the visual system and visual disorders is justified.

The visual system of the mouse serves many functions, ranging from adjusting pupillary diameter in response to changes in light levels to tracking moving targets and discerning spatial details of objects in the environment (Pinto and Enroth-Cugell, 2000). For this reason, no one behavioral task provides a comprehensive test of visual function in mice, and different techniques have been used to assess gross visual ability, visual detection, visual pattern discrimination, and visual acuity.

Many mouse strains, especially albino mice such as A/J, AKR/J, BALB/cByJ, and BALB/cJ, suffer from light-induced retinal degeneration, while other strains, such as C57BL/6J, do not (LaVail et al., 1987a, 1987b). This means that when mice are housed under bright lights or under 24-hour light conditions, some strains of mice experience retinal degeneration while others will not, and as they age, the retinal degeneration becomes more severe (Danciger et al., 2000, 2003, 2007). Thus, the lighting conditions under which mice are housed constitute an environmental factor that interacts with genetic differences between strains to alter visual ability, and it is important that the lighting conditions under which mice are housed be reported.

Gross Measures of Visual Ability Reflex responses to visual stimuli such as the eye blink reflex and pupillary constriction in response to light can be used to measure gross visual function (Crawley, 2000; Pinto and Enroth-Cugell, 2000). The visual cliff test (Fox, 1965) measures the ability of a mouse to detect the appearance of a drop-off at the edge of a horizontal plane and was designed to detect depth perception, and thus provides only a crude measure of visual acuity (Crawley, 2000).

Brightness/Visual Detection The ability of mice to detect visual stimuli as ascertained by behavioral testing was pioneered by Yerkes (1907), who developed a special discrimination box in which mice were trained to discriminate between black and white stimulus cards (figure 2.1*A*). The mice were trained to choose the box with the white card and received a mild electrical shock when they entered the box with the black card (Yerkes and Dodson, 1908). Mice achieved a perfect score (100% correct choices) after only 50 trials (Yerkes, 1907).

Many adaptations of the Yerkes apparatus have been used to test black versus white discrimination in mice. One of these was a modified water T-maze with rounded arms, one of which was painted black and the other white (Wimer and Weller, 1965). Mice were trained to escape from the black or the white arm using an escape ladder, and the correct number of responses in the 10 trials on the fourth day served as the learning measure. On this procedure, AKR/J, C57BL/6J, DBA/2J, and RF/J strains exhibited significant learning, but A/HeJ mice did not. The performance of mice with retinal degeneration (C3H/HeJ, SJL/J, SWR/J) was significantly inferior to that of all other stains tested except A/HeJ mice. Since A/J mice are the strain most sensitive to light-induced retinal degeneration (Danciger et al., 2007), and since A/J and A/HeJ mice are from the same stock (Fox and Witham, 1997), their performance may be related to light-induced retinal degeneration.

An adaptation of the water T-maze, the six-choice water maze (Balkema et al., 1983), was used to investigate brightness discrimination. The maze was painted white, and mice were trained to detect a black stimulus placed at the end of one of the six arms, which contained an escape ramp. Under normal lighting conditions, mice were trained for 10 trials per day to swim to the black stimulus. Once they reached a criterion of 90% correct, the room luminance was lowered until the success criterion was no longer achievable. C57BL/6J pe/pe mice have decreased dark-adaptive sensitivity but no photoreceptor degeneration (Balkema et al., 1983), and when tested on the six-choice water maze, these mice performed as well as the wild-type mice in the light-adapted state ($>10^{-3}$ cd/m^2), but their performance was significantly impaired in the dark-adapted state. This suggests that C57BL/6J pe/pe mice may provide a good model for some forms of human stationary night blindness.

The visual water box, developed by Prusky, West, and Douglas (2000a), assesses visual detection (Wong and Brown,

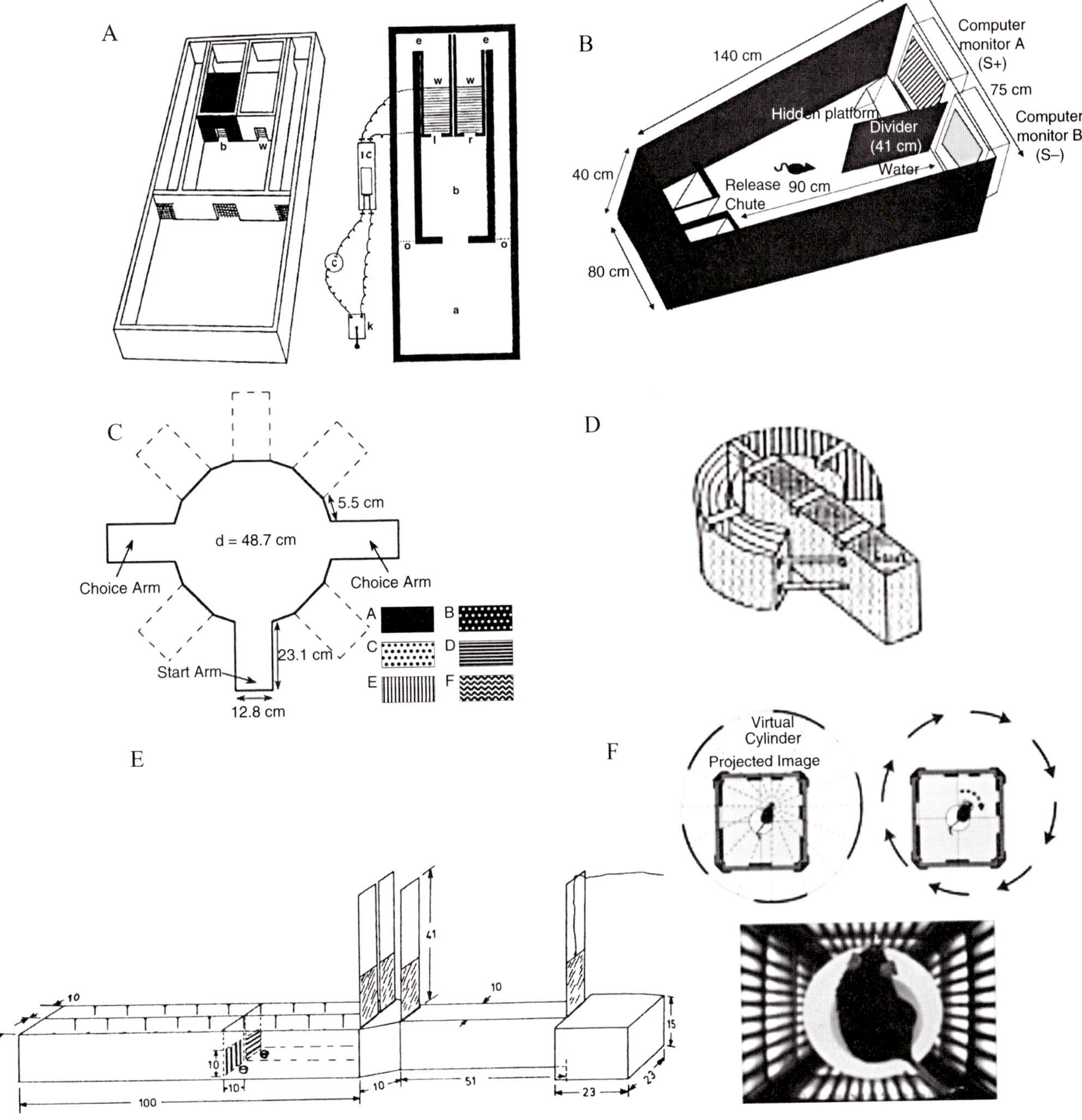

FIGURE 2.1 Examples of apparatus used to test for visual ability in mice. *A*, The discrimination box developed by Yerkes (1907) to test for black (b)-white (w) discriminations in mice. This box was 94 cm long, 30 cm wide, and 11.5 cm deep and was divided into a nest box (*a*), an entrance chamber (*b*), and two boxes (*l*, *r*) with wires (*w*) on the floor connected to a battery (*c*) and a switch (*k*), which could deliver foot shocks if mice entered the wrong compartment. Mice exited (*e*) from the boxes into an alley (*o*), which led back to the nest box. *B*, The visual water box designed to test vision in rodents by Prusky et al. (2000a) as used by Wong and Brown (2006, 2007). *C*, The radial maze used by Hyde and Denenberg (1999) to test pattern vision in mice and the six patterns used as stimuli. *D*, The modified water T-maze used for horizontal-vertical discriminations by Balogh et al. (1999). *E*, The two-alternative-choice apparatus used by Gianfranceschi et al. (1999) to measure visual acuity in mice. (From Wiesenfeld and Branchek, 1976.) *F*, The optomotor test apparatus used by Prusky et al. (2004) to test visual acuity in mice.

2006) on a task requiring mice to swim to a hidden platform, the location of which is predicted by a visual cue displayed on a computer screen (see figure 2.1*B*). Mice were trained for eight trials per day to discriminate between a low spatial frequency (0.17 c/deg) sinusoidal vertical grating (S+), and a gray screen (S–). The percentage of correct choices on each day was used as a measure of visual ability, with 70% correct set as the learning criterion. Using this procedure, Wong and Brown (2006) tested 14 strains of mice with different visual abilities as predicted by the physiology of their visual system (figure 2.2). Mice with reportedly normal vision at 3–4 months of age (129S1/SvImJ, C57BL/6J, DBA/2J) performed very well on this task, and mice with poor visual abilities due to albinism (AKR/J, A/J, BALB/cByJ, BALB/cJ) performed worse than mice with normal vision except AKR/J, which performed as well as mice with normal vision. Mice with retinal degeneration (C3H/HeJ, FVB/NJ, MOLF/EiJ, SJL/J) performed at chance levels, as did mice with uncharacterized visual abilities (CAST/EiJ, SM/J, SPRET/EiJ).

Pattern Discrimination Behavioral tasks have also been used to study pattern discrimination in mice. Using a modified version of the eight-arm radial maze, Ammassari-Teule and de Marsanich (1996) trained mice to collect food from four baited arms displaying distinctive visual patterns. CD-1 mice adopted a 45-degree angle turn strategy to locate the food instead of associating the visual patterns with the presence of food; however, C57BL/6NCrlBR and DBA/2NCrlBR mice successfully learned this pattern discrimination task, and there was no difference in performance between these strains (Passino and Ammassauri-Teule, 1999). The results of these experiments indicate there are strain differences in visual pattern discrimination ability, but discrimination ability could have been masked by the complexity of the task.

Using escape from an eight-arm water maze modified into a T-maze, Hyde and Denenberg (1999) found that BXSB mice could learn to discriminate between different pairs of visual patterns and could reach a criterion of 80% correct after 5 days of training with 10 trials per day with each of the nine pattern discrimination tasks (see figure 2.1*C*). On a probe trial in which all six patterns were available in the eight-arm maze, the mice showed a preference for the S+ over the S– patterns, indicating they were capable of complex pattern discrimination. The modified radial arm maze protocol employed by Hyde and Denenberg (1999) exploited the natural inclination for the mouse to escape from water, and the results on this task suggest that escape from water is a more successful motivation than food reward as used by Passino and Ammassauri-Teule (1999) for visual discrimination tasks in mice.

Balogh et al. (1998, 1999) found that C57BL/6J, ectopic BXSB mice, which have neocortical malformations and are used as a model of developmental learning difficulties, nonectopic BXSB mice, and 129/SvEvTac mice, which have the pink-eyed dilution allele, could be trained to discriminate between horizontal and vertical patterns in a water-escape T maze (see figure 2.1*D*). The 129/SvEvTac mice, however, did not perform as well as the BXSB and C57BL/6J strains, presumably because of deficits in visual acuity.

Using the visual water box, Wong and Brown (2006) trained mice of 14 strains to discriminate between vertical and horizontal gratings. Mice with reportedly normal vision (129S1/SvImJ, C57BL/6J, DBA/2J) were capable of pattern discrimination as they reached the criterion of 70% correct within the 8 days of testing. Albino mice (AKR/J, A/J, BALB/cByJ, and BALB/cJ) performed worse than mice with normal vision, taking longer to reach criterion, while mice with retinal degeneration (C3H/HeJ, FVB/NJ, MOLF/EiJ and SJL/J) and mice with uncharacterized visual abilities (CAST/EiJ, SM/J and SPRET/EiJ) performed at chance levels, a finding indicating they could not differentiate between the vertical and horizontal grating patterns (see figure 2.2).

Visual Acuity Visual acuity is the ability to detect small distances separating two points, and the threshold for visual acuity is reached when the observer can no longer determine a separation between the two points. Spatial frequency is defined by how rapidly a stimulus changes across space and is measured in term of cycles per degree (c/deg). For a grating stimulus, spatial frequency refers to the frequency with which the grating repeats itself per degree of visual angle (Goldstein, 1999).

One procedure for determining the visual acuity of mice is a two-alternative forced choice apparatus (see figure 2.1*E*) consisting of a start box that leads to a choice area with two parallel alleys, each with a food cup and a stimulus card at the end (Wiesenfeld and Branchek, 1976). Food-deprived mice were trained for 80 trials per day to discriminate

Figure 2.2 Mean (± SEM) percent correct for each of the 14 mouse strains on each of the eight days of testing in the visual detection task (*left column*) and the pattern discrimination task (*middle column*) and calculation of visual acuity threshold from mean (± SEM) percent correct for each strain on each of the eight spatial frequencies that were tested in the visual acuity task (*right column*). For clarity, mice were grouped into those with normal vision (*A*), albinos (*B*), those with retinal degeneration (*C*), and those of unknown visual abilities (*D*). (From Wong and Brown, 2006, p. 394.)

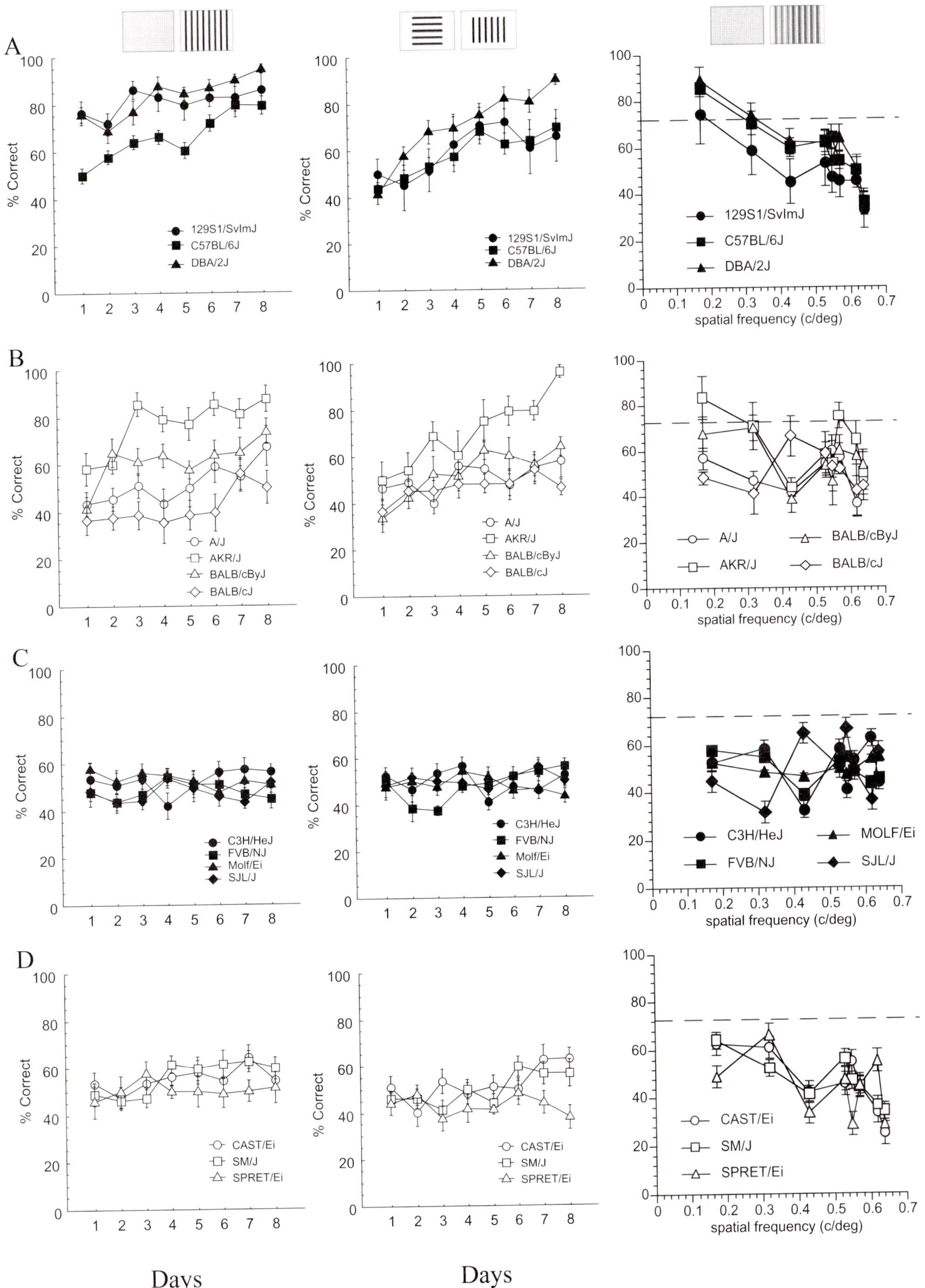

A
% Correct
129S1/SvImJ
C57BL/6J
DBA/2J
spatial frequency (c/deg)
B
A/J
AKR/J
BALB/cByJ
BALB/cJ
C
C3H/HeJ
FVB/NJ
Molf/Ei
SJL/J
MOLF/Ei
D
CAST/Ei
SM/J
SPRET/Ei
Days
Days

between pairs of vertical and horizontal stripes of the same spatial frequency (0.15 c/deg) using a food reward. During testing, the spatial frequencies were increased or decreased by 0.1 c/deg until the mouse reached a criterion of 90% correct choices. Using this protocol, Gianfranceschi et al. (1999) determined that the visual acuity of C57BL/6J mice was between 0.5 and 0.6 c/deg.

Using their visual water box, Prusky, West, and Douglas (2000a) trained mice as young as 40 days of age to swim to an escape platform signaled by a sinusoidal wave grating (S+) versus a homogeneous gray screen (S–). During testing, the spatial frequency of the grating was increased by one cycle at a time until the mouse made an incorrect response. A visual acuity threshold was obtained when the mouse performed below 70% correct at a particular spatial frequency. With this protocol, it was determined that C57BL/6J mice had a visual acuity of 0.51 c/deg.

Different test procedures, however, result in different visual acuity thresholds in the same strains of mice. Wong and Brown (2006) modified the procedure of Prusky et al. (2000a) by employing a standard set of eight spatial frequencies that were tested daily for 8 days. Using this procedure, mice with no known visual defects (129S1/SvImJ, C57BL/6J, DBA/2J) and two albino strains (AKR/J and BALB/cByJ) had defined visual acuity thresholds of 0.375, 0.245, 0.375, 0.375, and 0.320 c/deg, respectively. The other albino strains (A/J, BALB/cByJ, BALB/cJ) did not reach the criterion of 70% correct and so had thresholds below 0.17 c/deg (the largest stimulus used), whereas mice with retinal degeneration (C3H/HeJ, FVB/NJ, MOLF/EiJ, SJL/J) and mice with uncharacterized visual abilities (CAST/EiJ, SM/J, SPRET/EiJ) performed at chance levels. Using the same apparatus and procedure, however, Wong and Brown (2007) determined the visual acuity of 6-month-old C57BL/6J mice as 0.48 c/deg and that of DBA/2J mice as 0.54 c/deg.

There are also age-related differences in visual acuity within strains. As DBA/2J mice age, they develop glaucoma-like visual defects, and after 12 months of age they perform at chance, and no visual acuity threshold can be measured. C57BL/6J mice, on the other hand, retain their visual ability to at least 24 months of age, when it was measured at 0.38 c/deg (Wong and Brown, 2007) (figure 2.3). Because BALB/cByJ albino mice also show age-related retinal degeneration (Danciger et al., 2000, 2003), measurements of visual acuity obtained in young mice (3–6 months) may change as these mice age (see discussion in Wong and Brown, 2007).

Using the virtual optokinetic system, which records head movements in response to the "movement" of computer-generated vertical gratings in an optical cylinder (see figure 2.1*F*), Prusky et al. (2004) determined that C57BL/6J mice had a visual acuity threshold of 0.39 c/deg. The virtual optokinetic system is much less time-consuming than the visual water box, as it can provide reliable, consistent visual acuity thresholds in a single 25- to 40-minute test. Because it measures a reflex response and does not rely on swimming ability or involve the stress of immersion in water, as occurs with the visual water box, it seems to be a better way of measuring visual acuity, but this method is less sensitive than the visual water box in determining visual acuity thresholds in mice. Using an optokinetic drum, Abdeljalil et al. (2005) determined the visual acuity of C57BL/6J mice as 0.26 c/deg under scotopic conditions and 0.52 c/deg under photopic conditions, while 129/SvPas mice had a visual acuity threshold of 0.52 c/deg under both conditions. These measures are only crude estimates, because the steps were 0.26, 0.52, and 1.25 c/deg. CD-1 albino mice and C3HeB/FeJ mice, which have retinal degeneration, had no observable optomotor responses; thus their visual acuity was not measurable.

In general, behavioral tests indicate that mice without visual defects (C57BL/6J) have a visual acuity between 0.5 and 0.6 c/deg and albino mice have reduced visual acuity thresholds of 0.17–0.38 c/deg (Gianfranceschi et al., 1999; Prusky et al., 2000a; Sinex et al., 1979; Wong and Brown, 2006). This is relatively low compared to the visual acuity of 0.92 c/deg for the rat (Prusky et al., 2000a), 6–7 c/deg for cats (Blake et al., 1974; Smith, 1936), and 60 c/deg for humans (Oyster, 1999).

Hearing

The most sensitive and objective measure of hearing ability in mice is the measurement of the auditory evoked brainstem response (ABR), which is an evoked potential measurement of activity in the auditory nerve, fiber tracts, and nuclei within the auditory brainstem pathways. The ABR is a useful measure for determining hearing sensitivity in mice (Zhou et al., 2006), because analysis of ABR threshold, amplitude, and latency provides important information regarding the peripheral hearing status and the integrity of the brainstem pathways. The ABR is elicited using clicks and tones of varying frequency and intensity that are channeled through the ear canals of the mouse. Measurement of the ABR requires mice to be deeply anesthetized and subcutaneously implanted with a recording electrode below the pinna, superficial to the auditory nerve. Various clicks and tones ranging from 8 to 32 kHz are presented through earphones on both ears and the loudness of each tone is varied in 5-dB steps. Auditory nerve responses are filtered through a pre-amplifier and amplified 25,000–100,000 fold. The ABR is presented as a waveform for each stimulus, and an auditory threshold is defined as the lowest stimulus intensity that will evoke a normal ABR wave.

In a survey of 80 inbred mouse strains, Zheng et al. (1999) found that 61 strains had normal ABR thresholds and 19

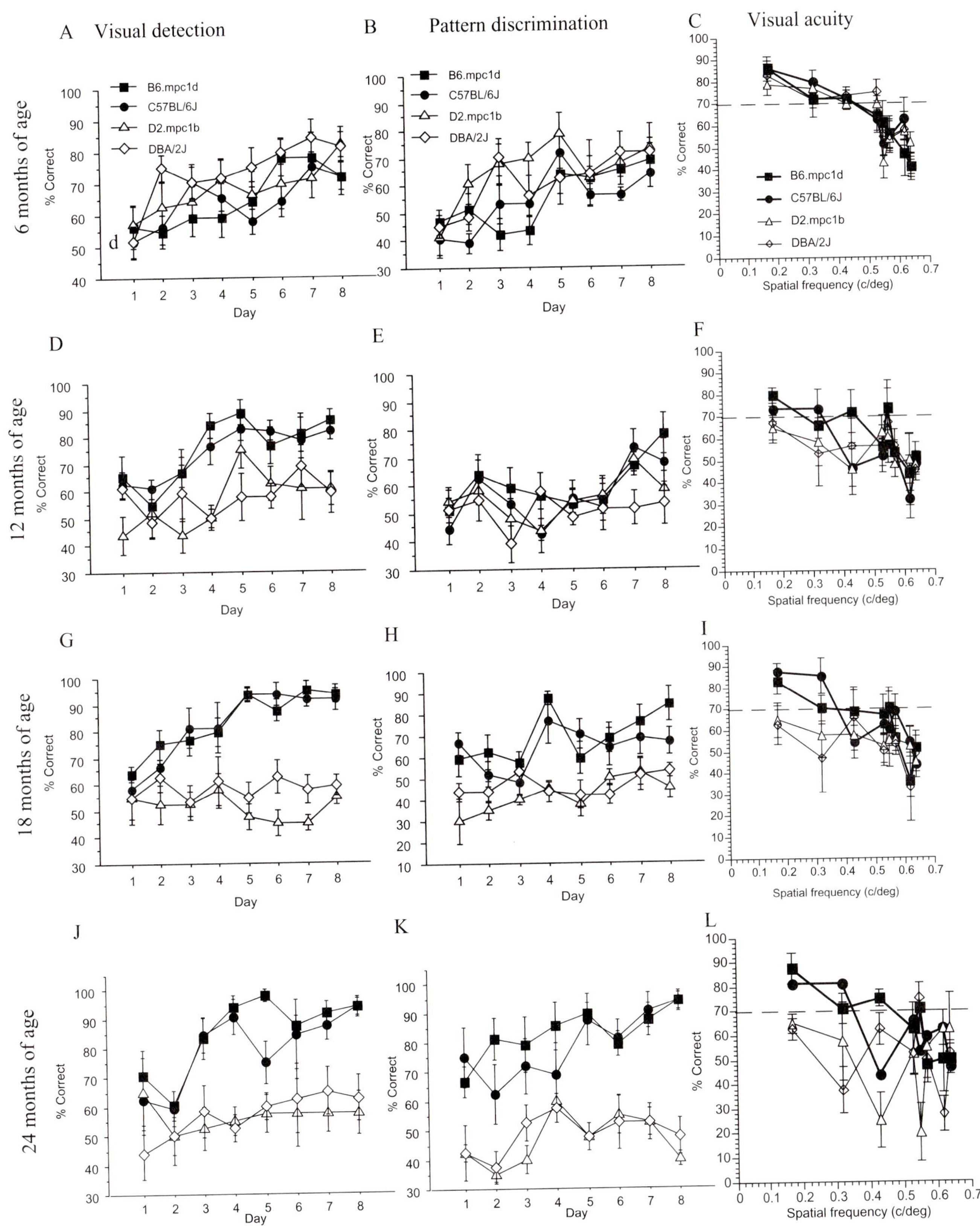

FIGURE 2.3 Mean (± SEM) percent correct for each strain on each of the eight days of testing in the visual detection task (*A*, *D*, *G*, and *J*) and the pattern discrimination task (*B*, *E*, *H*, and *K*) when mice were 6, 12, 18, and 24 months old. Visual acuity curves (*C*, *F*, *I*, and *L*) from mean (± SEM) percent correct for each strain on each of the eight spatial frequencies that were tested in the visual acuity task. (From Wong and Brown, 2007.)

strains had elevated ABR thresholds before 13 weeks of age. The 129/J, 129/ReJ, 129SvJ, C57BR/cdJ, C57L/J, DBA/2HaSmn, I/LnJ, and MA/MyJ strains had a mild hearing impairment (defined as 20–40 dB sound pressure level [SPL] above normal threshold); the A/J, DBA/2J, and SKH2/J strains had an intermediate impairment (41–60 dB SPL above normal threshold), and the BUB/BnJ, NOR/LtJ, and NOD/LtJ strains had a severe hearing impairment (>60 dB SPL above normal threshold). They also found that 16 strains with normal hearing when measured before 13 weeks of age exhibited age-related hearing loss. ABR thresholds for all hearing impaired strains increased with age, and for some strains, ABR thresholds varied significantly, depending on stimulus frequency (Zheng et al., 1999).

Tone detection thresholds have been evaluated behaviorally in mice using a testing cage divided into two compartments: a listening area, which has a speaker above it, and a response area, containing a water dipper. A water-deprived mouse is placed in the listening area, and when it hears a sequence of 250 ms tone bursts presented at a rate of two bursts per second, it must move into the response area within 3 s to receive a water reward. Tone detection thresholds are determined by gradually decreasing the tone levels in intervals of 5 dB. A tone detection threshold is calculated in terms of d' values, where d' = (z score for the percentage of hits for particular tone level) – (z score for the percentage of false alarms). An absolute threshold is defined as the sound pressure level that elicits a d' value of 1. Using this procedure, age-related hearing loss for high-frequency tones (16 kHz) in C57BL/6J mice was shown to develop between 21 and 33 weeks of age, while hearing loss for low-frequency tones (8 kHz) developed between 27 and 50 weeks of age. CBA/CaJ mice did not develop age-related hearing loss (Prosen et al., 2003).

Another widely used behavioral test for measuring auditory ability in the mouse is the acoustic startle test, which measures the startle response to a sudden loud noise. The startle reflex is measured by the amplitude of the whole-body flinch, and the acoustic startle amplitude is defined as the minimum decibel level that elicits a flinch (Crawley, 2000). Mice are placed in a small restraining tube in a chamber with white noise of 75–120 dB present as background noise. Brief tones of 70–120 dB are randomly delivered through a speaker on the wall of the chamber. Mice with normal hearing will show a startle response to tones of 100 dB or more, mice with impaired hearing will respond only to louder tones (100–120 dB), and deaf mice will respond only to acoustic stimuli of 120 dB or louder owing to their vibrational effects (Crawley, 2000).

A more sensitive measure of hearing is the prepulse inhibition of the acoustic startle response, which is also used as a behavioral measure of sensorimotor gating. First, a weak tone of 70–90 dB of varying frequencies (4, 12, or 20 kHz) is delivered, followed by a loud 100–120 dB tone 100 ms later. If mice can hear the weaker tone, they will inhibit their response to the louder tone, thus providing a measure of auditory ability. Willott et al. (2003) found significant differences among 40 inbred strains of mice tested for both acoustic startle and prepulse inhibition of acoustic startle. For example, DBA/2J mice, which have a hearing impairment, and C3H/HeJ mice had the smallest acoustic startle responses, BALB/c and FVB/NJ mice, which have normal hearing, had relatively large acoustic startle responses, and the responses of AKR/J mice fell in the middle.

Willott et al. (2003), however, demonstrated that there is only a weak relationship between hearing sensitivity as measured by the ABR and acoustic startle and prepulse inhibition of acoustic startle responses. Some strains of mice that demonstrate hearing loss at an early age (BUB/BnJ, A/J) show large acoustic startle amplitudes and relatively good prepulse inhibition, and conversely, some strains of mice that hear well (MOLF/Ei, C3H/HeJ, SJL/J) exhibit very small acoustic startle responses and weak prepulse inhibition. This could be due to the fact that measures of acoustic startle and prepulse inhibition of acoustic startle are not pure measures of hearing but have emotional and motor components that may confound the interpretation of the results. Also, a large body of literature suggests that dopamine is involved in sensory gating and prepulse inhibition (for a review, see Geyer, 2006). Strain differences in dopaminergic function could thus be responsible for this contradictory relationship between different measures of hearing ability.

Olfaction

The simplest behavioral test of olfactory ability in mice is the buried food test, in which the time taken for a food-deprived mouse to locate a piece of food buried in bedding material is recorded (Crawley, 2000). Using this test, Luo et al. (2002) showed that mice deficient in the G protein (G_o) were unable to locate a piece of food buried in 3 cm of bedding, while CD-1 hybrid and 129Sv-ter/C57BL/6 hybrid mice were able to do so. The buried food test is a measure of olfactory ability and cannot be used to measure strain differences in olfactory acuity or discrimination.

Odor discrimination ability can be tested using habituation-dishabituation or the habituation-discrimination tests, which are based on the observation that mice decrease their investigatory behavior when presented with a familiar odor and increase their investigatory behavior when presented with a novel odor (Slotnick et al., 2005). The habituation-dishabituation test involves the presentation of odor A for multiple trials (the habituation phase) and then a novel odor B is introduced (the dishabituation phase). In the habituation-discrimination test, odors A and B are both presented following habituation to odor A. Using the habituation-dishabituation test, Luo et al. (2002) found that mice deficient in G_o were unable to discriminate between geraniol (a flower odor) and citralua (lemon odor), whereas CD-1 hybrid and 129Sv-ter/C57BL/6 hybrid mice were able to discriminate between the two odors. Likewise, Macknin et al. (2004) found that transgenic mice overexpressing human tau protein (Tα1-3RT τTG mice) were unable to discriminate between vanilla and peach odors or between peppermint and vanilla orange spice odors in a habituation-dishabituation test, while their wild-type littermates were able to make this discrimination. Staggerer mutant (sg/sg) mice and their nonmutant littermates on a C57BL/6 background were both able to discriminate vanillin from amyl acetate odors in the habituation-dishabituation test (Deiss and Baudoin, 1999). Using the habituation-dishabituation test to determine olfactory acuity, Lee et al. (2003) showed that BALB/c mice could discriminate between conspecific urine odors at lower concentrations than C57BL/6J or 129/S1 mice. A criticism of these tests is that they depend on the intrinsic motivation of the mouse to investigate odors, and failure to show discrimination or dishabituation does not lead to the conclusion that the mice are unable to discriminate between odor A and odor B. They may be able to discriminate but may not show a motor investigatory response (Slotnick et al., 2005).

A more powerful method for studying the ability of mice to detect and discriminate between odors is to use an operant olfactometer, which delivers odors with controlled concentration, flow, and temporal parameters and measures operant responses (Slotnick et al., 2005). Water-deprived mice are trained to nose-poke into a glass odor port to sample the odor stimuli and receive a water reward when they detect the correct odor by licking the water spout (Bodyak and Slotnick, 1999). After the initial odor–no odor training, mice are trained in a go/no-go discrete trials procedure to discriminate between an odor that results in a water reward (CS+) and an odor that is not associated with reward (CS–). The operant olfactometer can also be used in mice to test odor detection thresholds, odor sampling behavior, discrimination between odor mixtures, odor masking, and odor memory. Using this protocol, it was shown that CF-1 mice readily acquired four separate two-odor discrimination tasks, and when all eight odors were randomly presented in the same session, the mice continued to perform well. Furthermore, memory for the eight odors after a 32-day rest period was at least 90% correct (Bodyak and Slotnick, 1999).

Mice with retinal degeneration, albino mice, and mice with age-related blindness are all able to learn to discriminate between odors in a conditioned odor preference task and remember these odors for up to 6 months (Brown and Schellinck, 2007; Brown and Wong, 2007; Schellinck et al., 2001; Wong and Brown, 2007).

Taste

The ability to discriminate different tastes is usually detected using a two-bottle choice test, in which two different taste solutions are presented in identical bottles in the home cage (Crawley, 2000; Ritchter 1939). To control for place preference, the position of the two bottles is switched over testing days and the volume of each taste solution consumed is measured over a fixed period of days. A difference between the volumes of each taste solution consumed is an index of taste discrimination ability, because mice will drink more of the preferred taste solution. Usually, a sweet (saccharin) or a bitter (quinine) solution is paired with normal tap water to investigate flavor discrimination ability; however, a two-bottle test of two different concentrations of the same flavor can be used to evaluate taste acuity.

In a survey of 28 mouse strains that were tested in a two-bottle preference test with different concentrations of NaCl, KCl, $CaCl_2$, or NH_4Cl versus water, Bachmanov et al. (2002) found significant strain differences in solution intakes and preferences. For example, CBA/J, C3H/HeJ, and AKR/J mice showed the strongest avoidance of NaCl solutions, while CAST/Ei, BUB/BnJ, and NZB/BINJ mice demonstrated the highest preference for NaCl solutions. AKR/J mice had the highest avoidance scores for KCl solutions, and C57BL/6J and SM/J mice had the highest preference scores for these solutions. All strains avoided the highest concentration of $CaCl_2$ solutions, with 129P3/J mice displaying the highest intake of $CaCl_2$. All strains also avoided the strongest concentration of NH_4Cl solution, with NZB/B1NJ and C57L/J mice having the highest intakes of NH_4Cl (Bachmanov et al., 2002).

There have been modifications of the two-bottle test that use three or six bottles (Owings et al., 1967). Tordoff and Bachmanov (2003) compared C57BL/6J and 129X1/SvJ mice on the standard two-bottle test and two forms of the three-bottle test, one in which the middle bottle contained flavored solution and the bottles on either side contained water and one in which two bottles of flavored solution were placed on either side of a bottle in the middle containing water. The results indicated that taste solution preferences were highest on the three-bottle test containing two flavored solutions and lowest on the standard two-bottle test. Similar results were found when the two-bottle test was compared with a six-bottle test, when more than half of the bottles on the six-bottle test contained a flavored solution. Thus, the relative availability of taste solution seems to determine taste preference scores, and Tordoff and Bachmanov (2003) suggest that the three-bottle test is more sensitive than the two-bottle test.

The two-bottle test is also subject to other confounds such as position preference, postingestional influences, and strain differences in thirst demand and water deprivation (Kotlus and Blizard, 1998). To avoid these confounds, one can use a short-term test that measures fluid intake in a 6-hour period from a single graduated cylinder given to non-water-deprived mice. Mice can be given a variety of flavored solutions over consecutive days, and water intake is measured three times before flavored solutions are introduced and twice after the last flavored solution is introduced. Using this protocol, Kotlus and Bizard (1998) found that among 10 inbred strains of mice (AKR/J, A/J, C3H/HeJ, C57BL/6J, C57/L, DBA/2J, NZB/BINJ, SJL/J, SM/J, SWR/J), there were significant strain differences in the intake of all flavored solutions (sucrose, saccharin, quinine, HCl, NaCl, and monosodium glutamate). Interestingly, unlike all other strains tested, DBA/2J and A/J mice did not increase their consumption of the sucrose- or saccharin-flavored solution, and DBA/2J mice were the only strain that did not decrease their intake of the quinine solution. DBA/2J mice (quinine insensitive) and C57BL/6J mice (quinine sensitive) have been used to study the genetic basis of bitter taste (Nelson et al., 2005).

Glendinning et al. (2002) developed a brief-access taste test that involves repeatedly presenting various flavor stimuli for 5–30 s to food- and water-deprived mice. This paradigm requires the use of a gustometer, an apparatus equipped with a taste stimulus delivery system that records the licking behavior of the mouse. When they tested C57BL/6J mice on three different flavored solutions (quinine hydrochloride, NaCl, and sucrose), Glendinning et al. (2002) demonstrated that a concentration–response curve for NaCl or sucrose could be generated in a single 30-minute session, and for quinine hydrochloride in three 30-minute sessions. This method is high throughput and can be used as a screening protocol to identify mice with either enhanced or diminished gustatory responsiveness. Furthermore, the data can be used to compare the gustatory responses of mutant mice maintained on a C57BL/6J background with wild-type C57BL/6J mice.

Tactile and vibrissae sensitivity

Tactile sensitivity can be measured by placing mice on a wire mesh platform and pushing von Frey monofilaments (e.g., bending forces of 0.3, 0.7, 1.6. 4.0, 9.8, 22.0, and 53.9 nM) through the mesh onto their hind feet from below using a single, steady application of more than 1 s. The median foot withdrawal threshold is a measure of tactile sensitivity (Crawley, 2000). In the von Frey filament test of mechanical sensitivity, C57BL/6J, CBA/J, and SM/J mice showed a below-average foot withdrawal threshold, 129/J, C3H/HeJ, C58/J, DBA/2J, and RIIIS/J mice showed an average response, and A/J, AKR/J, and BALB/cByJ mice showed an elevated foot withdrawal threshold (Mogil et al., 1999a). The tactile version of the startle reflex can also be used to measure the flinch response to a puff of air (Plappert et al., 2006).

To test tactile discrimination, two different types of textures can be placed on the floor in the arms of a Y-maze, and differences in the amount of time a mouse spends in each arm are recorded as an indication of tactile discrimination preference (Lipp and van der Loos, 1991). Tactile discrimination learning can also be tested using a Y-shaped modified Lashley jumping stand. A start platform is located approximately 6 cm away from the two choice platforms, which are lined with different textures (e.g., diamond vs. square wire mesh). Using only their vibrissae to detect these textures, mice are trained to jump to one of the platforms to receive a food reward (Cybulska-Klosowicz and Kossut, 2001; Mazarakis et al., 2005). Using this test, it was demonstrated that presymptomatic transgenic Huntington disease mice (R6/1) had a severe impairment of tactile discrimination learning compared with wild-type CBA × C57BL/6 mice (Mazarakis et al., 2005).

Visual-Somatosensory Interaction The topographic maps of visual input and somatosensory input from the vibrissae of mice in the superior colliculus (SC, optic tectum) are highly correlated (Drager and Hubel, 1975). In fact, the vibrissae projections to the SC follow "the roles dictated by the visual projections" (Drager and Hubel, 1976, p. 99), and in blind mice, the use of vibrissae and the somatosensory representation of the whiskers in the SC are both increased (Benedetti, 1992; Raushecker et al., 1992). This suggests that mice may be able to develop a tactile as well as a visual "cognitive map" of their environment, and that this vibrissae "map" may allow blind mice to perform many behavioral tasks.

Pain sensitivity

Pain sensitivity in mice can be measured in response to thermal, chemical, or neuropathic pain-inducing procedures.

Thermal Nociception The latency to withdraw from a hot or cold stimulus can be used as a measure of pain sensitivity. In the tail flick test, a mouse is placed on a platform with its tail positioned under a hot light beam and the latency to flick the tail out of the light beam is used as a measure of pain sensitivity. Adaptations of the tail flick test, such as the Hargreaves test (Hargreaves et al., 1988), involve directing the beam of light onto the skin of the hind paw instead of the tail. The hot water tail flick and cold water tail flick tests measure the latency to remove the tail from a beaker of hot (49.0–52.5°C) or ice water, respectively (Janssen et al., 1963). The hot-plate test involves placing the mouse on a metal plate that has been heated to 52–55°C.

The latency to lick or shake the paw or to jump in response to the heat is used as a measure of pain sensitivity (Crawley, 2000).

Chemical Nociception The formalin test consists of injecting formalin subcutaneously into the dorsal surface of the hind paw and scoring the responses to the affected paw (lifting, shaking, licking) as measures of pain sensitivity (Crawley, 2000; Tjolsen et al., 1992). Hind paw sensitivity to subcutaneous carrageenan injections is another method used to measure chemical pain sensitivity in mice. Carrageenan is a mucopolysaccharide that produces inflammation, hypersensitivity, and spontaneous pain (Tonussi and Ferreira, 1992). Four hours after injection, mice are observed for changes in sensitivity of the injected paw, using the Hargreaves test as previously described (Mogil et al., 1999a).

Neuropathic Pain Pain resulting from hind limb denervation is used as an animal model of anesthesia dolorosa (numbness accompanied by constant pain) or phantom limb (Mogil et al., 1999a; Wall et al., 1979). The Chung peripheral nerve injury model (Kim and Chung, 1992) is also used to produce neuropathic pain in mice. One of the three spinal nerves serving the hind limb is ligated, leaving partial innervation of the hind limb. Mice can be evaluated for hypersensitivity of the operate paw using the Hargreaves test of thermal nociception to compare paw withdrawal latencies in the operate paw and nonoperate paw (Mogil et al., 1999a).

There are strain differences in responses to all of these different pain-inducing stimuli (Kazdoba et al., 2007; Mogil et al., 1999a, 1999b), but strains have different rankings in pain sensitivity on each test. Thus, the comparisons of inbred mouse strains in terms of their sensitivity to pain depends on the type of pain stimulus used. For example, BALB/cJ, FVB/NJ, and DBA/2J mice are more sensitive to foot shock pain than C57BL/6J, 129X1/SvJ and C3H/HeJ mice (Kazdoba et al., 2007) and C57BL/6J and 129/J mice are more sensitive than C3H/He and DBA/2 mice to thermal pain on the hot-plate test (Mogil et al., 1999a). C57BL/6J mice are more sensitive than 129/J, BALB/c, C3H/HeJ, and DBA/2 mice on the tail withdrawal test of thermal sensitivity, but 129/J, BALB/cJ, C57BL/6J and DBA/2J mice are less sensitive than C3H/HeJ mice on the acute response to formalin injection test (Mogil et al., 1999a).

There is considerable evidence that pain responses are influenced by laboratory environmental variables such as experimenter effects, housing, time of day, seasonal effects, and test order (Chesler et al., 2002), as well as by differences in stimuli used to elicit pain, but there is no evidence from these studies that pain responses are influenced by visual ability in mice. However, if pain such as shock is used as punishment on a vision test, as in the Yerkes discrimination box (see figure 2.1*A*), strain differences in pain responsiveness may confound measures of strain differences in visual ability.

The importance of vision in tasks evaluating higher order cognitive functions

Behavioral tasks used to study higher order cognitive functions, such as learning and memory and anxiety-related behaviors, are crucial in the search for the genetic, neural, and molecular bases of these complex behaviors. These tasks, however, are dependent on the sensory abilities of the mouse, and if it is to be demonstrated that strain differences in complex behavioral responses are due to differences in cognitive function, it must be shown that these differences are not confounded by strain differences in sensory functions (Bailey et al., 2006; Brown and Wong, 2007; Crawley, 1999). The following section reviews of some of the tasks commonly used to study complex behavior, with examples of how performance on these tasks can be confounded by visual impairments.

Learning and memory tasks

Some learning and memory tasks depend on visual ability, others do not (see table 2.2). The following descriptions are divided into tasks that depend on visual ability and tasks that involve other sensory abilities to execute the task correctly.

Visually Dependent Tasks

The Morris water maze task. The Morris water maze (Morris, 1984) has become the most widely used task to evaluate spatial learning and memory in mice. It consists of a circular pool filled with opaque water, with a submerged platform in a hidden location. Over multiple trials, mice are trained to locate the hidden platform using spatial information from distal visual cues around the testing room, and the latency to find the platform is recorded. There are many different protocols for using the Morris water maze (Crawley, 2000). To evaluate reversal learning, the position of the platform can be moved to the opposite quadrant after 3 days of training, and to evaluate cued learning, a visible platform can be used (Wong and Brown, 2007). To evaluate memory, mice are tested in a probe trial in which the platform is removed from the pool and the time spent swimming in the quadrant where the platform was previously located is used as an index of spatial memory.

The Morris water maze relies on visual ability because the mouse must locate the hidden platform using visual cues. Thus, the experimenter must be sure that the mice being tested do not have any vision problems that would result in poor performance in the Morris water maze. Although researchers often use a visual platform test to control for visual deficits, the visual platform may not be adequate for detecting small differences in visual ability that may be responsible for poor performance (Prusky et al., 2000b; Robinson et al., 2001). For example, visual ability, as measured in the visual water box, was highly correlated with learning (swim latency and distance to find the platform) and memory (number of annulus crossings in the probe trial), indicating that mice with poor visual ability also performed poorly in the Morris water maze (Brown and Wong, 2007) (figure 2.4). Furthermore, when the performance of C3H/HeJ and CBA/J mice, which have the *rd1* mutation of the *Pde6b* gene causing retinal degeneration, on the Morris water maze task was compared with the performance of two *Pde6b* wild-type strains that do not have retinal degeneration (C3A.BLiA-*Pde6b*$^{+}$/J and CBA/CaJ), only the wild-type strains showed spatial learning (Clapcote et al., 2005). Transgenic anophthalmic mice displayed persistent thigmotaxic behavior and severe spatial learning impairments on the Morris water maze task when compared to their wild-type counterparts (Buhot et al., 2001). Likewise, Garcia et al. (2004) demonstrated that the presence of the retinal degeneration gene in three strains of transgenic Alzheimer's disease mice (App_{sw}, Tau, and Tau + APP_{sw}) and their wild-type controls resulted in profound impairment in learning the Morris water maze.

The Morris water maze also relies on adequate motor ability, because mice may have to swim for up to 60 s to find the platform. Thus, researchers who use the Morris water maze to evaluate learning and memory in the mouse must be sure that their mice are healthy enough to perform the task and have no obvious abnormalities in motor ability that would affect task performance. For example, many transgenic mice are smaller than their wild-type littermates, and smaller body weight could result in hypothermia in the Morris water maze (Iivonen et al., 2003).

The radial arm maze. The radial arm maze consists of a central start box with 8 or 12 radiating arms. Food-restricted mice are trained to find a food reward in one or more of the arms of the maze (Crusio et al., 1995; Olton and Samuelson, 1976). Different training protocols can be used, depending on the type of memory being evaluated (MacDonald and

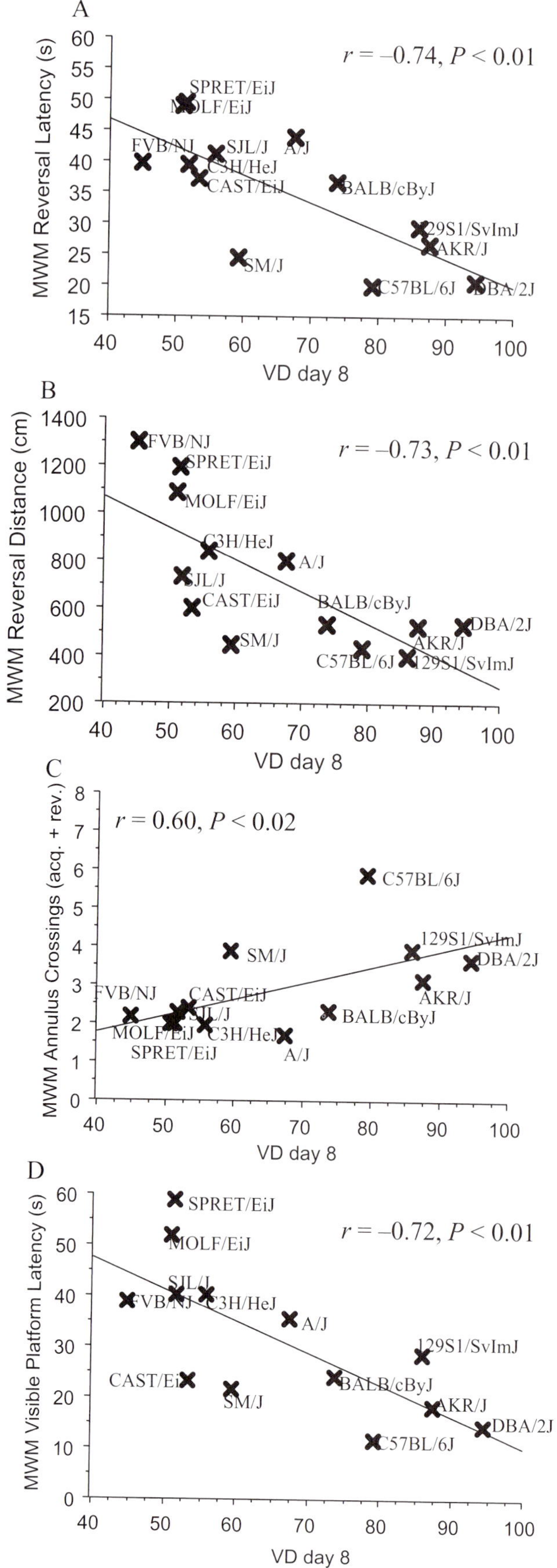

FIGURE 2.4 Regression plots showing the correlation of strain means between percent correct on day 8 of the visual detection task (VD 8) and mean reversal latency (s) (*A*), mean reversal swim distance (cm) (*B*), number of annulus crossings (*C*), and mean visible platform latency (s) (*D*) on the Morris water maze task. Visual ability was significantly correlated with all four measures of performance in the water maze. (From Brown and Wong, 2007, p. 141.)

White, 1993). For example, to assess working memory, every arm is baited with food, and errors are scored when the mouse visits arms more than once (win-shift). To assess reference memory, only particular arms contain food, with the same arms being baited over successive trials (win-stay). The mouse is required to learn the location of the baited arms, and errors are scored when mice enter nonbaited arms. To assess conditioned-cue preference, only two arms of the radial arm maze are used. Each arm has a cue (such as a light versus no light) and mice are trained to receive food reward in either the "light" or the "dark" arm. The stimulus-reward association memory is assessed by the time spent in each arm in a preference test in which neither arm contains food. Mice that remember the stimulus–reward association should spend more time in the arm that was previously paired with food. The radial arm maze relies on visual ability because researchers often place visual cues, such as lights, patterns, or small objects, between arms to orient the mouse. Mice with poor vision (CBA, C3H/He, BALB/c) exhibited poor performance in a radial arm maze using distal visual cues to signal food reward, whereas mice with normal vision (C57BL/6 and DBA/2) were able to learn the task (Roullet and Lassalle, 1995). Mice with retinal degeneration were impaired in learning to find the platform in a six-arm radial swim maze (Garcia et al., 2004).

The Barnes maze. The Barnes maze was developed to evaluate spatial learning and memory in rats (Barnes, 1979) and has been modified for use with mice (Bach et al., 1995; Holmes et al., 2002). It consists of a circular, white, brightly lit platform with 12 or more holes around the periphery, one of which leads to a small enclosed escape box. The mouse must learn to escape the bright light by finding the location of the escape hole using distal visual cues placed around the testing room. Thus the Barnes maze relies on visual ability as well as auditory ability, as many researchers use a buzzer to make the task more aversive. Many mice suffer from noise-induced hearing loss, so it is important to test mice in the Barnes maze after all other behavioral tasks that rely on hearing ability are completed. Although the Barnes maze relies on adequate motor ability to execute the task, it is less stressful than the Morris water maze, because swimming is not necessary. Furthermore, it offers an advantage over the radial arm maze task in that mice are not required to undergo food deprivation.

CBA/J mice (a strain of mice with retinal degeneration) and DBA/2J mice (a strain that is deaf by 3 months of age) were significantly worse at locating the escape hole in the Barnes maze than C57BL/6J or 129/SvEms mice (Nguyen et al., 2000). Garcia et al. (2004) found that performance in the Barnes maze was not affected by homozygosity of the retinal degeneration gene in three strains of transgenic Alzheimer's disease mice (App_{sw}, Tau, and Tau + APP_{sw}) and their wild-type controls, although there were clear trends for an rd effect in each genotype. However, this study used an adaptation of the original Barnes maze design, in which a black wall was placed around the periphery of the maze (Pompl et al., 1999), and the addition of this wall causes mice to adopt a nonvisual search strategy, as mice use tactile information rather than visual cues to navigate around the wall (O'Leary and Brown, 2005).

Cued and contextual fear conditioning. Cued and contextual fear conditioning measures the ability of the mouse to learn and remember environmental cues associated with an aversive experience (Fanselow, 1980; LeDoux, 1995). The major advantage of using the cued and context conditioning paradigm is that it provides a measure of learning and memory in only two test days. Each type of conditioning (cued versus contextual) places different sensory demands on the mouse, allowing the researcher to determine whether sensory deficits are the underlying cause for poor performance. The standard cued and contextual conditioning procedure entails placing the mouse in a visually distinct conditioning chamber and exposing it to an auditory stimulus followed by a mild foot shock. Approximately 24 hours later, the mouse is returned to the same conditioning chamber and observed for bouts of freezing. The number of seconds that the mouse spends freezing is a measure of memory for the context in which fear was conditioned. This task relies on visual, tactile, and olfactory ability, because the mouse must be able to recognize that it has been placed in the same chamber that had previously delivered the foot shock.

To test for memory of the auditory cue, mice are placed in a novel chamber with different visual, tactile, and/or odor cues from the conditioning chamber, and the auditory cue used in the conditioning phase is presented. The number of seconds spent freezing is an indication of memory for the auditory cue to which fear was conditioned. This task depends on auditory ability, because the mouse must be able to hear the auditory cue, and deaf mice will fail to freeze to the tone. Although visual ability plays some role in cued conditioning, changes in odor and texture of the chamber may be robust enough to elicit fear behavior in blind mice.

Strain differences have been reported in both cued and context conditioning, and three strains of mice with retinal degeneration (C3H/HeIbg, CBA/J, and SJL/J) had impaired memory for the context, while DBA/2J mice (which have age-related hearing loss) displayed memory impairment on the cued version of the task (Balogh and Wehner, 2003; Owen et al., 1997). However, Bolivar et al. (2001) found no influence of vision on cued or contextual fear conditioning.

Active and passive avoidance learning. Active and passive avoidance tasks require the mouse to avoid the location where it received a mild foot shock, either by exiting the chamber where it received the foot shock (active avoidance) or by refraining from entering the chamber in which the foot shock was delivered (passive avoidance) (Crawley, 2000; Mathis et al., 1994; McGaugh, 1966).

Testing active avoidance entails placing the mouse in the dark compartment of a two-compartment chamber and giving foot shock until the mouse enters the light compartment to escape the foot shock. Twenty-four hours later, the mouse is reintroduced to the dark compartment and latency to enter the light compartment is used as a measure of memory. In the passive avoidance task, the mouse is placed in the light compartment, and when the door between the two compartments is lifted the mouse enters the dark chamber. Once the mouse has entered the dark compartment, the door is closed and a single foot shock is administered. Twenty-four hours later, the mouse is reintroduced to the light compartment and latency to enter the dark compartment is used as a measure of memory (Crawley, 2000). Adaptations of the avoidance paradigms include step-down passive avoidance, in which the mouse must learn that stepping down from a small platform will elicit a foot shock, and Y-maze or T-maze avoidance learning, in which mice must learn to avoid or escape the arm of the maze that delivers a foot shock.

Avoidance learning requires mice to have normal pain perception and motor abilities to execute the task. Although visual ability is required for mice to differentiate between the two compartments, mice with retinal degeneration are capable of brightness detection (Nagy and Misinin, 1970). Blind mice are not impaired in learning an active avoidance response in a T-maze (Farr et al., 2002), but mice with retinal degeneration (C3H and CBA strains) were impaired in learning a one-way active avoidance task (Wahlsten, 1973). FVB/NJ mice (which have retinal degeneration), 129S6/SvEvTac mice (which have visual impairment), and C3H mice (which also have retinal degeneration) were the poorest learners in a lever press escape/avoidance task (Brennan, 2004).

Visually Independent Tasks

Conditioned odor preference. Schellinck et al. (2001) developed an olfactory discrimination task that entails training mice to associate an odor with a sugar reward. Food-deprived mice are presented with a rose odor paired with a sugar reward and a lemon odor paired with no reward (or vice versa) for four training trials per day over 4 days. They are then tested for a conditioned odor preference by presenting both odors with no reward, and the time spent digging in each odor pot is measured. Mice able to discriminate between a rose odor and a lemon odor will dig in the odor pot that was associated with the sugar reward (CS+) during training. Mice of three strains (CD-1, C57BL/6NCrlBR, and DBA/2NCrlBR) have been shown to learn this task (Schellinck, 2001), and both C57BL/6J and DBA/2J mice, a strain of mice that exhibits age-related blindness, can perform this task at 12–24 months of age, indicating that blind mice can perform this task as well as sighted mice (Wong and Brown, 2007). Indeed, blind mice appear to have a better memory for odors than sighted mice (Brown and Wong, 2007).

The olfactory tubing maze. The olfactory tubing maze is an ethologically relevant way to study learning and memory in mice, independent of their visual ability (Roman et al., 2002). The olfactory tubing maze consists of four chambers joined together by plastic elbow tubes. The testing chambers are composed of two plastic tubes connected in a plus shape and having an odor port, water well, and buzzer at one end and a fan above the center to exhaust the odor stimuli from the maze. After habituation to the apparatus, water-deprived mice are placed in the maze and a CS+ odor stimulus (associated with a drop of water in the water well) and a CS− odor stimulus (associated with a 3-second buzzer) are presented. The mouse is required to enter the tube with the CS+ odor in order to get a water reward. The mouse must then move to the second testing chamber to start the next trial. During the intertrial interval, clean air is flushed through the apparatus. Mice are tested for 20 trials per day for 7 days, and the percentage of correct responses and the latency to respond to an odor stimulus are analyzed to evaluate performance.

Using this protocol, Restivo et al. (2006) tested five strains of mice (BALB/c, CD-1, 129/SvPasCrl, C57BL/6, and DBA/2J) and found that all strains except DBA/2J mice were able to successfully acquire the odor–reward associations by the seventh day of testing. Because it has been previously demonstrated that DBA/2J mice are able to acquire simple odor discriminations (Schellinck et al., 2001; Wong and Brown, 2007), the poor performance of DBA/2J mice in the olfactory tubing maze may reflect an impairment of the odor–reward associations. However, DBA/2J mice suffer from hearing loss at an early age (see table 2.1), and therefore poor performance in the olfactory tubing maze could result from inability to hear the buzzer associated with an incorrect choice.

Conditioned taste aversion. Conditioned taste aversion is a classic conditioning paradigm that relies on the ability of the mouse to remember and avoid the taste of foods that had been associated with sickness (Palmerino et al., 1980). In this test, a novel taste, such as saccharin or sucrose, is added to the drinking water and paired with an intraperitoneal injection of a malaise-inducing agent such as lithium chloride.

The suppression of drinking liquid containing the taste paired with illness versus water in a two-bottle choice test is used as a measure of associative learning and memory. The advantages of using the conditioned taste aversion paradigm is that it has a short training period of one or two trials, associative learning is maintained after long delays between consumption of the novel taste and administration of the malaise-inducing drug, and performance relies mainly on normal taste perception.

Mice readily learn the conditioned taste aversion to a variety of malaise-inducing agents, including lithium chloride (Ingram, 1982), nicotine (Risinger and Brown, 1996), and ethanol (Broadbent et al., 2002). There is no evidence that visual impairment influences conditioned taste aversion ability, as mice with retinal degeneration (C3H, SJL) and albino mice with poor vision (BALB/cJ and A/J) perform as well as sighted mice (Broadbent et al., 2002).

Anxiety-related behavior tasks

Three different behavioral tasks, the elevated plus or zero maze, the open field test, and the light-dark transition test, are commonly used to assess anxiety-related behavior. All involve some form of visual cues.

The Elevated Plus and Elevated Zero Mazes The elevated plus maze is based on the principle that mice that are more anxious should avoid open, brightly lit areas and prefer dark, enclosed compartments. The elevated plus maze consists of two enclosed arms and two open arms, joined at the middle in the shape of a plus. All four arms of the maze are divided into equal areas, in order to determine activity levels. The maze is elevated approximately 1 m from the floor to emphasize the aversiveness of the open arms. Mice are placed in the middle compartment and observed for locomotor activity (line crosses, rears), risk assessment (head dips, stretch-attend postures), and anxiety-related behaviors (closed-arm duration, urinations, defecations) (Brown et al., 1999; Podhorna and Brown, 2002).

The elevated plus maze relies on visual ability because the aversive stimuli used to provoke anxiety-related behaviors entail visual cues such as height and light. Nontransgenic mice with retinal degeneration showed less anxiety on the elevated plus maze than those with normal vision (Garcia et al., 2004), as did transgenic anophthalmic mice (Buhot et al., 2001). C3H/HeJ, a strain with retinal degeneration, showed the least anxiety (spent the most time in the open arms of an elevated plus maze) compared to 129S2/Sv, BALB/c, C57BL/6J, CBA/Ca, and DBA/2 mice (Brooks et al., 2005). Mice with retinal degeneration also spent more time in the open areas of an elevated zero maze (an adaptation of the elevated plus maze) than mice with normal vision (Cook et al., 2001).

The Open Field Test The open field test consists of a square or circular arena, brightly lit from above, with the floor divided into a grid of equal squares with lines or photocells. Mice are placed in the apparatus for 5 minutes per day for 2 days, and the frequency of spontaneous behaviors such as line crosses, rearing, grooming, stretch-attend postures, time spent in the center square, urinations, and defecations are measured (Brown et al., 1999; Podhorna and Brown, 2002). From these behaviors, measures of locomotion (number of line crosses and rearing), risk assessment (frequency of stretch-attend postures), and anxiety (frequency of entries, duration in the center square, and number of defecations) can be obtained. Anxious mice have fewer entries into and duration in the center square. The open field test involves visual ability, because the apparatus must be seen by the mouse to provoke anxious behaviors. For example, among 13 strains of mice, Wong and Brown (2004) found a significant negative correlation between visual ability (as measured by performance on the visual water box) and frequency of center square entries, indicating that mice with poor visual ability (e.g., strains of mice with retinal degeneration: C3H/HeJ, FVB/NJ, MOLF/EiJ, SJL/J) entered the center square in the open field more often than mice that performed well in the visual water box. Thus, blind mice may venture into the center square because they are unaware that it is aversive. Albino mice behave differently from pigmented mice in the open field owing to differences in their visual system, and these strain differences depend on the light levels used during testing (DeFries et al., 1966).

The Light-Dark Transition Task The light-dark transition task exploits the natural inclination of the mouse to avoid brightly lit areas. The apparatus consists of a box with a smaller, dark compartment and a larger, brightly lit compartment, and an opening between the two compartments. Mice are placed in the center of the brightly lit compartment facing the opening and allowed to explore the apparatus for 5 minutes. A mouse that is more anxious will spend less time in the illuminated compartment and make fewer transitions between the two compartments (Bou.in and Hascoet, 2003). The benefit of using the light-dark transition task to test anxiety in mice is that even mice with retinal degeneration are capable of brightness detection (Nagy and Misanin, 1970) and modify their activity levels in response to pulses of bright light (Mrosovsky et al., 2000). This may be due to the presence of melanopsin in photosensitive retinal ganglion cells (Panda et al., 2003). Wong and Brown (2004) found there was no significant correlation between visual ability (as measured by performance in the visual water box) and time spent in the light zone of the light-dark transition test among 13 strains of mice, some of which had retinal degeneration (C3H/HeJ, FVB/NJ, MOLF/EiJ, SJL/J).

Future directions for using behavioral tasks in mice with normal visual ability and with deficits in visual ability: Exploiting the natural abilities of mice

It is important to develop behavioral tasks that exploit the natural abilities of the mouse, which can be used to test cognitive functions independently of visual ability. Although olfactory-based tasks seem to be the best suited for the mouse, tasks that rely on olfactory ability present problems in the generation, control, and measurement of the odor stimuli that are not encountered with stimuli for other sensory modalities (Slotnick et al., 2005). A behavioral test battery in which many tasks are used to measure the same underlying cognitive function is probably the best approach. In this way, scores from tasks that measure the same higher order functions but rely on different sensory abilities can be compared. For example, discrimination learning and memory ability can be measured on tasks that use visual, auditory, olfactory, gustatory, or tactile stimuli. Mice with visual impairments but normal cognitive ability will fail on the visual discrimination task but learn auditory, olfactory, gustatory, and tactile discriminations.

Bailey et al. (2006) recommend a multitiered approach to phenotyping transgenic mice that begins with evaluating basic measures of general health, followed by examining neurological, sensory, and motor functions. The last stages of the phenotyping strategy involve testing mice on behavioral tasks that are aimed to address the hypothesized function of the gene of interest, such as tests for anxiety-related behaviors, drug abuse, motor function, social interactions, learning and memory, and nociception. By determining sensory and motor abilities first, one can select complex tests of cognitive function that are not confounded by sensory or motor impairments (Bailey et al., 2006). Similarly, the SHIRPA test battery (Rodgers et al., 1997) is a systematic and hierarchical protocol used to detect mouse mutants. It consists of a primary screen of approximately 30 rapid tests for neurological and neuropsychological deficits, such as deficits in muscle and lower motor neuron function, spinocerebellar function, sensory function, neuropsychiatric function, and autonomic function. The secondary screen consists of a comprehensive behavioral screening battery and pathological analysis. Finally, the tertiary screen involves more sophisticated tests to assess behavior, such as the Morris water maze, electroencephalography, and nerve conduction. However, many mouse test batteries do not have systematic tests for sensory function (e.g., Takao et al., 2007).

Behavioral paradigms that are used to phenotype mice should be standardized and validated. Standardization is necessary to increase replicability within a given laboratory and is also required for comparison of results between laboratories (Wahlsten et al., 2003, 2006). Tasks for a specific behavioral domain should also be assessed for construct validity (how well a measure of a particular trait, process, or state reflects theoretical assumptions), predictive validity (how well a manipulation predicts performance in the condition that is to be modeled), and face validity (the degree of similarities between the model and the actual disorder) (van der Staay and Steckler, 2001, 2002). Furthermore, behavioral tasks that were originally developed for rats and adapted for mice require extensive validation (Arndt and Surjo, 2001).

Conclusions

Many of the behavioral tasks that are used to measure cognitive functions in mice depend on normal visual function. Thus, it is critical to first evaluate the sensory functioning of the mouse, and then compare the data with results obtained on behavioral tasks to determine higher order cognitive function. This is especially true for studies in transgenic mice that aim to determine the genetic contribution of human neurological diseases. Transgenic and knockout mice have the phenotypic traits of the background strain, and differences between inbred strains, which are independent of the gene of interest, may significantly affect the behavioral phenotype of a mouse. For this reason, it is important to examine phenotypic differences between inbred strains of mice used as background strains for transgenic mice (Bothe et al., 2005; Brooks et al., 2005; Gerlai 1996; Nguyen and Gerlai, 2002; Tarantino et al., 2000). In addition, the background strain used to maintain the genetic disruption must be carefully selected, so that noncognitive factors such as sensory deficits do not affect task performance and thus decrease the usefulness of a particular animal model.

REFERENCES

Abdeljalil, J., Hamid, M., Abdel-mouttalib, O., Stephane, R., Raymond, R., Johan, A., Jose, S., Pierre, C., and Serge, P. (2005). The optomotor response: A robust first-line visual screening method for mice. *Vision Res.* 45:1439–1446.

Ammassari-Teule, M., and de Marsanich, B. (1996). Spatial and visual discrimination in CD1 mice: Partial analogy between the effect of lesions to the hippocampus and the amygdala. *Physiol. Behav.* 60:265–271.

Arndt, S. S., and Surjo, D. (2001). Methods for the behavioural phenotyping of mouse mutants: How to keep the overview. *Behav. Brain Res.* 125:39–42.

Bach, M. E., Hawkins, R. D., Osman, M., Kandel, E. R., and Mayford, M. (1995). Impairment of spatial but not contextual memory in CaMKII mutant mice with a selective loss of hippocampal LTP in the range of θ frequency. *Cell* 81:905–915.

Bachmanov, A. A., Beauchamp, G. K., and Tordoff, M. G. (2002). Voluntary consumption of NaCl, KCl, $CaCl_2$ and NH_4Cl solutions by 28 mouse strains. *Behav. Genet.* 32:445–457.

Bailey, K. R., Rustay, N. R., and Crawley, J. N. (2006). Behavioral phenotyping of transgenic and knockout mice: Practical concerns and potential pitfalls. *ILAR J.* 47:124–131.

Balkema, G. W., Mangini, N. J., and Pinto, L. H. (1983). Discrete visual defects in pearl mutant mice. *Science* 219:1085–1087.

Balogh, S. A., McDowell, C. S., Stavnezer, A. J., and Denenberg, V. H. (1999). A behavioral and neuroanatomical assessment of an inbred substrain of 129 mice with behavioral comparisons to C57BL/6J mice. *Brain Res.* 836:38–48.

Balogh, S. A., Sherman, G. F., Hyde, L., and Denenberg, V. H. (1998). Effects of neocortical ectopias upon the acquisition and retention of a non-spatial reference memory task in BXSB mice. *Dev. Brain Res.* 111:291–293.

Balogh, S. A., and Wehner, J. M. (2003). Inbred mouse strain differences in the establishment of long-term fear memory. *Behav. Brain Res.* 140:97–106.

Barnes, C. A. (1979). Memory deficits associated with senescence: A neurophysiological and behavioral study in the rat. *J. Comp. Physiol. Psychol.* 93:74–104.

Beck, J. A., Lloyd, S., Hafezparast, M., Lennon-Pierce, M., Eppig, J. T., Festing, M. F. W., and Fisher, E. M. C. (2000). Genealogies of mouse inbred strains. *Nat. Genet.* 24:23–25.

Benedetti, F. (1992). The development of the somatosensory representation in the superior colliculus of visually deprived mice. *Brain Res. Dev. Brain Res.* 65:173–178.

Blake, R., Cool, S. J., and Crawford, M. L. J. (1974). Visual resolution in the cat. *Vision Res.* 14:1211–1217.

Bodyak, N., and Slotnick, B. (1999). Performance in an automated olfactometer: Odor detection, discrimination and odor memory. *Chem. Senses* 24:637–645.

Bolivar, V. J., Pooler, O., and Flaherty, L. (2001). Inbred strain variation in contextual and cued fear conditioning behavior. *Mamm. Genome* 12:651–656.

Bothe, G. W. M., Bolivar, V. J., Vedder, M. J., and Geistfeld, J. G. (2005). Behavioral differences among fourteen inbred mouse strains commonly used as disease models. *Comp. Med.* 55:326–334.

Bourin, M., and Hascoet, M. (2003). The mouse light/dark box test. *Eur. J. Pharmacol.* 463:55–65.

Brennan, F. X. (2004). Genetic differences in leverpress escape/avoidance conditioning in seven mouse strains. *Genes Brain Behav.* 3:110–114.

Broadbent, J., Muccino, K. J., and Cunningham, C. L. (2002). Ethanol-induced conditioned taste aversion in 15 inbred mouse strains. *Behav. Neurosci.* 116:138–148.

Brooks, S. P., Pask, T., Jones, L., and Dunnett, S. B. (2005). Behavioral profiles of inbred mouse strains used as transgenic backgrounds. II. Cognitive tests. *Genes Brain Behav.* 4:307–317.

Brown, R. E., Corey, S. C., and Moore, A. K. (1999). Differences in measures of exploration and fear in MHC-congenic C57BL/6J and B6-H-2K mice. *Behav. Genet.* 29:263–271.

Brown, R. E., and Schellinck, H. M. (2007). Spatial learning, motor learning and memory. MPD: 225. Mouse Phenome Database Web site, Jackson Laboratory, Bar Harbor, ME. www.jax.org/phenome (accessed July 9, 2007).

Brown, R. E., and Wong, A. A. (2007). The influence of visual ability on learning and memory performance in 13 strains of mice. *Learn. Mem.* 13:134–144.

Buhot, M. C., Dubayle, D., Malleret, G., Javerzat, S., and Segu, L. (2001). Exploration, anxiety, and spatial memory in transgenic anophthalmic mice. *Behav. Neurosci.* 115:455–467.

Chesler, E. J., Wilson, S. G., Lariviere, W. R., Rodriguez-Zas, S. L., and Mogil, J. S. (2002). Influences of laboratory environment on behavior. *Nat. Neurosci.* 5:1101–1102.

Clapcote, S. J., Lazar, N. L., Bechard, A. R., and Roder, J. C. (2005). Effect of the rd1 mutation and host strain on hippocampal learning in mice. *Behav. Genet.* 35:591–601.

Cook, M. N., Williams, R. W., and Flaherty, L. (2001). Anxiety-related behaviors in the elevated zero-maze are affected by genetic factors and retinal degeneration. *Behav. Neurosci.* 115:468–476.

Crawley, J. N. (1999). Behavioral phenotyping of transgenic and knockout mice: Experimental design and evaluation of the general health, sensory functions, motor abilities, and specific behavioral tests. *Brain Res.* 835:18–26.

Crawley, J. N. (2000). *What's wrong with my mouse?* New York: Wiley-Liss.

Crusio, W. E., Schwegler, H., and Brust, I. (1995). Covariations between hippocampal mossy fibers and working and reference memory in spatial and non-spatial radial maze tasks in mice. *Eur. J. Neurosci.* 5:1413–1420.

Cybulska-Klosowicz, A., and Kossut, M. (2001). Mice can learn roughness discrimination with vibrissae in a jump stand apparatus. *Acta Neurobiol. Exp.* (Wars.) 61:73–76.

Danciger, M., Lyon, J., Worrill, D., LaVail, M. M., and Yang, H. (2003). A strong and highly significant QTL on chromosome 6 that protects the mouse from age-related retinal degeneration. *Invest. Ophthalmol. Vis. Sci.* 44:2442–2449.

Danciger, M., Matthes, M. T., Yasamura, D., Akhmedov, N. B., Rickabaugh, T., Gentleman, S., Redmond, T. M., LaVail, M. M., and Farber, D. B. (2000). A QTL on distal chromosome 3 that influences the severity of light-induced damage to mouse photoreceptors. *Mamm. Genome* 11:422–427.

Danciger, M., Yang, H., Ralston, R., Liu, Y., Matthes, M. T., Peirce, J., and LaVail, M. M. (2007). Quantitative genetics of age-related retinal degeneration: A second F1 intercross between the A/J and C57BL/6 strains. *Mol. Vis.* 13:79–85.

DeFries, J. C., Hegmann, J. P., and Weir, M. W. (1966). Open-field behavior in mice: Evidence for a major gene effect mediated by the visual system. *Science* 154:1577–1579.

Deiss, V., and Baudoin, C. (1999). Olfactory learning abilities in staggerer mutant mice. *C R Acad. Sci.*, ser. 3, 322:467–471.

Drager, U. C., and Hubel, D. H. (1975). Physiology of visual cells in mouse superior colliculus and correlation with somatosensory and auditory input. *Nature* 253:203–204.

Drager, U. C., and Hubel, D. H. (1976). Topography of visual and somatosensory projections to mouse superior colliculus. *J. Neurophysiol.* 39:91–101.

Errijgers, V., Van Dam, D., Gantois, I., Van Ginneken, C. J., Grossman, A. W., D'Hooge, R., De Deyn, P. P., and Kooy, R. F. (2006). FVB.129P2-Pde6b^{+}Tyr$^{c\text{-}ch}$/ANT, a sighted variant of the FVB/N mouse strain suitable for behavioral analysis. *Gene Brain Behav.* epub, doi: 10.1111/j.1601-183X.2006.00282.x, Nov. 3, 2006.

Fanselow, M. S. (1980). Conditional and unconditional components of post-shock freezing. *Pavlov J. Biol. Sci.* 15:177–182.

Farr, S. A., Banks, W. A., La Scola, M. E., and Morley, J. E. (2002). Blind mice are not impaired in T-maze footshock avoidance acquisition and retention. *Physiol. Behav.* 76:531–538.

Festing, F. W., Simpson, E. M., Davisson, M. T., and Mobraaten, L. E. (1999). Revised nomenclature for strain 129 mice. *Mamm. Genome* 10:836.

Fox, M. W. (1965). The visual cliff test for the study of visual depth perception in the mouse. *Anim. Behav.* 13:232–233.

Fox, R. R., and Witham, B. A. (Eds.). (1997). *Handbook on genetically standardized JAX mice* (5th ed.). Bar Harbor, ME: Jackson Laboratory.

Garcia, M. F., Gorden, M. N., Hutton, M., Lewis, J., McGowan, E., Dickey, C. A., Morgan, D., and Arendash, G. W. (2004). The retinal degeneration (*rd*) gene seriously impairs spatial cognitive performance in normal and Alzheimer's transgenic mice. *Neuroreport* 15:73–77.

Gerlai, R. (1996). Gene-targeting studies of mammalian behavior: Is it the mutation or the background genotype? *Trends Neurosci.* 19:177–181.

Gerlai, R. (2001). Gene targeting: Technical confounds and potential solutions in behavioral brain research. *Behav. Brain Res.* 125:13–21.

Geyer, M. A. (2006). The family of sensorimotor gating disorders: Comorbidities or diagnostic overlaps? *Neurotox. Res.* 10: 211–220.

Gianfranceschi, L., Fiorentini, A., and Maffei, L. (1999). Behavioral visual acuity of wild type and *bcl2* transgenic mouse. *Vision Res.* 39:569–574.

Glendinning, J. I., Gresack, J., and Spector, A. C. (2002). A high-throughput screening procedure for identifying mice with aberrant taste and oromotor function. *Chem. Senses* 27:461–474.

Goldstein, B. F. (1999). *Sensation and perception.* Pacific Grove, CA: Brook/Cole.

Hargreaves, K., Dubner, R., Brown, F., Flores, C., and Joris, J. (1988). A new and sensitive method for measuring thermal nociception in cutaneous hyperalgesia. *Pain* 32:77–88.

Holmes, A., Wrenn, C. C., Harris, A. P., Thayer, K. E., and Crawley, J. N. (2002). Behavioral profiles of inbred mice strains on novel olfactory, spatial and emotional tests for reference memory in mice. *Genes Brain Behav.* 1:55–69.

Hyde, L. A., and Denenberg, V. H. (1999). BXSB mice can learn complex pattern discrimination. *Physiol. Behav.* 66:437–439.

Iivonen, H., Nurminen, L., Harri, M., Tanila, H., and Puolivali, J. (2003). Hypothermia in mice tested in Morris water maze. *Behav. Brain Res.* 141:207–213.

Ingram, D. K. (1982). Lithium chloride–induced taste aversion in C57BL/6J and DBA/2J mice. *J. Gen. Psychol.* 106:233–249.

Jackson Laboratory. (2007). Facts about the Jackson Laboratory, a non-profit institution. www.jax.org/about/jax_facts.html (accessed May 18, 2007).

Janssen, P. A. J., Niemegeers, C. J. E., and Dony, J. G. H. (1963). The inhibitory effect of fentanyl and other morphine-like analgesics on the warm water-induced tail withdrawal reflex. *Arzneimittelforschung* 13:502–507.

Kazdoba, T. M., Del Vecchio, R. A., and Hyde, L. A. (2007). Automated evaluation of sensitivity to foot shock in mice: Inbred strain differences and pharmacological validation. *Behav. Pharmacol.* 18:89–102.

Kim, S. H., and Chung, J. M. (1992). An experimental model for peripheral neuropathy produced by segmental spinal nerve ligation in the rat. *Pain* 50:355–363.

Kotlus, B. S., and Blizard, D. A. (1998). Measuring gustatory variation in mice: A short-term fluid intake test. *Physiol. Behav.* 64:37–47.

LaVail, M. M., Gorrin, G. M., and Repaci, M. A. (1987a). Strain differences in sensitivity to light-induced photoreceptor degeneration in albino mice. *Curr. Eye Res.* 6:825–834.

LaVail, M. M., Gorrin, G. M., Repaci, M. A., Thomas, L. A., and Ginsberg, H. M. (1987b). Genetic regulation of light damage to photoreceptors. *Invest. Ophthalmol. Vis. Sci.* 28:1043–1048.

LeDoux, J. E. (1995). Emotion: Clues from the brain. *Annu. Rev. Psychol.* 46:209–235.

Lee, A. W., Emsley, J. G., Brown, R. E., and Hagg, T. (2003). Marked differences in olfactory sensitivity and apparent speed of forebrain neuroblast migration in three inbred strains of mice. *Neuroscience* 118:263–270.

Linder, C. C. (2006). Genetic variables that influence phenotype. *ILAR J.* 47:132–140.

Lipp, H. P., and van der Loos, H. (1991). A computer-controlled Y-maze for the analysis of vibrissotactile discrimination learning in mice. *Behav. Brain Res.* 45:135–145.

Luo, A. H., Cannon, E. H., Wekesa, K. S., Lyman, R. F., Vandenbergh, J. G., and Anhold, R. R. H. (2002). Impaired olfactory behavior in mice deficient in the α subunit of G_o. *Brain Res.* 941:62–71.

MacDonald, R. J., and White, N. M. (1993). A triple dissociation of memory systems: Hippocampus, amygdala and dorsal striatum. *Behav. Neurosci.* 107:3–22.

Macknin, J. B., Higuchi, M., Lee, V. M. Y., Trojanowski, J. Q., and Doty, R. L. (2004). Olfactory dysfunction occurs in transgenic mice overexpressing human τ protein. *Brain Res.* 1000:174–178.

Mathis. C., Paul, S. M., and Crawley, J. N. (1994). Characterization of benzodiazepine-sensitive behaviors in the A/J and C57BL/6J inbred strains of mice. *Behav. Genet.* 24: 171–180.

Mazarakis, N. K., Cybulska-Klosowicz, A., Grote, H., Pang, T., Van Dellen, A., Kossut, M., Blakemore, C., and Hannan, A. J. (2005). Deficits in experience-dependent cortical plasticity and sensory discrimination learning in presymptomatic Huntington's disease mice. *J. Neurosci.* 25:3059–3066.

McGaugh, J. L. (1966). Time-dependent processes in memory storage. *Science* 153:1351–1358.

Mogil, J. S., Wilson, S. G., Bon, K., Lee, S. E., Chung, K., Raber, P., Pieper, J. O., Hain, H. S., Belknap, J. K., et al. (1999a). Heritability of nociception. I. Responses of 11 inbred mouse strains on 12 measures of nociception. *Pain* 80:67–82.

Mogil, J. S., Wilson, S. G., Bon, K., Lee, S. E., Chung, K., Raber, P., Pieper, J. O., Hain, H. S., Belknap, J. K., et al. (1999b). Heritability of nociception. II. "Types" of nociception revealed by genetic correlation analysis. *Pain* 80:83–93.

Morris, R. (1984). Developments of a water-maze procedure for studying spatial learning in the rat. *J. Neurosci. Methods.* 11: 47–60.

Mouse genome resources. (2006). www.ncbi.nih.gov/genome/guide/mouse/ (accessed May 31, 2007).

Mrosovsky, N., Salmon, P. A., Foster, R. G., and McCall, M. A. (2000). Responses to light after retinal degeneration. *Vision Res.* 40:575–578.

Nagy, Z. M., and Misanin, J. R. (1970). Visual perception in the retinal degenerate C3H mouse. *J. Comp. Physiol. Psychol.* 72:306–310.

Nelson, T. M., Munger, S. D., and Boughter, J. D., Jr. (2005). Haplotypes at the Tas2r locus on distal chromosome 6 vary with quinine taste sensitivity in inbred mice. *BMC Genet.* 6:32.

Nguyen, P. V., Abel, T., Kandel, E. R., and Bourtchouladze, R. (2000). Strain-dependent differences in LTP and hippocampus-dependent memory in inbred mice. *Learn. Mem.* 7: 170–179.

Nguyen, P. V., and Gerlai, R. (2002). Behavioural and physiological characterization of inbred mouse strains: Prospects for elucidating the molecular mechanisms of mammalian learning and memory. *Genes Brain Behav.* 1:72–81.

O'Leary, T. P., and Brown, R. E. (2005). Is the Barnes maze a test of spatial learning in mice? Program No. 995.13.2005, online. Washington, DC: Society for Neuroscience, 2005.

Olton, D. S., and Samuelson, R. J. (1976). Remembrance of places passed: Spatial memory in rats. *J. Exp. Psychol. Anim. Behav. Process.* 2:97–116.

Owen, E. H., Logue, S. F., Rasmussen, D. L., and Wehner, J. M. (1997). Assessment of learning by the Morris water task and fear conditioning in inbred mouse strains and F_1 hybrids: Implications of genetic background for single gene mutations and quantitative trait loci analyses. *Neuroscience* 80:1087–1099.

Owings, D. H., Haerer, H. A., and Lockard, R. B. (1967). Sucrose intake functions of rat and cockroach for single and six solution presentations. *Psychon. Sci.* 73:125–127.

Oyster, C. W. (1999). *The human eye: Structure and function.* Sunderland, MA: Sinauer.

Palmerino, C. C., Rusiniak, K. W., and Garcia, J. (1980). Flavor-illness aversions: The peculiar role of odor and taste in memory for poison. *Science* 4445:753–755.

Panda, S., Provencio, I., Tu, D. C., Pires, S. S., Rollag, M. D., Castrucci, A. M., Pletcher, M. T., Sato, T. K., Wiltshire, T., et al. (2003). Melanopsin is required for non-image-forming photic responses in blind mice. *Science* 301:525–527.

Passino, E., and Ammassari-Teule, M. (1999). Visual discrimination in inbred mice: Strain-specific involvement of hippocampal regions. *Physiol. Behav.* 67:393–399.

Peters, L. L. (2007). The mouse as a model for human biology: A resource guide for complex trait analysis. *Nat. Rev. Genet.* 8: 58–69.

Pinto, L. H., and Enroth-Cugell, C. (2000). Tests of the mouse visual system. *Mamm. Genome* 11:531–536.

Plappert, C. F., Schachner, M., and Pilz, P.K.D. (2006). Neural cell adhesion molecule ($NCAM^{-/-}$) null mice show impaired sensitization of the startle response. *Genes Brain Behav.* 5:46–52.

Podhorna, J., and Brown, R. E. (2002). Strain differences in activity and emotionality do not account for differences in learning and memory performance between C57BL/6 and DBA/2 mice. *Genes Brain Behav.* 1:96–110.

Pompl, P. N., Mullan, M. J., Bjugstad, K., and Arendash, G. W. (1999). Adaptation of the circular platform spatial memory task for mice: Use in detecting cognitive impairment in the APP_{sw} transgenic mouse model for Alzheimer's disease. *J. Neurosci. Methods* 27:87–95.

Prosen, C. A., Dore, D. J., and May, B. J. (2003). The functional age of hearing loss in a mouse model of prebycusis. *Hear. Res.* 183:44–56.

Prusky, G. T., Alam, N. M., Beekman, S., and Douglas, R. M. (2004). Rapid quantification of adult and developing mouse spatial vision using a virtual optomotor system. *Invest. Ophthalmol. Vis. Sci.* 45:4611–4616.

Prusky, G. T., West, P. W. R., and Douglas, R. M. (2000a). Behavioral assessment of visual acuity in mice and rats. *Vision Res.* 40:2201–2209.

Prusky, G. T., West, P. W. R., and Douglas, R. M. (2000b). Reduced visual acuity impairs place but not cued learning in the Morris water task. *Behav. Brain Res.* 116:135–140.

Rauschecker, J. P., Tian, B., Korte, M., and Egert, U. (1992). Crossmodal changes in the somatosensory vibrissa/barrel system of visually deprived animals. *Proc. Natl. Acad. Sci. U.S.A.* 89: 5063–5067.

Restivo, L., Chaillan, F. A., Ammassari-Teule, M., Roman, F. S., and Marchetti, E. (2006). Strain differences in rewarded discrimination learning using the olfactory tubing maze. *Behav. Genet.* 36:923–934.

Richter, C. P. (1939). Salt taste thresholds of normal and adrenalectomized rats. *Endocrinology* 24:367–371.

Risinger, F. O., and Brown, M. M. (1996). Genetic differences in nicotine-induced conditioned taste aversion. *Life Sci.* 58: 223–229.

Robinson, L., Bridge, H., and Riedel, G. (2001). Visual discrimination learning in the water maze: A novel test for visual acuity. *Behav. Brain Res.* 119:77–84.

Rodgers, D. C., Fisher, E. M., Brown, S. D., Peters, J., Hunter, A. J., and Martin, J. E. (1997). Behavioral and functional analysis of mouse phenotype: SHIRPA, a proposed protocol for comprehensive phenotype assessment. *Mamm. Genome* 8:711–713.

Roman, F. S., Marchetti, E., Bouquerel, A., and Soumireu-Mourat, B. (2002). The olfactory tubing maze: A new apparatus for studying learning and memory processes in mice. *J. Neurosci. Methods* 117:173–181.

Roullet, P., and Lassalle, J. M. (1995). Radial maze learning using exclusively distant visual cues reveals learners and nonlearners among inbred mouse strains. *Physiol. Behav.* 58:1189–1195.

Schellinck, H. M., Forestell, C. A., and Lolordo, V. M. (2001). A simple and reliable test of olfactory learning and memory in mice. *Chem. Senses* 26:663–672.

Shupe, J. M., Kristan, D. M., Austad, S. N., and Stenkamp, D. L. (2006). The eye of the laboratory mouse remains anatomically adapted for natural conditions. *Brain Behav. Evol.* 67:39–52.

Silver, L. M. (1995). *Mouse genetics.* New York: Oxford University Press.

Simpson, E. M., Linder, C. C., Sargent, E. E., Davisson, M. T., Mobraaten, L. E., and Sharp, J. J. (1997). Genetic variation among 129 substrains and its importance for targeted mutagenesis in mice. *Nat. Genet.* 16:19–27.

Sinex, D. G., Burdette, L. J., and Pearlman, A. L. (1979). A psychophysical investigation of spatial vision in the normal and reeler mutant mouse. *Vision Res.* 19:853–857.

Slotnick, B., Schellinck, H., and Brown, R. (2005). Olfaction. In I. Whishaw and B. Kolb (Eds.), *The behavior of the laboratory rat: A handbook with tests.* (pp. 90–104). New York: Oxford University Press.

Smith, K. (1936). Visual discrimination in the cat. IV. The visual acuity of the cat in relation to stimulus distance. *J. Gen. Psychol.* 49:297–313.

Staats, J. (1968a). The laboratory mouse. In E. L. Green (Ed.), *Biology of the laboratory mouse* (pp. 1–9). New York: Dover Publications.

Staats, J. (1968b). Standardized nomenclature for inbred strains of mice: Fourth listing. *Cancer Res.* 28:391–420.

Taft, R. A., Davisson, M., and Wiles, M. V. (2006). Know thy mouse. *Trends Genet.* 22:649–653.

Takao, K., Yamasaki, N., and Miyakawa, T. (2007). Impact of brain-behavior phenotyping of genetically-engineered mice on research of neuropsychiatric disorders. *Neurosci. Res.* 58: 124–132.

Tarantino, L. M., Gould, T. J., Druhan, J. P., and Bucan, M. (2000). Behavior and mutagenesis screens: The importance of baseline analysis of inbred strains. *Mamm. Genome* 11:555–564.

Tecott, L. H. (2003). The genes and brains of mice and men. *Am. J. Psychiatry* 160:646–656.

Tjolsen, A., Berge, O. G., Hunskaar, S., Rosland, J. H., and Hole, K. (1992). The formalin test: An evaluation of the method. *Pain* 51:5–17.

Tonussi, C. R., and Ferreira, S. H. (1992). Rat knee-joint carageenin incapacitation test: An objective screen for central and peripheral analgesics. *Pain* 48:421–427.

Tordoff, M. G., and Bachmanov, A. A. (2003). Mouse preference tests: Why only two bottles? *Chem. Senses* 28:315–324.

van der Staay, F. J., and Steckler, T. (2001). Behavioral phenotyping of mouse mutants. *Behav. Brain Res.* 125:3–12.

van der Staay, F. J., and Steckler, T. (2002). The fallacy of behavioral phenotyping without standardization. *Genes Brain Behav.* 1:9–13.

Vitaterna, M. H., Pinto, L. H., and Takahashi, J. S. (2006). Large scale mutagenesis and phenotypic screens for the nervous system and behavior in mice. *Trends Neurosci.* 29:233–240.

Wahlsten, D. (1973). Contributions of the genes albinism (c) and retinal degeneration (rd) to a strain-by-training procedure interaction in avoidance learning. *Behav. Genet.* 3:303–316.

Wahlsten, D., Bachmanov, A., Finn, D. A., and Crabbe, J. C. (2006). Stability of inbred mouse strain differences in behavior and brain size between laboratories and across decades. *Proc. Natl. Acad. Sci. U.S.A.* 103:16364–16369.

Wahlsten, D., Metten, P., Phillips, T. J., Boehm, S. L., II, Burkhart-Kasch, S., Dorow, J., Doerksen, S., Downing, C., Fogarty, J., et al. (2003). Different data from different labs: Lessons from studies of gene-environment interaction. *J. Neurobiol.* 54:283–311.

Wall, P. D., Devor, M., Inbal, R., Scadding, J. W., Schonfeld, D., Selzer, Z., and Tomkiewicz, M. M. (1979). Autonomy following peripheral nerve lesions: Experimental anesthesia dolorosa. *Pain* 7:103–113.

Wiesenfeld, Z., and Branchek, T. (1976). Refractive state and visual acuity in the hooded rat. *Vision Res.* 16:823–827.

Willott, J. F., Tanner, L., O'Steen, J., Johnson, K. R., Bogue, M. A., and Gagnon, L. (2003). Acoustic startle and prepulse inhibition in 40 inbred strains of mice. *Behav. Neurosci.* 117:716–727.

Wimer, R., and Weller, S. (1965). Evaluation of a visual discrimination task for the analysis of the genetics of a mouse behavior. *Percept. Mot. Skills* 20:203–208.

Wong, A. A., and Brown, R. E. (2004). The influence of visual ability on the behaviour of 13 strains of mice in a battery of tests. *Soci. Neurosci. Abstr.* 83.7, 2004.

Wong, A. A., and Brown, R. E. (2006). Visual detection, pattern discrimination and visual acuity in 14 strains of mice. *Genes Brain Behav.* 5:389–403.

Wong, A. A., and Brown, R. E. (2007). Age-related changes in visual acuity, learning and memory in C57BL/6J and DBA/2J mice. *Neurobiol. Aging* 28:1577–1593.

Yerkes, R. M. (1907). *The dancing mouse.* New York: Arno Press.

Yerkes, R. M., and Dodson, J. D. (1908). The relation of strength of stimulus to rapidity of habit information. *J. Comp. Neurol. Psychol.* 18:459–482.

Zheng, Q. Y., Johnson, K. R., and Erway, L. C. (1999). Assessment of 80 inbred strains of mice by ABR threshold analyses. *Hear. Res.* 130:94–107.

Zhou, X., Jen, P. H. S., Seburn, K. L., Frankel, W. N., and Zheng, Q. Y. (2006). Auditory brainstem responses in 10 inbred strains of mice. *Brain Res.* 1091:16–26.

3 Comparative Survey of the Mammalian Visual System with Reference to the Mouse

CATHERINE A. LEAMEY, DARIO A. PROTTI, AND BOGDAN DREHER

Until very recently, the house mouse (*Mus musculus*) was not a preferred model for study of the mammalian visual system. However, the power of transgenic and knockout mice as models for the study of the central nervous system (CNS) has led to important questions concerning the overall properties of the visual system of the house mouse compared with those of other mammalian species. Indeed, the power of knockout mice models was formally recognized by the award of the Nobel Prize in Physiology or Medicine for 2007 to Mario R. Capecchi, Martin J. Evans, and Oliver Smithies, the principal developers of the knockout mouse model.

This chapter addresses similarities and differences between the visual system of the mouse and that of other mammalian (especially eutherian) species. Available information indicates great similarity to other species, especially the closely related laboratory rat (*Rattus norvegicus*; see Arnason et al., 2002). However, substantial differences do exist between the visual systems of nocturnal rodents and those of more highly visual mammals, such as primates (including humans) and carnivores. Thus, although transgenic and knockout mice can provide useful and elegant models with which to assess visual function, there is sound justification to maintain a comparative approach.

The eye, the retina, and visual acuity

The adult house mouse is a very small nocturnal mammal with a relatively small eye having an axial length from anterior cornea to anterior choroid of about 3.4 mm (Remtulla and Hallett, 1985). As is typical for nocturnal mammals (see Walls, 1942), the mouse eye is characterized by a relatively large cornea and lens, the latter accounting for 60% of the axial length (Remtulla and Hallett, 1985).

Apart from limitations imposed by the optical properties of the eye, the limits of visual acuity depend on the arrays of neurons in the retinal network. Several factors determine the limits of the retinal acuity. These factors include the retinal sampling frequency, which is determined by the size and density of photoreceptors and their degree of convergence onto retinal ganglion cells (RGCs), the output cells of the retina. As is characteristic of nocturnal mammals, the mouse retina is strongly rod-dominated, with rods making up 97% of all photoreceptors. Cones constitute a much smaller proportion of photoreceptors (Carter-Dawson and LaVail, 1979; Jeon et al., 1998) in the house mouse than in diurnal rodents such as the ground squirrel (*Spermophilus beecheyi*; Kryger et al., 1998), diurnal primates such as macaque monkeys or humans, or nocturno-diurnal carnivores such as the domestic cat (*Felis catus*). Nevertheless, the cones appear to play an important role in mouse vision. A high degree of convergence combined with the small size of the eye results in rather small numbers of RGCs (48,000–65,000: Dräger and Olsen, 1980; ca. 45,000 RGCs out of 110,000 neurons in the ganglion cell layer: Jeon et al., 1998). Despite their relatively small numbers, the peak RGC density is about 8,000 cells/mm^2 (Dräger and Olsen, 1981). This figure is not only higher than the peak RGC density in the rabbit (*Oryctolagus cuniculus*, a crepuscular lagomorph with only partially vascularized retina; Robinson et al., 1990); it is also higher than that in other nocturnal rodents with strongly vascularized retinas, such as the rat (McCall et al., 1987) or the golden hamster (*Mesocricetus auratus*; Tiao and Blakemore, 1976b; Métin et al., 1995). Indeed, the peak RGC density in the mouse appears rather similar to that of the domestic cat (Stone, 1978; Hughes, 1981).

The structure of the mouse retina has been thoroughly studied anatomically using Golgi staining (Ramón y Cajal, 1972), Nissl staining, electron microscopy (Carter-Dawson and LaVail, 1979; Dräger and Olsen, 1981; Jeon et al., 1998; Tsukamoto et al., 2001), and differential interference contrast microscopy (Jeon et al., 1998). Apart from the photoreceptors and retinal neurons, three types of glial cells are found in the mouse retina (as in other mammals with vascularized retinas): astrocytes are found in the optic nerve fiber layer, microglial cell bodies form a regular array in the inner nuclear layer (INL), and Müller cells span the entire retina vertically (Haverkamp and Wässle, 2000). The Müller cells described in mice are morphologically similar to those in other mammals (Dreher, Robinson, et al., 1992).

As in all mammals other than primates (see Walls, 1942; Rowe and Dreher, 1982; Rowe, 1991; Provis et al., 1998), the mouse retina does not have a *fovea centralis* (a pitted region in the center of the retina with the highest density of cones, but no rods or other retinal neurons). In nonfoveate mammals, including mice, the density of rods and cones, as well as the density of the RGCs, peaks in the *area centralis* (Dräger and Olsen, 1980) and decreases more peripherally. In mice, the peak rod density is about 100,000/mm^2 and the peak cone density is 16,000/mm^2 (Jeon et al., 1998), similar to the average densities of rods and cones in the peripheral retina of macaque monkey (Packer et al., 1989) and domestic cat (Steinberg et al., 1973). The centroperipheral RGC density ratio in the mouse, at around 3.5 : 1 (Dräger and Olsen, 1980), is somewhat smaller than that in other murid rodents such as laboratory rat (McCall et al., 1987) or a critecid rodent, the golden hamster, in which it is approximately 5 : 1 (Tiao and Blakemore, 1976b; Métin et al., 1995).

PHOTORECEPTORS The spectral sensitivity of mouse rod photoreceptors (estimated using three different methods: rhodopsin absorption, the b-wave of electroretinograms [ERGs], and recordings of ganglion cell activity), peaks at 497–500 nm (Soucy et al., 1998; Toda et al., 1999; Fan et al., 2005). There are two types of cone photoreceptors, differing in their photopigments and their absorption spectra. One is maximally responsive to ultraviolet (UV) light (peak sensitivity at 360 nm); the other is to medium (M)-wavelength light (peak sensitivity at 508 nm; Nikonov et al., 2006). Most cones express both UV and M photopigments but are maximally sensitive at 360 nm (Nikonov et al., 2006). In the dorsal retina, however, cones are maximally sensitive at 508 nm, while the highest density of UV-sensitive cones occurs in the ventral retina (Szél et al., 1992, 1993).

RETINAL NETWORK The basic functional organization of the mouse retina is largely similar to that of other mammalian species (figure 3.1*A*). Scotopic signals are transmitted via the classical rod pathway, in which rod photoreceptors synapse onto rod bipolar cells. These bipolar cells do not transmit light signals directly to RGCs but rather piggyback them via AII amacrine cells onto the evolutionary preexisting cone pathways by making sign-inverting synapses with OFF cone bipolar cells and sign-conserving synapses with ON cone bipolar cells. Cone bipolar cells in turn synapse onto RGCs.

In addition, both anatomical and physiological evidence indicates the existence of alternative pathways for the transmission of scotopic signals. A second pathway by which rod signals could "leak" into the cone pathway via gap junctions between the two classes of photoreceptors has been described anatomically (Tsukamoto et al., 2001). This pathway has been shown to exist both anatomically and functionally in the cat (Kolb, 1977; Nelson, 1977) and macaque monkey (Raviola and Gilula, 1973; Schneeweis and Schnapf, 1995).

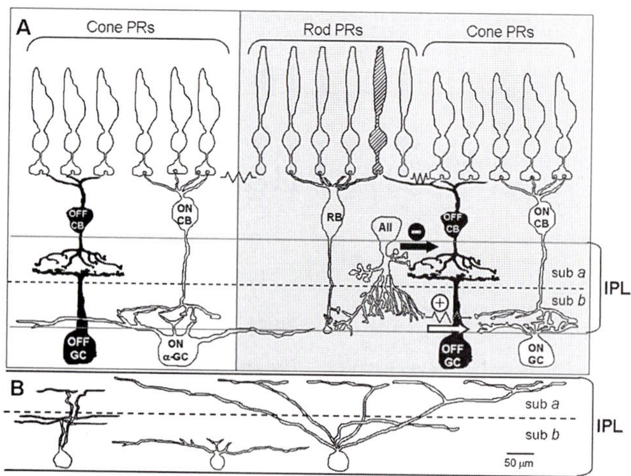

FIGURE 3.1*A* Signaling pathways in the mouse retina. Cone circuit: cone photoreceptors contact both ON and OFF bipolar cells. ON bipolar cells synapse onto ON ganglion cells (an α-like ganglion cell with a large dendritic tree is represented here). OFF bipolar cells synapse onto OFF ganglion cells. In the rod circuit, light signals can follow three different pathways: in the classical rod pathway, signals initiated in rod photoreceptors (Rod PRs) are transferred to a single type of bipolar cell, the rod bipolar cell (RB). RB cells transmit their signal to AII amacrine cells (AII), which split the signal into the ON and OFF channels by making gap junctions with the axons of ON cone bipolar cells (ON CB) in sublamina b (sub b) of the inner plexiform layer (IPL) and inhibitory synapses (glycinergic) in sublamina a (sub a) with the axons of OFF cone bipolar cells (OFF CB), respectively. ON CBs and OFF CBs synapse with ON and OFF ganglion cells, respectively. Alternatively, rod signals may flow via gap junctions into cone photoreceptors (Cone PRs), from which they are fed into ON CB and OFF CB cells and subsequently onto their respective ganglion cells. A third pathway has been described in which some rod PRs (*shaded* Rod PR) synapse directly onto the dendrites of a particular type of OFF CB cell, which transfers this signal to OFF ganglion cells. These pathways are likely to operate under different lighting conditions. (Modified from Protti et al., 2005, with permission.) *B*, Schematic drawing of three morphologically and physiologically identified ganglion cell types in the mouse retina. *Left*, Bistratified ON-OFF direction-selective ganglion cell with one dendritic plexus branching in the ON sublamina and the other in the OFF sublamina. (Based on Weng et al., 2005.) *Center*, ON α–ganglion cell with a large soma and several robust, radiating primary dendrites that expand to form a relatively wide dendritic tree covering between 6° and 12°. (Based on Pang et al., 2003.) *Right*, Melanopsin-containing ganglion cell with dendritic tree covering a large area of retina (>15°) and branching mainly in the outermost part of the inner plexiform layer. Scale bar in *B* corresponds only to part *B*. (*B*, Based on Berson et al., 2002.)

A third pathway involving direct synaptic contacts between rods and one type of OFF cone bipolar cell has also been described for the flow of scotopic signals (Soucy et al., 1998; Hack et al., 1999; Tsukamoto et al., 2001; Protti et al., 2005), although the relative contribution of this mechanism remains to be established. The anatomical basis for such a pathway has also been demonstrated in the cat (Fyk-Kolodziej et al., 2003), although thus far there are no reports of a similar circuit in primates. Tsukamoto and colleagues (2001) proposed that in nocturnal rodents, the transmission of scotopic light OFF rather than light ON signals might be favored because when these animals are active in twilight conditions, objects would appear dark on a brighter background and consequently would be most efficiently detected by the OFF pathway.

The structure of the photopic pathways in the mouse is also typical of that in other mammals. Cone photoreceptors connect to cone bipolar cells, which pass light signals directly to RGCs. Cone bipolar cells are subdivided into ON and OFF cells, according to their level of stratification in the inner plexiform layer (figure 3.1*B*). The generation of the ON and OFF channels of the visual system, optimized to respond to light increments and light decrements, respectively, relies on different types of glutamate receptors expressed in the dendritic tips of bipolar cells. ON bipolar cells express the metabotropic glutamate receptor mGluR6 (group 3) in the outer plexiform layer postsynaptic to photoreceptors (Masu et al., 1995), while OFF bipolar cells express AMPA/KA ionotropic glutamate receptors (Hack et al., 2001; Sun and Kalloniatis, 2006). So far, nine different types of cone bipolar cells, comprising four OFF and five ON cone bipolar cells, have been morphologically identified (Ghosh et al., 2004). Light-evoked responses also indicate the existence of two functionally distinct cone bipolar cell types, one responding to light by depolarizing, the other displaying hyperpolarizing light responses (Berntson and Taylor, 2000; Pang et al., 2004), consistent with their morphological identity. Recently, a bipolar cell type with morphological characteristics similar to the blue ON bipolar cells of the primate retina (Mariani, 1984; Kouyama and Marshak, 1992; Ghosh et al., 1997) has been identified in the mouse (Haverkamp et al., 2005). As postulated for the primate (Boycott and Wässle, 1999; Wässle, 2004), bipolar cell diversity may constitute the basis for segregation of parallel pathways of information. Although currently there is no precise information regarding the nature of these pathways in the mouse visual system, the wiring of the mouse retina could, therefore, provide higher visual centers with information concerning different aspects of the visual world carried by parallel channels via different classes of RGCs.

Retinal Ganglion Cells A number of different morphological types of RGCs have been distinguished in the mouse retina. This diversity seems to reflect a similar pattern to that observed in other mammals, including primates and domestic cats. Whereas earlier studies (Dräger and Olsen, 1981; Doi et al., 1995) distinguished only three to four principal morphological classes of RGCs, more recent surveys (Jeon et al., 1998; Sun et al., 2002; Kong, 2005; Coombs et al., 2006) indicate greater morphological diversity, with up to 11–14 morphological types identified. Similar trends in the classification of RGCs are present in the literature for the domestic cat and macaque monkey (Boycott and Wässle, 1974; Wässle and Boycott, 1991; Rowe, 1991; Rodieck and Watanabe, 1993; Pu, 1999; O'Brien et al., 2002; Dacey and Packer, 2003).

In the cat (Boycott and Wässle, 1974; Peichl and Wässle, 1979; Rowe and Dreher, 1982; Rowe, 1991) and macaque monkey (Leventhal et al., 1981; Rowe, 1991; Wässle and Boycott, 1991), the sizes of the somata and dendritic trees of RGCs increase with eccentricity concomitantly with a reduction in RGC density. This trend is present, although substantially weaker, in the ferret (Vitek et al., 1985) and rat (Perry and Linden, 1982; Dreher et al., 1985). In contrast, Sun and colleagues (2002) reported that in the mouse, neither somal sizes nor dendritic tree sizes of RGCs increase significantly with a reduction in RGC density.

Consistent with the aforementioned cone spectral sensitivity, in photopic conditions mouse RGCs are driven by signals originating from UV- and M-wavelength-sensitive cones. The majority of RGCs receive mixed cone input, with a preponderance of RGCs in ventral retina receiving UV cone input, while 18% of RGCs receive input from only UV and 3% from only M cones (Ekesten et al., 2000; Ekesten and Gouras, 2005). Interestingly, a small number of cells (ca. 2%) receive mixed input from UV and M cones of opposite polarity (ON vs. OFF), suggesting the existence of a pathway capable of carrying chromatic information (Ekesten and Gouras, 2005).

The functional properties of some mouse RGCs have been characterized both in vivo and in vitro (Stone and Pinto, 1993; Sagdullaev and McCall, 2005). Overall, mouse RGCs have relatively large receptive fields, 2–10° in diameter, with antagonistic center-surround organization (Stone and Pinto, 1992). Stone and Pinto (1993) identified mouse RGCs as X-like when they displayed linear spatial summation (compare X cells in cat retina; Enroth-Cugell and Robson, 1966; Hochstein and Shapley, 1976) or as Y-like when they displayed nonlinear spatial summation dynamics (compare Y cells in cat retina; Enroth-Cugell and Robson, 1966; Hochstein and Shapley, 1976). The high cutoff spatial frequency of both X-like and Y-like cells' RGCs in the central retina was found to be rather low, about 0.2 c/deg (Stone and Pinto, 1993). A more recent study found no clear separation between linear and nonlinear modes of operation in mouse RGCs but rather a continuum characterized by different degrees of nonlinearity (Carcieri et al., 2003). Since a correlation with their morphological identity has not yet been done, it is unknown whether Y-like cells in mice correspond to a type similar to α-like ganglion cells of other mammals (see Peichl et al., 1987), but RGCs with morphological characteristics similar to those of α-cells have been described in the mouse (Sun et al., 2002; Pang et al., 2003).

Both ON and ON-OFF direction-selective (DS) ganglion cells with functional and morphological characteristics similar to the rabbit DS ganglion cell have been described in the mouse (Yoshida et al., 2001; Weng et al., 2005; Sun et al., 2006). Furthermore, the mechanisms involved in the generation of DS responses seem to be similar to those in the well-characterized rabbit DS RGCs (Weng et al., 2005).

The recently described non-image-forming retinofugal pathway constituted by melanopsin-containing RGCs is also present in the mouse. A total of about 700 intrinsically photosensitive melanopsin-containing ganglion cells (ipRGCs), which are involved in the regulation of circadian rhythms and pupillary reflexes, has been reported in the mouse (Hattar et al., 2002). These cells project to the suprachiasmatic nucleus (SCN) of the hypothalamus, the ventral lateral geniculate nucleus (vLGN), and the intergeniculate leaflet (IGL) of the ventral thalamus (i.e., structures involved in the regulation of circadian rhythms). Other target regions of ipRGCs include the preoptic region, the hypothalamic subparaventricular zone, the superior colliculus (SC) in the midbrain, and the nucleus of the optic tract (NOT) in the pretectum (Gooley et al., 2003; Hattar et al., 2003; Hannibal and Fahrenkrug, 2004). Recently, projections to the perisupraoptic nucleus of the hypothalamus, medial amygdala, margin of the lateral habenula, posterior limitans nucleus, and periaqueductal gray have also been described (Hattar et al., 2006). Moreover, projections to the margins of the dorsal lateral geniculate nucleus (dLGN) were also observed, a finding consistent with the reported projection of ipRGCs to the dLGN in primates (Dacey et al., 2005). In knockout mice in which the melanopsin gene has been deleted, RGCs that normally express melanopsin are no longer intrinsically photosensitive, and both the pupillary light reflex (Lucas et al., 2003) and the circadian clock (Ruby et al., 2002; Panda et al., 2003) are severely impaired. Interestingly, despite great differences in the total number of RGCs among different mammalian species (see Dreher et al., 1985; Robinson and Dreher, 1990b), the total number of melanopsin-expressing RGCs seems to be highly conserved (ca. 2,300–2,600 ipRGCs per retina in the rat, corresponding to ca. 2.3%–2.6% of RGCs: Hattar et al., 2002; ca. 1,700 ipRGCs per retina in the cat, corresponding to ca. 1% of RGCs: Semo et al., 2005; ca. 3,000 ipRGCs per retina in humans, corresponding to 0.2%–0.3% of RGCs: Dacey et al., 2005).

Spatial Resolution Using the focal length of the eye, the retinal magnification factor (RMF), and assumptions of the sampling theorem, it is possible to derive the limits of animals' spatial acuity from the peak density of the RGC mosaic (e.g., Hughes, 1986; compare Pettigrew et al., 1988). Applying these calculations gives theoretical upper limits of visual acuity (in cycles/degree) of 1.3 in the mouse (Remtulla and Hallett, 1985; Hallett, 1987), and 9.1–9.8 in cats (Vakkur et al., 1963; Stone, 1978; Hughes, 1981). Since there are no RGCs in the fovea, estimates of visual acuity in primates are based on peak cone density, which give values of 42 in macaques (Perry and Cowey, 1985) and 56.5 in humans (Østerberg, 1935; Duke-Elder, 1953).

In carnivores and primates, the estimates based on the peak ganglion cell or cone densities and the RMF are close to those obtained behaviorally (7–9 c/deg in cat: Blake et al., 1974; Jacobson et al., 1976; Mitchell et al., 1977; 46 c/deg in macaque: De Valois et al., 1974; 50–64 c/deg in humans: Reymond and Cook, 1984). Estimates obtained behaviorally in mice, using either optokinetic reflexes (Sinex et al., 1979; Abdeljalil et al., 2005; Schmucker et al., 2005) or visual discrimination tasks (Gianfranceschi et al., 1999; Prusky et al., 2000) at 0.4.–0.5 c/deg (with peak sensitivities at 0.125–0.26 c/deg), are, however, substantially lower than the theoretical limits estimated on the basis of peak RGC density and RMF. It is possible that the current estimates of RGC density in the mouse are overestimates due to the relatively large amount of shrinkage of the small retina during histological processing. The discrepancy between the theoretical estimates of acuity based on the peak RGC density and RMFs and behavioral data may also be related to the fact that in mice (Hofbauer and Dräger, 1985) as in other nocturnal rodents (rat: Linden and Perry, 1983; Dreher et al., 1985; hamster: Chalupa and Thompson, 1980) and rabbit (Vaney et al., 1981), virtually all RGCs project to the SC, whereas only a subpopulation projects to the visual cortex via relays in the dLGN; this is different from what is seen in carnivores and primates, where the majority of RGCs project to the geniculocortical system. Indeed, estimates of visual acuity based on peak RCG density and RMF for a number of nocturnal rodents are substantially higher than estimates derived from behavioral testing (see Pettigrew et al., 1988). In contrast, there is a good correlation between measurements of visual acuity based on behavioral studies and those extrapolated from the visually evoked potentials (VEPs) recorded from area 17 in mouse (Porciatti et al., 1999), rat (Boyes and Dyer, 1983), and rabbit (Kulikowski, 1978). It is likely, therefore, that estimates of visual acuity based on the peak density of the RGCs contributing to the geniculocortical system may be a better predictor of behavioral acuity than peak RGC density per se. Interestingly, the behaviorally determined acuity in the mouse also correlates well with visual acuity in the mouse estimated on the basis of RMF and the spatial extent of the smallest dendritic trees of RGCs (ca. 30 μm, equivalent to ca. 1°; Sun et al., 2002; Coombs et al., 2006). Spatial resolution in the mouse may be limited at an early stage of the visual system by the low spatial resolution of the array of retinal bipolar cells (0.3 c/deg; Berntson and Taylor, 2000).

Ipsilateral and contralateral retinofugal projections and the visual field

In all mammals studied so far, the optic nerves meet at the optic chiasm. In all mammalian species, the majority of RGC axons carrying information from a given retina cross at the chiasm and project to the contralateral retinorecipient nuclei. The proportion of RGC axons that do not cross and thus project to the ipsilateral retinorecipient nuclei, however, varies considerably among species and is closely related to the position of the eyes in the skull. The visual field in virtually all mammals contains at least some region of binocular overlap. Table 3.1 lists the proportion of ipsilaterally projecting RGCs in a variety of mammalian species for comparison. In species with laterally positioned eyes and therefore a relatively small binocular field, the proportion of ipsilaterally projecting RGCs tends to be small. In particular, in the rabbit, with its very laterally positioned eyes, the binocular portion of the visual field is correspondingly small (ca. 25° out of the large 360° panoramic visual field; Hughes, 1971; Hughes and Vaney, 1982). In this species, only about 0.6% of RGCs project ipsilaterally (Robinson and Dreher, 1990a). In the mouse as in other nocturnal rodents (for a review, see Rhoades et al., 1991; see also table 3.1), the eyes are more frontally positioned, the binocular field is larger (30–40°; Dräger, 1978; Dräger and Olsen, 1980; Wagor et al., 1980), and the proportion of RGCs projecting ipsilaterally is slightly higher (2%–3%; Dräger and Olsen, 1980). The correlation between the extent of binocular visual field and the proportion of RGCs that project ipsilaterally is also apparent in carnivores. The eyes of the ferret are positioned more laterally than those of the cat. In ferrets, only about 7% of RGCs project ipsilaterally (Morgan et al., 1987), while in domestic cats, with their frontally positioned eyes and large binocular visual field (ca. 90° out of a ca. 180° visual field; Vakkur et al., 1963), the proportion of RGCs projecting ipsilaterally is much higher (ca. 25%–30%; Stone and Fukuda, 1974; Wässle and Illing, 1980; Illing and Wässle, 1981; Mastronarde, 1984; FitzGibbon and Burke, 1989; Tassinari et al., 1997). The proportion of ipsilaterally projecting RGCs is very high (ca. 40%) in diurnal primates with frontally positioned eyes, such as the Old World macaque monkey (Perry and Cowey, 1984; Perry et al., 1984).

Table 3.1

Proportions of ipsilaterally and contralaterally projecting RGCs in different mammalian species relative to proportions of binocular cells, proportions of cells receiving exclusive or dominant input from the contralateral eye and the presence or absence of ocular dominance columns

Species	% Ipsilaterally Projecting RGCs	% Binocular Cells in Binocular Region of V1	% Cells in Binocular Region of V1 Driven Exclusively or Dominated by Contralateral Inputs	Ocular Dominance Columns Present?	References*
Mouse	2–3	66	65	No	1–3
Rat	3	85	68	No	4–6
Syrian hamster	1–2.5	89	56	No	7–9
Rabbit	0.6	80	65	No	10–12
Opossum		85	37	?	13
Brushtail possum		65	46	?	14
Sheep		6.5	54	Maybe	15 (but see 16)
Ferret	7	72	53	Yes	17–19
Mink		57	64	Yes	20, 21
Cat	25–30	63	43	Yes	22–27
Cat (area 18)	25–30	64	57	Yes	28
Tree shrew		71	73	No	29, 30
Macaque	40	72	33	Yes	31–35

* *1*, Dräger, 1974, *2*, Gordon and Stryker, 1996; *3*, Antonini et al., 1999; *4*, Jeffery, 1984; *5*, Dreher et al., 1985; *6*, Fagiolini et al., 1994; *7*, Tiao and Blakemore, 1976a; *8*, Hsiao et al., 1984; *9*, Métin et al., 1995; *10*, Robinson et al., 1990; *11*, Van Sluyters and Stewart, 1974; *12*, Holländer and Hälbig, 1980; *13*, Rocha-Miranda et al., 1976; *14*, Crewther et al., 1984; *15*, Clarke et al., 1976; *16*, Pettigrew et al., 1984; *17*, Morgan et al., 1987; *18*, Law et al., 1988; *19*, White et al., 1999; *20*, McConnell and LeVay, 1986; *21*, LeVay et al., 1987; *22*, Stone and Fukuda, 1974; *23*, Illing and Wässle, 1981; *24*, Mastronarde, 1984; *25*, FitzGibbon and Burke, 1989; *26*, Burke et al., 1992; *27*, Tassinari et al., 1997; *28*, Dreher, Michalski, et al., 1992; *29*, Hubel, 1975; *30*, Humphrey et al., 1977; *31*, Hubel and Wiesel, 1968; *32*, Stone et al., 1973; *33*, Leventhal et al., 1988; *34*, Fukuda et al., 1989; *35*, Chalupa and Lia, 1991.

In all mammalian species studied so far, almost all ipsilaterally projecting RGCs are located within the temporal retina. In the mouse, virtually all ipsilaterally projecting RGCs are located in the peripheral ventrotemporal region known as the ventrotemporal crescent (VTC). Only a minority (ca. 15%) of RGCs located within the VTC project ipsilaterally, however, with the great majority projecting contralaterally (see figure 3.2; Dräger and Olsen, 1980). Because of the position of the eyes in the mouse skull, this means that the binocular field is approximately the central 30% of visual space contained within the receptive fields of RGCs in the VTC of both eyes (Dräger, 1978; Dräger and Olsen, 1980; figures 3.2 and 3.3). Since the ipsilateral projection arises from the VTC region, in mice the binocular field widens dorsally (see figure 3.2). This is not the case in carnivores with frontally positioned eyes, such as the domestic cat (Illing and Wässle, 1981), where ipsilateral projections arise from all dorsoventral levels of the temporal retina. Overall, in carnivores, such as the domestic cat or ferret, unlike in nocturnal rodents, contralaterally projecting cells constitute a significant minority of RGCs located in the temporal retina (Cooper and Pettigrew, 1979; Leventhal, 1982; Vitek et al., 1985; Tassinari et al., 1997). By contrast, in macaques (Chalupa and Lia, 1991) and humans, virtually all RGCs in the temporal retina project ipsilaterally. Thus, in primates, and to a lesser extent in carnivores, the region of binocular overlap is viewed by the nasal retina of one eye and the temporal retina of the other eye. In primates and carnivores there is also a more clearly defined line of decussation that passes through the region of highest acuity, the *fovea centralis* (Stone et al., 1973; Leventhal et al., 1988; Fukuda et al., 1989; Chalupa and Lia, 1991) or *area centralis* (Illing and Wässle, 1981), respectively. This is different from the situation in mice, in which RGCs from all regions of the retina project contralaterally and the ipsilateral projection arises exclusively from a subregion of peripheral retina (Dräger and Olsen, 1980).

Retinorecipient nuclei

In the mouse, there are direct retinal projections to the SCN of the hypothalamus, the dLGN of the dorsal thalamus, and the vLGN and IGL of the ventral thalamus (Dräger, 1974; Provencio et al., 1998). There is also a direct retinal projection to several nuclei in the pretectal complex of the epithalamus (Provencio et al., 1998). The most massive direct retinal

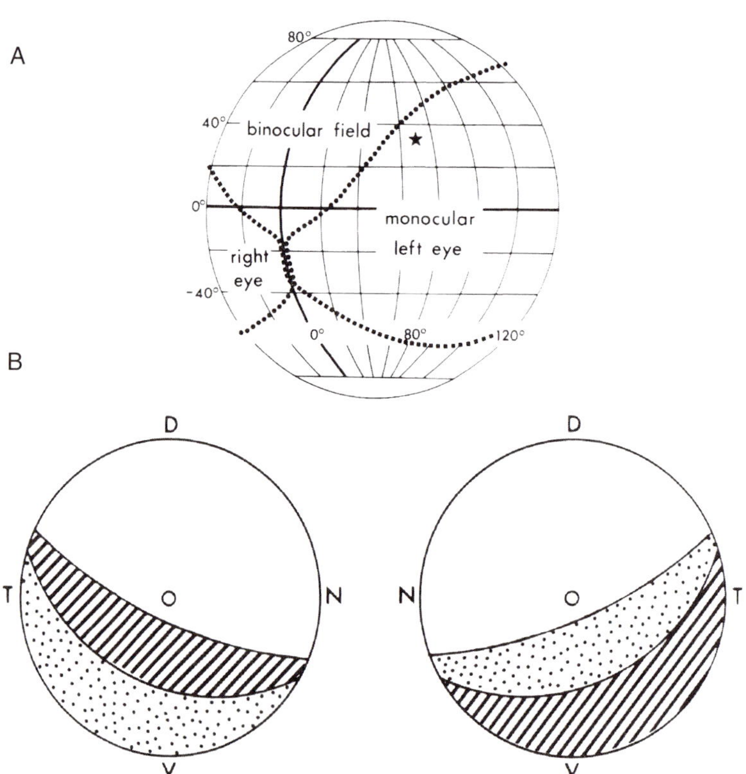

FIGURE 3.2*A* The visual field of the mouse. Projection of the mouse visual field onto a sphere, assuming that the mouse is sitting inside the sphere and facing intersection of zero vertical and zero horizontal meridian. *Star* indicates location of the optic disc. Note that the binocular field widens dorsally. (From Dräger, 1978, with permission.) *B*, Approximate positions of binocularly corresponding regions in mouse retinas. The small ipsilateral retinofugal projection originates from these regions. (From Dräger and Olsen, 1980, with permission.)

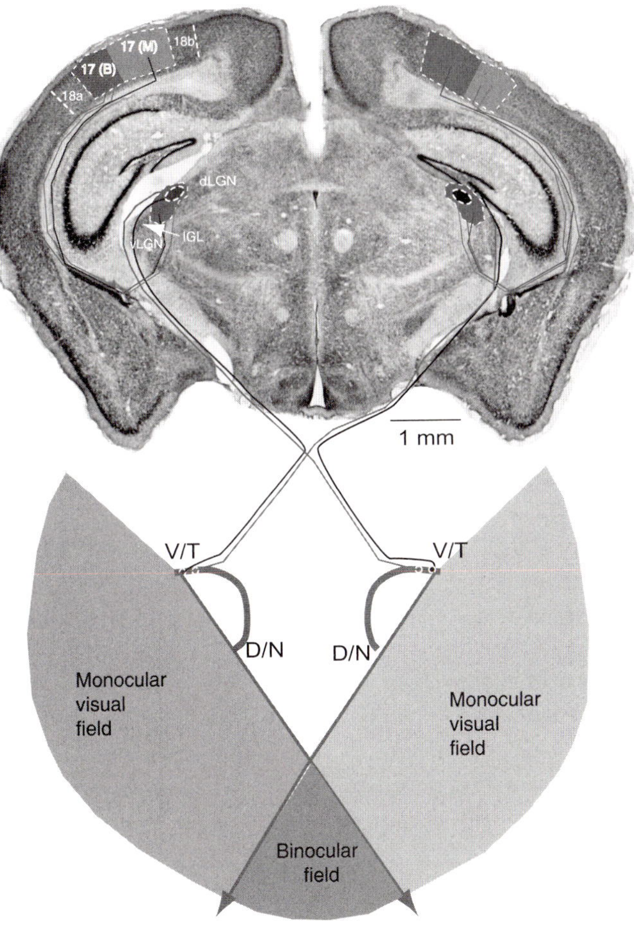

FIGURE 3.3 Schematic diagram showing the organization of the ipsilateral and contralateral visual pathways in mice. As shown in color plate 1, blue and red indicate fibers and regions representing the left and right eyes, respectively. Purple indicates binocular regions. Ipsilateral projections arising from the ventrotemporal retina terminate in dorsomedial dLGN. Contralateral retinal projections fill the rest of the dLGN. The locations of other retinorecipient nuclei in the dorsal thalamus, the intergeniculate leaflet (IGL), and ventral LGN (vLGN) are also shown. The dLGN projects topographically to primary visual cortex (area 17). The medial two-thirds of area 17 receives monocular input from the contralateral eye (17M). The lateral one-third receives binocular inputs (17B). Adjacent to area 17 laterally is area 18a; area 18b is medial. See color plate 1.

projection, however, is to the SC in the midbrain (Dräger, 1974; Hofbauer and Dräger, 1985; Provencio et al., 1998). Overall, the pattern of retinal projections in mouse is remarkably similar to that in the laboratory rat (Arnason et al., 2002; for a review, see Sefton et al., 2004). A schematic diagram illustrating the retinal projection to the thalamus is given in figure 3.3.

SUPRACHIASMATIC NUCLEUS, INTERGENICULATE LEAFLET, AND VENTROLATERAL GENICULATE NUCLEUS In nocturnal rodents, the SCN, IGL, and vLGN appear to be associated with circadian responses to light (Cassone et al., 1988; Sefton et al., 2004). Furthermore, the IGL and vLGN jointly with olivary pretectal nuclei (OPT) are also involved in the pupillary light reflex (for a review, see Sefton et al., 2004). Unlike the retinal input to the SC, the proportions of contralateral and ipsilateral RGCs that innervate the SCN are very similar (ca. 50/50; Abrahamson and Moore, 2001; Youngstrom and Nunez, 1986; Balkema and Drager, 1990; see also Dräger, 1974). The SCN, IGL, and vLGN receive direct retinal input from small but distinct subpopulations of RGCs (Provencio et al., 1998). Most of the direct retinal input to these nuclei is provided by melanopsin-expressing RGCs, which are thought to function as luminosity detectors (Berson, 2003; Dacey et al., 2005). By contrast, RGCs that express the Brn3a transcription factor do not project to these nuclei and innervate the SC and dLGN (Quina et al., 2005).

PRETECTUM AND ACCESSORY OPTIC TRACT NUCLEI There is a direct retinal input to the anterior and posterior OPT that originates mainly but not exclusively from the contralateral retina (Pak et al., 1987). In the anterior OPT the terminals from the contralateral and ipsilateral retinas occupy distinct parts of the nucleus. The anterior OPT is larger than the posterior OPT (Pak et al., 1987). In rat (Trejo and Cicerone, 1984), carnivores (Distler and Hoffmann, 1989), and primates (Gamlin et al., 1995), the OPT is the principal nucleus involved in the pupillary light reflex and receives its principal retinal input most from the melanopsin-expressing RGCs.

Two other pretectal nuclei, the posterior pretectal nucleus (PP) and the nucleus of optic tract (NOT), also receive direct retinal input, but only from the contralateral retina (Pak et al., 1987). In the mouse, all the accessory optic tract terminal nuclei—that is, the dorsal, lateral, and medial terminal nuclei (DTN, LTN, and MTN, respectively)—receive retinal input from the contralateral but not the ipsilateral eye (Pak et al., 1987). The DTN is located caudolateral to the NOT of pretectum between the *stratum griseum superficiale* of the SC and the medial geniculate nucleus (Pak et al., 1987). The LTN is a very small group of cells located just at the border of the medial geniculate nucleus and cerebral peduncles, while the MTN, the largest of the accessory optic tract nuclei, is located in the ventral midbrain tegmentum medial to the cerebral peduncle and the substantia nigra (Pak et al., 1987). The overall plan of organization of mouse accessory optic tract nuclei conforms well to that of other mammals (Cooper and Magnin, 1986). The accessory optic tract nuclei are strongly interconnected with each other as well as with the NOT. In all mammals studied so far, the DTN and NOT appear to play crucial roles in driving horizontal optokinetic nystagmus, while the LTN and MTN are associated with vertical optokinetic nystagmus (reviewed in Grasse and Cynader, 1991; Sefton et al., 2004; Ibbotson and Dreher, 2005).

SUPERIOR COLLICULUS The SC constitutes a part of the tectum of the mesencephalon (midbrain) and is the mammalian homologue of the optic tectum of other vertebrates. In all mammals, including the mouse, seven distinct alternating cellular and fibrous layers are apparent in Nissl-stained and myelin-stained coronal or sagittal sections through the SC (Paxinos and Franklin, 2004). In the mouse (Dräger and Hubel, 1975b) as in other nocturnal rodents (Sefton et al., 2004) and in virtually all other mammals studied so far (for reviews, see Rhoades et al., 1991; Stein and Meredith, 1991), the retinal input terminates almost exclusively in the three superficial layers of the SC, that is, the most superficial, thin, and relatively cell-poor *stratum zonale* (zonal layer), the adjacent thicker and cell-rich *stratum griseum superficiale* (superficial gray layer), and the white fibrous layer, the *stratum opticum* (optic layer). As mentioned earlier, the ipsilateral projection in mice arises from a minority of RGCs in the VTC; these terminate in distinct clumps in the lower *stratum griseum superficiale* and *stratum opticum* in the rostral and medial parts of the SC (Dräger and Hubel, 1975b; Godement et al., 1984).

In the mouse (Hofbauer and Dräger, 1985) as in the laboratory rat (Linden and Perry, 1983; Dreher et al., 1985), hamster (Chalupa and Thompson, 1980), rabbit (Vaney et al., 1981), and polyprotodont marsupials such as North American opossum (Rapaport et al., 2004), virtually all RGCs (and thus presumably all morphological and functional classes of RGCs) project to the SC. On the other hand, in carnivores such as the domestic cat only about 50% of RGCs project to the SC, while 80% project to the dLGN (Illing and Wässle, 1981). Of the RGCs that project to the SC, about half (25% of all RGCs) also send a collateral to the dLGN (Wässle and Illing, 1980; Illing and Wässle, 1981). In primates such as macaque monkeys, while most, if not all, RGCs project to the dLGN, only a small minority (<10%) project to the SC (Rodieck and Watanabe, 1993).

The overall pattern of the retinotopic organization of the mouse SC is very similar to that in other mammals (see Rhoades et al., 1991; Stein and Meredith, 1991; Ibbotson and Dreher, 2005). Thus, in all retinorecipient layers, the zero vertical meridian is represented rostrally (anteriorly), with more peripheral parts of the contralateral visual field (nasal retina) represented caudally (posteriorly), the lower visual field (dorsal retina) represented laterally, and the upper visual field (ventral retina) represented medially (cf. Dräger and Hubel, 1975b, 1976; figure 3.4). In the mouse, there is a fairly extensive representation of the ipsilateral hemifield in the most rostral (anterior) part of the SC and at an elevation of 20–30° above horizontal meridian the representation of the ipsilateral hemifield extends for about 35° (Dräger and Hubel, 1975b, 1976; see figure 3.4). Overall, the representation of the ipsilateral hemifield in the rostral SC is especially extensive in nocturnal rodents. There is some representation of the ipsilateral hemifield in the rostral SC, however, in virtually all nonprimate mammals (Rhoades et al., 1991; Stein and Meredith, 1991), with the possible exception of megachiropteran bats (Pettigrew, 1986; but see Thiele et al., 1991).

In the SC of the mouse, an excitatory convergence of signals driven by UV and M cones and/or rods (Ekesten and Gouras, 2001) has been recorded by means of local VEPs. In a number of other cases, however, VEPs recorded from mouse SC were driven exclusively by UV or M cones and/or rods, but not by both. The exclusively UV-cone-driven VEPs were most common in the medial part of the SC, where the ventral retina (upper visual field) is represented (see figure 3.4). By contrast, the VEPs driven exclusively by M cones and/or rods were most common in the lateral part of the SC, where the upper retina (the lower visual field) is represented. The spatial distribution of exclusively UV-cone-driven responses is consistent with the concentration of UV-sensitive cones in the lower retina (Calderone and Jacobs, 1995).

Apart from the retinal input to the SC layers, in mice as in other mammals (for reviews, see Rhoades et al., 1991;

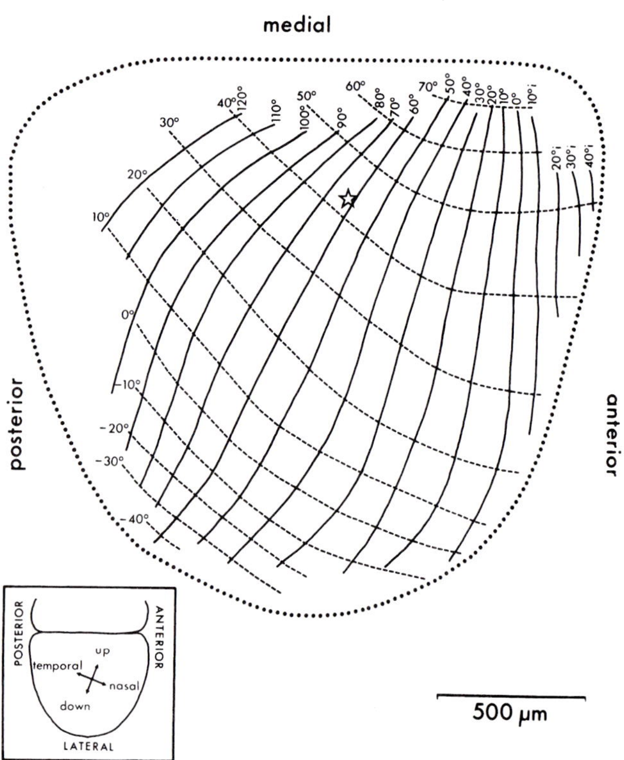

FIGURE 3.4 Retinotopic map projected onto the right superior colliculus of the mouse. *Dashed lines* represent constant elevation; *solid lines* indicate constant azimuth. *Star* indicates the projection of the optic disc of the contralateral (left) eye. *Inset* shows the overall plan of visual field representation in the superior colliculus. (From Dräger and Hubel, 1975.)

Stein and Meredith, 1991) there is also a strong input to these layers from lamina V of the ipsilateral visual cortex (especially from cytoarchitectonic area 17). In other mammals at least, the visuotopic maps based on corticotectal projections are in close alignment with the retinotopic map based in the topography of the retinal input (for a review, see Stein and Meredith, 1991). Substantial evidence indicates that in some mammals corticotectal input modulates receptive field (RF) properties of cells in the SC layers (reviewed in Stein and Meredith, 1991; Hashemi-Nezhad et al., 2003).

The excitatory (classical) RFs of neurons recorded from the most superficial layers of SC of the anesthetized mouse vary in size from 4° to 15°, with a mean size of about 9° (Dräger and Hubel, 1975b). These cells tend to respond optimally to stimuli substantially smaller than their discharge fields. They give ON/OFF responses to stationary stimuli positioned anywhere in their discharge fields and exhibit fairly low (ca. 3 spikes/s) spontaneous (background) activity (Dräger and Hubel, 1975b). Only a minority (25%) of neurons exhibit clear directional selectivity (Dräger and Hubel, 1975b). Very few cells (all of them recorded in the anteromedial SC) have binocular discharge fields, and monocular cells that could be activated by stimuli presented to the ipsilateral eye were not encountered (Dräger and Hubel, 1975b). Even though in nocturnal rodents virtually all RGCs project to the SC, selective ablation of the SC in laboratory rats results in only a transient disruption of the animal's ability to detect high-contrast square-wave gratings, and behaviorally measured visual acuity is not affected by collicular ablation (Dean, 1978).

A recent study by Girman and Lund (2007) in which sharp tungsten-in-glass electrodes were used to record from the upper part of the *stratum griseum superficiale* of anaesthetized laboratory rat suggests that in nocturnal murid rodents at least, the cells in that layer might be involved in "contour" perception. Girman and Lund (cf. Prévost et al., 2007) found that most cells recorded in the upper part of the *stratum griseum superficiale* exhibited fairly sharp orientation tuning (<60° width at half height) when the large (20°) luminance-contrast-modulated gratings were used. Furthermore, in all orientation selective collicular neurons, annulus gratings restricted to the silent suppressive RF surrounds strongly modulated in orientation specific manner the responses to stimulation of the classical RFs (Girman and Lund, 2007). Overall, the proportion of orientation selective and orientation biased cells (80%) in the upper part of the rat *stratum griseum superficiale* is very similar to that in rat's striate cortex (see Table 3.2).

Cells located in the deeper layers, the *stratum opticum* and *stratum griseum intermediale* (intermediate gray), tend to have larger discharge fields (often exceeding 20°), exhibit directional selectivity, and tend to prefer upward movements; in addition, they habituate, that is, responses decline to repeated stimulation with the same stimulus (Dräger and Hubel, 1975b). Most SC neurons located just below the intermediate gray layer are bimodal or trimodal cells that respond not only to visual stimuli (large discharge regions) but also to somatosensory and auditory stimuli. Bimodal neurons that respond to visual and somatosensory stimuli and those that respond to visual and auditory stimuli tend to be congregated into separate clusters. Finally, neurons located at deeper locations usually do not respond to visual stimuli but respond to either somatosensory or auditory stimuli (Dräger and Hubel, 1975b). The tactile RFs of neurons in this region of the SC are located exclusively on the contralateral side of the body. They most often involve the whiskers, and, in electrode penetrations made perpendicular to the collicular surface, the tactile RFs encountered in deep layers tend to correspond to the same region of space as the visual RFs of neurons encountered more superficially (Dräger and Hubel, 1975b, 1976; figure 3.5). Finally, the most effective auditory stimuli seem to be high-frequency clicks emanating from the contralateral space (Dräger and Hubel, 1975b).

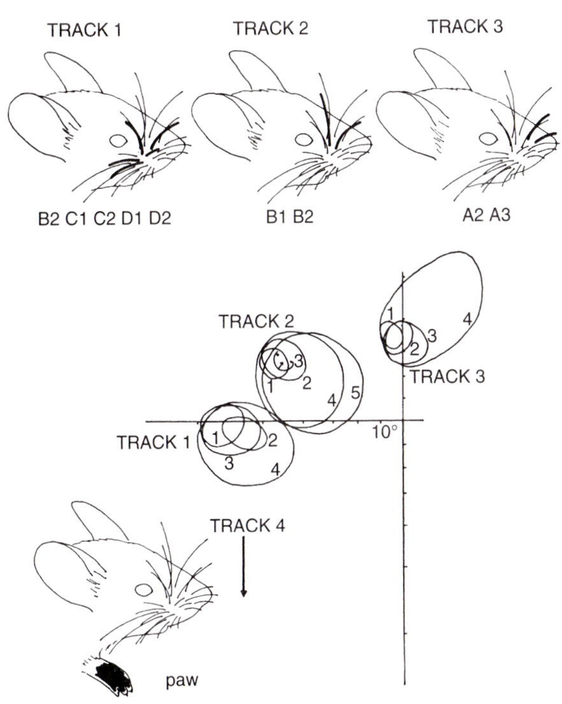

FIGURE 3.5 Location of somatosensory and visual RFs of neurons recorded in four successive vertical electrode tracks through the mouse SC. Note that representation of specific contralateral whiskers in the deep parts of tracks 1–3 corresponds with particular locations of visual RFs of cells encountered in the more superficial parts of a given track. In the case of the fourth track, the somatosensory RF was on the dorsum of the contralateral forepaw, whereas the visual RFs were in the inferotemporal part of the contralateral visual field. (From Dräger and Hubel, 1975, with permission.)

The neurons in the intermediate and deep collicular layers of other mammals often have somatosensory and/or auditory RFs spatially overlapping with visual RFs (Stein and Meredith, 1991; Stein et al., 2001; Gandhi and Sparks, 2003). Furthermore, these neurons are characterized by a high degree of cross-modal sensory integration, and the responses to visual stimuli can be strongly affected (enhanced or reduced) by cues from other sensory modalities (Stein and Meredith, 1991; Stein et al., 2001). The multisensory integration in the SC of other mammals such as domestic cats appears to be largely dependent on the corticotectal input from the "polysensory" cortical areas (Stein and Wallace, 1996; Stein et al., 2001). Interestingly, in the mouse there are visual cortical areas that are polysensory and that could provide input to the SC.

In mammals with retinal areas specialized for high-acuity vision such as the *fovea centralis* (in virtually all primates) or a well-developed *area centralis* (in the cat), the intermediate and deep collicular layers are strongly involved in the generation of saccadic eye movements, which bring the image of object of interest into areas specialized for high-acuity vision (for reviews, see Rhoades et al., 1991; Stein and Meredith, 1991; Stein and Wallace, 1996). Very little is known about the involvement of intermediate and deep collicular layers in generating exploratory saccadic eye movements in mammals with a poorly developed *area centralis*, such as the mouse and other nocturnal rodents.

Dorsal Lateral Geniculate Nucleus   As in other mammals, the dLGN of the mouse is a specific dorsal thalamic nucleus that relays visual information from the retina to cortical area V1. Indeed, it receives a substantial direct retinal input and projects heavily to V1. As in other nocturnal rodents, the mouse dLGN occupies the dorsolateral part of the dorsal thalamus and is separated from the vLGN by the IGL (Provencio et al., 1998; Paxinos and Franklin, 2004).

The mouse dLGN is organized retinotopically in a pattern similar to that of the rat (see Sefton et al., 2004). In particular, the temporal visual field (contralateral nasal retina) is represented in the rostrolateral part of the nucleus, while the ventronasal visual field is represented in the caudal region in close proximity of the optic tract (Wagner et al., 2000). In all species of Carnivora and Primata studied so far (see Casagrande and Norton, 1991; Garey et al., 1991), as well as in Order Scandentia (tree shrews; Conley et al., 1984; Holdefer and Norton, 1995) and in a diurnal, highly visual rodent, the gray squirrel (Kaas et al., 1972; Van Hooser et al., 2003), the dLGN cells that receive contralateral retinal inputs and those that receive ipsilateral retinal inputs are clustered into cellular layers apparent in Nissl-stained sections through the nucleus. By contrast, although the projection from the ipsilateral retina occupies 14%–18% of the mouse dLGN in the dorsomedial region of the nucleus (LeVay et al., 1978; Godement et al., 1984), no cellular layers can be discerned (Paxinos and Franklin, 2004). There is a similar lack of cellular lamination corresponding to ipsilateral and contralateral inputs in the rat (see Sefton et al., 2004).

In addition to cellular lamination, the dLGN of virtually all species of Carnivora and Primata (for reviews, see Garey et al., 1991; Casagrande and Norton, 1991), tree shrews (Conley et al., 1984; Holdefer and Norton, 1995), as well as the gray squirrel (Van Hooser et al., 2003), are characterized by functional heterogeneity of dLGN cells. Functional heterogeneity is also apparent, although to a lesser extent, in the dLGN of the rat (reviewed in Sefton et al., 2004) and rabbit (Swadlow and Weyand, 1985). By contrast, despite substantial morphological and functional heterogeneity of mouse RGCs, from the functional point of view the mouse dLGN appears to be extremely homogeneous (Grubb and Thompson, 2003).

All mouse dLGN neurons whose RFs have been plotted so far exhibited Kuffler-type (Kuffler, 1953) RF organization with a single, approximately circular region in the center that responded to either increases (ON-center) or decreases (OFF-center) in luminance of the stimulus covering the region as well as antagonistic surround regions, stimulation of which produced weaker responses (OFF discharges in case of ON-center cells and ON discharges in case of OFF-center cells; Grubb and Thompson, 2003). Virtually all mouse dLGN cells appear to sum spatial information linearly (Grubb and Thompson, 2003; see also Enroth-Cugell and Robson, 1966; Hochstein and Shapley, 1976). Nevertheless, when stimulated with stationary flashing full-screen black (OFF-center cells) or white (ON-center cells) stimuli, the dLGN cells respond in a fairly tonic or fairly phasic manner, allowing them to be categorized as distinct sustained or transient groups, respectively (Grubb and Thompson, 2003). The RF centers are usually large (ca. 11°) and tend to increase with eccentricity (Grubb and Thompson, 2003). Most dLGN cells exhibit low spatial resolution (ca. 0.2 c/deg) of luminance-contrast sinusoidally modulated gratings and respond maximally at temporal frequencies of 4 Hz (Grubb and Thompson, 2003). Although for most dLGN cells, the peak spatial performance was around 0.03 c/deg, a small proportion of them exhibited a spatial cutoff of 0.5 c/deg (Grubb and Thompson, 2003). This latter value is in good agreement with the behaviorally determined spatial resolution (Gianfranceschi et al., 1999; Prusky et al., 2000).

Despite the fact that the small "shell" region, located in the vicinity of the optic tract (in the dorsolateral part of the dLGN), contains the majority of cells positive for the antibody against the calcium-binding protein calbindin-D28k (Grubb and Thompson, 2004), there is no evidence of functional specialization of neurons located in this region (Grubb and Thompson, 2003). Interestingly, RGCs that express the Brn3a transcription factor also project to this region, as do most of the inputs from the ipsilateral SC (Grubb and Thompson, 2004). The apparent functional homogeneity of mouse dLGN might be at least partially related to the fact that, unlike in carnivores and primates, in the mouse (Hofbauer and Dräger, 1985) virtually all RGCs project to the SC. In the rat, in which virtually all RGCs project to the SC (Linden and Perry, 1983; Dreher et al., 1985), only about a third of RGCs project to the dLGN (Dreher et al., 1985). It is likely that in the mouse the retinal projection to the dLGN is also limited and that only particular types of RGCs project to the dLGN.

Visual cortex

Mouse visual cortex, like the visual cortices of all mammals studied so far, constitutes a part of the six-layer neocortex and consists of a number of cytoarchitectonically, visuotopically, and hodologically defined areas (Caviness, 1975; Olavarria et al., 1982; Simmons et al., 1982; Wagor et al., 1980; Olavarria and Montero, 1989; Wang and Burkhalter, 2007). Cytoarchitectonically defined areas that constitute V1 in mouse are areas 17, 18a, and 18b (Wagor et al., 1980; Simmons et al., 1982; Olavarria and Montero, 1989; Caviness and Frost, 1980).

Anatomy of Primary Visual Cortex In the mouse, cytoarchitectonic area 17 (striate cortex, area V1) occupies an area of about 2–3 mm^2 in the middle third of the posterior part of the occipital lobe (Caviness and Frost, 1980; Paxinos and Franklin, 2004). As in the rat (Krieg, 1946), area 17 of the mouse is surrounded rostrolaterally by area 18a and medially by area 18b (Caviness, 1975, Valverde, 1968; figure 3.6). In Nissl-stained sections, area 17 of the mouse, as in other mammalian species, is characterized by a high density of granule cells and substantial relative widths of the principal geniculorecipient layer, layer IV (granular layer; Caviness, 1975; Valverde, 1968). Furthermore, area 17 can be distinguished from the surrounding cortical areas 18a and 18b by the low density of cells in sublaminae Va and Vc and greater width of sublamina VIa (Caviness, 1975; Valverde, 1968), high acetylcholinesterase activity in layers IV and III, and strong staining for myelin (Antonini et al., 1999). Since area 17 of the mouse is the only cortical area that receives its principal dorsal thalamic input from the dLGN (Caviness and Frost, 1980; Frost and Caviness, 1980; Simmons et al., 1982), this area, as in other rodents (see Sefton et al., 2004) and primates (Valverde, 1991) but unlike in carnivores (cat: Payne and Peters, 2002; ferret: Baker et al., 1998; mink: McConnell and LeVay, 1986), constitutes the entire primary V1. However, in addition to massive dLGN projection to area 17 there is a small but distinct dLGN projection to area 18a (Antonini et al., 1999).

Visuotopic organization. Area 17 contains one complete representation of the contralateral visual hemifield with the zero vertical meridian represented close to the border with area 18a (located laterally to area 17; see figure 3.6), and with gradually more peripheral vertical meridians represented

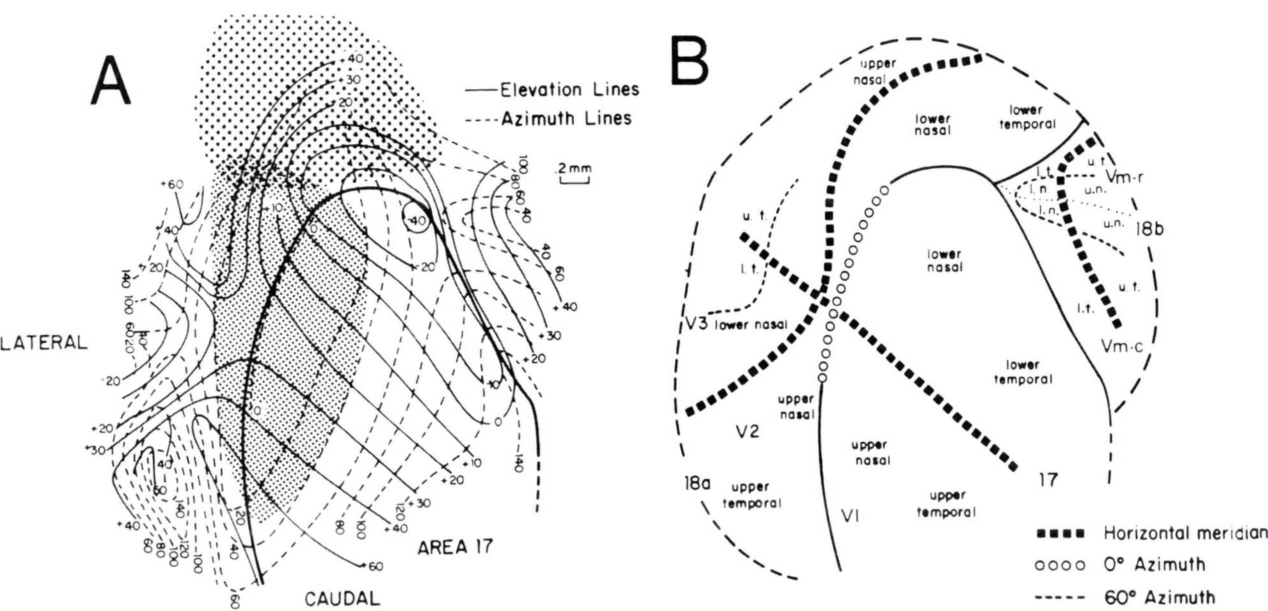

Figure 3.6 Dorsal view of the visuotopic organization of primary visual cortex (cytoarchitectonic area 17) and several extrastriate visual cortices in cytoarchitectonic areas 18a and 18b of the mouse. *Finely stippled area* in *A* indicates the region in which binocular neurons were encountered; *coarsely stippled area* indicates the region in which cells had both visual and somatosensory (vibrissal) RFs. *B*, Overall visuotopic organization of several visual cortical areas. (From Wagor et al. 1980, with permission.)

more medially toward the border with area 18b (Dräger, 1975; Wagor et al., 1980; Simmons et al., 1982; Kalatsky and Stryker, 2003; Wang and Burkhalter, 2007). Despite the relatively small number of ipsilaterally projecting RGCs, the binocular region of visual cortex occupies approximately the lateral one-third of area 17. In addition, a small (about 10°) part of the ipsilateral hemifield is represented in a small region of area 17 between the representation of the zero vertical meridian and the border with area 18a (Dräger, 1975; Wagor et al., 1980, Gordon and Stryker, 1996). As in other rodents, such as the laboratory rat (reviewed in Sefton et al., 2004) and golden hamster (Tiao and Blakemore, 1976a), or carnivores, such as the cat (Tusa et al., 1978; Payne, 1990) and ferret (Law et al., 1988), the lower contralateral visual field (dorsal retina) is represented rostrally while the upper contralateral visual field (ventral retina) is represented caudally (Dräger, 1975; Dräger and Olsen, 1980; Simmons et al., 1982; Wagor et al., 1980; Wang and Burkhalter, 2007). Overall, the topographic location and the visuotopic organization of mouse striate cortex are remarkably similar to those of the laboratory rat (see Sefton et al., 2004) and golden hamster (Tiao and Blakemore, 1976a).

Connections with the dorsal thalamus. The optic radiation fibers originating in the dLGN enter the cerebral hemisphere at the rostral end of the lateral geniculate body and constitute the thickest of the fibers entering area 17 from the white matter (Valverde and Ruiz-Marcos, 1969). The geniculocortical fibers terminate mainly in layer IV, with fewer fibers terminating in the layer III, the lower part of layer V, and the entire layer VI (Valverde and Ruiz-Marcos, 1969; Ruiz-Marcos and Valverde, 1970; Caviness and Frost, 1980; Frost and Caviness, 1980; Dräger, 1981). Furthermore, a few dLGN fibers terminate in lamina I (Frost and Caviness, 1980). As in other mammals, the geniculocortical terminals in the mouse appear to form asymmetric (i.e., excitatory) synapses, predominantly on the shafts of smooth or sparsely spinous dendrites of so-called stellate cells in layer IV or the spines of the proximal dendrites of pyramidal cells whose bodies lie in layers III and V. Interestingly, there appears to be a functional dependence of pyramidal cells on their dorsal thalamic input, since in mice raised in darkness there is a significant reduction in the number of dendritic spines on the apical shafts of layer V pyramidal cells (for a review, see Valverde, 1991).

Apart from its input from the dLGN, mouse area 17 receives direct inputs from the lateral posterior (LP) and lateral (L) dorsal thalamic nuclei and sends reciprocal connections to all these dorsal thalamic nuclei (Simmons et al., 1982; Olavarria and Montero, 1989). Overall, the laminar pattern of termination of projections from LP is similar to that of projections from dLGN, with an additional focus of termination in upper layer V (Frost and Caviness, 1980).

Connections with the ventral thalamus and mesencephalon. Striate cortex projects to presumably visuotopically corresponding parts of the ipsilateral vLGN (located in close proximity to the dLGN; Olavarria and Montero, 1989). Furthermore, cells in layer V project to visuotopically corresponding (Dräger and Hubel, 1975a, 1975b) parts of the superficial layers of the ipsilateral SC (Olavarria et al., 1982; Olavarria and Montero, 1989). However, the connections with vLGN and SC are not reciprocal.

Intrinsic associational corticocortical connections. The lamina IV cells provide the principal input to pyramidal cells in the supragranular layers II and III (Frost and Caviness, 1980).

Long-range associational corticocortical connections. Area 17 has strong reciprocal connections with visuotopically corresponding parts of ipsilateral areas 18a and 18b (Simmons et al., 1982; Olavarria et al., 1982; Olavarria and Montero, 1989). More specifically, area 17 projects to nine visuotopically organized areas within cytoarchitectonic areas 18a (six visuotopic areas) and 18b (three visuotopic areas; Olavarria and Montero, 1989; Wang and Burkhalter, 2007). Particularly dense connections were noted with a subregion of area 18a called the lateromedial (LM) area, which abuts the border of area 17 and has recently been suggested to constitute the mouse homologue of V2 (Wang and Burkhalter, 2007; see figure 3.9). Associational connections between areas 17 and 18a and 18b terminate mainly in layers II and III, and to a lesser extent in the upper half of layer IV (Olavarria and Montero, 1989). In addition, area 17 projects to the posteromedial border of the forehead and earlobe representation (Olavarria and Montero, 1989) as well as to the caudal whisker representation (Wang and Burkhalter, 2007) in the primary somatosensory cortex (area S1). In barrel cortex, axons originating from the part of area 17 (V1) in which the upper visual field is represented innervate preferentially A-row barrels, while axons originating from the part of area 17 where the lower visual field is represented innervate preferentially C-row barrels. Connections between the areas V1 and S1, however, do not appear to be reciprocal (Wang and Burkhalter, 2007). Area 17 also sends sparse projections to (1) the posterior cytoarchitectonic area, 36p; (2) the lateral entorhinal area located lateral to area 18a; (3) retrosplenial agranular cortex located medial to area 18b, and (4) the primary motor cortex. The V1 projections to these areas are not topographically organized (Wang and Burkhalter, 2007).

Callosal connections. The border region between areas 17 and 18a is strongly interhemispherically interconnected via the corpus callosum (Yorke and Caviness, 1975; Cusick and Lund, 1981; Olavarria and Van Sluyters, 1984; Olavarria et al., 1988; figure 3.7). In view of the relative paucity of the

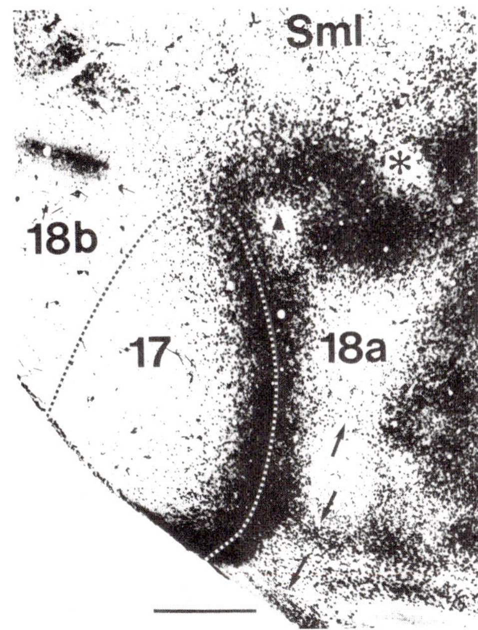

FIGURE 3.7 Pattern of callosal connections in the dorsal view of mouse visual cortex. Dark areas indicate high density of callosal cells and terminals following multiple injections of horseradish peroxidase. Note the high concentration of callosal cells and terminals at the border of cytoarchitectonic areas 17 and 18a. Note also several concentrations of callosal cells and terminals within cytoarchitectonic areas 18a and 18b. This, in turn, suggests that areas 18a and 18b contain several visuotopically organized areas. *Arrows* indicate callosal bridges across cytoarchitectonic area 18a. *Arrowhead* indicates the anterior callosal ring. *Asterisk* indicates "the ring-like callosal configuration" in the primary somatosensory cortex. Sml, primary somatosensory cortex. Scale bar = 0.5 mm. (From Olavarria and Montero, 1989, with permission.)

RGC projections to the ipsilateral dLGN and the high degree of binocular convergence in the binocular segment of area 17 in proximity of area 18a, it is likely that binocular convergence in the mouse striate cortex is mainly due to the interhemispheric callosal connections. Indeed, all transcallosal area 17 cells are binocular cells that could be activated by stimuli presented through either eye (Simmons and Pearlman 1983).

PHYSIOLOGY OF PRIMARY VISUAL CORTEX As in carnivores (cat: Hubel and Wiesel, 1962), primates (macaque monkeys: Hubel and Wiesel, 1968), or other nocturnal rodents (golden hamster: Tiao and Blakemore, 1976a), neurons in the mouse striate cortex tend to respond poorly to changes in overall level of illumination (Dräger, 1975). Unlike in the striate cortices of carnivores and primates, however, most cells in the mouse striate cortex are reported not to be orientation selective (Dräger, 1975; Mangini and Pearlman, 1980; Métin et al., 1988; table 3.2). Even though in the mouse, cones constitute only about 3% of photoreceptors, the VEPs recorded from mouse area 17 are primarily driven by cones, and low-luminance (scotopic range) visual stimuli do not produce detectable VEPs (Porciatti et al., 1999).

Nonoriented cells. Among the nonoriented cortical cells that respond to spatially restricted, flashing stationary stimuli, three distinct groups are commonly distinguished on the basis of the spatial organization of their RFs: (1) cells with ON discharge centers and antagonistic OFF discharge surrounds, (2) cells with OFF discharge centers and antagonistic ON discharge surrounds, and (3) cells with spatially overlapping ON and OFF discharge regions (Dräger, 1975; Mangini and Pearlman, 1980; Dräger, 1981; Métin et al., 1988). Some of the nonoriented cells with spatially overlapping ON and OFF discharge regions exhibit weak, spatially distinct, antagonistic ON, OFF, or ON/OFF surrounds (Dräger, 1975). Furthermore, a substantial proportion of nonoriented cells exhibit silent suppressive surrounds in their RFs (Mangini and Pearlman, 1980; Simmons and Pearlman, 1983; see also Schuett et al., 2002). The nonoriented cells that respond vigorously to flashing stationary stimuli tend to respond vigorously to spots or elongated bars of any orientation moving over a wide range of stimulus velocities (Métin et al., 1988), with peak velocity sensitivities in the range of 25–1,000 deg/s (most of them in the range of 50–100 deg/s; Mangini and Pearlman, 1980). The responses to stationary flashing stimuli are invariably transient (Dräger, 1975). A subgroup of nonoriented cells responds poorly to flashing stationary stimuli but vigorously to stimuli moving in both directions along a particular axis of movement or to stimuli moving in only one direction along a particular axis of movement (Mangini and Pearlman, 1980; Métin et al., 1988). With the exception of corticotectal cells, the nonoriented cells tend to have very low spontaneous (background) activity (0–2 spikes/s; Mangini and Pearlman, 1980).

The nonoriented cells are located in all layers, with most located in layer IV (Mangini and Pearlman, 1980). The sizes of minimum discharge fields of nonoriented cells vary from about 4° to 80°, while the mean size is around 15–20° (Dräger, 1975; Mangini and Pearlman, 1980; Métin et al., 1988; Kalatsky and Stryker, 2003; Wang and Burkhalter, 2007). There is a weak and not statistically significant trend for an increase in RF size with eccentricity of RF position (Dräger, 1975; Mangini and Pearlman, 1980; Wang and Burkhalter, 2007). The lack of a clear eccentricity-related increase in the size of classic RFs of cortical cells correlates with a similar lack of eccentricity (ganglion cell density)-related increase in the size of the dendritic trees of the RGCs (see Sun et al., 2002).

Corticotectal cells. A distinct group of nonoriented cells was found almost exclusively in layer V, the layer in which corticotectal cells projecting to the SC are located (Mangini and Pearlman, 1980). Irrespective of eccentricity of RF location,

Table 3.2

Orientation tunings and their relationships to presence or absence of orientation columns in different species

Species	Orientation Columns Present?	% of Orientation-Selective or Orientation-Biased Cells	Orientation Tuning Range	Mean Orientation Tuning Range	References[†]
Mouse	No	40–43	60–180°	60–180°	1–3
Rat	No	70–80 to 93	30–120°*	30–60°	4–5
Squirrel	No	68	10–70°*		6
Hamster	No	30	~30–~130°	50–80°	7
Rabbit	No	72	10–<160°	Most 40–130°	8
Mink	Yes	98	7.5–90°	29	9
Ferret	Yes	75	60–180°*	60–180°	10–12
Cat	Yes	91	<10–<160°*	Most common 20–60°	13–18
Cat (area 18)	Yes	90–95	20–140°	40–60°	19, 20
Tree shrew	Yes	75	10–80°	20–40°	21
Macaque	Yes	87	10–120°*	Most common 30–40°	22–24
Tammar wallaby	Probably no	70	30–180°*		25
Brush-tailed possum	Probably no	30			26

*Values given are half-width at half-height.

[†] *1*, Dräger, 1975; *2*, Mangini and Pearlman, 1980; *3*, Métin et al., 1988; *4*, Burne et al., 1984; *5*, Girman et al., 1999a; *6*, Van Hooser et al., 2005; *7*, Tiao and Blakemore, 1976a; *8*, Murphy and Berman, 1979; *9*, LeVay et al., 1987; *10*, Chalupa, 2006; *11*, Chapman et al., 1991; *12*, Rao et al., 1997; *13*, Henry et al., 1974b; *14*, Hammond and Andrews, 1978; *15*, Murphy and Berman, 1979; *16*, Hübener and Bonhoeffer, 2002; *17*, Löwell, 2002; *18*, Ohki et al., 2006; *19*, Hammond and Andrews, 1978; *20*, Dreher, Michalski, et al., 1992; *21*, Humphrey et al., 1977; *22*, Hubel and Wiesel, 1974; *23*, Schiller et al., 1976a; *24*, Hubel et al., 1978; *25*, Ibbotson and Mark, 2003; *26*, Crewther et al., 1984.

the presumptive corticotectal cells are characterized by larger than average RFs (Mangini and Pearlman, 1980). Apart from the lack of orientation and direction selectivities, identified corticotectal cells are characterized by very large RFs (mean, 66.5°; range, 30–95°), high background activity (6 spikes/s; range, 4–17 spikes/s), good responsiveness over a wide range of stimulus velocities (10–1,000 deg/s; mean preferred velocity ca. 250 deg/s), and relatively little spatial summation (Mangini and Pearlman 1980; Lemmon and Pearlman, 1981). RF characteristics of the corticotectal cells of the mouse (with the exception of apparent lack of orientation selectivity) are remarkably similar to those of the cat (Palmer and Rosenquist, 1974). Overall, corticotectal cells in the mouse (Mangini and Pearlman, 1980), as in the rat (see Sefton et al., 2004) and cat, are large pyramidal neurons located in layer V. This is in contrast to the situation in primates, where corticotectal cells are located in both layers V and VI (Finlay et al., 1976; Fries et al., 1985; Cusick and Lund, 1981; Lia and Olavarria, 1996).

Orientation selectivity. A substantial minority of cells in mouse striate cortex are orientation selective (34%–43%; Dräger, 1975; Mangini and Pearlman, 1980; Métin et al., 1988). They tend to have a very low level (0–1 spikes/s) of spontaneous activity (Mangini and Pearlman, 1980), and about half of them exhibit a substantial degree of direction selectivity (Métin et al., 1988). Applying the criteria developed for classification of oriented cortical cells in cats and primates (Hubel and Wiesel, 1962, 1968; Gilbert, 1977; Henry, 1977), orientation-selective cells in the mouse are classified as simple if they contain spatially distinct, mutually antagonistic ON and OFF discharge regions in their classical RFs or as complex if the ON and OFF discharge regions in their classical RFs spatially overlap (Dräger, 1975; Mangini and Pearlman, 1980; Métin et al., 1988). Simple and complex cells constitute respectively about half of orientation-selective cells, that is, about 20% of all neurons in the mouse striate cortex (Dräger, 1975; Métin et al., 1988). The diameter of simple RFs varies from 6° to 55° (mean, 23.5°; Dräger, 1975). It is worth pointing out that simple and complex cells have been reported in V1 in virtually all orders of mammals, both eutherian and noneutherian (for a review, see Van Hooser et al., 2005). The only known exception is the tree shrew, in which simple cells appear to be lacking (Mooser et al., 2004).

As indicated in table 3.2, in the striate cortex of carnivores, virtually all primates, including both Old World (Hubel and Wiesel, 1968; Leventhal et al., 1995, Schiller et al., 1976b) and New World diurnal monkeys (Forte et al., 2005), tree shrews (Humphrey et al., 1977), and in highly visual diurnal rodents such as gray squirrel (Van Hooser et al., 2005), the majority of cells are orientation selective. The relative paucity of orientation-selective cells in the mouse striate cortex is consistent with the relative paucity (ca. 30%) of orientation-selective neurons in the striate cortex of the golden hamster (Tiao and Blakemore, 1976a) and the rabbit (Chow et al., 1971, Murphy and Berman, 1979). Surprisingly, however, in the closely related murid rodent, the laboratory rat, at least 70%–80% of neurons in area 17 exhibit a clear orientation selectivity (Burne et al., 1984; Girman et al., 1999) and if one includes cells broadly tuned for orientation (orientation biased), about 93% of neurons in rat's striate cortex exhibit orientation tuning (Girman et al., 1999). In a number of species, cells that prefer a range of similar orientations are grouped together in radial columns referred to as orientation columns (or domains). This type of organization is present in cats and primates but has not been found in rodents, including the highly visual diurnal squirrels (see table 3.2).

The range of contour orientations over which orientation-selective, simple or complex cells in mouse striate cortex respond (orientation tuning width) varies from 60° to 180°, with an average of 120° (Métin et al., 1988). The overall range and average values of the orientation tuning width are rather similar to those for orientation-selective cells in the striate cortex of the rat (Girman et al., 1999) but broader than those of orientation-selective cells in striate cortex of the hamster (Tiao and Blakemore, 1976a). Large proportions of orientation selective simple (orientation tuning range 10–180°, with a median of 55°) or complex (orientation tuning range 15–180°, with a median of 68°) cells in cat's striate cortex (Payne and Berman, 1983) exhibit a substantially higher degree of orientation selectivity than those observed in the striate cortex of the mouse. The range of orientation tuning widths and the average orientation tuning widths of cells in the striate cortex of the mouse are also greater than those for neurons recorded from area 18 in the cat (range, 20–140°, with the 40–60° range most common; Dreher, Michalski, et al., 1992). Another measure of orientation selectivity (half-width at half-height of orientation tuning curves) also suggests that the orientation selectivity in carnivores (cat: Henry et al., 1974a, 1974b; Rose and Blakemore, 1974; ferret: Usrey et al., 2003) and primates (Ringach et al., 2002; Schiller et al., 1976a; De Valois et al., 1982; Leventhal et al., 1995) is sharper than that in mice.

Substantial evidence indicates that orientation selectivity of neurons in the striate cortex of the cat at least, is determined by a network of excitatory feedforward thalamocortical and intrinsic recurrent connections as well as intrinsic GABAergic inhibitory connections (for reviews, see Henry et al., 1994; Vidyasagar et al., 1996; Eysel, 2002; Somers et al., 2002). It is worth noting in this context that in the mouse striate cortex, almost all of the cortical neurons expressing γ-aminobutyric acid (GABA) are orientation insensitive, while most of the excitatory neurons are orientation selective (Sohya et al., 2007).

The reported difference in proportion of orientation-selective cells between rats and mice might, however, be more apparent than real, and could be related to the fact that the classical RFs of cells recorded from the mouse striate cortex tend to be much larger than the elongated bars used to determine cells' orientation selectivity (Dräger, 1975, 1981; Mangini and Pearlman, 1980; Métin et al., 1988). First, it has been clearly demonstrated in the striate cortex of cat (see Henry et al., 1974a, 1974b; Chen et al., 2005) and macaque (Schiller et al., 1976a) that when elongated stimuli shorter than the minimum discharge field (classical RF) of the cell, and therefore not encroaching onto the silent, extraclassical area surrounding the classical RF, were used to determine the orientation selectivity, orientation tuning became rather broad. As mentioned earlier, a substantial proportion of nonoriented cells in mouse area 17 have silent, suppressive regions in their RFs (Mangini and Pearlman, 1980; Simmons and Pearlman, 1983; Schuett et al., 2002; see also the discussion of hypercomplex cells in Dräger, 1975). Girman and colleagues (1999) determined the sharpness of orientation tuning of cells in the striate cortex of the rat using luminance-contrast-sinusoidally modulated gratings, presumably encroaching onto the silent, extraclassical RFs. Second, in both cats (Andrews and Pollen, 1979) and ferrets (Chapman et al., 1991; but see Usrey et al., 2003) the orientation tuning tends to be sharper when gratings rather than single elongated bars are used. Third, in the case of macaque striate cortex, the cells located in the "blobs" (regions in the supragranular layers II and III that express high levels of activity of mitochondrial enzyme cytochrome oxidase) tend to show very little orientation selectivity when elongated bars are used (Livingstone and Hubel, 1984; Leventhal et al., 1995). However, when luminance-contrast, sinusoidally modulated gratings were used, the cells located in the blobs exhibited a substantial degree of orientation selectivity (Leventhal et al., 1995).

Binocularity in the Primary Visual Cortex The binocular segment of mouse area 17, in which the binocular part of the visual field (nasal 30–40° of the visual field) is represented, occupies the lateral third of area 17 (see figure 3.3). It can be distinguished histologically from the more medial monocular segment by its more intense staining for acetylcholinesterase activity (Antonini et al., 1999). As mentioned in the section on dLGN, virtually all cells in the mouse dLGN are monocular. By contrast, about 70% of cells recorded from the binocular segment of the striate cortex respond to appropriate visual stimuli presented via either eye (Dräger, 1975, 1978; Métin et al., 1988; see table 3.1). This is somewhat surprising given that in mice, the overall proportion of all RGCs projecting ipsilaterally is very small (2%–3%; Dräger and Olsen, 1980; Godement et al., 1984). The ipsilateral projection to the dLGN is relatively enhanced, however, as 14%–18% of the dLGN volume is occupied by terminals from the ipsilateral eye (LaVail, 1991; Godement et al., 1984). Not surprisingly, as indicated in figure 3.8, the proportion of monocular cells in the binocular region of area 17 that can be activated only by stimuli presented through the contralateral eye is much larger than the proportion of monocular cells that can be activated only by the stimuli presented through the ipsilateral eye (ca. 25% vs. ca. 5%; Dräger, 1975, 1978; Métin et al., 1988). The amplitude of VEPs recorded from the binocular segment of area 17 is approximately threefold greater than when the stimuli are presented via the ipsilateral eye (Porciatti et al., 1999). Similarly, the magnitude of signals recorded using intrinsic optical imaging in the binocular segment of area V1 generated by square-wave gratings of low spatial frequency presented to the contralateral eye is about twice that generated by stimuli presented to the ipsilateral eye (Kalatsky and Stryker, 2003).

As indicated in table 3.1, in the striate cortex of mammals with frontally positioned eyes, such as most primates or cats, monocular cells responding only to stimuli presented via a particular eye or binocular cells responding preferentially to visual stimuli presented via a particular eye, cluster in radially oriented ocular dominance columns (see table 3.1; for reviews, see LeVay and Nelson, 1991; Casagrande and Kaas, 1994). Ocular dominance columns are also apparent in ferrets (Law et al., 1988), even though ferrets, unlike cats, have fairly laterally positioned eyes and a relatively small proportion of RGCs (ca. 7%) project ipsilaterally (Morgan et al., 1987). Similarly, in the striate cortex of ungulates such as sheep, with their relatively laterally positioned eyes, there appear to be clear eye dominance columns (Clarke et al., 1976). By contrast, in the striate cortex of small nocturnal murid rodents with laterally positioned eyes (and a small proportion of ipsilaterally projecting RGCs), such as the mouse (Dräger, 1975, 1978) and rat (Fagiolini et al., 1994; Sefton et al., 2004), there is no evidence of clustering of cells into radial columns based on eye preference. This is also the case for small diurnal mammals with laterally positioned eyes such as tree shrews (Humphrey et al., 1977). Indeed, in these species, monocular cells responding only to the stimuli presented to one eye, or binocular cells dominated by one eye, are intermingled with cells that preferentially (or solely) respond to stimuli presented to the other eye. In the mouse, the lack of ocular dominance columns reported physiologically is consistent with the results of transneuronal tracing (Dräger, 1974; Antonini et al., 1999). Even though mice and other rodents do not have anatomically distinct ocular dominance columns, they do, nevertheless, have a critical period during early postnatal life in which the relative representations of the two eyes in the binocular region of cortex are sensitive to monocular deprivation (Dräger, 1978; Gordon and Stryker, 1996; Antonini et al., 1999). This bears many similarities to the phenomenon of ocular dominance plasticity, which has been extensively studied in cats (Wiesel and Hubel, 1963, 1965; LeVay et al., 1978; Shatz and Stryker, 1978) and primates (LeVay et al., 1975, 1980; Hubel and Wiesel, 1977).

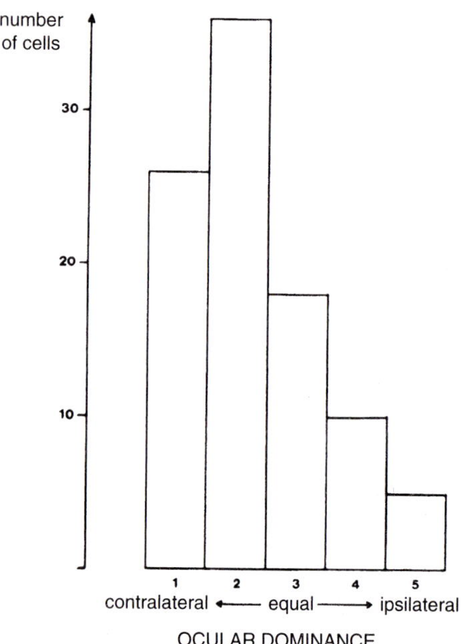

FIGURE 3.8 Ocular dominance distribution of cells recorded from cortical area 17 of the mouse. Class 1 and class 5 cells are monocular cells that could be activated by appropriate visual stimuli presented via the contralateral or ipsilateral eyes, respectively. Class 2 and class 4 cells are binocular cells dominated by the contralateral and ipsilateral eyes, respectively. Class 3 cells are binocular cells that respond equally strongly to stimuli presented via either eye. (From Dräger, 1975, with permission.)

Transcallosal cells. Transcallosal cells in area 17 can be activated antidromically by electrical stimulation of the contralateral visual cortex. They are predominantly located in layer III and to a lesser extent in layer II and in layers V and VI in the binocular part of area 17 in close vicinity of the border between areas 17 and 18a (Simmons and Pearlman, 1983). Transcallosal cells can be activated by visual stimuli presented through either eye, but tend to respond more vigorously to stimuli presented via the contralateral eye and their RFs were within 20° on either side of the representation of the vertical meridian (Simmons and Pearlman, 1983). Unlike the general population of mouse area 17 neurons, most transcallosal cells are orientation selective or orientation biased. They also have silent suppressive surround regions in their RFs and therefore respond poorly to large stimuli (Simmons and Pearlman, 1983).

Spatial Acuity and Temporal Resolution Probably only about a third of the RGCs project to the dLGN in the mouse, and hence V1 receives information only from a subpopulation of the RGCs. Nevertheless, visual acuity as determined by recording pattern VEPs from the binocular segment of mouse area 17 is about 0.6 c/deg (Porciatti et al., 1999). Similarly, the visual acuity of adult pigmented mice as determined by transcranial imaging of intrinsic signal in mouse area 17 is about 0.5 c/deg (Heimel et al., 2007). Those values are in very good agreement with the high cutoff limits of spatial resolution of the mouse visual system as determined by testing optokinetic reflexes (Sinex et al., 1979) or using behavioral techniques (Gianfranceschi et al., 1999, Prusky et al., 2000). This agreement is consistent with the fact that the visual acuity determined by recording VEPs to temporally countermodulated sine-wave gratings from area 17 of anesthetized macaque monkeys was virtually identical to that determined by recording the pattern electroretinogram responses (Ver Hoeve et al., 1999).

The VEPs recorded from the surface of the mouse area 17 are generated by a major dipole localized toward pyramidal cells in layers II and III (Porciatti et al., 1999). It is not surprising, then, that the peak spatial frequency of pattern VEPs recorded from the binocular segment of mouse area 17 at 0.06 c/deg (grating bars of ca. 8°) corresponds closely to the average size of RFs of neurons recorded from binocular segment of area 17 (Dräger, 1975; Mangini and Pearlman, 1980; Métin et al., 1988; Gordon and Stryker, 1996; Hensch et al., 1998). It is worth noting that in the rat, ablation of area 17 (plus some extrastriate cortices), with accompanying retrograde degeneration of the dLGN, results in transient disruption of animal's ability to detect high-contrast, low spatial frequency square-wave gratings, and after extensive retraining behaviorally measured visual acuity is reduced to about a third of the preablation value (Dean, 1978).

Based on the pattern VEP (to sinusoidally modulated luminance grating), the cells in binocular segment of mouse striate cortex appear to be most sensitive to temporal frequencies in the 2–4 Hz range, with a high cutoff at about 12 Hz and poor responsiveness at frequencies below 1 Hz (Porciatti et al., 1999). A high temporal frequency cutoff determined by transcranial imaging of intrinsic signal in mouse area 17 is even higher (16 Hz; Heimel et al., 2007). Consistent with the small axial length of mouse eye and its relatively large lens (Remtulla and Hallett, 1985), area 17 is more strongly activated strongly by fast rather than slowly moving visual stimuli, whether activity is measured by single unit recordings or VEPs (Dräger, 1975; Mangini and Pearlman, 1980, Porciatti et al., 1999). To our knowledge, the spatiotemporal tuning of single neurons in mouse visual cortex has not been examined, so we do not know if there is a spatial frequency invariant representation of stimulus velocity in mouse area 17.

Extrastriate visual cortices. In highly visual mammals such as primates (Payne, 1993; Rosa, 1997) or carnivores such as cats (for reviews, see Rosenquist, 1985; Burke et al., 1998) and ferrets (Manger et al., 2002a, 2002b, 2004), a large proportion of neocortex processes visual information. Furthermore, in both primates and carnivores (for reviews, see Maunsell and Newsome, 1987; Rosa, 1997; Burke et al., 1998), there are a large number of topographically organized cortical visual areas. These are generally considered to constitute the parts of at least two distinct streams, which process information about visual motion or pattern (and color in case of diurnal primates), respectively. In rodents, two cytoarchitectonically distinct areas, 18a and 18b, abut area 17 (see Sefton et al., 2004). Area 18a abuts area 17 laterally and rostrally, whereas area 18b abuts area 17 medially and rostrally. These areas also differ in terms of their primary thalamic input, which in the case of area 18a arises from the rostral part of the LP nucleus and in the case of area 18b arises from the L nucleus (Caviness and Frost, 1980). Wagor and colleagues (1980) distinguished at least two distinct topographically organized representations of parts of the contralateral visual fields in area 18a and two distinct topographic representations in area 18b (see figure 3.6). When combined, two representations within area 18a appear to form one complete representation of the contralateral visual field. As in the rat (Sefton et al., 2004), the border between area 17 and area 18a located lateral to area 17 contains dense aggregates of callosal cells and terminals (Olavarria and Montero, 1989). Since it was originally believed that the vertical meridian is represented along the entire border between area 17 and area 18a, the part of area 18a immediately abutting area 17 was designated area V2 (Wagor et al., 1980; Rosa and Krubitzer, 1999). Recently, however, evidence has been presented that the vertical meridian is represented only at the part of the border between areas 17 and 18a, that is, at the border of area V1 and one of the visuotopically organized areas within area 18a, the lateromedial (LM) area (Wang and Burkhalter, 2007). Since in almost all mammalian species studied to date, including some rodents (Rosa and Krubitzer, 1999; Sefton et al., 2004; Rosa and Tweedale, 2005), the representation of the vertical meridian delineates the border between areas V1 and V2, it appears that in the mouse only area LM, rather than the entire area V2 as designated by Wagor and colleagues (1980), is homologous to area V2 in other mammals (Wang and Burkhalter, 2007; figure 3.9). Thus, area V1 is adjoined laterally not only by area V2 (area LM) but also by several other visuotopically organized areas, specifically, the anterior (A), rostrolateral (RL), and posterior (P) areas (Wang and Burkhalter, 2007). As the zero horizontal meridian rather than the zero vertical meridian is represented at the border of presumptive V2 and the more lateral part of area 18a, the lateral part of area 18a has been designated area V3 (Wagor et al., 1980; see also Rosa and Manger, 2005, for presumptive homologous areas in other mammals). The area designated by Wagor and colleagues as area V3 appears to correspond to the laterointermediate (LI) area of Wang and Burkhalter (2007). The cortical neurons in 18a that are just rostral rather than lateral to area 17 (presumably corresponding to areas A and RL of Wang and Burkhalter, 2007) are bimodal, that is, they have clearly defined visual RFs and somewhat less well-defined somatosensory (vibrissal) RFs (Wagor et al., 1980). Rostrally, area 18a abuts somatosensory cortex, and bimodal area 18a neurons located in close proximity to somatosensory cortices are characterized by clearly defined vibrissal RFs and poorly defined visual RFs.

Similarly, in area 18b, which abuts area 17 medially and rostrally, two topographically organized areas were designated areas Vm-r and Vm-c (Wagor et al., 1980). Both of

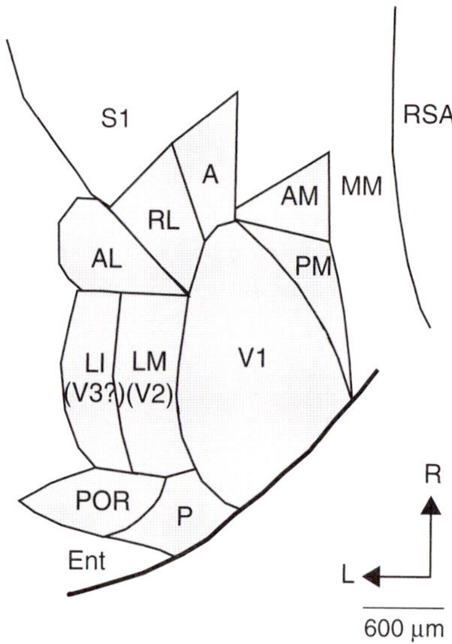

FIGURE 3.9 Schematic diagram depicting the relationship between striate and extrastriate visual cortical areas in the mouse. The cytoarchitectonically defined areas 18a (lateral to V1) and 18b (medial to V1) contain nine distinct, visuotopically organized areas. The lateromedial area (LM) abuts V1 laterally and is considered the homologue of V2. The laterointermediate area (LI) is probably the homologue of V3. Other areas are the posterior (P), postrhinal (POR), anterolateral (AL), rostrolateral (RL), anterior (A), anteromedial (AM), and posteromedial (PM). A number of other regions also receive V1 input but are not visuotopically organized. These regions include but are not limited to the mediomedial (MM), retrosplenial (RSA), and primary somatosensory (S1) areas shown. The entorhinal area (Ent) does not have direct connections with V1. (Figure based on Wang and Burkhalter, 2007.)

these areas contain distinct, approximately mirror representations of the temporal but not the nasal parts of the visual hemifield, and the visual RFs of neurons in both areas are poorly defined (Wagor et al., 1980). Consistent with the visuotopic subdivision of area 18b into areas Vm-r and Vm-c, each area receives partially distinct inputs from different parts of the lateral nucleus. Thus, while the lateral part of caudal lateral nucleus projects to area Vm-c, the medial part of caudal lateral nucleus projects mainly to area Vm-r (Caviness and Frost, 1980). Whereas in both carnivores and primates the polysensory cortical areas also abut purely visual cortices, unlike in the mouse, they appear to be separated from area 17 by numerous purely visual areas (see Stein and Meredith, 1993). However, it has recently been shown that multisensory integration in primates such as common marmosets occurs in the visual, somatosensory, and auditory cortical areas that were previously believed to be unisensory (Cappe and Barone, 2005).

As mentioned earlier, the visuotopic subdivisions of cytoarchitectonic areas 18a and 18b of the mouse are strongly supported by the patterns of associational corticocortical connections between area 17 and clusters of cells within area 18a and 18b (Olavarria and Montero, 1989; Wang and Burkhalter, 2007). Furthermore, the callosally projecting cells and callosal terminals concentrate not only at the border between areas 17 and 18a but also in several distinct regions within area 18a and, to a lesser extent, within area 18b (see figure 3.7 after Olavarria and Montero, 1989). Since the number and general location of callosally connected regions in the mouse extrastriate visual cortices are similar to those in the laboratory rat (for a review, see Sefton et al., 2004), it has been suggested that multiple visual cortical areas in murid rodents are arranged according to a common plan (Olavarria and Montero, 1989). Indeed, the pattern of callosal and associational striate-extrastriate connections in mice and rats is also very similar to that in hamsters (Olavarria and Montero, 1990). Consistent with findings in carnivores and primates, at any given eccentricity, the classical excitatory RFs of cells in all visuotopically organized extrastriate areas of the mouse tend to be larger than those of neurons in area V1 (Wang and Burkhalter, 2007). Furthermore, there is a type of receptive field size hierarchy in mouse extrastriate areas, with the mean size of RFs of area LM or V2 neurons being smallest, about 30°, and that of area A being largest, at around 60° (Wang and Burkhalter, 2007). Interestingly, as in V1, the RF sizes of neurons located in a given putative extrastriate visual area do not increase with eccentricity (Wang and Burkhalter, 2007). The paucity of detailed information concerning the RF properties (other than size) of these putative extrastriate visual cortical areas, however, prevents us from speculating about the possible homologues of these areas in carnivores and primates.

REFERENCES

Abdeljalil, J., Hamid, M., Abdel-mouttalib, O., Stéphane, R., Raymond, R., Johan, A., Jose, S., Pierre, C., and Serge, P. (2005). The optomotor response: A robust first-line visual screening method for mice. *Vision Res.* 45(11):1439–1446.

Abrahamson, E. E., and Moore, R. Y. (2001). Suprachiasmatic nucleus in the mouse: Retinal innervation, intrinsic organization and efferent projections. *Brain Res.* 916(1–2):172–191.

Andrews, B. W., and Pollen, D. A. (1979). Relationship between spatial frequency selectivity and receptive field profile of simple cells. *J. Physiol. (Lond.)* 287(1):163–176.

Antonini, A., Fagiolini, M., and Stryker, M. P. (1999). Anatomical correlates of functional plasticity in mouse visual cortex. *J. Neurosci.* 19(11):4388–4406.

Arnason, U., Adegoke, J. A., Bodin, K., Born, E. W., Esa, Y. B., Gullberg, A., Nilsson, M., Short, R. V., Xu, X. F., and Janke, A. (2002). Mammalian mitogenomic relationships and the root of the eutherian tree. *Proc. Natl. Acad. Sci. U.S.A.* 99(12): 8151–8156.

Baker, G. E., Thompson, I. D., Krug, K., Smyth, D., and Tolhurst, D. J. (1998). Spatial-frequency tuning and geniculocortical projections in the visual cortex (areas 17 and 18) of the pigmented ferret. *Eur. J. Neurosci.* 10(8):2657–2668.

Balkema, G. W., and Dräger, U. C. (1990). Origins of uncrossed retinofugal projections in normal and hypopigmented mice. *Vis. Neurosci.* 4(6):595–604.

Berntson, A., and Taylor, W. R. (2000). Response characteristics and receptive field widths of on-bipolar cells in the mouse retina. *J. Physiol. (Lond.)* 524(3):879–889.

Berson, D. M. (2003). Strange vision: Ganglion cells as circadian photoreceptors. *Trends Neurosci.* 26(6):314–320.

Berson, D. M., Dunn, F. A., and Takao, M. (2002). Phototransduction by retinal ganglion cells that set the circadian clock. *Science* 295(5557):1070–1073.

Blake, R., Cool, S. J., and Crawford, M. L. J. (1974). Visual resolution in the cat. *Vision Res.* 14(11):1211–1217.

Boycott, B., and Wässle, H. (1974). The morphological types of ganglion cells of the domestic cat's retina. *J. Physiol. (Lond.)* 240(2):397–419.

Boycott, B., and Wässle, H. (1999). Parallel processing in the mammalian retina: The Proctor Lecture. *Invest. Ophthalmol. Vis. Sci.* 40(7):1313–1327.

Boyes, W. K., and Dyer, R. S. (1983). Pattern reversal visual evoked potentials in awake rats. *Brain Res. Bull.* 10(6):817–823.

Burke, W., Dreher, B., Michalski, A., Cleland, B. G., and Rowe, M. H. (1992). Effects of selective pressure block of Y-type optic nerve fibers on the receptive field properties of neurons in the striate cortex of the cat. *Vis. Neurosci.* 9(1):47–64.

Burke, W., Dreher, B., and Wang (1998). Selective block of conduction in Y optic nerve fibres: Significance for the concept of parallel processing. *Eur. J. Neurosci.* 10(1):8–19.

Burne, R. A., Parnavelas, J. G., and Lin, C. S. (1984). Response properties of neurons in the visual cortex of the rat. *Exp. Brain Res.* 53(2):374–383.

Calderone, J. B., and Jacobs, G. H. (1995). Regional variations in the relative sensitivity to UV light in the mouse retina. *Vis. Neurosci.* 12(3):463–468.

Cappe, C., and Barone, P. (2005). Heteromodal connections supporting multisensory integration at low levels of cortical processing in the monkey. *Eur. J. Neurosci.* 22(11):2886–2902.

Carcieri, S. M., Jacobs, A. L., and Nirenberg, S. (2003). Classification of retinal ganglion cells: A statistical approach. *J. Neurophysiol.* 90(3):1704–1713.

Carter-Dawson, L. D., and LaVail, M. M. (1979). Rods and cones in the mouse retina. I. Structural analysis using light and electron microscopy. *J. Comp. Neurol.* 188(2):245–262.

Casagrande, V. A., and Kaas, J. H. (1994). The afferent, intrinsic, and efferent connections of primary visual cortex in primates. In A. Peters and K. S. Rockland (Eds.), *Primary visual cortex in primates*, Vol. 10 (pp. 201–259). New York: Plenum Press.

Casagrande, V. A., and Norton, T. T. (1991). Lateral geniculate nucleus: A review of physiology and function. In A. G. Leventhal (Ed.), *The neural basis of visual function*, Vol. 4 (pp. 41–84). Basingstoke, Hampshire, UK: Macmillan.

Cassone, V. M., Speh, J. C., Card, J. P., and Moore, R. Y. (1988). Comparative anatomy of the mammalian hypothalamic suprachiasmatic nucleus. *J. Biol. Rhythms* 3(1):71–91.

Caviness, V. S. (1975). Architectonic map of neocortex of normal mouse. *J. Comp. Neurol.* 164(2):247–263.

Caviness, V. S., and Frost, D. O. (1980). Tangential organization of thalamic projections to the neocortex in the mouse. *J. Comp. Neurol.* 194(2):335–367.

Chalupa, L. M. (2006). Developing dendrites demonstrate unexpected specificity. *Neuron* 52(4):567–568.

Chalupa, L. M., and Lia, B. (1991). The nasotemporal division of retinal ganglion cells with crossed and uncrossed projections in the fetal rhesus monkey. *J. Neurosci.* 11(1):191–202.

Chalupa, L. M., and Thompson, I. (1980). Retinal ganglion cell projections to the superior colliculus of the hamster demonstrated by the horseradish peroxidase technique. *Neurosci. Lett.* 19(1):13–19.

Chapman, B., Zahs, K. R., and Stryker, M. P. (1991). Relation of cortical cell orientation selectivity to alignment of receptive-fields of the geniculocortical afferents that arborize within a single orientation column in ferret visual cortex. *J. Neurosci.* 11(5):1347–1358.

Chen, G., Dan, Y., and Li, C.-Y. (2005). Stimulation of non-classical receptive field enhances orientation selectivity in the cat. *J. Physiol. (Lond.)* 564(1):233–243.

Chow, K. L., Masland, R. H., and Stewart, D. L. (1971). Receptive field characteristics of striate cortical neurons in rabbit. *Brain Res.* 33(2):337–352.

Clarke, P. G., Donaldson, I. M., and Whitteridge, D. (1976). Binocular visual mechanisms in cortical areas I and II of the sheep. *J Physiol. (Lond.)* 256(3):509–526.

Conley, M., Fitzpatrick, D., and Diamond, I. T. (1984). The laminar organization of the lateral geniculate-body and the striate cortex in the tree shrew (*Tupaia glis*). *J. Neurosci.* 4(1): 171–197.

Coombs, J., van der List, D., Wang, G. Y., and Chalupa, L. M. (2006). Morphological properties of mouse retinal ganglion cells. *Neuroscience* 140(1):123–136.

Cooper, H. M., and Magnin, M. (1986). A common mammalian plan of accessory optic system organization revealed in all primates. *Nature* 324 (6096):457–459.

Cooper, M. L., and Pettigrew, J. D. (1979). The decussation of the retinothalamic pathway in the cat, with a note on the major meridians of the cat's eye. *J. Comp. Neurol.* 187(2):285–311.

Crewther, D. P., Crewther, S. G., and Sanderson, K. J. (1984). Primary visual cortex in the brushtailed possum: Receptive field properties and corticocortical connections. *Brain Behav. Evol.* 24(4):184–97.

Cusick, C. G., and Lund, R. D. (1981). The distribution of the callosal projection to the occipital visual-cortex in rats and mice. *Brain Res.* 214(2):239–259.

Dacey, D. M., Liao, H. W., Peterson, B. B., Robinson, F. R., Smith, V. C., Pokorny, J., Yau, K. W., and Gamlin, P. D. (2005). Melanopsin-expressing ganglion cells in primate retina signal colour and irradiance and project to the LGN. *Nature* 433(7027):749–754.

Dacey, D. M., and Packer, O. S. (2003). Colour coding in the primate retina: Diverse cell types and cone-specific circuitry. *Curr. Opin. Neurobiol.* 13(4):421–427.

Dean, P. (1978). Visual acuity in hooded rats: Effects of superior collicular or posterior neocortical lesions. *Brain Res.* 156(1): 17–31.

De Valois, R. L., Morgan, H., and Snodderly, D. M. (1974). Psychophysical studies of monkey vision. III. Spatial luminance contrast sensitivity tests of macaque and human observers. *Vision Res.* 14(1):75–81.

De Valois, R. L., Yund, E. W., and Hepler, N. (1982). The orientation and direction selectivity of cells in macaque visual-cortex. *Vision Res.* 22(5):531–544.

Distler, C., and Hoffmann, K. P. (1989). The pupillary light reflex in normal and innate microstrabismic cats. I. Behavior and receptive field analysis in the nucleus praetectalis olivaris. *Vis. Neurosci.* 3(2):127–138.

Doi, M., Uji, Y., and Yamamura, H. (1995). Morphological classification of retinal ganglion cells in mice. *J. Comp. Neurol.* 356(3):368–386.

Dräger, U. C. (1974). Autoradiography of tritiated proline and fucose transported transneuronally from eye to visual-cortex in pigmented and albino mice. *Brain Res.* 82(2):284–292.

Dräger, U. (1975). Receptive fields of single cells and topography in mouse visual cortex. *J. Comp. Neurol.* 160(3): 269–290.

Dräger, U. C. (1978). Observations on monocular deprivation in mice. *J. Neurophysiol.* 41(1):28–42.

Dräger, U. C. (1981). Observations on the organization of the visual cortex in the reeler mouse. *J. Comp. Neurol.* 201(4):555–570.

Dräger, U. C., and Hubel, D. H. (1975a). Physiology of visual cells in mouse superior colliculus and correlation with somatosensory and auditory input. *Nature* 253(5488):203–204.

Dräger, U. C., and Hubel, D. H. (1975b). Responses to visual stimulation and relationship between visual, auditory, and somatosensory inputs in mouse superior colliculus. *J. Neurophysiol.* 38(3):690–713.

Dräger, U. C., and Hubel, D. H. (1976). Topography of visual and somatosensory projections to mouse superior colliculus. *J. Neurophysiol.* 39(1):91–101.

Dräger, U. C., and Olsen, J. (1980). Origins of crossed and uncrossed retinal projections in pigmented and albino mice. *J. Comp. Neurol.* 191(3):383–412.

Dräger, U., and Olsen, J. (1981). Ganglion cell distribution in the retina of the mouse. *Invest. Ophthalmol. Vis. Sci.* 20(3):285–293.

Dreher, B., Michalski, A., Cleland, B. G., and Burke, W. (1992). Effects of selective pressure block of Y-type optic nerve fibers on the receptive field properties of neurons in area 18 of the visual cortex of the cat. *Vis. Neurosci.* 9(1):65–78.

Dreher, B., Sefton, A. J., Ni, S. Y. K., and Nisbett, G. (1985). The morphology, number, distribution and central projections of class I retinal ganglion cells in albino and hooded rats. *Brain Behav. Evol.* 26(1):10–48.

Dreher, Z., Robinson, S. R., and Distler, C. (1992). Müller cells in vascular and avascular retinae: A survey of seven mammals. *J. Comp. Neurol.* 323(1):59–80.

Duke-Elder, S. (1953). The eye in evolution. In *System of ophthalmology*, Vol. 1. London: Kimpton.

Ekesten, B., and Gouras, P. (2001). Identifying UV-cone responses in the murine superior colliculus. *Vision Res.* 41(22):2819–2825.

Ekesten, B., and Gouras, P. (2005). Cone and rod inputs to murine retinal ganglion cells: evidence of cone opsin specific channels. *Vis. Neurosci.* 22(6):893–903.

Ekesten, B., Gouras, P., and Yamamoto, S. (2000). Cone inputs to murine retinal ganglion cells. *Vision Res.* 40(19):2573–2577.

Enroth-Cugell, C., and Robson, J. (1966). The contrast sensitivity of retinal ganglion cells of the cat. *J. Physiol. (Lond.)* 18(2): 517–552.

Eysel, U. T. (2002). Pharmacological studies on receptive field architecture. In B. R. Payne and A. Peters (Eds.), *The cat primary visual cortex* (pp. 427–470). San Diego: Academic Press.

Fagiolini, M., Pizzorusso, T., Berardi, N., Domenici, L., and Maffei, L. (1994). Functional postnatal development of the rat primary visual cortex and the role of visual experience: Dark rearing and monocular deprivation. *Vision Res.* 34(6):709–720.

Fan, J., Woodruff, M. L., Cilluffo, M. C., Crouch, R. K., and Fain, G. L. (2005). Opsin activation of transduction in the rods of dark-reared Rpe65 knockout mice. *J. Physiol. (Lond.)* 568(1):83–95.

Finlay, B. L., Schiller, P. H., and Volman, S. F. (1976). Quantitative studies of single-cell properties in monkey striate cortex. IV. Corticotectal cells. *J. Neurophysiol.* 39(6):1352–1361.

FitzGibbon, T., and Burke, W. (1989). Representation of the temporal raphe within the optic tract of the cat. *Vis. Neurosci.* 2(3):255–267.

Forte, J. D., Hashemi-Nezhad, M., Dobbie, W. J., Dreher, B., and Martin, P. R. (2005). Spatial coding and response redundancy in parallel visual pathways of the marmoset *Callithrix jacchus*. *Vis. Neurosci.* 22(4):479–491.

Fries, W., Keizer, K., and Kuypers, H. G. (1985). Large layer VI cells in macaque striate cortex (Meynert cells) project to both superior colliculus and prestriate visual area V5. *Exp. Brain Res.* 58(3):613–616.

Frost, D. O., and Caviness, V. S. (1980). Radial organization of thalamic projections to the neocortex in the mouse. *J. Comp. Neurol.* 194(2):369–393.

Fukuda, Y., Sawai, H., Watanabe, M., Wakakuwa, K., and Morigiwa, K. (1989). Nasotemporal overlap of crossed and uncrossed retinal ganglion cell projections in the Japanese monkey (*Macaca fuscata*). *J. Neurosci.* 9(7):2353–2373.

Fyk-Kolodziej, B., Qin, P., and Pourcho, R. G. (2003). Identification of a cone bipolar cell in cat retina which has input from both rod and cone photoreceptors. *J. Comp. Neurol.* 464(1): 104–113.

Gamlin, P. D., Zhang, H., and Clarke, R. J. (1995). Luminance neurons in the pretectal olivary nucleus mediate the pupillary light reflex in the rhesus monkey. *Exp. Brain Res.* 106(1): 169–176.

Gandhi, N. J., and Sparks, D. L. (2003). Changing views of the role of the superior colliculus in the control of gaze. In L. M. Chalupa, and J. S. Werner (Eds.), *The visual neurosciences*, Vol. 2 (pp. 1449–465). Cambridge, MA: MIT Press.

Garey, L. J., Dreher, B., and Robinson, S. R. (1991). The organization of the visual thalamus. In B. Dreher, and S. R. Robinson (Eds.), *Neuroanatomy of the visual pathways and their development*, Vol. 3 (pp. 176–234). Basingstoke, Hampshire, UK: Macmillan.

Ghosh, K. K., Bujan, S., Haverkamp, S., Feigenspan, A., and Wässle, H. (2004). Types of bipolar cells in the mouse retina. *J. Comp. Neurol.* 469(1):70–82.

Ghosh, K. K., Martin, P. R., and Grünert, U. (1997). Morphological analysis of the blue cone pathway in the retina of a New World monkey, the marmoset *Callithrix jacchus*. *J. Comp. Neurol.* 379(2):211–225.

Gianfranceschi, L., Fiorentini, A., and Maffei, L. (1999). Behavioural visual acuity of wild type and bcl2 transgenic mouse. *Vision Res.* 39(3):569–574.

Gilbert, C. D. (1977). Laminar differences in receptive field properties of cells in cat primary visual cortex. *J. Physiol.* (*Lond.*) 268(2):391–421.

Girman, S. V., and Lund, R. D. (2007). Most superficial sublamina of rat superior colliculus: Neuronal response properties and correlates with perceptual figure-ground segregation. *J Neurophysiol.* 98(1):161–177.

Girman, S. V., Sauvé, Y., and Lund, R. D. (1999). Receptive field properties of single neurons in rat primary visual cortex. *J. Neurophysiol.* 82(1):301–311.

Godement, P., Salaun, J., and Imbert, M. (1984). Prenatal and postnatal development of retinogeniculate and retinocollicular projections in the mouse. *J. Comp. Neurol.* 230(4):552–575.

Gooley, J. J., Lu, J., Fischer, D., and Saper, C. B. (2003). A broad role for melanopsin in nonvisual photoreception. *J. Neurosci.* 23(18):7093–106.

Gordon, J. A., and Stryker, M. P. (1996). Experience-dependent plasticity of binocular responses in the primary visual cortex of the mouse. *J. Neurosci.* 16(10):3274–3286.

Grasse, K., and Cynader, M. (1991). The accessory optic system in frontal eyed animals. In A. G. Leventhal (Ed.), *The neural basis of visual function*, Vol. 4 (pp. 111–139). Basingstoke, Hampshire, U.K.: Macmillan.

Grubb, M. S., and Thompson, I. D. (2003). Quantitative characterization of visual response properties in the mouse dorsal lateral geniculate nucleus. *J Neurophysiol.* 90(6):3594–3607.

Grubb, M. S., and Thompson, I. D. (2004). Biochemical and anatomical subdivision of the dorsal lateral geniculate nucleus in normal mice and in mice lacking the beta 2 subunit of the nicotinic acetylcholine receptor. *Vision Res.* 44(28):3365–3376.

Hack, I., Frech, M., Dick, O., Peichl, L., and Brandstätter, J. H. (2001). Heterogeneous distribution of AMPA glutamate receptor subunits at the photoreceptor synapses of rodent retina. *Eur. J. Neurosci.* 13(1):15–24.

Hack, I., Peichl, L., and Brandstätter, J. H. (1999). An alternative pathway for rod signals in the rodent retina: Rod photoreceptors, cone bipolar cells, and the localization of glutamate receptors. *Proc. Natl Acad. Sci. U.S.A.* 96(24):14130–14135.

Hallett, P. E. (1987). The scale of the visual pathways of mouse and rat. *Biol. Cybern.* 57(4–5):275–286.

Hammond, P., and Andrews, D. P. (1978). Orientation tuning of cells in areas 17 and 18 of the cat's visual cortex. *Exp. Brain Res.* 31(3):341–351.

Hannibal, J., and Fahrenkrug, J. (2004). Target areas innervated by PACAP-immunoreactive retinal ganglion cells. *Cell Tissue Res.* 316(1):99–113.

Hashemi-Nezhad, M., Wang, C., Burke, W., and Dreher, B. (2003). Area 21a of cat visual cortex strongly modulates neuronal activities in the superior colliculus. *J. Physiol.* (*Lond.*) 550(2): 535–552.

Hattar, S., Kumar, M., Park, A., Tong, P., Tung, J., Yau, K. W., and Berson, D. M. (2006). Central projections of melanopsin-expressing retinal ganglion cells in the mouse. *J. Comp. Neurol.* 497(3):326–349.

Hattar, S., Liao, H. W., Takao, M., Berson, D. M., and Yau, K. W. (2002). Melanopsin-containing retinal ganglion cells: Architecture, projections, and intrinsic photosensitivity. *Science* 295(5557):1065–1070.

Hattar, S., Lucas, R. J., Mrosovsky, N., Thompson, S., Douglas, R. H., Hankins, M. W., Lem, J., Biel, M., Hofmann, F., et al. (2003). Melanopsin and rod-cone photoreceptive systems account for all major accessory visual functions in mice. *Nature* 424(6944):75–81.

Haverkamp, S. and Wässle, H. (2000). Immunocytochemical analysis of the mouse retina. *J. Comp. Neurol.* 424(1):1–23.

Haverkamp, S., Wässle, H., Duebel, J., Kuner, T., Augustine, G. J., Feng, G., and Euler, T. (2005). The primordial, blue-cone color system of the mouse retina. *J. Neurosci.* 25(22):5438–5445.

Heimel, J. A., Hartman, R. J., Hermans, J. M. and Levelt, C. N. (2007). Screening mouse vision with intrinsic signal optical imaging. *Eur. J. Neurosci.* 25(3):795–804.

Henry, G. H. (1977). Receptive field classes of cells in the striate cortex of the cat. *Brain Res.* 133(1):1–28.

Henry, G. H., Bishop, P. O., and Dreher, B. (1974a). Orientation, axis and direction as stimulus parameters for striate cells. *Vision Res.* 14(9):767–777.

Henry, G. H., Dreher, B., and Bishop, P. O. (1974b). Orientation specificity of cells in cat striate cortex. *J. Neurophysiol.* 37(6): 1394–409.

Henry, G. H., Michalski, A., Wimborne, B. M., and McCart, R. J. (1994). The nature and origin of orientation specificity in neurons of the visual pathways. *Prog. Neurobiol.* 43(4–5):381–437.

Hensch, T. K., Fagiolini, M., Mataga, N., Stryker, M. P., Baekkeskov, S., and Kash, S. F. (1998). Local GABA circuit control of experience-dependent plasticity in developing visual cortex. *Science* 282(5393):1504–1508.

Hochstein, S., and Shapley, R. M. (1976). Quantitative analysis of retinal ganglion cell classifications. *J. Physiol.* (*Lond.*) 262 (2):237–264.

Hofbauer, A., and Dräger, U. C. (1985). Depth segregation of retinal ganglion cells projecting to mouse superior colliculus. *J. Comp. Neurol.* 234(4):465–474.

Holdefer, R. N., and Norton, T. T. (1995). Laminar organization of receptive field properties in the dorsal lateral geniculate nucleus of the tree shrew (*Tupaia glis belangeri*). *J. Comp. Neurol.* 358(3):401–413.

Holländer, H., and Hälbig, W. (1980). Topography of retinal representation in the rabbit cortex: an experimental study using transneuronal and retrograde tracing techniques. *J. Comp. Neurol.* 193(3):701–710.

Hubel, D. H. (1975). An autoradiographic study of the retinocortical projections in the tree shrew (*Tupaia glis*). *Brain Res.* 96(1):41–50.

Hubel, D. H., and Wiesel, T. N. (1962). Receptive fields, binocular interaction and functional architecture in the cat's visual cortex. *J. Physiol.* (*Lond.*) 160(1):106–154.

Hubel, D. H., and Wiesel, T. N. (1968). Receptive fields and functional architecture of monkey striate cortex. *J. Physiol.* (*Lond.*) 195(1):215–243.

Hubel, D. H., and Wiesel, T. N. (1974). Uniformity of monkey striate cortex: a parallel relationship between field size, scatter, and magnification factor. *J. Comp. Neurol.* 158(3):295–305.

Hubel, D. H., and Wiesel, T. N. (1977). Ferrier Lecture. Functional architecture of macaque monkey visual cortex. *Proc. R. Soc. Lond. B Biol. Sci.* 198(1130):1–59.

Hubel, D. H., Wiesel, T. N., and Stryker, M. P. (1978). Anatomical demonstration of orientation columns in macaque monkey. *J. Comp. Neurol.* 177(3):361–380.

Hübener, M., and Bonhoeffer, T. (2002). Optical imaging of functional architecture in cat primary visual cortex. In B. R. Payne and A. Peters (Eds.), *The cat primary visual cortex* (pp. 131–165). San Diego: Academic Press.

Hughes, A. (1971). Topographical relationships between the anatomy and physiology of the rabbit visual system. *Doc. Ophthalmol.* 30:33–159.

Hughes, A. (1981). Cat retina and the sampling theorem; the relation of transient and sustained brisk unit cut-off frequency to alpha and beta mode cell density. *Exp. Brain Res.* 42(2): 196–202.

Hughes, A. (1986). The schematic eye comes of age. In J. D. Pettigrew, K. J. Sanderson, and W. R. Levick (Eds.), *Visual neuroscience* (pp. 60–89). Cambridge: Cambridge University Press.

Hughes, A., and Vaney, D. I. (1982). The organization of binocular cortex in the primary visual area of the rabbit. *J. Comp. Neurol.* 204(2):151–164.

Humphrey, A. L., Albano, J. E., and Norton, T. T. (1977). Organization of ocular dominance in tree shrew striate cortex. *Brain Res.* 134(2):225–236.

Ibbotson, M. R., and Dreher, B. (2005). Visual functions of the retinorecipient nuclei in the midbrain, pretectum, and ventral thalamus of primates. In J. Kremers (Ed.), *The primate visual system: A comparative approach* (pp. 213–265). West Sussex, U.K.: John Wiley and Sons.

Ibbotson, M. R., and Mark, R. F. (2003). Orientation and spatiotemporal tuning of cells in the primary visual cortex of an Australian marsupial, the wallaby *Macropus eugenii*. *J. Comp. Physiol. A Neuroethol. Sens. Neural Behav. Physiol.* 189(2):115–123.

Illing, R. B., and Wässle, H. (1981). The retinal projection to the thalamus in the cat: A quantitative investigation and a comparison with the retinotectal pathway. *J. Comp. Neurol.* 202(2): 265–285.

Jacobson, S. G., Franklin, K. B. J., and McDonald, W. I. (1976). Visual acuity of the cat. *Vision Res.* 16(10):1141–1143.

Jeffery, G. (1984). Retinal ganglion cell death and terminal field retraction in the developing rodent visual system. *Dev. Brain Res.* 13:81–96.

Jeon, C. J., Strettoi, E., and Masland, R. H. (1998). The major cell populations of the mouse retina. *J. Neurosci.* 18(21): 8936–8946.

Kaas, J. H., Guillery, R. W., and Allman, J. M. (1972). Some principles of organization in the dorsal lateral geniculate nucleus. *Brain Behav. Evol.* 6(1):253–299.

Kalatsky, V. A., and Stryker, M. P. (2003). New paradigm for optical imaging: temporally encoded maps of intrinsic signal. *Neuron* 38(4):529–545.

Kolb, H. (1977). The organization of the outer plexiform layer in the retina of the cat: Electron microscopic observations. *J. Neurocytol.* 6(2):131–153.

Kong, J., Fish, D. R., Rockhill, R. L., and Masland, R. H. (2005). Diversity of ganglion cells in the mouse retina: Unsupervised morphological classification and its limits. *J. Comp. Neurol.* 489(3):293–310.

Kouyama, N., and Marshak, D. (1992). Bipolar cells specific for blue cones in the macaque retina. *J. Neurosci.* 12(4):1233–1252.

Krieg, W. J. S. (1946). Connections of the cerebral cortex. I. The albino rat. B. Structure of the cortical areas. *J. Comp. Neurol.* 84(3):277–323.

Kryger, Z., Galli-Resta, L., Jacobs, G. H., and Reese, B. E. (1998). The topography of rod and cone photoreceptors in the retina of the ground squirrel. *Vis. Neurosci.* 15(4):685–891.

Kuffler, S. W. (1953). Discharge patterns and functional organization of mammalian retina. *J. Neurophysiol.* 16(1):37–68.

Kulikowski, J. J. (1978). Pattern and movement detection in man and rabbit: Separation and comparison of occipital potentials. *Vision Res.* 18(2):183–189.

LaVail, M. M., Rapaport, D. H., and Rakic, P. (1991). Cytogenesis in the monkey retina. *J. Comp. Neurol.* 309(1):86–114.

Law, M. I., Zahs, K. R., and Stryker, M. P. (1988). Organization of primary visual cortex (area 17) in the ferret. *J. Comp. Neurol.* 278(2):157–180.

Lemmon, V., and Pearlman, A. L. (1981). Does laminar position determine the receptive field properties of cortical neurons? A study of corticotectal cells in area 17 of the normal mouse and the reeler mutant. *J. Neurosci.* 1(1):83–93.

LeVay, S., Hubel, D. H., and Wiesel, T. N. (1975). The pattern of ocular dominance columns in macaque visual cortex revealed by a reduced silver stain. *J. Comp. Neurol.* 159(4):559–576.

LeVay, S., McConnell, S. K., and Luskin, M. B. (1987). Functional organization of primary visual cortex in the mink (*Mustela vison*), and a comparison with the cat. *J. Comp. Neurol.* 257(3): 422–441.

LeVay, S. and Nelson, S. B. (1991). Columnar organization of the visual cortex. In A. G. Leventhal (Ed.), *The neural basis of visual function*, Vol. 4 (pp. 266–315). Basingstoke, Hampshire, U.K.: Macmillan Press.

LeVay, S., Stryker, M. P., and Shatz, C. J. (1978). Ocular dominance columns and their development in layer IV of the cat's visual cortex: A quantitative study. *J. Comp. Neurol.* 179(1): 223–244.

LeVay, S., Wiesel, T. N., and Hubel, D. H. (1980). The development of ocular dominance columns in normal and visually deprived monkeys. *J. Comp. Neurol.* 191(1):1–51.

Leventhal, A. G. (1982). Morphology and distribution of retinal ganglion cells projecting to different layers of the dorsal lateral geniculate nucleus in normal and Siamese cats. *J. Neurosci.* 2(8):1024–1042.

Leventhal, A. G., Ault, S. J., and Vitek, D. J. (1988). The nasotemporal division in primate retina: the neural bases of macular sparing and splitting. *Science* 240(4848):66–67.

Leventhal, A. G., Rodieck, R. W., and Dreher, B. (1981). Retinal ganglion cell classes in the Old World monkey: morphology and central projections. *Science* 213(4512):1139–1142.

Leventhal, A. G., Thompson, K. G., Liu, D., Zhou, Y., and Ault, S. J. (1995). Concomitant sensitivity to orientation, direction, and color of cells in layers 2, 3, and 4 of monkey striate cortex. *J. Neurosci.* 15(3):1808–1818.

Lia, B., and Olavarria, J. F. (1996). The distribution of corticotectal projection neurons correlates with the interblob compartment in macaque striate cortex. *Vis. Neurosci.* 13(3):461–466.

Linden, R., and Perry, V. H. (1983). Massive retinotectal projection in rats. *Brain Res.* 272(1):145–149.

Livingstone, M. S., and Hubel, D. H. (1984). Anatomy and physiology of a color system in the primate visual cortex. *J. Neurosci.* 4(1):309–356.

Löwel, S. (2002). 2-Deoxyglucose architecture of primary visual cortex. In B. R. Payne and A. Peters (Eds.), *The cat primary visual cortex* (pp. 167–193). San Diego: Academic Press.

Lucas, R. J., Hattar, S., Takao, M., Berson, D. M., Foster, R. G. and Yau, K. W. (2003). Diminished pupillary light reflex at high irradiances in melanopsin-knockout mice. *Science* 299(5604):245–247.

Manger, P. R., Kiper, D., Masiello, I., Murillo, L., Tettoni, L., Hunyadi, Z., and Innocenti, G. M. (2002a). The representation of the visual field in three extrastriate areas of the ferret (*Mustela putorius*) and the relationship of retinotopy and field boundaries to callosal connectivity. *Cereb. Cortex* 12(4):423–437.

Manger, P. R., Masiello, I., and Innocenti, G. M. (2002b). Areal organization of the posterior parietal cortex of the ferret (*Mustela putorius*). *Cereb. Cortex* 12(12):1280–1297.

Manger, P. R., Nakamura, H., Valentiniene, S., and Innocenti, G. M. (2004). Visual areas in the lateral temporal cortex of the ferret (*Mustela putorius*). *Cereb. Cortex* 14(6):676–689.

Mangini, N. J., and Pearlman, A. L. (1980). Laminar distribution of receptive field properties in the primary visual cortex of the mouse. *J. Comp. Neurol.* 193(1):203–222.

Mariani, A. P. (1984). Bipolar cells in monkey retina selective for the cones likely to be blue-sensitive. *Nature* 308(5955):184–186.

Mastronarde, D. N. (1984). Organization of the cat's optic tract as assessed by single-axon recordings. *J. Comp. Neurol.* 227(1):14–22.

Masu, M., Iwakabe, H., Tagawa, Y., Miyoshi, T., Yamashita, M., Fukuda, Y., Sasaki, H., Hiroi, K., Nakamura, Y., et al. (1995). Specific deficit of the ON response in visual transmission by targeted disruption of the mGluR6 gene. *Cell* 80(5):757–765.

Maunsell, J. H., and Newsome, W. T. (1987). Visual processing in monkey extrastriate cortex. *Annu. Rev. Neurosci.* 10:363–401.

McCall, M. J., Robinson, S. R., and Dreher, B. (1987). Differential retinal growth appears to be the primary factor producing the ganglion cell density gradient in the rat. *Neurosci. Lett.* 79(1–2):78–84.

McConnell, S. K., and LeVay, S. (1986). Anatomical organization of the visual system of the mink, *Mustela vison*. *J. Comp. Neurol.* 250(1):109–132.

Métin, C., Godement, P., and Imbert, M. (1988). The primary visual cortex in the mouse: Receptive field properties and functional organization. *Exp. Brain Res.* 69(3):594–612.

Métin, C., Irons, W. A., and Frost, D. O. (1995). Retinal ganglion cells in normal hamsters and hamsters with novel retinal projections. I. Number, distribution, and size. *J. Comp. Neurol.* 353(2):179–199.

Mitchell, D. E., Giffin, F. and Timney, B. (1977). A behavioural technique for the rapid assessment of the visual capabilities of kittens. *Perception* 6(2):181–193.

Mooser, F., Bosking, W. H., and Fitzpatrick, D. (2004). A morphological basis for orientation tuning in primary visual cortex. *Nat. Neurosci.* 7(8):872–879.

Morgan, J. E., Henderson, Z., and Thompson, I. D. (1987). Retinal decussation patterns in pigmented and albino ferrets. *Neuroscience* 20(2):519–535.

Murphy, E. H., and Berman, N. (1979). The rabbit and the cat: A comparison of some features of response properties of single cells in the primary visual cortex. *J. Comp. Neurol.* 188(3):401–427.

Nelson, R. (1977). Cat cones have rod input: A comparison of the response properties of cones and horizontal cell bodies in the retina of the cat. *J. Comp. Neurol.* 172(1):109–135.

Nikonov, S. S., Kholodenko, R., Lem, J., and Pugh, E. N., Jr. (2006). Physiological features of the S- and M-cone photoreceptors of wild type mice from single cell recordings. *J. Gen. Physiol.* 127(4):359–374.

O'Brien, B. J., Isayama, T., Richardson, R., and Berson, D. M. (2002). Intrinsic physiological properties of cat retinal ganglion cells. *J. Physiol.* (*Lond.*) 538(3):787–802.

Ohki, K., Chung, S., Kara, P., Hubener, M., Bonhoeffer, T., and Reid, R. C. (2006). Highly ordered arrangement of single neurons in orientation pinwheels. *Nature* 442(7105):925–928.

Olavarria, J., Mignano, L. R., and Van Sluyters, R. C. (1982). Pattern of extrastriate visual areas connecting reciprocally with striate cortex in the mouse. *Exp. Neurol.* 78(3):775–779.

Olavarria, J., and Montero, V. (1989). Organization of visual cortex in the mouse revealed by correlating callosal and striate-extrastriate connections. *Vis. Neurosci.* 3(1):59–69.

Olavarria, J., and Montero, V. (1990). Elaborate organization of visual cortex in the hamster. *Neurosci. Res.* 8(1):40–47.

Olavarria, J., Serra-Oller, M. M., Yee, K. T., and Van Sluyters, R. C. (1988). Topography of interhemispheric connections in neocortex of mice with congenital deficiencies of the callosal commissure. *J. Comp. Neurol.* 270(4):575–590.

Olavarria, J., and Van Sluyters, R. C. (1984). Callosal connections of the posterior neocortex in normal-eyed, congenitally anophthalmic, and neonatally enucleated mice. *J. Comp. Neurol.* 230(2):249–268.

Østerberg, G. (1935). Topography of the layer of rods and cones in the human retina. *Acta Ophthal. Scand.* 437(suppl. 6):1–103.

Packer, O., Hendrickson, A. E., and Curcio, C. A. (1989). Photoreceptor topography of the retina in the adult pigtail macaque (*Macaca nemestrina*). *J. Comp. Neurol.* 288(1):165–183.

Pak, M. W., Giolli, R. A., Pinto, L. H., Mangini, N. J., Gregory, K. M., and Vanable, J. W., Jr. (1987). Retinopretectal and accessory optic projections of normal mice and the OKN-defective mutant mice beige, beige-J, and pearl. *J. Comp. Neurol.* 258(3):435–446.

Palmer, L. A., and Rosenquist, A. C. (1974). Visual receptive fields of single striate cortical units projecting to superior colliculus in cat. *Brain Res.* 67(1):27–42.

Panda, S., Provencio, I., Tu, D. C., Pires, S. S., Rollag, M. D., Castrucci, A. M., Pletcher, M. T., Sato, T. K., Wiltshire, T., et al. (2003). Melanopsin is required for non-image-forming photic responses in blind mice. *Science* 301(5632):525–257.

Pang, J. J., Gao, F., and Wu, S. M. (2003). Light-evoked excitatory and inhibitory synaptic inputs to ON and OFF alpha ganglion cells in the mouse retina. *J. Neurosci.* 23(14):6063–6073.

Pang, J. J., Gao, F., and Wu, S. M. (2004). Light-evoked current responses in rod bipolar cells, cone depolarizing bipolar cells and AII amacrine cells in dark-adapted mouse retina. *J. Physiol.* (*Lond.*) 558(3):897–912.

Paxinos, G., and Franklin, K. B. J. (2004). *The mouse brain in stereotaxic coordinates.* Oxford: Academic Press.

Payne, B. R. (1990). Representation of the ipsilateral visual field in the transition zone between areas 17 and 18 of the cat's cerebral cortex. *Vis. Neurosci.* 4(5):445–474.

Payne, B. R. (1993). Evidence for visual cortical area homologs in cat and macaque monkey. *Cereb. Cortex* 3(1):1–25.

Payne, B. R., and Berman, N. (1983). Functional organization of neurons in cat striate cortex: variations in preferred orientation and orientation selectivity with receptive-field type, ocular dominance, and location in visual field map. *J. Neurophysiol.* 49(4):1051–1072.

Payne, B. R., and Peters, A. (2002). The concept of cat primary visual cortex. In B. R. Payne and A. Peters (Eds.), *The cat primary visual cortex* (pp. 1–129). San Diego: Academic Press.

Peichl, L., Ott, H., and Boycott, B. B. (1987). Alpha ganglion cells in mammalian retinae. *Proc. R. Soc. Lond. B Biol. Sci.* 231(1263):169–197.

Peichl, L., and Wässle, H. (1979). Size, scatter and coverage of ganglion cell receptive field centres in the cat retina. *J. Physiol.* (*Lond.*) 291(1):117–141.

Perry, V. H., and Cowey, A. (1984). Retinal ganglion cells that project to the superior colliculus and pretectum in the macaque monkey. *Neuroscience* 12(4):1125–1137.

Perry, V. H., and Cowey, A. (1985). The ganglion cell and cone distributions in the monkey's retina: Implications for central magnification factors. *Vision Res.* 25(12):1795–810.

Perry, V. H., and Linden, R. (1982). Evidence for dendritic competition in the developing retina. *Nature* 297(5868):683–685.

Perry, V. H., Oehler, R., and Cowey, A. (1984). Retinal ganglion cells that project to the dorsal lateral geniculate nucleus in the macaque monkey. *Neuroscience* 12(4):1101–1123.

Pettigrew, J. D. (1986). Flying primates? Megabats have the advanced pathway from eye to midbrain. *Science* 231(4743): 1304–1306.

Pettigrew, J. D., Dreher, B., Hopkins, C. S., McCall, M. J., and Brown, M. (1988). Peak density and distribution of ganglion cells in the retinae of microchiropteran bats: Implications for visual acuity. *Brain Behav. Evol.* 32(1):39–56.

Pettigrew, J. D., Ramachandran, V. S., and Bravo, H. (1984). Some neural connections subserving binocular vision in ungulates. *Brain Behav. Evol.* 24(2–3):65–93.

Porciatti, V., Pizzorusso, T., and Maffei, L. (1999). The visual physiology of the wild type mouse determined with pattern VEPs. *Vision Res.* 39(18):3071–3081.

Prévost, F., Lepore, F., and Guillemot, J-P. (2007). Spatio-temporal receptive field properties of cells in the rat superior colliculus. *Brain Res.* 1142:80–91.

Protti, D. A., Flores-Herr, N., Li, W., Massey, S. C., and Wässle, H. (2005). Light signaling in scotopic conditions in the rabbit, mouse and rat retina: A physiological and anatomical study. *J. Neurophysiol.* 93(6):3479–3488.

Provencio, I., Cooper, H. M., and Foster, R. G. (1998). Retinal projections in mice with inherited retinal degeneration: Implications for circadian photoentrainment. *J. Comp. Neurol.* 395(4): 417–439.

Provis, J. M., Diaz, C. M., and Dreher, B. (1998). Ontogeny of the primate fovea: A central issue in retinal development. *Prog. Neurobiol.* 54(5):549–580.

Prusky, G. T., West, P. W., and Douglas, R. M. (2000). Behavioral assessment of visual acuity in mice and rats. *Vision Res.* 40(16):2201–2209.

Pu, M. (1999). Dendritic morphology of cat retinal ganglion cells projecting to suprachiasmatic nucleus. *J. Comp. Neurol.* 414(2):267–274.

Quina, L. A., Pak, W., Lanier, J., Banwait, P., Gratwick, K., Liu, Y., Velasquez, T., O'Leary, D. D., Goulding, M., and Turner, E. E. (2005). Brn3a-expressing retinal ganglion cells project specifically to thalamocortical and collicular visual pathways. *J. Neurosci.* 25(50):11595–11604.

Ramón y Cajal, S. (1972). *The structure of the retina.* Springfield, IL: Charles C. Thomas.

Rao, S. C., Toth, L. J., and Sur, M. (1997). Optically imaged maps of orientation preference in primary visual cortex of cats and ferrets. *J. Comp. Neurol.* 387(3):358–370.

Rapaport, D. H., Wong, L. L., Wood, E. D., Yasumura, D., and LaVail, M. M. (2004). Timing and topography of cell genesis in the rat retina. *J. Comp. Neurol.* 474(2):304–324.

Raviola, E., and Gilula, N. B. (1973). Gap junctions between photoreceptor cells in the vertebrate retina. *Proc. Natl. Acad. Sci. U.S.A.* 70(6):1677–1681.

Remtulla, S., and Hallett, P. E. (1985). A schematic eye for the mouse, and comparisons with the rat. *Vision Res.* 25(1):21–31.

Reymond, L., and Cook, M. (1984). Relation between simultaneous spatial-discrimination thresholds and luminance in man. *Behav. Brain Res.* 14(1):51–59.

Rhoades, R. W., Mooney, R. D., and Fish, S. E. (1991). Retinotopic and visuotopic representations in the mammalian superior colliculus. In B. Dreher and S. R. Robinson (Eds.), *Neuroanatomy of the visual pathways and their development*, Vol. 3 (pp. 150–175). Basingstoke, Hampshire, U.K.: Macmillan Press.

Ringach, D. L., Shapley, R. M., and Hawken, M. J. (2002). Orientation selectivity in macaque V1: Diversity and laminar dependence. *J. Neurosci.* 22(13):5639–5651.

Robinson, S. R., and Dreher, B. (1990a). Müller cells in adult rabbit retinae: Morphology, distribution and implications for function and development. *J. Comp. Neurol.* 292(2):178–192.

Robinson, S. R., and Dreher, Z. (1990b). The visual pathways of eutherian mammals and marsupials develop according to a common timetable. *Brain Behav. Evol.* 36(4):177–195.

Robinson, S. R., Sung, L., Dreher, B., and Taylor, I. (1990). The distribution of ipsilaterally projecting retinal ganglion cells in adult and neonatal rabbits. *Proc. Aust. Physiol. Soc.* 21(1):28P.

Rocha-Miranda, C. E., Linden, R., Volchan, E., Lent, R., and Bombar-Dieri, R. A., Jr. (1976). Receptive field properties of single units in the opossum striate cortex. *Brain Res.* 104(2): 197–219.

Rodieck, R. W., and Watanabe, M. (1993). Survey of the morphology of macaque retinal ganglion cells that project to the pretectum, superior colliculus, and parvicellular laminae of the lateral geniculate nucleus. *J. Comp. Neurol.* 338(2):289–303.

Rosa, M. G. (1997). Extrastriate cortex in primates. In K. S. Rockland, J. H. Kaas, and A. Peters (Eds.), *Cerebral cortex*, Vol. 12 (pp. 127–203). New York: Plenum Press.

Rosa, M. G., and Krubitzer, L. A. (1999). The evolution of visual cortex: Where is V2? *Trends Neurosci.* 22(6):242–248.

Rosa, M. G., and Manger, P. R. (2005). Clarifying homologies in the mammalian cerebral cortex: The case of the third visual area (V3). *Clin. Exp. Pharmacol. Physiol.* 32(5–6):327–339.

Rose, D., and Blakemore, C. (1974). An analysis of orientation selectivity in the cat's visual cortex. *Exp. Brain Res.* 20(1):1–17.

Rosenquist, A. C. (1985). Connections of visual cortical areas in the cat. In A. Peters and E. G. Jones (Eds.), *Visual cortex*, Vol. 3 (pp. 81–116). New York: Plenum Press.

Rowe, M. H. (1991). Functional organization of the retina. In B. Dreher and S. R. Robinson (Eds.), *Neuroanatomy of the visual pathways and their development*, Vol. 3 (pp. 1–168). Basingstoke, Hampshire, U.K.: Macmillan.

Rowe, M. H., and Dreher, B. (1982). Functional morphology of beta cells in the area centralis of the cat's retina: A model for the evolution of central retinal specializations. *Brain Behav. Evol.* 21(1):1–23.

Ruby, N. F., Brennan, T. J., Xie, X., Cao, V., Franken, P., Heller, H. C., and O'Hara, B. F. (2002). Role of melanopsin in circadian responses to light. *Science* 298(5601):2211–2213.

Ruiz-Marcos, A., and Valverde, F. (1970). Dynamic architecture of visual cortex. *Brain Res.* 19(1):25–39.

Sagdullaev, B. T., and McCall, M. A. (2005). Stimulus size and intensity alter fundamental receptive field properties of mouse retinal ganglion cells in vivo. *Vis. Neurosci.* 22(5):649–659.

Schiller, P. H., Finlay, B. L., and Volman, S. F. (1976a). Quantitative studies of single-cell properties in monkey striate cortex. II. Orientation specificity and ocular dominance. *J. Neurophysiol.* 39(6):1320–1333.

SCHILLER, P. H., FINLAY, B. L., and VOLMAN, S. F. (1976b). Short-term response variability of monkey striate neurons. *Brain Res.* 105:347–349.

SCHMUCKER, C., SEELIGER, M., HUMPHRIES, P., BIEL, M., and SCHAEFFEL, F. (2005). Grating acuity at different luminances in wild-type mice and in mice lacking rod or cone function. *Invest. Ophthalmol. Vis. Sci.* 46(1):398–407.

SCHNEEWEIS, D., and SCHNAPF, J. (1995). Photovoltage of rods and cones in the macaque retina. *Science* 268(5213):1053–1056.

SCHUETT, S., BONHOEFFER, T., and HUBENER, M. (2002). Mapping retinotopic structure in mouse visual cortex with optical imaging. *J. Neurosci.* 22(15):6549–6559.

SEFTON, A. J., DREHER, B., and HARVEY, A. (2004). Visual system. In G. Paxinos (Ed.), *The rat nervous system* (pp. 1083–1165). Amsterdam: Elsevier; London: Academic Press.

SEMO, M., MUNOZ LLAMOSAS, M., FOSTER, R. G., and JEFFERY, G. (2005). Melanopsin (Opn 4) positive cells in the cat retina are randomly distributed across the ganglion cell layer. *Vis. Neurosci.* 22(1):111–116.

SHATZ, C. J., and STRYKER, M. P. (1978). Ocular dominance in layer IV of the cat's visual cortex and the effects of monocular deprivation. *J. Physiol. (Lond.)* 281(1):267–283.

SIMMONS, P. A., LEMMON, V., and PEARLMAN, A. L. (1982). Afferent and efferent connections of the striate and extrastriate visual cortex of the normal and reeler mouse. *J. Comp. Neurol.* 211 (3):295–308.

SIMMONS, P. A., and PEARLMAN, A. L. (1983). Receptive-field properties of transcallosal visual cortical neurons in the normal and reeler mouse. *J. Neurophysiol.* 50(4):838–848.

SINEX, D. G., BURDETTE, L. J., and PEARLMAN, A. L. (1979). A psychophysical investigation of spatial vision in the normal and reeler mutant mouse. *Vision Res.* 19(8):853–857.

SOHYA, K., KAMEYAMA, K., YANAGAWA, Y., OBATA, K., and TSUMOTO, T. (2007). GABAergic neurons are less selective to stimulus orientation than excitatory neurons in layer II/III of visual cortex, as revealed by *in vivo* functional Ca^{2+} imaging in transgenic mice. *J. Neurosci.* 27(8):2145–2149.

SOMERS, D., DRAGOI, V., and SUR, M. (2002). Orientation selectivity and its modulation by local and long-range connections in visual cortex. In B. R. Payne and A. Peters (Eds.), *The cat primary visual cortex* (pp. 471–520). San Diego: Academic Press.

SOUCY, E., WANG, Y., NIRENBERG, S., NATHANS, J., and MEISTER, M. (1998). A novel signaling pathway from rod photoreceptors to ganglion cells in mammalian retina. *Neuron* 21(3):481–493.

STEIN, B. E., JIANG, W., WALLACE, M. T., and STANFORD, T. R. (2001). Nonvisual influences on visual-information processing in the superior colliculus. *Prog. Brain Res.* 134:143–156.

STEIN, B. E., and MEREDITH, M. A. (1991). Functional organization of the superior colliculus. In A. G. Leventhal (Ed.), *The neural basis of visual function*, Vol. 4 (pp. 85–110). Basingstoke, Hampshire, U.K.: Macmillan.

STEIN, B. E., and MEREDITH, M. A. (1993). *The merging of the senses.* Cambridge, MA: MIT Press.

STEIN, B. E., and WALLACE, M. T. (1996). Comparisons of cross-modality integration in midbrain and cortex. *Prog. Brain Res.* 112:289–299.

STEINBERG, R. H., REID, M., and LACY, P. L. (1973). The distribution of rods and cones in the retina of the cat (*Felis domesticus*). *J. Comp. Neurol.* 148(2):229–248.

STONE, C., and PINTO, L. H. (1992). Receptive field organization of retinal ganglion cells in the spastic mutant mouse. *J. Physiol. (Lond.)* 456(1):125–142.

STONE, C., and PINTO, L. H. (1993). Response properties of ganglion cells in the isolated mouse retina. *Vis. Neurosci.* 10(1): 31–39.

STONE, J. (1978). The number and distribution of ganglion cells in the cat's retina. *J. Comp. Neurol.* 180(4):753–771.

STONE, J., and FUKUDA, Y. (1974). The naso-temporal division of the cat's retina re-examined in terms of Y-, X- and W-cells. *J. Comp. Neurol.* 155(4):377–394.

STONE, J., LEICESTER, J., and SHERMAN, S. M. (1973). The naso-temporal division of the monkey's retina. *J. Comp. Neurol.* 150(3):333–348.

SUN, D., and KALLONIATIS, M. (2006). Mapping glutamate responses in immunocytochemically identified neurons of the mouse retina. *J. Comp. Neurol.* 494(4):686–703.

SUN, W., DENG, Q., LEVICK, W. R., and HE, S. (2006). ON direction selective ganglion cells in the mouse retina. *J. Physiol. (Lond.)* 576(1):197–202.

SUN, W., LI, N., and HE, S. (2002). Large scale morphological survey of mouse retinal ganglion cells. *J. Comp. Neurol.* 451(2):115–126.

SWADLOW, H. A., and WEYAND, T. G. (1985). Receptive field and axonal properties of neurons in the dorsal lateral geniculate nucleus of awake unparalyzed rabbits. *J. Neurophysiol.* 54(1): 168–183.

SZÉL, A., ROHLICH, P., CAFFE, A. R., JULIUSSON, B., AGUIRRE, G., and VAN VEEN, T. (1992). Unique topographic separation of two spectral classes of cones in the mouse retina. *J. Comp. Neurol.* 325(3):327–342.

SZÉL, A., ROHLICH, P., MIEZIEWSKA, K., AGUIRRE, G., and VAN VEEN, T. (1993). Spatial and temporal differences between the expression of short- and middle-wave sensitive cone pigments in the mouse retina: A developmental study. *J. Comp. Neurol.* 331(4):564–577.

TASSINARI, G., BENTIVOGLIO, M., CHEN, S., and CAMPARA, D. (1997). Overlapping ipsilateral and contralateral retinal projections to the lateral geniculate nucleus and superior colliculus in the cat: A retrograde triple labelling study. *Brain Res. Bull.* 43(2):127–139.

THIELE, A., VOGELSANG, M., and HOFFMANN, K.-P. (1991). Pattern of retinotectal projection in the megachiropteran bat *Rousettus aegyptiacus*. *J. Comp. Neurol.* 314(4):671–683.

TIAO, Y. C., and BLAKEMORE, C. (1976a). Functional organization in the visual cortex of the golden hamster. *J. Comp. Neurol.* 168(4):459–481.

TIAO, Y. C., and BLAKEMORE, C. (1976b). Regional specialization in golden hamster's retina. *J. Comp. Neurol.* 168(4):439–457.

TODA, K., BUSH, R. A., HUMPHRIES, P., and SIEVING, P. A. (1999). The electroretinogram of the rhodopsin knockout mouse. *Vis. Neurosci.* 16(2):391–398.

TREJO, L. J., and CICERONE, C. M. (1984). Cells in the pretectal olivary nucleus are in the pathway for the direct light reflex of the pupil in the rat. *Brain Res.* 300(1):49–62.

TSUKAMOTO, Y., MORIGIWA, K., UEDA, M., and STERLING, P. (2001). Microcircuits for night vision in mouse retina. *J. Neurosci.* 21(21):8616–8623.

TUSA, R. J., PALMER, L. A., and ROSENQUIST, A. C. (1978). The retinotopic organization of area 17 (striate cortex) in the cat. *J. Comp. Neurol.* 177(2):213–235.

USREY, W. M., SCENIAK, M. P., and CHAPMAN, B. (2003). Receptive fields and response properties of neurons in layer 4 of ferret visual cortex. *J. Neurophysiol.* 89(2):1003–1015.

VAKKUR, G. J., BISHOP, P. O., and KOZAK, W. (1963). Visual optics in the cat, including posterior nodal distance and retinal landmarks. *Vision Res.* 3:289–294.

Valverde, F. (1968). Structural changes in the area striata of the mouse after enucleation. *Exp. Brain Res.* 5(4):274–292.

Valverde, F. (1991). The organization of the striate cortex. In B. Dreher and S. R. Robinson (Eds.), *Neuroanatomy of the visual pathways and their development* (pp. 235–277). Basingstoke, Hampshire, U.K.: Macmillan.

Valverde, F., and Ruiz-Marcos, A. (1969). Dendritic spines in visual cortex of mouse: Introduction to a mathematical model. *Exp. Brain Res.* 8(3):269–283.

Vaney, D. I., Peichl, L., Wässle, H., and Illing, R. B. (1981). Almost all ganglion cells in the rabbit retina project to the superior colliculus. *Brain Res.* 212(2):447–453.

Van Hooser, S. D., Heimel, J. A., and Nelson, S. B. (2003). Receptive field properties and laminar organization of lateral geniculate nucleus in the gray squirrel (*Sciurus carolinensis*). *J. Neurophysiol.* 90(5):3398–3418.

Van Hooser, S. D., Heimel, J. A., and Nelson, S. B. (2005). Functional cell classes and functional architecture in the early visual system of a highly visual rodent. *Prog. Brain Res.* 149:127–145.

Van Sluyters, R. C., and Stewart, D. L. (1974). Binocular neurons of the rabbit's visual cortex: Receptive field characteristics. *Exp. Brain Res.* 19(2):166–195.

Ver Hoeve, J. N., Danilov, Y. P., Kim, C. B., and Spear, P. D. (1999). VEP and PERG acuity in anesthetized young adult rhesus monkeys. *Vis. Neurosci.* 16(4):607–617.

Vidyasagar, T. R., Pei, X., and Volgushev, M. (1996). Multiple mechanisms underlying the orientation selectivity of visual cortical neurones. *Trends Neurosci.* 19(7):272–277.

Vitek, D. J., Schall, J. D., and Leventhal, A. G. (1985). Morphology, central projections, and dendritic field orientation of retinal ganglion cells in the ferret. *J. Comp. Neurol.* 241(1):1–11.

Wagner, E., McCaffery, P., and Dräger, U. C. (2000). Retinoic acid in the formation of the dorsoventral retina and its central projections. *Dev. Biol.* 222(2):460–470.

Wagor, E., Mangini, N. J., and Pearlman, A. L. (1980). Retinotopic organization of striate and extrastriate visual cortex in the mouse. *J. Comp. Neurol.* 193(1):187–202.

Walls, G. L. (1942). *The vertebrate eye and its adaptive radiation.* Bloomfield Hills, MI: Cranbrook Institute of Science.

Wang, Q., and Burkhalter, A. (2007). Area map of mouse visual cortex. *J. Comp. Neurol.* 502(3):339–357.

Wässle, H. (2004). Parallel processing in the mammalian retina. *Nat. Rev. Neurosci.* 5(10):747–757.

Wässle, H., and Boycott, B. B. (1991). Functional architecture of the mammalian retina. *Physiol. Rev.* 71(2):447–480.

Wässle, H., and Illing, R. B. (1980). The retinal projection to the superior colliculus in the cat: A quantitative study with HRP. *J. Comp. Neurol.* 190(2):333–356.

Weng, S., Sun, W., and He, S. (2005). Identification of ON-OFF direction-selective ganglion cells in the mouse retina. *J. Physiol. (Lond.)* 562(3):915–923.

White, L. E., Bosking, W. H., Williams, S. M., and Fitzpatrick, D. (1999). Maps of central visual space in ferret V1 and V2 lack matching inputs from the two eyes. *J. Neurosci.* 19(16):7089–7099.

Wiesel, T. N., and Hubel, D. H. (1963). Single cell responses in striate cortex of kittens deprived of vision in one eye. *J. Neurophysiol.* 26(6):1003–117.

Wiesel, T. N., and Hubel, D. H. (1965). Comparison of the effects of unilateral and bilateral eye closure on cortical unit responses in kittens. *J. Neurophysiol.* 28(6):1029–1040.

Yorke, C. H., Jr., and Caviness, V. S., Jr. (1975). Interhemispheric neocortical connections of the corpus callosum in the normal mouse: a study based on anterograde and retrograde methods. *J. Comp. Neurol.* 164(2):233–245.

Yoshida, K., Watanabe, D., Ishikane, H., Tachibana, M., Pastan, I., and Nakanishi, S. (2001). A key role of starburst amacrine cells in originating retinal directional selectivity and optokinetic eye movement. *Neuron* 30(3):771–780.

Youngstrom, T. G., and Nunez, A. A. (1986). Comparative anatomy of the retino-hypothalamic tract in photoperiodic and non-photoperiodic rodents. *Brain Res. Bull.* 17(4):485–492.

4 Survey of the Research Opportunities Afforded by Genetic Variation in the Mouse Visual System

LAWRENCE H. PINTO AND JOHN B. TROY

Historical perspective: Use of the mouse to study retinal diseases, neurogenesis, and cell biology

Although the mouse has long been the experimental mammalian genetic model system of choice (Paigen, 1995), and although one of the earliest mammalian genetic mapping studies was performed with the mouse visual system (Sidman and Green, 1965), early studies focused more on retinal diseases (Searle and Fielder, 1990), neurogenesis (LaVail, 1973; Young, 1985), and cell biology (Sidman and Green, 1965; Young, 1984). Only recently has the mouse been used to study the normal visual system or the processes involved in visual perception. As a result, less is known about its visual system than about the visual systems of other mammals. Another reason that earlier work did not focus on the normal visual system of the mouse was the widely held belief that the mouse was not a "visual animal."

It is ironic that one reason that the mouse was not generally considered to be a visual animal stemmed from the widespread occurrence of a mutation that was very useful for understanding the basis for one form of a severe blinding disease, retinitis pigmentosa. The retinal degeneration (*rd*, now *Pde6b*^{rd1}) mutation of the phosphodiesterase 6b enzyme occurs in many common laboratory strains and renders all the mice in these strains incapable of normal responses to light (Chang et al., 2002) (table 4.1).

There is ample historical reason for researchers to be wary of using mice for studies of the visual system. In 1924, Keeler, while examining mouse retinas histologically, found the retinas of some mice to be deficient in photoreceptors. This mutation was named rodless (*r*), and the mutant mice were distributed to many laboratories. A similar phenotype was found by Bruckner in 1951 among wild mice from the Basel and Zurich areas that were probably interbred with some laboratory strains; this mutation was named retinal degeneration (*rd*). The similarity between the phenotypes of the *r*/*r* and *rd*/*rd* mutants led to speculation that they might be the same mutation. This question was resolved in Baehr's laboratory by using PCR to amplify DNA from archival microscope slides containing the *r*/*r* mutant retinas (Pittler et al., 1993). In these experiments, both the sequences of the coding region of *Pde6b* and intronic polymorphisms were characterized to "fingerprint" the DNA of this region of the fifth chromosome. The results showed that both *r*/*r* and *rd*/*rd* retinas, the latter from many strains, contained not only the same missense mutation but also the same polymorphisms (differences in one or more nucleotides that usually do not result in deleterious effects but can be used to "fingerprint" the DNA to determine its origin). This led to the conclusion that the mutations are genetically identical and supported the interpretation that the retinal degeneration mutation present in many laboratory strains had its origin in Keeler's rodless mutation. Since so many strains are affected with the same blinding mutation, it is understandable that researchers dismissed the mouse as a model for visual studies beyond studies of degeneration.

The *rd* mutation is not the only mutation that has been of help in understanding the function of the visual system. In addition to the strains that carry the *rd* mutation, some strains of mice bear mutations in genes other than *Pde6b* that affect vision (see table 4.1). For example, many laboratory strains are albino (*Tyr*^{c}) or hypopigmented, so that under the bright illumination of a research laboratory they may not be able to see properly; this mutation is useful for understanding low vision due to albinism and other disorders. Older DBA mice undergo ocular changes that lead to glaucoma (John et al., 1998; Libby et al., 2005). The fact that a number of common laboratory strains have genetic alterations impairing their vision does not mean, of course, that the majority of strains of mice without these mutations are also blind. However, it undoubtedly contributed to the earlier perception that all mice generally have poor vision, and may have inhibited earlier interest in studying the visual process in normal mice.

TABLE 4.1

Useful mutations in common laboratory mouse strains

Strain	Mutation	Effect	Reference
C3H, FVB, CBA, BUB, SJL, SB, others	*rd1* mutation of phosphodiesterase 6 beta: *Pde6b*^{rd1}	Loss of rods and cones, outer nuclear layer	Chang et al., 2002
BALB, A, BUB, FVB, SJL, NZW, others	Albino (*c*) mutation of tyrosinase: *Tyr*^{c}	Lacks pigment in the retinal pigment epithelium, scattering light impairs vision; altered visual "map" impairs nystagmus	Balkema et al., 1984
129P3/J, P/J; spontaneous and induced mutations on other strain backgrounds	Pink-eyed dilution (*p*)	Lacks pigment in the retinal pigment epithelium, scattering light impairs vision; altered visual "map" impairs nystagmus	Balkema et al., 1984; Vitaterna et al., 1994
SB	Beige mutation of lysosomal trafficking regulator: *Lyst*^{bg}	Lacks pigment in the retinal pigment epithelium, scattering light impairs vision; altered visual "map" impairs nystagmus	Balkema et al., 1984
Spontaneous mutations maintained in C57BL and C3H substrains	Pale ear (*ep*) mutation of Hermansky-Pudlak syndrome 1 homologue: *Hps1*^{ep}	Lacks pigment in the retinal pigment epithelium, scattering light impairs vision; altered visual "map" impairs nystagmus	Balkema et al., 1984
DBA	Dilute	Decreased pigment in the retinal pigment epithelium, scattering light impairs vision; altered visual "map" impairs nystagmus; glaucoma	Balkema et al., 1984; John et al., 1998

Mice in fact use their sense of vision under conditions of dim lighting—perhaps another reason that mice might not be considered visual animals. Nocturnal animals, they are most active at night under low illumination, not during the day under the bright illumination of a laboratory, when they are usually observed. Another reason that the vision of mice is discounted may be that their most obvious behaviors seen in the laboratory are sniffing and touching objects with whiskers. However, ethologists who have observed mice in more natural settings have long known that mice engage in exploratory, feeding, and aggressive behaviors that clearly depend on vision (Crowcroft, 1966).

Even though many mouse strains harbor mutations that affect vision adversely, most strains have normal visually guided behaviors. These behaviors include optokinetic nystagmus (Balkema et al., 1984), optomotor responses (Prusky et al., 2004), water maze performance (Balkema et al., 1983; Hayes and Balkema, 1993; Prusky and Douglas, 2004), and performance on forced choice touchscreen tasks (Bussey et al., 2001). The strain that researchers have settled on as a standard strain is C57BL/6J ("B6") because it is pigmented, lacks degeneration in any part of the nervous system, and exhibits all of the cited visually guided behaviors. In addition to these benefits, the genomic DNA sequence of C57BL/6J has been determined. Finally, polymorphisms between the B6 strain and many other strains have been characterized, making it possible to map mutations and the genes that are responsible for the differences in various traits between strains.

The mutations that are widespread among inbred strains can be used to study important pathological processes such as those that cause degenerations. This can be done by selectively breeding an affected strain with a normal strain, usually B6. This process is repeated a number of times until every chromosome except that carrying the mutant allele comes from B6. The latter chromosome will contain a small region surrounding the mutant allele, the size of which decreases with the number of generations of breeding. There are two ways in which this process, called making the mutant allele congenic, can be achieved. First, the breeding process can be repeated for 20 generations, and the result will be a segment on the mutation-carrying chromosome that derives from the mutation-bearing strain and is about 5 centimorgans (2–10 megabases) long. The second way is to use polymorphic markers to choose the desired animals at each generation and use only these animals for breeding. This is called making a "speed congenic." The same result that is obtained in the traditional way can be achieved in approximately five generations. Thus, even strains that carry an allele undesirable for vision can be used to study the process that makes the allele undesirable.

Exploiting differences among mouse strains to find the genes that control vision

Most inherited familial diseases are the result of a mutation that affects a single gene and has a strong effect on the phenotype of the affected individuals. Two examples that affect vision are mutations in *Pde6b* and rhodopsin that cause photoreceptor degeneration. However, many diseases, such as high blood pressure, type 2 diabetes, and stroke, are believed to result from the interactions between many genes (Hirschhorn and Daly, 2005). Similarly, retinal diseases are likely to result from the interactions of separate genes or gene products. For example, a variant of complement factor H (CFH-Y_{402}H) has been shown to be a major risk factor for the dry form of age-related macular degeneration (AMD) (Klein et al., 2005), and variants of a different gene, the serine protease HTRA1, have been proposed to be risk factors for the wet form of AMD in several populations (Dewan et al., 2006; Yang et al., 2006). It would seem only logical that interactions between these genes should determine the final disease state in patients (Dewan et al., 2006). Similarly, other properties of biological systems are often the result of the combined effects of several genes. A useful strategy to help identify these genes is to make comparisons among inbred strains. The process by which this comparison is started is called quantitative trait locus (QTL) analysis. This process is the subject of chapter 54 in this volume. One way in which the approximate location of the relevant genes is determined is illustrated in figure 4.1.

For QTL analysis to work in finding genes that control vision, strains must differ in some property of the visual system. The earliest example was the number of ganglion cells found in the retina, which was found to differ between the B6 strain and the DBA/2J strain. Williams and co-workers took advantage of the difference between this interstrain difference to identify the region of the genome where a gene that controls ganglion cell number is located, the quantitative trait locus (Williams et al., 1998). They did this by exploiting a genetic resource of great power, the set of recombinant inbred strains, or RI strains (see figure 4.1), which are made by creating F_1 hybrids between these two strains and then breeding each of many brother-sister pairs to form breeding lines, each of which constitutes a strain after 20 generations. Each RI line will have a different assortment of chromosomal segments from the two parent strains, and thus each RI line will have a different assortment of alleles. For this particular combination of strains, more than 80 RI lines are available. Williams and co-workers measured the ganglion cell number in many of these RI strains. To identify the chromosomal segments carrying the important genes, they searched the genomes of the RI strains with the greatest number of ganglion cells for segments that had their origin in the parent strain with the greater number of ganglion cells. In fact, the process is more complicated, because among these RI strains there are members with both higher and lower numbers of ganglion cells than contained in either parental strain. A mapping program that accounts for the intergene interactions necessary to cause this wide range of ganglion cell number is used to identify the interacting loci containing interacting genes (www.mapmanager.org). Thus, interstrain differences and RI strains can be used to identify the location of genes that are important for vision.

It is not necessary to use RI strains to identify a QTL. Instead, the investigator can make many F_2 mice from a cross between two strains having differences in the trait to be studied. However, in this case the burden of genotyping falls on the investigator, whereas the DNA polymorphisms between each RI strain have already been characterized (www.genenetwork.org).

Interstrain differences can also be used to map QTLs (figure 4.2). The presently used inbred laboratory strains derive from very few wild-caught mice, and thus their genomes are mosaics of the chromosomes of these founder mice (Wade et al., 2002; Wiltshire et al., 2003). The genetic diversity of the founder mice allows the DNA derived from them to be identified by characterizing their polymorphisms. The polymorphisms between many standard laboratory strains have been characterized (Pletcher et al., 2004) at more than 150,000 locations in the genome. These polymorphisms have been used to identify known genes that affect vision. The investigator measures the phenotype in each of many strains and then applies the data in a mapping program designed for this purpose. The program establishes associations between the DNA segments of each strain (from the small number of founder mice) and the phenotype. A program for this purpose is available on the Web (http://snpster.gnf.org/cgi-bin/snpster_ext.cgi). Thus, naturally occurring variation among strains of mice provides a resource for vision researchers that can be exploited readily at the present time with available resources.

Using targeted mutagenesis to test hypotheses regarding specific, known proteins in the visual process

Targeted mutagenesis is often used to study the function of proteins, such as enzymes, receptors, and ion channels. Many proteins have been identified in the visual system, and these proteins can be studied in several ways by altering their primary amino sequence or by preventing their expression altogether. Fortunately, these manipulations are possible for most proteins in the mouse. The process requires the use of homologous recombination to introduce a mutant DNA into the mouse genome. This process can be done with efficiency using embryonic stem cells of only "129" strains; variation among these strains has been described (Simpson et al., 1997). The 129 strains differ in many ways from the B6 strain that is usually used for functional studies. For example, there are thousands of DNA polymorphisms between the two strains, and the electroretinogram (ERG) of the two strains differ considerably. Thus, interstrain differences need

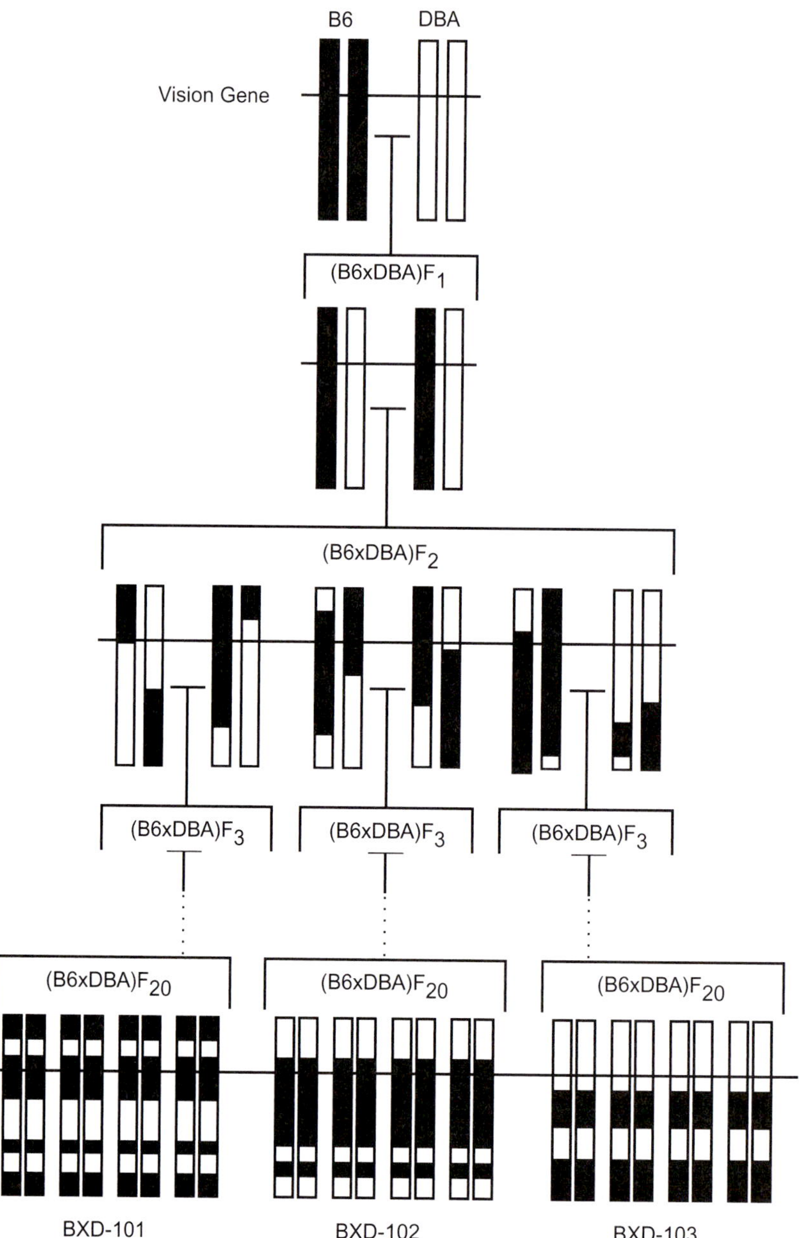

FIGURE 4.1 Recombinant inbred (RI) strains can be used to localize genes that are important for vision. A hypothetical vision-related gene is located at the same place on the chromosomes of two inbred strains (C57BL/6J or B6 and DBA/2J or DBA), but the alleles differ for the two strains, and this allelic difference results in a different vision phenotype for the two strains. The process of localizing this gene (QTL analysis) can be assisted by employing RI strains, which are created by the breeding process shown. For the two parental strains shown, more than 80 RI strains exist. In the absence of interactions with other genes, the hypothetical phenotype of the BXD-101 and BXD-102 strains will be equal to that of the B6 parental strain because they both inherited the B6 allele of the vision gene (black). On the other hand, the hypothetical phenotype of the BXD-103 strain will be equal to that of the parental DBA strain (white). The mosaic pattern of the DNA of many RI strains has been well characterized (www.genenetwork.org). By using at least 20 RI strains, it is usually possible to localize genes that have different alleles in the parental strains to a relatively small portion of the chromosome. Further effort is required to identify the actual gene. In general, interactions among genes occur, but these interactions can be identified with available analytical tools (see www.mapmanager.org). Genes can also be localized by analyzing F_2 animals, but each F_2 animal has a unique pattern of inheritance, and thus the investigator must perform analysis for each F_2. This task has already been done for the RI strains.

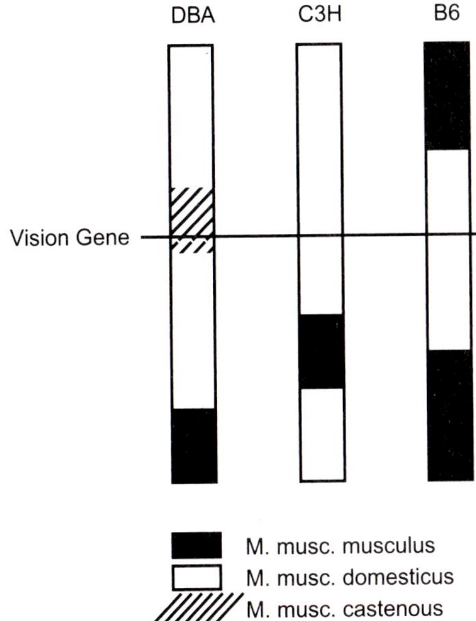

FIGURE 4.2 Differences among inbred strains can be used to identify genes that are important for vision. A hypothetical vision gene is present in the same location on the chromosomes of the strains shown, but the alleles of this gene differ, and these differences result in different phenotypes for the strains. The set of inbred laboratory strains has been derived from relatively few founder mice, and each strain's genome can be considered to be a mosaic of DNA from a few hypothetical founders. These hypothetical founders are believed to be similar to contemporary strains, three of which are shown. The DNA mosaic of the laboratory strains has been characterized with high resolution (http://snpster.gnf.org/cgi-bin/snpster_ext.cgi). By characterizing the phenotype in many strains and searching for the DNA segments that all the strains with a particular phenotype have in common, it is possible to identify the segment of the chromosome in which the vision gene lies. In fact, several genes usually contribute to a phenotype, and the available analytical tools allow the genomic segments in which they are found to be identified. Further studies are needed to identify each gene.

to be considered in comparing targeted mouse mutants with a wild-type mouse. This comparison is made more difficult by the fact that the successfully mutated embryonic stem cells are used to make chimeras with mice of a strain other than 129 (usually B6). Thus, several generations of selective breeding to make the targeted mutation congenic on B6 are necessary before quantitative comparisons will be valid. However, the use of polymorphic markers between strains can speed this process (an example of making speed congenics).

One of the most frequently used targeted mutations is the null mutation or knockout. For knockouts, the first exon of the target gene is often replaced with a marker. Caution needs to be exercised with this type of mutation, for several reasons. First, about one-third of knockout mice experience lethal changes early in development. Second, about one-third of knockout mice in which a known important gene is targeted are only mildly affected. An example of this is the *Clock* gene, which plays a central role in generating circadian rhythms, as evidenced by the severe effect of truncation mutations (Vitaterna et al., 1994; King et al., 1997). However, deletion of the *Clock* gene results in much less severe alterations in the phenotype than the truncation mutation, probably because substitute genes are expressed in its stead (Debruyne et al., 2006). Third, it is possible for a knockout allele to have a more severe phenotype than a simple point mutation. For example, an active site mutation of the kinase PI3Kγ results in a less severe phenotype than the null allele because the kinase protein forms part of a complex with another enzyme, PDE3B. The absence of the kinase interferes with the second enzyme's activity, resulting in elevated cAMP levels. Thus, for several reasons, care must be exercised in the interpretation of results obtained with null alleles.

The importance of strain background cannot be overstressed. Examples of the importance of strain background abound, but two striking examples are the following. On the B6 background, the diabetes (*db*) and obese (*ob*) mutations cause obesity and transient diabetes, but on the C57BLKS/J background they cause obesity and overt diabetes (Coleman and Hummel, 1973). The second example comes from combined effects of the multiple intestinal neoplasia mutation (Min) and the adenomatous polyposis coli (*ApcMin*) gene (Su et al., 1992; Moser et al., 1993). B6 mice heterozygous for the mutation are very susceptible to developing intestinal polyps, but offspring mated with several other strains (AKR/J, MA/MyJ, and CAST) are significantly less susceptible because the latter strains possess an allele of a modifier locus (*Mom1*) that ameliorates the effect of the *Min* mutation (Dietrich et al., 1993).

We are fortunate that targeted disruption of genes is possible in the mouse. Unfortunately, the technology for targeted mutation has not been developed to the point of being convenient for several other organisms that are also useful for genetic studies.

Transgenic mice are useful for studying the effects of exogenous genes and for determining the effects of gene dosage (the number of copies of the normal allele of a gene). Transgenic mice are also useful for confirming the identity of genes that have been mutated either naturally or by chemical means, or by other methods of mutagenesis. There is one very important point to bear in mind when using transgenes: the location where the transgene is inserted affects the strength and distribution of its expression. Perhaps the clearest example of this is the distribution of expression of GFP under the control of the *Thy1* promoter (Feng et al., 2000): in each of 25 independently generated lines, the pattern of expression of GFP and its spectral variants was unique.

Various neurons, or regions of retina, were labeled in each different line. This unique pattern of expression of the very same transgene can be attributed to variation in the location of insertion of the transgene within the genome. Thus, care must be exercised in the interpretation of results obtained in mice that have been generated by genetic manipulation such as transgenesis or site-directed mutation, especially mutations that cause the null allele.

Forward genetics: An approach for discovering novel genes that are essential for vision

The mouse is also a useful model in which to apply the forward genetics approach, in which genes important for vision can be discovered. This approach starts with the random or spontaneous mutagenesis of genes whose identity is unknown, proceeds with the discovery of visually affected mutants by screening for mice with abnormal vision, and continues with identification of the mutated gene and study of the mechanism by which the mutated gene results in abnormal vision. This approach offers several advantages. (1) It requires no prior knowledge of the mechanism, components, or genes involved. (2) A number of mutant alleles can often be isolated that alter gene function in a number of ways. (3) This approach usually identifies point mutations, which in some instances can be more informative than targeted null mutations because gain of function and dominant negative mutations can be isolated. (4) Finding a single essential gene opens the door to finding other genes in the affected pathway. (5) This approach parallels most closely natural mutagenesis.

Forward genetics has been useful in vision research by discovering genes of importance to vision. A number of these genes were discovered in the invertebrate visual system and were later found to be important for the function of the vertebrate nervous system. Several of the proteins involved in the invertebrate phototransduction cascade were identified with forward genetic screens in *Drosophila.* Among them were the Trp (transient receptor potential) ion channel (Minke, 1982); phospholipase C (Bloomquist et al., 1988), mutation of which can eliminate the receptor potential; and the cyclophilin NinaA (Schneuwly et al., 1989; Stamnes et al., 1991; Ferreira et al., 1996), mutation of which alters the receptor potential time inactivation and recovery. These proteins all have mammalian orthologues, and two of them were discovered as a result of research on the *Drosophila* eye.

Forward genetics has also helped to identify proteins involved in mammalian vision (figure 4.3). More than 80 genes that, when mutated, result in human retinal degeneration have been identified (Pacione et al., 2003). The following examples show the wide variety of essential retinal genes that have been identified using forward genetics in mammals. The *rd* mutation in mouse occurs in a gene in the phototransduction cascade ($Pde6^{rd1}$) (Bowes et al., 1993), and the *rdy* mutation in rats disrupts the receptor tyrosine kinase *Mertk* and impairs phagocytosis of shed rod outer segments by the retinal pigment epithelium, resulting in degeneration of the retina (D'Cruz et al., 2000). The protein nyctalopin, essential for bipolar cell function, was identified by cloning the *nob* gene (Gregg et al., 2003). Mutation of nyctalopin eliminates the b-wave of the ERG (Pardue et al., 1998) and results in congenital stationary night blindness in humans (Bech-Hansen et al., 2000). Genes have been identified that modify the effects of deleterious mutations. The tubby (*tub*) gene in the mouse, named for its effect on body weight, also results in retinal degeneration. However, when mice of the C57BL/6J strain bearing this mutation are intercrossed with mice of the AKR strain, some of the resulting homozygous mutant mice are spared. Those mice that are spared have inherited the AKR allele of a defined region of chromosome 2 (Ikeda et al., 2002), suggesting the presence of a modifying allele on chromosome 2.

Recently, a forward genetic screen for visual mutants was completed by three research centers (Vitaterna et al., 2006). Each center screened the eye or the retina using a combination of morphological and functional criteria, and many mutants were produced. A catalogue of the visual mutants that was produced in this forward genetic screen is available on the Internet (www.neuromice.org). Of note, many mutations that affected histology were found, and some fewer mutations that affected retinal function were also found. The reason is probably that screening for functional mutations took much longer per mouse than a morphological screen, required working with anesthetized mice, and had to produce a severe effect to be reliably detected in the offspring of the founder mutant mice. No mice with primary defects in the brain were identified, to complement the large number of spontaneous decussation-deficient mutants that are available (LaVail et al., 1978; Balkema et al., 1984; Pak et al., 1987). The reason for this is probably that the vision tests that were used would not have detected brain defects. Indeed, detecting brain defects requires either imaging technology or behavioral measurements that are not yet well enough developed to be applied individually to a large number of mice.

Special Features of the Mouse Visual System That Need to Be Kept in Mind by Investigators For optimal vision to occur, the retinal image must be in focus, a condition that requires a correct state of refraction. Because the posterior nodal distance of the mouse (Remtulla and Hallett, 1985) is small (ca. 3 mm), the distance between the photoreceptors and the structures that are usually used to assess the refractive state of the eye is significant, and the mouse thus appears to be hyperopic by the usual means of measurement (Glickstein

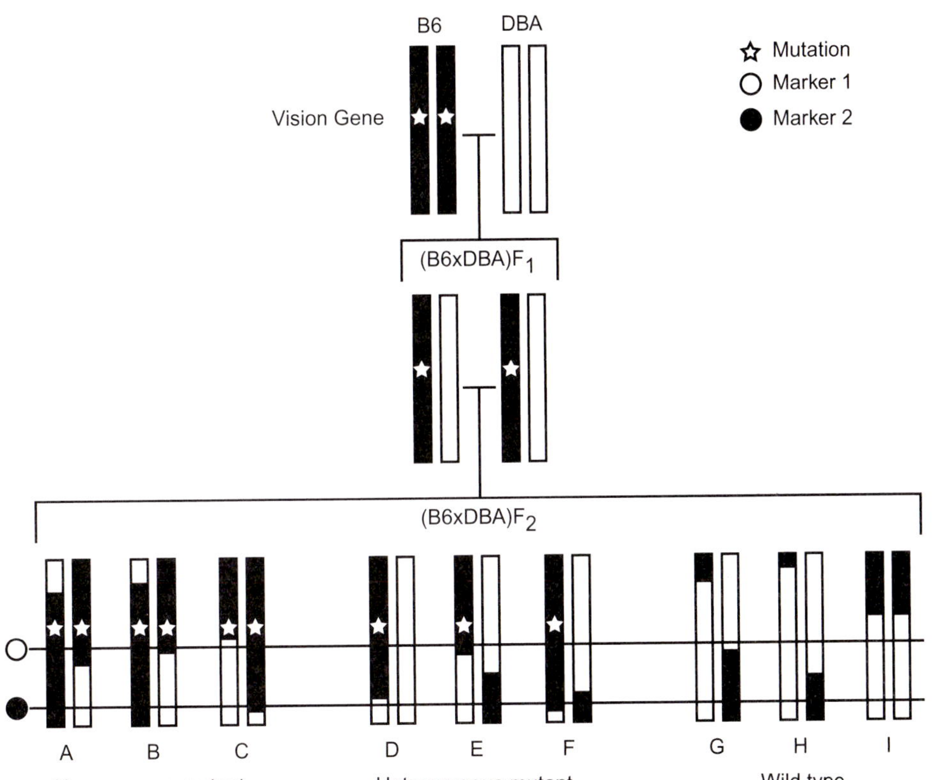

FIGURE 4.3 A vision-related gene that was mutated using the forward genetic approach is localized. The B6 mouse in the first row has been mutagenized with a chemical mutagen, and it is assumed that the mutation is autosomal recessive (this animal would have to be the third-generation offspring of a mutagenized male in order to be homozygous for the mutation). The mutant is bred with a mouse from a strain with many DNA polymorphisms (a counterstrain); in this case, DBA/2J is illustrated. Each F_1 mouse will be heterozygous for the mutation, and, most important, the mutation continues to lie in a B6 background. Intercrossing the F_1 mice to produce F_2s will result in mice having the chromosomes shown in the third row; each of these mice has a mosaic of B6 and DBA chromosomes. Only those F_2s that inherit two chromosomal segments from B6 in the region that bears the mutation will be affected (homozygous mutant). Markers such as marker 1 will often be coinherited with the mutant phenotype if they are close to the mutagenized gene, whereas more distant markers such as marker 2 will be less frequently coinherited. In practice, the haplotype of the affected chromosome is determined to localize the gene, because determining the haplotype takes advantage of information from many markers. This approach requires careful selection of the counterstrain, as alleles of genes from the counterstrain might modify the effect of the mutation under study (see the example from the *Min* mutation).

and Millodot, 1970). The spectrum of the light stimulus for the mouse needs to be considered as well. Mice are very sensitive to ultraviolet light (Calderone and Jacobs, 1995; Lyubarsky et al., 1999) and thus might respond to stimuli that the investigator cannot see. Finally, the dorsal-ventral gradient in M cone distribution found in the mouse retina (Applebury et al., 2000) needs to be kept in mind when designing stimuli for testing visual function.

Conclusion

Experiments in a number of fields with transgenic and targeted mutant mice have demonstrated that this organism has unique uses for testing hypotheses regarding the function of proteins within the nervous system. However, the misconception that the mouse is not a visual animal has prevented it from being fully exploited in studies of the visual system, save studies of processes that are affected by mutations widespread among inbred strains. This situation should now change. The realization that mice of most inbred strains are visual animals with normal visual behaviors will make it possible to use the recent advances in forward genetics and in our understanding of the diversity among inbred strains to identify genes that are important for vision and to elucidate the mechanisms by which they function.

ACKNOWLEDGMENT Work was supported by grants U01-MH61915 and R01 EY06669 from the National Institutes of Health.

REFERENCES

Applebury, M. L., Antoch, M. P., Baxter, L. C., Chun, L. L., Falk, J. D., Farhangfar, F., Kage, K., Krzystolik, M. G., Lyass, L. A., et al. (2000). The murine cone photoreceptor: A single cone type expresses both S and M opsins with retinal spatial patterning. *Neuron* 27:513–523.

Balkema, G. W., Mangini, N. J., and Pinto, L. H. (1983). Discrete visual defects in pearl mutant mice. *Science* 219:1085–1087.

Balkema, G. W., Mangini, N. J., Pinto, L. H., and Vanable, J. W., Jr. (1984). Visually evoked eye movements in mouse mutants and inbred strains: A screening report. *Invest. Ophthalmol. Vis. Sci.* 25:795–800.

Bech-Hansen, N. T., Naylor, M. J., Maybaum, T. A., Sparkes, R. L., Koop, B., Birch, D. G., Bergen, A. A., Prinsen, C. F., Polomeno, R. C., et al. (2000). Mutations in NYX, encoding the leucine-rich proteoglycan nyctalopin, cause X-linked complete congenital stationary night blindness. *Nat. Genet.* 26:319–323.

Bloomquist, B. T., Shortridge, R. D., Schneuwly, S., Perdew, M., Montell, C., Steller, H., Rubin, G., and Pak, W. L. (1988). Isolation of a putative phospholipase C gene of *Drosophila*, *norpA*, and its role in phototransduction. *Cell* 54:723–733.

Bowes, C., Li, T., Frankel, W. N., Danciger, M., Coffin, J. M., Applebury, M. L., and Farber, D. B. (1993). Localization of a retroviral element within the *rd* gene coding for the beta subunit of cGMP phosphodiesterase. *Proc. Natl. Acad. Sci. U.S.A.* 90: 2955–2959.

Bruckner, R. (1951). [Slit-lamp microscopy and ophthalmoscopy in rat and mouse.] *Doc. Ophthalmol.* 5–6:452–554.

Bussey, T. J., Saksida, L. M., and Rothblat, L. A. (2001). Discrimination of computer-graphic stimuli by mice: A method for the behavioral characterization of transgenic and gene-knockout models. *Behav. Neurosci.* 115:957–960.

Calderone, J. B., and Jacobs, G. H. (1995). Regional variations in the relative sensitivity to UV light in the mouse retina. *Vis. Neurosci.* 12:463–468.

Chang, B., Hawes, N. L., Hurd, R. E., Davisson, M. T., Nusinowitz, S., and Heckenlively, J. R. (2002). Retinal degeneration mutants in the mouse. *Vision Res.* 42:517–525.

Coleman, D. L., and Hummel, K. P. (1973). The influence of genetic background on the expression of the obese (*Ob*) gene in the mouse. *Diabetologia* 9:287–293.

Crowcroft, P. (1966). *Mice all over.* London: Foulis.

D'Cruz, P. M., Yasumura, D., Weir, J., Matthes, M. T., Abderrahim, H., LaVail, M. M., and Vollrath, D. (2000). Mutation of the receptor tyrosine kinase gene *Mertk* in the retinal dystrophic RCS rat. *Hum. Mol. Genet.* 9:645–651.

Debruyne, J. P., Noton, E., Lambert, C. M., Maywood, E. S., Weaver, D. R., and Reppert, S. M. (2006). A clock shock: Mouse *CLOCK* is not required for circadian oscillator function. *Neuron* 50:465–477.

Dewan, A., Liu, M., Hartman, S., Zhang, S. S., Liu, D. T., Zhao, C., Tam, P. O., Chan, W. M., Lam, D. S., et al. (2006). HTRA1 promoter polymorphism in wet age-related macular degeneration. *Science* 314:989–992.

Dietrich, W. F., Lander, E. S., Smith, J. S., Moser, A. R., Gould, K. A., Luongo, C., Borenstein, N., and Dove, W. (1993). Genetic identification of Mom-1, a major modifier locus affecting *Min*-induced intestinal neoplasia in the mouse. *Cell* 75: 631–639.

Feng, G., Mellor, R. H., Bernstein, M., Keller-Peck, C., Nguyen, Q. T., Wallace, M., Nerbonne, J. M., Lichtman, J. W., and Sanes, J. R. (2000). Imaging neuronal subsets in transgenic mice expressing multiple spectral variants of GFP. *Neuron* 28:41–51.

Ferreira, P. A., Nakayama, T. A., Pak, W. L., and Travis, G. H. (1996). Cyclophilin-related protein RanBP2 acts as chaperone for red/green opsin. *Nature* 383:637–640.

Glickstein, M., and Millodot, M. (1970). Retinoscopy and eye size. *Science* 168:605–606.

Gregg, R. G., Mukhopadhyay, S., Candille, S. I., Ball, S. L., Pardue, M. T., McCall, M. A., and Peachey, N. S. (2003). Identification of the gene and the mutation responsible for the mouse nob phenotype. *Invest. Ophthalmol. Vis. Sci.* 44: 378–384.

Hayes, J. M, and Balkema, G. W. (1993). Elevated dark-adapted thresholds in hypopigmented mice measured with a water maze screening apparatus. *Behav. Genet.* 23:395–403.

Hirschhorn, J. N., and Daly, M. J. (2005). Genome-wide association studies for common diseases and complex traits. *Nat. Rev. Genet.* 6:95–108.

Ikeda, A., Naggert, J. K., and Nishina, P. M. (2002). Genetic modification of retinal degeneration in tubby mice. *Exp. Eye. Res.* 74:455–461.

John, S. W., Smith, R. S., Savinova, O. V., Hawes, N. L., Chang, B., Turnbull, D., Davisson, M., Roderick, T. H., and Heckenlively, J. R. (1998). Essential iris atrophy, pigment dispersion, and glaucoma in DBA/2J mice. *Invest. Ophthalmol. Vis. Sci.* 39: 951–962.

Keeler, C. E. (1924). The inheritance of a retinal abnormality in white mice. *Proc. Natl. Acad. Sci. U.S.A.* 10:329–333.

King, D. P., Zhao, Y., Sangoram, A. M., Wilsbacher, L. D., Tanaka, M., Antoch, M. P., Steeves, T. D., Vitaterna, M. H., Kornhauser, J. M., et al. (1997). Positional cloning of the mouse circadian *Clock* gene. *Cell* 89:641–653.

Klein, R. J., Zeiss, C., Chew, E. Y., Tsai, J. Y., Sackler, R. S., Haynes, C., Henning, A. K., SanGiovanni, J. P., Mane, S. M., et al. (2005). Complement factor H polymorphism in age-related macular degeneration. *Science* 308:385–389.

LaVail, J. H., Nixon, R. A., and Sidman, R. L. (1978). Genetic control of retinal ganglion cell projections. *J. Comp. Neurol.* 182:399–421.

LaVail, M. M. (1973). Kinetics of rod outer segment renewal in the developing mouse retina. *J. Cell Biol.* 58:650–661.

Libby, R. T., Anderson, M. G., Pang, I. H., Robinson, Z. H., Savinova, O. V., Cosma, I. M., Snow, A., Wilson, L. A., and Smith, R. S. (2005). Inherited glaucoma in DBA/2J mice: Pertinent disease features for studying the neurodegeneration. *Vis. Neurosci.* 22:637–648.

Lyubarsky, A. L., Falsini, B., Pennesi, M. E., Valentini, P., and Pugh, E. N., Jr. (1999). UV- and midwave-sensitive cone-driven retinal responses of the mouse: A possible phenotype for coexpression of cone photopigments. *J. Neurosci.* 19:442–455.

Minke, B. (1982). Light-induced reduction in excitation efficiency in the *trp* mutant of *Drosophila*. *J. Gen. Physiol.* 79:361–385.

Moser, A. R., Mattes, E. M., Dove, W. F., Lindstrom, M. J., Haag, J. D., and Gould, M. N. (1993). *ApcMin*, a mutation in the murine *Apc* gene, predisposes to mammary carcinomas and focal alveolar hyperplasias. *Proc. Natl. Acad. Sci. U.S.A.* 90: 8977–8981.

Pacione, L. R., Szego, M. J., Ikeda, S., Nishina, P. M., and McInnes, R. R. (2003). Progress toward understanding the genetic and biochemical mechanisms of inherited photoreceptor degenerations. *Annu. Rev. Neurosci.* 26:657–700.

Paigen, K. (1995). A miracle enough: The power of mice. *Nat. Med.* 1:215–220.

Pak, M. W., Giolli, R. A., Pinto, L. H., Mangini, N. J., Gregory, K. M., and Vanable, J. W., Jr. (1987). Retinopretectal and accessory optic projections of normal mice and the OKN-defective mutant mice beige, beige-J, and pearl. *J. Comp. Neurol.* 258:435–446.

Pardue, M. T., McCall, M. A., LaVail, M. M., Gregg, R. G., and Peachey, N. S. (1998). A naturally occurring mouse model of X-linked congenital stationary night blindness. *Invest. Ophthalmol. Vis. Sci.* 39:2443–2449.

Pittler, S. J., Keeler, C. E., Sidman, R. L., and Baehr, W. (1993). PCR analysis of DNA from 70-year-old sections of rodless retina demonstrates identity with the mouse *rd* defect. *Proc. Natl. Acad. Sci. U.S.A.* 90:9616–9619.

Pletcher, M. T., McClurg, P., Batalov, S., Su, A. I., Barnes, S. W., Lagler, E., Korstanje, R., Wang, X., Nusskern, D., et al. (2004). Use of a dense single nucleotide polymorphism map for in silico mapping in the mouse. *PLoS Biol.* 2:e393.

Prusky, G. T., Alam, N. M., Beekman, S., and Douglas, R. M. (2004). Rapid quantification of adult and developing mouse spatial vision using a virtual optomotor system. *Invest. Ophthalmol. Vis. Sci.* 45:4611–4616.

Prusky, G. T., and Douglas, R. M. (2004). Characterization of mouse cortical spatial vision. *Vision Res.* 44:3411–3418.

Remtulla, S., and Hallett, P. E. (1985). A schematic eye for the mouse, and comparisons with the rat. *Vision Res.* 25:21–31.

Schneuwly, S., Shortridge, R. D., Larrivee, D. C., Ono, T., Ozaki, M., and Pak, W. L. (1989). *Drosophila ninaA* gene encodes an eye-specific cyclophilin (cyclosporine A binding protein). *Proc. Natl. Acad. Sci. U.S.A.* 86:5390–5394.

Searle, A. E., and Fielder, A. R. (1990). Screening for ocular disease and visual impairment. *Curr. Opin. Ophthalmol.* 1:654–659.

Sidman, R. L., and Green, M. C. (1965). Retinal degeneration in the mouse: Location of the Rd locus in linkage group Xvii. *J. Hered.* 56:23–29.

Simpson, E. M., Linder, C. C., Sargent, E. E., Davisson, M. T., Mobraaten, L. E., and Sharp, J. J. (1997). Genetic variation among 129 substrains and its importance for targeted mutagenesis in mice. *Nat. Genet.* 16:19–27.

Stamnes, M. A., Shieh, B. H., Chuman, L., Harris, G. L., and Zuker, C. S. (1991). The cyclophilin homolog ninaA is a tissue-specific integral membrane protein required for the proper synthesis of a subset of *Drosophila* rhodopsins. *Cell* 65: 219–227.

Su, L. K., Kinzler, K. W., Vogelstein, B., Preisinger, A. C., Moser, A. R., Luongo, C., Gould, K. A., and Dove, W. F. (1992). Multiple intestinal neoplasia caused by a mutation in the murine homolog of the APC gene. *Science* 256:668–670.

Vitaterna, M. H., King, D. P., Chang, A. M., Kornhauser, J. M., Lowrey, P. L., McDonald, J. D., Dove, W. F., Pinto, L. H., Turek, F. W., et al. (1994). Mutagenesis and mapping of a mouse gene, *Clock*, essential for circadian behavior. *Science* 264:719–725.

Vitaterna, M. H., Pinto, L. H., and Takahashi, J. S. (2006). Large-scale mutagenesis and phenotypic screens for the nervous system and behavior in mice. *Trends Neurosci.* 29:233–240.

Wade, C. M., Kulbokas, E. J. III, Kirby, A. W., Zody, M. C., Mullikin, J. C., Lander, E. S., Lindblad-Toh, K., and Daly, M. J. (2002). The mosaic structure of variation in the laboratory mouse genome. *Nature* 420:574–578.

Williams, R. W., Strom, R. C., and Goldowitz, D. (1998). Natural variation in neuron number in mice is linked to a major quantitative trait locus on Chr 11. *J. Neurosci.* 18:138–146.

Wiltshire, T., Pletcher, M. T., Batalov, S., Barnes, S. W., Tarantino, L. M., Cooke, M. P., Wu, H., Smylie, K., Santrosyan, A., et al. (2003). Genome-wide single-nucleotide polymorphism analysis defines haplotype patterns in mouse. *Proc. Natl. Acad. Sci. U.S.A.* 100:3380–3385.

Yang, Z., Camp, N. J., Sun, H., Tong, Z., Gibbs, D., Cameron, D. J., Chen, H., Zhao, Y., and Pearson, E. (2006). A variant of the *HTRA1* gene increases susceptibility to age-related macular degeneration. *Science* 314:992–993.

Young, R. W. (1984). Cell death during differentiation of the retina in the mouse. *J. Comp. Neurol.* 229:362–373.

Young, R. W. (1985). Cell proliferation during postnatal development of the retina in the mouse. *Brain Res.* 353:229–239.

II OPTICS, PSYCHOPHYSICS, AND VISUAL BEHAVIORS OF MICE

5 The Mouse as a Model for Myopia, and Optics of Its Eye

FRANK SCHAEFFEL

Like a number of small mammals, mice are not predominantly "visual animals." Duke-Elder (1958, p. 639) wrote, "Mice are nocturnal in type and obviously depend visually on the appreciation of differences in luminosity and movement, rather than on the very imperfect pattern vision of which their eyes are capable." Had researchers not advanced beyond these assumptions, mice might never have been proposed as a model to study the mechanisms of myopia. As it happens, the visual control of eye growth in the mouse appears to be marginal. On the other hand, the findings from numerous knockout models and microarrays and extensive knowledge of the physiology, biochemistry, and genetics of the mouse cannot be ignored. Furthermore, spontaneous ocular mutations such as the albino locus and the p locus caught the attention of eye researchers long before knockout animals were known. These two eye color mutations represent the first gene loci that were ever mapped in vertebrates, in this case to chromosome 7. For these reasons, attempts to establish the mouse as a new model for myopia studies may be worthwhile.

How good can spatial resolution be in a mouse eye?

The eye of an adult mouse has an axial length of little more than 3 mm (Remtulla and Hallett, 1985; Schmucker and Schaeffel, 2004a). At this size, the mouse eye is comparable to the eyes of other mammals of similar weight, as illustrated in an impressive figure by A. Hughes (1977, p. 654). Hughes showed eye length versus body weight for many different vertebrates. If eye weight is scaled to body weight, the mouse eye is five times larger than the human eye. Thus, the mouse eye cannot be considered vestigial.

To focus an image of the environment onto the retina of a mouse eye, the refractive power of cornea and lens must be more than 500 diopters (D) in air (a third of power is lost because the backside of the eye's optics is, as in all vertebrate eyes, filled with water-like fluid). Because of this high power, a refractive error of a few diopters—most disturbing for humans, who have only about 60 D of total power in the eye—is not so relevant for the mouse. For the same reason, small imperfections in the optics of the mouse eye are less important than in the human eye.

Even if optically optimal, small vertebrate eyes generally have lower visual acuity (Kirschfeld, 1984). This is because the image projected onto the retina is proportionally smaller. To sample the fine details in a tiny image, the sampling units—the photoreceptors—should also be proportionally smaller. However, this is not possible, for physical reasons: when photoreceptor diameters approach the range of the wavelength of light, "optical crosstalk" between receptors occurs since light energy "leaks out" (Kirschfeld and Snyder, 1976). This phenomenon limits further increase in sampling density. Probably for this reason, vertebrate photoreceptors are not thinner than about 1 μm—two times the wavelength of visible light.

In a human eye, 1° of the visual field maps on 0.29 mm linear distance on the retina. In a 28-day-old mouse, the image magnification is only a tenth (0.03 mm/deg). Accordingly, even with the best possible optics, a mouse eye can achieve only a tenth of the human eye's spatial resolution. As shown in chapter 7 in this volume, the spatial resolution of the mouse eye is even lower, by almost another factor of 10, in part as a result of optical aberrations but mainly because of the large photoreceptor diameters (>2–3 μm; Carter-Dawson and LaVail, 1979) and neuronal spatial processing (de la Cera et al., 2006). Given this poor visual acuity, it seems likely that emmetropization (the developmental matching of axial eye length to the focal length of the optics) may not be as precise as in some birds or primates that have high visual acuity and are, in part, not limited by ocular optical aberrations but rather by physics—the diffraction of light.

Schematic eye modeling

The first schematic eye for the adult C57B1/6J mouse was presented by Remtulla and Hallett in 1985. It was developed based on frozen sections of 14 eyes of 20- to 23-week-old animals. Schmucker and Schaeffel (2004a) developed a paraxial schematic eye model for C57BL/6J mice at different ages, also based on frozen sections (figure 5.1). Although frozen sections have limited resolution because of the distortions that can occur during freezing and sectioning, it is possible to average measurements from several eyes and to

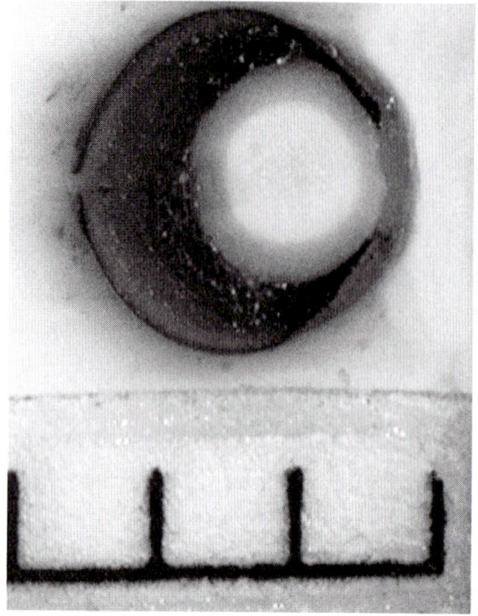
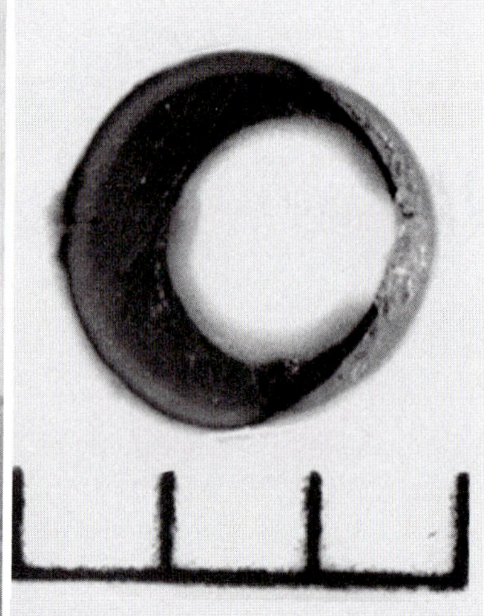

Figure 5.1 Frozen sections of mouse eyes at age 26 and 44 days. (Replotted from Schmucker and Schaeffel, 2004a.) The overproportional growth of the lens reduces the depth of the vitreous chamber with age. Such large lenses make it unlikely that accommodation is present in the eye, because these lenses cannot be easily deformed. Note the relative thickness of the retina, which should give rise to a large "small eye artifact" in retinoscopic measurements (Glickstein and Millodot, 1970). Scale bars denote millimeters.

fit the biometrical data from different ages by polynomials. The averaging procedure reduces the impact of measurement variability, and a few general statements can be made about the optics of the mouse eye:

1. In line with an observation by Zhou and Williams (1999), the eyes grow linearly over the first 100 days, with no signs of saturation. Axial length increases from 3.0 mm at 22 days of age, by 4.4 μm/day.

2. Interestingly, because the lens increases in thickness from 1.74 mm at 22 days of age by 5.5 μm/day, the vitreous chamber actually declines in depth from 0.83 mm at 22 days, by 3.2 μm/day.

3. A recent study using video photokeratometry in *Egr-1* −/− mice and their wild-type littermates (Schippert et al., 2007) showed that the corneal radius of curvature increases from 1.35 mm to 1.53 mm from day 22 to 100.

4. To make a mouse eye more myopic by 1 D, axial length must be increased by 5.41 μm at the age of 22 days and by 6.49 μm at the age of 100 days.

5. Retinal image magnification increases from 0.032 mm/deg at 22 days to 0.034 mm/deg at 100 days.

6. As in other animals (e.g., chicken: Schaeffel et al., 1986; barn owl: Schaeffel and Wagner, 1996), the retinal image brightness increases with age. Image brightness is proportional to the inverse squared f-number, the ratio of anterior focal length to pupil size. Typical for humans are f-numbers around 5 (for a 3.3-mm pupil), but for the mouse, the f-number is 1.02 already at day 22. This produces a 25 times brighter retinal image than in humans. Until the age of 100 days, the f-number in mouse declines even further, to about 0.92, providing another 20% more brightness. Even owls do not have such a low f-number (1.13; Schaeffel and Wagner, 1996). The mouse probably has one of the brightest retinal images among vertebrates.

7. The thickness of the retina, relative to axial length (which increases from 0.178 mm at 22 days of age, by 0.6 μm/day), should give rise to a large difference in the position of the photoreceptor layer and of the light reflecting layer(s) in retinoscopy—resulting in large amounts of apparently measured hyperopia (the "small eye artifact"; Glickstein and Millodot, 1970). From the schematic eye, the small eye artifact was calculated to more than 30 D (Schmucker and Schaeffel, 2004a). Since infrared photorefraction and even streak retinoscopy did not show such large amounts of hyperopia, either mice must be myopic (but see the discussion of behavioral depth-of-field measurements in the next section) or the light-reflecting layer(s) is (are) not at the vitreoretinal interface but rather deeper in the retina.

New techniques to measure optical parameters in very small eyes like the mouse's

To study the mechanisms of visual control of eye growth and myopia in a mouse, optical parameters of the eye must be measured in vivo. Standard optometric techniques generally fail, owing to the tiny size of the eye.

Infrared Photoretinoscopy First, refractive state must be determined. In a number of previous studies, this was done by white light streak retinoscopy (e.g., Drager, 1975;

Remtulla and Hallett, 1985; Beuerman et al., 2003; Tejedor and de la Villa, 2003). In streak retinoscopy, a slightly defocused light streak is projected onto the eye from the retinoscope, which is held at about arm's length distance from the subject, the mouse. A small fraction of this light is reflected from the back of the eye, the fundus, and is visible in the pupil. The movement of the reflection in the pupil is compared to the movement of the light streak on the fur surrounding the eye as the streak retinoscope is titled up and down. If the reflection in the pupil appears stationary with no clear direction of movement, the "reversal point" is reached, where the eye is assumed to be in focus with the observer. Otherwise, trial lenses of different power are held in front of the eye until the reversal point is reached, and the lens power then provides the information about refractive state. The procedure works well in animals with large pupils, but it is very difficult to judge the direction of the movement of the light bar in small pupils (1 mm in diameter, or smaller if the pupil constricts due to the white light emitted by the retinoscope). In a trial carried out by a certified optometrist, no correlation could be found between streak retinoscopy and infrared photoretinoscopy in 52 alert, noncyclopleged mouse eyes (refraction measured with streak retinoscopy = 0.276 × refraction measured with infrared [IR] photoretinoscopy + 15.988, $R^2 = 0.047$; Schmucker, 2004). The range of refractions measured with IR photoretinoscopy was from +2 and +12 D, but the values obtained with streak retinoscopy ranged between +12 and +22 D. As can be seen, streak retinoscopy also provides considerably more hyperopic readings than IR photoretinoscopy. High hyperopia was also found in other studies using streak retinoscopy (+20 D: Drager, 1975; +13.5 D: Tejedor and de la Villa, 2003; +15 D: Beuerman et al., 2003).

A more powerful technique for refracting small vertebrates may be IR photoretinoscopy. This technique is video-based, uses IR light, and has been successfully applied in a variety of vertebrate eyes (e.g., toads and tadpoles: Mathis et al., 1988; frogs and salamanders: Schaeffel et al., 1994; water snakes: Schaeffel and Mathis, 1991; barn owls: Schaeffel and Wagner, 1996). Because IR light is used, the animal is not disturbed by the measurement and the pupil does not constrict. To measure a mouse, it is sufficient to slightly restrain it by holding its tail while it rests on a small platform. An IR-sensitive video camera is positioned at about 60 cm distance. Attached to the camera lens is an arrangement of IR light-emitting diodes (IR LEDs; figure 5.2*A*, *white arrow* at top right). A small fraction of this light enters the pupil, is diffusely reflected from the fundus of the eye, and returns to the camera. Because the IR LEDs are positioned directly below the camera aperture, they produce a brightly illuminated pupil, like the red eye effect seen with flash cameras. Furthermore, the brightness distribution in the vertical pupil meridian displays a gradient, with more light in the top in the case of a hyperopic eye (figure 5.2*A*) and more light in the bottom in a myopic eye (figure 5.2*B*). The measured brightness profiles are shown to the right of the pupils in figures 5.2*A* and 5.2*B*, together with a linear regression line fit through the pixel brightness values (*arrows* in the figures). The refractions can be determined from the slopes of these regression lines. The only unknown variable then is the conversion factor from slope of the brightness profile in the pupil into refraction. This factor can be determined by placing trial lenses of known optical power in front of the mouse eye, inducing known refractive errors, and recording the slopes (Schaeffel et al., 2004). The temporal sampling rate of this technique is determined by the video frame rate (analogue cameras: 25 Hz [PAL] or 30 Hz [NTSC], and 30 Hz or more with firewire cameras). As soon as the mouse eye appears in the video frame, the image-processing software detects the pupil—which is a simple task, because it is brightly illuminated over a dark background—and fits a linear regression through the pixel brightness values in the vertical pupil meridian.

Even though the measurements are easy to perform, some limitations have to be considered: (1) Because of the excavation of the optic disc (nicely visible in the frozen section of the mouse eye presented by Remtulla and Hallett, 1985), the eye is more myopic (or less hyperopic) close to the pupillary axis and appears considerably more hyperopic in the periphery due to the thickness of the retina (Schaeffel et al., 2004). Therefore, for consistent refractions, it is important to align the eye with the camera axis. (2) Mice sometimes change their refractive state for a few seconds and become a few diopters more myopic. The mechanism behind this optical change has not yet been systematically studied, but it is clear that it occurs without visual stimulation and most likely is not accommodation. It was also observed under cycloplegia with tropicamide (Schaeffel et al., 2004), and Woolf (1956) was unable to find a ciliary muscle for accommodation in the mouse eye. Also, Smith et al. (2002) state that the ciliary muscle in the mouse eye is weak and accommodation lacking. An alternative explanation for this change in refraction is that it is produced by the activity of the retractor bulbi muscles (Lorente de No, 1933; Pachter et al., 1976), which can pull the globe back into the orbit, causing a temporary change in intraocular pressure that, in turn, could affect refractive state. Therefore, it is important to observe mice for several seconds to ensure their eyes are in relaxed condition. (3) Mice were measured more hyperopic when they had larger pupils (about 0.9 D more hyperopia per 0.1 mm increase in pupil size; Schaeffel et al., 2004). This effect could result from negative spherical aberration (more hyperopic refractions in the pupil periphery). On the other hand, positive spherical aberration was found in mouse eyes by Hartmann-Shack aberrometry (de la Cera et al., 2006), and it is more likely that the increasing hyperopia results from non-

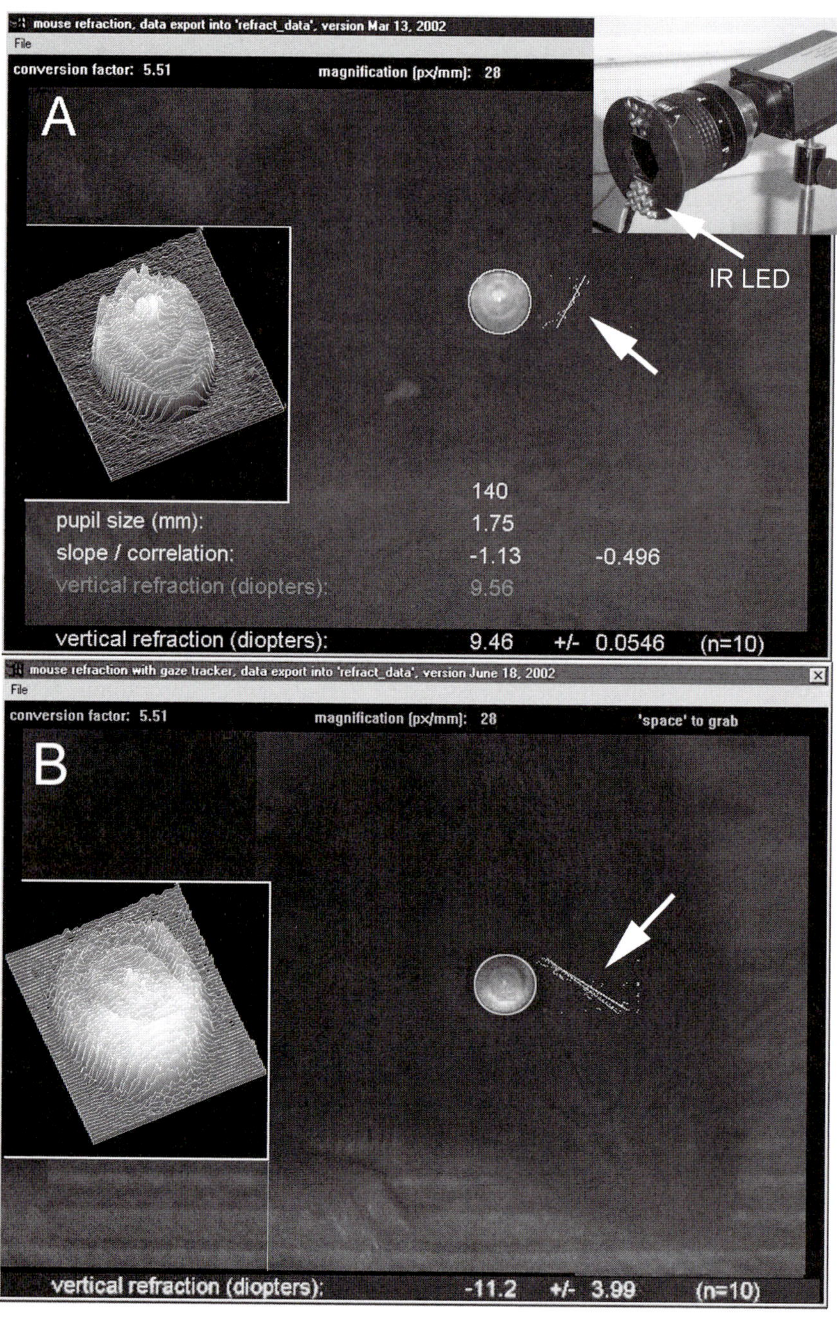

FIGURE 5.2 Infrared photorefraction in alert mice. *A*, Hyperopic eye. *B*, Myopic eye. The IR LED arrangement (*A*, *inset*, *white arrow*) causes brightly illuminated pupils. The brightness gradient in the vertical pupil meridian can be fit by linear regression (*white lines* indicated by *arrow* to right of pupil). Calibration with trial lenses showed that the slopes of the regression lines are linearly related to refractive error of the eye. The brightness distributions in the pupils (see 3D brightness profile of the pupil, *left*, and brightness profile, *right*) are quite heterogeneous in eyes with poor optics, such as in the mouse, but smooth in eyes with high optical quality, such as in humans (not shown). (Replotted from Schaeffel et al., 2004.)

linearities in the video system. Larger pupils return more light, proportional to pupil area, and pixel values are not perfectly log-linear to the absolute brightness. A more extensive calibration with different camera aperture sizes would be necessary to control for this factor. The standard deviation typically obtained in the same eyes on repeated measurement was about 2.7 D (Schaeffel et al., 2004)—much less than the optical depth of focus.

PHOTOKERATOMETRY The corneal surface is the optically most powerful surface of the eye—in most vertebrates it generates more than 60% of the total optical power.

Therefore, it is important to measure its radius of curvature. This can be done by IR photokeratometry in alert mice. Mice are placed on a platform (figure 5.3*A*, *white arrow*) and slightly restrained by holding their tail. The platform is positioned about 15 cm from a metal ring with a diameter of 300 mm that carries eight IR LEDs (figure 5.3*A*). The reflections of the IR LEDs on the corneal surface, the first Purkinje images, are also arranged in a circular pattern (figure 5.3*B*). In a digital video image of the eye, the reflections can be detected by an image-processing program and fit by a circle in real time (at 25–60 Hz, depending on the hardware platform). The diameter of the fitted circle is proportional to the curvature of the cornea—small circles for steep corneas with small radius of curvature and larger circles for flat corneas. Although the equations to calculate corneal curvature from camera distance, distance of the IR LEDs of the keratometer, distance of the keratometer to the mouse, and camera magnification have been worked out (Howland and Sayles, 1985), it is easier just to measure a few ball bearings with a known radius of curvature (figure 5.3*C*) and extrapolate to the corneal radius of curvature of the animal under study. The standard deviation of this procedure is about 1%, with the major source of variability the depth of focus of the video camera. The video camera depth of field ultimatively determines how precisely the distance of the mouse to the keratometer and the camera are controlled.

Low-Coherence Interferometry Perhaps the most important variable in myopia studies is axial length. Human myopia is axial in most cases (Curtin, 1985), which means that the eye is growing too long in the anteroposterior axis compared to an eye of an emmetropic control group. In a few cases myopia develops because the refractive power of the lens increases (e.g., when diabetes or cataract develops),

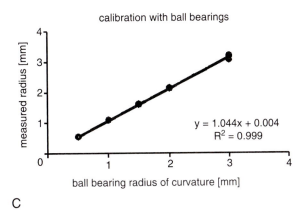

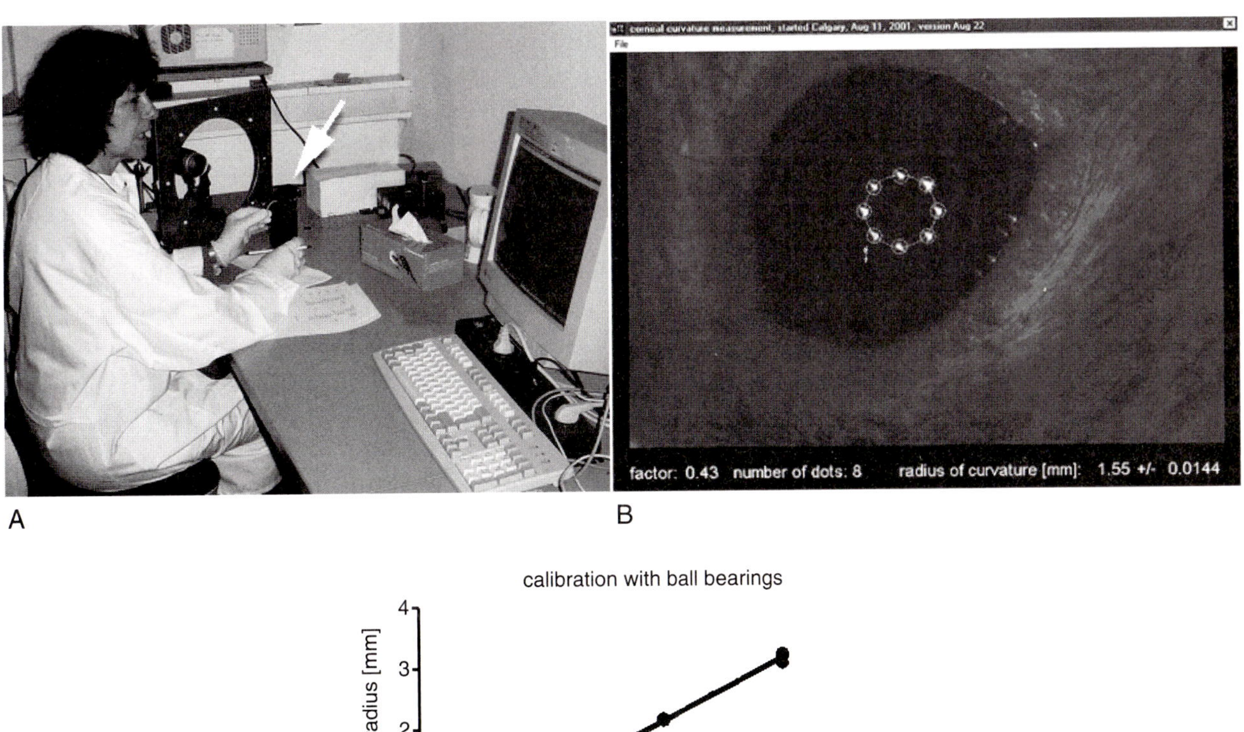

Figure 5.3 Infrared photokeratometry. *A*, The alert mouse is positioned on a wooden platform and is slightly restrained by the tester holding its tail (*white arrow*). The block is slowly moved back and forth until the reflections from eight IR LEDs are visible in a highly magnified video image of the eye (*B*). Once the first Purkinje images are in focus, the software detects their centers and fits a circle through them. This occurs at a video frequency between 25 and 60 Hz, depending on the hardware. The high-speed measurements also provide the current standard deviations of the radii. The diameter of this circle is proportional to the curvature of the cornea. *C*, The calibration factor can be determined by comparing the measured radius to the radius of ball bearings.

and this is referred to as refractive myopia (Curtin, 1985). The type of myopia that is experimentally induced in animal models is almost always axial.

Therefore, the first question is about the axial length changes. Several attempts have been made to measure axial eye lengths in mice using various techniques, such as video imaging of freshly enucleated eyes (Fernandes et al., 2004; Schaeffel et al., 2004), analysis of histological sections of eyes (Tejedor and de la Villa, 2003), highly enlarged photographs of frozen sections (Schmucker and Schaeffel, 2004a), and eye weight measurements (Zhou and Williams, 1999). All techniques could be used only post-mortem, and all probably have insufficient resolution to show that experimentally induced myopia is, in fact, axial. Attempts to measure axial eye length in vivo with A-scan ultrasonography (which is typically used in other animal models of myopia) failed in the mouse (Schaeffel, et al., 2004). The curvature of the cornea is so steep that little sound energy can be transmitted into the eye when the sound transducer is placed on the cornea; also, sound waves are focused at about 20 mm distance from the transducer. A water-filled rubber tube is attached to the transducer to mimic a longer eye if short, nonhuman eyes are measured (Schaeffel and Howland, 1991), but this procedure was not successful in mouse eyes. A major advance came when a commercial low-coherence interferometer was adapted to measure short-range optical distances. The goal was to measure corneal thickness and anterior chamber depth in humans (the Carl Zeiss AC Master [www.meditec.zeiss.com/], Jena, Germany; figure 5.4). A test showed that this device was also able to measure the intraocular distances in living mouse eyes (Schmucker and Schaeffel, 2004b). Unfortunately, Zeiss decided not to market the AC Master, so that only prototypes are currently used in a few laboratories.

The optical principle of low-coherence interferometry is based on a Michelson interferometer. A low-coherence superluminescent laser diode (SLD) that emits IR light with a peak emission at 850 nm and a half-bandwidth of 10 nm serves as light source. As a result of the broadened bandwidth, the coherence length is rather short (about 10 μm), compared to standard laser diodes, in which it is about 160 μm. The IR laser beam emerging from the LED is divided into two perpendicular beams via a semisilvered mirror. One part is transmitted through the semisilvered mirror and reaches a stationary mirror. The other part reaches a second mirror that can be moved along the light path with high positional precision. After reflecting from the mirrors, the two coaxial beams propagate to the eye, where they are reflected off the cornea, the lens, and the fundal layers. Interference between beams can occur only when their optical path lengths are matched with extreme precision, within the coherence length. The occurrence of interference is detected by a photocell and recorded as a function of the displacement of the movable mirror. Because of the coaxial beams, the measurements are largely insensitive against longitudinal eye movements. The scanning time of the movable mirror is about 0.3 s. In the human eye, a measurement precision in the range of 2 μm has been achieved in corneal thickness measurements, and a precision of 5–10 μm has been achieved for the anterior chamber depth and lens thickness measurements (R. Bergner, pers. comm., 2004). On repeated measurement of mouse eyes, a standard

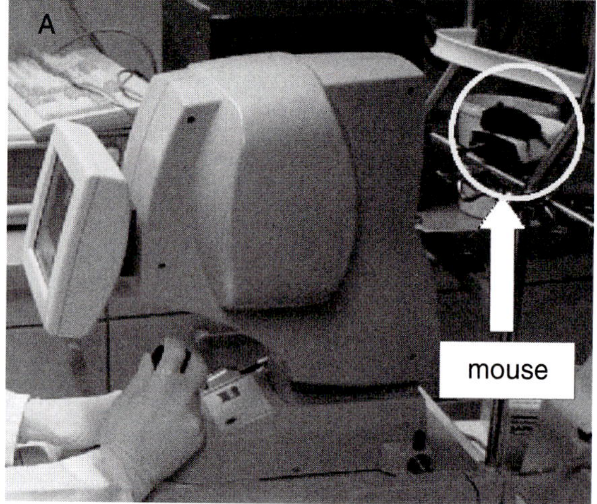

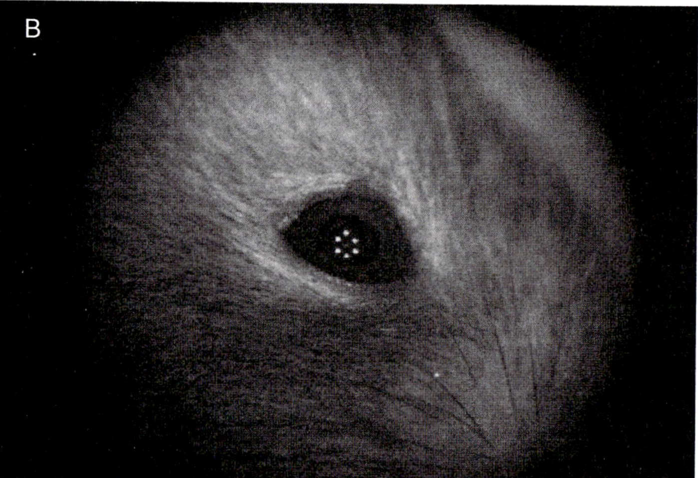

Figure 5.4 The AC Master during measurements of a mouse eye. *A*, The slightly anesthetized mouse, positioned on an adjustable platform attached to the chin rest of the device, is encircled. *B*, Close-up view used to adjust the eye in the measurement beam. The first Purkinje images of six infrared LEDs, built into the device, are used to align the eye. (Replotted from Schmucker and Schaeffel, 2004b.)

deviation of 8 µm was found for axial length, equivalent to less than 2 D (Schmucker and Schaeffel, 2004b).

This technique measures optical path lengths, which need to be converted into geometrical path lengths. The conversion requires that the refractive indices for the ocular media be known. The problem has been analyzed by Schmucker and Schaeffel (2004b). The errors are generally small even if the refractive indices are not exactly known. Also, in most cases, the differences of interest are those between the treated and control eyes, rather than absolute axial lengths.

Measurements of the Optical Aberrations of the Mouse Eye with a Custom-Built Hartmann-Shack Sensor Given the low spatial acuity of the mouse (see chapter 7 in this volume), the question arises as to whether visual acuity is limited by optics or by neural factors, such as the pooling of photoreceptor signals. New optical techniques have recently been developed to describe the optical quality of the human eye in vivo. Perhaps the most successful technique currently used, Hartmann-Shack aberrometry, has been adapted for measurements in mice (de la Cera et al., 2006). For Hartmann-Shack measurements, an SLD at 676 nm produces a bright spot on the retina. A fraction of the light is reflected from the fundus and returns from the eye through the pupil. This light reaches a microlens array of 65 × 65 square lenslets with a 400 µm aperture and a focal length of 24 mm. The lenslets create a pattern of focal spots on a CCD chip of a video camera. If an eye has no aberrations and is focused at infinity, the spot pattern is perfectly regular, and each of the foci is exactly along the optical axes of the lenslets. However, if the wavefront is distorted due to optical aberrations in cornea and lens, the focal spots are laterally displaced and form irregular patterns (figure 5.5; the left columns show the original Hartmann-Shack images). The displacement of each of the foci is proportional to the tilt of

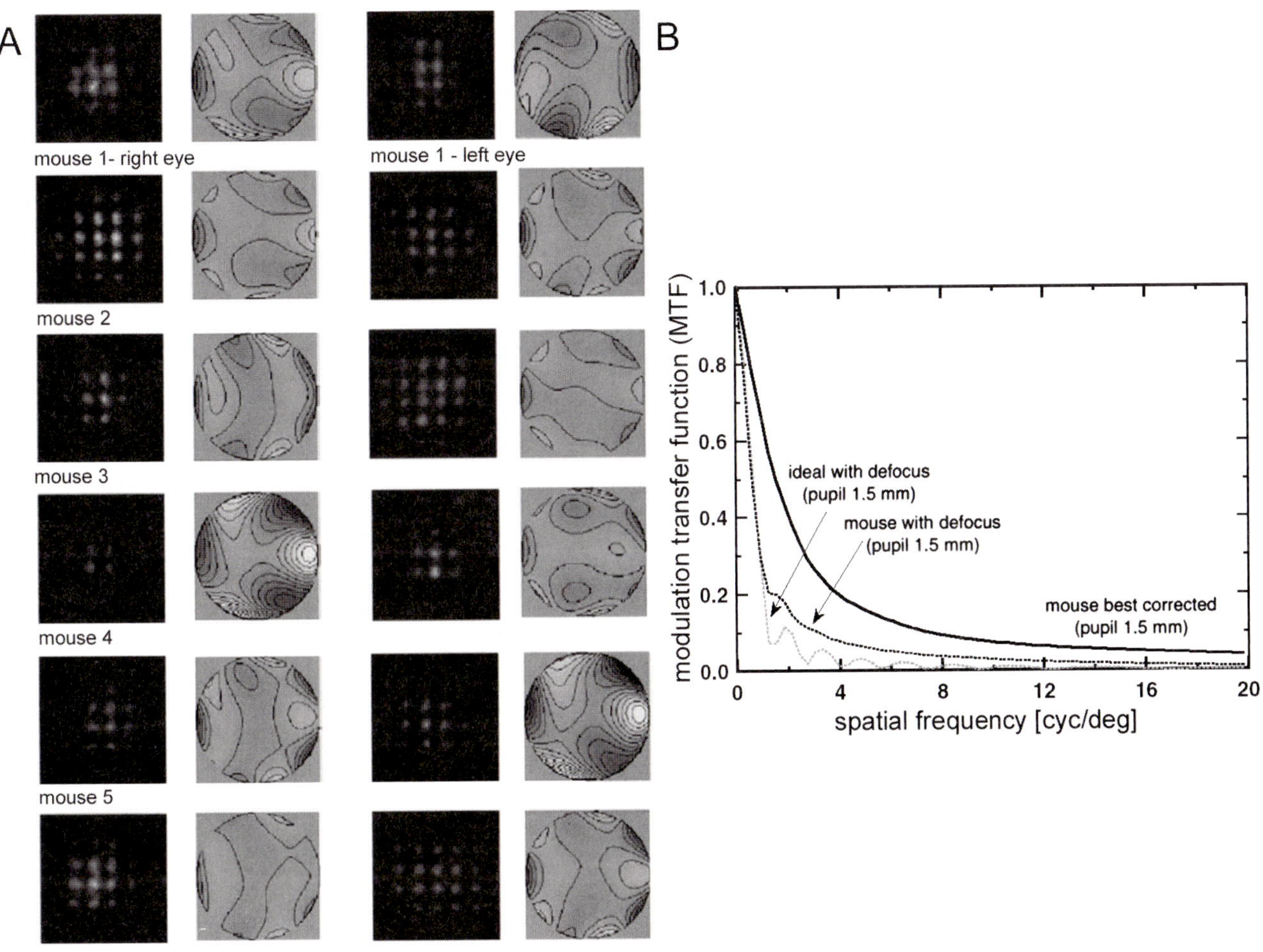

Figure 5.5 *A*, Original Hartmann-Shack images, and reconstructions of the wavefronts recorded from 12 eyes of alert mice. Wave aberration maps are for the third- and higher-order aberrations, and contour lines are plotted in 0.1 µm steps. *B*, Calculations of the average modulation transfer functions of the mouse eyes. The contrast transfer drops off steeply with increasing spatial frequency, but the contrast transfer is still around 20% at 4 c/deg. (Replotted from de la Cera et al., 2006.)

the wavefront at the respective position. To reconstruct the three-dimensional shape of the wavefront, the centers of the focal spots are detected by image-processing software—a demanding task if they are as diffuse, as shown in figure 5.5A (de la Cera et al., 2006). The shape of the wavefront is typically described as a polynomial expansion, as proposed by Zernike. The coefficients describe the magnitude of known optical aberrations, such as defocus, astigmatism, spherical aberration, and so on. In the mouse, defocus was the most dominant aberration (average hyperopia +10.12 ± 1.41 D), but astigmatism (3.64 ± 3.7 D) and positive spherical aberration (wavefront error 0.15 ± 0.07 μm for a 1.5-mm pupil) were also highly significant.

The Zernike coefficients also permit the calculation of how much contrast the optics of the eye transfers at the different spatial frequencies. The transfer function is called modulation transfer function. The mouse eye's optics transfers about 20% of the contrast at 4 c/deg (see figure 5.5). Compared to the behavioral limit of spatial resolution of the mouse at around 0.5 c/deg, it is unlikely that the optics of the eye are the limiting factor for visual acuity in mice.

It turned out that alert mice could be accurately positioned for Hartmann-Shack aberrometry by holding their tails, moving the platform, and waiting until they calmed down. They did not close their eyes as chickens do. Attempts were also made to obtain measurements under anesthesia. However, the optical quality of the eyes was then much poorer (de la Cera et al., 2006). This could explain why such low optical quality was described in rodent eyes in a previous study in mouse and rat (Artal et al., 1998).

Depth of focus: Optical and behavioral measurements

Remtulla and Hallett (1985) estimated the depth of field of the mouse as large as ±56 D, based on photoreceptor diameters and using the equations provided by Green et al. (1980). But they also stated that this number may be unrealistic. They noted that behavioral visual acuity may be five times higher, as calculated from anatomical variables (Birch and Jacobs, 1979), and finally estimated the depth of field as ±11 D.

Recently, aberrometric techniques have permitted more direct estimations of the optical depth of field. De la Cera et al. (2006) calculated the contrast transfer (modulation) of the mouse optics for a sine wave grating of 2 c/deg, at different amounts of defocus. The modulation drops to 50% at about 5 D of defocus (figure 5.6*A*). But since the spatial acuity of the mouse is only about one-fourth of this value in behavioral studies, the depth of field must accordingly be several times larger. Optomotor responses elicited by drifting 0.03 c/deg square wave gratings were measured in mice wearing trial lenses. They showed significant responses with up to at least ±10 D of imposed defocus (figure 5.6*B*). In summary, the depth of field in the mouse must be larger than ±10 D, and this suggests that neither accommodation nor precise emmetropization is very important for the mouse.

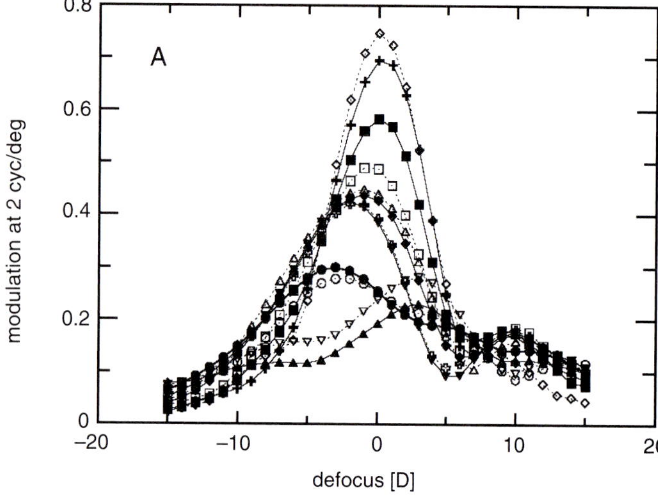

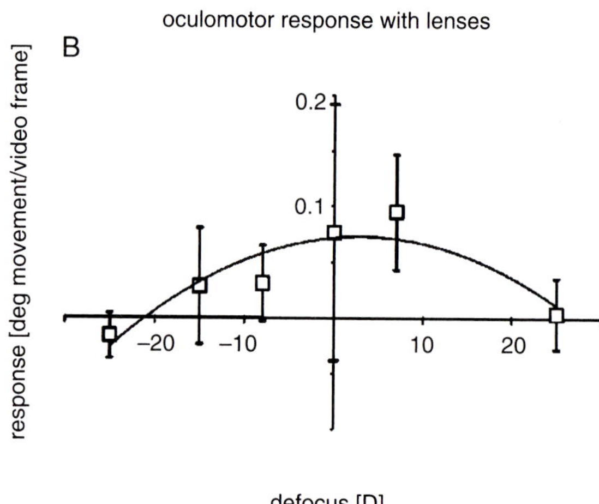

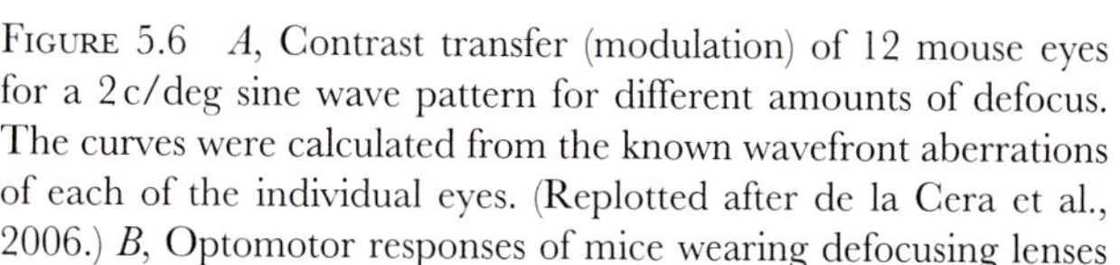

FIGURE 5.6 *A*, Contrast transfer (modulation) of 12 mouse eyes for a 2 c/deg sine wave pattern for different amounts of defocus. The curves were calculated from the known wavefront aberrations of each of the individual eyes. (Replotted after de la Cera et al., 2006.) *B*, Optomotor responses of mice wearing defocusing lenses in front of both eyes. The optomotor response was elicited by a drifting 0.03 c/deg square wave pattern. Significant responses could be elicited with at least ±10 D of defocus. (Replotted from Schmucker and Schaeffel, 2006.)

Spatial vision at different illuminances and the contribution of rods and cones

It could be expected from the extremely bright retinal images that mice have good spatial vision also at low ambient illuminances. However, optomotor experiments in an automated optomotor drum suggested that this is not the case. In these experiments, individual mice were placed in a small perspex drum in the center of a larger drum that was rotated with vertical square wave patterns of adjustable fundamental spatial frequency (figure 5.7). Their movements were recorded from above by a small surveillance video camera. Movement analysis was fully automated. Both the angular movement of the center of mass of the mouse and angular changes in the orientation of the body axis were tracked by image-processing software and automatically statistically analyzed. Even though the mice often ignored the visual stimuli when they cleaned themselves, the objective video tracking procedure produced statistically meaningful results. An advantage of the procedure is that the mice experienced no further behavioral restriction, causing little stress. Disadvantages are that the "whole body optomotor response" is less reliable than the eye (Faulstich et al., 2006) or head (Abdeljalil et al., 2005) optomotor response, and the data are therefore more noisy. In yet other studies, whole animal body movements were also evaluated, but in this case they were subjectively judged. A "virtual drum" was used that permitted better control of the stimulus variables (Prusky et al., 2004, 2006; Douglas et al., 2005; see also descriptions of these techniques in chapter 7 in this volume). Finally, optomotor experiments measure "visual acuity" of the extracortical accessory optic system, which may be different from cortically processed acuity for stationary targets. Nevertheless, in the mouse, there is no indication that the two types of acuity are particularly different (Prusky and Douglas, 2004).

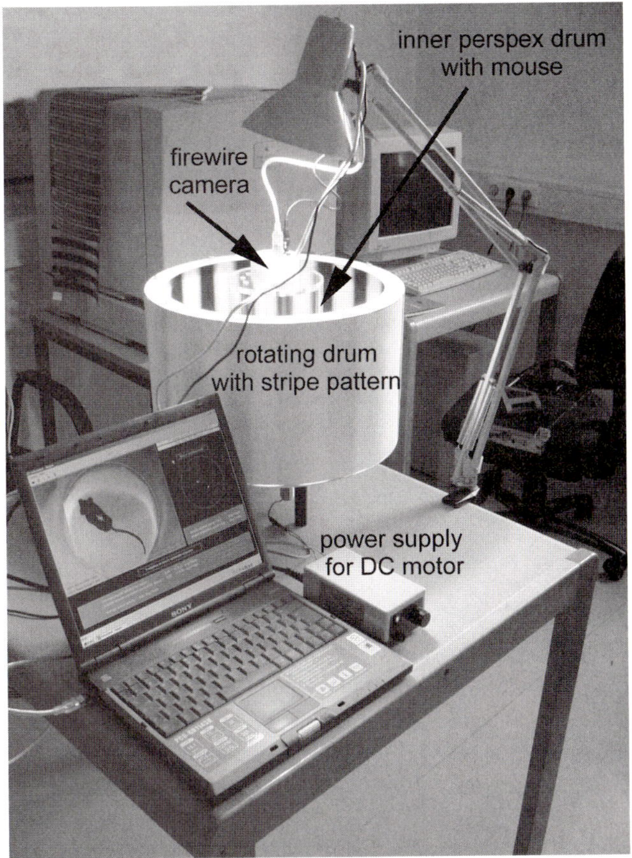

FIGURE 5.7 Automated optomotor drum. The mouse is placed in a small inner perspex drum in the center of a larger drum that is covered inside with the square wave stripe pattern (*long black arrow*). The large drum is mechanically rotated by a DC motor. Both the center of mass of the mouse and the angular orientation of its body axis are automatically tracked by a video system (*short black arrow*: small surveillance firewire camera that images the mouse; see also the screen of the laptop). The net angular movement is statistically evaluated and compared to the direction of movement of the stripe pattern. (From Schmucker et al., 2005.)

The automated version of the "whole body optomotor analysis" used by Schmucker et al. (2005) provided some new results:

1. Grating acuity reached its limit at about 0.4–0.5 c/deg, slightly less than in other behavioral techniques (see chapter 7 in this volume).
2. It declined continuously when the illuminance (or luminance) was reduced: the "relative responses" were 100% at 400 lux (about 30 cd/m^2), 76% at 40 lux (about 0.1 cd/m^2), and 46% at 4 lux (about 0.005 cd/m^2). A similar decline was not observed in an older study in the hooded rat (Birch and Jacobs, 1979), where grating acuity at 1.2 c/deg remained similar between 3.4 and 0.0034 cd/m^2 in a three-choice discrimination apparatus. On the other hand, a 2005 study in mice found an increase in spatial acuity with higher illuminances (Abdeljalil et al., 2005).
3. An optomotor analysis of mutant mice lacking rods or cones, or both, showed reduced visual acuity in cone-only models (0.10 c/deg in *Rho–/–* and 0.20 c/deg in *CNGB1–/–*, compared to 0.30 c/deg in C57BL/6 wild-type mice). The "all-rod mouse" (*CNGA3–/–*) performed similarly on the optomotor test as the wild-type mouse, under both photopic and scotopic conditions. This observation suggests that the rod system is not saturated, even at illuminances of 400 lux (about 30 cd/m^2). It should also be kept in mind that rods represent about 95% of the photoreceptors in most vertebrates (Sterling, 2003), including the mouse. Since the remaining 5% of cones are not clustered in a fovea but are more evenly distributed across the retina, they may not reach a sampling density necessary for good spatial vision. In mice without any functional photoreceptors (*CNGA3 –/–*,

Rho −/−), no optomotor response could be elicited, suggesting that the light-sensitive, melanopsin-containing ganglion cells do not contribute to spatial vision.

Induction of refractive errors by frosted diffusers or spectacle lenses

The large depth of field and the relatively low visual acuity of the mouse suggest that retinal image degradation must become quite severe before it is detectable for the retina, and before it can potentially trigger changes in eye growth.

Deprivation Myopia Induced by Hemispherical Plastic Diffusers Glued to the Fur around the Eye Deprivation myopia refers to the type of myopia that develops by default when the retinal image clarity is experimentally degraded. Studies on the regulation of the retinal mRNA of *Egr-1* by light and retinal image contrast in mice showed surprisingly high sensitivity to the changes in retinal image contrast, despite their low acuity and large depth of field. Even if the retinal illumination was matched in the fellow eye by using neutral density filters that had similar light attenuation as the diffusers, the minor difference in image contrast had clear effects on *Egr-1* mRNA concentrations in the retina (Brand et al., 2005). Furthermore, a microarray analysis of gene expression under the same visual stimulation conditions showed surprisingly clear transcription changes of a number of genes (Brand et al., 2007). This shows that even minor differences in image contrast were detected. If eye growth were as tightly regulated by vision as in other animal models, like chicken (Wallman et al., 1978), tree shrew (Norton, 1990), guinea pig (Howlett and McFadden, 2006), or rhesus monkey (Wiesel and Raviola, 1977), the image degradation imposed by the diffusers should have been sufficient to produce deprivation myopia also in the mouse. Unfortunately, this standard treatment was not very effective even when extended to 2 weeks (Schaeffel and Burkhardt, 2002; Schaeffel et al., 2004) or even 8 weeks (Fernandes et al., 2004). There was a significant myopic shift in refraction when data from many animals were pooled, but it was quite small compared to the total power of the eyes—only about 4–5 D (Fernandes et al., 2004; Schaeffel et al., 2004). More reliable effects and fewer ocular side effects, such as inflammation, were described if the diffusers were not glued to the fur but rather were attached to head-mounted pedestals (Faulkner et al., 2007b).

The large variability in the diffuser experiments cannot be explained by poor measurement resolution; it must result from low sensitivity of the emmetropization mechanism to changes in visual experience, and from the fact that axial eye growth is rather slow in mice (Schaeffel et al. 2004). Somehow, one might expect poor responsiveness due to the large depth of focus (more than ±10 D). But then it remains unclear why the variability of the refractions among untreated animals is considerably less than the depth of focus (about ±3 D: Schaeffel et al., 2004; or even less, ±1.14 D: de la Cera et al., 2006). This raises the question as to what keeps the refractions in such close range when emmetropization is so insensitive to visual input.

Deprivation Myopia from Lid Suture Lid suture seems to be more effective in producing deprivation myopia. Both Tejedor and de la Villa (2003) and Beuerman et al. (2003) found significant changes in axial eye growth and refraction with lid suture for 20 days or 4 weeks, respectively. However, in those cases, nonvisual effects on eye growth could be excluded, such as increased mechanical pressure on the globe, which might cause a rebound effect after lid reopening, or changes in the metabolic conditions due to reduced oxygen supply or elevated ocular temperature. Another complication is that the changes in refraction were not well predicted by the changes in axial length (Beuerman et al., 2003; Tejedor and de la Villa, 2003), using the schematic eye by Remtulla and Hallett (Schaeffel and Howland, 2003).

Attempts to Induce Refractive Errors by Spectacle Lenses A few studies have been performed in mice with spectacle lenses. Although Beuerman et al. (2003) induced myopia and considerable axial elongation by 8 weeks of treatment with −10 D contact lenses glued to fur around the eye, no consistent effect on eye growth could be observed in another study in which +15 D or −15 D spectacle lenses were attached to the fur for 2 weeks (Burkhardt and Schaeffel, 2006). In chicken (Bitzer and Schaeffel, 2002) and monkey retina (Zhong et al., 2004), the expression of the transcription factor *ZENK* (or *Egr-1* in mammals) is controlled by the sign of imposed defocus. Such a sign of defocus-dependent regulation of *Egr-1* was not (yet) observed in the mouse retina (Burkhardt and Schaeffel, 2006).

Effects of Continuous Light on Refractive Development Continuous light rearing, which causes severe flattening of the cornea and large hyperopic refractive errors in chickens (Li et al., 2000), had no effect on corneal curvature in C57BL/6 mice. After 37 days in continuous white light with about 500 lux ambient illuminance, corneal radius was 1.42 ± 0.04 mm (n = 25 eyes), versus 1.401 ± 0.05 mm (n = 20 eyes) in animals kept under a regular 12/12 hour light/dark cycle. There were significant differences in refraction (+3.11 ± 3.60, n = 40, vs. +6.36 ± 4.29, n = 51; $P < 0.001$), but these small changes were in the opposite direction as in chickens (Howland and Schaeffel, 2004).

Other Differences between the Chicken and the Mouse Glucagon, released from glucagon-containing amacrine cells, seems to act as a stop signal for eye growth in chickens (Feldkaemper et al., 2004; Vessey et al., 2005). Glucagon amacrine cells also express *ZENK* in a sign of defocus-dependent fashion. Unfortunately, this type of glucagon-containing amacrine cells could not be found in mouse retina (Mathis and Schaeffel, 2007) or in monkey retina (Zhong et al., 2004), even though the glucagon receptor was detected in the mouse retina (Feldkaemper et al., 2004). These observations suggest that biochemical differences between birds and mammals may exist in the retinal signaling cascade for the visual control of eye growth.

Refractive errors in knockout mouse models, and experiments with drugs

Few data have been published on the refractive errors of knockout mouse models. Schippert et al. (2007) found that mice lacking a functional gene for the transcription factor *Egr-1* were more myopic than their heterozygous and wild-type littermates. The homozygous knockout animals also had significantly longer eyes, but they showed no differences in corneal curvature or anterior chamber depth. They also had normal optomotor responses. This suggests that the effect of *Egr-1* knockout is surprisingly selective for axial eye growth. That these knockout animals were more myopic fits the idea that the EGR-1 protein appears to be associated with an inhibition signal for axial eye growth: in chickens, the protein is upregulated when hyperopia is induced and downregulated when myopia is induced (Fischer et al., 1999; Bitzer and Schaeffel, 2002).

Genetic knockouts may also result in changed sensitivity to deprivation myopia. Fernandes et al. (2005) found that deprivation myopia could be more easily induced in *nob* knockout mice (lacking the ERG b-wave due to a defect in the rod ON pathway). A more extended screening for refractive errors in mutant mice was recently presented by Faulkner et al. (2007a). Significant refraction differences were detected between C57BL/6J mice, which had refractive errors ranging from +6.9 ± 0.5 to +8.5 ± 0.3 D, *nob* and *rd1* mice, which were about 2 D more hyperopic, and *GABAC* null mice, which were about 5 D more myopic than C57 mice. A next step would be to find out which morphological changes determine the changes in refraction. It could even be that retinal thickness changes are responsible.

There are no published data on the effects of drugs on refractive development in mice. Atropine is currently the most powerful drug against myopia development in both humans and animal models (e.g., Diether et al., 2007). Also in mice, it was found that daily application of one 0.1% atropine eyedrop for 2 weeks in one eye reduced axial eye growth compared to that in the vehicle-treated fellow eye, although the significance levels were not very impressive ($P < 0.04$ in six atropine-treated and six control mice; Burkhardt and Schaeffel, 2006).

Summary

The mouse is probably not a very powerful model to study the visually controlled mechanisms of axial eye growth. This is in line with a conclusion by Guggenheim et al. (2004) for the rat. It may, however, be promising to study knockout models lacking certain elements of the signaling cascade translating the output of retinal image processing into growth commands to the sclera. Microarray analyses of retinal and scleral transcripts following alterations in visual experience or in knockout models may help to identify new pharmacological targets for myopia inhibition. Finally, a mouse model may be feasible for screening drugs against myopia, because the drug can be given as eyedrops (not as intravitreal injection, as in chickens) and can reach retinal and scleral targets in sufficient concentrations, owing to the small volume of the globe.

ACKNOWLEDGMENTS Work was supported by grant no. DFG-Scha 518/13-1 from the German Research Council. I thank Christine Schmucker for providing data on the correlation of IR photoretinoscopy and streak retinoscopy; Howard Howland for data on corneal curvatures and refractions in mice raised in continuous light; and Marita Feldkaemper, Ute Mathis, and Susana Marcos for commenting on an earlier version of the manuscript.

REFERENCES

Abdeljalil, J., Hamid, M., Abdel-Mouttalib, O., Stephane, R., Raymond, R., Johan, A., Jose, S., Pierre, C., and Serge, P. (2005). The optomotor response: A robust first-line visual screening method for mice. *Vision Res.* 45:1439–1446.

Artal, P., Herreros de Tejada, P., Munoz Tedo, C., and Green, D. G. (1998). Retinal image quality in the rodent eye. *Vis. Neurosci.* 15:597–605.

Beuerman, R. W., Barathi, A., Weon, S. R., and Tan, D. (2003). Two models of experimental myopia in the mouse. *Invest. Ophthalmol. Vis. Sci.*; ARVO e-abstract 4338.

Birch, D., and Jacobs, G. H. (1979). Spatial contrast sensitivity in albino and pigmented rats. *Vision Res.* 19:933–938.

Bitzer, M., and Schaeffel, F. (2002). Defocus-induced changes in ZENK expression in the chicken retina. *Invest. Ophthalmol. Vis. Sci.* 43:246–252.

Brand, C., Burkhardt, E., Schaeffel, F., Choi, J. W., and Feldkaemper, M. P. (2005). Regulation of Egr-1, VIP, and Shh mRNA and Egr-1 protein in the mouse retina by light and image quality. *Mol. Vis.* 11:309–320.

Brand, C., Schaeffel, F., and Feldkaemper, M. (2007). A microarray analysis of retinal transcripts that are controlled by retinal image contrast in mice. *Mol. Vis.* 13:920–932.

Burkhardt, E., and Schaeffel, F. (2006). Unpublished raw results.

Carter-Dawson, L. D., and LaVail, M. M. (1979). Rods and cones in the mouse retina. I. Structural analysis using light and electron microscopy. *J. Comp. Neurol.* 15:245–262.

Curtin, B. J. (1985). *The myopias: Basic science and clinical management.* Philadelphia: Harper and Row.

de la Cera, E. G., Rodriguez, G., Llorente, L., Schaeffel, F., and Marcos, S. (2006). Optical aberrations in the mouse eye. *Vision Res.* 46:2546–2553.

Diether, S., Schaeffel, F., Lambrou, G. N., Fritsch, C., and Trendelenburg, A. U. (2007). Effects of intravitreally and intraperitoneally injected atropine on two types of experimental myopia in chicken. *Exp. Eye Res.* 84:266–274.

Douglas, R. M., Alam, N. M., Silver, B. D., McGill, T. J., Tschetter, W. W., and Prusky, G. T. (2005). Independent visual threshold measurements in the two eyes of freely moving rats and mice using a virtual-reality optokinetic system. *Vis. Neurosci.* 22:677–684.

Drager, U. C. (1975). Receptive fields of single cells and topography in mouse visual cortex. *J. Comp. Neurol.* 160: 269–290.

Duke-Elder, S. (1958). *System of ophthalmology: The eye in evolution* (Vol. 1). London: Henry Kimpton.

Faulkner, A. E., Choi, H. Y., Kim, M. K., McCall, M. A., Iuvone, P. M., and Pardue, M. T. (2007a). Retinal defects influence unmanipulated refractive development in mice. *Invest. Ophthalmol. Vis. Sci.* 48; ARVO e-abstract 4419.

Faulkner, A. E., Kim, M. K., Iuvone, P. M., and Pardue, M. T. (2007b). Head-mounted goggles for murine form deprivation myopia. *J. Neurosci. Methods* 161:96–100.

Faulstich, M., van Alphen, A. M., Luo, C., du Lac, S., and De Zeeuw, C. I. (2006). Oculomotor plasticity during vestibular compensation does not depend on cerebellar LTD. *J. Neurophysiol.* 96:1187–1195.

Feldkaemper, M. P., Burkhardt, E., and Schaeffel, F. (2004). Localization and regulation of glucagon receptors in the chick eye and preproglucagon and glucagon receptor expression in the mouse eye. *Exp. Eye Res.* 79:321–329.

Fernandes, A., Yin, H., Byron, E. A., Iuvone, P. M., Schaeffel, F., Williams, R. W., and Pardue, M. T. (2004). Effects of form deprivation on eye size and refraction in C57BL/6J mouse. *Invest. Ophthalmol. Vis. Sci.* 45; ARVO e-abstract 4280.

Fernandes, A., Yin, H., Faulkner, A. E., Iuvone, P. M., Williams, R. W., Schaeffel, F., and Pardue, M. T. (2005). Mouse model with ON pathway defect has increased susceptibility to form deprivation myopia. *Invest. Ophthalmol. Vis. Sci.* 46; ARVO e-abstract 2281.

Fischer, A. J., McGuire, J. J., Schaeffel, F., and Stell, W. K. (1999). Light- and focus-dependent expression of the transcription factor ZENK in the chick retina. *Nat. Neurosci.* 2: 706–712.

Glickstein, M., and Millodot, M. (1970). Retinoscopy and eye size. *Science* 168:605–606.

Green, D. G., Powers, M. K., and Banks, M. S. (1980). Depth of focus, eye size and visual acuity. *Vision Res.* 20:827–835.

Guggenheim, J. A., Creer, R. C., and Qin, X. J. (2004). Postnatal refractive development in the brown Norway rat: Limitations of standard refractive and ocular component dimensions measurement techniques. *Curr. Eye Res.* 29:369–376.

Howland, H. C., and Sayles, N. (1985). Photokeratometric and photorefractive measurements of astigmatism in infants and young children. *Vision Res.* 25:73–81.

Howland, H. C., and Schaeffel, F. (2004). Unpublished raw results.

Howlett, M. H., and McFadden, S. A. (2006). Form-deprivation myopia in the guinea pig (*Cavia porcellus*). *Vision Res.* 46:267–283.

Hughes, A. (1977). The topography of vision in mammals of contrasting life style: Comparative optics and retinal organization. In F. Crescitelli (Ed.), *Handbook of sensory physiology* (Vol. 8, Sect. 5, pp. 613–756). Berlin: Springer-Verlag.

Kirschfeld, K. (1984). Linsen und Komplexaugen: Grenzen ihrer Leistung [Lens and complex eyes: Limits of their performance]. *Naturwissensch. Rund.* 37:352–362.

Kirschfeld, K., and Snyder, A. W. (1976). Measurement of a photoreceptor's characteristic waveguide parameter. *Vision Res.* 16:775–778.

Li, T., Howland, H. C., and Troilo, D. (2000). Diurnal illumination patterns affect the development of the chick eye. *Vision Res.* 40:2387–2393.

Lorente de No, R. (1933). The interaction of the corneal reflex and vestibular nystagmus. *Am. J. Physiol.* 103:704–711.

Mathis, U., and Schaeffel, F. (2007). Glucagon-related peptides in the mouse retina and the effects of deprivation of form vision. *Graefes. Arch. Clin. Exp. Ophthalmol.* 245:267–275.

Mathis, U., Schaeffel, F., and Howland, H. C. (1988). Visual optics in toads (*Bufo americanus*). *J. Comp. Physiol.* A 163:201–213.

Norton, T. T. (1990). Experimental myopia in tree shrews. *Ciba Found. Symp.* 155:178–194.

Pachter, B. R., Davidowitz, J., and Breinin, G. M. (1976). Morphological fiber types of retractor bulbi muscle in mouse and rat. *Invest. Ophthalmol.* 15:654–657.

Prusky, G. T., Alam, N. M., Beekman, S., and Douglas, R. M. (2004). Rapid quantification of adult and developing mouse spatial vision using a virtual optomotor system. *Invest. Ophthalmol. Vis. Sci.* 45:4611–4616.

Prusky, G. T., Alam, N. M., and Douglas, R. M (2006). Enhancement of vision by monocular deprivation in adult mice. *J. Neurosci.* 26:11554–11561.

Prusky, G. T., and Douglas, R. M. (2004). Characterization of mouse cortical spatial vision. *Vision Res.* 44:3411–3418.

Remtulla, S., and Hallett, P. E. (1985). A schematic eye for the mouse, and comparisons with the rat. *Vision Res.* 25:21–31.

Schaeffel, F., and Burkhardt, E. (2002). Measurement of refractive state and deprivation myopia in the black wildtype mouse. *Invest. Ophthalmol. Vis. Sci.* 43; ARVO e-abstract 182.

Schaeffel, F., Burkhardt, E., Howland, H. C., and Williams, R. W. (2004). Measurement of refractive state and deprivation myopia in two strains of mice. *Optom. Vis. Sci.* 81:99–110.

Schaeffel, F., Hagel, G., Eikermann, J., and Collett, T. (1994). Lower-field myopia and astigmatism in amphibians and chickens. *J. Opt. Soc. Am. A* 11:487–495.

Schaeffel, F., and Howland, H. C. (1991). Properties of the feedback loops controlling eye growth and refractive state in the chicken. *Vision Res.* 31:717–734.

Schaeffel, F., and Howland, H. C. (2003). Axial lengths changes in myopic mouse eyes. *Invest. Ophthalmol. Vis. Sci.*, e-letter to the editor. Apr. 25, 2003.

Schaeffel, F., Howland, H. C., and Farkas, L. (1986). Natural accommodation in the growing chicken. *Vision Res.* 26:1977–1993.

Schaeffel, F., and Mathis, U. (1991). Underwater vision in semi-aquatic European snakes. Naturwissenschaften 78:373–375.

Schaeffel, F., and Wagner, H. (1996). Emmetropization and optical development in the eye of the barn owl (*Tyto alba*). *J. Comp. Physiol. A* 178:717–734.

Schippert, R., and Burkhardt, E., Feldkaemper, M., and Schaeffel, F. (2007). Relative axial myopia in an *EGR-1* (ZENK) knock-out mouse. *Invest. Ophthalmol. Vis. Sci.* 48:11–17.

Schmucker, C. (2004). Unpublished raw results.

Schmucker, C., and Schaeffel, F. (2004a). A paraxial schematic eye model for the growing C57BL/6 mouse. *Vision Res.* 44: 1857–1867.

Schmucker, C., and Schaeffel, F. (2004b). In vivo biometry in the mouse eye with low coherence interferometry. *Vision Res.* 44:2445–2456.

Schmucker, C., and Schaeffel, F. (2006). Contrast sensitivity of wild-type mice wearing diffusers or spectacle lenses, and the effect of atropine. *Vision Res.* 46:678–687.

Schmucker, C., Seeliger, M., Humphries, P., Biel, M., and Schaeffel, F. (2005). Grating acuity at different luminances in wild-type mice and in mice lacking rod or cone function. *Invest. Ophthalmol. Vis. Sci.* 46:398–407.

Smith, S. S., Sundberg, J. P., and John S. W. M. (2002). The anterior segment and ocular adnexae. In R. S. Smith (Ed.), *Systematic evaluation of the mouse eye: Anatomy, pathology and biomethods* (pp. 3–24). Boca Raton, FL: CRC Press.

Sterling, P. (2003). How retinal circuits optimize the transfer of visual information. In L. M. Chalupa and J. S. Werner (Eds.), *The visual neurosciences.* (Vol. 1, pp 234–259). Cambridge, MA: MIT Press.

Tejedor, J., and de la Villa, P. (2003). Refractive changes induced by form deprivation in the mouse eye. *Invest. Ophthalmol. Vis. Sci.* 44:32–36.

Vessey, K. A., Rushforth, D. A., and Stell, W. K. (2005). Glucagon- and secretin-related peptides differentially alter ocular growth and the development of form-deprivation myopia in chicks. *Invest. Ophthalmol. Vis. Sci.* 46:3932–3942.

Wallman, J., Turkel, J., and Trachtman, J. (1978). Extreme myopia produced by modest change in early visual experience. *Science* 201:1249–1251.

Wiesel, T. N., and Raviola, E. (1977). Myopia and eye enlargement after neonatal lid fusion in monkeys. *Nature* 266: 66–68.

Woolf, D. (1956). A comparative cytological study of the ciliary muscle. *Anat. Rec.* 124:145–163.

Zhong, X., Ge, J., Smith, E. L. III, and Stell, W. K. (2004). Image defocus modulates activity of bipolar and amacrine cells in macaque retina. *Invest. Ophthalmol. Vis. Sci.* 45:2065–2074.

Zhou, G., and Williams, R. W. (1999). Eye1 and Eye2: Gene loci that modulate eye size, lens weight, and retinal area in the mouse. *Invest. Ophthalmol. Vis. Sci.* 40:817–825.

6 Characteristics and Applications of Mouse Eye Movements

JOHN S. STAHL

To see clearly, the eyes must be properly oriented and held stable with respect to the visual world. Visual motion across the retina at as little as 1–4 deg/s degrades acuity and contrast sensitivity in humans (Barnes and Smith, 1981; Carpenter, 1988; Flipse and Maas, 1996). Thus, control of eye movements is critical to vision, and reciprocally, the visual system continuously monitors and optimizes the function of the oculomotor system. Oculomotor control is one of the best understood aspects of brain function, reflecting some five decades of research conducted primarily in rabbits, cats, and nonhuman primates. Although recordings of mouse eye movements have been reported periodically for decades (e.g., Grusser-Cornehls and Bohm, 1988; Mangini et al., 1985; Mitchiner et al., 1976), the data were only semiquantitative or imprecise in comparison with data available from larger animals. However, this situation changed within the past decade as the technique of magnetic search coil oculography was adapted for use in mice (Boyden and Raymond, 2003; De Zeeuw et al., 1998b; Killian and Baker, 2002; van Alphen et al., 2001) and as new methods of recording mouse eye movements using infrared video-oculography were developed (Stahl, 2002, 2004a; Stahl et al., 2000). This chapter reviews the rapidly expanding state of knowledge of mouse ocular motility and compares mouse eye movements with those of other mammals that, like the mouse, lack a retinal area devoted to high-acuity vision (species I loosely refer to as "afoveate mammals"). Although the eye movements of foveate and afoveate mammals share much in common, there are also significant differences in behaviors, as well as in the physiology underlying apparently similar behaviors (e.g., optokinetic nystagmus). Thus, scant mention is made of the voluminous literature on well-studied foveate species such as the cat, nonhuman primates, and humans. Likewise, a comprehensive review of the physiological principles and analysis of ocular motility would exceed the scope of this chapter. Interested readers are directed to primers on ocular motility that have appeared elsewhere (Leigh and Zee, 2006; Robinson, 1981; Stahl, 2004b).[1]

Three forces have impelled the growing interest in mouse eye movements. First, the broad range of genetic techniques and genetic resources developed for the laboratory mouse can be applied to study the oculomotor system. For instance, transgenics, knockouts, or strains carrying mutations of genes of interest can be used to test the contribution of specific structures, cell types, or biochemical processes to oculomotor functions. Examples of such applications are provided at the end of this chapter. Second, an ultimate goal of neurophysiology is to determine how the electrophysiological properties of individual neurons and local neural circuits contribute to the function of larger neural circuits and, ultimately, animal behavior. This goal is particularly realistic in the mouse oculomotor system, in which the physiology and pharmacology of individual neurons can be assessed in vitro using the brain slice preparation and these observations can then be considered together with precise analyses of single-neuron activity and concomitant eye movement behaviors in the intact animals. Third, eye movements are a powerful tool for assessing the function of many regions of the brain, and analyzing eye movements can therefore serve as a method of testing mutant strains, even when the primary motivation for their study is not oculomotor research (Stahl, 2004b). For example, a demonstration that optokinetically driven eye movements in the Ames waltzer mouse are normal suggested that the mutant's profound vestibular deficits stemmed from abnormalities of hair cell function rather than abnormalities of central vestibular circuitry. The oculomotor findings encouraged further study of hair cell function, despite earlier structural studies that argued that the vestibular periphery was normal (Alagramam et al., 2005).

Eye movements comprise a collection of behaviors that can be divided into two classes: movements that stabilize the retina with respect to the stationary world and movements that shift the retina with respect to the world. The latter "gaze-shifting" movements include saccades (rapid eye movements that shift the direction of the point of regard), vergence movements (slower movements that orient the eyes independently to adjust the distance at which the lines of sight of the two eyes converge), and smooth pursuit (slow eye movements that shift the point of regard to keep pace with a visual target moving with respect to the background). An

[1]One of these references (Leigh and Zee, 2006) includes, in CD-ROM form, D. A. Robinson's classic lecture notes on the application of control systems analysis to oculomotor physiology.

additional fixation mechanism allows the retina-stabilizing reflexes to be overridden when they would take the point of regard off the target (for instance, during attempts to pursue an object by moving the eyes and head together), and this fixation mechanism is conceptually and probably mechanistically related to gaze-shifting movements. Gaze-shifting movements rely on many of the same brainstem and cerebellar circuits that support gaze-stabilizing movements, but also employ a variety of cerebral circuits related to the perception, selection, and memorization of targets of visual interest. Gaze-shifting movements are robust in foveate mammals. In afoveate mammals, the evidence for equivalent gaze-shifting mechanisms is more limited or conjectural. Convergence eye movements have been documented in rabbits engaged in feeding or visual discrimination behaviors (van Hof, 1966; Zuidam and Collewijn, 1979), and the combined eye-head saccades of freely moving rabbits (Collewijn, 1977) may conceivably rely on the same neural machinery (or at least the evolutionary precursors of the machinery) used by foveates to control their fovea-directing saccades. On the other hand, when either a rabbit or mouse is held stationary with its head fixed in place, it executes only rare eye movements (Collewijn, 1977; van Alphen et al., 2001), arguing against the existence of any mechanism designed to use eye movements to explore the visual world. Head-fixed rats do execute up to 20 rapid eye movements per minute (Fuller, 1985; Hess et al., 1988), but whether these eye movements are intended to orient the eyes to a specific visual target (as is the case for the saccades of foveate mammals) or merely to reorient the visual fields within the larger visual surround has not been determined. Smooth pursuit has never been convincingly demonstrated in any afoveate mammal.

In contrast to their rudimentary gaze-shifting behaviors, afoveate mammals exhibit robust behaviors that stabilize and orient the eyes with respect to the visual world. These phylogenetically ancient "compensatory eye movements" include the angular vestibulo-ocular reflex (aVOR, which counterrotates the eyes to prevent image motion during rotational head movements), the linear vestibulo-ocular reflex (lVOR, which rotates the eyes to prevent image motion during translation head movements, and also shifts the eyes during sustained head tilts to maintain a particular orientation of the eyes with respect to gravity), and the optokinetic reflex (OKR, which shifts the eyes in response to motion of large portions of the visual field that may occur during head movements). Additionally, during large-amplitude compensatory eye movements, afoveate mammals exhibit fast phases of nystagmus, rapid eye movements whose purpose is to prevent the eyes becoming so eccentric within the orbits that further compensatory eye movements are impossible. These fast phases (which are also present in foveate mammals) rely on some of the same brainstem mechanisms utilized to generate foveate saccades, but unlike saccades they do not bring the eyes into alignment with a specific visual target. The following sections consider the characteristics of the afoveate compensatory eye movements in more detail.

The angular vestibulo-ocular reflex

To prevent head rotations from causing retinal image motion, the aVOR must process the head movement signals generated by the semicircular canals so as to engender an eye rotation about the correct axis, with the correct amplitude and timing. The eye rotational axis must parallel that of the head rotation. In the simplest geometric condition, that is, when the axis of head rotation is located much closer to the eyes than the objects producing the images that are to be stabilized on the retina, the amplitude of the angular eye velocity must equal the amplitude of the head velocity (Snyder and King, 1992); in other words, the ratio of eye velocity to head velocity (gain) must be 1.0. The eye movements must also be temporally synchronized with the head movements. For the case of a sinusoidal oscillation of head angle,[2] the phase of the compensatory sinusoidal eye movement must lead the phase of the head by 0°.[3] In fact, the aVOR alone fails to be fully compensatory. Figure 6.1 shows

---

[2]The quantitative analysis of eye movements draws heavily on the techniques of linear control systems analysis (Robinson, 1981), and consequently emphasizes the response to sinusoidal inputs. All continuous waveforms can be decomposed into a sum of sine waves of various frequencies, amplitudes, and phase angles, where the value of the component of frequency ω (in rad/s) at time t is given as $y_\omega(t) = A_\omega \sin(\omega t + \varphi_\omega)$, where A_ω is the component amplitude and φ_ω is the component phase. Two required properties of a linear system are (1) the output of a linear system in response to a sinusoidal input is a sinusoid of the same frequency, altered only by a scaling of amplitude or shifting of phase angle, and (2) the system's response to any continuous waveform is merely a linear sum of the responses to each of the sine waves into which the input waveform can be decomposed. It follows from these two principles that the signal-transforming effects of a linear system can be completely summarized by plotting its amplitude-scaling (gain) and phase-shifting effects as functions of input (stimulus) frequency. The pair of gain versus frequency and phase versus frequency plots is referred to as a Bode plot. As the goal of the aVOR is to minimize retinal image velocity (the difference between head velocity and eye velocity), gain is customarily calculated as the ratio of eye velocity to head velocity, and phase as the difference between the phases of eye and head velocity. Gain and phase could also be calculated with reference to other quantities, such as eye acceleration and head acceleration.

[3]A system producing an equal and opposite eye movement could be considered to have either a gain of −1.0 and a phase of 0° or, equivalently, a gain of 1.0 and a phase lead (or lag) of 180°. However, for greater conceptual simplicity, the head movement signal is generally inverted, so that a perfectly compensatory eye movement would have a gain of 1.0 and a phase of 0°.

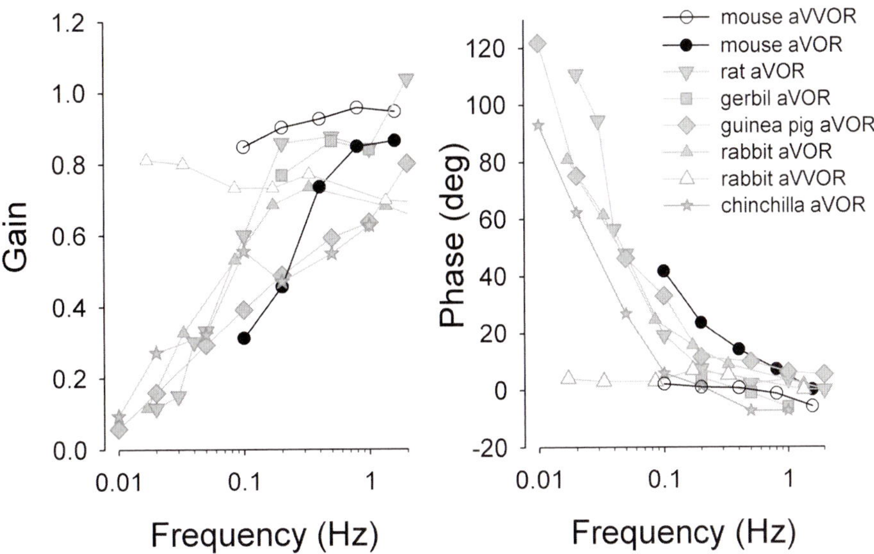

FIGURE 6.1 Horizontal aVOR and aVVOR gain and phase versus stimulus frequency for the mouse and five other afoveate mammals for which data are available. For data sources, see note 5.

the Bode plot for the horizontal aVOR of the mouse (*solid circles*) derived by averaging video-oculography data from 11 2- to 8-month-old C57BL/6 animals (Stahl, 2004a). The plot demonstrates that at higher stimulus frequencies, the aVOR approaches ideal behavior. However, as frequency decreases, gain falls, and the phase of the sinusoidal eye movement progressively leads with respect to the head movement. This incompletely compensatory behavior reflects the properties of the semicircular canals, which report head velocity accurately only around a certain range of stimulus frequencies (Fernandez and Goldberg, 1971). At lower frequencies, the canals progressively shift to reporting head acceleration. Head acceleration leads head velocity by 90°, and its amplitude falls more rapidly as a function of frequency than does the amplitude of head velocity. Thus, eye velocity response progressively leads, and diminishes in proportion to, head velocity. It should be noted that there is no acceleration during a constant-velocity rotation, and so, during prolonged rotations at constant velocity, the canal signal—and thus the aVOR—decays to nil. In the natural situation, rotation occurs in the presence of vision. As such, the aVOR is supplemented by visually driven eye movements (the OKR), particularly at lower stimulus frequencies, where the canal-derived head movement signal is deficient. The gain and phase curves for the same animals during rotation in the light (visual-vestibulo-ocular reflex, VVOR) are plotted as *open circles* in figure 6.1 and demonstrate that the VVOR of the mouse approaches ideal performance across the entire range of tested frequencies. The slight reduction in aVVOR gain at lower frequencies may be an effect of the particular video recording setup, which incorporates visible apparatus that moves with the rotating animal and thus conflicts with the gain-augmenting effects of the stationary visual surround (Stahl, 2004a). Data gathered using a similar video technique but less intrusive apparatus lacked this attenuation at lower frequencies (Faulstich et al., 2004, 2006). Data gathered using a still less visually intrusive magnetic search coil apparatus also lacked the low-frequency attenuation, but gains were lower at all stimulus frequencies, an effect attributed to the coil impeding eye movement (Stahl et al., 2000; van Alphen et al., 2001).[4]

Figure 6.1 also plots aVOR and aVVOR curves for other afoveate mammals for which Bode plots have been pub-

[4]Magnetic search coil oculography has traditionally been considered the gold standard of oculography. However, implanting a search coil on the mouse eye reduces gain, possibly because the coil impedes free movement of the eye (Stahl et al., 2000). Although the eye movement amplitudes recorded using search coils have greatly improved since the earliest search coil studies (i.e., De Zeeuw et al., 1998a; Koekkoek et al., 1997), they remain consistently lower than those obtained using video-oculography, irrespective of whether the coils were implanted (Boyden and Raymond, 2003; Kimpo et al., 2005; van Alphen et al., 2001) or temporarily glued to the cornea (Harrod and Baker, 2003; Killian and Baker, 2002). Pupil-tracking video-oculography introduces its own problems, mostly related to the assumptions and approximations that must be made when converting the raw signals from position within the video image to eye angle. Ideally, this conversion process takes into account both the horizontal and the vertical position of the pupil, as well as pupil diameter and the position of a reference corneal reflection (Stahl, 2004a; Stahl et al., 2000, 2006). For these reasons, where absolute gain is critical to our argument, we cite studies in which eye movements were obtained using the most precise video-oculography technique in preference to studies performed using other techniques.

lished.[5] aVOR phase curves exhibit configurations similar to those of the mouse, but appear to be shifted toward lower frequencies. This shift is consistent with the proposition that the frequency of natural head movements increases with smaller animal size, and semicircular canal dynamics are also shifted to match the head movement frequency range (Wilson and Melvill Jones, 1979). The gain curves exhibit more scatter than the phase curves, a difference that likely arises in part from the wide variety of oculography techniques employed in their acquisition. However, if each animal's curve is normalized to its value at the highest tested stimulus frequency, the mouse curve again appears to be shifted to the right of all but the guinea pig curve (plot not shown).

Bode plots such as those shown in figure 6.1 are most informative when applied to systems that are linear, at least over the range of stimulus frequencies and amplitudes at which the system was probed (see note 2). In fact, the horizontal aVOR, like many biological systems, is only approximately linear. Two types of aVOR nonlinearity have been described, a variation of gain with stimulus amplitude and a variation of gain with stimulus direction. Figure 6.2 replots aVOR data from four studies in which sinusoidal eye movements of C57BL/6 mice were acquired at different stimulus amplitudes.[6] The gains and the degree of nonlinearity vary considerably, in part due to significant differences in the oculography techniques (which included search coil oculography and video-oculography with and without the use of a corneal reflection to minimize artifacts resulting from the eye rotating about points other than its geometric center [Stahl et al., 2000]). Nevertheless, in all studies and at all stimulus frequencies, aVOR gain increased and phase lead decreased as stimulus amplitude increased. Similar effects of amplitude have been reported in mice recorded with search coils (van Alphen et al., 2001) and in rabbits (Baarsma and Collewijn, 1974). Another nonlinearity of the mouse aVOR is an increase in gain of up to 0.1 when the eye moves in the temporal-nasal direction (Stahl et al., 2006). This asymmetry implies that the aVOR causes the eyes to move in a dysconjugate fashion. A similar dependence of gain on direction has been reported in the gerbil (Kaufman, 2002). The aVVOR shows considerably less dependence on stimulus amplitude, based on the two studies used in figure 6.2 that provided both aVOR and aVVOR data (Iwashita et al., 2001; Katoh et al., 2005). The aVOR directional asymmetry, however, was essentially unchanged by the addition of vision (Stahl et al., 2006). In sum, the aVOR exhibits significant nonlinearities that must be considered, for instance, when comparing data produced in different laboratories using different stimulus amplitudes. Particular care must be taken when interpreting data produced using very small

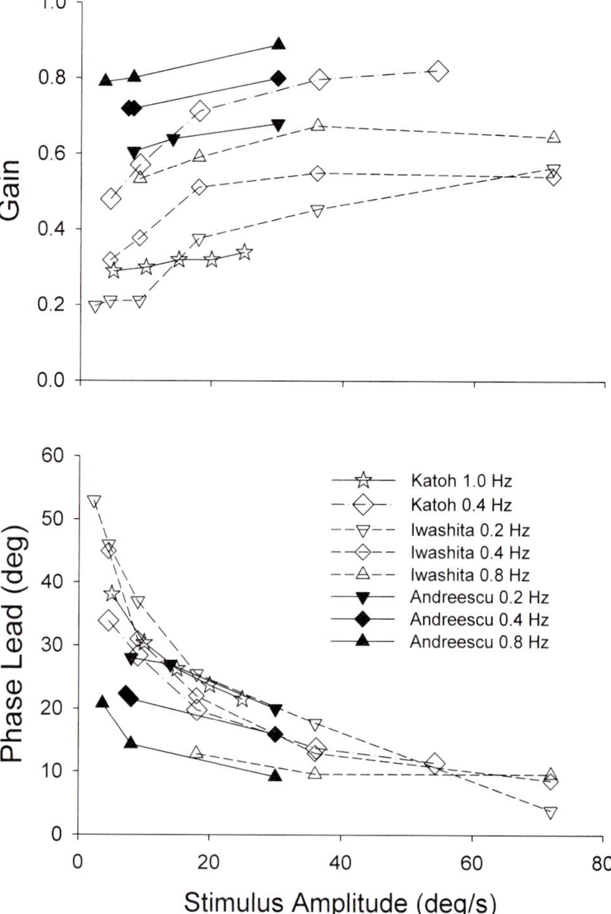

FIGURE 6.2 Amplitude-related nonlinearities of the mouse horizontal aVOR. Gain decreases and phase lead increases markedly at lower stimulus amplitudes. For details on sources of data and full references, see note 6.

[5]Sources and oculography technique for the data plotted in figure 6.1 for species other than the mouse are as follows: Rabbit, implanted search coil (van der Steen and Collewijn, 1984). Rat, glued-on search coil (Brettler et al., 2000). As this rat study reported all gains relative to the response at 0.2 Hz, we converted the normalized curve to absolute gains based on the assumption that the gain at 0.1 Hz would have been equivalent to the absolute value reported by Rabbath et al. (2001), in which the rat eye movements were similarly recorded using glued-on search coils. Gerbil, video (Kaufman, 2002). Guinea pig, search coil (Escudero et al., 1993). Chinchilla, electro-oculography (Merwin et al., 1989).

[6]Sources of data plotted in figure 6.2 are as follows: Data from Andreescu et al. (2005) extracted from their figure 4b and c. Data from their figure 4a (6, 13, and 25 deg/s at 0.2, 0.4, and 0.8 Hz, respectively) were excluded, because the gains in that figure fall conspicuously below the curves generated from the data in figure 4b and c. The 0.4 Hz data from Katoh et al. (2005) were extracted from their figure 7c and d, and the 0 Hz data from Katoh et al. (2006) were obtained from their figure 1a. Data from Iwashita et al. (2001) were extracted from their figure 5a–e.

position and velocity amplitudes. Visual reflexes compensate to some extent for the aVOR nonlinearities, resulting in a more linear aVVOR response.

The optokinetic reflex

During rotation in the light, any residual image motion due to a less than perfectly compensatory aVOR is transduced by slip-sensitive retinal ganglion cells, and, after processing by the accessory optic system (AOS) and vestibular nuclei, the image velocity signal ultimately drives a compensatory eye movement response, the optokinetic reflex (Simpson, 1984). In the laboratory, the OKR is usually elicited by enclosing the experimental animal in a cylinder (drum) whose interior is painted with stripes or a similar high-contrast pattern and rotating the drum about the animal. Alternatively, a moving pattern of stars can be projected onto a featureless background using a rotating projection planetarium (Leonard et al., 1988). Whereas the aVOR is approximately linear over restricted ranges of stimulus frequency and amplitude, the OKR is grossly nonlinear, because the gain of the AOS's image velocity signals declines rapidly with increasing image velocity. Consequently, the performance of the OKR is better captured by its speed tuning curve, that is, a plot of OKR gain as a function of drum velocity, than by the Bode plots that are so useful in describing the aVOR and aVVOR. Figure 6.3 shows a speed tuning curve constructed from an average of the individual curves for 20 C57BL/6 mice. The OKR gain falls off rapidly as drum velocity exceeds approximately 5 deg/s. The gain curve recalculated from sinusoidal, gain versus frequency data (Faulstich et al., 2006) is quite similar, supporting Collewijn's observation that the speed-dependent nonlinearity is a major factor in determining the eye movement response to sinusoidal stimuli (Collewijn, 1981). Figure 6.3 also plots the speed tuning curves for the three other afoveate species for which comparable data are available.[7] All the curves exhibit a similar rapid decline in gain above 2–5 deg/s. The mouse exhibits the highest overall gains. As in the case of the aVOR/aVVOR data, some of the variations in gain across species may reflect differences in recording techniques, as well as the visual characteristics of the optokinetic stimulus. Both sets of mouse data, in contrast, were obtained using similar recording apparatus and analysis techniques. It should be noted that in many species, OKR gain increases in the course of a prolonged, unidirectional optokinetic stimulation (due to velocity storage). It is the initial gain in response to a constant-velocity stimulus, or the gain in response to the changing velocities of a sinusoidal stimulus, that most accurately reflects the output of the afoveate AOS. Consequently, all the curves in figure 6.3 are based on either the initial responses to constant-velocity stimuli or the responses to sinusoidal stimuli.

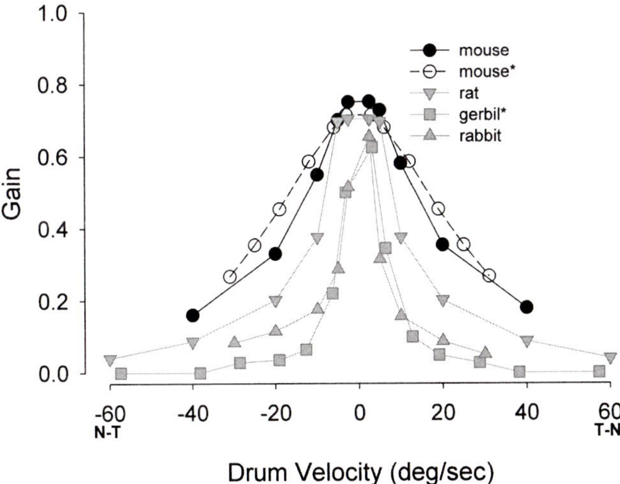

FIGURE 6.3 Horizontal OKR speed tuning curve for the mouse, rat, gerbil, and rabbit. For data sources, see note 7. All responses are for binocular stimulation. Curves denoted by an *asterisk* in the key were obtained from the response to sinuoidal (rather than constant velocity) stimuli. For mouse sinusoid and rat data, separate gains for nasally and temporally directed stimuli (with respect to the recorded eye) were not available, and consequently the available values were mirror-imaged. T-N and N-T denote temporal-to-nasal and nasal-to-temporal stimuli with respect to the recorded eye.

As the OKR gain in response to sinusoidal stimuli is strongly influenced by the nonlinearity of the AOS, so too the response phase is dominated by the long delays engendered in processing the image velocity signals. In the mouse, the lag between the onset of a visual stimulus and the oculomotor response averages 70 ms (van Alphen et al., 2001), comparable to the value of 75 ms reported for the rabbit (Collewijn, 1972). This 70 ms "dead time" would account for 25° of the 26° by which the eye lags the optokinetic stimulus at 1 Hz, and 40° of the 62° lag at 1.6 Hz shown in two published phase-versus-stimulus-frequency plots (Faulstich et al., 2006; van Alphen et al., 2001).

The otolith-ocular reflexes

Linear acceleration stimulating the otolith organs (the utricle and saccule) can arise from either translational acceleration or from tilt with respect to the gravity vector (Angelaki et al.,

[7]Sources of data plotted in figure 6.3 are as follows: Mouse response to constant velocity stimuli (Stahl, 2004b). Mouse response to sinusoids (Faulstich et al., 2006). Rat (Hess et al., 1988). Gerbil (Kaufman, 2002; data extracted from his figure 6e and f). Note that Kaufman's values are normalized gains, but the difference between the normalized and absolute values was claimed to be less than 2%. Rabbit (Collewijn, 1969).

1999; Paige and Tomko, 1991). The appropriate compensatory ocular response to the two perturbations differs. For instance, the appropriate response of a frontal-eyed animal to a leftward translation along an interaural axis would be a rightward eye movement, whereas the response to a rightward head roll (which would generate the same stimulus to the utricle), would be a counterclockwise, "orienting" eye movement. Consequently the otolith-ocular reflexes can actually be viewed as two overlapping reflexes, the translational VOR (transVOR) and the tilt, or orienting, VOR (tiltVOR). Foveate and afoveate mammals exhibit considerable differences in the strength of their transVOR and tiltVOR. Whereas the tiltVOR in response to maintained tilts is weak in humans (Collewijn et al., 1985), it is robust in afoveates. Conversely, the transVOR is strong in foveate mammals, but in the rabbit and rat (the only afoveate mammals in which transVOR has been tested to date), the responses to translation on a linear sled are weak and have actually been ascribed to inappropriate tiltVOR responses to the illusory tilt (Baarsma and Collewijn, 1975b; Hess and Dieringer, 1991). The weakness of true transVOR responses in the rabbit and rat supports the idea that this reflex evolved specifically to serve the stabilization demands of foveal vision (Angelaki et al., 2003). In contrast, the robust tiltVOR responses of afoveates may reflect the desirability of aligning retinal specializations other than a fovea (e.g., the visual streak) with the features of the overall visual surround such as the horizon (Maruta et al., 2001).

The response of the mouse to static tilt has been reported for roll angles over ±30° (Andreescu et al., 2005). Figure 6.4 demonstrates the performance of the static tiltVOR for both pitch (*left plots*) and roll (*right plots*) over a wider, ±180° range in the C57BL/6 mouse. We measured horizontal and vertical equilibrium eye positions in the light in four C57BL/6 mice using 2D video-oculography. Eye positions of the four animals were averaged and have been plotted versus tilt angle, where the 0° pitch position corresponds to the bregma-lambda axis being horizontal. Both pitch and roll engendered strong vertical responses. Both downward pitch and ipsilateral roll, for instance, shifted the rest position of the eye upward. When replotted (plots not shown) against the fraction of the gravity vector that lay in the plane of the utricle (i.e., against the sine of the tilt angle), the eye position was a nearly perfect linear function of

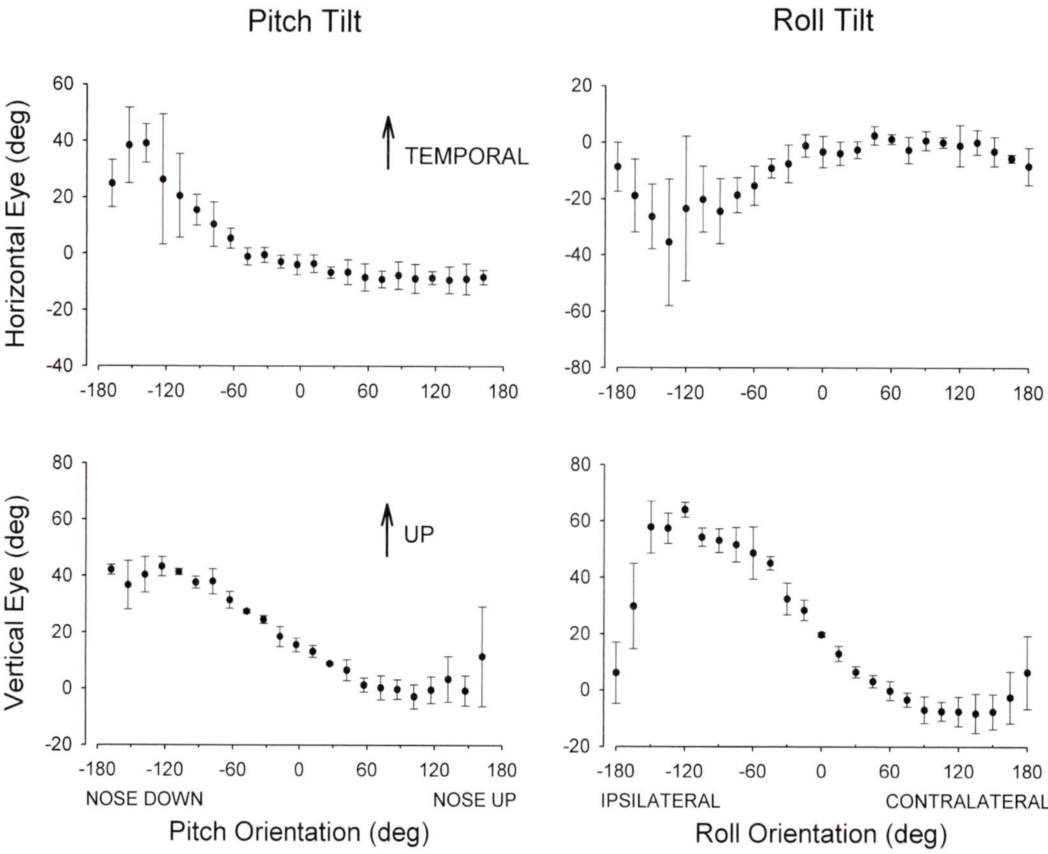

FIGURE 6.4 Horizontal and vertical equilibrium positions of the eye in response to pitch (*left plots*) and roll (*right plots*) tilts. Results are the averages of data from four C57BL/6 mice recorded in the light. Error bars are ±1 SD. Roll direction (ipsilateral or contralateral) is given with respect to the recorded eye.

gravity over the central ±90° tilt range. Vertical sensitivities measured 18.4 deg/g for pitch and 28.9 deg/g for roll movements. Since the mouse optic axes are angled approximately 62° from the midline (Walls, 1942), the appropriate vertical ocular responses to pitch and roll are 0.47 (cos62°) and 0.88 (sin62°) times the tilt angle, respectively. Taking these factors into account, the gains (degrees of eye rotation per degree of tilt about the eye's up-down axis) of the pitch and roll responses were 0.44 and 0.36, respectively. For comparison, the pitch sensitivity of the rabbit recorded with search coils in darkness is 17 deg/g and the gain is 0.28, and the roll sensitivity and gain values are 16 deg/g and 0.26 (Maruta et al., 2001). Higher values for the rabbit's roll tiltVOR (0.5–0.6) have also been reported, obtained using prolonged transverse linear accelerations with the eyes covered to prevent vision (Baarsma and Collewijn, 1975b). A practical consequence of these observations is that when horizontal eye movements are measured in afoveates using video-oculography, the calibration scheme must be adjusted to account for vertical movements whenever the head is reoriented with respect to gravity (Stahl, 2004a).

Pitch and roll movements also engender horizontal movements, although weaker and having a less linear relationship to gravity. In the mouse (figure 6.4, *top plots*), nose-down pitch generated a temporal movement of the recorded eye. Assuming the eyes move symmetrically, the eyes must diverge during downward and converge during upward pitch. Roll tilts generated a more irregular response, with a tendency for the eye to move nasally during inclination to the same side. Identical directions of horizontal eye movement have been observed in the rabbit during tilts (Maruta et al., 2001) and the rat (Hess and Dieringer, 1991) during sled accelerations about the naso-occipital and transverse axes (simulating pitch and roll tilts, respectively). These motions have been interpreted as an appropriate response to changing viewing distance during translation (Hess and Dieringer, 1991), although this interpretation seems to assume that an afoveate mammal can fixate a specific point in the visual world. An alternative and more compelling interpretation (Maruta et al., 2001) is that the horizontal movements produce advantageous repositionings of the visual fields of the two eyes with respect to the entire surround. Thus, when the animal pitches its head down to feed, the eyes diverge, maximizing the ability to detect predators approaching from overhead or behind. When the head pitches up, the eyes converge, increasing the degree of binocular overlap and thereby potentially improving vision of the terrain ahead. Similarly, during head roll, the eyes would rotate to better survey the world overhead.

While the static properties of the mouse tiltVOR are clearly well suited to maintaining the static orientation of the retina with respect to the visual surround, the tiltVOR can also play a role during dynamic stimuli, since any reorienting movements executed to counteract tilt with respect to gravity would also be appropriate to reduce the image motion engendered during the tilting motion. Thus the tiltVOR synergizes with the aVOR during rotations about earth-horizontal axes. The low-pass characteristics of the afoveate otolith system are particularly suitable to complement the semicircular canals' reflexes, which perform poorly at low stimulus frequencies (Baarsma and Collewijn, 1975b; Fernandez and Goldberg, 1971). The augmentation of the aVOR by the dynamic tiltVOR in afoveate mammals has been demonstrated in the mouse (Andreescu et al., 2005; Harrod and Baker, 2003), rat (Brettler et al., 2000), and rabbit (Barmack, 1981) by comparing the responses to rotation about an earth-vertical axis (i.e., the horizontal movements during upright yaw, or the vertical movements during nose-up roll) to the responses during rotations about earth-horizontal axes (vertical eye movements during upright roll or horizontal movements during nose-up yaw). In all cases, the response to horizontal axis rotation (which stimulates both canals and otoliths) exhibited higher gains and lower degrees of phase lead than the vertical axis rotation (which stimulates the canals alone). This improvement was absent in mutant mouse strains congenitally deficient in otoconia, proving that the otolith signals are the origin of the improvement in normal animals (Andreescu et al., 2005; Harrod and Baker, 2003).

Off-vertical axis stimulation

As addressed in the previous section, two methods of studying the otolith system in isolation from the canal system are to use static tilts or linear translations. A third method is to record eye movements during constant-velocity yaw rotations of the animal about an axis that is tilted from the vertical (off-vertical axis rotation, OVAR). The tilt projects a portion of the gravity vector into the plane of the utricle, and the rotation causes this component of the gravity vector to sweep around the utricle once per revolution of the animal. Commonly, 30° is selected for the tilt angle, perhaps because this angle is easy to achieve with minimal modification to the stimulation apparatus, and also because, conveniently, the 30° tilt projects exactly one-half of the gravity vector into the plane of the utricle (sin30° = 0.5). Since the rotation is performed at a constant angular velocity, it produces no effect on the semicircular canals, once the transient response to the startup of rotation has decayed.

OVAR produces qualitatively similar responses in all foveate and afoveate species studied to date, including the mouse (Killian and Baker, 2002), rat (Hess and Dieringer, 1990), guinea pig (Jones et al., 2003), rabbit (Maruta et al., 2001), rhesus macaque (Kushiro et al., 2002), and humans (Darlot et al., 1988). Figure 6.5 shows the horizontal eye movements of a C57BL/6 mouse being yawed at a 90° tilt

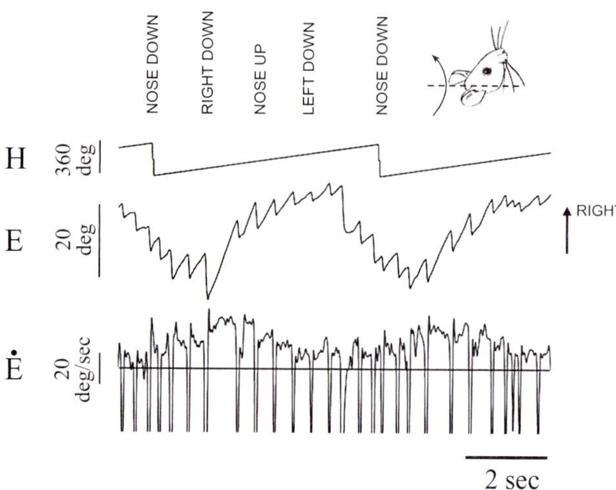

FIGURE 6.5 Horizontal eye movements of OVAR in the mouse during leftward yaw rotation. The head position trace resets as the animal crosses through the nose-down position. Note the sinusoidal oscillation in average eye position, as well as the systematic variation in horizontal eye velocity about a positive bias velocity. (Adapted from Killian and Baker, 2002, with permission.)

angle. As in other species, the rotation engenders a horizontal nystagmus, with the slow phases directed opposite the direction of rotation (i.e., in the appropriate direction to stabilize retinal image velocity). There is also a sinusoidal variation of the average position of the eye during each slow phase, that is, a modulation of the "beating field" of the nystagmus. If one ignores the prominent downward-directed spikes related to the fast phases of nystagmus in the eye velocity plot, one can see that the slow phase velocity, like the eye position, also fluctuates in a systematic but somewhat irregular fashion about the "bias velocity." In this case the highest velocities correspond approximately with the nose-up position. Three-dimensional eye movement recordings performed in rat (Hess and Dieringer, 1990), rabbit (Maruta et al., 2001), and monkey (Kushiro et al., 2002) demonstrate that vertical and torsional positions, like horizontal position, also vary sinusoidally. In afoveates, the variations in eye torsion, elevation, and the beating field of the horizontal nystagmus are in the same directions as the orienting responses to static tilt, and are believed to arise from the tiltVOR (Hess and Dieringer, 1990; Maruta et al., 2001). The shift of the horizontal beating field in the rhesus, however, is opposite to an orienting response (for instance, the eyes deflect rightward in the right-ear-down position) (Kushiro et al., 2002) and presumably arises from a different mechanism. Each utricular afferent encodes only the strength of the gravity vector lying in its individual preferred direction (Goldberg and Fernandez, 1982), and thus the entire utricle provides only a population-encoded measure of instantaneous tilt. The horizontal bias velocity signal is constructed from this distributed representation by central vestibular circuitry in a process termed velocity estimation (Schnabolk and Raphan, 1994). As would be desired for an eye movement intended to compensate for rotation about the yaw axis, the magnitude of the bias component depends on rotation velocity, not the angle of tilt, for any tilt steeper than approximately 15–20° (Kushiro et al., 2002). Thus, the bias velocities in the mouse, which have only been recorded to date at 90° tilts (Harrod and Baker, 2003; Killian and Baker, 2002), can be compared to values obtained in other mammals at the more customary 30° tilt value. In the mouse, rotations in darkness at 64 deg/s produced bias velocities of 10–25 deg/s, corresponding to gains of 0.16–0.39 (Harrod and Baker, 2003; Killian and Baker, 2002). These values are comparable to the gains obtained at 60 deg/s in the rat (0.40: Hess and Dieringer, 1990, their figure 6) and guinea pig (0.23: Jones et al., 2003, their figure 5b). They are appreciably greater than an example in the rabbit (ca. 0.08: Maruta et al., 2001) but lower than the values in the cat (0.73: Harris, 1987), rhesus macaque (0.78: Kushiro et al., 2002, their figure 2e), and squirrel monkey (0.53, obtained at 30 deg/s: Goldberg and Fernandez, 1982). In sum, the response to OVAR of the mouse is typical for afoveate mammals studied to date.

After-nystagmus and the velocity storage integrator

In many mammalian species, continuous horizontal optokinetic stimulation engenders a compensatory horizontal nystagmus whose slow phase velocity gradually builds as the stimulus continues. If the lights are extinguished after this velocity buildup, the nystagmus continues for a few seconds as "optokinetic after-nystagmus" (OKAN). OKAN is one of several manifestations of the vestibular system's "velocity storage integrator," so called because it appears to store the stimulus velocity, charging and discharging in the manner of a "leaky" electronic integrator (Raphan et al., 1979). Another manifestation of velocity storage is that if rotation is suddenly halted after a prolonged head rotation in darkness, a postrotatory nystagmus (PRN) is generated whose decay matches the rate of decay of OKAN, rather than the considerably more rapid decay of the postrotatory signals emanating from the semicircular canals (Collewijn et al., 1980). Thus the velocity storage integrator effectively increases the time constant of the semicircular canal signal, shifting toward lower stimulus frequencies the point at which the aVOR gain begins to decline and the phase lead begins to increase (see earlier discussion of aVOR). This action is particularly important during rotations about an earth-vertical axis, during which the aVOR cannot be assisted by the dynamic tiltVOR (since in this case the utricle is not activated by any rotating gravity vector, in contrast to the situation during earth-horizontal or off-vertical rotations). Thus, velocity storage has been regarded as the substitute for the utricle during rotations about the vertical axis. Its special relationship to vertical axis rotations is emphasized by the fact that after-nystagmus is most intense for rotational stimuli about an earth-vertical axis, whether the stimulus (and resulting after-nystagmus) is about the yaw axis in an upright animal or about the pitch axis of an animal lying on its side (Dai et al., 1991). Still further, an animal that is optokinetically stimulated about its yaw axis while lying on its side will rapidly develop a pitch nystagmus (i.e., nystagmus about an earth-vertical axis) once the lights are extinguished (Dai et al., 1991). An additional role for storage unrelated to any substitution for the utricle is that the optokinetic signal that is stored during prolonged head rotations in the light is appropriate to assist in canceling the postrotatory vestibular signals emanating from the semicircular canals, thus minimizing the duration and intensity of the undesirable PRN (Collewijn et al., 1980).

Velocity storage, as evidenced by OKAN, can be observed to varying degrees in a number of species, including the rabbit (Collewijn, 1969), cat (Maioli and Precht, 1984), monkey (Cohen et al., 1977), and human (Fletcher et al., 1990). The *left panel* of figure 6.6 shows the OKN/OKAN response of the rabbit produced by 15 deg/s optokinetic stimulation. Note the gradual buildup of the slow phase velocity consistent with charging of velocity storage. After the lights were extinguished, the nystagmus continued for approximately 15 s, declining in an approximately linear fashion (Collewijn et al., 1980). In some circumstances, the initial OKAN (OKAN I) may be followed by a period of reversed OKAN (OKAN II), and still further reversals can occur (OKAN III, IV, etc.) (Maioli, 1988). The *right panel* of figure 6.6 shows the typical response of a mouse recorded with video-oculography during and after a horizontal optokinetic stimulus at 25 deg/s. The response differs markedly from that of the rabbit. After a slight buildup of velocity during the first 10 s of stimulation, the response declined to zero, reappearing briefly in the context of a flurry of fast phases of nystagmus toward the end of the lights-on period. Immediately after extinction of the lights, a weak, oppositely directed slow phase appeared, consistent with an OKAN II. Search coil recordings have produced similar results, including the slight buildup of OKN and absence of OKAN I, although the per-stimulus habituation and OKAN II phenomena were not described (van Alphen et al., 2001).

To date, no definitive evidence of significant velocity storage in mice has been reported. The time constant of the aVOR has been reported to be 3.8 s, based on the duration of PRN (Killian and Baker, 2002), while a time constant of just 1.4 s is calculated from the phase lead of the aVOR at 0.1 Hz (41° in 2- to 14-month-old animals; Stahl et al., 2006), given the rough assumption that the aVOR can be modeled as a first-order high-pass system. These values are

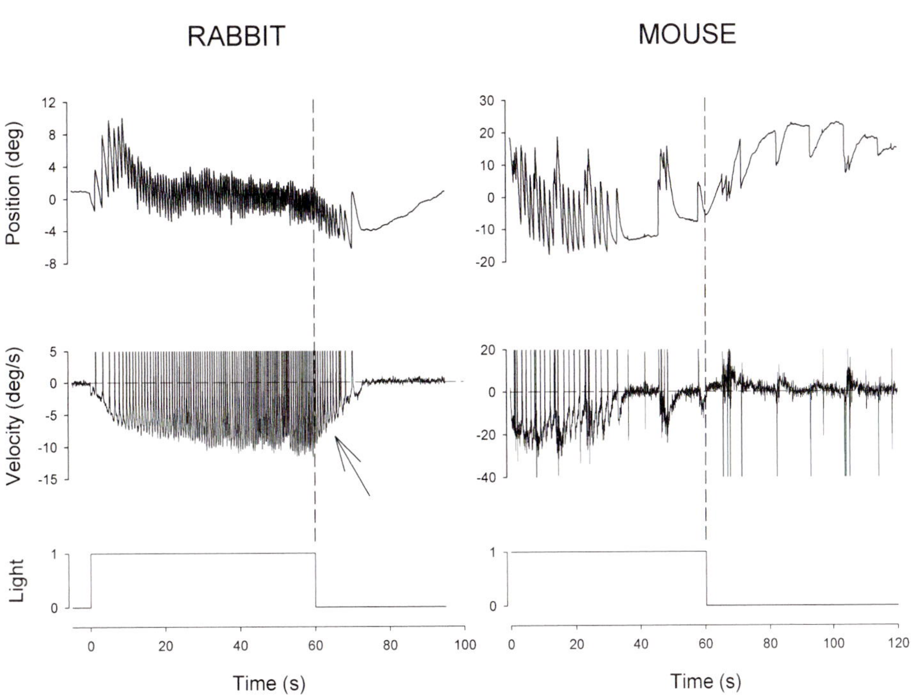

FIGURE 6.6 OKN and OKAN in rabbit (*left*) and mouse (*right*). Each panel shows horizontal eye position and velocity during constant-velocity optokinetic stimulation (15 deg/s for rabbit or 25 deg/s for mouse). Velocity scale truncates the positive-going spikes of the fast phases of OKN and OKAN. *Arrow* indicates OKAN in rabbit. (Rabbit data courtesy of Maarten Frens and Beerend Winkelman, Erasmus MC, Rotterdam, The Netherlands.)

close to the 2–4 s peripheral time constant derived from recordings of more than 200 primary vestibular afferents in anesthetized mice (Lloyd Minor and David Lasker, pers. comm., November 2006). Thus, one of the two goals of velocity storage discussed earlier—extending the bandwidth of the compensatory response to low-frequency, sinusoidal stimuli about the vertical axis—does not appear to be achieved in mice. The other goal, storing an optokinetic signal during rotation in the light that can be used to shorten the duration of PRN, would be difficult to reconcile with the failures to demonstrate OKAN, as OKAN is the usual basis for the claim that the optokinetic signal is stored. Whether the presence of OKAN II in figure 6.6 supports the existence of a velocity storage integrator is unclear. The exact mechanism underlying OKAN II remains unknown, and many published theoretical models do not account for it (Maioli, 1988). OKAN II and OKAN I often appear to have a reciprocal relationship, with factors that augment OKAN II (e.g., repetitive stimulation) tending to reduce OKAN I (Maioli, 1988). But whether a reciprocal relationship between OKAN I and II indicates that OKAN II is a manifestation of velocity storage or an entirely separate phenomenon that happens to consistently antagonize velocity storage is unknown. Further experiments are needed to assess the degree to which mice can perform velocity storage. If they bear out the impression that velocity storage is absent or weak in this species, it would be necessary to reevaluate commonly held assumptions that storage is a necessary and universal attribute of the mammalian vestibular system.

Gaze holding and the velocity-to-position neural integrator

To maintain the eyes in any eccentric position, the oculomotor system must generate a constant activation of extraocular muscles to counteract the elastic forces that would tend to recenter the eyes. The continuous neural activity, proportional to desired eye position, is generated by a process of mathematical integration of eye velocity command signals by a mechanism referred to as the oculomotor neural integrator (Cannon and Robinson, 1987; Robinson, 1968). Because the neural integrator is imperfect, in the absence of visual cues and further gaze shifts the eyes will gradually recenter with a roughly exponential time course, from which the time constant of the neural integrator can be measured. In normal foveates, including humans, monkeys, and cats, this time constant exceeds 20 s (Becker and Klein, 1973; Cannon and Robinson, 1987; Kaneko, 1997). In contrast, the integrator time constant in the mouse has been reported as 2–5 s (Stahl et al., 2006; van Alphen et al., 2001), comparable to the 1.6–4 second range reported for rats (Chelazzi et al., 1990). The inferior performance of the integrators in these afoveates likely reflects the lesser need in afoveate vision for precise position control. For the purposes of afoveate vision, it is sufficient to maintain retinal image velocity at a low value, which can be achieved in a stationary animal by the OKR in conjunction with a relatively weak integrator. Moreover, in the head-free condition, afoveates usually couple eye movements with head movements (Collewijn, 1977; Meier and Dieringer, 1993), so the final eye position is likely to be close to a central orbital position, where the elastic restoring forces, and the need for a counteracting neural integrator signal, are less. In contrast, the foveate animal must maintain retinal *position* stable, often at eccentric orbital positions.

Adaptive properties of compensatory eye movements

An important feature of the vestibulo-ocular system is its ability to use visual signals to monitor its own performance, and to adapt so that compensatory eye movements remain of appropriate amplitude, timing, and direction. Studies of the plasticity of the vestibulo-ocular system have figured importantly in the history of oculomotor physiology, in part because they have been looked to as a way to study motor learning in a system that is peculiarly experimentally and analytically tractable (Boyden et al., 2004; Gittis and du Lac, 2006; Highstein, 1998; Ito, 1982; Miles and Lisberger, 1981). Gain and response axis of the aVOR can be adapted using combinations of optokinetic and visual stimulation. For instance, if an animal is oscillated on a turntable while the visual surround is oscillated at the same rate but in the opposite direction, the compensatory responses would need a gain of 2.0 (instead of the usual gain of 1.0) to maintain the eyes stable with respect to the visual surround. Under such circumstances, the resulting image velocity causes the gain of the aVOR to gradually increase over a period of minutes to hours. Similarly, the gain of the aVOR can be shifted toward zero by exposing the animal to a situation in which the optokinetic surround moves with the oscillating animal (0× condition), or inverted by oscillating the surround in the same direction but at twice the amplitude of the turntable rotation (−1× condition). Gain can also be manipulated by fixing magnifying, minifying, or reversing spectacles over an animal's eyes (Gonshor and Jones, 1976; Miles and Eighmy, 1980). The direction of the aVOR can be manipulated by coupling turntable rotation to rotation of the visual surround about a different axis (Schultheis and Robinson, 1981).

The adaptability of mouse compensatory eye movements has already received extensive attention, since one of the incentives of working with this species has been the opportunity to use genetic tools to dissect the synaptic and cellular mechanisms through which the plasticity is achieved. Table 6.1 summarizes the results of nine studies in which aVOR gain was manipulated in C57BL/6 mice (or strains extensively backcrossed to the C57BL/6 reference) by combined

Table 6.1

Results of studies of adaptation of horizontal aVOR gain in C57BL/6 mice

Source, year	Gain goal	Stimulus	$Gain_0$	ΔGain, %	$Phase_0$	ΔPhase, %	Oculography Method
Iwashita et al., 2001	2×	0.4 Hz, 7.2° × 40 min	.41	+29%	29°	−79%	Video
van Alphen and De Zeeuw, 2002	2×, staged	0.6 Hz, 5° × 90 min × 8 sessions	.31	+58%	32	−16%	Implanted coil
Boyden and Raymond, 2003	1.5×	1.0 Hz, 10° × 30 min	.40	+40%	23	−1%	Implanted coil
	1.5×	1.0 Hz, 10° × 30 min × 3 sessions	.40	+61%	23	−17%	
Faulstich et al., 2004	2×	0.5 Hz, 5° × 30 min	0.66	+23%	24	+17%	Video
Kimpo et al., 2005	2×	0.5 Hz, 3.2° × 30 min	0.14	+29%	27	+7%	Implanted coil
	2×	2 Hz, 0.8° × 30 min	0.29	+38%	9	+11%	
Katoh et al., 2005	1.25×	0.4 Hz, 7.2° × 40 min	0.72	+31%	—	—	Video
Hansel et al., 2006	2×	1.0 Hz, 1.6° × 50 min	0.81	+33%	13	−18%	Video
Boyden et al., 2006	1.5×	0.5 Hz, 3.2° × 30 min	0.30	+15%	—	—	Implanted coil
	1.5×	0.66 Hz, 2.4° × 30 min	0.28	+24%	—	—	
	1.5×	1.0 Hz, 1.6° × 30 min	0.39	+37%	—	—	
	1.5×	1.0 Hz, 1.6° × 30 min × 3 sessions	0.39	+49%	—	—	
	1.5×	2.0 Hz, 0.8° × 30 min	0.44	+36%	—	—	
Iwashita et al., 2001	0×	0.4 Hz, 7.2° × 40 min	0.40	−42%	25	+48%	Video
van Alphen and De Zeeuw, 2002	−1×, staged	0.6 Hz, 5° × 90 min × 8 sessions	0.44	−43%	29	+228%	Implanted coil
Boyden and Raymond, 2003	0×	1.0 Hz, 10° × 30 min	0.42	−40%	23	+9%	Implanted coil
	0×	1.0 Hz, 10° × 30 min × 3 sessions	0.42	−76%	23	+143%	
Faulstich et al., 2004	0×	0.5 Hz, 5° × 30 min	0.7	−28%	24	+29%	Video
Kimpo et al., 2005	0×	0.5 Hz, 3.2° × 30 min	0.16	−38%	30	+27%	Implanted coil
	0×	2.0 Hz, 0.8° × 30 min	0.30	−33%	10	−10%	
Katoh et al., 2005	0×	0.4 Hz, 7.2° × 40 min	0.72	−31%	—	—	Video
Hansel et al., 2006	0×	1.0 Hz, 1.6° × 50 min	0.81	−40%	13	−5%	Video
Boyden et al., 2006	0×	1.0 Hz, 1.6° × 30 min	0.40	−44%	—	—	Implanted coil
Katoh et al., 2006	−1×	1.0 Hz, 1.6° × 30 min	0.29	−20%	32	+97%	Video

Note: Most values have been measured from published figures and are thus approximate. In some cases baseline and gain/phase change data were obtained in different animals or samples. Stimulus column lists stimulus frequency, 0–peak amplitude, and minutes of training in each training session. $Gain_0$, $Phase_0$ are baseline values prior to training. Positive phase values denote phase lead. All gain and phase values are determined at the training frequency. Note that van Alphen et al. approached their final training goal gradually; the relationship between optokinetic and vestibular stimulation was adjusted in each daily training session. Boyden et al. (2003) used both 2-hour and 24-hour rest intervals in their multisession training paradigms. Where results differed appreciably, the 24-hour data are tabulated.

vestibular and optokinetic stimulation (Boyden and Raymond, 2003; Boyden et al., 2006; Faulstich et al., 2004; Hansel et al., 2006; Iwashita et al., 2001; Katoh et al., 2006; Katoh et al., 2005; Kimpo et al., 2005; van Alphen and De Zeeuw, 2002). The degree to which gain was modified varied widely for both "gain-up" and "gain-down" training. For training performed in a single 30- to 40-minute session, gain increases have ranged from 15% to 40% for gain-up training, and decreases have ranged from 20% to 42% of the pre-adaptation value. The variation reflects in part the broad range of adapting parameters (target gain, frequency, amplitude, training duration). Of these differences, duration of a single session is probably the least important factor, since gain tends to plateau after 30 minutes of training (Boyden and Raymond, 2003; Boyden et al., 2006; Katoh et al., 1998), and all the tabulated studies used session lengths of at least that duration. Rotation frequency, amplitude, and the target gain (i.e., 1.5×, 2×) are more critical, because these, along with the animal's initial gain, determine the magnitude of the retinal image velocities available to drive the adaptive process. Additionally, gain adaptation at different stimulus frequencies may engage different mechanisms (Kimpo et al., 2005) with potentially different susceptibility to adaptation. In three of the tabulated studies, adaptation was performed in multiple sessions separated by rest periods of hours or a day, during which the animals were maintained in darkness to prevent the natural visual-vestibular synergies from reversing the previous training (Boyden and Raymond, 2003; Boyden et al., 2006; van Alphen and De Zeeuw, 2002). Such multisession training produced the largest increases and decreases in aVOR gain. Gain changes from the previous session were retained, and subsequent training built on the new baseline. However, in two of the studies, the gain increments beyond that of the first day were not retained (Boyden and Raymond, 2003; Boyden et al., 2006), so the cumulative effect of multisession gain-up training was less than that of multisession gain-down training. It is interesting to note, however, that in both of those studies, the gain-up target was 1.5× and the increase in aVOR gain actually reached or surpassed 150% of the baseline value. If the system sought to multiply its baseline aVOR gain by 1.5, rather than to achieve an actual absolute gain of 1.5, then the target was met, and one would not expect further increments to be retained. In contrast, for gain-down training the goal of 0× was never met, which may explain why each daily gain decrement was retained.

Visual-vestibular training paradigms engender effects beyond the intended modulation of aVOR gain. Both gain-up and gain-down aVOR training augmented the gain of the OKR (Faulstich et al., 2004; van Alphen and De Zeeuw, 2002). In contrast, increases in OKR gain induced by prolonged exposure to the optokinetic stimulus alone did not engender changes in aVOR gain (Faulstich et al., 2004). aVOR gain training also produces changes in aVOR phase. Table 6.1 tabulates these changes, where available. In general, phase lead increased following gain-down training and decreased (or increased to a lesser extent) following gain-up training. However, as with the gain changes engendered by training, the magnitude of the results was highly variable. The variability likely reflects all the causes suggested for the gain data. Additionally, larger degrees of phase shift are expected for gain reversal (−1×) training (Gonshor and Jones, 1976). Phase values following gain reduction may also be more variable owing to the inherent unreliability of phase angle measurements made from waveforms in which the sinusoidal modulation is very weak. Finally, studies in which the effects of training were assessed at stimulus frequencies other than the training frequency (Iwashita et al., 2001; Kimpo et al., 2005; van Alphen and De Zeeuw, 2002) have demonstrated that in many cases, the phase effect crossed over from a relative phase lead to a relative phase lag near the training frequency. Thus, minor shifts of the frequency at which crossover occurred could change the observed effect on phase from lead to lag (or vice versa) when tested only at the training frequency. Even in the three studies that provided phase data over multiple frequencies, the form, magnitude, and even sign of the frequency effects on phase varied. Given the wide variation in the effects of training on phase, caution is warranted when attempting to employ current phase data to draw conclusions about underlying mechanisms of adaptation.

Three other types of eye movement adaptation have been explored in mice to date. OKR can be adapted directly by exposing the stationary animal to an oscillating optokinetic stimulus. Gain increases of 13%–40% have been reported in response to 60-minute training sessions (Katoh et al., 2000; Shutoh et al., 2003), and average gain increases of 116% were reported when animals were trained for multiple sessions (Shutoh et al., 2006). Figure 6.7 shows how the gain change built up in the course of the multiple sessions. Another type of aVOR manipulation is cross-axis adaptation, in which the direction of the aVOR is altered by rotating the animal about one axis while exposing it to an optokinetic stimulus rotating about a different axis (Schultheis and Robinson, 1981). Cross-axis adaptation in mice has been accomplished by combining a vertical axis turntable oscillation with a roll optokinetic stimulus, timed to induce downward eye movement during nasally directed eye movements (Stahl, 2004a; Stahl et al., 2006). As shown in the insets in figure 6.8, prior to the training period, turntable rotation in darkness evoked an essentially horizontal eye movement.

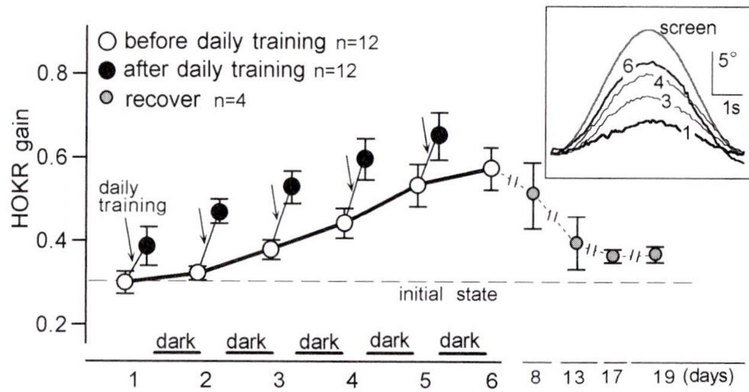

FIGURE 6.7 Direct adaptation of the horizontal OKR by daily sessions in which the animals were exposed to sustained 0.17 Hz, ±7.5° optokinetic stimulation. Gain increased during each session, and some fraction of that increase was retained until the following day, resulting in a gradual buildup of OKR gain. *Inset* shows the stimulus (screen) waveform and typical averaged eye movement responses obtained at the start of each day's session. Gain gradually reverted toward baseline in animals held in normal, lighted conditions after the training had concluded. (From Shutoh et al., 2006, with permission.)

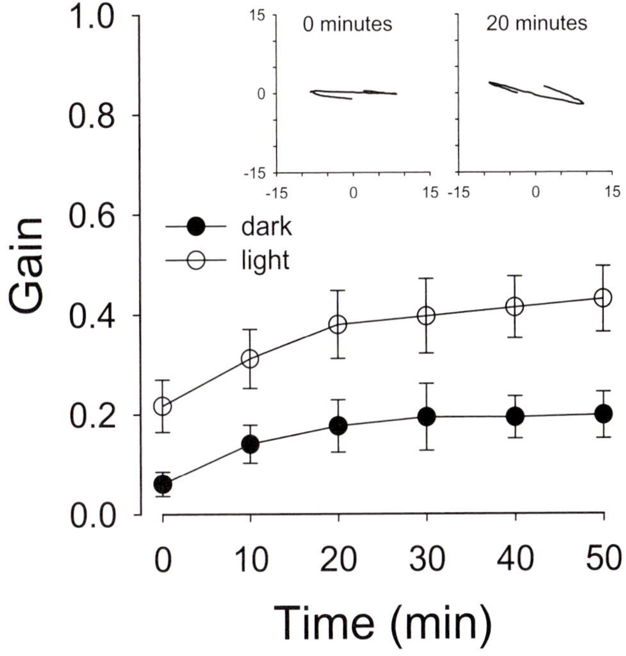

FIGURE 6.8 Time course of cross-axis adaptation in 30 C57BL/6 mice (Stahl, 2004a). Each *inset* plots vertical versus horizontal eye position for one typical cycle of aVOR and shows how, after 20 minutes of exposure to the training stimulus, development of a vertical response component renders the response trajectory diagonal. *Main panel* plots vertical gain (calculated as ratio of the amplitudes of vertical eye velocity and horizontal head velocity) over the course of the 50-minute adaptation period. Gain in light is the response in the presence of the training stimulus. Error bars are ±1 SD.

After 20 minutes of training, a vertical (roll axis) eye movement component had developed, rendering the eye position trajectory diagonal. Cross-coupling developed rapidly, plateauing around 20 minutes, although the vertical response to the training stimulus continued to grow for the duration of the training period. Cross-axis adaptation has some advantages over simple gain-up or gain-down training as an experimental paradigm. Among these, the appearance of the training effect can be detected by the experimenter "online," without quantitative analysis. In the case of simple gain training, the effects of training can be confounded by variations in gain due to changes in alertness or habituation to the vestibular stimulus (Stahl, 2004a). In contrast, the axis of the response is less likely to be shifted by a global increase or decrease in vestibular responsiveness.

A final form of experimental vestibular plasticity is vestibular compensation, or the adaptive response to the destruction of the vestibular nerve or labyrinth on one side (Curthoys and Halmagyi, 1995; Vidal et al., 1998). While extreme, this paradigm is biologically relevant, since acute, unilateral dysfunction of the peripheral vestibular apparatus is a clinical situation commonly encountered by neurologists (Leigh and Zee, 2006). The oculomotor phenomena of vestibular compensation have been explored in multiple afoveate mammalian species, including rats, gerbils, guinea pigs, and rabbits (Hamann et al., 1998). In all species, the lesion acutely engenders a spontaneous eye deviation and nystagmus, a head tilt, and a dramatic reduction in compensatory eye movements. Over a period of days, the spontaneous nystagmus recovers. Head tilt normalizes to a degree that varies across species (e.g., rapidly in the rat: Hamann et al., 1998; never in the rabbit: Baarsma and Collewijn, 1975a). In contrast, recovery of compensatory eye movements is universally weak, suggesting that most of the functional improvement following peripheral vestibular lesions is due to suppression of the debilitating static vestibular imbalance rather than to alteration of the function of the intact side to compensate for the lesion (Curthoys, 2000). Unilateral labyrinthectomy in mice has effects similar to those seen in other species, including induction of a head tilt, circling, and eye deviation, but only intermittent nystagmus (Faulstich et al., 2006). aVOR drops to 29%–54% of baseline (Faulstich et al., 2006; Murai et al., 2004), recovering to a plateau of only 39%–75% within 10 days of the lesion. The response in the light recovers to a greater degree, likely facilitated by a concomitant increase in OKR gain. Thus, vestibular compensation in mice as in other species is characterized by a recovery of the static vestibular imbalance and enhancement of alternative compensatory reflexes.

Fast phases of nystagmus

While not technically a compensatory eye movement, fast phases are critical to the operation of the compensatory reflexes because they prevent the eyes from reaching the limits of their range during large-amplitude head rotations. Unlike saccades, fast phases are intended to reset the position of the eyes within the orbit, rather than to aim the eyes at a specific point in space. However, they are orchestrated by much of the same brainstem circuitry as saccades and exhibit the same highly regular relationship between their peak velocities and amplitudes, and so for convenience we refer loosely to both types of rapid eye movements as "saccades." Saccades are the most rapid of eye movements, and, owing to the viscous properties of the extraocular tissues, achieving these high velocities requires the highest level of extraocular muscle forces of any eye movement. Thus, saccade dynamics provide an index of the ability of the oculomotor system to generate force (Leigh and Zee, 2006; Stahl et al., 2006). Saccade dynamics have been studied in C57BL/6 mice using video-oculography (Stahl, 2004a; Stahl et al., 2006). As in other species, the horizontal saccades exhibited consistent relationships between peak velocity and amplitude (a relationship sometimes referred to as a "saccade main sequence"; Bahill et al., 1975). The relationship was linear as in guinea pigs (Escudero et al., 1993) and rats (Fuller, 1985), rather than exponential or saturating as in rabbits (Collewijn, 1977), cats (Evinger and Fuchs, 1978), and humans (Bahill et al., 1981). Adducting saccades were approximately 13% faster than abducting saccades. Recently, mouse saccade dynamics have been reassessed using search coil recording, which permitted a much higher filtering frequency (1.5 kHz, vs. the 100 Hz employed in the later of the two mouse video studies), with a commensurate increase in the ability to resolve the peak velocity (Baker, 2004; Killian and Baker, 2006). The velocity-amplitude relationship for one animal is plotted in figure 6.9, superimposed on published curves for rats (Fuller, 1985), guinea pigs (Escudero et al., 1993), rabbits (Collewijn, 1977), cats (Evinger and Fuchs, 1978), rhesus (Fuchs, 1967), and humans (Baloh et al., 1975). Reaching velocities of up to 1,500 deg/s and having velocity-amplitude slopes of approximately 50 deg/s-deg, the mouse saccades are the fastest mammalian eye movements recorded to date.

Applications of the mouse eye movement recordings

Studies employing mouse oculography are being reported at an ever-increasing rate, and any summary of this literature would be doomed to rapid obsolescence. A sample of the literature is presented here with the goal of illustrating how techniques or resources specific to mice are providing new ways to study the oculomotor system, as well as how oculography can be applied as a tool in fields other than oculomotor physiology.

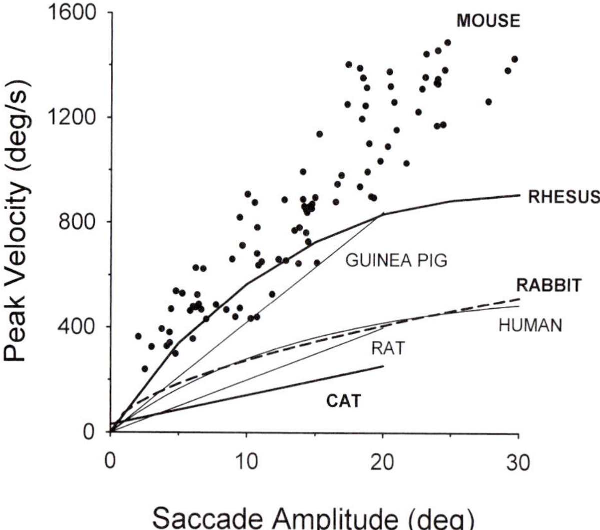

FIGURE 6.9 Plot of peak velocity versus amplitude for horizontal saccades or fast phases of vestibular nystagmus for several species. Relationship for a typical mouse recorded with a 0.8 mg, glued-on search coil is plotted as *solid circles*. Other species (plotted as *lines*) are based on published best-fit relationships. Directions (abducting or adducting) are unavailable for most sources and thus are not distinguished. (See the text for sources.)

To date, the single most common application of mice has been in the study of the molecular mechanisms underlying plasticity of the compensatory eye movement system.

One mechanism that has been proposed to mediate changes in aVOR gain is long-term depression (LTD) at the synapse between parallel fibers and Purkinje cells within the cerebellar flocculus (Ito, 1982, 2001). LTD can be blocked by inhibiting protein kinase C, one of the enzymes of the underlying signaling cascade. In a study that exemplifies the advantages of studying ocular motility in mice, De Zeeuw and colleagues performed a critical test of the involvement of both LTD and the cerebellum in aVOR plasticity through the use of a transgenic mouse that expresses a protein kinase C inhibitor in cerebellar Purkinje cells, but not in other cells of the oculomotor circuitry (De Zeeuw et al., 1998a). They demonstrated that the transgenics had normal baseline compensatory eye movements, but their aVOR gains could neither be increased nor decreased with 1-hour sessions of visual-vestibular training. They concluded that Purkinje cell LTD was indeed involved in rapid forms of motor learning, although other, slower mechanisms must exist that allowed the animals to achieve and maintain their normal baseline performance. The latter prediction was upheld when this same transgenic mutant was shown able to adjust its gain when training was continued for several days (van Alphen and De Zeeuw, 2002) and able to exhibit normal vestibular compensation following destruction of one labyrinth (Faulstich et al., 2006). Other receptors or enzymes whose role in vestibular plasticity has been investigated using genetically engineered mutant mice include the ionotropic glutamate receptor δ2 subunit (GluRδ2) (Katoh et al., 2005; Murai et al., 2004; Yoshida et al., 2004), nitric oxide synthase (Katoh et al., 2000), α-calcium/calmodulin-dependent protein kinase II (αCaMKII) (Hansel et al., 2006), and calcium/calmodulin-dependent protein kinase IV (CaMKIV) (Boyden et al., 2006). The studies of GluRδ2 demonstrate some of the interpretive hazards of using knockout mutants to study vestibular plasticity. Although the gene product is restricted to the Purkinje cell and its absence blocks LTD, the knockout also induces changes in baseline eye movements, Purkinje cell firing patterns, and activity in extracerebellar circuitry, obscuring the link between the function of GluRδ2 and vestibular adaptation.

Although many of the mutants studied to date have been knockouts of a gene of interest, mutations leading to expression of an altered gene product have also received attention. An advantage here is that multiple allelic mutants can be studied, and the oculomotor performance of the different mutants can be compared. For instance, multiple strains of mice are known to carry different mutations of *Cacna1a*, the gene encoding the ion pore subunit of the P/Q calcium channel. Comparison between two of these strains allowed hypotheses to be advanced regarding the minimum numbers of pathological processes that could explain the eye movement abnormalities (Stahl et al., 2006). Exploration of Purkinje cell activity in two of the P/Q mutants led to the idea that one of these pathological processes is the induction of irregularities in firing rates, which in turn stem ultimately from reduced calcium entry through the mutated channels (Hoebeek et al., 2005; Walter et al., 2006).

Mutant mouse strains have also been put to use by oculomotor physiologists as a method of producing a complete lesion of a specific structure. Both lurcher and Purkinje cell degeneration (*pcd*) mice undergo spontaneous postnatal degeneration of the cerebellar cortex. Studies have employed lurcher as a "disease control" for another strain bearing a mutation that results in a more focused alteration of cerebellar physiology (Katoh et al., 2005; Koekkoek et al., 1997). *Pcd* was used to demonstrate that the process of velocity estimation, previously hypothesized to rely on nodulo-uvular cerebellum, could also be accomplished in the absence of a functional cerebellar cortex (Killian and Baker, 2002). Two mutants characterized by their congenital absence of otoconia, head tilt (*het*) and tilted (*tlt*), have been employed to test the relative contributions of otolith and semicircular canal inputs to the response to rotations about earth-horizontal axes (Andreescu et al., 2005; Harrod and Baker, 2003).

Another attraction of studying the mouse oculomotor system is the potential to address a question using combinations of in vivo and in vitro techniques that would be impractical in animals such as rabbits, cats, and monkeys, formerly the customary models for oculomotor research. For instance, the influence of visual experience on the maturation of the extraocular muscles has been explored in dark-reared mice using a combination of eye movement recordings, recordings of contractility of isolated extraocular muscles, and gene expression profiling within the extraocular motor nuclei (McMullen et al., 2004). The origin of behavioral abnormalities in patients with paraneoplastic syndromes traced to autoantibodies against a metabotropic glutamate receptor has been explored using a combination of recordings from mouse cerebellar slices, cultured Purkinje cells, and recordings of eye movements during intrafloccular infusions of the antibodies (Coesmans et al., 2003). The ability to manipulate the mouse genome can also generate tools that facilitate the combination of in vitro and in vivo investigations. For instance, Sekirnjak and colleagues generated a mouse whose Purkinje cells express green fluorescent protein, allowing the Purkinje cells and their synaptic targets to be visualized when recording in vitro from brain slices from the vestibular nuclei (Sekirnjak et al., 2003). Brain slices from such animals obtained before and after aVOR gain training could be used to explore interactions between Purkinje cells and their targets related to vestibular plasticity.

Mouse oculography has also been used as a tool in studies not primarily concerned with oculomotor physiology. Thus, studies of mutations affecting the structure or physiology of the peripheral vestibular system have used measurements of eye movements to prove both the absence of a functioning vestibular periphery and the integrity of central vestibular circuitry (Alagramam et al., 2005; Sun et al., 2001). Eye movement recordings have also been used in investigations of the retinal circuitry as assays of the ability to process visual motion (Iwakabe et al., 1997; Yoshida et al., 2001). The precise, quantitative nature of eye movement recordings makes them a particularly sensitive assay for function of any part of the brain whose operation bears on ocular motility (Stahl, 2004b). Thus, oculomotor indices were among the measures used to assess whether genetically knocking out inferior olive gap junctions alters motor behavior (Kistler et al., 2002). The gap junctions electrotonically couple inferior olive cells, and have been hypothesized to play a role in motor coordination by synchronizing Purkinje cell activity within the cerebellar cortex (Blenkinsop and Lang, 2006). The power of eye movement recordings as an assay of brain function is, however, somewhat offset by the time-consuming nature of preparing animals for oculography, conducting the testing, and properly analyzing the data. Thus it has, to date, been impractical for use in high-throughput screening of mutants (Stahl, 2004b). However, assessing postural responses to optokinetic or vestibular stimuli in partially restrained or unrestrained animals is simpler, provides data sufficient for detecting gross optokinetic or vestibular deficits, and may provide a useful surrogate for eye movement recording in screening protocols (Prusky et al., 2004; Takemura and King, 2005).

Concluding remarks

Work to date has demonstrated that mouse eye movements are typical of the oculomotor repertoire of afoveate mammals. With some exceptions (notably the apparent lack of velocity storage, a particularly weak velocity-to-position neural integrator, and a tendency of response gains to decline during prolonged vestibular stimulation), the oculomotor performance is as good as, and in some cases superior to, that of animals with a longer history in oculomotor research. Some aspects of mouse ocular motility remain entirely unexplored, in particular the three-dimensional geometry of the compensatory movements. This absence reflects the additional technical challenges of recording torsional eye movements in this species. However, techniques for recording torsional movements with the aid of markers placed on the cornea have been employed in other afoveate mammals (Maruta et al., 2006; Migliaccio et al., 2005) and will likely be adapted for the mouse. Reliable recordings of eye movements in head-free animals will be a more challenging problem. The rapidly expanding literature on the eye movements of genetically altered mice illustrates the potential for genetic tools to create new ways to study the oculomotor system.

ACKNOWLEDGMENTS I am grateful to Brian Oommen for conducting the mouse static tilt experiments, as well as assisting in preparing several of the figures. Maarten Frens and Beerend Winkelman conducted recordings expressly to provide me with examples of rabbit OKAN. Jim Baker provided as yet unpublished saccade dynamics data, and Lloyd Minor and David Lasker provided primary afferent data. Jim Baker and Jerry Simpson both made helpful comments on an early version of the manuscript. Finally, I thank Bruce Cumming, Gary Paige, David Solomon, and Ted Raphan for their correspondence on issues related to afoveate vision, lVOR, and velocity storage.

REFERENCES

Alagramam, K. N., Stahl, J. S., Jones, S. M., Pawlowski, K. S., and Wright, C. G. (2005). Characterization of vestibular dysfunction in the mouse model for Usher syndrome 1F. *J. Assoc. Res. Otolaryngol.* 6:106–118.

Andreescu, C. E., De Ruiter, M. M., De Zeeuw, C. I., and De Jeu, M. T. (2005). Otolith deprivation induces optokinetic compensation. *J. Neurophysiol.* 94:3487–3496.

Angelaki, D. E., McHenry, M. Q., Dickman, J. D., Newlands, S. D., and Hess, B. J. (1999). Computation of inertial motion: Neural strategies to resolve ambiguous otolith information. *J. Neurosci.* 19:316–327.

Angelaki, D. E., Zhou, H. H., and Wei, M. (2003). Foveal versus full-field visual stabilization strategies for translational and rotational head movements. *J. Neurosci.* 23:1104–1108.

Baarsma, E., and Collewijn, H. (1974). Vestibulo-ocular and optokinetic reactions to rotation and their interaction in the rabbit. *J. Physiol.* 238:603–625.

Baarsma, E. A., and Collewijn, H. (1975a). Changes in compensatory eye movements after unilateral labyrinthectomy in the rabbit. *Arch. Otorhinolaryngol.* 211:219–230.

Baarsma, E. A., and Collewijn, H. (1975b). Eye movements due to linear accelerations in the rabbit. *J. Physiol.* 245:227–247.

Bahill, A. T., Brockenbrough, A., and Troost, B. T. (1981). Variability and development of a normative data base for saccadic eye movements. *Invest. Ophthalmol. Vis. Sci.* 21:116–125.

Bahill, A. T., Clark, M. R., and Stark, L. (1975). The main sequence, a tool for studying human eye movements. *Math. Biosci.* 24:191–204.

Baker, J. F. (2004). Large and small eye movements in mice. *Soc. Neurosci. Abstr.* 30:990.913.

Baloh, R. W., Sills, A. W., Kumley, W. E., and Honrubia, V. (1975). Quantitative measurement of saccade amplitude, duration, and velocity. *Neurology* 25:1065–1070.

Barmack, N. H. (1981). A comparison of the horizontal and vertical vestibulo-ocular reflexes of the rabbit. *J. Physiol.* 314: 547–564.

Barnes, G. R., and Smith, R. (1981). The effects of visual discrimination of image movement across the stationary retina. *Aviat. Space Environ. Med.* 52:466–472.

Becker, W., and Klein, H. M. (1973). Accuracy of saccadic eye movements and maintenance of eccentric eye positions in the dark. *Vision Res.* 13:1021–1034.

Blenkinsop, T. A., and Lang, E. J. (2006). Block of inferior olive gap junctional coupling decreases Purkinje cell complex spike synchrony and rhythmicity. *J. Neurosci.* 26:1739–1748.

Boyden, E. S., Katoh, A., Pyle, J. L., Chatila, T. A., Tsien, R. W., and Raymond, J. L. (2006). Selective engagement of plasticity mechanisms for motor memory storage. *Neuron* 51:823–834.

Boyden, E. S., Katoh, A., and Raymond, J. L. (2004). Cerebellum-dependent learning: The role of multiple plasticity mechanisms. *Annu. Rev. Neurosci.* 27:581–609.

Boyden, E. S., and Raymond, J. L. (2003). Active reversal of motor memories reveals rules governing memory encoding. *Neuron* 39:1031–1042.

Brettler, S. C., Rude, S. A., Quinn, K. J., Killian, J. E., Schweitzer, E. C., and Baker, J. F. (2000). The effect of gravity on the horizontal and vertical vestibulo-ocular reflex in the rat. *Exp. Brain Res.* 132:434–444.

Cannon, S. C., and Robinson, D. A. (1987). Loss of the neural integrator of the oculomotor system from brain stem lesions in monkey. *J. Neurophysiol.* 57:1383–1409.

Carpenter, R. H. S. (1988). *Movements of the eyes.* London: Pion.

Chelazzi, L., Ghirardi, M., Rossi, F., Strata, P., and Tempia, F. (1990). Spontaneous saccades and gaze-holding ability in the pigmented rat. II. Effects of localized cerebellar lesions. *Eur. J. Neurosci.* 2:1085–1094.

Coesmans, M., Smitt, P. A., Linden, D. J., Shigemoto, R., Hirano, T., Yamakawa, Y., van Alphen, A. M, Luo, C., van der Geest, J. N., et al. (2003). Mechanisms underlying cerebellar motor deficits due to mGluR1-autoantibodies. *Ann. Neurol.* 53:325–336.

Cohen, B., Matsuo, V., and Raphan, T. (1977). Quantitative analysis of the velocity characteristics of optokinetic nystagmus and optokinetic after-nystagmus. *J. Physiol.* 270:321–344.

Collewijn, H. (1969). Optokinetic eye movements in the rabbit: Input-output relations. *Vision Res.* 9:117–132.

Collewijn, H. (1972). Latency and gain of the rabbit's optokinetic reactions to small movements. *Brain Res.* 36:59–70.

Collewijn, H. (1977). Eye and head movements in freely moving rabbits *J. Physiol.* 266:471–498.

Collewijn, H. (1981). *The oculomotor system of the rabbit and its plasticity.* New York: Springer-Verlag.

Collewijn, H., Van der Steen, J., Ferman, L., and Jansen, T. C. (1985). Human ocular counterroll: Assessment of static and dynamic properties from electromagnetic scleral coil recordings. *Exp. Brain Res.* 59:185–196.

Collewijn, H., Winterson, B. J., and van der Steen, J. (1980). Post-rotary nystagmus and optokinetic after-nystagmus in the rabbit linear rather than exponential decay. *Exp. Brain Res.* 40:330–338.

Curthoys, I. S. (2000). Vestibular compensation and substitution. *Curr. Opin. Neurol.* 13:27–30.

Curthoys, I. S., and Halmagyi, G. M. (1995). Vestibular compensation: A review of the oculomotor, neural, and clinical consequences of unilateral vestibular loss. *J. Vestib. Res.* 5:67–107.

Dai, M. J., Raphan, T., and Cohen, B. (1991). Spatial orientation of the vestibular system: Dependence of optokinetic after-nystagmus on gravity. *J. Neurophysiol.* 66:1422–1439.

Darlot, C., Denise, P., Droulez, J., Cohen, B., and Berthoz, A. (1988). Eye movements induced by off-vertical axis rotation (OVAR) at small angles of tilt. *Exp. Brain Res.* 73:91–105.

De Zeeuw, C. I., Hansel, C., Bian, F., Koekkoek, S. K. E., van Alphen, A. M., Linden, D. J., and Oberdick, J. (1998a). Expression of a protein kinase C inhibitor in Purkinje cells blocks cerebellar LTD and adaptation of the vestibulo-ocular reflex. *Neuron* 20:495–508.

De Zeeuw, C. I., van Alphen, A. M., Koekkoek, S. K., Buharin, E., Coesmans, M. P., Morpurgo, M. M., and van den Burg, J. (1998b). Recording eye movements in mice: A new approach to investigate the molecular basis of cerebellar control of motor learning and motor timing. *Otolaryngol. Head Neck Surg.* 119: 193–203.

Escudero, M., de Waele, C., Vibert, N., Berthoz, A., and Vidal, P. P. (1993). Saccadic eye movements and the horizontal vestibulo-ocular and vestibulo-collic reflexes in the intact guinea-pig. *Exp. Brain Res.* 97:254–262.

Evinger, C., and Fuchs, A. F. (1978). Saccadic, smooth pursuit, and optokinetic eye movements of the trained cat. *J. Physiol.* 285:209–229.

Faulstich, B. M., Onori, K. A., and du Lac, S. (2004). Comparison of plasticity and development of mouse optokinetic and vestibulo-ocular reflexes suggests differential gain control mechanisms. *Vision Res.* 44:3419–3427.

Faulstich, M., van Alphen, A. M., Luo, C., du Lac, S., and De Zeeuw, C. I. (2006). Oculomotor plasticity during vestibular compensation does not depend on cerebellar LTD. *J. Neurophysiol.* 96:1187–1195.

Fernandez, C., and Goldberg, J. M. (1971). Physiology of peripheral neurons innervating semicircular canals of the squirrel monkey. II. Response to sinusoidal stimulation and dynamics of peripheral vestibular system. *J. Neurophysiol.* 34:661–675.

Fletcher, W. A., Hain, T. C., and Zee, D. S. (1990). Optokinetic nystagmus and afternystagmus in human beings: Relationship to nonlinear processing of information about retinal slip. *Exp. Brain Res.* 81:46–52.

Flipse, J. P., and Maas, A. J. (1996). Visual processing during high frequency head oscillation. *Aviat. Space Environ. Med.* 67:625–632.

Fuchs, A. F. (1967). Saccadic and smooth pursuit eye movements in the monkey. *J. Physiol.* 191:609–631.

Fuller, J. H. (1985). Eye and head movements in the pigmented rat. *Vision Res.* 25:1121–1128.

Gittis, A. H., and du Lac, S. (2006). Intrinsic and synaptic plasticity in the vestibular system. *Curr. Opin. Neurobiol.* 16:385–390.

Goldberg, J., and Fernandez, C. (1982). Eye movements and vestibular-nerve responses produced in the squirrel monkey by rotations about an earth-horizontal axis. *Exp. Brain Res.* 46:393–402.

Gonshor, A., and Jones, G. M. (1976). Extreme vestibulo-ocular adaptation induced by prolonged optical reversal of vision. *J. Physiol.* 256:381–414.

Grusser-Cornehls, U., and Bohm, P. (1988). Horizontal optokinetic ocular nystagmus in wildtype (B6CBA+/+) and weaver mutant mice. *Exp. Brain Res.* 72:29–36.

Hamann, K. F., Reber, A., Hess, B. J., and Dieringer, N. (1998). Long-term deficits in otolith, canal and optokinetic ocular reflexes of pigmented rats after unilateral vestibular nerve section. *Exp. Brain Res.* 118:331–340.

Hansel, C., de Jeu, M., Belmeguenai, A., Houtman, S. H., Buitendijk, G. H., Andreev, D., De Zeeuw, C. I., and Elgersma, Y. (2006). alphaCaMKII Is essential for cerebellar LTD and motor learning. *Neuron* 51:835–843.

Harris, L. R. (1987). Vestibular and optokinetic eye movements evoked in the cat by rotation about a tilted axis. *Exp. Brain Res.* 66:522–532.

Harrod, C. G., and Baker, J. F. (2003). The vestibulo ocular reflex (VOR) in otoconia deficient head tilt (*het*) mutant mice versus wild type C57BL/6 mice. *Brain Res.* 972:75–83.

Hess, B. J., and Dieringer, N. (1990). Spatial organization of the maculo-ocular reflex of the rat: Responses during off-vertical axis rotation. *Eur. J. Neurosci.* 2:909–919.

Hess, B., and Dieringer, N. (1991). Spatial organization of linear vestibuloocular reflexes of the rat: Responses during horizontal and vertical linear acceleration. *J. Neurophysiol.* 66:1805–1818.

Hess, B. J. M., Savio, T., and Strata, P. (1988). Dynamic characteristics of optokinetically controlled eye movements following inferior olive lesions in the brown rat. *J. Physiol.* 397:349–370.

Highstein, S. M. (1998). Role of the flocculus of the cerebellum in motor learning of the vestibulo-ocular reflex. *Otolaryngol. Head Neck Surg.* 119:212–220.

Hoebeek, F. E., Stahl, J. S., van Alphen, A. M., Schonewille, M., Luo, C., Rutteman, M., van den Maagdenberg, A. M., Molenaar, P. C., Goosens, H. H., et al. (2005). Increased noise level of Purkinje cell activities can cancel impact of their modulation during sensorimotor control. *Neuron* 45:953–965.

Ito, M. (1982). Cerebellar control of the vestibulo-ocular reflex: Around the flocculus hypothesis. *Annu. Rev. Neurosci.* 5:275–296.

Ito, M. (2001). Cerebellar long-term depression: characterization, signal transduction, and functional roles. *Physiol. Rev.* 81:1143–1195.

Iwakabe, H., Katsuura, G., Ishibashi, C., and Nakanishi, S. (1997). Impairment of pupillary responses and optokinetic nystagmus in the mGluR6-deficient mouse. *Neuropharmacology* 36:135–143.

Iwashita, M., Kanai, R., Funabiki, K., Matsuda, K., and Hirano, T. (2001). Dynamic properties, interactions and adaptive modifications of vestibulo-ocular reflex and optokinetic response in mice. *Neurosci. Res.* 39:299–311.

Jones, G. E., Balaban, C. D., Jackson, R. L., Wood, K. A., and Kopke, R. D. (2003). Effect of trans-bullar gentamicin treatment on guinea pig angular and linear vestibulo-ocular reflexes. *Exp. Brain. Res.* 152:293–306.

Kaneko, C. R. S. (1997). Eye movement deficits after ibotenic acid lesions of the nucleus prepositus hypoglossi in monkeys. I. Saccades and fixation. *J. Neurophysiol.* 78:1753–1768.

Katoh, A., Jindal, J. A., and Raymond, J. L. (2007). Motor deficits in homozygous and heterozygous P/Q-type calcium channel mutants. *J. Neurophysiol.* 97:1280–1287.

Katoh, A., Kitazawa, H., Itohara, S., and Nagao, S. (1998). Dynamic characteristics and adaptability of mouse vestibulo-ocular and optokinetic response eye movements and the role of the flocculo-olivary system revealed by chemical lesions. *Proc. Natl. Acad. Sci. U.S.A.* 95:7705–7710.

Katoh, A., Kitazawa, H., Itohara, S., and Nagao, S. (2000). Inhibition of nitric oxide synthesis and gene knockout of neuronal nitric oxide synthase impaired adaptation of mouse optokinetic response eye movements. *Learn. Mem.* 7:220–226.

Katoh, A., Yoshida, T., Himeshima, Y., Mishina, M., and Hirano, T. (2005). Defective control and adaptation of reflex eye movements in mutant mice deficient in either the glutamate receptor delta2 subunit or Purkinje cells. *Eur. J. Neurosci.* 21:1315–1326.

Kaufman, G. D. (2002). Video-oculography in the gerbil. *Brain Res.* 958:472–487.

Killian, J. E., and Baker, J. F. (2002). Horizontal vestibuloocular reflex (VOR) head velocity estimation in Purkinje cell degeneration (*pcd/pcd*) mutant mice. *J. Neurophysiol.* 87:1159–1164.

Killian, J. E., and Baker, J. F. (2006). Quick-phase three-dimensional eye velocity in roll and pitch vestibulo-ocular reflex during whole-body rotation about an earth-vertical axis follow a saccade-like "main sequence" in the mouse. *Soc. Neurosci. Abstr.* 32:48.13.

Kimpo, R. R., Boyden, E. S., Katoh, A., Ke, M. C., and Raymond, J. L. (2005). Distinct patterns of stimulus generalization of increases and decreases in VOR gain. *J. Neurophysiol.* 94:3092–3100.

Kistler, W. M., De Jeu, M. T., Elgersma, Y., Van Der Giessen, R. S., Hensbroek, R., Luo, C., Koekkoek, S. K., Hoogenraad, C. C., Hamers, F. P., et al. (2002). Analysis of Cx36 knockout does not support tenet that olivary gap junctions are required for complex spike synchronization and normal motor performance. *Ann. N. Y. Acad. Sci.* 978:391–404.

Koekkoek, S. K. E., Alphen, A. M., van der Burg, J., Grosveld, F., Galjart, N., and de Zeeuw, C. I. (1997). Gain adaptation and phase dynamics of compensatory eye movements in mice. *Genes Function* 1:175–190.

Kushiro, K., Dai, M., Kunin, M., Yakushin, S. B., Cohen, B., and Raphan, T. (2002). Compensatory and orienting eye movements induced by off-vertical axis rotation (OVAR) in monkeys. *J. Neurophysiol.* 88:2445–2462.

Leigh, R. J., and Zee, D. S. (2006). *The neurology of eye movements.* New York: Oxford University Press.

Leonard, C. S., Simpson, J. I., and Graf, W. (1988). Spatial organization of visual messages of the rabbit's cerebellar flocculus. I. Typology of inferior olive neurons of the dorsal cap of Kooy. *J. Neurophysiol.* 60:2073–2090.

Maioli, C. (1988). Optokinetic nystagmus: Modeling the velocity storage mechanism. *J. Neurosci.* 8:821–832.

Maioli, C., and Precht, W. (1984). The horizontal optokinetic nystagmus in the cat. *Exp. Brain Res.* 55:494–506.

Mangini, N. J., Vanable, J. W. J., Williams, M. A., and Pinto, L. H. (1985). The optokinetic nystagmus and ocular pigmentation of hypopigmented mouse mutants. *J. Comp. Neurol.* 241:191–209.

Maruta, J., MacDougall, H. G., Simpson, J. I., Raphan, T., and Cohen, B. (2006). Eye velocity asymmetry, ocular orientation, and convergence induced by angular rotation in the rabbit. *Vision Res.* 46:961–969.

Maruta, J., Simpson, J. I., Raphan, T., and Cohen, B. (2001). Orienting otolith-ocular reflexes in the rabbit during static and dynamic tilts and off-vertical axis rotation. *Vision Res.* 41:3255–3270.

McMullen, C. A., Andrade, F. H., and Stahl, J. S. (2004). Functional and genomic changes in the mouse ocular motor system in response to light deprivation from birth. *J. Neurosci.* 24:161–169.

Meier, R. K., and Dieringer, N. (1993). The role of compensatory eye and head movements in the rat for image stabilization and gaze orientation. *Exp. Brain Res.* 96:54–64.

Merwin, W. H. J., Wall, C. R., and Tomko, D. L. (1989). The chinchilla's vestibulo-ocular reflex. *Acta. Otolaryngol.* 108:161–167.

Migliaccio, A. A., Macdougall, H. G., Minor, L. B., and Della Santina, C. C. (2005). Inexpensive system for real-time 3-dimensional video-oculography using a fluorescent marker array. *J. Neurosci. Methods.* 143:141–150.

Miles, F. A., and Eighmy, B. B. (1980). Long-term adaptive changes in primate vestibuloocular reflex. I. Behavioral observations. *J. Neurophysiol.* 43:1406–1425.

Miles, F. A., and Lisberger, S. G. (1981). Plasticity in the vestibulo-ocular reflex: A new hypothesis. *Annu. Rev. Neurosci.* 4:273–299.

Mitchiner, J. C., Pinto, L. H., and Vanable, J. W. J. (1976). Visually evoked eye movements in the mouse (*Mus musculus*). *Vision Res.* 16:1169–1171.

Murai, N., Tsuji, J., Ito, J., Mishina, M., and Hirano, T. (2004). Vestibular compensation in glutamate receptor delta-2 subunit knockout mice: Dynamic property of vestibulo-ocular reflex. *Eur. Arch. Otorhinolaryngol.* 261:82–86.

Paige, G., and Tomko, D. (1991). Eye movement responses to linear head motion in the squirrel monkey. I. Basic characteristics. *J. Neurophysiol.* 65:1170–1182.

Prusky, G. T., Alam, N. M., Beekman, S., and Douglas, R. M. (2004). Rapid quantification of adult and developing mouse spatial vision using a virtual optomotor system. *Invest. Ophthalmol. Vis. Sci.* 45:4611–4616.

Rabbath, G., Necchi, D., de Waele, C., Gasc, J.-P., Josset, P., and Vidal, P.-P. (2001). Abnormal vestibular control of gaze and posture in a strain of a waltzing rat. *Exp. Brain Res.* 136:211–223.

Raphan, T., Matsuo, V., and Cohen, B. (1979). Velocity storage in the vestibulo-ocular reflex arc (VOR). *Exp. Brain Res.* 35:229–248.

Robinson, D. A. (1968). Eye movement control in primates. *Science* 161:1219–1224.

Robinson, D. A. (1981). The use of control systems analysis in the neurophysiology of eye movements. *Annu. Rev. Neurosci.* 4:463–503.

Schnabolk, C., and Raphan, T. (1994). Modeling three-dimensional velocity-to-position transformation in oculomotor control. *J. Neurophysiol.* 71:623–638.

Schultheis, L., and Robinson, D. (1981). Directional plasticity of the vestibuloocular reflex in the cat. *Ann. N.Y. Acad. Sci.* 374:504–512.

Sekirnjak, C., Vissel, B., Bollinger, J., Faulstich, M., and du Lac, S. (2003). Purkinje cell synapses target physiologically unique brainstem neurons. *J. Neurosci.* 23:6392–6398.

Shutoh, F., Katoh, A., Ohki, M., Itohara, S., Tonegawa, S., and Nagao, S. (2003). Role of protein kinase C family in the cerebellum-dependent adaptive learning of horizontal optokinetic response eye movements in mice. *Eur. J. Neurosci.* 18:134–142.

Shutoh, F., Ohki, M., Kitazwa, H., Itohara, S., and Nagao, S. (2006). Memory trace of motor learning shifts transsynaptically from cerebellar cortex to nuclei for consolidation. *Neuroscience* 139:767–777.

Simpson, J. I. (1984). The accessory optic system. *Annu. Rev. Neurosci.* 7:13–41.

Snyder, L., and King, W. (1992). Effect of viewing distance and location of the axis of head rotation on the monkey's vestibuloocular reflex. I. Eye movement responses. *J. Neurophysiol.* 67:861–874.

Stahl, J. S. (2002). Calcium channelopathy mutants and their role in ocular motor research. *Ann. N.Y. Acad. Sci.* 956:64–74.

Stahl, J. S. (2004a). Eye movements of the murine P/Q calcium channel mutant rocker, and the impact of aging. *J. Neurophysiol.* 91:2066–2078.

Stahl, J. S. (2004b). Using eye movements to assess brain function in mice. *Vision Res.* 44:3401–3410.

Stahl, J. S., James, R. A., Oommen, B. S., Hoebeek, F. E., and De Zeeuw, C. I. (2006). Eye movements of the murine p/q calcium channel mutant tottering, and the impact of aging. *J. Neurophysiol.* 95:1588–1607.

Stahl, J. S., van Alphen, A. M., and De Zeeuw, C. I. (2000). A comparison of video and magnetic search coil recordings of mouse eye movements. *J. Neurosci. Methods.* 99:101–110.

Sun, J. C., van Alphen, A. M., Wagenaar, M., Huygen, P., Hoogenraad, C. C., Hasson, T., Koekkoek, S. K., Bohne, B. A., and De Zeeuw, C. I. (2001). Origin of vestibular dysfunction in Usher syndrome type 1B. *Neurobiol. Dis.* 8:69–77.

Takemura, K., and King, W. M. (2005). Vestibulo-collic reflex (VCR) in mice. *Exp. Brain Res.* 167:103–107.

van Alphen, A. M., and De Zeeuw, C. I. (2002). Cerebellar LTD facilitates but is not essential for long-term adaptation of the vestibulo-ocular reflex. *Eur. J. Neurosci.* 16:486–490.

van Alphen, A. M., Stahl, J. S., Koekkoek, S. K. E., and De Zeeuw, C. I. (2001). The dynamic characteristics of the mouse vestibulo-ocular and optokinetic response. *Brain Res.* 890: 296–305.

van der Steen, J., and Collewijn, H. (1984). Ocular stability in the horizontal, frontal and sagittal planes in the rabbit. *Exp. Brain Res.* 56:263–274.

van Hof, M. W. (1966). Discrimination between striated patterns of different orientation in the rabbit. *Vision Res.* 6:89–94.

Vidal, P. P., de Waele, C., Vibert, N., and Muhlethaler, M. (1998). Vestibular compensation revisited. *Otolaryngol. Head Neck Surg.* 119:34–42.

Walls, G. L. (1942). *The Vertebrate eye and its adaptive radiation.* Bloomfield Hills, MI: Cranbrook Press.

Walter, J. T., Alvina, K., Womack, M. D., Chevez, C., and Khodakhah, K. (2006). Decreases in the precision of Purkinje cell pacemaking cause cerebellar dysfunction and ataxia. *Nat. Neurosci.* 9:389–397.

Wilson, V. J., and Melvill Jones, G. (1979). *Mammalian vestibular physiology.* New York: Plenum Press.

Yoshida, K., Watanabe, D., Ishikane, H., Tachibana, M., Pastan, I., and Nakanishi, S. (2001). A key role of starburst amacrine cells in originating retinal directional selectivity and optokinetic eye movement. *Neuron* 30:771–780.

Yoshida, T., Katoh, A., Ohtsuki, G., Mishina, M., and Hirano, T. (2004). Oscillating Purkinje neuron activity causing involuntary eye movement in a mutant mouse deficient in the glutamate receptor delta2 subunit. *J. Neurosci.* 24:2440–2448.

Zuidam, I., and Collewijn, H. (1979). Vergence eye movements of the rabbit in visuomotor behavior. *Vision Res.* 19:185–194.

7 Measuring Vision in the Awake Behaving Mouse

GLEN T. PRUSKY AND ROBERT M. DOUGLAS

Three blind mice, three blind mice,
See how they run, see how they run.
They all ran after the farmer's wife,
Who cut off their tails with a carving knife.
Did you ever see such a sight in your life,
As three blind mice?

Even though the "Three Blind Mice" nursery rhyme was not composed as a sleight to mouse vision but as an allegorical reference to the brutality of Queen Mary I ("Bloody Mary"), it has probably done more than anything else to diminish the reputation of the mouse as a visual mammal. The general public seems to accept without question that mice are both witless and sightless, and, as a nocturnal animal with diminutive eyes, the laboratory mouse has historically not been an animal of choice for vision research. With the emergence of the mouse as the most powerful mammalian model for molecular genetic manipulations, however, cellular and physiological studies of the mouse visual system have gained acceptance, even prominence, in visual neuroscience. Behavioral studies of mouse vision, on the other hand, have lagged behind, for at least two reasons: (1) methods to quantify mouse vision have been lacking, and (2) many consider measures of vision as an adjunct to corroborate cellular and physiological studies rather than as a powerful and necessary tool to comprehensively understand the visual system. As a result of the lack of effective testing methods, the vast majority of experimental studies of mouse vision have employed no behavioral measure of vision at all. There is also little basic information available on normal mouse visual behavior, and mice with genetic modifications affecting the visual system are being produced but not screened for vision. In addition, many of the mutations that target the visual system will have developmental consequences, and interpretations of the experiments would benefit from knowledge about the early development of vision. Fortunately, there has been progress on the methodological front, and the quantification of mouse vision is now practicable. Demonstrations of the experimental value of measuring mouse vision have followed and are now available in the literature.

This chapter discusses the rationale for measuring vision, explores available methods for measuring mouse vision, presents some pertinent data on mouse visual behavior, and suggests strategies for incorporating mouse visual behavior into vision studies. The goal is to enable vision scientists to effectively evaluate and use behavioral measurements of mouse vision, as well as to provide a general primer on mouse visual behavior.

Why measure mouse visual behavior?

One of the defining principles of neuroscience is that the evolutionary selection and survival of neural mechanisms occur only as their effects are manifested in behavior. As a consequence, the eventual aim of all physiological research is the understanding of behavior, whether or not individual researchers choose to study behavior. It was visual *function*, then, that was the grist of the natural selection of the visual system, and studies aimed at understanding the structure and physiology of the visual system are ultimately aimed at understanding vision. Measures of visual behavior can therefore provide a unifying perspective for studies of the mouse visual system because they measure the function that is most relevant to the evolutionary history of the system.

Behavioral measures of vision also have important experimental advantages that enable the measurement of visual functions in ways not feasible with other methods. For example, experiments that would benefit from repeated-measures design are often precluded when using methods that are practically limited to a single session (e.g., unit recording) or end with euthanasia (e.g., histology). Many neurophysiological measurements also require the use of anesthetics, which can alter cellular responses (Pham et al., 2004) and produce detrimental cumulative effects when used repeatedly. Another advantage of behavioral measures is that they are often more sensitive than physiological methods in detecting visual function or dysfunction. For example, behavioral methods are able to measure visual thresholds long after the electroretinogram (ERG) is measurable (McGill et al., 2004). The reasons for this disparity include the nature of vision as a systemwide product, not solely a function of the retina—that is, we "see" with our visual system, not with our eyes—and the wide distribution of the circuitry underlying most visual functions, such that most physiological methods sample function in only a subset of these circuits. In addition, anesthetic, analgesic, and paralytic agents can dampen cellular responses.

An important experimental advantage of visual behavior is that it is the measure of visual system function most relevant to the identification and treatment of visual diseases. Many diseases of the visual system are manifested as, and defined by, abnormalities in vision (e.g., age-related macular degeneration, amblyopia, retinitis pigmentosa, glaucoma, myopia), and it is almost always the lack of normal vision that brings individuals to the clinic. This has both practical and conceptual implications. Practically, it means that an animal model of a visual disease must include a measure of vision to ensure that it is relevant to the human condition. For example, many visual diseases are characterized by great variability in the presentation of symptoms (i.e., expressivity), and an animal model that does not have this feature may not be the best model, or the definition of the human disease may need to be revised. Conceptually, it means that a successful treatment for a visual disorder is defined not solely as a gain or replacement of circuits or physiological function but as a benefit to, or replacement of, vision: it does not help a patient to hear that the visual system has been "fixed" if that fix does not translate into improved vision.

Considerations when testing mouse vision

Although there are distinct experimental advantages to measuring vision, there are also idiosyncrasies associated with whole animal behavior that cannot be ignored. When behavioral signals are the dependent variables in an experiment, the environmental circumstances under which the experiment is conducted and the physiology and genotype of the animal are important concerns. For example, mice are nocturnal rodents that almost certainly use their visual systems to solve different problems under light and dark conditions. As light levels decrease from daylight conditions, receptive fields (RFs) in the retina are thought to be transformed from bandpass filters, which trade off light sensitivity for spatial sensitivity, to low-pass filters, which favor the opposite. Consequently, scotopic vision (roughly approximated with rod-dominated, dark-cycle vision) is characterized by enhanced light detection at the expense of pattern detection, whereas photopic vision (roughly approximated with cone-dominated vision during the light cycle) is characterized by the ability to detect patterned stimuli at the expense of light sensitivity. Asking pattern vision questions under scotopic conditions or light sensitivity questions in photopic conditions, then, should be carefully considered. It should be noted that almost all visuobehavioral experiments (i.e., memory tasks) in mice are conducted under photopic conditions.

Mice are also most active around the transition between light and dark phases of the circadian cycle. In most rodent vivaria, the transition between light and dark is not gradual but abrupt, and the ability to measure behavior effectively under these "hyperactive" conditions is often difficult. In addition, mice are social animals that function at a high metabolic level and need social contact and regular sustenance to maintain normal behavioral function. Novel odors and sounds, an animal's sex, age, housing conditions, position in the estrous cycle, and so on should also be brought under experimental control. Genotype is also an important factor that can affect behavioral measures of vision. Gene products almost always support functions beyond the visual system, and so-called performance effects on behavior can occlude the ability to measure vision. For example, if a mutation affects the motor system and a visual task relies on competent motor function, measures of vision may be impossible, or the data may be misleading.

Measuring visual behavior is also not a one-size-fits-all proposition. An informative example is the measurement of visual acuity. The operational definition of acuity is the maximal perceptual ability to distinguish two high-contrast items as distinct (traditionally, in humans, the ability to distinguish Mizar and Alcor, a double star system on the handle of the Big Dipper, as separate stars). Many think of visual acuity as the best measure of vision that captures in one number the function of the visual system. Of course, the visual system is not one system but a collection of many systems, and acuity measures only a subset of the functions of those systems. Consequently, measures of acuity should be considered one of many possible measures of function, and the appropriate measure should be tailored to the experimental question. Additionally, measuring the spatial frequency (SF) thresholds of different visual behaviors does not necessarily measure acuity. In a related vein, experimental questions are often explicitly directed at a specific visual system structure and are not compatible with a systemwide measure of function. If a manipulation of the lateral geniculate nucleus (LGN) is the critical variable in an experiment, a measurement of vision that depends on the collective integrity of the retina, LGN, and visual cortex (V1) may not provide meaningful information because manipulations of any of the structures may result in the same behavioral result. Likewise, a freely moving and unanesthetized animal is not compatible with many techniques that require stability of the visual system (e.g., electrophysiological recordings, optical imaging) or when temporal and spatial restriction of a visual stimulus is required (e.g., mapping cellular RF properties). Technical advances may enable such techniques to be applied in awake, behaving animals in the future, but at present, a moving animal is irreconcilable with such techniques.

As with any useful technique, measuring visual behavior also requires an investment in equipment and technical expertise. There is an attitude among some that measuring behavior is easy, that generating data should be fast and simple, and that the measurement of behavior can be easily automated. Although behavioral measurements of vision can be relatively fast and simple, and technological advances have been applied effectively, this is usually the result of the hard work of talented and trained people and the development of sophisticated technology; fast and simple measurements of vision carried out poorly can be worse than not measuring vision at all. As a consequence, anyone deciding to include measures of visual behavior in his or her experimental repertoire should be prepared to invest significant resources in the effort. There are good grounds for including measures of vision in many experiments today, and this rationale will not go away in the future. Consequently, a laboratory that makes a long-term investment in the methodology and that endeavors to use behavioral measures appropriately will undoubtedly reap significant rewards.

Testing methodologies

Most would probably agree that vision is the act or power of seeing. The apparent simplicity of this definition, however, is at variance with the multiplicity of ways the word is applied in the scientific literature, where everything from a light avoidance response to hyperacuity has been represented as "vision." One practical way to deal with this ambiguity when it comes to testing mouse vision is to distinguish between behavioral tests that measure *whether* an animal can see and those that test *what* it can see. In many cases, the test of a hypothesis requires only an endpoint measure of whether an animal's visual system can detect light, and simple tests such as measuring the pupillary reflex, light avoidance response, or light-induced circadian phase shift may suffice. More often, however, a measure of the quality of vision is desirable, and more sophisticated tests are required. The balance of this chapter deals primarily with this later category and examines measures of vision that quantify the degree of *what* a mouse can see.

Measures of Visual Perception in Reinforcement-Based Tasks A common strategy in the experimental analysis of behavior is to use a reward (reinforcer; e.g., food, water, escape) as a means to shape a desired behavior; increasingly accurate approximations of a desired behavioral response are reinforced, such that the response becomes more like the desired behavior. The classic reinforcement-based task for measuring vision in rodents is the Lashley jumping stand (Lashley, 1930). The task had many pitfalls as a practical method for the measurement of rat vision and is probably no longer used with rodents; to our knowledge, it was never successfully adapted for the measurement of mouse vision. Many other attempts have been made to convert rat tasks to mouse versions, apparently on the assumption that mice are small versions of rats. However, mice and rats are very different animals with different adaptive traits, and mice seem to be less prepared to learn many behavioral tasks (Whishaw, 1995) than rats. As a consequence, far fewer intricate behavioral methods have been successfully applied in mice than in rats.

Despite this, a number of clever instrumental learning tasks have been used with success in mice. One is an adaptation of a three-alternative, forced choice discrimination task (Jacobs et al., 1999). In this task, lights are projected onto three test panels on the wall of a testing chamber, and through an operant shaping procedure, mice are trained to touch the stimulus panel illuminated by a test light, and correct choices are reinforced with a liquid. The task has been used to measure spectral sensitivities in mice by identifying the threshold ability to detect a difference between the test light and background light (Jacobs et al., 2004). In another task (Gianfranceschi et al., 1999), mice are food deprived and trained to discriminate between pairs of stimuli. A correct choice is rewarded with a pellet, and the animal is then allowed to walk through a swinging door to a start box, where it is again rewarded with a pellet. Following a wrong choice, the food reward is omitted, the return path is blocked, and the mouse is placed back in the start box. Grating acuity, measured as the SF threshold to discriminate a vertical from a horizontal square wave grating, has been measured with this task. Although each of these tasks has been used with some success, none has gained wide popularity, probably because the shaping and testing procedures, even in the most obliging mice, require a considerable amount of time (weeks to months), and in our hands, many animals are effectively untrainable in such appetitive-based tasks.

The Morris water maze (Morris et al., 1982), which was originally developed as a rat visuospatial learning task, has also been adapted to measure mouse vision. The now classic configuration of the task to measure spatial learning takes advantage of the fact that laboratory rodents are instinctive swimmers and are motivated to escape from the water to a solid, submerged platform in a large circular pool of water, the position of which is stable in reference to the constellation of surrounding visual cues. Since animals can readily learn to use the configuration of visual cues outside the pool to locate the platform and swim to it, and no appetitive motivation is required, adaptations of the task provide for the possibility of accelerating the efficiency of visual measures.

The initial water maze experiments, which measured place learning and memory (Morris et al., 1982), anticipated that interpretations of the data could be confounded by abnormal visual function. One configuration of the task that was developed to control for reduced visual function and that has been used widely with mice is the cued platform task. The rationale was that if animals could not learn to swim directly to a visible platform in the pool, they probably had visual impairments, and conversely, if animals could swim directly to the cued platform, they were relatively free of visual deficits. We performed a set of experiments in rats to explicitly test this hypothesis by measuring place learning in animals with a 30% reduction in vision (Prusky et al., 2000b) and found they had a significant impairment in learning the task. The same animals, however, were not impaired in their ability to locate a cued platform. Together, these results showed that identifying animals with at least 30% reduced acuity, a reduction that significantly affects adaptive function, is not possible using a cued platform version of the Morris water task—a clear example of a performance effect.

The major limitations of the cued platform task as a measure of vision are the relative lack of stimulus control and the difficulty of monitoring viewing distances in a moving animal. In addition, the task is essentially a signal detection task, not a visual discrimination task. For example, any image can be analyzed as if it were formed by a set of sine waves of different SFs, and the RF organization of mammalian retinal and cortical cells appear to measure the magnitude and location of the different SF components. The ability to identify cues and locate a place in visual space is limited by sensitivity to the highest spatial frequencies. In a typical cued platform task, the single platform cue usually appears dark against a white pool wall. That object can be decomposed into many frequencies, any of which can be used to identify the platform. That is, in the absence of distractors or multiple visual cues that must be discriminated, detection of a single large cue may be possible with vision consisting of only the lowest SF detectors. Moreover, performance on the cued platform task is not an accurate measure of visual acuity because the cue is usually too large and there is little control of the viewing distance. Even from the farthest viewing position in a 1.5-m pool, a 10-cm cue will subtend about 5° of visual angle, corresponding to a grating acuity of 0.1 cycles/degree (c/deg), well below the threshold that normal mice can discriminate. In other words, the cued-platform task is capable of determining *whether* a mouse can see but not *what* it can see.

In an effort to mitigate these problems, a different configuration of the Morris water task and an accompanying training procedure were developed to measure visual acuity in mice (Robinson et al., 2001). Animals are trained to discriminate between two cue cards displaying very different vertical square-wave gratings. Cards are presented in two adjacent quadrants of the pool separated by a barrier, with the escape platform located in front of the card displaying the higher SF. When cards were systematically exchanged to make the discrimination more difficult and the swimming pattern of the animals was analyzed, the threshold for mice was estimated to be approximately 1.3 c/deg (Robinson et al., 2004).

Although swimming to an exit platform and using visual cues in the Morris water maze seem to come naturally to the mouse, enabling more rapid training and testing of visual thresholds, this modification of the task to measure visual acuity still has significant drawbacks. Even with the analysis of swimming patterns, viewing distances to the stimuli are difficult to control, and the reported acuity of mice in this task is about twice that reported with other tasks (Gianfranceschi et al., 1999; Prusky et al., 2000c), indicating that animals are making decisions much closer to the stimuli than the video analysis indicates. In addition, printed cards restrict the range of stimulus options, and the manual exchanging of the cards practically limits the efficiency with which an experiment can be carried out.

The possibility that the motivation and reward structure of a water-based escape task could enable more efficient training and testing of animals, and that computer-controlled stimulus presentation could better manage an experiment, prompted us to develop the visual water task (Prusky et al., 2000c). As shown in figure 7.1*A*, a trapezoidal tank is made into a Y-maze with a central divider, and computer monitors are placed behind a glass wall at the end of each arm. A platform is submerged below a positive (reinforced) stimulus displayed on one of the two monitors. Once mice learn that the images on the screens are clues to where the platform is, the animals either stop at the end of the divider and inspect both screens or swim slowly near the divider while looking at the two screens alternately, before making their choices. At no time have we had to explicitly reinforce this scanning behavior, because animals appear to spontaneously compare the screens before taking a chance on going the wrong way. The end of the divider, therefore, sets a choice point that is as close as the mice can get to the screens without entering one of the two arms, and the length of the divider sets the effective SF of the stimuli. The water aids in dispersing odor trails, which can be a problem in terrestrial reinforcement-based tasks, and also focuses the mouse's attention on the computer monitors without generating a great deal of stress. On land, mice have multiple sensory inputs to consider, but in water, they seem to know that vision is the best modality to use and that the visual cues will be some distance away. Besides the task exploiting an ecologically relevant behavior, using computer-generated stimuli is also advantageous, since it allows stimuli to be presented that are impossible to produce with printed cards. In addition, software control facilitates the automatic interleaving of stimuli and animals, which greatly increases throughput in the laboratory. The collective benefit of these features is that the measurement of many different visual thresholds can be completed with relative efficiency.

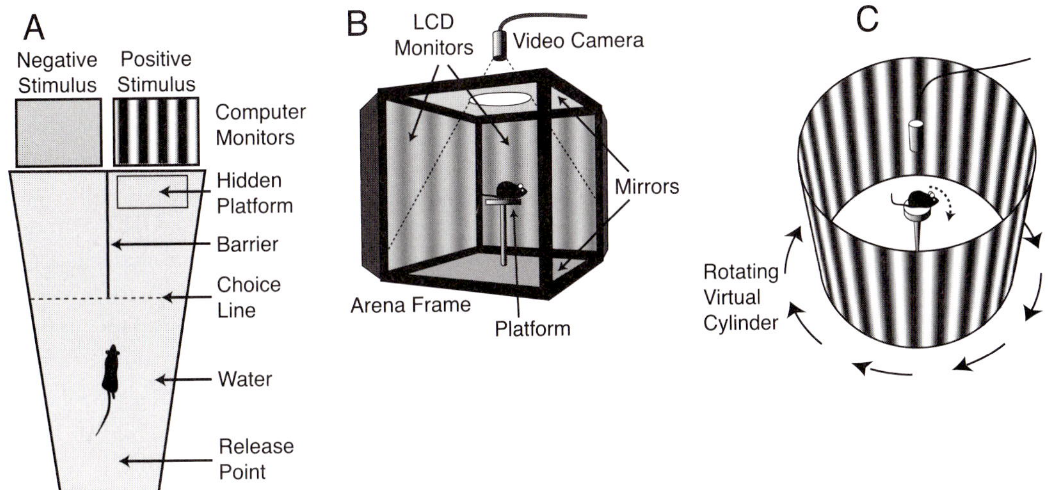

FIGURE 7.1 *A*, Schematic view of the visual water task. Apparatus consists of a trapezoidal tank containing water with a midline barrier, creating a Y-maze. Two monitors face into the arms of the maze and display either a positive (+, reinforced [i.e., grating]) or a negative (–, nonreinforced [i.e., gray]) stimulus. A platform is always submerged below the + stimulus, regardless of its left or right position, which is varied randomly over trials. Mice are released into the pool at the narrow end and then swim to the divider. They inspect each screen from this vantage point and then choose to swim toward one of them. If they select the + stimulus, they are rewarded quickly with escape from water, and the trial is scored as correct. If they choose the – stimulus (by crossing the choice line on the side with the – stimulus), they are compelled to swim until they find the escape platform on the opposite side, and the trial is scored as incorrect. (Adapted from Prusky and Douglas, 2004.) *B*, Cutaway schematics of OptoMotry (CerebralMechanics Inc.), a virtual optokinetic system (VOS). A testing chamber is created by attaching four inward-facing LCD computer monitors to a frame. Gratings on the monitors are reflected in floor and ceiling mirrors that extend the stimulus above and below. A mouse is placed on a small circular platform on a stand at the center of the chamber, where it is free to move. A camera mounted above is used to image the animal. *C*, Optokinetic stimulus. A virtual cylinder is calculated by a computer in a three-dimensional coordinate system and projected onto the monitors. From the animal's point of view, an illusory cylinder rotates outside the chamber. The spatial frequency, contrast, and direction of rotation of the grating on the cylinder can be changed in real time. An experimenter uses the video image to maintain the hub of cylinder between the eyes as the animal moves about the platform and to judge when the animal tracks the cylinder movement. (Adapted from Douglas et al., 2005.)

The task has been used with stimuli that consist of different patterns, contrasts and movement in order to measure mouse visual thresholds. For example, we have measured spatial contrast sensitivity (see figure 7.4*A*) as well as grating acuity with two different sets of discriminanda, and have shown that the thresholds are limited by the function of visual cortex (figure 7.2*A*; Prusky and Douglas, 2004). Others have used the task to screen mouse strains for spatial visual function or dysfunction (Wong and Brown 2006, 2007). We have also used the discrimination of moving dot kinematograms to show that mice possess local and global visual motion-processing systems (Douglas et al., 2006) analogous to those in higher mammals. In addition, we have measured the threshold for mice to discriminate the size (visual angle) of sine wave gratings to gain insight into areal processing in the retina (figure 7.2*B*). Our work and the work of others have also used the visual water task to map plasticity associated with developmental enrichment (Prusky et al., 2000a; Sale et al., 2004) and the visual "critical period" (figure 7.2*C*; Cancedda et al., 2004; Gianfranceschi et al., 2003; Prusky and Douglas, 2003).

That mouse acuity at approximately 0.56 c/deg is more than 50 times worse than human 20/20 visual acuity of 30 c/deg appears, on face value, to confirm the preconception that mice are effectively blind. However, the relatively low acuity does not mean that mouse vision is not useful. Much of what is relevant for a mouse to look at is inside 30 cm, much closer than the distance at which humans routinely fixate. More distant objects may not be as clearly seen, but large ones may be helpful for navigation in photopic conditions. In figure 7.3 we consider an intermediate distance, 1 m, and illustrate what a cat and a mouse might see of each other by removing all SFs above each species's threshold. Although the cat's view of the mouse (figure 7.3*C*) is better than the mouse's view of the cat (figure 7.3*B*), the mouse can still see the cat quite well. Furthermore, figure 7.3*C* also presents what a mouse might see of another mouse 10 cm away: vision could well be used by mice in their social interactions.

MEASURES OF AUTOMATED VISUAL RESPONSES The visual system is often termed a sensory system, but from a functional

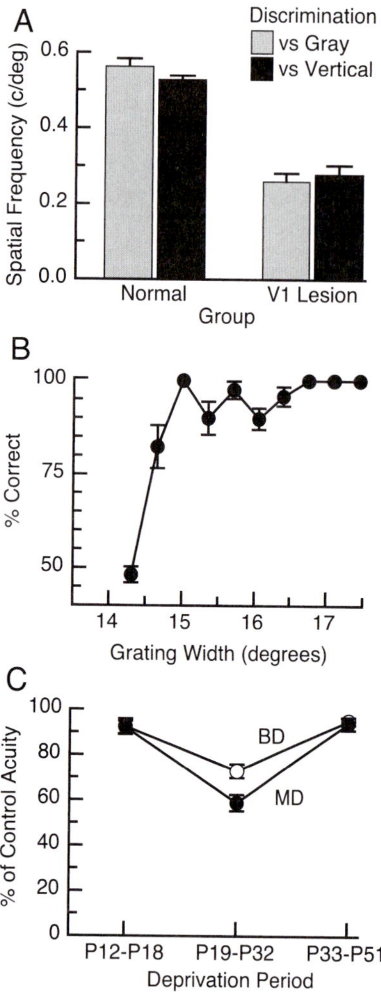

FIGURE 7.2 Examples of visual water task data. *A*, Grating (+, reinforced stimulus) versus gray (unreinforced stimulus) and vertical grating (+) versus horizontal grating (–) discrimination SF thresholds in intact adult C57BL/6 mice, and the effect of bilateral V1 lesions. Thresholds were comparable between the tasks and were substantially reduced following lesions. Bars in this and other figures represent ±SEM. (Adapted from Prusky and Douglas, 2004.) *B*, Effect of varying the size of the discriminanda (grating [0.315 c/deg] vs. gray) on task performance. Performance declined when the dimensions of the grating fell below 15°, revealing the likely minimum retinal surface area required for computations related to spatial frequency processing. *C*, Effect of binocular deprivation (BD) and monocular deprivation (MD) on acuity. Only deprivation during the "critical period" for ocular dominance plasticity results in amblyopia, with MD having a more severe effect than BD. (From Prusky and Douglas, 2003.)

point of view it is really an integrated sensorimotor system: normal function is not possible without a variety of visuomotor reflexes to ensure that a relatively stable image of the visual field is maintained on the retina. Because these reflexes are essentially automated, they provide an opportunity to test visual function without reinforcement-based training of an animal, and they hold the promise of enabling the measurement of vision in experiments in which reinforcement training and testing are either impractical or precluded. One of these reflexes, the optokinetic response (OKR), compensates for the motion of the visual field, using the relative velocity of the image on the retina to induce in rodents head movements in the same direction and at about the same velocity as in the external world. OKRs in rodents have been studied for some time using a mechanical apparatus (Cowey and Franzini, 1979) consisting of a drum with printed stimuli on the inside wall; the drum rotates around the animal, generating compensatory head movements that track the rotation. A variation of this task has been used as a tool to screen for visual abnormalities in mice (Abdeljalil et al., 2005) by using post hoc video analysis to estimate the SF threshold to elicit tracking under scotopic and photopic conditions. Another variant of the task has been developed to automatically track the angular speed of mice in relation to the center of the drum, using the angular orientation of the snout-tail body axis. Research using this task has reported that the mouse visual system is most responsive to bright luminance, as well as the surprising finding that rods are not saturated in the mesopic or low photopic range (Schmucker et al., 2005). Other research has shown that the mouse OKR system has sufficient spatial vision to respond to refractive errors induced with spectacle lenses or diffusers (Schmucker and Schaeffel, 2006).

Notwithstanding the reported success of the tasks using the drum, the difficulty of controlling the speed of the drum and its position in relation to the animal, combined with the problem of printing precise visual stimuli and exchanging them rapidly, has limited the popularity of the device. We have addressed these obstacles by developing a virtual OKR system (VOS; Prusky et al., 2004; see figure 7.1*B* and *C*). A virtual cylinder comprised of a vertical sine wave grating is projected in 3D coordinate space on a quadrangle of computer monitors around a testing arena. Individual mice are placed on a circular elevated platform in the center of the arena, where they are allowed to move freely. The mouse is imaged from above and the animal's head is tracked continuously with the aid of a computer mouse and a crosshair superimposed on a video image of the arena. The *x-y* positional coordinates of the crosshair in the video frame center the hub of the virtual cylinder, enabling the cylinder wall to be maintained at a constant virtual distance from the animal's eyes and thereby clamping the SF of the stimulus at the animal's viewing position. When the cylinder is rotated and the mouse follows with corresponding horizontal head and neck movements (OKR), it is judged in real time by an observer that the animal's visual system can distinguish the grating. We have used a cylinder velocity of 12°/s for most of our experiments because it generates a robust response, but it is in a range in which variations in velocity (and hence temporal frequency) have little effect on the final threshold

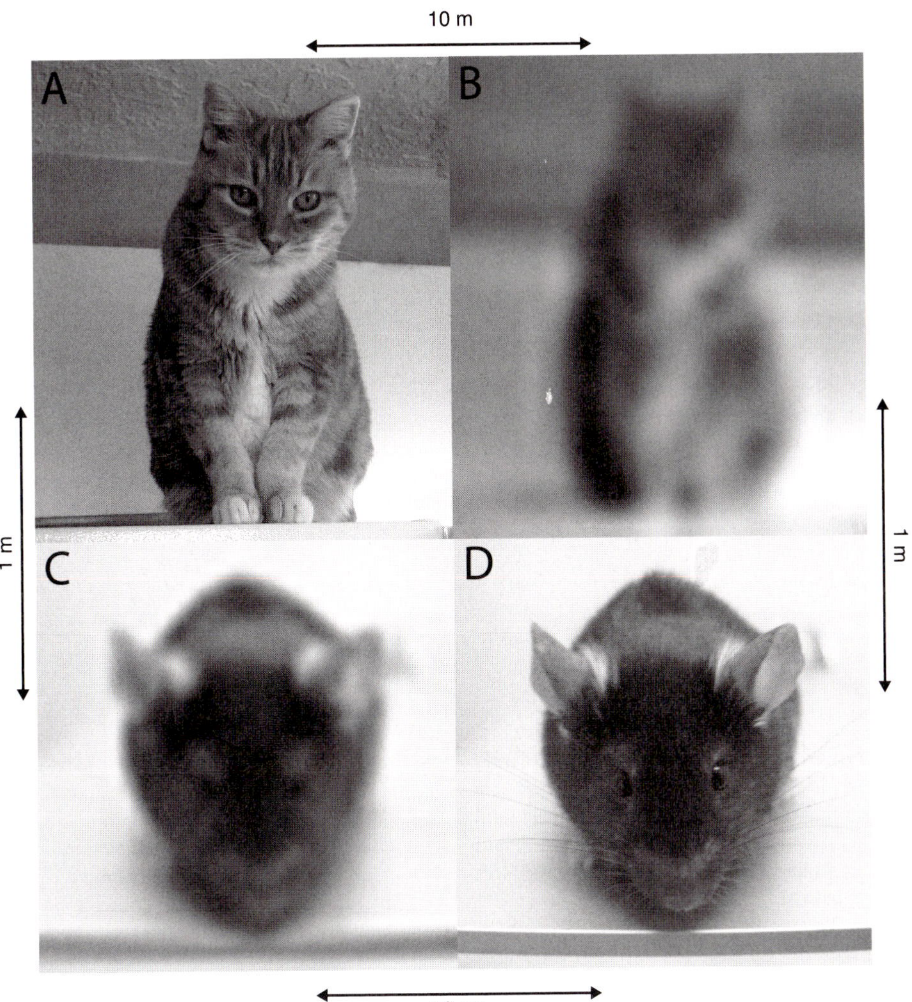

FIGURE 7.3 Model of what the mouse and a common predator, the cat, can see. Mouse acuity is about 10 times worse than cat acuity. *A* and *D* are the original photographs, printed with an effort to maintain as much resolution as possible. *B* and *C* have had all the spatial frequencies (SFs) above the two species' acuities removed, assuming a viewing distance of 1 m, about the distance that a cat strikes a mouse. This was created in Photoshop by reducing the size in pixels of each image to 2×(width in degrees)/SF and then expanding the image to the original size using bicubic interpolation. This method ignores changes in contrast sensitivity as a function of SF, so it overestimates what each can see, but it allows comparison of what the two animals can see. As shown in *B*, the image of the cat is discernible to the mouse. A second set of comparisons can be made across the rows. *C* shows what a mouse would look like to another mouse at 10 cm, whereas *B* is what a cat would look like to another cat 10 m away. As these simple simulations suggest, vision is quite useful to the mouse in dealing with its local environment.

(figure 7.4*C*). The tracking behavior is stereotyped, and the variability in thresholds is very low (Douglas et al., 2005).

To measure the SF threshold of the OKR, a homogeneous gray stimulus is projected on the cylinder at the beginning of each testing session, and the experimenter waits until the animal stops moving, at which time the gray is switched to a low-SF (e.g., 0.04 c/deg), high-contrast sine wave grating moving in one direction. The animal is then assessed for tracking behavior for a few seconds, after which the gray stimulus is restored. The procedure is repeated until unambiguous examples of tracking are observed. The SF of the grating is then increased incrementally until the animal no longer tracks the stimulus. We have reported that the SF threshold of the OKR of normal C57BL/6 mice is about 0.4 c/deg (figure 7.5*A*; Prusky et al., 2004, 2006). This value is lower than that obtained with the visual water task, but it probably reflects the characteristics of the subcortical retinal efferents. It does not, however, reflect a lower sensitivity: contrast sensitivity measurements in the VOS are significantly higher than those seen on the visual water task (see figure 7.4*A*).

Thresholds through each eye can be measured independently by reversing the rotation of the cylinder. When one eye is temporarily occluded, only rotation in the

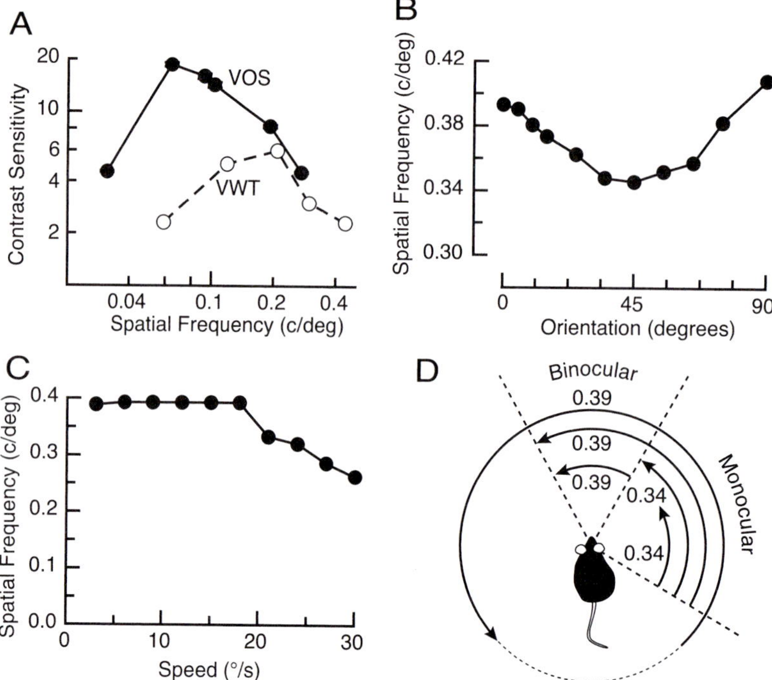

FIGURE 7.4 Examples of visual thresholds in a virtual optokinetic system (VOS). *A*, Contrast sensitivity curve generated in intact adult C57BL/6 mice. (Adapted from Prusky et al., 2004.) *Dashed line* represents contrast sensitivity curve generated with the visual water task. (Adapted from Prusky and Douglas, 2004.) General and peak sensitivity and SF thresholds (predicted points at which curves intersect the *x*-axis) differ between tasks. *B*, Effect of varying the orientation of the optokinetic stimulus from vertical (0°) through oblique (45°) to horizontal (90°) on SF threshold; gratings were always moved on a stationary drum surface in the direction perpendicular to the orientation. The threshold is reduced from vertical to oblique orientations and is slightly higher at horizontal orientations, indicating orientation tuning of the OKR. *C*, Effect of stimulus velocity on SF threshold. Threshold does not vary between 2 and 20°/s but decreases thereafter, indicating that variations in the SF threshold at 12°/s (the typical velocity used for OKR experiments) represent SF sensitivity, not changes in temporal frequency tuning. *D*, Selective visual field responses of normal C57BL/6 mice in schematic illustration. (Adapted from Prusky et al., 2006.) *Arrow length* represents the segment of the visual field in which the grating was present during testing (binocular or monocular field), and the associated numbers represent SF thresholds in c/deg. Full-field (*outside arrow*: *dashed segment* represents the region of the field not visible to the eyes) stimulation generated a threshold of 0.39 c/deg. Limiting the stimulus to the binocular field resulted in the same threshold as full-field stimulation (0.39 c/deg); monocular field responses (0.34 c/deg) were lower regardless of the size of the stimulus within the field. Combining monocular and binocular stimulation resulted in the same threshold (0.39 c/deg) as binocular-alone or full-field stimulation. The data indicate that the temporal retina (which sees the binocular field) may have a higher acuity than the nasal retina.

temporal-to-nasal direction for the other eye evokes tracking; when the maximal SF capable of driving a response is measured separately under monocular and binocular viewing conditions, the monocular threshold is identical to the binocular threshold measured with the same direction of rotation (Douglas et al., 2005).

Although mice lack a specialized fovea, they regularly "foveate" (move their head to place information of interest in their binocular field), indicating that binocular and monocular visual functions differ. To quantify behavioral correlates of this bias, we have used the VOS to measure SF thresholds within restricted segments of the visual field. The general procedures described earlier are used, with the addition that the drifting grating is limited to only part of the visual field. Although mice are unrestrained during testing, their OKRs are effectively limited to a plane parallel to the horizon. We take advantage of this and monitor gaze by continuously tracking the horizontal orientation of the head with the aid of a line superimposed on the video frame and oriented along the snout. The vector generated by this procedure is then used to maintain in real time the grating patch at a constant angle relative to the head. The central 30–40° of the upper portion of each visual hemifield in mice has the potential to receive input from both eyes (Wagor et al., 1980). Since cells in V1 with RFs outside the central 25° in each hemifield are less likely to be driven by the ipsilateral eye (Gordon and Stryker, 1996), for binocular field testing we conservatively define the binocular zone as, and limit our stimulation to, 50° straddling the midline. For measuring thresholds within the monocular zone we center a patch of

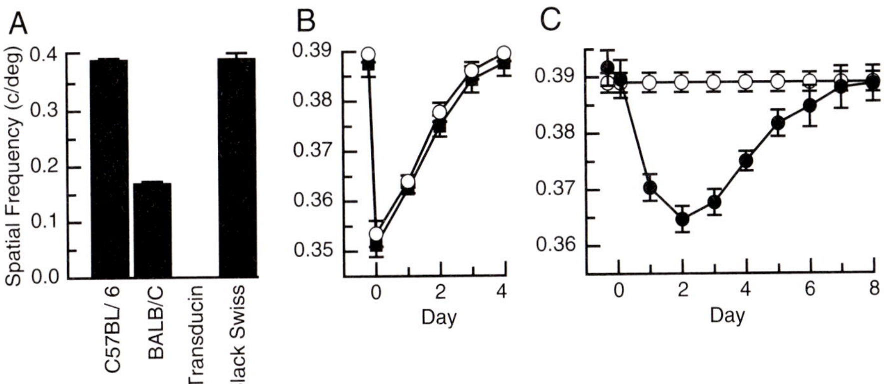

FIGURE 7.5 Use of OptoMotry, a virtual optokinetic system, to screen mouse visual function/dysfunction. *A*, SF thresholds for adult C57BL/6, BALB/C (albino), transducin−/−, and Black Swiss mice. Normal pigmented mouse SF thresholds are approximately 0.4 c/deg. Albinism results in reduced SF thresholds, as does retinal degeneration. *B*, SF thresholds in C57BL/6 mice following a single intraperitoneal injection of scopolamine hydrobromide (0.03 mL; 2.5 mg/mL). Thresholds in both eyes (*open circles*, left eye; *solid circles*, right eye) decreased about 0.04 c/deg from baseline within 1 hour of the injection (second set of points at day 0). Thresholds returned to baseline only after 4 days. *C*, Effect of a single drop of 1% atropine in the right eye (*solid circles*) of C57BL/6 mice. Although the pupil was dilated within a few minutes of treatment and remained dilated for 1 week, the threshold was not affected when measured 1 hour after the treatment (second point at day 0). Over the course of 2 days, thresholds in the treated eye decreased by about 0.03 c/deg and then recovered to baseline over the following 5 days. The untreated eye (*left*, *open circles*) was unaffected.

varying widths, 65° from the midline (Prusky et al., 2006). Figure 7.4*D* illustrates measurements of SF thresholds in various visual fields in normal adult C57BL/6 mice, showing that the monocular field threshold is lower than the binocular field threshold.

Since the virtual cylinder can be rotated in any orientation around the animal, we have also used the VOS to measure the orientation sensitivity of the OKR. Figure 7.4*B* shows there is a clear "oblique effect" in the SF threshold; it is decreased at 45° from horizontal or vertical. In addition, even with suboptimal viewing conditions for scoring vertical tracking, the SF threshold at vertical (measured with horizontally oriented gratings) is clearly higher than at horizontal (measured with vertically oriented gratings), indicating there may be a specialization in the OKR system for RFs tuned to vertical motion.

In summary, perceptual and reflexive measures of mouse vision evaluate different visual functions, and each has its strengths and weaknesses. Perceptual measures, such as the visual water task, assess thresholds most comparable to clinical measures of vision, and the SF threshold (i.e., acuity) is limited by visual cortex. These reinforcement-based tasks, however, require a significant investment of time (on the order of weeks for each threshold), and training young animals and animals with low vision is problematic. With the measurement of automated responses, such as the OKR, SF thresholds are normally mediated through subcortical circuits, and multiple thresholds can be generated in a few minutes and repeated daily. The methodology, however, is not a measure of visual perception, and SF thresholds are lower than those seen on the visual water task. Computer control of visual stimuli in both perceptual and OKR tasks has enabled, and will continue to facilitate in the future, the measurement of novel visual thresholds.

Applied measurement of mouse vision

The development of practical behavioral methods to measure mouse vision has facilitated a recent surge of research that has shown that the mouse has sophisticated visual function. It is difficult to overestimate the significance of the mouse for future research in vision, simply because it is the animal model in which the widest range of experimental manipulations and measures can be brought to bear on a research problem.

One of the most important applications of behavioral tests of mouse vision in the future will be for screening visual phenotypes in mutant animals. Screening often involves large numbers of animals, and there is a trade-off between the time it takes to test an individual animal and the rigor of testing; it is simply not feasible to test every animal over the course of weeks. We suggest a "staircase" approach to the screening process in which it is first determined *whether* a mouse can see, and then the stringency of the tests is incrementally increased to ultimately determine *what* it can see. Optokinetic tests are probably best suited to the question of whether an animal can see, because if an animal is placed in an OKR device and the animal tracks a salient stimulus (e.g., low SF grating), it is clear that the animal can see. The process is fast (seconds to minutes) and can identify animals

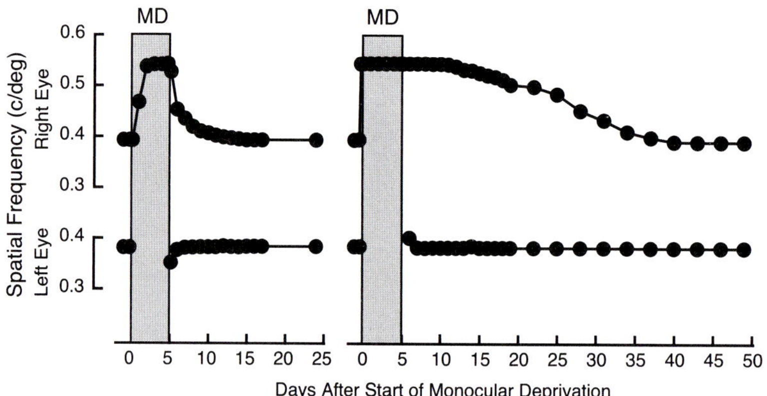

FIGURE 7.6 Effect of two periods of monocular deprivation (MD; *shading*), each lasting 5 days, on SF threshold in adult C57BL/6 mice. *Left*, Sensitivity through nondeprived (right) eye was increased and reached a maximum over 3–4 days of the first MD. Opening the deprived (left) eye initiated a gradual decline to baseline over 5–6 days. *Right*, A second 5-day period of MD resulted in an immediate maximal enhancement that was maintained at maximal values and remained above baseline far longer than after the first MD. Deprived (left) eye responses were not affected after the first day. (Adapted from Prusky et al., 2006.)

with gross visual or motor abnormalities. Once an animal is determined to have functional vision, more rigorous testing can then be undertaken, such as testing over a gradation of preselected SFs or contrasts, or possibly measuring a full contrast sensitivity function or SF threshold. If no visual abnormalities are identified at this point, then tests of visual perception, such as acuity, or other higher order tests might be appropriate. The strategy avoids spending valuable time on animals with obvious abnormalities, which can significantly improve throughput. Another application of the staircase strategy could be in drug safety tests, for which current practice often involves only crude tests of orienting to a visual cue, which are not able to grade an effect on vision. In addition, evaluations of potential treatments for visual disorders, such as retinal degeneration, would benefit from clinically relevant measures of vision.

The methods outlined in this chapter have been used to measure both gains and losses of visual function (i.e., figure 7.5) and demonstrate that such techniques can be valuable tools for experimental research in vision. An elegant demonstration of the ability of behavioral measures to enable the discovery of a novel visual system function, not just to corroborate the results of cellular or physiological studies, comes from a recent study. In it, we showed that monocular deprivation in adult mice causes an enhancement of vision through the nondeprived eye that was restricted to the monocular field (Prusky et al., 2006). In addition, we showed that varying the duration and pattern of deprivation could enable both a learning-like enhancement of cortex-dependent function (figure 7.6), and a permanent trace of a prior deprivation. Not only is this kind of study not feasible with current physiological techniques (extensive repeated threshold measures), but the data can guide clear, hypothesis-driven experiments at other levels of analysis (Are there physiological differences between the plasticity in monocular and binocular cortex? What are the cellular mechanisms underlying the various forms of plasticity?). That this kind of information can be gleaned from a mouse, the only animal model that provides an opportunity to address research questions from molecules to behavior, makes the mouse the most powerful mammalian model system for vision research.

REFERENCES

ABDELJALIL, J., HAMID, M., ABDEL-MOUTTALIB, O., STEPHANE, R., RAYMOND, R., JOHAN, A., JOSE, S., PIERRE, C., and SERGE, P. (2005). The optomotor response: A robust first-line visual screening method for mice. *Vision Res.* 45:1439–1446.

CANCEDDA, L., PUTIGNANO, E., SALE, A., VIEGI, A., BERARDI, N., and MAFFEI, L. (2004). Acceleration of visual system development by environmental enrichment. *J. Neurosci.* 24:4840–4848.

COWEY, A., and FRANZINI, C. (1979). The retinal origin of uncrossed optic nerve fibres in rats and their role in visual discrimination. *Exp. Brain Res.* 35:443–455.

DOUGLAS, R. M., ALAM, N. M., SILVER, B. D., MCGILL, T. J., TSCHETTER, W. W., and PRUSKY G. T. (2005). Independent visual threshold measurements in the two eyes of freely moving rats and mice using a virtual-reality optokinetic system. *Vis. Neurosci.* 22:677–684.

DOUGLAS, R. M., NEVE, A., QUITTENBAUM, J. Q., ALAM, N. M., and PRUSKY, G. T. (2006). Perception of visual motion coherence by rats and mice. *Vision Res.* 46:2842–2847.

GIANFRANCESCHI, L., FIORENTINI, A., and MAFFEI, L. (1999). Behavioural visual acuity of wild type and bcl2 transgenic mouse. *Vision Res.* 39:569–574.

GIANFRANCESCHI, L., SICILIANO, R., WALLS, J., MORALES, B., KIRKWOOD, A., HUANG, Z. J., TONEGAWA, S., and MAFFEI, L. (2003). Visual cortex is rescued from the effects of dark rearing by overexpression of BDNF. *Proc. Natl. Acad. Sci. U.S.A.* 100: 12486–12491.

GORDON, J. A., and STRYKER, M. P. (1996). Experience-dependent plasticity of binocular responses in the primary visual cortex of the mouse. *J. Neurosci.* 16:86.

JACOBS, G. H., FENWICK, J. C., CALDERONE, J. B., and DEEB, S. S. (1999). Human cone pigment expressed in transgenic mice yields altered vision. *J. Neurosci.* 19:3258–3265.

JACOBS, G. H., WILLIAMS, G. A., and FENWICK, J. A. (2004). Influence of cone pigment coexpression on spectral sensitivity and color vision in the mouse. *Vision Res.* 44:1615–1622.

LASHLEY, K. S. (1930). The mechanism of vision. I. A method for rapid analysis of pattern vision in the rat. *J. Gen. Psychol.* 37:453–460.

MCGILL, T. J., LUND, R. D., DOUGLAS, R. M., WANG, S., LU, B., and PRUSKY, G. T. (2004). Preservation of vision following cell-based therapies in a model of retinal degenerative disease. *Vision Res.* 44:2559–2566.

MORRIS, R. G., GARRUD, P., RAWLINS, J. N., and O'KEEFE J. (1982). Place navigation impaired in rats with hippocampal lesions. *Nature* 297:681–683.

PHAM, T. A., GRAHAM, S. J., SUZUKI, S., BARCO, A., KANDEL, E. R., GORDON, B., and LICKEY, M. E. (2004). A semi-persistent adult ocular dominance plasticity in visual cortex is stabilized by activated CREB. *Learn. Memory* 11:738–747.

PRUSKY, G. T., ALAM, N. M., BEEKMAN, S., and DOUGLAS, R. M. (2004). Rapid quantification of adult and developing mouse spatial vision using a virtual optomotor system. *Invest. Ophthalmol. Vis. Sci.* 45:4611–4616.

PRUSKY, G. T., ALAM, N. M., and DOUGLAS, R. M. (2006). Enhancement of vision by monocular deprivation in adult mice. *J. Neurosci.* 26:11554–11561.

PRUSKY, G. T., and DOUGLAS, R. M. (2003). Developmental plasticity of mouse visual acuity. *Eur. J. Neurosci.* 17:167–173.

PRUSKY, G. T., and DOUGLAS, R. M. (2004). Characterization of mouse cortical spatial vision. *Vis. Res.* 44:3411–3418.

PRUSKY, G. T., REIDEL, C., and DOUGLAS, R. M. (2000a). Environmental enrichment from birth enhances visual acuity but not place learning in mice. *Behav. Brain Res.* 114:11–15.

PRUSKY, G. T., WEST, P. W. R., and DOUGLAS, R. M. (2000b). Reduced visual acuity impairs place but not cued learning in the Morris water task. *Behav. Brain Res.* 116:135–140.

PRUSKY, G. T., WEST, P. W. R., and DOUGLAS, R. M. (2000c). Behavioral assessment of visual acuity in mice and rats. *Vision Res.* 40:2201–2209.

ROBINSON, L., BRIDGE, H., and RIEDEL, G. (2001). Visual discrimination learning in the water maze: A novel test for visual acuity. *Behav. Brain Res.* 119:77–84.

ROBINSON, L., HARBARAN, D., and RIEDEL, G. (2004). Visual acuity in the water maze: Sensitivity to muscarinic receptor blockade in rats and mice. *Behav. Brain Res.* 151:277–286.

SALE, A., PUTIGNANO, E., CANCEDDA, L., LANDI, S., CIRULLI, F., BERARDI, N., and MAFFEI, L. (2004). Enriched environment and acceleration of visual system development. *Neuropharmacology* 47:649–660.

SCHMUCKER, C., and SCHAEFFEL, F. (2006). Contrast sensitivity of wildtype mice wearing diffusers or spectacle lenses, and the effect of atropine. *Vision Res.* 46:678–687.

SCHMUCKER, C., SEELIGER, M., HUMPHRIES, P., BIEL, M., and SCHAEFFEL, F. (2005). Grating acuity at different luminances in wild-type mice and in mice lacking rod or cone function. *Invest. Ophthalmol. Visual Sci.* 46:398–407.

WAGOR, E., MANGINI, N. J., and PEARLMAN, A. L. (1980). Retinotopic organization of striate and extrastriate visual cortex in the mouse. *J. Comp. Neurol.* 193:187–202.

WHISHAW, I. Q. (1995). A comparison of rats and mice in a swimming pool place task and matching to place task: Some surprising differences. *Physiol. Behav.* 58:687–693.

WONG, A. A., and BROWN, R. E. (2006). Visual detection, pattern discrimination and visual acuity in 14 strains of mice. *Genes Brain Behav.* 5:389–403.

WONG, A. A., and BROWN, R. E. (2007). Age-related changes in visual acuity, learning and memory in C57BL/6J and DBA/2J mice. *Neurobiol. Aging* 28(10):1577–1593. (Accessed online September 28, 2006.)

8 Electroretinographic Correlates of Normal and Abnormal Retinal Ganglion Cell Activity

VITTORIO PORCIATTI

Optic nerve diseases include a variety of blinding disorders such as glaucoma, optic neuritis, ischemic optic neuropathy, and mitochondrial optic neuropathy. Mouse models for these diseases are being developed at an increasing rate to investigate specific pathophysiological mechanisms. Experimental mouse models of optic nerve transection and crush injury are also widely used to better understand molecular mechanisms of retinal ganglion cell (RGC) and axon death, as well as to explore neuroprotective treatments, including gene therapy (Levkovitch-Verbin, 2004). The use of these models may be greatly enhanced by the availability of noninvasive methods able to monitor RGC function longitudinally.

The pattern electroretinogram as a tool to measure retinal ganglion cell function

The pattern electroretinogram (PERG) is a particular kind of ERG obtained in response to contrast reversal of patterned visual stimuli (gratings, checkerboards) rather than traditional flashes of diffuse light (figure 8.1), and has characteristics fundamentally different from the flash ERG.

The pattern stimulus consists of two sets of elements of equal areas whose luminances increase and decrease at a given frequency F_{Hz} (flicker). At the retinal level, flickering pattern elements generate local flicker ERGs at frequency F_{Hz}. Because adjacent pattern elements generate local flicker ERGs 180 degrees out of phase, these are summed and canceled at the distant electrode. An ERG is recordable in response to pattern reversal because additional, nonlinear ERG components are generated (mainly at $2\,F_{Hz}$ frequency, corresponding to the contrast reversal rate) that are in-phase and do not cancel at the electrode. This is what constitutes the PERG. The main generators of local flicker ERGs at F_{Hz} are likely the photoreceptors, which have approximately linear behavior, whereas the PERG generators at $2\,F_{Hz}$ are likely postreceptoral elements with center-surround receptive field (RF) organization and nonlinear behavior (Baker and Hess, 1984). In sum, photoreceptor activity is necessary for PERG generation but it is not apparent in the PERG waveform because of cancellation at the electrode. Since RGCs have RFs with strong center-surround antagonism, these seem the best candidates for PERG generation. RGCs are expected to be maximally activated by pattern elements whose dimensions match the average size of the RGC RF center. In keeping with this prediction, the PERG amplitude displays a maximum at a specific spatial frequency that approximately corresponds to the average RGC RF size (Hess and Baker, 1984; Drasdo et al., 1987; Porciatti, 2007). In addition, for a given retinal eccentricity and stimulus area, the PERG amplitude to the peak spatial frequency is linearly proportional to the expected volume of RGCs (Drasdo et al., 1990).

RGC activity is indeed necessary for PERG generation, since RGC retrograde degeneration after optic nerve transection abolishes the response in all mammals tested so far. These include cat (Maffei and Fiorentini, 1981), monkey (Maffei et al., 1985), rat (Berardi et al., 1990), and mouse (Porciatti et al., 1996; Chierzi et al., 1998) (see figure 8.1). In the same experimental animals the a- and b-waves of the conventional bright flash ERG, which originate in the outer retina, are little or not affected. PERG generation also requires physiological integrity of anatomically present RGCs. The PERG amplitude can be reversibly reduced, though not abolished, by intravitreal injections of tetrodotoxin, which block Na^+-dependent spiking activity in the inner retina (Trimarchi et al., 1990; Viswanathan et al., 2000). Short-term, moderate elevation of intraocular pressure (IOP) reversibly reduces the PERG amplitude while leaving the flash ERG intact (Siliprandi et al., 1988; Feghali et al., 1991). A reduction in PERG amplitude may therefore reflect both the reduced activity of nonfunctional RGCs and the lack of activity of lost RGCs.

Thus, the PERG may represent an important tool for monitoring the onset and progression of RGC dysfunction in mouse models of optic nerve disease, as well as for probing the effects of neuroprotective treatments. Strong evidence supports the view that functional RGCs are necessary to generate the PERG, whereas less is known about what aspects of RGC activity relate to the response. Although a

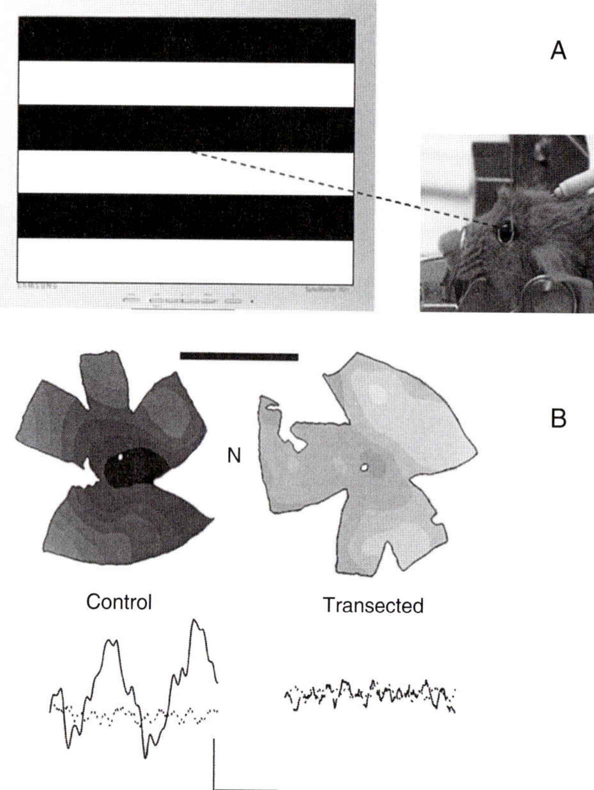

FIGURE 8.1 *A*, The PERG is recorded from anesthetized mice by means of corneal electrodes, allowing unobstructed viewing of alternating grating patterns. *B*, Two months after intracranial optic nerve transection, isodensity maps of cell bodies in the retinal ganglion cell layer of flat mount retinas show massive depletion of neurons and loss of PERG response compared with the control eye. Calibration bar = 3 mm. N, nasal quadrant of each retina. For the PERG, calibration is 0.5 μV (vertical) and 100 ms (horizontal). (Modified from Porciatti et al., 1996, 2007, and Chierzi et al., 1998.)

TTX-dependent component suggests that RGC axon spiking activity plays a role in PERG generation, slow electrical activity generated at the level of RGC dendrites, or electrical activity in the inner retina circuitry impinging on RGCs, cannot be excluded. Finally, a Müller cell component in the PERG generation cannot be excluded, since Müller cells can passively generate electric currents in response to extracellular modulation of K^+ ions produced by active retinal neurons (Kline et al., 1978).

Methods for pattern electroretinogram recording

An optimized protocol for mouse PERG recording has been recently described (Porciatti et al., 2007). In brief, mice are anesthetized with intraperitoneal (IP) injections (0.5–0.7 ml/kg) of a mixture of ketamine, 42.8 mg/mL; xylazine, 8.6 mg/mL; and acepromazine, 1.4 mg/mL. Mice are gently restrained using a mouth bite and a nose holder that allows unobstructed vision, and kept at constant body temperature at 37.0°C using a feedback-controlled heating pad. Under these conditions the eyes of mice are naturally wide open and in a stable position, with pupils pointing laterad and upward. The recording electrode is a thin (0.25 mm diameter) silver wire configured in a semicircular loop of 2 mm radius. It is gently leaned on the corneal surface in such a way as to encircle the undilated pupil without interfering with vision (see figure 8.1). Electrode positioning entails minimal corneal stimulation, which might otherwise induce cataract (Fraunfelder and Burns, 1970) and preclude further PERG testing. Reference and ground electrodes—small stainless steel needles—are inserted into the skin of the back of the head and the back of the body, respectively. Instillations of BSS drops every 30 minutes are sufficient to maintain the cornea and lens in excellent condition for many hours. Pattern stimuli consist of horizontal bars of variable spatial frequency and contrast that alternate at different temporal frequency. Stimuli are displayed on a television monitor whose center is aligned with the projection of the pupil and presented from short distance (typically 20 cm) to stimulate a large retinal area (typically 50–60°) centered on the optic disc (see figure 8.1). Eyes are not refracted for the viewing distance because the mouse eye has a large depth of focus due to the pinhole pupil (Remtulla and Hallett, 1985). PERGs (Porciatti et al., 1996) and pattern visual evoked potentials (VEPs; Porciatti et al., 1999b) are not modified by trial lenses of ±10 spherical diopters placed before the eyes. Compared to the traditional ERG, the amplitude of the PERG is smaller by a factor of about 100. Therefore, robust averaging (1,000–2,000 sweeps) is needed to isolate the response from background noise and reduce variability. At optimal spatial frequency (0.05 c/deg), temporal frequency (1 Hz), and contrast (100%), the PERG signal-to-noise ratio is of the order of 10 : 1 (Porciatti et al., 2007), which represents an adequate dynamic range for application in mouse models of optic nerve disease.

Pattern electroretinogram correlates of visual behaviors

Being an RGC-driven electrical response, the PERG represents an index of the retinal output. By changing the spatial-temporal characteristics of the pattern stimulus, it is possible to obtain estimates of retinal resolution (acuity) (Porciatti et al., 1996; Rossi et al., 2001), contrast threshold (Porciatti et al., 1996), and temporal resolution (Porciatti and Falsini, 2003) (figure 8.2).

Visual thresholds determined at retinal level with PERG have a counterpart in corresponding measures of visual acuity and contrast sensitivity determined with VEPs (Porciatti et al., 1999b), operant psychophysical behavior (Gianfranceschi et al., 1999; Prusky and Douglas, 2004), and passive optomotor responses (Prusky et al., 2004; Schmucker

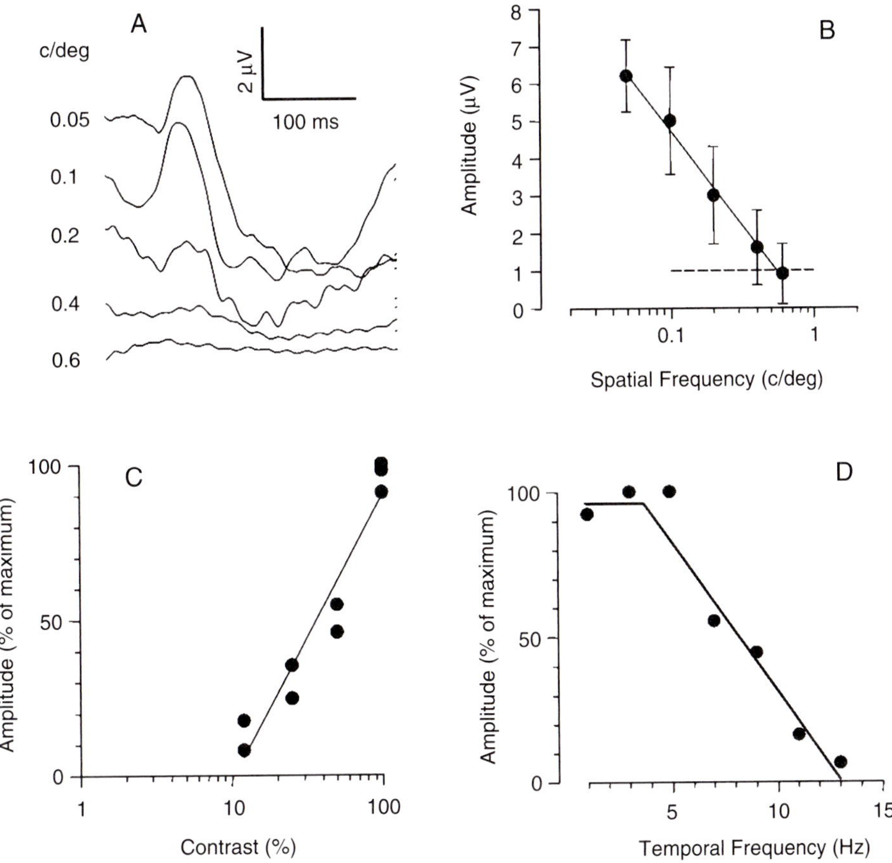

FIGURE 8.2 Spatial-temporal properties of the mouse PERG. *A*, Examples of PERG responses recorded in young adult C57BL/6J mice in response to 1 Hz alternating gratings of high contrast (95%) and different spatial frequency (numbers to the left of each waveform expressed in c/deg). *B*, The mean (±SEM) PERG amplitude in six different mice decreases with increasing spatial frequency and reaches the noise level (*dashed line*) at 0.6 c/deg, which represents the retinal acuity. For gratings of 0.05 c/deg, the PERG amplitude decreases with decreasing contrast (*C*) and increasing temporal frequency (*D*). The contrast threshold is about 10%, and the temporal resolution is about 13 Hz (26 reversals/s). (From Porciatti and Falsini, 2003.)

et al., 2005). PERG acuity develops postnatally (Porciatti and Falsini, 2000; Porciatti et al., 2002) in parallel with visual acuity determined with either VEPs (Huang et al., 1999) or optomotor responses (Prusky et al., 2004). Around eye opening (postnatal day 14–15), the PERG acuity is of the order of 0.2 c/deg and matures during the next 2 weeks to reach the adult acuity (0.6 c/deg) by about 1 month of age (figure 8.3). By combining PERG measures with VEPs, optomotor responses, or psychophysical visual behavior, it is possible to evaluate the relative contribution of retinal and postretinal stages to a particular disease or condition.

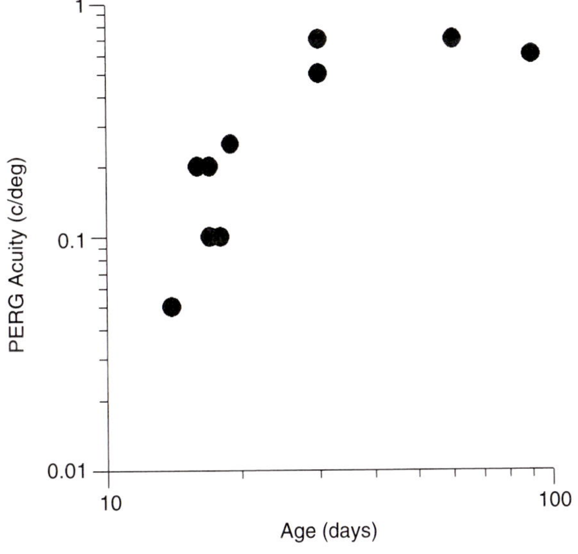

FIGURE 8.3 Postnatal maturation of PERG acuity in C57BL/6J mice. (From Porciatti and Falsini, 2000.)

Examples of pattern electroretinogram application to study central nervous system plasticity and degeneration

ROLE OF DEVELOPMENTAL SPONTANEOUS ACTIVITY In the mammalian visual system the formation of eye-specific layers at the thalamic level depends on retinal waves of spontaneous activity (Wong, 1999), which rely on nicotinic acetylcholine receptor activation (Feller et al., 1996). In mutant mice lacking the β_2 subunit of the neuronal nicotinic receptor (Picciotto et al., 1995), but not in mice lacking the α_4 subunit, retinofugal projections do not form eye-specific layers in the dorsolateral geniculate nucleus (Rossi et al., 2001; Muir-Robinson et al., 2002). Still, retinogeniculate projections segregate into a patchy distribution (Muir-Robinson et al., 2002), indicating that segregation of left eye and right eye axons can be uncoupled from macroscopic patterning in the visual system. β_2−/− mice show an expansion of the binocular subfield of the primary visual cortex and a decrease in visual acuity at the cortical level (VEP) (Rossi et al., 2001). This indicates that the β_2 subunit of the nicotinic acetylcholine receptor is necessary for the anatomical and functional development of the postretinal visual system. The retinal acuity determined with PERG, however, is identical in β_2−/− and wild-type mice (Rossi et al., 2001). In addition, detailed anatomical analysis of different RGC classes does not reveal significant differences between wild-type and β_2−/− animals (Van der List et al., 2006). These results indicate that cholinergic-mediated activity in the developing retina is not required for the normal postnatal development of retinal ganglion cells (figure 8.4).

Role of Developmental Cell Death The BCL2 protein is a potent inhibitor of apoptotic cell death. Transgenic mice have been generated with overexpression of the human *Bcl-2* gene in RGCs and in most neurons of the central nervous system (CNS) (Martinou et al., 1994). As a result of inhibition of apoptotic cell death during development, adult *Bcl-2*-overexpressing mice have 2.6 times more RGCs and optic nerve fibers than normal, and have larger brains (Cenni et al., 1996). Despite the marked neuronal redundancy of the retinal and postretinal visual pathway, the retinal acuity (as determined by PERG) of the *Bcl-2*-overexpressing mouse is normal (Porciatti et al., 1996). The cortical (VEP) visual acuity (Porciatti et al., 1999a) and the behavioral visual acuity (Gianfranceschi et al., 1999) are also normal. A detailed anatomical study of the *Bcl-2* transgenic mouse (Strettoi and Volpini, 2002) indicates that a compensatory growth of axonal arborizations of bipolar cells ultimately results in an increased divergence on RGCs, thus neutralizing the effect of their higher density. At cortical level, neuronal redundancy causes expansion of the brain, which keeps neuronal density in the normal range (Porciatti et al., 1999a). To account for brain expansion, the cortical representation of the visual coordinates (i.e., the vertical meridian) is shifted laterally (Porciatti et al., 1999a).

Survival of Retinal Ganglion Cells after Lesion CNS neurons of adult *Bcl-2* mice are little altered after lesions. The great majority of RGCs survive for a long time after optic nerve section (Cenni et al., 1996), and their physiological response (P-ERG) is spared (Porciatti et al., 1996; Chierzi et al., 1998) (figure 8.5). This suggests that neuroprotective strategies aimed at targeting the apoptotic cascade at mitochondrial level may successfully rescue from death a high number of RGCs with normal physiological response. Mice deficient in BCL2-associated X protein (BAX) can be also used to investigate the role of BAX-mediated cell death in optic nerve lesions. BAX deficiency protects RGCs after axon injury by optic nerve crush (Libby et al., 2005c). BAX deficiency in DBA/2J mice with spontaneous glaucoma (discussed in the next section) protect RGCs from death (Libby et al., 2005c). It remains to be established whether protected RGCs retain normal function.

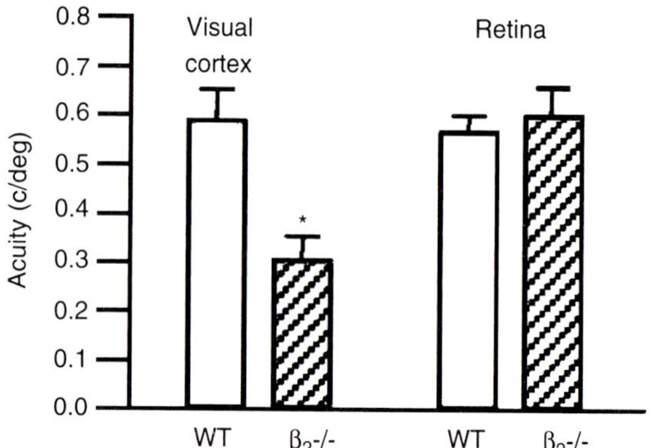

Figure 8.4 Comparison between cortical and retinal acuity in adult C57BL/6J mice (WT) and in mutant mice lacking the beta2 subunit of the neuronal nicotinic receptor (β_2−/−). In β_2−/− mice, visual acuity is reduced at cortical level but not at retinal level. (Modified from Rossi et al., 2001, fig. 4.)

Pattern electroretinogram application in mouse models of glaucoma

The DBA/2J mouse is a well-established model of spontaneous glaucoma. Recessive mutations in two genes, *Gpnmb* and *Tyrp1*, cause iris atrophy and pigment dispersion (John et al., 1998). The iris disease is apparent at 6 months and progresses with age, resulting in elevated intraocular pressure (IOP) (Libby et al., 2005a). Young (2- to 4-month-old) DBA/2J mice have normal IOP, a normal PERG, and normal histological appearance of RGCs and optic nerve. Glaucoma damage in the optic nerve is apparent in about 60% of eyes by 10–11 months of age, and in about 90% of eyes by 18 months (Libby et al., 2005a). Between 10 and 11 months of age, the PERG amplitude is markedly reduced in 100% of eyes, including eyes with no signs of nerve damage (figure 8.6). Between 2 and 13 months of age, the outer retina is histologically intact (Jakobs et al., 2005) and the light-adapted flash ERG displays only minor

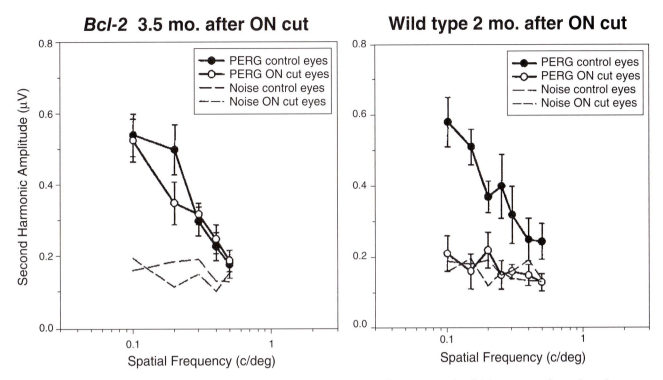

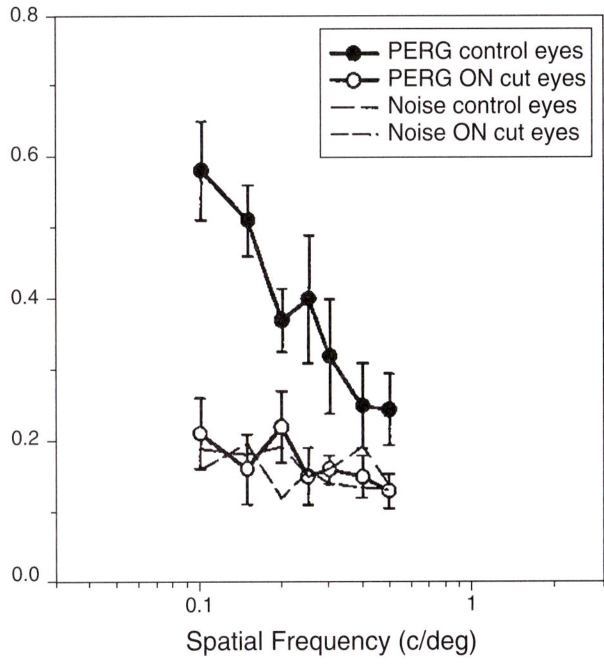

FIGURE 8.5 Effect of intracranial section of one optic nerve on the PERG. In C57BL/6J mice, the mean (±SEM, n = 3) PERG amplitude of axotomized eyes is at noise level (*dashed lines*) 2 months after surgery. By contrast, in *Bcl-2*-overexpressing mice, the mean (±SEM, n = 3) PERG amplitude is at control values 3.5 months after axotomy. (Modified from Porciatti et al., 1996, fig. 4.)

changes (Porciatti et al., 2007; Libby et al., 2006) (see figure 8.6). Taken together, these results suggest that DBA/2J mice develop a progressive functional damage in the inner retina (abnormal PERG) but not in the outer retina (normal flash ERG) that seems to precede anatomical damage of the RGC layer and of the optic nerve. This may suggest that surviving RGCs may not be functional. Therefore, neuroprotection studies using mouse models of glaucoma should include functional endpoints in addition to anatomical endpoints.

The noninvasive nature of PERG allows serial recordings as a function of changing conditions (e.g., age, IOP levels). Recently, we have been able to characterize the natural history of RGC dysfunction and its relationship with IOP in a 12-month longitudinal study of BDA/2J mice (Saleh et al., 2007). On average, the IOP increases moderately between 2 and 6 months, with a progression of 0.92 mm Hg/month. After 6 months the IOP displays a steeper increase, and tends to level off by 11 months at a value of about 30 mm Hg (Saleh et al., 2007). After 3 months, the PERG amplitude decreases linearly with age to reach the noise level at about 10–11 months (Saleh et al., 2007). Histological analysis of eyes with abolished PERG shows that the retinal nerve fiber layer is largely preserved. Between 2 and 11 months the cone-flash ERG does not show significant changes (Saleh et al., 2007). We were also able to characterize the changes

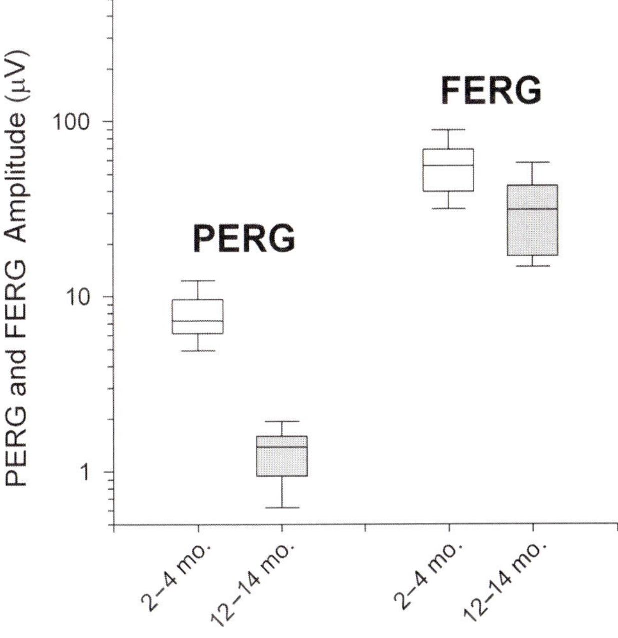

FIGURE 8.6 Amplitude of PERG and light-adapted flash ERG in DBA/2J mice of different ages. The PERG of glaucomatous 12- to 14-month-old mice, compared with that of preglaucomatous 2- to 4-month-old mice, is reduced to the noise range (mean 1.18 ± 0.35 μV). The light-adapted flash ERG displays minor changes in glaucomatous 12- to 14-month-old mice. (Replotted from Porciatti et al., 2007, fig. 5.)

in IOP and PERG that occur when DBA/2J mice are put in a head-down (60-degree) body position (Aihara et al., 2003). Postural changes cause substantial (+30%–35%) reversible IOP increases in DBA/2J mice of different ages (3–10 months) (Nagaraju et al., 2007). Postural changes also cause PERG amplitude reductions that are strongly age dependent (3-month-old: no change; 5-month-old: −48%; 10-month-old: −67%) (Nagaraju et al., 2007). Finally, when 10-month-old mice with reduced PERG amplitude are treated with mannitol, the IOP decreases by about 50% and the PERG amplitude increases by 80% (Nagaraju et al., 2007). These results indicate that RGC vulnerability in the DBA/2J mouse model of glaucoma is age and IOP dependent, and that existing RGC dysfunction can be restored by reducing the level of IOP.

Use of the pattern electroretinogram in human clinical research

Since Maffei and Fiorentini reported that the ERG with contrast reversal was abolished by optic nerve section in the cat (Maffei and Fiorentini, 1981), PERG has received considerable attention for clinical application in a wide spectrum of optic nerve disorders (reviewed in Holder, 2001; Parisi, 2003; Ventura and Porciatti, 2006). Applications in glaucoma have received by far the largest consideration; the spontaneous DBA/2J mouse model of glaucoma described above, together with mouse genetics and noninvasive functional tests such as PERG, may represent a powerful link with the clinical condition to unlock the mechanisms of glaucoma (John et al., 1999; Libby et al., 2005b). Recent results in human glaucoma indicate that RGC dysfunction, as measured by PERG (Porciatti and Ventura, 2004), exceeds the proportion expected from loss of RGC axons (Ventura et al., 2006). This implies that the population of surviving axons is not functional. Additional results show that RGC dysfunction in patients with early glaucoma may at least in part be restored by reducing IOP with eye drops (Ventura and Porciatti, 2005). Taken together, these results suggest that in glaucoma, RGCs undergo a stage of reversible dysfunction before death, thereby offering a window of opportunity to detect and treat the condition before irreversible damage and loss of vision occur. As described earlier in the chapter, qualitatively similar results have been obtained in the DBA/2J model. The current standard for initiating glaucoma treatment is based on a repeatable abnormality of the psychophysical visual field sensitivity, which typically occurs when at least 30% of RGCs have already degenerated (e.g., Kerrigan-Baumrind et al., 2000). That in glaucomatous optic neuropathy RGCs undergo a phase of reversible dysfunction before irreversible damage and death occur has important implications for the early diagnosis and treatment of a wide variety of progressive neurological disorders.

Limitations of the pattern electroretinogram technique

The main limitation of the technique is that it requires the integrity of the eye optics to be properly recorded. Cataracts may develop in experimental mouse eyes as a result of drugs, cold, anoxia, stress, and dehydration (Fraunfelder and Burns, 1970). Careful manipulation of experimental mice, however, prevents cataract formation (Porciatti et al., 2007). Another potential shortcoming is that PERG is a relatively small signal, since generator sources are limited to cone-driven (light-adapted) postreceptoral activity. Robust averaging, however, permits obtaining PERGs with excellent signal-to-noise ratio and with a variability comparable to that of traditional ERG (Porciatti et al., 2007).

A component of full-field flash ERG, the scotopic threshold response (STR), has been shown to depend on RGCs activity in rats (Bui and Fortune, 2004) and is altered in rat models of glaucoma (Fortune et al., 2004). Compared with PERG, the STR is expected to depend less on eye optics and might represent an alternative to PERG. The STR is also recordable in mice (Saszik et al., 2002), but the contribution of normal and abnormal RGC activity to the response still needs to be demonstrated.

Conclusion

PERG is a valuable tool for characterizing the spatial-temporal retinal output in mice of different ages and genotypes. Its noninvasive nature allows serial recording to evaluate longitudinal changes of normal and abnormal RGC activity in mouse models of optic nerve disease, as well as their response to stress factors. Overall, PERG may represent a powerful tool for neuroprotection studies.

ACKNOWLEDGMENTS Work was supported by NIH grant no. RO1 EY014957, NIH grant no. RO3 EY016322, NIH center grant no. P30-EY14801, and an unrestricted grant to the University of Miami from Research to Prevent Blindness, Inc.

REFERENCES

Aihara, M., Lindsey, J. D., and Weinreb, R. N. (2003). Episcleral venous pressure of mouse eye and effect of body position. *Curr. Eye Res.* 27(6):355–362.

Baker, C. L., Jr., and Hess, R. F. (1984). Linear and nonlinear components of human electroretinogram. *J. Neurophysiol.* 51(5):952–967.

Berardi, N., Domenici, L., Gravina, A., and Maffei, L. (1990). Pattern ERG in rats following section of the optic nerve. *Exp. Brain Res.* 79(3):539–546.

Bui, B. V., and Fortune, B. (2004). Ganglion cell contributions to the rat full-field electroretinogram. *J. Physiol.* 555(Pt. 1):153–173.

Cenni, M. C., Bonfanti, L., Martinou, J.-C., Ratto, G. M., Strettoi, E., and Maffei, L. (1996). Long-term survival of retinal ganglion cells following optic nerve section in adult I *bcl-2* transgenic mice. *Eur. J. Neurosci.* 8:1735–1745.

Chierzi, S, Cenni, M. C., Maffei, L., Pizzorusso, T., Porciatti, V., Ratto, G. M., and Strettoi, E. (1998). Protection of retinal ganglion cells and preservation of function after optic nerve lesion in *bcl-2* transgenic mice. *Vision Res.* 38:1537–1543.

Drasdo, N., Thompson, D. A., and Arden, G. B. (1990). A comparison of pattern ERG amplitudes and nuclear layer thickness in different zones of the retina. *Clin. Vision Sci.* 5(4): 415–420.

Drasdo, N., Thompson, D. A., Thompson, C. M., and Edwards, L. (1987). Complementary components and local variations of the pattern electroretinogram. *Invest. Ophthalmol. Vis. Sci.* 28(1):158–162.

Feghali, J. G., Jin, J. C., and Odom, J. V. (1991). Effect of short-term intraocular pressure elevation on the rabbit electroretinogram. *Invest. Ophthalmol. Vis. Sci.* 32(8):2184–2189.

Feller, M. B., Wellis, D. P., Stellwagen, D., Werblin, F. S., and Shatz, C. J. (1996). Requirement for cholinergic synaptic transmission in the propagation of spontaneous retinal waves. *Science* 272(5265):1182–1187.

Fortune, B., Bui, B. V., Morrison, J. C., Johnson, E. C., Dong, J., Cepurna, W. O., Jia, L., Barber, S., and Cioffi, G. A. (2004). Selective ganglion cell functional loss in rats with experimental glaucoma. *Invest. Ophthalmol. Vis. Sci.* 45(6):1854–1862.

Fraunfelder, F. T., and Burns, R. P. (1970). Acute reversible lens opacity: Caused by drugs, cold, anoxia, asphyxia, stress, death and dehydration. *Exp. Eye Res.* 10(1):19–30.

Gianfranceschi, L., Fiorentini, A., and Maffei, L. (1999). Behavioural visual acuity of wild-type and *bcl2* transgenic mouse. *Vision Res.* 39(3):569–574.

Hess, R. F., and Baker, C. L., Jr. Human pattern-evoked electroretinogram. *J. Neurophysiol.* 51(5):939–951.

Holder, G. E. (2001). Pattern electroretinography (PERG) and an integrated approach to visual pathway diagnosis. *Prog. Retin. Eye Res.* 20(4):531–561.

Huang, Z. J., Kirkwood, A., Pizzorusso, T., Porciatti, V., Morales, B., Bear, M. F., Maffei, L., and Tonegawa, S. (1999). BDNF regulates the maturation of inhibition and the critical period of plasticity in mouse visual cortex. *Cell* 98(6): 739–755.

Jakobs, T. C., Libby, R. T., Ben, Y., John, S. W., and Masland, R. H. (2005). Retinal ganglion cell degeneration is topological but not cell type specific in DBA/2J mice. *J. Cell Biol.* 171(2): 313–325.

John, S. W., Anderson, M. G., and Smith, R. S. (1999). Mouse genetics: A tool to help unlock the mechanisms of glaucoma. *J. Glaucoma* 8(6):400–412.

John, S. W., Smith, R. S., Savinova, O. V., Hawes, N. L., Chang, B., Turnbull, D., Davisson, M., Roderick, T. H., and Heckenlively, J. R. (1998). Essential iris atrophy, pigment dispersion, and glaucoma in DBA/2J mice. *Invest. Ophthalmol. Vis. Sci.* 39(6):951–962.

Kerrigan-Baumrind, L. A., Quigley, H. A., Pease, M. E., Kerrigan, D. F., and Mitchell, R. S. (2000). Number of ganglion cells in glaucoma eyes compared with threshold visual field tests in the same persons. *Invest. Ophthalmol. Vis. Sci.* 41(3):741–748.

Kline, R. P., Ripps, H., and Dowling, J. E. (1978). Generation of b-wave currents in the skate retina. *Proc. Natl. Acad. Sci. U.S.A.* 75(11):5727–5731.

Levkovitch-Verbin, H. (2004). Animal models of optic nerve diseases. *Eye* 18(11):1066–1074.

Libby, R. T., Anderson, M. G., Pang, I. H., Robinson, Z. H., Savinova, O. V., Cosma, I. M., Snow, A., Wilson, L. A., Smith, R. S., et al. (2005a). Inherited glaucoma in DBA/2J mice: Pertinent disease features for studying the neurodegeneration. *Vis. Neurosci.* 22(5):637–648.

Libby, R. T., Gould, D. B., Anderson, M. G., and John, S. W. (2005b). Complex genetics of glaucoma susceptibility. *Annu. Rev. Genomic. Hum. Genet.* 6:15–44.

Libby, R. T., Li, Y., Savinova, O. V., Barter, J., Smith, R. S., Nickells, R. W., and John, S. W. (2005c). Susceptibility to neurodegeneration in a glaucoma is modified by Bax gene dosage. *PLoS. Genet.* 1(1):17–26.

Libby, R. T., Porciatti, V., Tapia, M., Lee, R. K., and John, S. W. M. (2006). PERG analysis detects physiological dysfunction prior to ganglion cell loss in DBA/2J glaucoma. ARVO e-abstract 4005.

Maffei, L., and Fiorentini, A. (1981). Electroretinographic responses to alternating gratings before and after section of the optic nerve. *Science* 211(4485):953–955.

Maffei, L., Fiorentini, A., Bisti, S., and Hollander, H. (1985). Pattern ERG in the monkey after section of the optic nerve. *Exp. Brain Res.* 59(2):423–425.

Martinou, J. C., Dubois-Dauphin, M., Staple, J. K., Rodriguez, I., Frankowski, H., Missotten, M., Albertini, P., Talabot, D., Catsicas, S., et al. (1994). Overexpression of BCL-2 in transgenic mice protects neurons from naturally occurring cell death and experimental ischemia. *Neuron* 13(4):1017–1030.

Muir-Robinson, G., Hwang, B. J., and Feller, M. B. (2002). Retinogeniculate axons undergo eye-specific segregation in the absence of eye-specific layers. *J. Neurosci.* 22(13):5259–5264.

Nagaraju, M., Saleh, M., and Porciatti, V. (2007). IOP-dependent retinal ganglion cell dysfunction in glaucomatous DBA/2J mice. *Invest. Ophthalmol. Vis. Sci.* 48:4573–4579.

Parisi, V. (2003). Correlation between morphological and functional retinal impairment in patients affected by ocular hypertension, glaucoma, demyelinating optic neuritis and Alzheimer's disease. *Semin. Ophthalmol.* 18(2):50–57.

Picciotto, M. R., Zoli, M., Lena, C., Bessis, A., Lallemand, Y., Le Novere, N., Vincent, P., Pich, E. M., Brulet, P., et al. (1995). Abnormal avoidance learning in mice lacking functional high-affinity nicotine receptor in the brain. *Nature* 374(6517): 65–67.

Porciatti, V. (2007). The mouse pattern electroretinogram. *Doc. Ophthalmol.*, epub ahead of print.

Porciatti, V., and Falsini, B. (2000). Maturation of flash-cone ERG and pattern ERG in the mouse. ARVO abstract 500.

Porciatti, V., and Falsini, B. (2003). Physiological properties of the mouse pattern electroretinogram. ARVO abstract 2705.

Porciatti, V., Pizzorusso, T., Cenni, M. C., and Maffei, L. (1996). The visual response of retinal ganglion cells is not altered by optic nerve transection in transgenic mice overexpressing *Bcl-2*. *Proc. Natl. Acad. Sci. U.S.A.* 93(25):14955–14959.

Porciatti, V., Pizzorusso, T., and Maffei, L. (1999a). Vision in mice with neuronal redundancy due to inhibition of developmental cell death. *Vis. Neurosci.* 16(4):721–726.

Porciatti, V., Pizzorusso, T., and Maffei, L. (1999b). The visual physiology of the wild type mouse determined with pattern VEPs. *Vision Res.* 39(18):3071–3081.

Porciatti, V., Pizzorusso, T., and Maffei, L. (2002). Electrophysiology of the postreceptoral visual pathway in mice. *Doc. Ophthalmol.* 104(1):69—82.

Porciatti, V., Saleh, M., and Nagaraju, M. (2007). The pattern electroretinogram as a tool to monitor progressive retinal ganglion cell dysfunction in the DBA/2J mouse model of glaucoma. *Invest. Ophthalmol.* 48(2):745–751.

Porciatti, V., and Ventura, L. M. (2004). Normative data for a user-friendly paradigm for pattern electroretinogram recording. *Ophthalmology* 111(1):161–168.

Prusky, G. T., Alam, N. M., Beekman, S., and Douglas, R. M. (2004). Rapid quantification of adult and developing mouse spatial vision using a virtual optomotor system. *Invest. Ophthalmol. Vis. Sci.* 45(12):4611–4616.

Prusky, G. T., and Douglas, R. M. (2004). Characterization of mouse cortical spatial vision. *Vision. Res.* 44(28):3411–3418.

Remtulla, S., and Hallett, P. E. (1985). A schematic eye for the mouse, and comparisons with the rat. *Vision Res.* 25(1): 21–31.

Rossi, F. M., Pizzorusso, T., Porciatti, V., Marubio, L. M., Maffei, L., and Changeux, J. P. (2001). Requirement of the nicotinic acetylcholine receptor beta 2 subunit for the anatomical and functional development of the visual system. *Proc. Natl. Acad. Sci. U.S.A.* 98(11):6453–6458.

Saleh, M., Nagaraju, M., and Porciatti, V. (2007). Longitudinal evaluation of retinal ganglion cell function and IOP in the DBA/2J mouse model of glaucoma. *Invest. Ophthalmol. Vis. Sci.* 48:4564–5472.

Saszik, S. M., Robson, J. G., and Frishman, L. J. (2002). The scotopic threshold response of the dark-adapted electroretinogram of the mouse. *J. Physiol.* 543(Pt. 3):899–916.

Schmucker, C., Seeliger, M., Humphries, P., Biel, M., and Schaeffel, F. (2005). Grating acuity at different luminances in wild-type mice and in mice lacking rod or cone function. *Invest. Ophthalmol. Vis. Sci.* 46(1):398–407.

Siliprandi, R., Bucci, M. G., Canella, R., and Carmignoto, G. (1988). Flash and pattern electroretinograms during and after acute intraocular pressure elevation in cats. *Invest. Ophthalmol. Vis. Sci.* 29(4):558–565.

Strettoi, E., and Volpini, M. (2002). Retinal organization in the *bcl-2*-overexpressing transgenic mouse. *J. Comp. Neurol.* 446(1):1–10.

Trimarchi, C., Biral, G., Domenici, L., Porciatti, V., and Bisti, S. (1990). The flash- and pattern electroretinogram generators in the cat: A pharmacological approach. *Clin. Vision Sci.* 6: 19–24.

Van der List, D. A., Coombs, J. L., and Chalupa, L. M. (2006). Normal development of retinal ganglion cell morphological properties in mice lacking the beta2 subunit of the nicotinic acetylcholine receptor. ARVO abstract 3313.

Ventura, L. M., and Porciatti, V. (2005). Restoration of retinal ganglion cell function in early glaucoma after intraocular pressure reduction: A pilot study. *Ophthalmology* 112(1):20–27.

Ventura, L. M., and Porciatti, V. (2006). Pattern electroretinogram in glaucoma. *Curr. Opin. Ophthalmol.* 17(2):196–202.

Ventura, L. M., Sorokac, N., De Los Santos, R., Fener, W. J., and Porciatti, V. (2006). The relationship between retinal ganglion cell function and retinal nerve fiber thickness in early glaucoma. *Invest. Ophthalmol. Vis. Sci.* 47(9):3904–3911.

Viswanathan, S., Frishman, L. J., and Robson, J. G. (2000). The uniform field and pattern ERG in macaques with experimental glaucoma: Removal of spiking activity. *Invest. Ophthalmol. Vis. Sci.* 41(9):2797–2810.

Wong, R. O. (1999). Retinal waves and visual system development. *Annu. Rev. Neurosci.* 22:29–47.

III ORGANIZATION OF THE ADULT MOUSE EYE AND CENTRAL VISUAL SYSTEM

9 Aqueous Humor Dynamics and Trabecular Meshwork

ERNST R. TAMM AND ANTONIA KELLENBERGER

Aqueous humor inflow

Aqueous humor in the anterior eye is a clear fluid that contains the nutrients needed by the lens and the cornea, tissues that need to be avascular to serve their respective optical functions. The site of aqueous humor formation is the ciliary body, where aqueous humor is secreted into the posterior chamber by an active, energy-dependent secretory process involving the ciliary epithelium. The structural details of the ciliary epithelium that enable its secretory function have been extensively studied in humans and traditional laboratory animal models of eye research, such as monkeys and rabbits, and have been reviewed elsewhere (Tamm and Lütjen-Drecoll, 1996). In contrast, the existing information on the structure of the ciliary epithelium in the mouse eye is limited. The available data, however, strongly indicate no major structural or functional differences between mouse ciliary epithelium and that of other mammalian species. Accordingly, the ciliary epithelium in the mouse eye consists of two layers (figure 9.1). The outer layer is formed by the pigmented ciliary epithelium (PE), which is continuous with the retinal pigmented epithelium in the back of the eye and derives from the outer layer of the optic cup during embryonic eye development (Pei and Rhodin, 1970). The inner layer is formed by the nonpigmented ciliary epithelium (NPE), which is continuous with the retina and shares its origin from the inner layer of the optic cup. The mouse ciliary epithelium expresses critical requirements for aqueous humor secretion such as tight junctions between NPE cells as the site of the blood-aqueous barrier (Calera et al., 2006), and Na^+/Ka^+-ATPase for secretory activity (Wetzel and Sweadner, 2001). As in other mammalian species (Tamm and Lütjen-Drecoll, 1996), both epithelial layers are extensively coupled by gap junctions (Calera et al., 2006) and work synergistically to achieve aqueous humor secretion by facilitating movement of NaCl and water between NPE and PE (Civan and Macknight, 2004). Accordingly, in mutant mice that express no gap junctions between NPE and PE, secretion of aqueous humor is critically impaired (Calera et al., 2006). The total volume of aqueous humor in the mouse eye has been reported at $5.9 \pm 0.5\,\mu l$, and the rate of aqueous humor formation as measured in the NIH Swiss White mouse has been reported at $0.18 \pm 0.05\,\mu l/min$ (Aihara et al., 2003a).

The ciliary processes covered by NPE and PE (pars plicata region) show a more irregular arrangement than that of other species, as they are not strictly parallel but rather overlap and intersect with each other (Napier and Kidson, 2005). As in other mammalian species, the fibers of the zonular apparatus are mainly attached to the NPE in the valleys between the ciliary processes and in the pars plana region, behind the ciliary processes and immediately adjacent to the sensory retina (figures 9.1 and 9.2).

The ciliary muscle in the mouse eye is localized in the posterior parts of the ciliary body, underneath the pars plana region of the ciliary epithelium (see figure 9.1). It is considerably smaller than in humans and higher primates (Tamm, 2002). In meridional or sagittal sections through the anterior eye, mouse ciliary muscle usually consists of only four to six smooth muscle cells, indicating there is no significant accommodative power in the mouse eye.

Aqueous humor outflow

After it is secreted into the posterior chamber, aqueous humor passes through the pupil into the anterior chamber. It leaves the eye via two outflow pathways, the conventional outflow pathway, through the trabecular meshwork, and the unconventional or uveoscleral outflow pathway, through the ciliary muscle, and the supraciliary and suprachoroidal spaces. The entrance to both outflow pathways is localized in the iridocorneal or chamber angle of the anterior chamber. The architecture of the outflow pathways in the mouse eye shows several distinct structural differences from that in humans or primates. The most obvious difference relates to the position of the ciliary body. In humans and primates, the ciliary body is localized posterior to the trabecular meshwork outflow pathways. In contrast, in the mouse eye, the root of the ciliary body completely covers the trabecular meshwork outflow pathways (see figure 9.1*A* and *B*). The ciliary body is attached to the cornea by pectinate ligaments that originate near the junction between iris and ciliary body and attach to the periphery of the cornea anterior to the trabecular meshwork. Aqueous humor passes through the pectinate

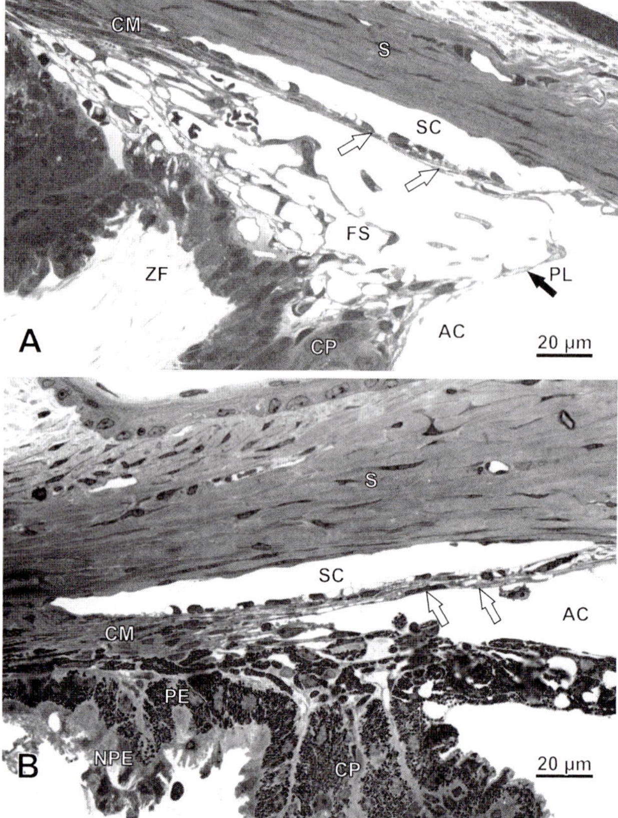

Figure 9.1 Light micrographs of Schlemm's canal (SC) and trabecular meshwork (*white arrows*) in the chamber angle of a Balb/c mouse (*A*) and a C57/Bl6 mouse (*B*) at 6 weeks of age. Internal to the trabecular meshwork is the root of the ciliary body, which is connected to the periphery of the cornea by strands of the pectinate ligament (PL, *black arrow*). Posterior to the pectinate ligament are uveal connective tissue strands with large spaces in between (Fontana's spaces [FS]), which are connected to the anterior chamber (AC) and filled with aqueous humor. At the apex of the ciliary body, ciliary processes (CP) are formed. Behind the ciliary processes, in the pars plana region, zonular fibers (ZF) take their origin from the nonpigmented ciliary epithelium. In the C57/Bl6 background, the chamber angle is somewhat narrower than in the Balb/c background, and Fontana's spaces are smaller. CM, ciliary muscle; NPE, nonpigmented ciliary epithelium; PE, pigmented ciliary epithelium.

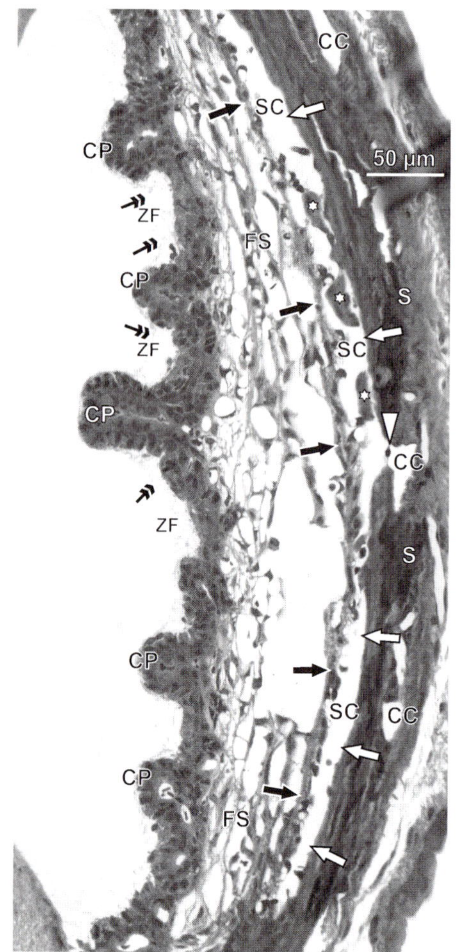

Figure 9.2 Frontal section through Schlemm's canal (SC) in a Balb/c mouse at 6 weeks of age. Schlemm's canal (*white arrows*) is clearly circumferentially oriented and covered along its entire length by the trabecular meshwork (*black arrows*). Collector channels (CC) in the sclera (S) are in places in contact with Schlemm's canal (*white arrowhead*). *White stars* mark connective tissue septa in the lumen of Schlemm's canal. Internal to the trabecular meshwork is the root of the ciliary body, consisting of a meshwork of uveal connective tissue strands. Large open spaces (Fontana's spaces [FS]) that are open to the anterior chamber and are filled with aqueous humor are localized between the strands. At the apex of the ciliary body, ciliary processes (CP) are found at regular intervals. In the valley between the processes, zonular fibers (ZF) take their origin from the nonpigmented ciliary epithelium (*double arrows*).

ligaments into a meshwork of uveal connective tissue strands that are covered by flat cells. Between the uveal strands are large empty spaces, termed "Fontana's spaces" (Duke-Elder, 1958; Franz, 1934; Rohen, 1964, 1982; Tripathi, 1977). The number of uveal strands and Fontana's spaces, as well as the width of the iridocorneal angle, differs between different mouse strains. Balb/c mice have usually a wide-open angle with numerous uveal strands (see figure 9.1*A*), whereas the angle is somewhat narrower in mice with a C57/Bl6 background (see figure 9.1*B*). A detailed analysis of the structural differences of the outflow pathways in different mouse strains is beyond the scope of this discussion. It should be noted, however, that in eyes fixed by immersion only, the iridocorneal angle of the mouse eye is usually considerably collapsed. To get an impression of the architecture of the outflow pathways under the normal condition of continuous flow of aqueous humor, eyes need to be fixed by perfusion via the heart, or, even better, by perfusion with fixative via the anterior chamber.

After entering the spaces between the uveal strands of the iridocorneal angle, aqueous humor either passes into Schlemm's canal via the trabecular meshwork or enters the ciliary muscle and the supraciliary spaces of the uveoscleral outflow pathways. It is reasonable to assume that, as in other mammalian species (Johnson, 2006; Johnson and Erickson, 2000), the mouse trabecular meshwork outflow pathways are the site that provides resistance to aqueous humor outflow. In response to this resistance, intraocular pressure (IOP) is generated, until the pressure is high enough to drive aqueous humor out of the eye, against the resistance. IOP varies considerably between individual mouse strains. In strains with low IOP, such as Balb/c, IOP is 10 mm Hg, whereas in strains with higher pressure, such as CBA/J, IOP has been measured at 18 mm Hg (Savinova et al., 2001). So far, no structural or molecular differences between the outflow pathways of strains with low or high IOP have been identified. IOP in the mouse eye shows a 24-hour pattern, with low levels at daytime and higher levels during nighttime (Aihara et al., 2003c).

Similar to the situation in humans and primates and very unlike to that in rabbits, pigs and cows, Schlemm's canal in the mouse eye is a circumferentially oriented vessel (see figure 9.2). Schlemm's canal is in contact with collector channels in the sclera (see figure 9.2), which will carry aqueous humor to the episcleral vessel system outside the eye (Aihara et al., 2003b). In places, there are connective tissue septa present in the lumen of Schlemm's canal that are in contact with the connective tissue of the adjacent sclera (see figure 9.2).

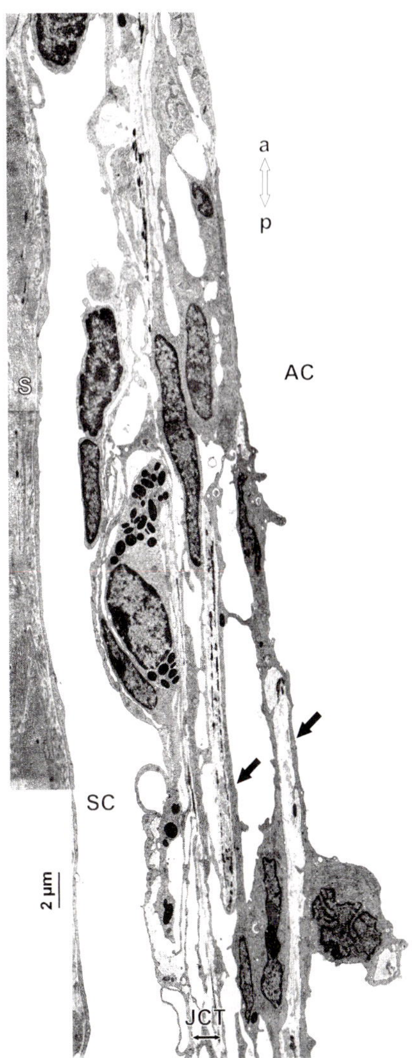

FIGURE 9.3 Electron micrograph of the trabecular meshwork in a C57/Bl6 mouse at 6 weeks of age. The meshwork consists of an inner part with two connective tissue lamellae (*arrows*) covered by flat trabecular meshwork cells, and the outer juxtacanalicular connective tissue (JCT) next to the endothelium of the inner wall of Schlemm's canal (SC).

The trabecular meshwork

As in humans and primates, the mouse trabecular meshwork is divided into an inner part, which consists of connective tissue strands or lamellae that are covered by flat trabecular cells, and an outer juxtacanalicular connective tissue (JCT; figure 9.3) (Tamm et al., 1999). The inner part usually does not form more than one or two lamellae, which are fixed posteriorly at the sclera behind Schlemm's canal and anteriorly at the periphery of the cornea. Accordingly, the inner part of the mouse trabecular meshwork resembles the corneoscleral meshwork in the human eye. The outer JCT does not form organized lamellae but resembles a loose connective tissue that is 1–2 µm wide in the mouse eye. In the JCT, there are trabecular cells that are in contact with the endothelial layer of Schlemm's canal and with the cells covering the strands of the outer corneoscleral meshwork. The intercellular spaces of the JCT are filled with sparse extracellular matrix components, mostly in the form of fine fibrillar material (Tamm et al., 1999). In the posterior spaces of the JCT, electron-dense fiber bundles are present that resemble the elastic-like fibers, which are a characteristic component of the JCT in the human eye (Lütjen-Drecoll and Rohen, 2001). In humans, the elastic-like fibers in the JCT are covered by a sheath of largely amorphous material that increases with age. In patients with advanced primary open-angle glaucoma (POAG), this increase is even more pronounced, and the sheath material forms the "sheath-derived plaque material," a hallmark of the JCT in eyes with POAG. Elastic-like fibers in the mouse trabecular meshwork appear not to be surrounded by a sheath material comparable to that in humans. The fetal development of the mouse trabecular meshwork has been reviewed recently (Cvekl and Tamm, 2004; Smith et al., 2001) and is not discussed here.

The cells of Schlemm's canal inner wall endothelium in the mouse eye are connected by tight junctions and adherens-type junctions, very similar to the situation that is found in the human eye (Ethier, 2002; Johnson, 2006; Johnson and Erickson, 2000). When eyes are fixed by perfusion, numerous outpouchings of the inner wall into the lumen of Schlemm's canal are found. The outpouchings, which form in response to aqueous humor flow, are characteristic of the inner wall endothelium in the mammalian eye and have been called giant vacuoles (Ethier, 2002; Johnson, 2006; Tripathi, 1977; Tripathi and Tripathi, 1972). A second characteristic feature of the inner wall endothelium is the presence of large intra- or intercellular pores that open in response to aqueous humor flow and are often associated with giant vacuoles. Although pores have not been systematically analyzed in the mouse inner wall endothelium, they can be readily observed (figure 9.4*D*), indicating there is no substantial difference between the mouse inner wall endothelium and that of other mammalian species.

In summary, the structural details of the trabecular meshwork outflow pathways are remarkably similar between the mouse eye and that of higher primates and humans, and the mouse appears to be an excellent animal model for molecular and experimental studies on the mechanisms that control aqueous humor outflow resistance.

Uveoscleral outflow pathways

In contrast to trabecular meshwork outflow, uveoscleral outflow is anatomically less well defined and understood. The pathway was first described by Anders Bill, who observed that large tracers, as markers of bulk flow, exited the anterior chamber through the ciliary body into the supraciliary space and out through the sclera into the extraocular tissues (Bill, 1975). Uveoscleral outflow is largely pressure independent and does not contribute substantially to the formation of IOP (Johnson and Erickson, 2000). Fluid in this pathway ultimately drains into the lymphatic system. Comparable findings have been reported for the mouse eye after injection of fluorescent 70-kDa dextran into the anterior chamber of NIH Swiss mice (Lindsey and Weinreb, 2002). After injection, tracer was observed first in the ciliary muscle and

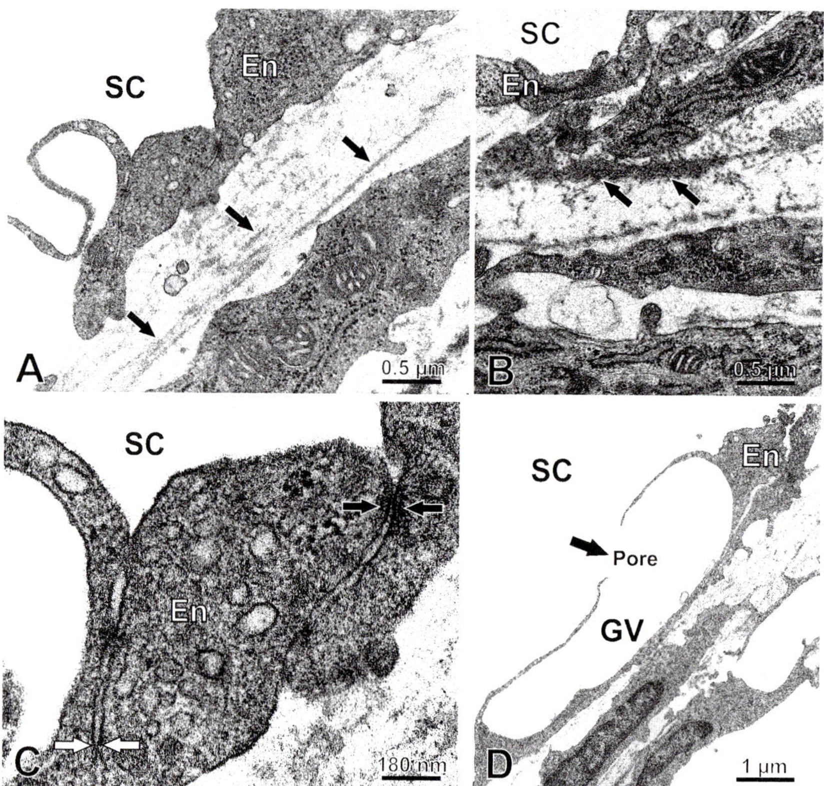

FIGURE 9.4 Ultrastructural details of the juxtacanalicular region in the trabecular meshwork of a C57/Bl6 mouse. The intercellular spaces in the JCT are filled with fine fibrillar material (*arrows* in *A*), and by electron-dense elastic-like fibers (*arrows* in *B*). The endothelial cells (En) of Schlemm's canal (SC) inner wall endothelium are connected with each other by tight junctions (*white arrows* in *C*) and adherens-type junctions (*black arrows* in *C*). When eyes are fixed by perfusion, numerous outpouchings ("giant vacuoles" [GV]) of the inner wall endothelium are present. Pores in the inner wall endothelium are often found at the apex of giant vacuoles (*arrow* in *D*).

anterior choroid, and later in the equatorial choroid and within the stroma of the adjacent equatorial sclera. According to data of Aihara and co-workers (2003a), almost 80% of the aqueous humor leaves the mouse eye via the uveoscleral pathways. Assuming these data are correct, uveoscleral outflow in the mouse eye would be considerably higher as in other mammalian species such as humans, monkeys, and rabbits (Bill, 1962, 1971, 1975; Bill and Phillips, 1971). In mutant mice with larger abnormalities of the chamber angle, such as heterozygous $Pax6^{-/+}$ mice that do not form a differentiated trabecular meshwork and in which Schlemm's canal is absent (Baulmann et al., 2002), aqueous humor outflow probably uses exclusively the uveoscleral outflow pathways.

ACKNOWLEDGMENTS Work was supported by a grant from the Deutsche Forschungsgemeinschaft (TA 115/15-1). We thank Margit Schimmel for expert technical assistance.

REFERENCES

Aihara, M., Lindsey, J. D., and Weinreb, R. N. (2003a). Aqueous humor dynamics in mice. *Invest. Ophthalmol. Vis. Sci.* 44: 5168–5173.

Aihara, M., Lindsey, J. D., and Weinreb, R. N. (2003b). Episcleral venous pressure of mouse eye and effect of body position. *Curr. Eye Res.* 27:355–362.

Aihara, M., Lindsey, J. D., and Weinreb, R. N. (2003c). Twenty-four-hour pattern of mouse intraocular pressure. *Exp. Eye Res.* 77:681–686.

Baulmann, D., Ohlmann, A., Flügel-Koch, C., Goswami, S., Cvekl, A., and Tamm, E. R. (2002). *Pax6* heterozygous eyes show defects in chamber angle differentiation that are associated with a wide spectrum of other anterior eye segment abnormalities. *Mech. Dev.* 118:3–17.

Bill, A. (1962). The drainage of blood from the uvea and the elimination of aqueous humor in rabbits. *Exp. Eye Res.* 1: 200–205.

Bill, A. (1971). Aqueous humor dynamics in monkeys (*Macaca irus* und *Cecopithecus ethiops*). *Exp. Eye Res.* 11:195–206.

Bill, A. (1975). Blood circulation and fluid dynamics in the eye. *Physiol. Rev.* 55:383–417.

Bill, A., and Phillips, C. (1971). Uveoscleral drainage of aqueous humor in human eyes. *Exp. Eye Res.* 12:275–281.

Calera, M. R., Topley, H. L., Liao, Y., Duling, B. R., Paul, D. L., and Goodenough, D. A. (2006). Connexin43 is required for production of the aqueous humor in the murine eye. *J. Cell Sci.* 119:4510–4519.

Civan, M. M., and Macknight, A. D. (2004). The ins and outs of aqueous humour secretion. *Exp. Eye Res.* 78:625–631.

Cvekl, A., and Tamm, E. R. (2004). Anterior eye development and ocular mesenchyme: New insights from mouse models and human diseases. *Bioessays* 26:374–386.

Duke-Elder, S. (1958). *System of ophthalmology: Vol. 1. The eye in evolution.* St. Louis: Mosby.

Ethier, C. R. (2002). The inner wall of Schlemm's canal. *Exp. Eye Res.* 74:161–172.

Franz, V. (1934). Vergleichende Anatomie des Wirbeltierauges. In L. Bolk, E. Göppert, E. Kallius, and W. Lubosch (Eds.), *Handbuch der vergleichenden Anatomie der Wirbeltiere: Vol. 2/2.* Berlin: Urban and Schwarzenberg.

Johnson, M. (2006). What controls aqueous humour outflow resistance? *Exp. Eye Res.* 82:545–557.

Johnson, M., and Erickson, K. (2000). Mechanisms and routes of aqueous humor drainage. In D. M. Albert and F. A. Jakobiec (Eds.), *Principles and practice of ophthalmology* (pp. 2577–2595). Philadelphia: Saunders.

Lindsey, J. D., and Weinreb, R. N. (2002). Identification of the mouse uveoscleral outflow pathway using fluorescent dextran. *Invest. Ophthalmol. Vis. Sci.* 43:2201–2205.

Lütjen-Drecoll, E., and Rohen, J. W. (2001). Functional morphology of the trabecular meshwork. In W. Tasman and E. A. Jaeger (Eds.), *Duane's foundations of clinical ophthalmology* (pp. 1–30). Philadelphia: Lippincott Williams & Wilkins.

Napier, H. R., and Kidson, S. H. (2005). Proliferation and cell shape changes during ciliary body morphogenesis in the mouse. *Dev. Dyn.* 233:213–223.

Pei, Y. F., and Rhodin, J. A. G. (1970). The prenatal development of the mouse eye. *Anat. Rec.* 168:105–126.

Rohen, J. W. (1964). Ciliarkörper (corpus ciliare). In W. von Möllendorf and W. Bargmann (Eds.), *Handbuch der mikroskopischen Anatomie des Menschen.* Vol. 3, Pt. 4. *Haut und Sinnesorgane. Das Auge und seine Hilfsorgane* (pp. 189–237). Heidelberg: Springer-Verlag.

Rohen, J. W. (1982). The evolution of the primate eye in relation to the problem of glaucoma. In E. Lütjen-Drecoll (Ed.), *Basic aspects of glaucoma research* (pp. 3–33). Stuttgart: Schattauer Verlag.

Savinova, O. V., Sugiyama, F., Martin, J. E., Tomarev, S. I., Paigen, B. J., Smith, R. S., and John, S. W. (2001). Intraocular pressure in genetically distinct mice: An update and strain survey. *B.M.C. Genet.* 2:12. (E-pub: doi 10.1186/1471-2156/2/12.)

Smith, R. S., Zabaleta, A., Savinova, O. V., and John, S. W. (2001). The mouse anterior chamber angle and trabecular meshwork develop without cell death. *B.M.C. Dev. Biol.* 1:3. (E-pub: doi 10.1186/1471-213x/1/3.)

Tamm, E. R. (2002). Myocilin and glaucoma: Facts and ideas. *Prog. Retin. Eye Res.* 21:395–428.

Tamm, E. R., and Lütjen-Drecoll, E. (1996). Ciliary body. *Microscop. Res. Tech.* 33:390–439.

Tamm, E. R., Russell, P., and Piatigorsky, J. (1999). Development and characterization of an immortal and differentiated murine trabecular meshwork cell line. *Invest. Ophthalmol. Vis. Sci.* 40:1392–1403.

Tripathi, R. C. (1977). The functional morphology of the outflow systems of ocular and cerebrospinal fluid. *Exp. Eye Res. (Suppl.),* 65–116.

Tripathi, R. C., and Tripathi, B. J. (1972). The mechanism of aqueous outflow in lower mammals. *Exp. Eye Res.* 14:73–79.

Wetzel, R. K., and Sweadner, K. J. (2001). Immunocytochemical localization of NaK-ATPase isoforms in the rat and mouse ocular ciliary epithelium. *Invest. Ophthalmol. Vis. Sci.* 42:763–769.

10 Recent Advances in the Investigation of Mouse Cone Photoreceptors

ARKADY LYUBARSKY, SERGEI S. NIKONOV, LAUREN L. DANIELE, AND EDWARD N. PUGH, JR.

Functions of cones

Cone photoreceptors subserve day vision; their most critical function is to enable the retina to generate signals in the presence of bright light, escaping the saturation that rods undergo at modest intensity (Rodieck, 1998). In addition to this primary function, cones in retinas expressing multiple cone opsins provide the signals necessary for discriminating objects on the basis of the spectral content of the light they reflect. In humans, cones are the dominant photoreceptor type in the macula, the portion of the retina corresponding to the central 5° of visual space, which projects massively to approximately $10\,cm^2$ (37%) of primary visual cortex (V1). Because of the distinct and critical roles that cones play in normal human vision, cone disease and death, such as occur in age-related macular degeneration, are devastating.

To investigate the molecular mechanisms that allow cones to perform their unique functions and the molecular mechanisms of cone-specific disease, there is a need for mammalian models that allow (1) manipulation of genes expressed in cones, (2) molecular and biochemical characterization of the protein products of such genes, and (3) electrophysiological analysis of cones and their neural circuits. The mouse has become the mammal of choice for the investigation of organ function and the molecular mechanisms of disease. There are a number of reasons for this choice, including the genomic proximity of mice to humans, the array of molecular tools for making targeted gene manipulations in mice, the vast knowledge base of molecular, cellular, and behavioral experimentation involving mice, the relatively short generation time, and the economics of mouse husbandry. Despite these compelling reasons, investigation of the functional consequences of molecularly manipulated cone-specific genes in mice has been an elusive goal. Our laboratory has been investigating mouse cones for a number of years, initially with electroretinographic (ERG) methods (Lyubarsky et al., 1999, 2000, 2001) and more recently with single-cell recordings (Nikonov et al., 2005, 2006). This chapter summarizes our progress and provides a prospectus. We begin with a summary of the basic features of mouse cones.

The anatomy of mouse cones

Numerosity and Retinal Disposition The adult C57BL/6 mouse eye is approximately a sphere of diameter 3.3 mm, and the retina a hemispheric surface of area of $18\,mm^2$ and average thickness of $200\,\mu m$; the photoreceptor layer itself is about $100\,\mu m$ thick (reviewed in Lyubarsky and Pugh, 2004). An excellent inventory of the major cell types of the C57BL/6 mouse retina has been provided, with rods shown to outnumber all other cell types by more than 20:1: at an average density of $4.4 \times 10^5\,mm^{-2}$, the adult C57BL/6 retina comprises 6.4×10^6 rod photoreceptors (Jeon et al., 1998). Cones constitute about 3% of the total photoreceptors in the C57BL/6 retina (Carter-Dawson and LaVail, 1979; Jeon et al., 1998), numbering approximately 200,000. Overall, the cone density in the mouse retina appears uniform (there being no fovea or retinal streak), and corresponds to about one cone per retinal pigment epithelium (RPE) cell. It might be thought that the relative paucity of cones implies that the mouse retina has minimal cone signaling capacity. However, several lines of evidence point to the contrary conclusion, among them the large number of cone bipolars (Jeon et al., 1998), whose depolarizing ("ON") subclass produces a large ERG b-wave (Lyubarsky et al., 1999).

Mouse cones have a disposition in the photoreceptor layer distinct from that of rods in at least three ways. First, the cell bodies of cones are invariably located at the outermost of the approximately 11–12 rows of nuclei in the outer nuclear layer (ONL), just vitread to the outer limiting membrane (OLM), whereas rod nuclei are distributed throughout the OLM. Second, cone outer segments (OSs) are shorter than those of rods, typically have their base (where disc synthesis occurs) closer to the OLM than rods do, and terminate on average about $10\,\mu m$ short of the tips of the rod OSs, which are in contact with the apical surface of RPE cells (Carter-Dawson and LaVail, 1979). Some of these distinctive features of mouse cones are illustrated in figure 10.1.

Ultrastructure of Mouse Cones The classic investigation of the ultrastructure of mouse cones is that of Carter-Dawson and LaVail (1979). These investigators found that on average, C57BL/6 mouse cone OSs are shorter than rod OSs (15 μm vs. 25 μm) and somewhat narrower (1.2 μm vs. 1.4 μm), and the cone disc repeat frequency is slightly lower ($38\,\mu m^{-1}$) than that of rods ($41\,\mu m^{-1}$). The intradiscal spaces of mouse cone OSs are not all "patent" (open to the extracellular space), as in the classic picture derived from nonmammalian vertebrates such as fishes and amphibia; however, the base of the mouse cone OS typically has 15 or more patent discs, while in the rod typically only five to seven are patent. Moreover, in the more distal OS, patent discs are occasionally seen in mouse cones, but never in rods. Similar ultrastructural details differentiating cones from rods are generally common among mammals (Arikawa et al., 1992).

Retinal Connectivity of Mouse Cones Before focusing further on mouse cones, it is useful to mention briefly some general issues in neuroscience that will be facilitated by their investigation. One such issue is synaptic transmission. The cone pedicle is arguably one of the most complex synaptic specializations in the CNS, comprising as it does 20–50 presynaptic ribbons, each flanked by numerous vesicles

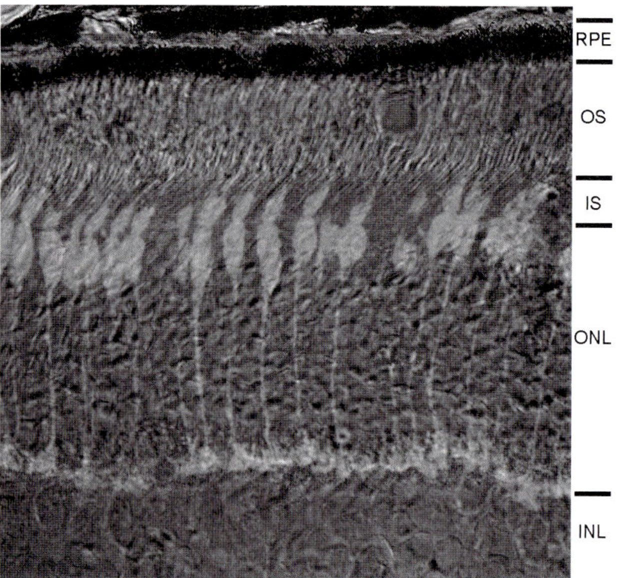

Figure 10.1 Disposition and numerosity of mouse cones. The image superimposes confocal DIC and fluorescence image of a frozen section of the photoreceptor and RPE cell layer of a mouse retina. The mouse from whose eye the section was made expressed EGFP under the human M/L cone promoter (Fei and Hughes, 2001). See color plate 2.

in preparation for synaptic release (Haverkamp et al., 2000; Wässle, 2004). The synaptic transmitter, glutamate, is released maximally in the dark-adapted state, when cones are most depolarized, and the release is suppressed when the cones hyperpolarize to light. Thus, the pedicle is specialized for massive packaging and delivery of synaptic vesicles, together with recycling of the membrane and transmitter. The full complexity of the cone pedicle, however, is manifest in the variety of postsynaptic contacts.

Mouse cone pedicles, like those of other mammals, make synaptic contact with nine morphologically distinct bipolar cells, which to some extent can also be distinguished by molecular markers (Haverkamp et al., 2003; Ghosh et al., 2004), as well as with several classes of horizontal cells. The nine bipolar types are divided into two principal classes, depolarizing bipolar cells (DBCs) and hyperpolarizing bipolar cells (HBCs), and each class likely appears further divided into "sustained" and "transient" subclasses (DeVries, 2000). DBCs make sign-inverting connections at ribbon synapses, while HBCs make sign-conserving synapses at flat junctions. The sign inversion of the cone → DBC synapse is effected by a GPCR cascade initiated by a metabotropic glutamate receptor (mGluR6) that activates a G protein, G_o (Dhingra et al., 2000), leading through yet undetermined signaling components to the opening of cation channels near the invaginating dendritic tips of the bipolars. The sign-conserving cone → HBC synapses are made via ionotropic (AMPA) receptors.

The significance of the cone synapses and cone bipolars, in the context of the work discussed here describing the physiology of mouse cones, is that the mouse now offers a valuable preparation for investigating the role of many specific molecules in these complex synapses. Thus, for example, synaptic vesicle protein 2 (SVP2) has three isoforms (Sv2a, b, c) expressed in the mouse retina: Sv2a is expressed only in cone synaptic terminals, Sv2b in the ribbon synapses of cones, rods, and bipolar cells, and Sv3c in starburst amacrine terminals (Wang et al., 2003). Genetic manipulations of Sv2s in mouse will be the most likely path to resolving the distinct roles of the different Sv2 isoforms. But assessing the functional consequences of such manipulations requires the investigator to have a clear understanding of the distinctive functional features of the mouse cone system, which we now describe.

Mouse Cone S- and M-opsins; Dorsoventral Gradient of M-Opsin Expression; Coexpression of S and M Cone Opsins The mouse retina, like that of most mammals, expresses, in addition to the rod pigment rhodopsin, two cone opsins, a mid-wavelength-sensitive opsin (M-opsin) and a short-wavelength-sensitive opsin (S-opsin) (Szel et al., 1992, 1993). (In many primates, including human, three distinct cone opsins are expressed, but two of the three are so closely homologous—ca. 98% in man [Nathans et al., 1986]—that only two distinct classes of cone opsin are considered to be present.) The two mouse cone opsins have λ_{max} values of approximately 510 nm (M-opsin) and approximately 360 nm (S-opsin), respectively (Jacobs et al., 1991; Sun et al., 1997; Yokoyama et al., 1998). Mouse S-opsin is a member of the SWS1 subfamily of opsins, to which human S-opsin also belongs, while mouse M-opsin belongs to the LW1 subfamily, whose members include the human L and M cone pigments (Yokoyama, 1996; Yokoyama and Yokoyama, 2000; Ebrey and Koutalos, 2001). In mice, M-opsin is expressed in a dorsoventral gradient, with a much higher level of M-opsin in cones of the most dorsal retina, and S-opsin is more purely expressed in the ventral retina (Szel et al., 1992, 1993; Applebury et al., 2000). Most cones of the mouse coexpress both S- and M-opsin, and this coexpression itself exhibits a dorsoventral gradient (Applebury et al., 2000). As discussed in the next section, in individual cones that coexpress them, both S- and M-opsins drive phototransduction.

Electroretinographic studies of mouse cone function

A full-field (*ganzfeld*) flash delivered to the eye evokes a light-dependent, massed potential, the ERG, which arises from light-driven changes in cellular currents flowing radially in the extracellular spaces of the retina. The initial, corneal-negative potential is known as the a-wave and the subsequent corneal-positive component is known as the b-wave. The a-wave originates primarily from suppression of the photoreceptor "dark" or circulating current (Hagins et al., 1970), while the b-wave has its origin primarily in activation of the light-driven, postsynaptic currents of depolarizing (ON) bipolar cells (DBCs), coupled to the photoreceptors by a metabotropic (mGluR6) receptor cascade (Robson and Frishman, 1995; reviewed in Pugh et al., 1998; Robson and Frishman, 1998).

The Mouse Cone-Driven (Photopic) b-Wave The flash-activated, rodent cone-driven b-wave was first characterized in albino rats by Green (1973). Peachey subsequently characterized aspects of the cone-driven b-wave in mice (Peachey et al., 1993). The ultraviolet (UV) sensitivity of mouse cones was discovered by Jacobs and colleagues, using the flicker ERG (Jacobs et al., 1991). Lyubarsky et al. (1999) extensively investigated the cone-driven b-wave of the C57BL/6 mouse: about one-third of the saturated amplitude (ca. 650 μV) of the dark-adapted mouse b-wave was found to arise from cone-driven cells, so that suppression of the rod a-wave and b-wave with steady background light or strong flashes completely isolates an approximately 180 μV cone component. If this component can be attributed to the complete activation of the postsynaptic current of DBCs, and if cone DBCs constitute approximately one-third of the total population (rod DBCs constituting the remaining two-thirds), then the maximum cone DBC postsynaptic current can be estimated to be 500–1,000 pA (Lyubarsky et al., 1999), using the rod a-wave and circulating current as a gauge (figure 10.2).

The b-wave action spectrum comprises two peaks, at approximately 360 nm and 510 nm, corresponding to the S and M cone opsins, respectively (see figure 10.2), with the S-opsin component fourfold more sensitive than the M-opsin component (Lyubarsky et al., 1999). The cone-driven b-wave is characterized by oscillatory potentials (Wachtmeister, 1998; Dong et al., 2004), which are negligible or minimal in purely scotopic b-waves. Reliable differences between oscillatory potentials associated with dim-flash responses driven by S-opsin and M-opsin suggest subtle differences in the light-evoked currents of cone DBCs and/or of subsequent retinal neurons with radial extent driven by these bipolar cells (see Lyubarsky et al., 1999, their figures 4 and 9).

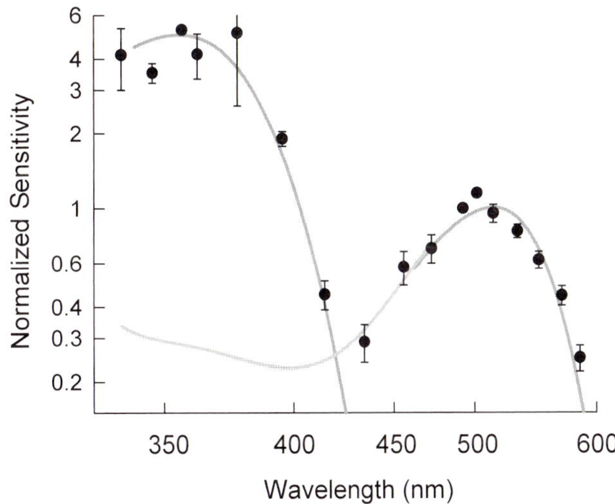

Figure 10.2 Spectral sensitivity of the mouse cone-driven ERG b-wave. Each point represents the sensitivity of the mouse cone-driven b-wave to brief (ca. 1 ms) flashes of light, expressed in photon units (mean ± SEM, n = 3 or more mice). The data have been normalized at 510 nm. The smooth curves are photopigment templates (Lamb, 1995), with λ_{max} values of 360 nm and 510 nm, respectively, corresponding to the λ_{max} values of the two mouse cone photopigments (see the text), but in the case of the M cone opsin, extended in the near UV, according to Lyubarsky et al. (1999). Note that the sensitivity at the secondary maximum at 510 nm is approximately one-fourth that of the primary maximum at 360 nm. The sensitivity of the secondary maximum at 510 nm varies with age, strain, and light-rearing conditions, varying from one-half to one-sixth that of the primary maximum (Lyubarsky et al., 2002). Other investigations have found systematic variation in the number and responsivity of cones with age and strain in mice (Gresh et al., 2003).

THE MOUSE CONE A-WAVE Under cone isolation conditions, a small corneal-negative a-wave component of approximately 15 μV saturating amplitude can be recorded and characterized (Lyubarsky et al., 1999); this is approximately the amplitude expected on the assumption that cones and rods have about the same magnitude circulating currents, given that cones are about 3% of the photoreceptors and that the rod a-wave recorded under similar conditions is approximately 400–500 μV. In sum, its sign, amplitude, kinetics, and behavior in wild-type mice and in mice null for genes expressed in cones all indicate that the mouse cone a-wave originates in the suppression of the cones' circulating current (Lyubarsky et al., 1999, 2000, 2001, 2002).

RAPID RECOVERY FROM BLEACHING STIMULI ERG recordings have revealed mouse cone responses to recover much faster than rods from strong flashes that completely suppress the circulating current. Thus, for example, the cone a- and b-waves recover from a flash estimated to isomerize 1% of cone M-opsin in 1 s (Lyubarsky et al., 1999), while the recovery of mouse rods measured with the ERG a-wave under similar conditions (including anesthetic) takes minutes (Lyubarsky and Pugh, 1996). These results are paralleled by extensive data in humans (Thomas and Lamb, 1999; Mahroo and Lamb, 2004).

ELECTRORETINOGRAPHIC PHENOTYPES OF MICE WITH CONE PHOTOTRANSDUCTION GENES INACTIVATED Though the mouse cone a-wave is difficult to isolate in practice because of its relatively small amplitude, in conjunction with the cone-driven b-wave it has proven valuable in establishing the function of several visual transduction proteins expressed in cones. Specifically, the greatly slowed recoveries of the a- and b-waves of *Grk1*$^{-/-}$ mice after a strong flash show Grk1 to be essential for normal inactivation of mouse cones (Lyubarsky et al., 2000), while the greatly slowed recoveries of the a- and b-waves in *Rgs9-1*$^{-/-}$ mice shows Rgs9-1 to be necessary for normal cone inactivation (Lyubarsky et al., 2001) (figure 10.3).

FUNCTIONAL COEXPRESSION OF S- AND M-OPSINS IN MOUSE CONES The very wide spectral separation (ca. 150 nm) of the two mouse cone opsins, together with steep fall-off in absorbance of visual pigments on their long-wave tail,[1] makes it possible to deliver an intense "orange" ($\lambda > 530$ nm) flash that isomerizes a substantial fraction (ca. 1%) of the M-opsin present in the retina while negligibly isomerizing S-opsin. Such an orange flash completely saturates the cone b-wave response to a UV flash for 200–300 ms, suggesting that virtually all mouse cones expressing S-opsin coexpress M-opsin to some degree (Lyubarsky et al., 1999). Confirmation of the hypothesis that the capacity of an orange flash to eliminate b-wave responsivity to UV flashes arises from the functional coexpression of M-opsin in "S cones" comes from

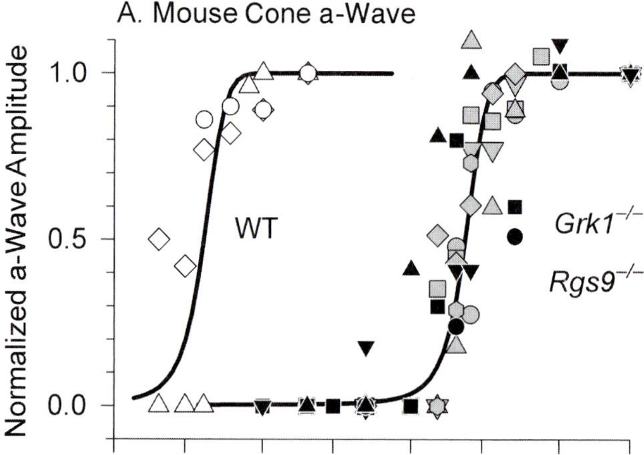

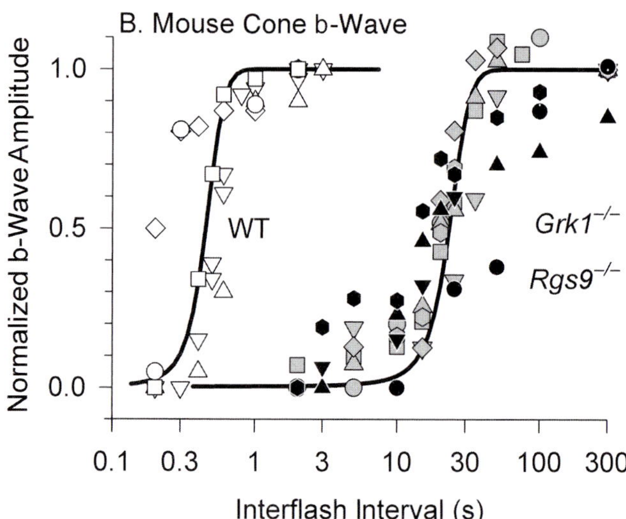

FIGURE 10.3 Recovery kinetics of components of cone ERGs of wild-type, *Grk1*$^{-/-}$, and *Rgs9*$^{-/-}$ mice in a paired-flash paradigm. Under conditions that isolate the cone components of the ERG, an intense "white" flash, estimated to isomerize 1.2% of the cone M-opsin and 0.09% of the S-opsin (Lyubarsky et al., 1999), was followed at various interflash intervals ranging from 0.2 s to 300 s by a second flash of comparable intensity and wavelength composition, which produced a saturated amplitude response. In the absence of Grk1 (rhodopsin kinase), which is the only GRK known to be expressed in the mouse retina and is expressed in both rods and cones, recovery to 50% of the initial amplitude is slowed roughly 60- to 70-fold (Lyubarsky et al., 2000). In the absence of Rgs9-1, the photoreceptor-specific regulator of transducin GTPase activity, recovery is similarly slowed (Lyubarsky et al., 2001). The a-wave and b-wave recoveries are comparably slowed.

[1]The long-wavelength sensitivity of visual pigments declines by about 5 $\log_{10}$ units per 0.2 units of the dimensionless abscissa, λ_{max}/λ (Lamb, 1995).

the work of Ekesten et al. (2002), who observed a similar phenomenon in the presence of pharmacological blockers of postreceptor neurons. The minimum fraction of coexpressed M-opsin required to explain complete b-wave suppression by an orange flash is quite small, no doubt undetectable by histochemical methods. In contrast, single-cone action spectra, which can detect in cones that predominantly express S-opsin M-opsin coexpressed at less than 1 part in 10,000 (Nikonov et al., 2005), confirm M-opsin coexpression in most mouse cones (Nikonov et al., 2006).

Functional features of wild-type mouse cones from single-cell recordings

A breakthrough in the characterization of the functional properties of mouse cones came with the development of a suction pipette method suitable for recording from them (Nikonov et al., 2005). This development rested on the well-established fact that the circulating or "dark" current of vertebrate photoreceptors, which "sinks" into the outer segment through the cGMP-activated channels, has its sources in K^+ channels distributed throughout the inner segment and remaining portions of the cell (reviewed in Pugh and Lamb, 2000). Indeed, it is the radial separation of the sources and sinks of the dark current that gives rise to the extracellular loop of the circulating current discovered by Hagins et al. (1970), and with its suppression, the a-wave of the ERG (reviewed in Pugh et al., 1998). Since the 1980s, many investigators have taken advantage of the radial separation of the sources and sinks of the circulating current to record photoresponses of amphibian rods whose "inner segments" are drawn into the suction pipette. The development of a suction pipette method suitable for recording from mouse cones was propelled by failure to record reliable responses from the OSs of *Nrl*$^{-/-}$ photoreceptors, leading to the hypothesis that their OSs are particularly fragile and not separable from the pigment epithelium with impunity (Nikonov et al., 2005). The novel method is characterized by two features: first, one to several nuclei from the ONL are carefully drawn under infrared viewing into a suction pipette with an appropriate-sized orifice; second, the circulating currents of rods whose perinuclear regions are also inevitably drawn into the pipette are suppressed by a steady 500 nm background).

Light response families obtained with this method (figure 10.4) have many features that identify them as originating in the suppression of the circulating current of cones rather than rods, including (1) their action spectra, which typically peaks around 360 nm (as expected for mouse cone S-opsin), and which also has a shoulder around 510 nm (as expected from functional coexpression of M-opsin) (see figure 10.6); (2) their approximately 100-fold lower flash sensitivity (0.02% vs. 2.7% current suppressed per photoisomerization) (figure 10.4*C*, *F*, *I*, and *L*); (3) their distinctive kinetics, including a shorter time to peak (t_{peak}) of the dim flash response than rods recorded under the same conditions (t_{peak} = 73 ms vs. 200 ms at 20 Hz bandwidth)[2] and smaller "Pepperberg" or dominant recovery time constants (τ = 70 vs. 230 ms) (figure 10.4*C*, *F*, *I*, and *L*; figure 10.5); and (4) their relatively greater immunity to the effects of bleaching exposures (see Nikonov et al., 2006, for details). Such recordings also confirm that most mouse cones also functionally coexpress both S- and M-opsin; that is, photoisomerization of either pigment in a cone drives phototransduction with similar kinetics (figures 10.5 and 10.6).

*Neural retina leucine zipper (*Nrl$^{-/-}$*) knockout mouse: An all-cone retina*

Background: Are *Nrl*$^{-/-}$ Photoreceptors Cones or "Cods"? In humans, mutations in the Maf-family transcription factor neural retina leucine (NRL) lead to a serious form of autosomal dominant retinitis pigmentosa (RP) (Bessant et al., 1999). In an effort to understand the effects of NRL mutations, Swaroop and colleagues generated an *Nrl*$^{-/-}$ mouse (Mears et al., 2001). The retina of this mouse exhibited a somewhat unexpected phenotype, a complete absence of a number of rod-specific proteins, including rhodopsin, and the rod-specific isoforms of other phototransduction proteins (Mears et al., 2001). A basic conclusion drawn by Mears et al. that has stood the test of additional investigations is that Nrl is necessary for a postmitotic, multipotent photoreceptor cell precursor to differentiate terminally into S cones (the default pathway) or rods (Mears et al., 2001; Corbo and Cepko, 2005; Oh et al., 2007). A critical question raised by the investigation of Mears et al. (2001) was whether the photoreceptors in the *Nrl*$^{-/-}$ retina are in fact cones, or whether they may be "cods," an intermediate, abnormal cell type exhibiting properties of both rods and cones. Among the reasons for this question were that some proteins generally thought to be rod-specific, such as "rhodopsin kinase" (Grk1) and "rod arrestin" (Arr1), were expressed in the *Nrl*$^{-/-}$ photoreceptors, and that the

---

[2]Use of 20 Hz bandwidth facilitates isolation of the relatively small and noisy cone responses obtained with the "inner-segment, loose-patch" method (Nikonov et al., 2005) but distorts their kinetics to some extent. We measured the delay produced by the 20 Hz lowpass filtering to be 22 ms, and further confirmed that with a much wider bandwidth, averaged dim-flash responses peaked instead at about 50 ms. Correction for the distortion of the filtering thus brings the time to peak the dim-flash response of single cones ($t_{peak,corrected}$ = 73 ms − 22 ms = 51 ms; Nikonov et al., 2005, 2006) into good correspondence with that (t_{peak} ~ 50 ms) extracted with the paired flash paradigm applied to the a-wave of the ERG of the *Nrl*$^{-/-}$ (Daniele et al., 2005).

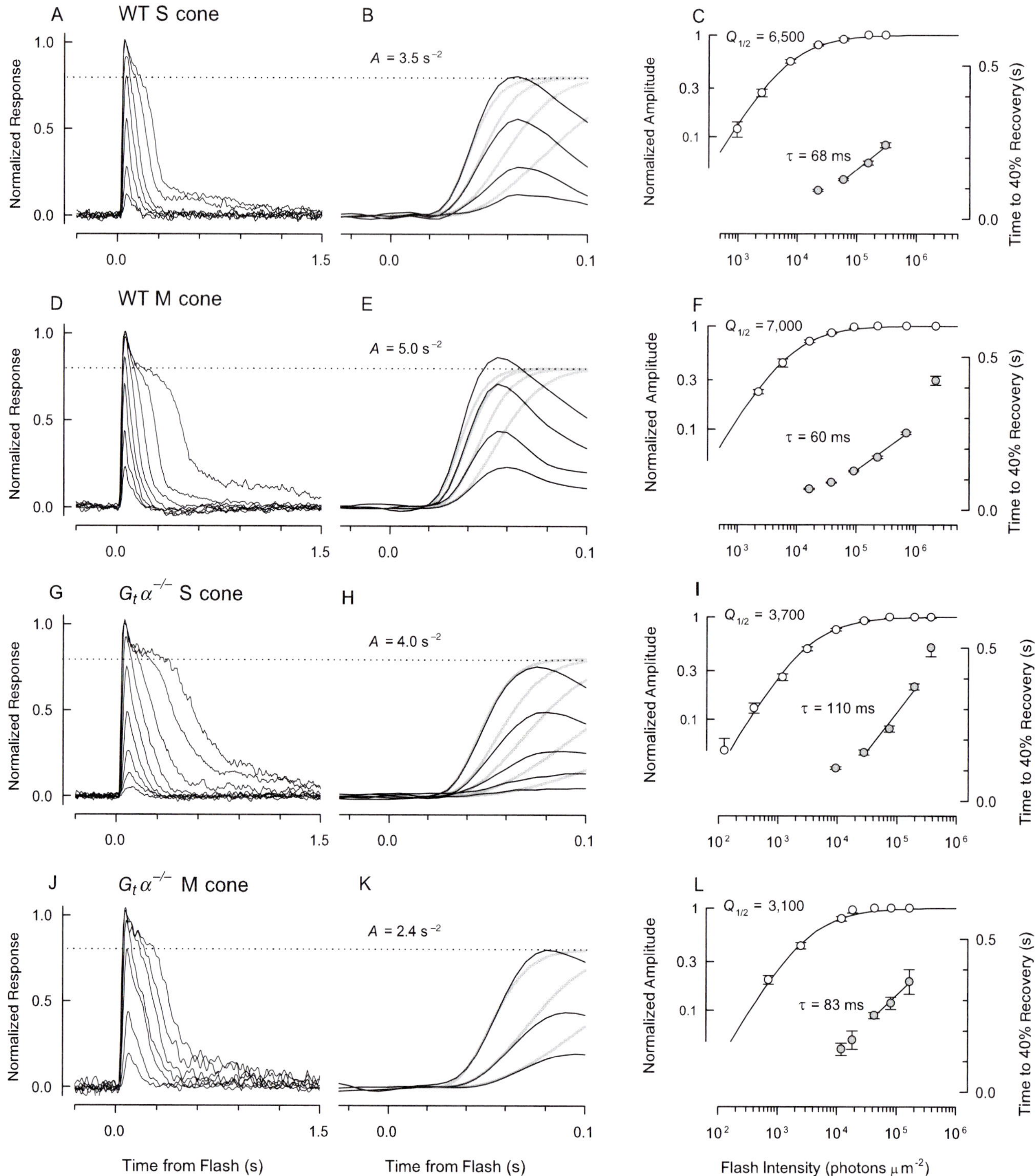

FIGURE 10.4 Kinetics, amplification, and sensitivity of single mouse cones recorded with suction pipettes (Nikonov et al., 2006). *A* and *D*, Shown are light response families of wild-type cones; the "S-dominant cone" was maximally sensitive at 360 nm, while the "M-dominant cone" was maximally sensitive at 510 nm. *G* and *J*, Shown are similar families obtained from cones of $G_t\alpha^{-/-}$ mice, whose rods have no electrical responses (Calvert et al., 2000). *B*, *E*, *H*, and *K*, Shown are the estimation of the amplification constant from the light responses of the corresponding panels to the left (the rising phase of the data shown on an expanded time base). *C*, *F*, *I*, and *L*, Plotted here are the response versus intensity functions derived from the flash response families and the extraction of the so-called dominant recovery time constant (τ) from the recoveries to saturating flashes (see Nikonov et al., 2006, for details).

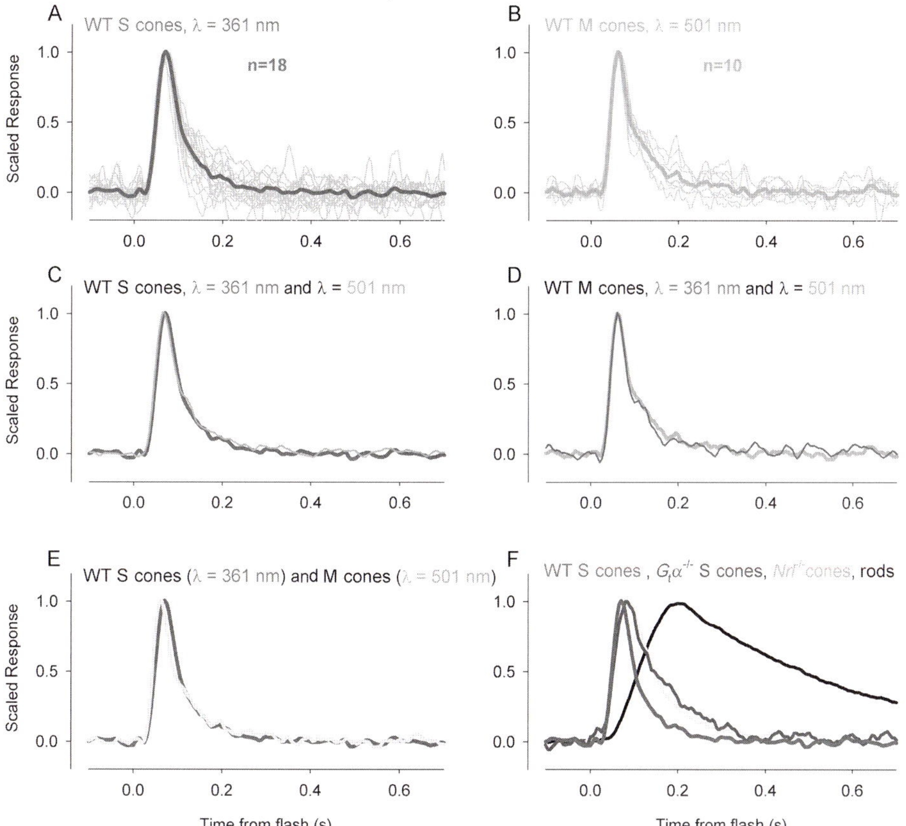

Figure 10.5 Dim-flash responses of single mouse cones. Average dim-flash response data of S-dominant (*A* and *C*) and M-dominant (*B* and *D*) cones, stimulated with either UV (361 nm) or midwave (501 nm) flashes, are shown. In each case, analysis of the action spectrum reveals that the UV flash activates only the S-opsin in the cone, while the midwave flash activates M-opsin (the two being coexpressed). *F*, The averaged responses in *A* and *B* are compared with those of the cones of $G_t\alpha^{-/-}$ and *Nrl*$^{-/-}$ mice and with responses from wild-type mouse rods recorded under the same conditions (Nikonov et al., 2006). The midwave background light required to suppress rod responses in the wild-type mouse is not needed in experiments with $G_t\alpha^{-/-}$ and *Nrl*$^{-/-}$ cones and is at least partially responsible for the faster response kinetics of the wild-type cones. See color plate 3.

outer segments did not exhibit an obvious conelike morphology. The identity of the cellular type—rods versus cods—was addressed in investigations in which *Nrl*$^{-/-}$ photoreceptors were compared with rods on a series of ultrastructural, histochemical, molecular, and physiological benchmarks (Daniele et al., 2005; Nikonov et al., 2005), as we now describe.

Histochemical and Ultrastructural Evidence that *Nrl*$^{-/-}$ Photoreceptors Are Cones Each *Nrl*$^{-/-}$ photoreceptor is associated with a "sheath" that binds (and can be stained by) the lectin peanut agglutinin, a classic marker of cones (Johnson et al., 1986; Blanks et al., 1988), and each also exhibits a clumping of chromatin characteristic of mouse cones but not rods (Carter-Dawson and LaVail, 1979). Each *Nrl*$^{-/-}$ photoreceptor also has an inner segment substantially wider than its outer segment, a feature generally exhibited by cones (which enhances their trapping and waveguiding of light), including those of wild-type mice, but not by rods. At the ultrastructural level, *Nrl*$^{-/-}$ photoreceptors have mitochondria that are distinctively conelike, being on average half the length of the mitochondria of rods. These various features of *Nrl*$^{-/-}$ photoreceptors are summarized in table 10.1, where they are compared with the corresponding features of rods and cones in wild-type mice. The conclusion is inescapable: *Nrl*$^{-/-}$ *photoreceptors are a species of cones*, and definitely not a cone-rod intermediate (Daniele et al., 2005).

Electrophysiological Recordings Confirm That *Nrl*$^{-/-}$ Photoreceptors Are Cones The electrical responses of *Nrl*$^{-/-}$ photoreceptors have been recorded with two methods: (1) ERG a-waves, including single- and paired-flash methods (Daniele et al., 2005) (figure 10.7), and (2) single-cell, suction pipette recordings (Nikonov et al., 2005) (see figure 10.5*F*). These measurements, viewed in the context of single-cell recordings of wild-type mouse cones (Nikonov et al., 2006), strongly confirm the identification of *Nrl*$^{-/-}$ photoreceptors

TABLE 10.1

Structural and histochemical features of wild-type rods, cones, and Nrl$^{-/-}$

Feature	*Nrl*$^{-/-}$ Photoreceptors	Wild-type Cones	Wild-type Rods
OS length (μm)	7.3 ± 1.3 (21)	13.4 ± 0.7*	23.6 ± 0.4*
OS width (μm)	1.2 ± 0.3 (21)	1.2 ± 0.03*	1.4 ± 0.1*
OS volume (μm^3)	8.3	14	36
Open discs	Up to 30	>15*	5–7*
Mitochondrial length (μm)	0.94 ± 0.38 (50)	1.31 ± 0.7 (13)*	2.20 ± 0.7 (15)
Chromatin clumping	Yes	Yes	No
PNA-stained OS sheath	Yes	Yes	No

*See Daniele et al., 2005, for additional details.

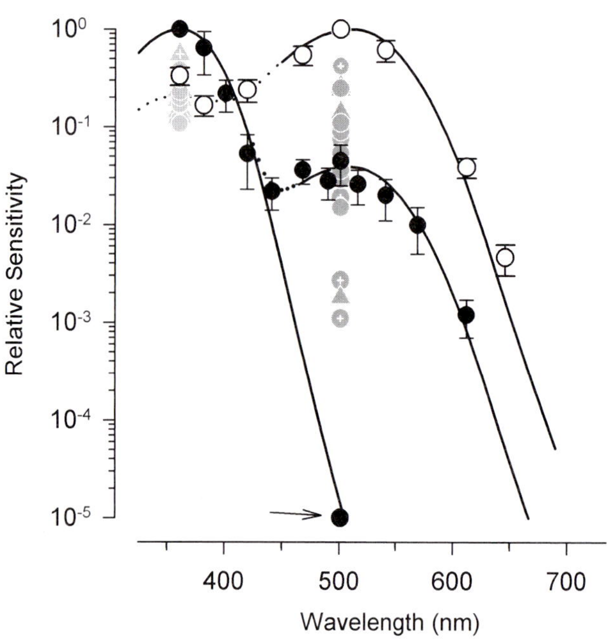

FIGURE 10.6 Spectral sensitivities of wild-type and $G_t\alpha^{-/-}$ mouse cones. Data from each cone have been normalized at the wavelength of maximal sensitivity, either 360 nm or 508 nm. The *black circles with error bars* plot the data of a single wild-type mouse cone and are characterized by a maximally sensitive S-opsin component, combined with an M-opsin component about 0.04 as sensitive at its maximum; the *white circles with error bars* are from a single wild-type M-dominant cone. For other cells, only a pair of symbols is plotted, one at 360 nm and one at 501 nm: for cones maximally sensitive at 360 nm, *light gray symbols* are used, whereas for cones maximally sensitive at 510 nm, *darker gray symbols* are used; the data pertaining to wild-type cones are plotted as *circles* and those of $G_t\alpha^{-/-}$ cones are plotted as *triangles*. Coexpression of M-opsin in all but one S-dominant cone is confirmed, but the coexpression of S-opsin in M-dominant cones cannot be detected at a level of sensitivity below the β band of the M-opsin near 360 nm (*dotted line*).

as cones. First, the average dim-flash response of *Nrl*$^{-/-}$ photoreceptors is very similar to that of both wild-type mouse cones and those of mice lacking the α-subunit of (rod) transducin ($G_t\alpha^{-/-}$) (see figure 10.4*F*) recorded under the same conditions. Second, *Nrl*$^{-/-}$ photoreceptor dim-flash responses in vivo, extracted with the paired flash method, peak at around 50 ms (Daniele et al., 2005), threefold faster than rods do under the same conditions (Hetling and Pepperberg, 1999).

CAVEATS FOR INVESTIGATIONS OF *NRL*$^{-/-}$ PHOTORECEPTORS Nonetheless, for the unequivocal identification of *Nrl*$^{-/-}$ photoreceptors as cones on structural and electrophysiological criteria, it cannot be asserted that these cones are identical to wild-type cones in all respects. Work to date shows that *Nrl*$^{-/-}$ cones differ from their wild-type counterparts in several features (Daniele et al., 2005): (1) the OSs are shorter (see table 10.1); (2) the expression of M-opsin is lower (compare figure 10.7*C* with figure 10.2); (3) the OSs tend to have irregularities in the organization of the disc stacks; and (4) the OSs degenerate, quite noticeably after 4–6 weeks. That the level of M-opsin—whose expression is regulated by thyroid hormone (TH) via the transcription factor/TH-binding receptor TRβ_2 (Ng et al., 2001; Roberts et al., 2006)—is relatively lower in *Nrl*$^{-/-}$ cones (figure 10.7*C*) suggests that at least some of these cells are not fully differentiated. This in turn suggests that other genes may be found to be differentially expressed in *Nrl*$^{-/-}$ and wild-type cones. Finally, degeneration of the *Nrl*$^{-/-}$ retina (Mears et al., 2001) (figure 10.7*D*), while unlikely to be explicable in terms of features of the retina directly affected by the deletion of the transcription factor Nrl,[3] calls for both care and caution in the investigation of this as an "all-cone retina."

[3]Daniele et al. (2005) discuss some hypotheses about the nature of the degeneration of the *Nrl*$^{-/-}$ retina.

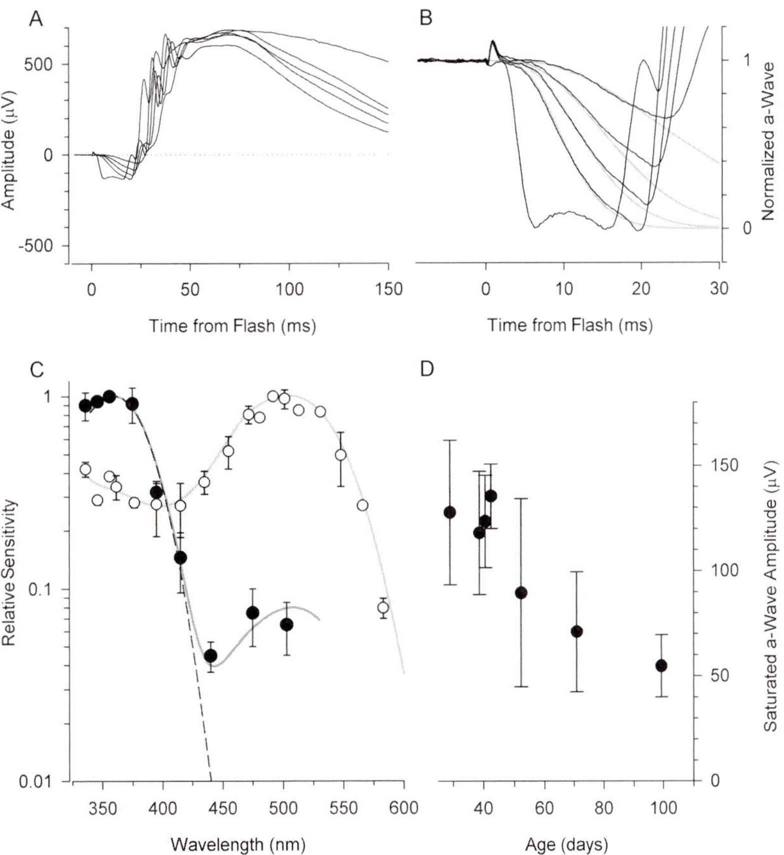

FIGURE 10.7 ERG a-waves of the *Nrl*$^{-/-}$ mouse: amplification and spectral sensitivity decline with age (Daniele et al., 2005). *A*, Full-field ERGs of an *Nrl*$^{-/-}$ mouse produced in response to a series of UV flashes. *B*, The nearly a-wave data of *A* are plotted on an expanded scale, normalized by the 150 μV saturated amplitude and fitted with the model of Lamb and Pugh (1992) to extract the amplification constant of phototransduction. *C*, Spectral sensitivity of the a-wave of the *Nrl*$^{-/-}$ mouse (*solid circles*). For comparison, the spectral sensitivity of the rod a-wave of the wild-type mouse is provided (*open circles*). Like the cone-driven b-wave of the wild-type mouse (see figure 10.2), the cone a-wave of the *Nrl*$^{-/-}$ mouse is maximally sensitive at 360 nm, with a secondary maximum around 510 nm; however, the relative sensitivity of the 510 nm peak is at least fivefold lower in the *Nrl*$^{-/-}$ mouse relative to that in the wild-type mouse, suggesting that M-opsin expression is relatively diminished in *Nrl*$^{-/-}$ cones. *D*, Decline of saturating a-wave amplitude in a population of *Nrl*$^{-/-}$ mice as a function of age. The amplitude is stable at less than 40 days but shows much greater variability and decline thereafter, indicating progressive deterioration.

PROSPECTS FOR INVESTIGATIONS EMPLOYING *NRL*$^{-/-}$ CONES

The prospects are great for use of the *Nrl*$^{-/-}$ mouse in elucidating the differentiation of photoreceptors, in identifying cone-specific genes, and in investigating the biochemistry of the protein products of such genes. Indeed, the first fruits of investigations using the *Nrl*$^{-/-}$ mouse have now appeared.

Photoreceptor differentiation. Swaroop and his colleagues have made great strides in uncovering the network of genes regulated by Nrl in the differentiation of rods (Akimoto et al., 2006; Khanna et al., 2006; Oh et al., 2007), with parallel advances in understanding the downstream transcriptional factor Nr2e3 (Cheng et al., 2004; Wright et al., 2004; Corbo and Cepko, 2005), whose mutation gives rise to enhanced S cone syndrome (Jacobson et al., 1990; Hood et al., 1995).

Cone-specific genes and their molecular function. An analysis of the genes whose message level in the retina is enhanced in the *Nrl*$^{-/-}$ mouse has been derived from a microarray analysis by Yoshida et al. (2004): the genes with elevated expression are candidates for cone-specific expression or for playing a role in cone cell biology. An interesting example is *JamC*, a gene whose expression in the retina would not have been suspected in the absence of microarray data from the *Nrl*$^{-/-}$ retina. *JamC*, whose message is threefold increased in the 8-week-old *Nrl*$^{-/-}$ retina over the level seen in the retina of wild-type mice, encodes a junctional adhesion molecule of the Ig superfamily that is typically associated with tight junctions in endo- and epithelia (Ebnet et al., 2004). Not surprisingly, JamC, along with another JAM isoform, JamA, is localized to the apical complexes of RPE tight junctions (Daniele et al., 2007). However, JamC was also found at the adherens junctions forming the OLM and at the base of the inner segments of cones, suggesting that it may play a novel role in the adhesion of cones and Müller cells at the OLM (Daniele et al., 2007). Perusal of the microarray data of Yoshida et al. (2004) suggests that a number of other novel cone-related genes will be similarly confirmed.

Mouse cone protein biochemistry. Craft and colleagues measured light-dependent phosphorylation of murine opsins using the *Nrl*$^{-/-}$ mouse and have begun characterizing some of its aspects, including the consequent binding of cone arrestin (Zhu et al., 2003). Such studies are possible only because of the biochemistry permitted by the absence of the large (30-fold) excess rod proteins and the abundance of cones. Similarly, our laboratory has begun investigating some biochemical aspects of the mammalian cone retinoid cycle using the *Nrl*$^{-/-}$ mouse (Lyubarsky et al., 2006).

Summary and conclusion

The field of rod photoreceptor biology rests on a firm foundation of four methodological cornerstones: anatomy, biochemistry, molecular genetics, and single-cell electrophysiology. Though data from rods of many species have contributed to the construction of this edifice, those from mouse rods have played a special role in elucidating the role of specific proteins, by dint of the power of mouse molecular genetics to accomplish targeted manipulations of genes (Burns and Baylor, 2001).

Several of the cornerstones of a similar edifice for cones have been laid for some time, with outstanding anatomy and physiology from many species, notably salamander, ground squirrel, and human retinas. However, only recently, with developments in ERG methods (Lyubarsky et al., 1999, 2000, 2001, 2002; Calvert et al., 2000)—and very recently, with suction pipette recording (Nikonov et al., 2005, 2006)—has it been possible to include investigations of mouse cones in all four methodological categories. As a consequence, the power of mouse molecular genetics can now be harnessed in the investigation of cones, as it has been for more than a decade in the investigation of mouse rods. Moreover, the second methodological cornerstone, biochemistry, now includes mouse, thanks to the all-cone *Nrl*$^{-/-}$ mouse (Mears et al., 2001; Daniele et al., 2005; Nikonov et al., 2005), whose retina can be used for identifying and purifying cone-specific proteins without the interference of the vast background of homologous rod proteins that are present in the wild-type mouse retina.

Many areas of science other than the investigation of mouse cones are expected to contribute to our rapidly expanding understanding of cone structure, function and disease. These include the spectacular anatomical characterization of living human cones by David Williams and his colleagues with adaptive optics (e.g., Roorda and Williams, 1999; Pallikaris et al., 2003; Hofer et al., 2005), genomic and microarray data (Yoshida et al., 2004), biochemistry of cones from other species such as ground squirrel (e.g., Zhang et al., 2003), and tremendous advances in the use of optical methods for probing living tissue, such as multiphoton microscopy, which allow imaging of specific cells functioning in their natural milieu.

As cones occupy a little more of the stage, the investigation of rods should not be abandoned, or even curtailed. In humans as in mice, rods outnumber cones by more than 20:1. The sheer numerosity of rods not only means that disease that leads to rod death also causes cone malfunction and demise, but also that the delivery and removal of metabolites needed by both types of photoreceptors—including generic substances such as oxygen and glucose, as well as specific molecules such as retinoids—are of potentially great significance to cone health. We must not lose sight of the fact that the human retina, like that of the mouse and most of our vertebrate relatives, is inherently duplex, having evolved both cones and rods to provide effective visual signals over the more than 8 $\log_{10}$ unit range of diurnal intensities (Rodieck, 1998). Rods and cones in the duplex retina have evolved to complement each other and cooperate, not only in their starring roles in signaling in night and day, but also in performing the many mundane chores of domestic cellular life. This chapter closes, then, with the hope that the vision community will see advances in understanding mouse cones not as "the next big thing" but rather as an opportunity to understand fully *both* types of vertebrate photoreceptors in their shared natural matrix, the retina.

ACKNOWLEDGMENTS Work was supported by NIH grant no. EY02660 and by the Research to Prevent Blindness Foundation.

REFERENCES

Akimoto, M., Cheng, H., Zhu, D., Brzezinski, J. A., Khanna, R., Filippova, E., Oh, E. C., Jing, Y., Linares, J. L., et al. (2006). Targeting of GFP to newborn rods by Nrl promoter and temporal expression profiling of flow-sorted photoreceptors. *Proc. Natl. Acad. Sci. U.S.A.* 103:3890–3895.

Applebury, M. L., Antoch, M. P., Baxter, L. C., Chun, L. L., Falk, J. D., Farhangfar, F., Kage, K., Krzystolik, M. G., Lyass, L. A., and Robbins, J. T. (2000). The murine cone photoreceptor: A single cone type expresses both S and M opsins with retinal spatial patterning. *Neuron* 27:513–523.

Arikawa, K., Molday, L. L., Molday, R. S., and Williams, D. S. (1992). Localization of peripherin/rds in the disk membranes of cone and rod photoreceptors: Relationship to disk membrane morphogenesis and retinal degeneration. *J. Cell Biol.* 116:659–667.

Bessant, D. A., Payne, A. M., Mitton, K. P., Wang, Q. L., Swain, P. K., Plant, C., Bird, A. C., Zack, D. J., Swaroop, A., and Bhattacharya, S. S. (1999). A mutation in NRL is associated with autosomal dominant retinitis pigmentosa. *Nat. Genet.* 21:355–356.

Blanks, J. C., Hageman, G. S., Johnson, L. V., and Spee, C. (1988). Ultrastructural visualization of primate cone photoreceptor matrix sheaths. *J. Comp. Neurol.* 270:288–300.

Burns, M. E., and Baylor, D. A. (2001). Activation, deactivation, and adaptation in vertebrate photoreceptor cells. *Annu. Rev. Neurosci.* 24:779–805.

Calvert, P. D., Krasnoperova, N. V., Lyubarsky, A. L., Isayama, T., Nicolo, M., Kosaras, B., Wong, G., Gannon, K. S., Margolskee, R. F., et al. (2000). Phototransduction in transgenic mice after targeted deletion of the rod transducin alpha-subunit. *Proc. Natl. Acad. Sci. U.S.A.* 97:13913–13918.

Carter-Dawson, L. D., and LaVail, M. M. (1979). Rods and cones in the mouse retina. I. Structural analysis using light and electron microscopy. *J. Comp. Neurol.* 188:245–262.

Cheng, H., Khanna, H., Oh, E. C., Hicks, D., Mitton, K. P., and Swaroop, A. (2004). Photoreceptor-specific nuclear receptor NR2E3 functions as a transcriptional activator in rod photoreceptors. *Hum. Mol. Genet.* 13:1563–1575.

Corbo, J. C., and Cepko, C. L. (2005). A hybrid photoreceptor expressing both rod and cone genes in a mouse model of enhanced S-cone syndrome. *PLoS Genet.* 1:140–153.

Daniele, L., Adams, R., Durante, D., Pugh, E. N., Jr., and Philp, N. (2007). Novel distribution of junctional adhesion molecule-C in the neural retina and retinal pigment epithelium. *J. Comp. Neurol.* 506:166–176.

Daniele, L. L., Lillo, C., Lyubarsky, A. L., Nikonov, S. S., Philp, N., Mears, A. J., Swaroop, A., Williams, D. S., and Pugh, E. N., Jr. (2005). Cone-like morphological, molecular, and electrophysiological features of the photoreceptors of the *Nrl* knockout mouse. *Invest. Ophthalmol. Vis. Sci.* 46:2156–2167.

DeVries, S. H. (2000). Bipolar cells use kainate and AMPA receptors to filter visual information into separate channels. *Neuron* 28:847–856.

Dhingra, A., Lyubarsky, A., Jiang, M., Pugh, E. N., Jr., Birnbaumer, L., Sterling, P., and Vardi, N. (2000). The light response of ON bipolar neurons requires $G_{\alpha}o$. *J. Neurosci.* 20: 9053–9058.

Dong, C. J., Agey, P., and Hare, W. A. (2004). Origins of the electroretinogram oscillatory potentials in the rabbit retina. *Vis. Neurosci.* 21(4):533–543.

Ebnet, K., Suzuki, A., Ohno, S., and Vestweber, D. (2004). Junctional adhesion molecules (JAMs): More molecules with dual functions? *J. Cell Sci.* 117:19–29.

Ebrey, T., and Koutalos, Y. (2001). Vertebrate photoreceptors. *Prog. Retin. Eye Res.* 20:49–94.

Ekesten, B., Gouras, P., and Hargitai, J. (2002). Co-expression of murine opsins facilitates identifying the site of cone adaptation. *Vis. Neurosci.* 19:389–393.

Fei, Y., and Hughes, T. E. (2001). Transgenic expression of the jellyfish green fluorescent protein in the cone photoreceptors of the mouse. *Vis. Neurosci.* 18(4):615–623.

Ghosh, K. K., Bujan, S., Haverkamp, S., Feigenspan, A., and Wässle, H. (2004). Types of bipolar cells in the mouse retina. *J. Comp. Neurol.* 469:70–82.

Green, D. G. (1973). Scotopic and photopic components of the rat electroetinogram. *J. Physiol.* 228:781–797.

Gresh, J., Goletz, P. W., Crouch, R. K., and Rohrer, B. (2003). Structure-function analysis of rods and cones in juvenile, adult, and aged C57bl/6 and Balb/c mice. *Vis. Neurosci.* 20:211–220.

Hagins, W. A., Penn, R. D., and Yoshikami, S. (1970). Dark current and photocurrent in retinal rods. *Biophys. J.* 10:380–412.

Haverkamp, S., Ghosh, K. K., Hirano, A. A., and Wassle, H. (2003). Immunocytochemical description of five bipolar cell types of the mouse retina. *J. Comp. Neurol.* 455:463–476.

Haverkamp, S., Grunert, U., and Wassle, H. (2000). The cone pedicle, a complex synapse in the retina. *Neuron* 27:85–95.

Hetling, J. R., and Pepperberg, D. R. (1999). Sensitivity and kinetics of mouse rod flash responses determined in vivo from paired-flash electroretinograms. *J. Physiol.* 516(Pt. 2):593–609.

Hofer, H., Carroll, J., Neitz, J., Neitz, M., and Williams, D. R. (2005). Organization of the human trichromatic cone mosaic. *J. Neurosci.* 25:9669–9679.

Hood, D. C., Cideciyan, A. V., Roman, A. J., and Jacobson, S. G. (1995). Enhanced S cone syndrome: Evidence for an abnormally large number of S cones. *Vision Res.* 35:1473–1481.

Jacobs, G. H., Neitz, J., and Deegan, J. F. (1991). Retinal receptors in rodents maximally sensitive to ultraviolet light. *Nature* 353:655–656.

Jacobson, S. G., Marmor, M. F., Kemp, C. M., and Knighton, R. W. (1990). SWS (blue) cone hypersensitivity in a newly identified retinal degeneration. *Invest. Ophthalmol. Vis. Sci.* 31: 827–838.

Jeon, C. J., Strettoi, E., and Masland, R. H. (1998). The major cell populations of the mouse retina. *J. Neurosci.* 18:8936–8946.

Johnson, L. V., Hageman, G. S., and Blanks, J. C. (1986). Interphotoreceptor matrix domains ensheath vertebrate cone photoreceptor cells. *Invest. Ophthalmol. Vis. Sci.* 27:129–135.

Khanna, H., Akimoto, M., Siffroi-Fernandez, S., Friedman, J. S., Hicks, D., and Swaroop, A. (2006). Retinoic acid regulates the expression of photoreceptor transcription factor NRL. *J. Biol. Chem.* 281:27327–27334.

Lamb, T. D. (1995). Photoreceptor spectral sensitivities: Common shape in the long-wavelength region. *Vision Res.* 35(22):3083–3091.

Lamb, T. D., and Pugh, E. N., Jr. (1992). A quantitative account of the activation steps involved in phototransduction in amphibian photoreceptors. *J. Physiol.* 449:719–758.

Lyubarsky, A. L., Chen, C., Simon, M. I., and Pugh, E. N., Jr. (2000). Mice lacking G-protein receptor kinase 1 have profoundly slowed recovery of cone-driven retinal responses. *J. Neurosci.* 20:2209–2217.

Lyubarsky, A. L., Falsini, B., Pennesi, M. E., Valentini, P., and Pugh, E. N., Jr. (1999). UV- and midwave-sensitive cone-driven retinal responses of the mouse: A possible phenotype for coexpression of cone photopigments. *J. Neurosci.* 19:442–455.

Lyubarsky, A. L., Feathers, K. L., Teofilo, K., Williams, D. S., Swaroop, A., Pugh, E. N., Jr., and Thompson, D. A. (2006). Nrl knockout mice lacking Rpe65 do not synthesize 11-cis retinal. *Invest. Ophthalmol. Vis. Sci.* 47:2966.

Lyubarsky, A. L., Lem, J., Chen, J., Falsini, B., Iannaccone, A., and Pugh, E. N. (2002). Functionally rodless mice: Transgenic models for the investigation of cone function in retinal disease and therapy. *Vision Res.* 42:401–415.

Lyubarsky, A. L., Naarendorp, F., Zhang, X., Wensel, T., Simon, M. I., and Pugh, E. N., Jr. (2001). RGS9-1 is required for normal inactivation of mouse cone phototransduction. *Mol. Vis.* 7:71–78.

Lyubarsky, A. L., and Pugh, E. N., Jr. (1996). Recovery phase of the murine rod photoresponse reconstructed from electroretinographic recordings. *J. Neurosci.* 16:563–571.

Lyubarsky, A. L., and Pugh, E. N., Jr. (2004). From candelas to photoisomerizations in the mouse eye by rhodopsin bleaching in situ, and the light-dependence of the major components of the mouse ERG. *Vision Res.* 44:3235–3251.

Mahroo, O. A., and Lamb, T. D. (2004). Recovery of the human photopic electroretinogram after bleaching exposures: Estimation of pigment regeneration kinetics. *J. Physiol.* 554(Pt. 2):417–437.

Mears, A. J., Kondo, M., Swain, P. K., Takada, Y., Bush, R. A., Saunders, T. L., Sieving, P. A., and Swaroop, A. (2001). Nrl is required for rod photoreceptor development. *Nat. Genet.* 29:447–452.

Nathans, J., Thomas, D., and Hogness, D. S. (1986). Molecular genetics of human color vision: The genes encoding blue, green, and red pigments. *Science* 232:193–202.

Ng, L., Hurley, J. B., Dierks, B., Srinivas, M., Salto, C., Vennstrom, B., Reh, T. A., and Forrest, D. (2001). A thyroid hormone receptor that is required for the development of green cone photoreceptors. *Nat. Genet.* 27:94–98.

Nikonov, S. S., Daniele, L. L., Zhu, X. M., Craft, C. M., Swaroop, A., and Pugh, E. N. (2005). Photoreceptors of Nrl(−/−) mice coexpress functional S- and M-cone opsins having distinct inactivation mechanisms. *J. Gen. Physiol.* 125:287–304.

Nikonov, S. S., Kholodenko, R., Lem, J., and Pugh, E. N. (2006). Physiological features of the S- and M-cone photoreceptors of wild-type mice from single-cell recordings. *J. Gen. Physiol.* 127:359–374.

Oh, E. C., Khan, N., Novelli, E., Khanna, H., Strettoi, E., and Swaroop, A. (2007). Transformation of cone precursors to functional rod photoreceptors by bZIP transcription factor NRL. *Proc. Natl. Acad. Sci. U.S.A.* 104:1679–1684.

Pallikaris, A., Williams, D. R., and Hofer, H. (2003). The reflectance of single cones in the living human eye. *Invest. Ophthalmol. Vis. Sci.* 44:4580–4592.

Peachey, N. S., Goto, Y., Al-Ubaidi, M. R., and Naash, M. I. (1993). Properties of the mouse cone-mediated electroretinogram during light adaptation. *Neurosci. Lett.* 162:9–11.

Pugh, E. N., Jr., Falsini, B., and Lyubarksy, A. L. (1998). The origin of the major rod- and cone-driven components of the rodent electroretinogram and the effect of age and light-rearing history on the magnitude of these components. In T. P. Williams and A. B. Thistle (Eds.), *Photostasis and related phenomena* (pp. 93–128). New York: Plenum Press.

Pugh, E. N., Jr., and Lamb, T. D. (2000). Phototransduction in vertebrate rods and cones: Molecular mechanisms of amplification, recovery and light adaptation. In D. G. Stavenga, W. J. de Grip, and E. N. Pugh, Jr. (Eds.), *Molecular mechanisms in visual transduction* (pp. 183–255). New York: Elsevier.

Roberts, M. R., Srinivas, M., Forrest, D., de Escobar, G. M., and Reh, T. A. (2006). Making the gradient: Thyroid hormone regulates cone opsin expression in the developing mouse retina. *Proc. Natl. Acad. Sci. U.S.A.* 103:6218–6223.

Robson, J. G., and Frishman, L. J. (1995). Response linearity and kinetics of the cat retina: The bipolar cell component of the dark-adapted electroretinogram. *Vis. Neurosci.* 12:837–850.

Robson, J. G., and Frishman, L. J. (1998). Dissecting the dark-adapted electroretinogram. *Doc. Ophthalmol.* 95:187–215.

Rodieck, R. W. (1998). *The first steps in seeing.* Sunderland, MA: Sinauer Associates.

Roorda, A., and Williams, D. R. (1999). The arrangement of the three cone classes in the living human eye. *Nature* 397:520–522.

Sun, H., Macke, J. P., and Nathans, J. (1997). Mechanisms of spectral tuning in the mouse green cone pigment. *Proc. Natl. Acad. Sci. U.S.A.* 94:8860–8865.

Szel, A., Rohlich, P., Caffe, A. R., Juliusson, B., Aguirre, G., and Van, V. T. (1992). Unique topographic separation of two spectral classes of cones in the mouse retina. *J. Comp. Neurol.* 325:327–342.

Szel, A., Rohlich, P., Mieziewska, K., Aguirre, G., and Van, V. T. (1993). Spatial and temporal differences between the expression of short- and middle-wave sensitive cone pigments in the mouse retina: A developmental study. *J. Comp. Neurol.* 331:564–577.

Thomas, M. M., and Lamb, T. D. (1999). Light adaptation and dark adaptation of human rod photoreceptors measured from the a-wave of the electroretinogram. *J. Physiol.* 518(Pt. 2):479–496.

Wachtmeister, L. (1998). Oscillatory potentials in the retina: What do they reveal? *Prog. Retin. Eye Res.* 17:485–521.

Wang, M. M., Janz, R., Belizaire, R., Frishman, L. J., and Sherry, D. M. (2003). Differential distribution and developmental expression of synaptic vesicle protein 2 isoforms in the mouse retina. *J. Comp. Neurol.* 460:106–122.

Wässle, H. (2004). Parallel processing in the mammalian retina. *Nat. Rev. Neurosci.* 5:747–757.

Wright, A. F., Reddick, A. C., Schwartz, S. B., Ferguson, J. S., Aleman, T. S., Kellner, U., Jurklies, B., Schuster, A., Zrenner, E., et al. (2004). Mutation analysis of NR2E3 and NRL genes in enhanced S cone syndrome. *Hum. Mutat.* 24:439.

Yokoyama, R., and Yokoyama, S. (2000). Comparative molecular biology of visual pigments. In D. G. Stavenga, W. J. de Grip, and E. N. Pugh, Jr. (Eds.), *Molecular mechanisms in visual transduction* (pp. 257–296). New York: Elsevier.

Yokoyama, S. (1996). Molecular evolution of retinal and nonretinal opsins. *Genes Cells* 1:787–794.

Yokoyama, S., Radlwimmer, F. B., and Kawamura, S. (1998). Regeneration of ultraviolet pigments of vertebrates. *FEBS Lett.* 423:155–158.

Yoshida, S., Mears, A. J., Friedman, J. S., Carter, T., He, S., Oh, E., Jing, Y., Farjo, R., Fleury, G., et al. (2004). Expression profiling of the developing and mature Nrl−/− mouse retina: Identification of retinal disease candidates and transcriptional regulatory targets of Nrl. *Hum. Mol. Genet.* 13:1487–1503.

Zhang, X., Wensel, T. G., and Kraft, T. W. (2003). GTPase regulators and photoresponses in cones of the Eastern chipmunk. *J. Neurosci.* 23:1287–1297.

Zhu, X., Brown, B., Li, A., Mears, A. J., Swaroop, A., and Craft, C. M. (2003). GRK1-dependent phosphorylation of S and M opsins and their binding to cone arrestin during cone phototransduction in the mouse retina. *J. Neurosci.* 23:6152–6160.

11 Mosaic Architecture of the Mouse Retina

BENJAMIN E. REESE

The various classes of nerve cell in the retina are each distributed as orderly arrays across the retinal surface, permitting a uniform distribution of labor in processing the visual image despite global variations in cellular density. This regularity in somal distribution is widely presumed to increase the uniformity by which the processes of these cells sample the retinal surface. Many cell types exhibit a corresponding increase in the size of their dendritic fields as cell density declines with eccentricity, yielding a constant dendritic coverage across the retina. The nerve cells in these patterned arrays, or *mosaics*, extend their dendrites to sample from a layer of afferent innervation, establishing a dendritic morphology and degree of dendritic overlap that are unique to each cell type (Wässle and Riemann, 1978). Both of these features are associated with the functional contribution carried out by each array, defined by the synaptic connectivity established within the plexiform layers. These network properties of retinal mosaics, their somal patterning and dendritic coverage, are largely conserved across the vertebrate retina, and have recently been reviewed (Reese, 2007). This chapter reviews current understanding of how this mosaic architecture is produced during development, in which application the mouse retina has proved particularly enlightening.

The development of mosaic architecture

While seemingly unique to the problem of building a functional retina, the establishment of such regularity in a retinal mosaic reduces to a common if fundamental issue in the field of developmental biology, that of pattern formation (Meinhardt, 1982; Lawrence, 1992). Numerous studies have shown that the patterning present in such retinal mosaics may be accounted for by exclusively local interactions constraining proximity between neighboring like-type cells (Galli-Resta et al., 1999; Eglen et al., 2003a; Cameron and Carney, 2004; Eglen and Galli-Resta, 2006); no grand architectural plan or protomap is required to generate the patterning that is so commonplace among cell types in the vertebrate retina.

The implementation of a local spacing rule preventing proximity between two cells is an attractively simple means for generating patterning within a mosaic, but defining the biological embodiment of this spacing rule has not been straightforward. Three different types of mechanism have been proposed (figure 11.1), but direct evidence for any of them has been hard to come by. Such patterning has been ascribed to fate determination events occurring periodically across the retina, whereby, for instance, a newly fated cell may inhibit surrounding neighbors from acquiring the identical fate (McCabe et al., 1999; Cameron and Carney, 2004; Tyler et al., 2005). Alternatively, the patterning could be sculpted from an initially disordered and overproduced mosaic, followed by a process of naturally occurring cell death in which closely positioned cells may compete for limited trophic support, leading to one or the other being eliminated (Jeyarasasingam et al., 1998; Eglen and Willshaw, 2002). Finally, closely spaced cells may repel one another, dispersing tangentially on the retina to minimize proximity with immediate neighbors (Reese et al., 1999; Eglen et al., 2000). Although any of these three types of mechanism could in principle underlie the establishment of regularity in a mosaic, and although there is ample evidence for the lateral inhibition of cell fate, for naturally occurring cell death, and for tangential dispersion of retinal neuroblasts (for reviews, see Reese and Galli-Resta, 2002; Agathocleous and Harris, 2006; Linden and Reese, 2006), the evidence in support of any of them as the basis for the patterning observed in mature retinal mosaics is scant and usually indirect.

To generate direct evidence, one would ideally like to assay the patterning associated with the spatial locations within the plane of the retina at which cells of a given type had acquired their fate; or to compare the patterning before and after naturally occurring cell death in the absence of any tangential dispersion occurring within the intervening period; or to observe, in a live preparation, the change in the patterning of a population produced by tangentially dispersing neuroblasts. None of these more direct assessments has been achieved, but some limited conclusions can still be made for certain nerve cell classes.

With respect to dendritic coverage, different cell types would appear to implement one of two different strategies to achieve their characteristic degree of dendritic overlap, either regulating their dendritic growth in direct proportion to proximity with their homotypic neighbors or through the use of cell-intrinsic mechanisms, otherwise oblivious to local

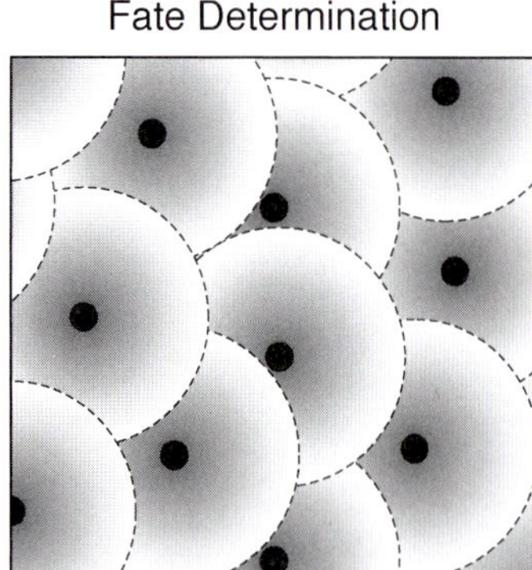

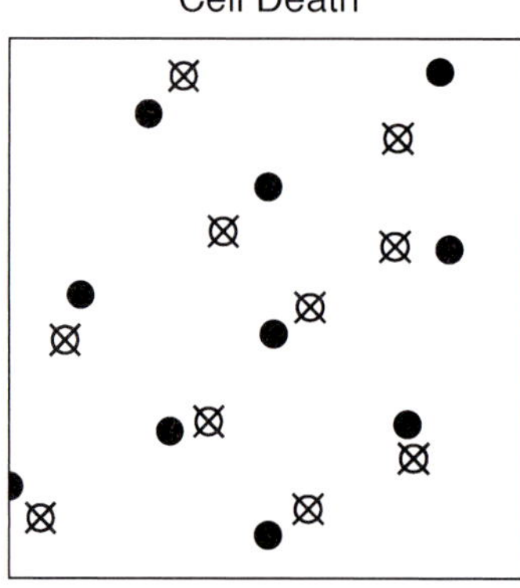

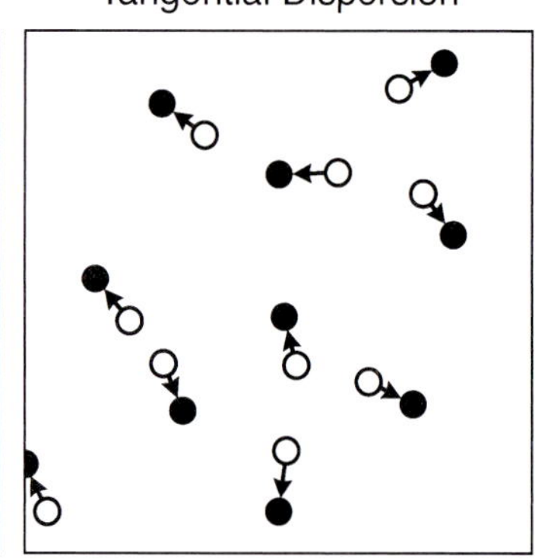

FIGURE 11.1 Three different hypothesized biological mechanisms underlying the local spacing rule that creates the patterning in retinal mosaics. *Left*, Fate determination events establish a minimal spacing between like-type cells, creating a template for the patterning found in the mature mosaic. *Center*, Cell death eliminates a subset of an initially overproduced population of neurons, preferentially killing those in close proximity. *Right*, Mutual repulsion between neighboring neurons propels them to disperse tangentially until they minimize proximity to like-type neighbors.

density, relying on the periodic distribution of somata to ensure a uniformity of coverage. In species where dendritic field extent and local cell density are inversely related (e.g., Wässle et al., 1978), it is not obvious which of these strategies is responsible, since a differential expansion of the retina that dilutes peripheral cell density as the eye grows may as well be responsible for a passive, or interstitial, elongation of the dendrites. Although experimental studies in fish and chick retina have attempted to analyze these competing accounts of the regulation of dendritic coverage among various types of retinal ganglion cell classes (Hitchcock and Easter, 1986; Hitchcock, 1989; Troilo et al., 1996), studies on the mouse retina have recently provided compelling evidence for or against particular types of cellular interactions playing a role in this process for a variety of retinal nerve cell classes. They have generally ruled out a third possible explanation, namely, that field extent depends on the afferent or target cells (Farajian et al., 2004; Lin et al., 2004; Reese et al., 2005).

This chapter focuses on three different types of retinal interneuron to consider the variation in mechanism responsible for the establishment of mosaic patterning and dendritic coverage. The discussion draws on recent studies that have all made use of the unique opportunities afforded by the mouse model, whether it is the natural variation that exists between different inbred strains, the induced variation that selective breeding strategies have allowed, the existence of mutations on those genetic backgrounds, or the genetic engineering of transgenic and knockout mice.

Horizontal cells

There is only one class of horizontal cell in the mouse retina, making it an attractive candidate for study for several reasons (Peichl et al., 1998). First, it is readily labeled with antibodies that do not label other cells at this depth within the retina, enabling the determination of its mosaic properties over large regions of retina (Raven and Reese, 2002). Second, it is an axon-bearing horizontal cell, permitting the ready labeling of dendritic or axonal arbors using tracers applied to the axon itself (Raven, Oh, et al., 2007). Third, it is sparsely distributed across the retina, accounting for less than 0.3% of all retinal neurons (Young, 1985), yet it extends processes to provide a coverage of the retinal surface well in excess of one (Reese et al., 2005). And fourth, the population of retinal horizontal cells exhibits a substantial variation between different strains of mice (Raven et al., 2005b), allowing analysis of the natural variation in mosaic regularity and dendritic coverage as a function of this variation in cellular density while in the absence of any differences in retinal growth. For example, the C57BL/6 and A strains of mice exhibit a nearly twofold difference in total horizontal cell number (C57BL/6J: 18,424 ± 279; A/J: 9835 ± 260, mean ± SE) while not differing in the size of their retinas.

If the patterning present in the horizontal cell mosaic were dependent on a local spacing rule of fixed distance, as has been shown for the photoreceptors in the ground squirrel's retina (Galli-Resta et al., 1999), different strains of mice might be expected to exhibit strain-specific spacing rules to maintain mosaic regularity at a comparable level between strains (figure 11.2, *top*). Alternatively, such a spacing rule might not vary between strains, so that variation in density would simply lead to a variation in the regularity of the mosaic, as exhibited in the ground squirrel's retina (Galli-Resta et al., 1999), and lower-density strains would show less efficient packing and less regularity than the higher-density strains (see figure 11.2, *bottom*). In fact, although a compari-

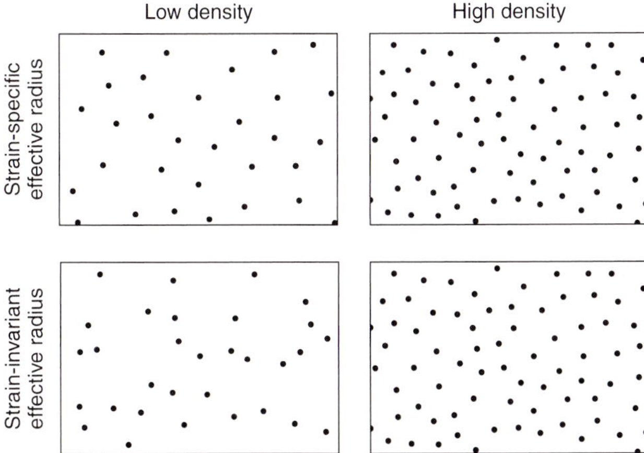

Figure 11.2 Different strains of mice (*left* and *right*) might exhibit different fixed spacing rules to achieve the same regularity despite variation in cell density (*top*). Alternatively, the identical fixed spacing rule may be employed in different strains, yielding lower-density strains with mosaics of lesser regularity (*bottom*).

son of horizontal cell mosaics between four different strains showed significant differences in average intercellular spacing, those strain differences were shown to be a by-product of the average difference in density; that is, the variation in density, even within individual strains, was shown to be a near perfect predictor of intercellular spacing, indicating the operation of a flexible rather than fixed spacing rule (Raven et al., 2005b). Horizontal cells appear to space themselves apart from one another, independent of genotype. If anything, mosaic regularity increases slightly with the decline in density, contrary to the prediction of a fixed spacing rule operating beneath maximally permissible packing.

How this flexible spacing rule is established during development is unclear. The number of horizontal cells is well below the number of clonal columns derived from single progenitors at the outset of neurogenesis (Williams and Goldowitz, 1992), but because the horizontal cells are one of the earliest generated retinal neurons (Sidman, 1961; Blanks and Bok, 1977; Hinds and Hinds, 1979), a lateral inhibitory mechanism could be envisioned to produce a local periodic distribution with a density that is subsequently diluted by clonal expansion (Reese et al., 1999). There is, however, no evidence bearing directly on the early patterning or spacing achieved immediately following the determination of the horizontal cell fate.

With respect to naturally occurring cell death, the horizontal cells stand out as being the best retinal exception to what had been regarded as a general rule, that nerve cell types are overproduced (Linden and Reese, 2006). There is no published evidence that horizontal cells undergo naturally occurring cell death (Young, 1984; Mayordomo, 2001), and no evidence that horizontal cell numbers are overproduced during normal development, at least postnatally (Raven et al., 2005a). Transgenic mice that overexpress the antiapoptotic gene *Bcl-2* have, however, been shown to exhibit 20% more horizontal cells, raising the possibility that there is some prenatal cell death that could in principle improve mosaic regularity from an initially less orderly mosaic. There is as well some indication that the neurotrophin nerve growth factor (NGF) signals through the tyrosine kinase A (trkA) receptor in the chick retina to maintain horizontal cell numbers during development (Karlsson et al., 1998).

Following birth, when all but the most peripherally situated horizontal cells have migrated to the future outer plexiform layer, after which no detectable horizontal cell loss occurs, in both the densest and sparsest populated retinas of these various strains, the regularity and packing efficiency of the horizontal cell mosaic increase significantly until postnatal day 5. Thereafter these indices of mosaic patterning remain largely unchanged into maturity (Raven et al., 2005a; see also Scheibe et al., 1995). During the period between birth and postnatal day 5, horizontal cells disperse tangentially for short distances within the retina, as evidenced through the use of X-inactivation transgenic mosaic mice to reveal clonal boundaries (Reese et al., 1999). Unlike with other means of identifying clonally related cells, in X-inactivation mosaic mice a known proportion of progenitor cells is labeled, permitting direct calculation of the proportion of dispersing cells among any cell class (Reese and Tan, 1998). For the horizontal cells, virtually all must engage in this tangential dispersion (Reese et al., 1999). Because this dispersion can only change the positioning of horizontal cell neuroblasts relative to their sites of birth and determination, and relative to any spatial relationships that were established by hypothesized cell death occurring prenatally, this dispersion must change the spatial patterning established by those other mechanisms. Since its occurrence coincides with an increase in regularity and packing, a relationship between the two would be implicated: tangential dispersion increases the patterning already present at birth (Raven et al., 2005a).

The difference in mosaic regularity or packing between the mosaic of horizontal cells on the day of birth and random (density-matched and soma-constrained) distributions is still significant, indicating that something else contributes to the patterning before birth. It could be that some degree of naturally occurring cell death leads to the patterning present at birth; it may be that fate determination events set a coarse grain to the mosaic that is subsequently refined by tangential dispersion; or it may be that tangential dispersion of horizontal cells also occurs between the time of fate determination and postnatal day 1, when the dispersing horizontal cells may be situated within the amacrine cell layer, masquerading as dispersed amacrine cells that are already present on the day of birth, before they translocate back to the future horizontal cell layer (Reese et al., 1999; Edqvist and Hallbook, 2004).

The final patterning of the horizontal cell mosaic is also independent of the afferents: transgenic mice carrying an attenuated diphtheria toxin gene under the control of a human L cone regulatory sequence lose nearly all of their cones prior to synaptogenesis with the horizontal cells (Soucy et al., 1998). Despite this loss of cone afferents, mosaic regularity shows no change relative to that seen in control littermates (Raven and Reese, 2003). These results are consistent with the finding that the patterning within retinal mosaics is largely independent of the patterning present in other mosaics, regardless of whether those mosaics are synaptic partners (Rockhill et al., 2000).

Like their intercellular spacing, the dendritic outgrowth of horizontal cells is related to local horizontal cell density (figure 11.3); higher-density strains have smaller dendritic fields than do lower-density strains, and the degree of dendritic growth appears to be modulated precisely to maintain dendritic overlap as a constant, being about six (Reese et al., 2005). This would suggest that the extent of dendritic growth is controlled by homotypic interactions between neighboring horizontal cells rather than by any cell-intrinsic program determining dendritic field size. Of course, each strain could have allelic variants of genes that drive dendritic growth. To discriminate between these possibilities, a *Lim1* mosaic-conditional knockout mouse has been used to modulate the density of horizontal cells. Lim1 is a transcription factor that is expressed exclusively within horizontal cells during development and plays a critical role in specifying their migratory endpoint: horizontal cells lacking Lim1 become mispositioned in the amacrine cell layer and stratify in the inner plexiform layer (Poché et al., 2007). Those remaining Lim1-positive horizontal cells, settling in their normal stratum and arborizing normally within the outer plexiform layer, show a nearly twofold increase in dendritic field area when the local density in this stratum is reduced by about 50% (Poché et al., in press), demonstrating that their field size is clearly dependent on homotypic interactions. This effect on the overall size of the dendritic field is to be contrasted with the patterning of the dendritic field, which is controlled primarily by afferent rather than homotypic interactions (Raven, Oh, et al., 2007).

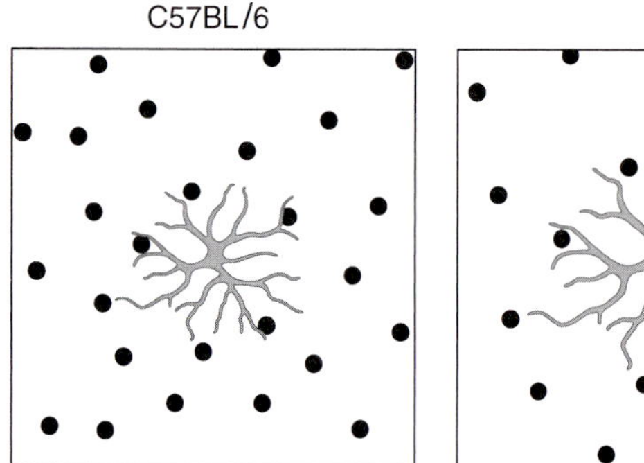

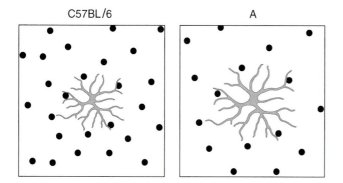

FIGURE 11.3 Horizontal cell spacing and dendritic field growth are each regulated by local horizontal cell density. Horizontal cells in the mouse retina are positioned to minimize proximity with neighboring horizontal cells. Mouse strains with lower average densities of horizontal cells (e.g., the A strain, *right*) extend their dendritic fields farther than those with higher average densities (e.g., C57BL/6, *left*) to maintain a constant dendritic coverage of roughly six cells.

Cholinergic amacrine cells

The cholinergic amacrine cells in the mouse retina are distributed to two strata within the ganglion cell and inner nuclear layers, extending their characteristic starburst dendritic arbors into an inner and an outer stratum within the inner plexiform layer, as in other mammalian retinas. The two populations are spatially independent of one another (Galli-Resta et al., 1997, 2002), as in all other species examined (Diggle, 1986; Rockhill et al., 2000). They have densities comparable to the population of horizontal cells, but unlike the horizontal cells, they extend their dendritic arbors far more extensively, yielding a dendritic overlap of about 30 (Farajian et al., 2004).

The mosaics of cholinergic amacrine cells, when compared with the horizontal cells (Raven et al., 2005b), are never as regularly distributed yet are still more regular than simulated random distributions (Whitney et al., 2008). Like the horizontal cell mosaics, the cholinergic mosaics show a decline in average intercellular spacing as density increases, although this relationship is perturbed for the mosaic in the ganglion cell layer (Whitney et al., 2008). Tangential dispersion of cholinergic amacrine cells is, as for the horizontal cells, nearly universal (Reese et al., 1999), and the intercellular spacing of cholinergic amacrine cells may be constrained solely by soma diameter prior to these cells settling within their mosaic layers, at least in the developing rat's retina (Galli-Resta et al., 1997). Although the presence of such immediate near-neighbor pairings during radial migration suggests these cells must move apart from one another as they arrive in the mosaic layer, this population of cells is also modulated by naturally occurring cell death (Galli-Resta and Novelli, 2000), with roughly 20% being overproduced. This naturally occurring cell death can be prevented by blocking ATP signaling via P2X receptors, and these denser mosaics contain more frequent near-neighbor pairings, but their regularity and packing have not yet been adequately described (Resta et al., 2005). Yet a comparison of mosaic regularity before and after naturally occurring cell death does not reveal any increase in regularity for this cell type at the latter time point, suggesting that cell death does not appreciably modulate the patterning associated with this population (Galli-Resta and Novelli, 2000). The presence of such closer near-neighbor pairings during the radial migratory phase of cholinergic amacrine cells (Galli-Resta et al., 1997) also suggests that the spacing present within the mosaic layers is not a passive consequence of a spacing established at the time of fate determination. But their presence is by no means an unambiguous demonstration that the patterning present at the time of fate determination or during migration is entirely random. For this cell class, there is currently no good estimate of the extent to which fate determination events contribute to the patterning achieved in maturity.

There is, however, additional evidence that neighboring cholinergic amacrine cells can modulate their intercellular spacing conspicuously during early postnatal development. Disruption of microtubule stability within the processes of cholinergic (and also horizontal) cells immediately after birth leads to a dramatic, and transient, redistribution of their somata within the mosaic layers (Galli-Resta et al., 2002). These results, in conjunction with the independent evidence for naturally occurring tangential dispersion, support the notion that neighboring cholinergic amacrine cells space themselves apart within the plane of the mosaic, mediated by some form of homotypic interaction via the dendrites. The interaction is unrelated to synaptic associations with retinal ganglion cells, since experimental or genetic manipulations that eliminate or double the latter population have no effect on the patterning of cholinergic cells (Galli-Resta, 2000). One result inconsistent with that former study is the finding that excitotoxic ablation of roughly 40% of the cholinergic amacrine cells on postnatal day 3 has no effect on the positioning of remaining cholinergic amacrine cells (Farajian et al., 2004), although it remains a possibility that this age is too late to alter the cell-cell interactions governing relative positioning.

The processes of cholinergic amacrine cells overlap one another extensively, generating dendritic coverage factors that range from 20 to 70, depending on the species. That same latter study demonstrated that the excitotoxic ablation of 40% of the cholinergic amacrine cells did not appear to harm those cells that survived into maturity; those cells went on to differentiate a normal starburst morphology, growing their dendritic fields sevenfold thereafter, well in excess of the extent of overall retinal growth. Interestingly, the fields achieved by those surviving cholinergic amacrine cells were virtually indistinguishable from those in the control condition, including their overall dendritic field area (Farajian et al., 2004). That is, cholinergic amacrine cells would appear to grow their dendrites to establish a dendritic field extent that is independent of the density of either the cholinergic somata or their processes (figure 11.4). These conclusions are supported by other results comparing the density and field area of cholinergic amacrine cells in the C57BL/6 and A strains of mice: despite there being 25% fewer cholinergic amacrine cells in the ganglion cell layer in the A strain, dendritic field size is no different (Keeley et al., 2008). The cholinergic amacrine cells would appear to operate a cell-intrinsic growth strategy, defining a field of a particular size rather than titrating growth precisely to yield a constant degree of dendritic overlap.

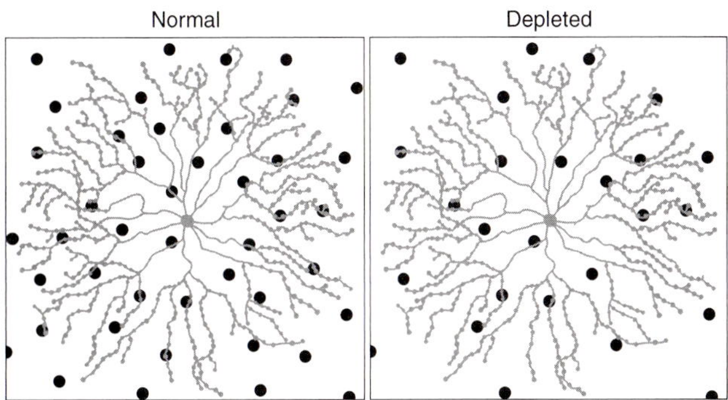

Figure 11.4 Cholinergic amacrine cells extend their dendritic fields to achieve a degree of dendritic overlap on the order of 30 (*left*). Early partial depletion of the mosaic, before appreciable dendritic growth has taken place, does not alter the subsequent dendritic growth of remaining cells (*right*).

Similar conclusions have recently been drawn for the dendritic growth of two types of retinal ganglion cells using *Brn3b* and *Math5* knockout mice, cells that normally establish a degree of dendritic coverage closer to one but which do not appear to modulate their dendritic growth in the absence of normal neighbor relationships (Lin et al., 2004). That result would appear to contradict the evidence that experimental manipulations altering neighbor relations in turn alter dendritic growth among ganglion cells (Perry and Linden, 1982; Eysel et al., 1985; Kirby and Chalupa, 1986; Leventhal et al., 1988). Although this discrepancy may simply indicate an intrinsic upper limit on the size of the dendritic field that can still be biased or restricted by neighbor relationships, it may alternatively indicate that different ganglion cell classes define their dendritic growth via intrinsic constraints versus extrinsic cellular interactions.

Dopaminergic amacrine cells

The dopaminergic amacrine cells are one of the sparsest classes of neuron found in the retina, accounting for less than one-hundredth of a percent of the total complement of retinal neurons (Versaux-Botteri et al., 1984). In the mouse retina, they are all situated in the inner nuclear layer immediately adjacent to the inner plexiform layer, unlike in some other species, where a sizable proportion is positioned in the ganglion cell layer (Peichl, 1991; Eglen et al., 2003b). Remarkably, their minuscule number is tightly regulated, so that there is minimal variation in the total number present in mice from the same strain (Masland et al., 1993), yet different strains of mice reveal a nearly fourfold variation in the size of this population (Raven, Whitney, et al., 2007). For example, the A strain contains 276 ± 9.5 dopaminergic amacrine cells, whereas the ALR strain contains 962 ± 11.9 cells. Indeed, an analysis of 25 recombinant inbred strains of mice (the AxB/BxA strain set) derived from the A and C57BL/6 strains (strains showing a twofold difference in dopaminergic amacrine cell number) indicates a putative locus for the control of dopaminergic amacrine cell number on chromosome 7 (Raven, Whitney, et al., 2007). These cells give rise to sparse and frequently asymmetric dendritic fields, plus extensive if also sparse axonal processes that may spread for millimeters within the plexiform layers, primarily within the substratum of the inner plexiform layer immediately adjacent to the inner nuclear layer (Versaux-Botteri et al., 1984; Oyster et al., 1985; Savy et al., 1989; Dacey, 1990; Zhang et al., 2004).

The somal patterning of the dopaminergic amacrine cells is close to that expected for a random distribution in nearly all species examined. The issue has been most thoroughly examined in the retina of the mouse, where the distribution of somata is found to be nonrandom using a variety of indices, although not much more regular than random (Raven et al., 2003). Modeling studies showed that a fixed spacing rule was effective at simulating a limited sample of four different fields of dopaminergic amacrine cells, although multiple spacing rules were found to be effective for some of those same sampled fields. In short, the distribution of dopaminergic amacrine cells loosely abides by a rule that reduces the frequency of pairings closer than 100 μm relative to what would be expected for a random distribution of cells at comparable density. Although such a spacing rule is large relative to those observed for most other cell types, this distance is still meager relative to the density of dopaminergic amacrine cells, the latter being far below the maximal packing limit for spheres of this size (Raven et al., 2003). The low-density mosaics generated by such a fixed spacing rule are, consequently, hardly regular.

The mechanism underlying this spacing rule is unlikely to be related to tangential dispersion, since minimal numbers of dopaminergic amacrine cells exhibit any dispersion from their clonal columns (Reese et al., 1999), rarely greater than a distance comparable to soma diameter (Raven et al., 2003). In the fish retina, the patterning of the dopaminergic amacrine cells is readily simulated by a lateral inhibitory fate determination model (Cameron and Carney, 2004), and additional observations in the fish retina are inconsistent with either dispersion or cell death accounts (Tyler et al., 2005). In the mouse, however, the *Bcl-2*-overexpressing transgenic retina has been particularly informative, for this cell type shows a nearly 10-fold increase in total number (Strettoi and Volpini, 2002), where their distribution is indiscriminable from random simulations matched in density and constrained by soma size (Raven et al., 2003). Unlike the wild-type (C57BL/6) retina, where side-by-side dopaminergic amacrine cell pairings are never detected, their frequency in the *Bcl-2*-overexpressing retina is exactly to be predicted from random distributions matched for density.

The transgene is driven by a neuron-specific enolase promoter that should ensure that the construct is expressed only after neuroblasts have undergone their final mitosis and begun differentiating. Accordingly, these results have been interpreted to indicate a role for this antiapoptotic gene in regulating dopaminergic amacrine cell survival (Strettoi and Volpini, 2002), although there exists no independent evidence that dopaminergic amacrine cells undergo naturally occurring cell death (Linden and Reese, 2006). These results are, however, consistent with other studies showing a role for BDNF-trkB receptor signaling in the control of dopaminergic amacrine cell number (Cellerino et al., 1998). These results, then, suggest that dopaminergic amacrine cells are normally overproduced and that the determinants of survival or death are at least partially influenced by proximity to other dopaminergic amacrine cells, perhaps through a competition for trophic factors provided by targets or other neighboring cells. Of course, if proximity were the sole rule for reducing this population by approximately 90%, far more regular mosaics could be sculpted from random distributions of cells with this degree of cell loss (Eglen and Willshaw, 2002). Clearly, other factors must play a role in the decision to survive or die within this population of cells.

The results from these *Bcl-2*-overexpressing mice would imply that there are no constraints on the production of dopaminergic amacrine cells residing immediately next to one another. Unless lateral inhibitory or other fate-determining mechanisms are somehow altered in these transgenic retinas, these results are perhaps the strongest available for ruling out any role for fate-determining events in creating the minimal distance spacing rule responsible for the patterning present in the dopaminergic amacrine cell mosaic, modest as that patterning may be for this cell type.

Little is known about the control of process outgrowth for the dopaminergic amacrine cells. In the rat retina, the dendritic fields are conspicuously asymmetric, and there may be a tendency for closer neighboring cells to extend their dendrites away from one another (Savy et al., 1989), suggesting that their growth is controlled by homotypic interactions. Given the nearly fourfold variation in dopaminergic amacrine cell number across different strains of mouse (Raven,

Whitney, et al., 2007), it would be interesting to see whether dendritic field growth scaled accordingly, as it does for the horizontal cells. But because this cell type plays a neuromodulatory role rather than a role in image-forming processes, one might predict no change in field size between the strains but rather a modulation in the release or reception of this neurotransmitter within the retina.

Outstanding issues

The studies just reviewed have implicated the differentiating processes as being the means by which horizontal and cholinergic amacrine cells may space themselves out during development, but exactly how they do so has yet to be determined. Do these cells define local domains as they first begin differentiating, when they have barely an overlap of one, shifting their somal position toward the center of this domain (Cook and Chalupa, 2000)? Might these cells establish contacts with homotypic neighbors that mediate tensile forces across the network, leading to uniform spacing (Galli-Resta, 2002)? Or are the somata truly repelled by the presence of close neighbors, engaging in active cellular migration (Reese et al., 1995)? Furthermore, what is the relationship between the interactions governing positioning and those governing constraints on dendritic overlap, for the horizontal cells? A simple contact inhibition at the tips of growing dendrites would be sufficient for establishing a dendritic coverage of one (and may be all that is required to trigger tangential dispersion), but mouse horizontal cells ultimately generate a coverage of around six. This degree of coverage approximates dendritic growth extending to neighboring somata, suggesting that the processes of each horizontal cell are inhibited from further growth on contacting those cell bodies. Given these differences in generating coverages of one versus six, one can envision symmetric versus asymmetric interactions that might mediate such contact-mediated events, but these arenas are largely unexplored for the moment (but see Tanabe et al., 2006).

The dopaminergic amacrine cell mosaic is itself puzzling, for even if it is sculpted from an initially denser mosaic, it is difficult to envision how fate determination mechanisms initially generate such a random distribution of overproduced neurons at such low density. Even more remarkable is the consistency with which developmental mechanisms yield a final number that is so reliably established among members of the same strain. Although dopaminergic amacrine cell number may depend on trophic relationships governed by the size of other populations, including the retinal ganglion cells, for which there is good evidence for allelic variants modulating neuronal number (Williams et al., 1998), it remains puzzling how such a dependency could produce precision in cellular number in the absence of any precision in cellular patterning.

Conclusion

Much of our understanding of the organizing principles of retinal mosaics had been established in other mammalian species long before the mouse came into vogue as a model for studying the retina and visual system. The use of the mouse as a model system has benefited our understanding of the development of this mosaic architecture, its coverage, and its connectivity, although so far implementation of the mouse model has largely clarified the role of cellular interactions in these processes rather than any details of the molecular mechanisms governing those interactions. Researchers may be well positioned to move in this direction as increasing numbers of genetically modified mouse resources become available. Other species traditionally associated with the field of experimental embryology (e.g., chick, frog, fish), permitting as they do the ready transfection or transplantation of progenitors to alter gene expression in known lineages of cells in order to dissect the cell-autonomous and environmental signaling controlling these interactions, have been the models of choice for addressing events that occur in utero in the mouse retina, but novel genetically engineered mice and experimental approaches are quickly overcoming such limitations (e.g., Badea et al., 2003; Matsuda and Cepko, 2007). To the extent that the processes involved in building the mosaic architecture of the retina prove to be related to more general processes associated with retinal growth, which in mammals does not proceed by an annular accumulation of cells characteristic of other vertebrates, the use of those other species may have only limited potential for understanding these systems features of the mammalian retina, further driving the application of new approaches for genetic manipulation within the developing mouse retina.

ACKNOWLEDGMENT Supported by grant no. EY-11087 from the National Institutes of Health.

REFERENCES

Agathocleous, M., and Harris, W. A. (2006). Cell determination. In E. Sernagor, S. Eglen, B. Harris, and R. Wong (Eds.), *Retinal development* (pp. 75–98). Cambridge: Cambridge University Press.

Badea, T. C., Wang, Y., and Nathans, J. (2003). A noninvasive genetic/pharmacologic strategy for visualizing cell morphology and clonal relationships in the mouse. *J. Neurosci.* 23:2314–2322.

Blanks, J. C., and Bok, D. (1977). An autoradiographic analysis of postnatal cell proliferation in the normal and degenerative mouse retina. *J. Comp. Neurol.* 174:317–328.

Cameron, D. A., and Carney, L. H. (2004). Cellular patterns in the inner retina of adult zebrafish: Quantitative analyses and a computational model of their formation. *J. Comp. Neurol.* 471:11–25.

Cellerino, A., Pinzon-Duarte, G., Carroll, P., and Kohler, K. (1998). Brain-derived neurotrophic factor modulates the

development of the dopaminergic network in the rodent retina. *J. Neurosci.* 18:3351–3362.
Cook J. E., and Chalupa, L. M. (2000). Retinal mosaics: New insights into an old concept. *Trends Neurosci.* 23:26–34.
Dacey, D. M. (1990). The dopaminergic amacrine cell. *J. Comp. Neurol.* 301:461–489.
Diggle, P. J. (1986). Displaced amacrine cells in the retina of a rabbit: Analysis of a bivariate spatial point pattern. *J. Neurosci. Meth.* 18:115–125.
Edqvist, P. H., and Hallbook, F. (2004). Newborn horizontal cells migrate bi-directionally across the neuroepithelium during retinal development. *Development* 131:1343–1351.
Eglen, S. J., and Galli-Resta, L. (2006). Retinal mosaics. In E. Sernagor, S. Eglen, B. Harris, and R. Wong (Eds.), *Retinal development* (pp. 193–207). Cambridge: Cambridge University Press.
Eglen, S. J., Galli-Resta, L., and Reese, B. E. (2003a). Theoretical models of retinal mosaic formation. In A. van Ooyen (Ed.), *Modelling neural development* (pp. 133–150). Cambridge, MA: MIT Press.
Eglen, S. J., Raven, M. A., Tamrazian, E., and Reese, B. E. (2003b). Dopaminergic amacrine cells in the inner nuclear layer and ganglion cell layer comprise a single functional retinal mosaic. *J. Comp. Neurol.* 466:343–355.
Eglen, S. J., van Ooyen, A., and Willshaw, D. J. (2000). Lateral cell movement driven by dendritic interactions is sufficient to form retinal mosaics. *Network Comput. Neural Syst.* 11: 103–118.
Eglen, S. J., and Willshaw, D. J. (2002). Influence of cell fate mechanisms upon retinal mosaic formation: A modelling study. *Development* 129:5399–5408.
Eysel, U. T., Peichl, L., and Wässle, H. (1985). Dendritic plasticity in the early postnatal feline retina: Quantitative characteristics and sensitive period. *J. Comp. Neurol.* 242:134–145.
Fadool, J. M., and Dowling, J. E. (2006). Zebrafish models of retinal development and disease. In E. Sernagor, S. Eglen, B. Harris, and R. Wong (Eds.), *Retinal development* (pp. 342–370). Cambridge: Cambridge University Press.
Farajian, R., Raven, M. A., Cusato, K., and Reese, B. E. (2004). Cellular positioning and dendritic field size of cholinergic amacrine cells are impervious to early ablation of neighboring cells in the mouse retina. *Vis. Neurosci.* 21:13–22.
Galli-Resta, L. (2000). Local, possibly contact-mediated signalling restricted to homotypic neurons controls the regular spacing of cells within the cholinergic arrays in the developing rodent retina. *Development* 127:1509–1516.
Galli-Resta, L. (2002). Putting neurons in the right places: Local interactions in the genesis of retinal architecture. *Trends Neurosci.* 25:638–643.
Galli-Resta L, and Novelli, E. (2000). The effects of natural cell loss on the regularity of the retinal cholinergic arrays. *J. Neurosci.* 20:61–65 (RC60).
Galli-Resta, L., Novelli, E., Kryger, Z., Jacobs, G. H., and Reese, B. E. (1999). Modelling the mosaic organization of rod and cone photoreceptors with a minimal-spacing rule. *Eur. J. Neurosci.* 11:1461–1469.
Galli-Resta, L., Novelli, E., and Viegi, A. (2002). Dynamic microtubule-dependent interactions position homotypic neurones in regular monolayered arrays during retinal development. *Development* 129:3803–3814.
Galli-Resta, L., Resta, G., Tan, S.-S., and Reese, B. E. (1997). Mosaics of islet-1 expressing amacrine cells assembled by short range cellular interactions. *J. Neurosci.* 17:7831–7838.
Hinds, J. W., and Hinds, P. L. (1979). Differentiation of photoreceptors and horizontal cells in the embryonic mouse retina: An electron microscopic, serial section analysis. *J. Comp. Neurol.* 187:495–512.
Hitchcock, P. F. (1989). Exclusionary dendritic interactions in the retina of the goldfish. *Development* 106:589–598.
Hitchcock, P. F., and Easter, S. S. (1986). Retinal ganglion cells in goldfish: A qualitative classification into four morphological types, and a quantitative study of the development of one of them. *J. Neurosci.* 6:1037–1050.
Jeyarasasingam, G., Snider, C. J., Ratto, G.-M., and Chalupa, L. M. (1998). Activity-regulated cell death contributes to the formation of ON and OFF alpha ganglion cell mosaics. *J. Comp. Neurol.* 394:335–343.
Karlsson, M., Clary, D.O., Lefcort, F. B., Reichardt, L. F., Karten, H. J., and Hallböök, F. (1998). Nerve growth factor receptor trkA is expressed by horizontal and amacrine cells during chicken retinal development. *J. Comp. Neurol.* 400:408–416.
Keeley, P. W., Whitney, I. E., Raven, M. A., and Reese, B. E. (2008). Dendritic spread and functional coverage of starburst amacrine cells. *J. Comp. Neurol.* 505:539–546.
Kirby, M. A., and Chalupa, L. M. (1986). Retinal crowding alters the morphology of alpha ganglion cells. *J. Comp. Neurol.* 251: 532–541.
Lawrence, P. A. (1992). *The making of a fly: The genetics of animal design.* Oxford: Blackwell.
Leventhal, A. G., Schall, J. D., and Ault, S. J. (1988). Extrinsic determinants of retinal ganglion cell structure in the cat. *J. Neurosci.* 8:2028–2038.
Lin, B., Wang, S. W., and Masland, R. H. (2004). Retinal ganglion cell type, size, and spacing can be specified independent of homotypic dendritic contacts. *Neuron* 43:475–485.
Linden, R., and Reese, B. E. (2006). Programmed cell death. In E. Sernagor, S. Eglen, B. Harris, and R. Wong (Eds.), *Retinal development* (pp. 208–241). Cambridge: Cambridge University Press.
Masland, R. H., Rizzo, J. F., and Sandell, J. H. (1993). Developmental variation in the structure of the retina. *J. Neurosci.* 13:5194–5202.
Matsuda, T., and Cepko, C. L. (2007). Controlled expression of transgenes introduced by in vivo electroporation. *Proc. Natl. Acad. Sci. U.S.A.* 104:1027–1032.
Mayordomo, R. (2001). Differentiated horizontal cells seem not to be affected by apoptosis during development of the chick retina. *Int. J. Dev. Biol.* 45:S79-S80.
McCabe, K. L., Gunther, E. C., and Reh, T. A. (1999). The development of the pattern of retinal ganglion cells in the chick retina: Mechanisms that control differentiation. *Development* 126:5713–5724.
Meinhardt, H. (1982). *Models of biological pattern formation.* London: Academic Press.
Oyster, C. W., Takahashi, E. S., Cillufo, M., and Brecha, N. (1985). Morphology and distribution of tyrosine hydroxylase-like immunoreactive neurons in the cat retina. *Proc. Natl. Acad. Sci. U.S.A.* 82:6445–6339.
Peichl, L. (1991). Catecholaminergic amacrine cells in the dog and wolf retina. *Vis. Neurosci.* 7:575–587.
Peichl, L., Sandmann, D., and Boycott, B. B. (1998). Comparative anatomy and function of mammalian horizontal cells. In L. M. Chalupa and B. L. Finlay (Eds.), *Development and organization of the retina.* New York: Plenum Press.
Perry, V. H., and Linden, R. (1982). Evidence for dendritic competition in the developing retina. *Nature* 297:683–685.

Poché, R. A., Kwan, K. M., Raven, M. A., Furuta, Y., Reese, B. E., and Behringer, R. R. (2007). Lim1 is essential for the correct laminar positioning of retinal horizontal cells. *J. Neurosci.* 27:14099–14107.

Poché, R. A., Raven, M. A., Kwan, K. M., Furuta, Y., Behringer, R. R., and Reese, B. E. (in press). Somal positioning and dendritic growth of horizontal cells are regulated by interactions with homotypic neighbors. *Europ. J. Neurosci.*

Raven, M. A., Eglen, S. J., Ohab, J. J., and Reese, B. E. (2003). Determinants of the exclusion zone in dopaminergic amacrine cell mosaics. *J. Comp. Neurol.* 461:123–136.

Raven, M. A., Oh, E. C. T., Swaroop, A., and Reese, B. E. (2007). Afferent control of horizontal cell morphology revealed by genetic respecification of rods and cones. *J. Neurosci.* 27:3540–3547.

Raven, M. A., and Reese, B. E. (2002). Horizontal cell density and mosaic regularity in pigmented and albino mouse retina. *J. Comp. Neurol.* 454:168–176.

Raven, M. A., and Reese, B. E. (2003). Mosaic regularity of horizontal cells in the mouse retina is independent of cone photoreceptor innervation. *Invest. Ophthalmol. Vis. Sci.* 44:965–973.

Raven, M. A., Stagg, S. B., Nassar, H., and Reese, B. E. (2005a). Developmental improvement in the regularity and packing of mouse horizontal cells: Implications for mechanisms underlying mosaic pattern formation. *Vis. Neurosci.* 22:569–573.

Raven, M. A., Stagg, S. B., and Reese, B. E. (2005b). Regularity and packing of the horizontal cell mosaic in different strains of mice. *Vis. Neurosci.* 22:461–468.

Raven, M. A., Whitney, I., Williams, R. W., and Reese, B. E. (2007). Regulation of dopaminergic amacrine cell number in the mouse retina. *ARVO Abs.* 48:5688.

Reese, B. E. (2007). Mosaics, tiling and coverage by retinal neurons. In A. Kaneko and R. H. Masland (Eds.), *Handbook of the senses: Vision*. Oxford: Elsevier.

Reese, B. E., and Galli-Resta, L. (2002). The role of tangential dispersion in retinal mosaic formation. *Prog. Ret. Eye Res.* 21:153–168.

Reese, B. E., Harvey, A. R., and Tan, S.-S. (1995). Radial and tangential dispersion patterns in the mouse retina are cell-class specific. *Proc. Natl. Acad. Sci. U.S.A.* 92:2494–2498.

Reese, B. E., Necessary, B. D., Tam, P. P. L., Faulkner-Jones, B., and Tan, S.-S. (1999). Clonal expansion and cell dispersion in the developing mouse retina. *Eur. J. Neurosci.* 11:2965–2978.

Reese, B. E., Raven, M. A., and Stagg, S. B. (2005). Afferents and homotypic neighbors regulate horizontal cell morphology, connectivity and retinal coverage. *J. Neurosci.* 25:2167–2175.

Reese, B. E., and Tan, S.-S. (1998). Clonal boundary analysis in the developing retina using X-inactivation transgenic mosaic mice. *Semin. Cell Dev. Biol.* 9:285–292.

Resta, V., Novelli, E., Di Virgilio, F., and Galli-Resta, L. (2005). Neuronal death induced by endogenous extracellular ATP in retinal cholinergic neuron density control. *Development* 132:2873–2882.

Rockhill, R. L., Euler, T., and Masland, R. H. (2000). Spatial order within but not between types of retinal neurons. *Proc. Natl. Acad. Sci. U.S.A.* 97:2303–2307.

Savy, C., Yelnik, J., Martin-Martinelli, E., Karpouzas, I., and Nguyen-Legros, J. (1989). Distribution and spatial geometry of dopamine interplexiform cells in the rat retina: I. Developing retina. *J. Comp. Neurol.* 289:99–110.

Scheibe, R., Schnitzer, J., Rohrenbeck, J., Wohlrab, F., and Reichenbach, A. (1995). Development of A-type (axonless) horizontal cells in the rabbit retina. *J. Comp. Neurol.* 354:438–458.

Sidman, R. L. (1961). Histogenesis of mouse retina studied with thymidine-H^3. In G. Smelser (Ed.), *The structure of the eye* (pp. 487–505). New York: Academic Press.

Soucy, E., Wang, Y., Nirenberg, S., Nathans, J., and Meister, M. (1998). A novel signaling pathway from rod photoreceptors to ganglion cells in mammalian retina. *Neuron* 21:481–493.

Strettoi, E., and Volpini, M. (2002). Retinal organization in the *bcl-2*-overexpressing transgenic mouse. *J. Comp. Neurol.* 446:1–10.

Tanabe, K., Takahashi, Y., Sato, Y., Kawakami, K., Takeichi, M., and Nakagawa, S. (2006). Cadherin is required for dendritic morphogenesis and synaptic terminal organization of retinal horizontal cells. *Development* 133:4085–4096.

Troilo, D., Xiong, M., Crowley, J. C., and Finlay, B. L. (1996). Factors controlling the dendritic arborization of retinal ganglion cells. *Vis. Neurosci.* 13:721–733.

Tyler, M. J., Carney, L. H., and Cameron, D. A. (2005). Control of cellular pattern formation in the vertebrate inner retina by homotypic regulation of cell-fate decisions. *J. Neurosci.* 25:4565–4576.

Versaux-Botteri, C., Nguyen-Legros, J., Vigny, A., and Raoux, N. (1984). Morphology, density and distribution of tyrosine hydroxylase-like immunoreactive cells in the retina of mice. *Brain Res.* 301:192–197.

Wässle, H., Peichl, L., and Boycott, B. B. (1978). Topography of horizontal cells in the retina of the domestic cat. *Proc. R. Soc. Lond. B. Biol. Sci.* 203:269–291.

Wässle, H., and Riemann, H. J. (1978). The mosaic of nerve cells in the mammalian retina. *Proc. R. Soc. Lond. B.* 200:441–461.

Whitney, I. E., Keeley, P. W., Raven, M. A., and Reese, B. E. (2008). Spatial patterning of cholinergic amacrine cells in the mouse retina. *J. Comp. Neurol.* 508:1–12.

Williams, R. W., and Goldowitz, D. (1992). Structure of clonal and polyclonal cell arrays in chimeric mouse retina. *Proc. Natl. Acad. Sci. U.S.A.* 89:1184–1188.

Williams, R. W., Strom, R. C., and Goldowitz, D. (1998). Natural variation in neuron number in mice is linked to a major quantitative trait locus on Chr 11. *J. Neurosci.* 18:138–146.

Young, R. W. (1984). Cell death during differentiation of the retina in the mouse. *J. Comp. Neurol.* 229:362–373.

Young, R. W. (1985). Cell differentiation in the retina of the mouse. *Anat. Rec.* 212:199–205.

Zhang, D. Q., Stone, J. F., Zhou, T., Ohta, H., and McMahon, D. G. (2004). Characterization of genetically labeled catecholamine neurons in the mouse retina. *Neuroreport* 15:1761–1765.

12 Synaptic Organization of the Mouse Retina

ENRICA STRETTOI

The fundamental plan of the mouse retina follows the blueprint common to all mammalians: rods largely predominate, as they represent 97% of the photoreceptor population (Carter-Dawson and LaVail, 1979; Jeon et al., 1998). In the common C57Bl6/J strain of mouse, there are approximately 6.4 million rods and 180,000 cones (figure 12.1). The first are presynaptic to a single type of bipolar cell, the rod bipolar cell; each cone, instead, is connected to a cohort of different cone bipolar cells, all together forming parallel, vertical channels across the retina and variably connecting to ganglion cells. Additional, mixed rod-cone pathways also exist. The signal is modulated in the outer retina by a single type of horizontal cell and, in the inner retina, by more than 20 different types of amacrine cells that are reciprocally connected to bipolar cells and are presynaptic to ganglion cell dendrites. Ganglion cells also occur in a variety of types and with different functional features.

The work of many laboratories and the use of state-of-the art neuroanatomical techniques have led to recognition of the cellular complexity of the retina, and the mouse visual system has been the object of many studies in recent years (because of the use of this species for transgenic and knockout experiments). Nevertheless, many functional issues remain unresolved. Yet the concept of a retinal fundamental circuit, constituted by a discrete number of neuronal types (about 50) and repeated across the retinal surface, with no single cell type playing a dominant role, is applicable to the retina of all mammals, including the mouse (Masland, 2001).

A quantitative analysis of the mouse inner nuclear layer (INL) demonstrated that its cells have a dome-shaped distribution, slightly more peaked than that of the photoreceptors, with a maximum density around 300 µm from the optic nerve head. The topography of cells in the ganglion cell layer is more peaked still, with a density relatively higher in the nasal quadrant of the retina (Jeon et al., 1998). All three distributions in the mouse, though, are flatter than those found in rat, rabbit, cat, or monkey (Hughes, 1975; Mitrofanis et al., 1988; Martin and Grünert, 1992; Strettoi and Masland, 1995); thus, the mouse retina is more homogeneous across its surface than is the retina of other mammals.

The relative fractions of various cell types in the INL is known: bipolar cells make up 41% of all cells in the layer, amacrines 39%, Müller cells 16%, and horizontal cells 3% (Jeon et al., 1998). Thus, although it is generally assumed that the retinas of lower mammals are more rich in amacrine cells, these numbers demonstrate that the bipolar-to-amacrine ratio is close to one in the retina of the mouse, exactly like that of the rabbit and very close to that of the monkey. Actually, the retina of higher mammals, such as macaque monkeys and humans, is made more complex by the presence of the fovea, with a dedicated circuit of midget neurons that is completely absent from the rodent retina. However, the fovea represents only 1% of all the retinal surface; hence, the fundamental plan of the retina is highly conserved among mammals.

The relative proportion of rod versus cone bipolar cells in the mouse retina has also been estimated. In the C57Bl6/J mouse, rod bipolar cells number approximately 208,000, while cone bipolar cells are twice as numerous (Strettoi and Volpini, 2002). This confirms another general rule of retinal architecture, in that even in a strongly rod-dominated retina (and rodents are among the mammals with the highest rod:cone ratio), cone bipolar cells outnumber rod bipolar cells (Strettoi and Masland, 1995). This is partly due to the fact that each cone diverges on several cone bipolar cells of different types, whereas multiple rods converge on individual rod bipolars, thus increasing the sensitivity of the scotopic pathway.

With the main features of the mouse retina now summarized, this chapter briefly reviews the architecture of the rod pathways and that of cone pathways to ganglion cells.

The rod pathway

Mice have classic rod bipolar cells. These well-known neurons have ovoid cell bodies (around 10 µm in diameter), usually located in the outer half of the INL, and bushy dendritic arborizations. The axons are thin and straight, while the axon terminals are large, each composed of three to five bulblike varicosities that reach the deepest part of sublamina b of the inner plexiform layer (IPL). Typically, rod bipolar cells can be stained with antibodies against the alpha isoform

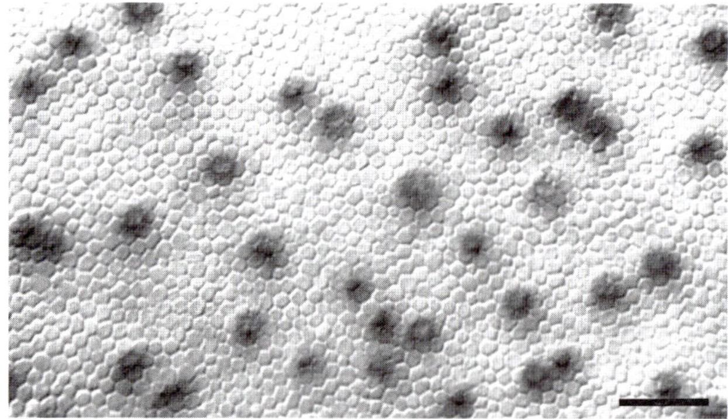

FIGURE 12.1 Light micrograph obtained with differential interference contrast illustrating the mosaic of rods and cones in the mouse retina. The matrix surrounding the cones has been stained with peanut lectins and appears dark. Cones make up only 3% of all the photoreceptors in the mouse retina. (From Jeon et al., 1998.)

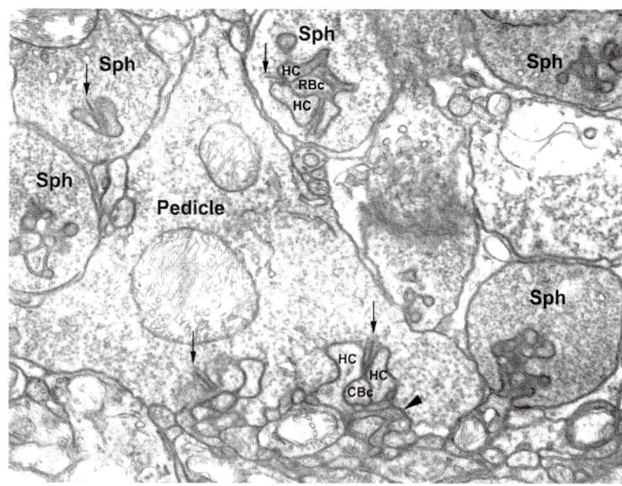

FIGURE 12.2 Electron micrograph of the mouse outer plexiform layer. A single cone pedicle of typical conical shape is surrounded by several rod spherules (Sph), each carrying one synaptic ribbon (*arrows*). Cone pedicles establish multiple ribbon synapses with cone bipolar (CBc) and horizontal cell dendrites (HC), as well as flat contacts (*arrowhead*) with cone bipolar cells. Spherules establish ribbon contacts with rod bipolar cells (RBc) and with axonal processes of horizontal cells (HC).

of protein kinase C, which allows their study as a population (Haverkamp and Wässle, 2000).

Electron microscopy of the outer plexiform layer (OPL) shows typical ribbon contacts between rod spherules and rod bipolar cell apical dendrites; these form the central elements of triads, while processes originating from the axonal arborizations of horizontal cells form the lateral processes (figure 12.2). Because rod spherules are small and densely packed, histological sections cut at a perfect right angle with respect to the retinal surface are not easy to obtain. This reason, along with the fact that each spherule makes connections to only one (rarely, two) triplet of processes (see figure 12.2), explains why typical triads can be observed in only a fraction of all the spherules encountered in conventional ultrathin sections. Most commonly, only one or two dendrites are visible, facing the ribbon of each spherule. Ribbon contacts are termed invaginated and represent the only kind of synapse established by rod spherules. At the postsynaptic site of the invagination, rod bipolar dendrites carry a retinal-specific type of metabotropic glutamate receptor, mGluR6 (Ueda et al., 1997). By means of mGluR6, the hyperpolarizing light response of rods is transformed into a graded depolarization of postsynaptic rod bipolar cells. Hence, invaginating synapses are called sign-inverting. On binding to mGluR6, glutamate released onto retinal ON bipolar neurons activates a heterotrimeric G protein, G_o, that ultimately closes a nonspecific cation channel (Dhingra et al., 2002). In particular, the light response of ON bipolar cells requires the strongly expressed splice variant of the G protein known as $G_{\alpha o1}$. The pathway ultimately leading from glutamate binding to mGluR6 to the final change in membrane potential in ON bipolar cells is still somewhat obscure, although recent studies suggest the existence of multiple transduction mechanisms (Huang et al., 2003).

Rod bipolar cells have circular receptive fields (RFs) and depolarize in response to light stimuli; hence, as in all mammals, they belong to the functional type of ON-center neurons. The average width of their RF is approximately 70 µm (Berntson and Taylor, 2000), slightly larger than the dendritic diameter. This suggests there is not extensive signal spread in the OPL through gap junction connections between the terminals of the photoreceptors. It also shows that each rod bipolar cell receives contacts from all the rods within reach (around 22; Tsukamoto et al., 2001). In addition, each rod terminal establishes gap junctions with processes (telodendria) originating from cone pedicles.

Mice have typical AII amacrine cells. These neurons were first described almost 30 years ago in the retina of the cat (Kolb, 1979) and are considered a hallmark of the mammalian retinal architecture. They are narrow-field cells with a distinctive bistratified morphology (figure 12.3). Their somata, localized to the innermost part of the INL, bulge into the IPL, giving rise to one or more sturdy primary dendrites from which large varicosities (1–4 µm in diameter) termed lobular appendages branch in sublamina a. Several thinner, bushy dendrites ramify further down in the IPL in sublamina b; these dendrites are thin and long and cover a diameter of 8–12 µm.

Electron microscopy of serial sections has shown that rod bipolar cells' axonal endings express ribbon synapses directed mostly at the AII amacrine cell's innermost dendritic branches. In turn, each AII cell sends conventional chemical synapses at the axon terminals of OFF cone bipolar cells (see figure 12.4) by means of the lobular appendages

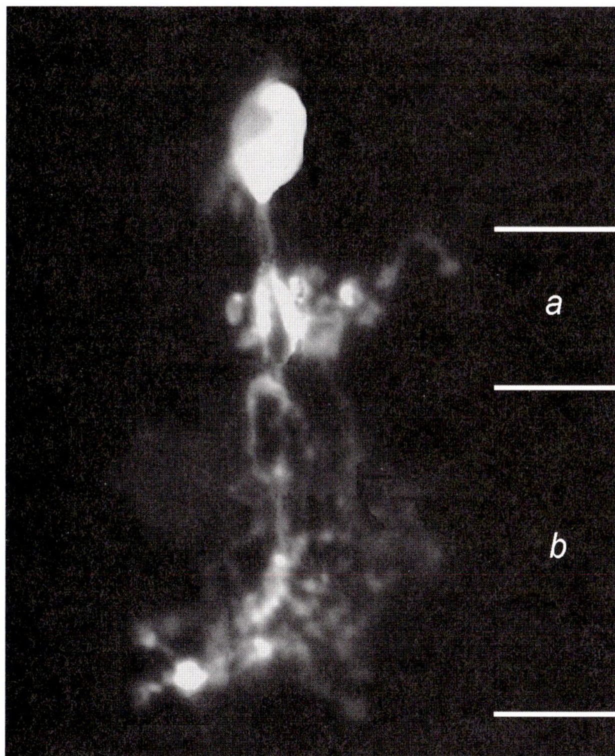

FIGURE 12.3 A typical AII amacrine cell of the mouse retina, stained with DiI, loaded on tungsten bullets and delivered with a gene gun. The sublaminae a and b of the IPL are indicated. The cell has a characteristic bistratified morphology.

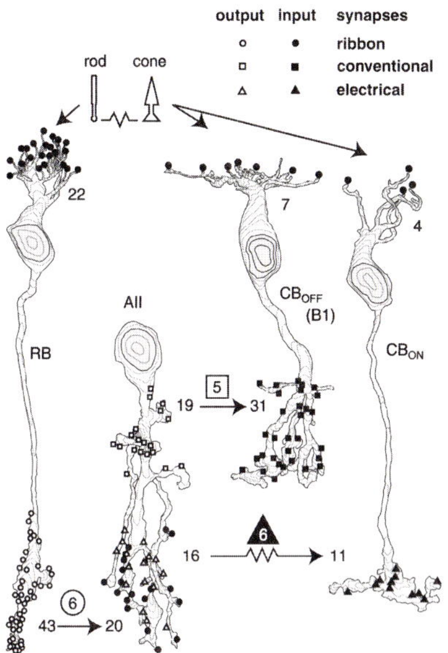

FIGURE 12.4 The rod pathway of the mouse retina reconstructed from electron micrographs of serial sections. Each rod diverges to one to two rod bipolar cells (RB); in turn, 22 rods converge onto one rod bipolar cell. The rod bipolar cell provides 43 ribbon synapses to AII amacrine cells. One AII amacrine cell forms 16 gap junctions with ON cone bipolar terminals (CB_{ON}) and 19 conventional synapses with the OFF cone bipolar terminals (CB_{OFF}). Numbers in a *circle*, *square*, and *triangle* represent the number of input or output synapses between a given pair of adjacent cells. (From Tsukamoto et al., 2001.)

(Tsukamoto et al., 2001). In addition, AII form large gap junctions with axon terminals of ON cone bipolar cells (figure 12.4).

Thus, as in all mammals, in the mouse retina too AII amacrine cells are the main postsynaptic target of rod bipolar cells (Strettoi et al., 1992).

Each rod bipolar axonal ending expresses approximately 40 ribbon synapses by which it contacts several AII amacrine cells. The AII cell, collecting from several rod bipolar cells, expresses many gap junctions and diverges onto several ON bipolar terminals. The AII cell also expresses many conventional synapses by which it diverges to several OFF bipolar terminals of homogeneous type. Finally, AII amacrines are electrically coupled through small gap junctions occurring among their dendrites in sublamina b (see figure 12.4).

Therefore, as in the cat, rabbit, rat, and monkey retina, the rod-generated signal is fed into the ON and OFF pathway through AII amacrine cells that establish sign-conserving electrical connections with the axonal endings of ON cone bipolar cells while forming sign-inverting, glycinergic synapses with OFF cone bipolars. Because neither rod bipolars nor AII amacrines form direct connections to ganglion cell dendrites, the largest part of the scotopic signal reaches ganglion cells through cone bipolar cells. In fact, the final transfer to the retinal exit occurs through sign-conserving ribbon synapses established between ON and OFF cone bipolar axonal endings and corresponding sets of ganglion cell dendrites in the ON and OFF laminae of the IPL. These synapses use glutamate as a neurotransmitter. The particular array by which rod signals exploit cone bipolar cells to gain access to ganglion cell is known as a piggyback arrangement.

AII amacrine cells can be stained selectively with antibodies against the cytoplasmic protein disabled-1 (Rice and Curran, 2000) and thus studied as a single population. There are approximately 49,000 AII amacrine cells in the retina of the C57Bl6/J mouse; their density shows a peak in the central retina. As in the rabbit, and probably as in all mammals, they constitute the largest population of amacrine cells, of which they represent around 12%.

The cell body and primary dendrite of each AII amacrines are surrounded by a ring of amacrine cell varicosities containing dopamine as well as γ-aminobutyric acid (Contini and Raviola, 2003). Dopaminergic rings are one of the sites of output of wide-field dopaminergic amacrine cells, which ramify in a narrow stratum at the INL/IPL border and also send processes to the OPL (they are also called interplexiform cells); these neurons can be visualized clearly with antibodies against tyrosine hydroxylase. There are fewer than 500 dopaminergic amacrine cells in the mouse retina;

however, their long, ramified processes cover the retina uniformly. From studies carried out in various mammals, it is known that dopaminergic amacrines receive input primarily from other amacrine cells and, to a lesser degree, from cone bipolar cells (Dowling and Ehinger, 1978; Hokoc and Mariani, 1988; Kolb et al., 1990). They are believed to modulate the light adaptation state of the retina by providing lateral inhibitory signals to AII amacrine cells. They spontaneously generate action potentials in a rhythmic fashion, and their molecular determinants have been studied in great detail by means of transgenic technology (Raviola, 2002).

In general, dopamine is a powerful modulator of gap junction permeability and a regulator of retinal sensitivity to light. Hence, dopamine is capable of influencing many components of the retinal circuitry. A well-known action is control of the conductance of gap junctions occurring between horizontal cells and between amacrine cells. In addiction, this transmitter increases the responses of ionotropic glutamate receptors on bipolar cells, and ultimately influences the center-surround balance of ganglion cells. Part of the dopamine action is exerted nonsynaptically, through a form of extrasynaptic, paracrine release. Various dopamine-dependent functions result in increased signal flow through cone circuits and a diminution in signal flow through rod circuits (Witkovsky, 2004). Variations in dopamine release are also responsible for the modulation of homologous electrical coupling between AII amacrine cells, as well as between AII amacrine cells and ON cone bipolar cells, in different conditions of illumination (Bloomfield et al., 1997). In total dark adaptation, the average size of the AII-AII network matches the size of AII cell ON-center RFs. However, as light increases, AII cells form much larger networks, comprising more than 300 amacrine cells, with a corresponding increase in RF size.

Additional rod pathways

Besides the standard mammalian circuit for night vision, two additional pathways exist that route rod-generated information to ganglion cells.

As mentioned earlier, cone pedicles have processes, called telodendria, that extend laterally in the OPL and are engaged in small gap junctions with neighboring photoreceptors (rods and cones) (Raviola and Gilula, 1975). Electrophysiological recordings have long shown that mammalian cones carry rod signals (Nelson, 1977). These appear as a slow hyperpolarization following the initial response to a brief flash of light. Through this additional pathway, rod signals can utilize the fast-tuned cone pathways to access the inner retina.

Recent recordings from mouse ganglion cells suggest a direct pathway from rods to cone bipolar cells (Soucy et al., 1998). In a mouse retina genetically modified to be "coneless," a fast rod signal was detected in OFF ganglion cells, suggesting the existence of direct connections between rods and OFF cone bipolar cells.

Confocal and electron microscopy have demonstrated the existence of symmetrical contacts involving rod spherules and the dendrites of OFF cone bipolar cells, which therefore collect direct input from rods (Hack et al., 1999; Tsukamoto et al., 2001). The dendrites of such cone bipolar cells express ionotropic glutamate receptors at the site of apposition to rod spherules. Hence, rod-generated signals can exit the retina through gap junctions between rods and cones, as well as through this third pathway using mixed cone-rod bipolar cells. Apparently, only 20% of all the rods are involved in this particular type of connection with OFF cone bipolar cells. However, it has been proposed that rod-generated signals can enter this pathway through rod-rod gap junctions, which are infrequent in most mammals but apparently common in the mouse retina (Tsukamoto et al., 2001).

It must be noted that, although the alternative rod pathway was first discovered in rodents, anatomical evidence for direct connections between rods and OFF cone bipolar cells has now been provided for the rabbit as well (Li et al., 2004). However, electrophysiological and pharmacological experiments have shown that, in the mouse retina, only a low proportion of OFF signals are carried in parallel to rod bipolar cells, and no ganglion cells at all in the rat retina display OFF responses attributable to direct contacts between rods and OFF cone bipolar cells (Protti et al., 2005). This observation suggests that the alternative rod pathway may be a common feature of the mammalian retina but that its relative importance and significance differ between species.

A multidisciplinary approach has demonstrated that all three rod pathways are functional in the mouse retina but operate under stimulus intensity ranges that are widely different, so that the primary rod pathway carries signals with the lowest threshold, whereas the secondary rod pathway (based on rod-cone gap junctions) is approximately 1 logarithmic unit less sensitive (Völgyi et al., 2004). Some ganglion cells receive signals preferentially from one pathway, while others exhibit convergent signals.

It is worth noting that all three rod pathways, the standard route and the two indirect ones, ultimately exploit cone bipolar axonal endings to gain access to ganglion cells. Thus, although in the beginning the neural network strictly associated with rods (composed of rods, rod bipolar cells, and AII amacrine cells) is quite minimal, ultimately the whole retinal machinery is shared by both the scotopic and the photopic pathways.

I am fond of the idea that the general use of the piggyback arrangement might be justified in evolutionary terms: cone-mediated vision and color vision evolved in parallel and before dim light vision (Bowmaker, 1998). Hence, the ancestral inner retina was shaped by cones. Insofar as each cone brings in several types of cone bipolar cells with various functional properties, it is tempting to speculate that the antique vertebrate retina was constituted by several types of cone bipolar cells and cone-driven amacrine cells that diversely made connections to ganglion cells. Later in evolution rhodopsin appeared, and the ancestors of modern rods emerged. The preexisting retinal network, with the already achieved computational capabilities, was made available to the newly evolved photoreceptors tout court and without undesirable duplication: rod bipolar cells (of a single type) ensured high convergence (and thus high sensitivity) of rods in the scotopic pathway; AII amacrines, which received the bulk of rod bipolar synapses, recruited the cone pathways, connecting to ON and OFF cone bipolar cells in the IPL. Among other advantages, the piggyback architecture ensures access of the scotopic signal to parallel processing, which originally evolved in the cone system.

The notion that rod and cone pathways are not only exquisitely balanced but also deeply integrated is reinforced by, among other things, the identification of secondary effects caused by various forms of inherited photoreceptor degeneration (such as retinitis pigmentosa) on neurons of the inner retina. In this family of diseases, even though the primary genetic defect occurs in rods, which die first, cones undergo secondary degeneration. Inner retinal cells, and particularly rod bipolar cells, horizontal cells, and cone bipolar cells, display abnormal morphologies and eventually die out, while gliosis and general atrophy are observed. Such a complex chain of events, called remodeling (Jones et al., 2003; Marc et al., 2003; Gargini et al., 2007), strongly suggests that maintaining a normal morphology, as well as the long-term survival of second-order neurons, requires the presence of viable photoreceptors. This brings to light the existence of (possibly trophic) interactions normally occurring between the outer and the inner retina and acting in parallel to the synaptic-related communication.

Horizontal cells

Cell bodies of horizontal cells form the outermost tier of the INL; their processes connect within the borders of the OPL. Each horizontal cell is postsynaptic to a large cohort of photoreceptors and has the important task of averaging their signals, feeding them back onto photoreceptor synaptic terminals, and at the same time feeding them forward onto the dendrites of bipolar cells. Horizontal cells are connected to each other by large gap junctions that provide electrical coupling. The strength of the coupling varies with the retinal adaptation to light and is modulated by, among other substances, dopamine released by amacrine cells. Horizontal cells therefore play a key role in the mechanism of neural adaptation, because through their feedback they adjust cone sensitivity and shape the RFs of bipolar and ganglion cells.

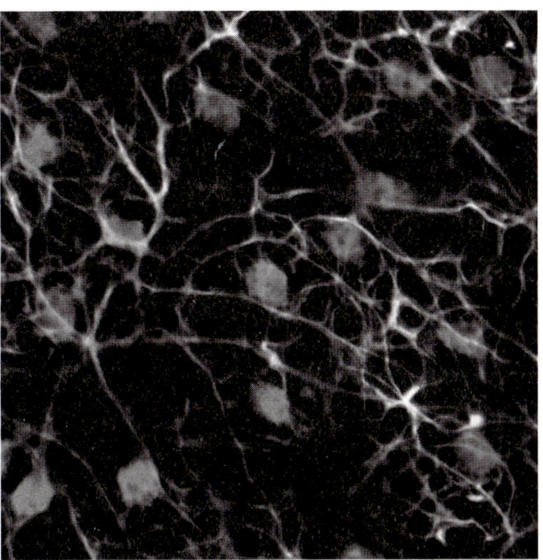

FIGURE 12.5 Confocal image of a whole mount mouse retina in which horizontal cells are revealed with antibodies against calbindin D (red signal), while their axonal complexes are labeled with antineurofilament antibodies (green staining). See color plate 4.

Although most vertebrates have at least two types of horizontal cells, rodents (and thus mice) are a noticeable exception in that they carry only a single variety (Peichl and Gonzalez-Soriano, 1994), the one with a long, thin axon that ramifies into an elaborate and rich axonal arborization. Although dendritic branches emerging from the cell somata are postsynaptic to cones, axonal arborizations connect to rod spherules exclusively. Electrophysiology has shown that cone input from the dendrites does not reach the axonal arborization, connected to rods (Suzuky and Pinto, 1986). Therefore, a single soma provides metabolic support to two sets of processes with completely different connections and virtually isolated. In the mouse retina, the whole plexus of horizontal cells can be stained by antibodies against the calcium-binding protein calbindin D. Antibodies against the heavy subunit of neurofilament proteins instead reveal only horizontal cell axonal arborizations (figure 12.5). There are approximately 18,000 horizontal cells in the retina of the C57Bl6/J mouse.

Cone pathways to ganglion cells

Retinal parallel processing begins at the first synapse between photoreceptors and different types of bipolar cells. These carry glutamate receptors of heterogeneous molecular composition that thereby give rise to a variety of parallel channels that run vertically across the retina (Wässle, 2004).

Cones respond to light stimuli with a graded hyperpolarization and release glutamate at multiple synaptic sites endowed in each pedicle. Glutamate release is higher in the dark and is reduced by light shed onto cones. Unlike rod spherules, which only make connections to the terminal process of one horizontal cell and to one to two dendrites of rod bipolar cells, each cone pedicle has numerous postsynaptic partners (see figure 12.2). As in all vertebrates, two types of bipolar cell contacts are typically found: flat (or basal) contacts and invaginating (or ribbon) contacts (Dowling and Boycott, 1966). The dendritic tips of invaginating bipolar cells are flanked by two lateral horizontal cell dendrites in the typical triad configuration, much like that described earlier for rod spherules. The dendritic terminals of flat bipolar cells make numerous contacts at the pedicle membrane facing the OPL (see figure 12.2). Basal contacts mediate sign-conserving synapses with cone bipolar cells, which therefore respond to light with graded hyperpolarizations (OFF cone bipolar cells); ribbon contacts, instead, mediate sign-inverting synapses with another group of cone bipolar cells that respond to light with graded depolarizations (ON cone bipolar cells). The molecular basis for the functional effects of these synaptic contacts is well known: cone bipolar cells establishing flat contacts carry ionotropic glutamate receptors on their dendritic tips, whereas those engaged in invaginating contacts instead mainly express mGluR6, exactly like rod bipolar cells. According to a general rule in retinal architecture that has no known exceptions, OFF bipolar cells have axonal endings that ramify in the outer third of the IPL, sublamina a; conversely, cone bipolar cells that respond to light with a depolarization end in the deepest part of the IPL, or sublamina b. The ON-OFF dichotomy, established at the first synaptic station in the retina, is maintained throughout the visual system.

Traditionally, the stratification and morphology of the axonal arborizations of bipolar cells have been used as main distinguishing criteria, more than the shape of their dendritic arbors or the size of the soma. Unfortunately, the molecular determinants of cone bipolar cells are very similar, and it is difficult to make a distinction among them using cell-type-specific antibodies, a method that has been largely used to visualize retinal neurons. Hence, population studies of types of cone bipolar cells are rare for the mouse retina. Antibodies against the neurokinin receptor 3 label a large population of OFF cone bipolar cells whose axonal arbors span the whole thickness of sublamina a. These cells number approximately 90,000 per retina in the C57Bl6/J mouse (Pignatelli and Strettoi, 2004), but it is not easy to tell whether they form a homogeneous or a mixed population. In addition, a subset of them can be stained with recoverin antibodies (Haverkamp and Wässle, 2000), but the intensity of the staining and the number of stained cells vary in degenerating retinas, making it difficult to assign a functional meaning to the immunolabeling. It is clear that at least a fraction of them coincide with the type called CBb1 by Tsukamoto et al. (2001), which receives multiple contacts from the lobular appendages of AII amacrine cells in the sublamina OFF of the IPL (see figure 12.4).

A transgenic mouse line (357) has been created that expresses GFP in all members of a single type of ON cone bipolar cell and coincides with that termed CB4a by Pignatelli and Strettoi (2004) and with type 7 of Ghosh et al. (2004). One type of monostratified ON ganglion cell and the inner dendrites of one bistratified ganglion cell tightly cofasciculate with axon terminals of the line 357 bipolar cells and are likely to receive synaptic input from them (Lin and Masland, 2005).

Superimposed on the ON/OFF dichotomy are four types of OFF and five types of ON cone bipolar cells (figure 12.6). We are just beginning to understand their distinguishing features and their functional roles (Euler and Wässle, 1995; Hartveit, 1997; Euler and Masland, 2000; Berntson and Taylor, 2000; Freed, 2000). For instance, different types of ON cone bipolar cells express at least two different connexins at their gap junctions with AII amacrine cells (Han and Massey, 2005; Lin et al., 2005). It is not unlikely that two types of gap junction have distinctive physiological or regulatory properties (Mills and Massey, 2000), optimized to meet the functions of particular subsets of cone bipolar cells. Hence, the visual signal could be differently processed by types of ON cone bipolar cells expressing different electric junctions.

Some of the bipolar cells select certain types of cones, such as the blue cone bipolar cells, and thus transfer a chromatic signal into the IPL. In the mouse, the type labeled 9 in the

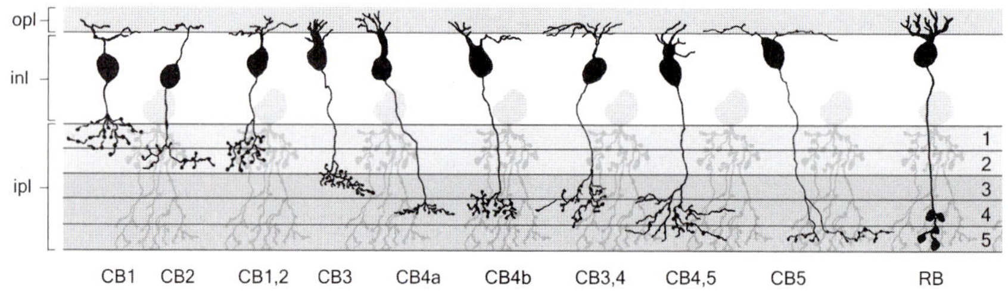

Figure 12.6 The various types of bipolar cells of the mouse retina, classified after labeling with fluorescent dyes delivered with a gene gun. AII amacrine cells are represented in light gray in the background. Nine types of cone bipolar cells (CB) and one type of rod bipolar cell (RB) have been identified. (From Pignatelli and Strettoi, 2004.) A classification produced by Ghosh et al. at the same time and based on intracellular injection is consistent with the types illustrated here.

classification of Ghosh et al. (2004) and CB5 in the classification of Pignatelli and Strettoi (2004) has sparsely branching and wide dendrites in the OPL; the axonal arborization is narrow and unistratified in the innermost tier of the IPL (see figure 12.6). This ON cell is strongly reminiscent of the blue cone bipolar cell described in other species (Boycott and Wässle, 1991; Euler and Wässle, 1995). Recently, blue cone bipolar cells have been labeled in a transgenic mouse expressing clomeleon, a chloride-sensitive fluorescent protein under the control of the Thy1 promoter. It was shown that blue cone bipolar cells constitute only 1%–2% of the bipolar cell population, and their dendrites selectively contact cones that express short-wavelength opsin (S cones) (Haverkamp et al., 2005).

Unlike the blue ON cone bipolar, most bipolar cells contact all the cones, usually five to ten, within their dendritic field; despite the nonselectivity in their synaptic input, these bipolar cells differ in intrinsic properties. For instance, OFF bipolar cells can be further subdivided according to the specific expression of AMPA or kainate receptors on their dendrites (DeVries, 2000). The physiological consequences of this molecular diversity are different temporal resolution and possibly different threshold sensitivity. It has been observed that the different types of OFF and ON cone bipolar cells can provide separate channels for high-frequency and low-frequency information.

Recent data support the notion that bipolar cells are capable of discriminating between the sustained and transient components of the light stimuli (Cohen and Sterling, 1992; Roska and Werblin, 2001; Werblin et al., 2001). This possibility would arise from the ordered and layered organization of the retina: each type of cone bipolar cell should be able to provide a characteristic stimulation of a selected type of ganglion cell that cofasciculates at the same level of the IPL. Inhibition, on the contrary, would take place more diffusely, by means of amacrine cells (Masland, 2001). The presence of a variety of cone bipolar cell types is thought to reflect a variety of parallel functions; although their different roles are only beginning to be understood, all the available evidence indicates that the various types transmit different representations of the visual scenery to the inner retina. The power of computation of the cone pathway is exploited by the rod pathway as well, which is "grafted" onto the cone system by means of the connections of AII amacrine cells.

In light of the similarities of the various types of cone bipolar cells, the use of transgenic mice that express fluorescent markers in one or more populations of bipolar and ganglion (or amacrine) cells appears to be the most promising method for understanding their specific pattern of connections. The small size of these neurons and their relatively high density make it difficult to use single-cell injection as a major tool to study bipolar cell circuitry. Because of the resolution limits of confocal microscopy, however, the assessment of true synaptic contacts remains to be identified at the electron microscopy level.

REFERENCES

Berntson, A., and Taylor, W. R. (2000). Response characteristics and receptive field widths of on-bipolar cells in the mouse retina. *J. Physiol.* 524 (Pt. 3):879–889.

Bloomfield, S. A., Xin, D., and Osborne, T. (1997). Light-induced modulation of coupling between AII amacrine cells in the rabbit retina. *Vis. Neurosci.* 14(3):565–576.

Bowmaker, J. K. (1998). Evolution of colour vision in vertebrates. *Eye* 12(Pt. 3b):541–547.

Boycott, B. B., and Wässle, H. (1991). Morphological classification of bipolar cells of the primate retina. *Eur. J. Neurosci.* 3(11):1069–1088.

Carter-Dawson, L. D., and LaVail, M. M. (1979). Rods and cones in the mouse retina. I. Structural analysis using light and electron microscopy. *J. Comp. Neurol.* 188(2):245–262.

Cohen, E., and Sterling, P. (1992). Parallel circuits from cones to the ON-beta ganglion cell. *Eur. J. Neurosci.* 4(6):506–520.

Contini, M., and Raviola, E. (2003). GABAergic synapses made by a retinal dopaminergic neuron. *Proc. Natl. Acad. Sci. U.S.A.* 100(3):1358–1363.

Dalke, C., and Graw, J. (2005). Mouse mutants as models for congenital retinal disorders. *Exp. Eye Res.* 81(5):503–512.

DeVries, S. H. (2000). Bipolar cells use kainate and AMPA receptors to filter visual information into separate channels. *Neuron* 28(3):847–856.

Dhingra, A., Jiang, M., Wang, T. L., Lyubarsky, A., Savchenko, A., Bar-Yehuda, T., Sterling, P., Birnbaumer, L., and Vardi, N. (2002). Light response of retinal ON bipolar cells requires a specific splice variant of Galpha(o). *J. Neurosci.* 22(12):4878–4884.

Dowling, J. E., and Boycott, B. B. (1966). Organization of the primate retina: Electron microscopy. *Proc. R. Soc. Lond. B. Biol. Sci.* 166(2):80–111.

Dowling, J. E., and Ehinger, B. (1978). Synaptic organization of the dopaminergic neurons in the rabbit retina. *J. Comp. Neurol.* 180(2):203–220.

Euler, T., and Masland, R. H. (2000). Light-evoked responses of bipolar cells in a mammalian retina. *J. Neurophysiol.* 83(4):1817–1829.

Euler, T., and Wässle, H. (1995). Immunocytochemical identification of cone bipolar cells in the rat retina. *J. Comp. Neurol.* 361(3):461–478.

Freed, M. A. (2000). Parallel cone bipolar pathways to a ganglion cell use different rates and amplitudes of quantal excitation. *J. Neurosci.* 20(11):3956–3963.

Gargini, C., Terzibasi, E., Mazzoni, F., and Strettoi, E. (2007). Retinal organization in the retinal degeneration 10 (rd10) mutant mouse: A morphological and ERG study. *J. Comp. Neurol.* 500(2): 222–238.

Ghosh, K. K., Bujan, S., Haverkamp, S., Feigenspan, A., and Wässle, H. (2004). Types of bipolar cells in the mouse retina. *J. Comp. Neurol.* 469(1):70–82.

Hack, I., Peichl, L., and Brandstatter, J. H. (1999). An alternative pathway for rod signals in the rodent retina: Rod photoreceptors, cone bipolar cells, and the localization of glutamate receptors. *Proc. Natl. Acad. Sci. U.S.A.* 96(24):14130–14135.

Han, Y., and Massey, S. C. (2005). Electrical synapses in retinal ON cone bipolar cells: Subtype-specific expression of connexins. *Proc. Natl. Acad. Sci. U.S.A.* 102(37):13313–13318.

Hartveit, E. (1997). Functional organization of cone bipolar cells in the rat retina. *J. Neurophysiol.* 77(4):1716–1730.

Haverkamp, S., and Wässle, H. (2000). Immunocytochemical analysis of the mouse retina. *J. Comp. Neurol.* 424(1):1–23.

Haverkamp, S., Wässle, H., Duebel, J., Kuner, T., Augustine, G. J., Feng, G., and Euler, T. (2005). The primordial, blue-cone color system of the mouse retina. *J. Neurosci.* 25(22):5438–5445.

Hokoc, J. N., and Mariani, A. P. (1988). Synapses from bipolar cells onto dopaminergic amacrine cells in cat and rabbit retinas. *Brain Res.* 461(1):17–26.

Huang, L., Max, M., Margolskee, R. F., Su, H., Masland, R. H., and Euler, T. (2003). The G protein subunit Gγ13 is co-expressed with Gαo and Gβ3 in retinal On bipolar cells. *J. Comp. Neurol.* 455:1–10.

Hughes, A. (1975). A quantitative analysis of the cat retinal ganglion cell topography. *J. Comp. Neurol.* 163(1):107–128.

Ivanova, E., Muller, U., and Wässle, H. (2006). Characterization of the glycinergic input to bipolar cells of the mouse retina. *Eur. J. Neurosci.* 23(2):350–364.

Jeon, C. J., Strettoi, E., and Masland, R. H. (1998). The major cell populations of the mouse retina. *J. Neurosci.* 18(21):8936–8946.

Jones, B. W., Watt, C. B., Frederick, J. M., Baehr, W., Chen, C. K., Levine, E. M., Milam, A. H., Lavail, M. M., and Marc, R. E. (2003). Retinal remodeling triggered by photoreceptor degenerations. *J. Comp. Neurol.* 464(1):1–16.

Kolb, H. (1979). The inner plexiform layer in the retina of the cat: Electron microscopic observations. *J. Neurocytol.* 8(3):295–329.

Kolb, H., Cuenca, N., Wang, H. H., and Dekorver, L. (1990). The synaptic organization of the dopaminergic amacrine cell in the cat retina. *J. Neurocytol.* 19(3):343–366.

Li, W., Keung, J. W., and Massey, S. C. (2004). Direct synaptic connections between rods and OFF cone bipolar cells in the rabbit retina. *J. Comp. Neurol.* 474(1):1–12.

Lin, B., Jacobs, T. C., and Masland, R. H. (2005). Different functional types of bipolar cells use different gap-junctional proteins. *J. Neurosci.* 25(28):6696–6701.

Lin, B., and Masland, R. H. (2005). Synaptic contacts between an identified type of ON cone bipolar cell and ganglion cells in the mouse retina. *Eur. J. Neurosci.* 21(5):1257–1270.

Marc, R. E., Jones, B. W., Watt, C. B., and Strettoi, E. (2003). Neural remodeling in retinal degeneration. *Prog. Retin. Eye Res.* 22(5):607–655.

Martin, P. R., and Grünert, U. (1992). Spatial density and immunoreactivity of bipolar cells in the macaque monkey retina. *J. Comp. Neurol.* 323(2):269–287.

Masland, R. H. (2001). Neuronal diversity in the retina. *Curr. Opin. Neurobiol.* 11(4):431–436.

Mills, S. L., and Massey, S. C. (2000). A series of biotinylated tracers distinguishes three types of gap junction in retina. *J. Neurosci.* 20(22):8629–8636.

Mitrofanis, J., Vigny, A., and Stone, J. (1988). Distribution of catecholaminergic cells in the retina of the rat, guinea pig, cat, and rabbit: Independence from ganglion cell distribution. *J. Comp. Neurol.* 267(1):1–14.

Nelson, R. (1977). Cat cones have rod input: A comparison of the response properties of cones and horizontal cell bodies in the retina of the cat. *J. Comp. Neurol.* 172(1):109–135.

Peichl, L., and Gonzalez-Soriano, J. (1994). Morphological types of horizontal cell in rodent retinae: A comparison of rat, mouse, gerbil, and guinea pig. *Vis. Neurosci.* 11(3):501–517.

Pignatelli, V., Cepko, C. L., and Strettoi, E. (2004). Inner retinal abnormalities in a mouse model of Leber's congenital amaurosis. *J. Comp. Neurol.* 469(3):351–359.

Pignatelli, V., and Strettoi, E. (2004). Bipolar cells of the mouse retina: A gene gun, morphological study. *J. Comp. Neurol.* 476(3): 254–266.

Protti, D. A., Flores-Herr, N., Li, W., Massey, S. C., and Wässle, H. (2005). Light signaling in scotopic conditions in the rabbit, mouse and rat retina: A physiological and anatomical study. *J. Neurophysiol.* 93(6):3479–3488.

Raviola, E. (2002). A molecular approach to retinal neural networks. *Funct. Neurol.* 17(3):115–119.

Raviola, E., and Gilula, N. B. (1975). Intramembrane organization of specialized contacts in the outer plexiform layer of the retina: A freeze-fracture study in monkeys and rabbits. *J. Cell Biol.* 65(1):192–222.

Rice, D. S., and Curran, T. A. (2000). Disabled-1 is expressed in type AII amacrine cells in the mouse retina. *J. Comp. Neurol.* 424(2):327–338.

Roska, B., and Werblin, F. (2001). Vertical interactions across ten parallel, stacked representations in the mammalian retina. *Nature* 410(6828):583–587.

Soucy, E., Wang, Y., Nirenberg, S., Nathans, J., and Meister, M. (1998). A novel signaling pathway from rod photoreceptors to ganglion cells in mammalian retina. *Neuron* 21(3): 481–493.

Strettoi, E., and Masland, R. H. (1995). The organization of the inner nuclear layer of the rabbit retina. *J. Neurosci.* 15:875–888.

Strettoi, E., and Pignatelli, V. (2000). Modifications of retinal neurons in a mouse model of retinitis pigmentosa. *Proc. Natl. Acad. Sci., U.S.A.* 97(20):11020–11025.

Strettoi, E., Porciatti, V., Falsini, B., Pignatelli, V., and Rossi, C. (2002). Morphological and functional abnormalities in the inner retina of the rd/rd mouse. *J. Neurosci.* 22(13):5492–5504.

Strettoi, E., Raviola, E., and Dacheux, R. F. (1992). Synaptic connections of the narrow-field, bistratified rod amacrine cell (AII) in the rabbit retina. *J. Comp. Neurol.* 325(2):152–168.

Strettoi, E., and Volpini, M. (2002). Retinal organization in the bcl-2-overexpressing transgenic mouse. *J. Comp. Neurol.* 446(1):1–10.

Suzuki, H., and Pinto, L. H. (1986). Response properties of horizontal cells in the isolated retina of wild-type and pearl mutant mice. *J. Neurosci.* 6(4):1122–1128.

Tsukamoto, Y., Morigiwa, K., Ueda, M., and Sterling, P. (2001). Microcircuits for night vision in mouse retina. *J. Neurosci.* 21(21):8616–8623.

Ueda, Y., Iwakabe, H., Masu, M., Suzuki, M., and Nakanishi, S. (1997). The mGluR6 5′ upstream transgene sequence directs a cell-specific and developmentally regulated expression in retinal rod and ON-type cone bipolar cells. *J. Neurosci.* 17(9):3014–3023.

Völgyi, B., Deans, M. R., Paul, D. L., and Bloomfield, S. A. (2004). Convergence and segregation of the multiple rod pathways in mammalian retina. *J. Neurosci.* 24(49):11182–11192.

Wässle, H. (2004). Parallel processing in the mammalian retina. *Nat. Neurosci.* 5:747–757.

Werblin, F., Roska, B., and Balya, D. (2001). Parallel processing in the mammalian retina: Lateral and vertical interactions across stacked representations. *Prog. Brain Res.* 131:229–238.

Witkovsky, P. (2004). Dopamine and retinal function. *Doc. Ophthalmol.* 108(1):17–40.

13 Distribution and Functional Roles of Neuronal Gap Junctions in the Mouse Retina

STEWART A. BLOOMFIELD AND BÉLA VÖLGYI

Just as for other CNS loci, the major mode of neuronal communication in the retina is chemically mediated synaptic transmission. However, it has been long known from serial reconstructions of electron micrographs that some neighboring retinal neurons form gap junctions between their closely opposed plasma membranes, suggesting a role for electrical transmission as well. In fact, coupling between horizontal cells was described more than 40 years ago by Yamada and Ishikawa (1965), some 5 years before Goodenough and Revel (1970) coined the term "gap junction."

Gap junctions, the morphological substrate of electrical synapses, are composed of two hemichannels or connexons that link across the extracellular space to form an intercellular pathway for diffusion of molecules up to about 1,000 daltons. Hemichannels are hexameric structures composed of six subunit transmembrane proteins called connexins. Twenty different connexin genes have been characterized in the mouse, and a number of connexin proteins are widely expressed in murine retinal neurons, including connexin 36 (Cx36), connexin 45 (Cx45), and connexin 57 (Cx57) (Söhl and Willecke, 2003; Söhl et al., 2005; Kamasawa et al., 2006). In fact, recent studies suggest that gap junctions are found in almost all of the approximate 60 subtypes of neuron in the retina, indicating that electrical synaptic transmission plays a significant role in retinal signal processing. The degree of coupling between retinal neurons does not appear to be a static process but shows high plasticity regulated by neuromodulators such as dopamine and nitric oxide, whose release is dependent on the adaptational state of the retina (Lasater and Dowling, 1985; Witkovsky and Dearry, 1991; DeVries and Schwartz, 1992; Hampson et al., 1992; Bloomfield et al., 1997; Xin and Bloomfield, 1999a, 1999b).

Still, the role of electrical transmission in the retina and brain has long been underestimated. Over the past decade, owing to recent technical advances in cell labeling techniques, particularly the advent of the gap junction permeable biotinylated tracers, electrophysiology, and molecular cloning, studies of electrical synaptic transmission in the retina have proliferated. The use of mouse mutants in which selective gap junctions are disrupted by targeting connexin genes has become a particularly important tool to characterize the function of these electrical synapses. In this chapter we review the distribution of gap junctions in the mouse retina and recent work detailing their significant and varied functional roles in visual processing.

Photoreceptor gap junctions

As shown in a variety of mammalian retinas (Raviola and Gilula, 1973; Kolb and Jones, 1985; Tsukamoto et al., 1992), direct gap junctional coupling occurs between the axon terminals of neighboring cone photoreceptors and also between rods and cones in the mouse (Tsukamoto et al., 2001). β-gal and PLAP reporters in heterozygous Cx36 knockout (KO) mouse lines were detected within cell bodies in the outer nuclear layer (ONL) and in processes extending distally to the region occupied by photoreceptor inner segments (Deans et al., 2002) (figure 13.1*A*). The widespread labeling of photoreceptors suggested that Cx36 was at least expressed by rods, which constitute 97% of all photoreceptors in the mouse (Jeon et al., 1998). However, a study of two Cx36 transgenic mutants indicated that Cx36 was expressed only in cone photoreceptors and thus subserved both the homologous cone-cone and heterologous rod-cone coupling (Feigenspan et al., 2004). The Cx36 expression limited only to murine cone photoreceptors was consistent with the distribution described in the guinea pig retina (Lee et al., 2003).

Electrical coupling between cones has been shown to increase the signal-to-noise ratio of their visually evoked responses (DeVries et al., 2002). Since the intrinsic noise produced in neighboring cones is independent, whereas their visual signals are partially shared, electrical coupling averages out the noisy fluctuations in voltage more than the response signals. The conductance of cone-to-cone gap junctions does result in a small blur, but this is lower than that of the eye's optics. Thus, the signal fidelity gained by electrical coupling between cones outweighs any compromise in visual acuity.

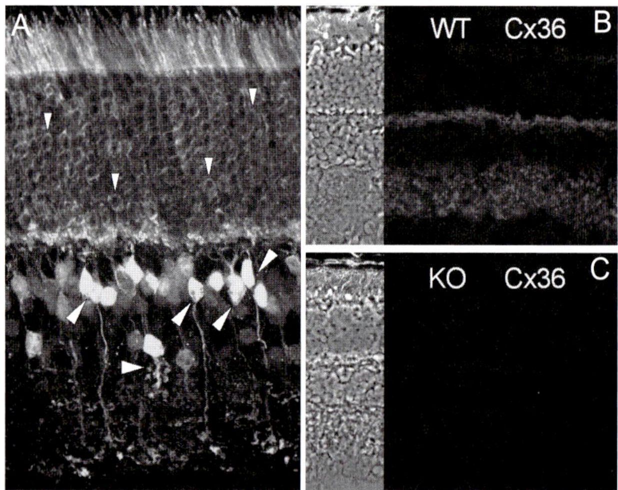

FIGURE 13.1 *A*, β-Gal reporter in transgenic mouse retina indicates that Cx36 is expressed by photoreceptors in the ONL and by bipolar cells and amacrine cells in the INL. *Small arrowheads* indicate photoreceptor somata; *large arrowheads* indicate somata of an AII amacrine cell and bipolar cells. *B*, Transverse view of immunolabeling of the wild-type mouse retina for Cx36. Labeling is confined to the plexiform layers, consistent with the known locations of gap junctions between retinal neurons. *C*, Immunolabeling for Cx36 is absent in the Cx36 KO mouse retina. See color plate 5. (*A*, Adopted from Deans et al., 2002, with permission. *B* and *C*, Adopted from Deans et al., 2001, with permission.)

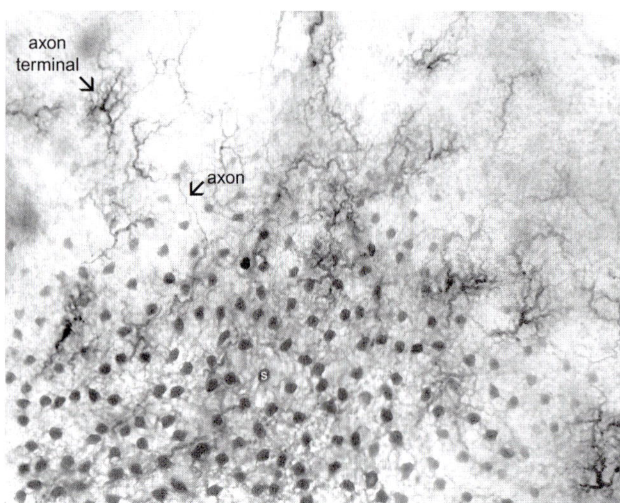

FIGURE 13.2 Tracer-coupled group of horizontal cells in the mouse retina following injection of single horizontal cell soma with Neurobiotin. The cluster of darkly labeled somata (s) are surrounded by axon terminals and connecting axons. Scale bar = 50 μm.

In contrast, the coupling between rods and cones is believed to form a secondary rod pathway in which scotopic signals can be communicated directly to cones and then relayed to ganglion cells via the cone bipolar cells. Evidence for the functionality of this pathway include demonstrations of rod signals within cone photoreceptors (Nelson, 1977; Schneeweis and Schnapf, 1995) and the survival of rod signals at the ganglion cell level after blockade of the principal rod pathway subserved by rod bipolar and AII amacrine cells (Strettoi et al., 1990, 1992; DeVries and Baylor, 1995). In addition, studies of the Cx36 KO mouse retina showed that disruption of rod-cone coupling resulted in a significant loss of rod signaling to ganglion cells (Deans et al., 2002). Consistent with human psychophysical evidence (Sharpe and Stockman, 1999), these studies further indicated that the primary rod pathway conveys the most sensitive rod signals to the ganglion cells, whereas the secondary pathway conveys higher threshold scotopic signals (Deans et al., 2002; Völgyi et al., 2004).

In contrast to larger mammals, rods are homologously coupled to each other via gap junctions in the mouse retina (Tsukamoto et al., 2001). Interestingly, approximately 20% of mouse rods form a chemical synapse with a mixed rod-cone bipolar cell, thus creating a third rod pathway for scotopic OFF signal transmission to the inner retina (Soucy et al., 1998; Tsukamoto et al., 2001). It has been proposed that rod-rod coupling pools the scotopic signals at the photoreceptor level for conveyance to the ganglion cells via the third pathway. This third rod pathway may thus be useful at dusk and dawn, when relatively greater numbers of photons are available than during starlight and the pooled signal may thereby more efficiently encode faintly backlit objects. Physiological evidence for this third pathway was recently provided by Völgyi et al. (2004), who described ganglion cells with scotopic sensitivities that were lower than those of signals conveyed by the primary and secondary rod pathways. Further, signals presumably transmitted via the third rod pathway survived in the Cx36 KO mouse retina, suggesting that pooling of scotopic signals via rod-rod coupling was still intact. This lends further support to the notion described earlier that Cx36 is not expressed at the gap junctions between rod photoreceptors in the mouse.

Horizontal cell gap junctions

Most vertebrate retinas contain two subtypes of horizontal cell, one that is axonless and a second that maintains an axon that typically extends for a few hundreds microns before ending in an elaborate terminal arbor (Fisher and Boycott, 1974; Kolb, 1974; Boycott et al., 1978). Only the axon-bearing subtype of horizontal cell is found in the mouse retina (He et al., 2000). Neighboring horizontal cells in mammalian retinas are extensively coupled via gap junctions (Kolb, 1974; Raviola and Gilula, 1975; Vaney, 1991; Bloomfield et al., 1995; He et al., 2000) (figure 13.2). The axonless and axon-bearing horizontal cells show only homologous coupling resulting in separate electrical syncytia. Likewise, the somatic and axon terminal endings of the axon bearing horizontal cells are segregated into homologously coupled networks.

The horizontal cell gap junctions form an efficient pathway for intercellular electrical communication whereby the receptive fields (RFs) of individual horizontal cells dwarf the size of their dendritic arbors (Tomita, 1965; Naka and Rushton, 1967; Bloomfield and Miller, 1982). Coupled with feedforward and/or feedback chemical synaptic transmission, the enlarged RFs of horizontal cells are thought to mediate the surround RFs of bipolar cells necessary for contrast discrimination (Naka and Nye, 1971; Naka and Witkovsky, 1971; Bloomfield et al., 1995).

There is abundant evidence that the gap junctions connecting horizontal cells are dynamically regulated by the neuromodulator dopamine as a mediator of light adaptation (Witkovsky and Dearry, 1991). Application of dopamine or cAMP reduces the coupling between the somatic endings of mouse horizontal cells, whereas the coupling is significantly increased by D1 receptor antagonists (He et al., 2000). Interestingly, these agents appear to have no effect on the coupling between horizontal cell axon terminals, suggesting that the subunit composition of their interconnecting gap junctions is different from that of the somatic junctions (He et al., 2000).

Mouse horizontal cells do not express either Cx26 or Cx36 (Deans and Paul, 2001). They do express Cx57, and tracer coupling is abolished in the Cx57 KO mouse retina, indicating that this connexin protein is critical for horizontal cell electrical coupling (Hombach et al., 2004). Indeed, horizontal cells in the Cx57 KO mouse retina show a significant reduction in their RF size compared with that seen in wild-type animals (Shelley et al., 2006). Coupling appears to be lost for both somatic and axon terminal endings, indicating that Cx57 is crucial for both sets of gap junctions. However, as mentioned earlier, the results of He et al. (2000) showing different pharmacological sensitivities of these junctions suggest that whereas they both express Cx57, they may be heteromeric, with different overall connexin composition.

Recently, Kamermans et al. (2001) posited that the feedback circuit from horizontal cells to cone photoreceptors in the fish retina may rely on ephaptic transmission via Cx26 hemichannels. In this scheme, electrical charge moving across hemichannels communicates with the extracellular space and modifies the activity of nearby cone photoreceptor axon terminals. Although this mechanism has not been confirmed in the mammal, it is possible that Cx57 could also form functional hemichannels on mouse horizontal cells for which Cx26 protein has not been detected (Deans and Paul, 2001).

Bipolar cell and amacrine cell gap junctions

Bipolar cells can be coupled either heterologously to amacrine cells or homologously to other bipolar cell neighbors. The different mosaics and coverage factors for the subtypes of bipolar cells in the mouse suggest that only a few may display the dendritic overlap necessary for homologous coupling (Mills and Massey, 1992; Massey and Mills, 1996; Lin et al., 2005). Indeed, the only evidence for homologous coupling of murine bipolar cell comes from a study of transgenic mice in which Cx36 expression was found on the dendrites of three subtypes of OFF bipolar cells just below the cone pedicles (Feigenspan et al., 2004). Interestingly, Cx45 expression has been found in all four types of OFF cone bipolar cells, suggesting that a subset may express more than one connexin (Maxeiner et al., 2005), although they may be spatially segregated to the outer and inner plexiform layers.

In contrast, a number of studies have been made of the heterologous gap junctions formed between ON cone bipolar cells and AII amacrine cells. To date, only the coupling of the AII subtype of amacrine cell has been studied in the mouse retina. The junctions formed by AII amacrine cells are discussed in detail in the next section.

Gap junctions in the proximal rod pathways

As mentioned, there are three rod pathways in the mammalian retina (Bloomfield and Dacheux, 2003). The role of rod-cone and rod-rod coupling in the secondary and tertiary rod pathways, respectively, was discussed earlier. The principal rod pathway for ON signaling is rods → rod bipolar cells → AII amacrine cells → ON cone bipolar cells → ON ganglion cells. There are two sets of gap junctions found in this pathway: homologous AII-AII cell junctions and heterologous AII-ON cone bipolar cell junctions. Cx36 is abundantly expressed by AII amacrine cells (Feigenspan et al., 2001; Deans et al., 2002) (see figure 13.1) and AII cell-AII cell coupling is lost in the Cx36 KO mouse retina (Deans et al., 2002) (see figure 13.3) indicating that Cx36 comprises the homologous junctions between these cells. Based on a computational model, Smith and Vardi (1995) speculated that AII cell-AII cell coupling serves to sum synchronous signals and subtract asynchronous noise, thereby preserving the fidelity of the high-sensitivity signals carried by the primary rod pathway. This function is similar to that described earlier for cone photoreceptor coupling in the outer retina. Consistent with this idea, the intensity-response profiles of the most sensitive ganglion cells in the mouse retina show a rightward shift in the Cx36 KO retina due to an approximate one log unit loss of sensitivity (Völgyi et al., 2004) (figure 13.4). This results in equal sensitivities for the rod signals carried by the primary and secondary rod

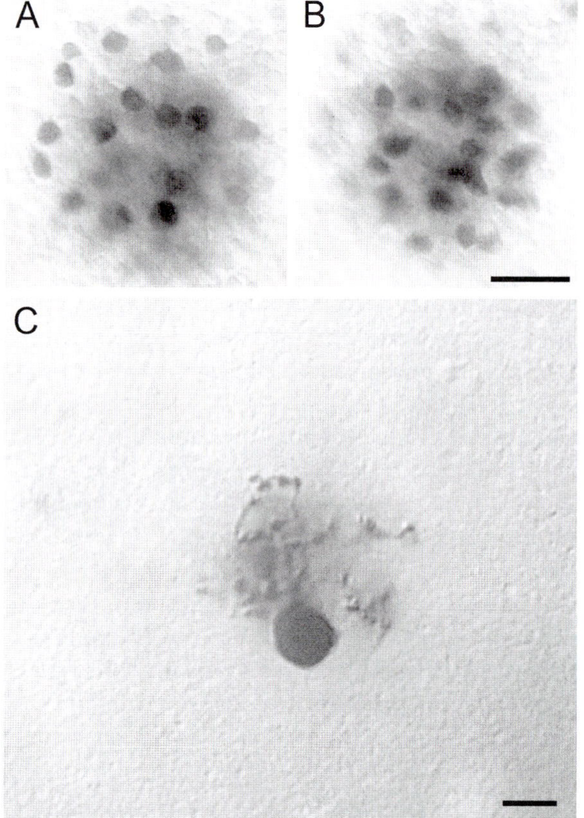

Figure 13.3 Tracer coupling pattern of AII amacrine cells in the mouse retina. *A*, Tracer-coupled group of AII amacrine cell somata following injection of an AII amacrine cell in the wild-type mouse retina. Tracer has moved through AII cell-AII cell gap junctions. *B*, Plane of focus shifted to the more distal INL to show the tracer-coupled somata of ON cone bipolar cells. Tracer has moved through AII cell-ON cone bipolar cell gap junctions as well. Scale bar for *A* and *B* = 50 μm. *C*, No tracer coupling is evident following injection of an AII amacrine cell with Neurobiotin in the Cx36 KO retina. This finding indicates that Cx36 is crucial for both AII cell-AII cell and AII cell-ON cone bipolar cell coupling. Scale bar = 10 μm. (*A* and *B*, Adopted from Deans et al., 2002, with permission.)

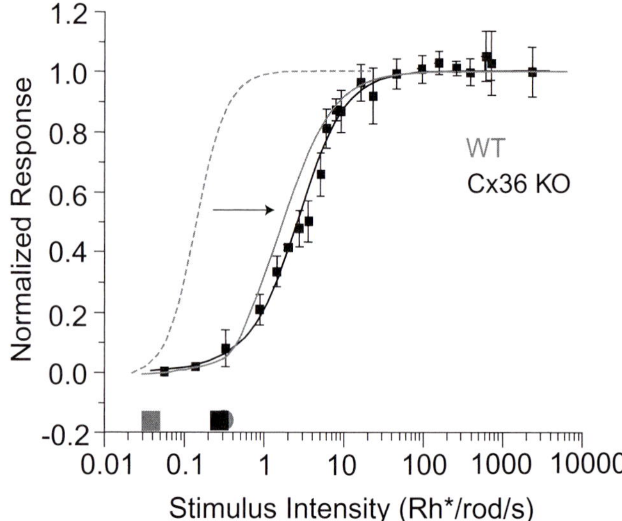

Figure 13.4 Intensity-response functions of ganglion cells in the wild-type and Cx36 KO mouse retina. *Dashed gray curve* indicates the averaged intensity-response function of the high-sensitivity OFF-center ganglion cells in the wild-type mouse retina. These signals are carried by the primary rod pathway. *Solid gray line* indicates the average intensity-response function of intermediate sensitivity OFF-center ganglion cells in the wild-type mouse retina. The signals are carried by the secondary rod pathway. In the Cx36 KO mouse retina, the intensity-response profile of the high-sensitivity ganglion cells (*black curve* and data points) is shifted rightward by about one log unit (*arrow*). Symbols along the abscissa indicate the response thresholds for high-sensitivity cells in the wild-type retina (*gray square*), intermediate-sensitivity cells in the wild-type retina (*gray circle*), and high-sensitivity cells in the Cx36 KO retina (*black square*). (Adapted from Völgyi et al., 2004, with permission.)

pathways. Taken together, these results indicate that the homologous coupling between AII cells maintains the high sensitivity of signals transmitted by the rod bipolar cells to the inner retina. In the rabbit retina, AII cell coupling is modulated by dopamine (Mills and Massey, 1995) and by changes in adapting background light conditions (Bloomfield et al., 1997), but this has not yet been studied in the mouse.

Scotopic signaling to ganglion cells is also compromised in the Cx36 KO animal, indicating that Cx36 plays a role in the heterologous AII amacrine cell-ON cone bipolar cell gap junctions as well (Guldenagel et al., 2001; Deans et al., 2002). This idea is supported by the finding that tracer coupling between AII amacrine cells and ON cone bipolar cells is disrupted in the Cx36 KO mouse retina (Deans et al., 2002) (see figure 13.3). Further, glycine accumulation in ON cone bipolar cells derived from diffusion across the gap junction made with AII amacrine cells is eliminated in the Cx36 KO mouse (Deans et al., 2002).

While Cx36 is almost certainly expressed by the AII amacrine cell hemichannel, the composition of the hemichannel on the cone bipolar cell side of the gap junction is less clear. Deans et al. (2002) showed expression of Cx36 reporters in a subset of bipolar cells in a transgenic mouse line (see figure 13.1). These bipolar cells showed axon terminations within sublamina b of the IPL, suggesting that they were ON cone bipolar cells. These data suggested that the AII amacrine cell-cone bipolar cell gap junctions were homotypic, both expressing Cx36. In contrast, Feigenspan et al. (2001) reported that ON cone bipolar cells in the rodent retina did not display Cx36 immunoreactivity, suggesting that the AII cell-cone bipolar cell gap junctions are heterotypic. Further, a study of a conditional Cx45 KO mouse showed that deletion of Cx45 resulted in a reduction of the b-wave of the scotopic ERG and elimination of glycine in Cx45-expressing bipolar cells (Maxeiner et al., 2005), similar to that shown in the Cx36 KO mouse retina (Guldenagel et al., 2001; Deans et al., 2002). These data suggested that at least some of the AII cell-cone bipolar cell gap junctions are heterotypic. A number of recent studies have confirmed that whereas certain ON cone bipolar cells express Cx36, others express Cx45 (Lin et al., 2005; Han and Massey, 2005; Dedek et al., 2006). Thus, the emerging scenario is that certain AII cell-cone bipolar cell gap junctions are homotypic, with both hemichannels expressing Cx36, whereas others are heterotypic, with Cx36 and Cx45 hemichannels. The existence of heterotypic junctions can explain the different conductances and pharmacology of the AII cell-AII cell and AII cell-cone bipolar cell gap junctions, as well as the rectifying properties of the latter (Mills and Massey, 2000; Veruki and Hartveit, 2002).

Why would different ON cone bipolar cells use different connexins for the gap junctions they form with the AII amacrine cells? Gap junctions assembled from different subunits express different biophysical properties, including gating, permeability, and conductance (reviewed by Bennett and Zukin, 2004). Clearly, the different gap junctions formed between AII cells and cone bipolar cells introduce an additional complexity in the transmission and modulation of signaling in the primary rod pathway. In this regard, it is interesting to note that whereas rod signals are passed from AII amacrine cells to cone bipolar cells under dark-adapted conditions, the direction of signal flow is reversed under light-adapted conditions during which cone signals move into the network of coupled AII cells (Xin and Bloomfield, 1999a). Perhaps the different connexin makeup of AII cell-cone bipolar cell gap junctions are related to their dualistic function related to scotopic and photopic vision.

Ganglion cell coupling

Perhaps the most unexpected result of recent studies on tracer coupling in the retina has been the extensive homologous and heterologous coupling patterns seen for ganglion cells in the proximal retina (Vaney, 1991, 1994; Xin and Bloomfield, 1997). At first glance, this extensive coupling appeared problematic, as it suggested lateral intercellular propagation of signals across the IPL, which would result in the reduction of visual acuity of neuronal signals just as they exit the retina. However, a study in the rabbit retina showed that the RFs of ganglion cells approximated the extent of their dendritic arbors, irrespective of the extent of tracer coupling (Bloomfield and Xin, 1997). Further, the tracer-coupling networks formed by ganglion cells with their ganglion and/or amacrine cell neighbors were highly circumscribed, in that coupled cells were usually within one gap junction of the injected neuron. Overall, these findings indicated that ganglion cell gap junctions underlie local operations rather than lateral transmission of signals across the inner retina. Clearly, ganglion cell coupling is not analogous to the electrical syncytia formed by horizontal cells in the outer retina.

Although the core of our knowledge about ganglion cell gap junctions comes from studies of rabbit and cat retinas (Vaney, 1991, 1994; Xin and Bloomfield, 1997), a number of recent studies have extended work to the mouse. Although only a few mouse ganglion cell subtypes have been studied so far, they each display stereotypic tracer coupling patterns. For example, the ON alpha subtype of ganglion cell displays tracer coupling to two populations of amacrine cells with somata displaced to the ganglion cells layer, whereas OFF alpha ganglion cells are coupled homologously to one another and heterologously to two to three subtypes of amacrine cells with somata lying in the INL (Schubert et al., 2005a; Völgyi et al., 2005) (figure 13.5*A* and *D*). Reconstruction of the tracer-coupled amacrine cells indicated that they displayed extensive dendritic arbors characteristic of wide-field amacrine cell morphology (Völgyi et al., 2005). In addition, Schubert et al. (2005b) found that two subtypes of bistratified ganglion cells in the mouse retina, including ON-OFF direction-selective cells, are homologously coupled to their neighbors (figure 13.5*G*). A number of other ganglion cell subtypes in the mouse also show characteristic tracer coupling (figure 13.5*I–L*), suggesting that electrical synaptic transmission is common to the microcircuitry in the inner retina and thereby likely plays a major role in shaping ganglion cell light responses.

Relatively little is known about the connexin makeup of murine ganglion cell gap junctions. Recent studies have shown that heterologous gap junctions formed between amacrine cells and both ON and OFF alpha ganglion cells are dependent on Cx36 in that tracer coupling is abolished in the Cx36 KO mouse retina (Schubert et al., 2005a; Völgyi et al., 2005) (see figure 13.4*A–E*). However, the subunit composition of the homologous gap junctions connecting alpha ganglion cells is less clear. Völgyi et al. (2005) found that alpha cell-alpha ganglion cell tracer coupling remains intact in the Cx36 KO mouse retina, whereas Schubert et al. (2005a) reported that it is abolished in their Cx36 KO strain. This discrepancy may be explained either by divergent phenotypes of the two mutant mouse strains or by the different histological methods employed by the two research groups. In any event, these conflicting data highlight the problems that may occur in interpreting data from mutant mouse models and stress that caution must be taken in drawing conclusions.

Most recently, Cx45 has emerged as a possible constituent of ganglion cell gap junctions (Petrasch-Parwez et al., 2004). So far, immunolabeled Cx45 puncta have been localized to the homologous gap junctions connecting neighboring ON-OFF direction-selective ganglion cells (Schubert et al., 2005b) (see figure 13.4*G–H*). However, as both Cx36 and Cx45 puncta are widely distributed in the IPL of the mouse retina, it is likely that many other ganglion cell subtypes express these connexins as well. In addition, other yet

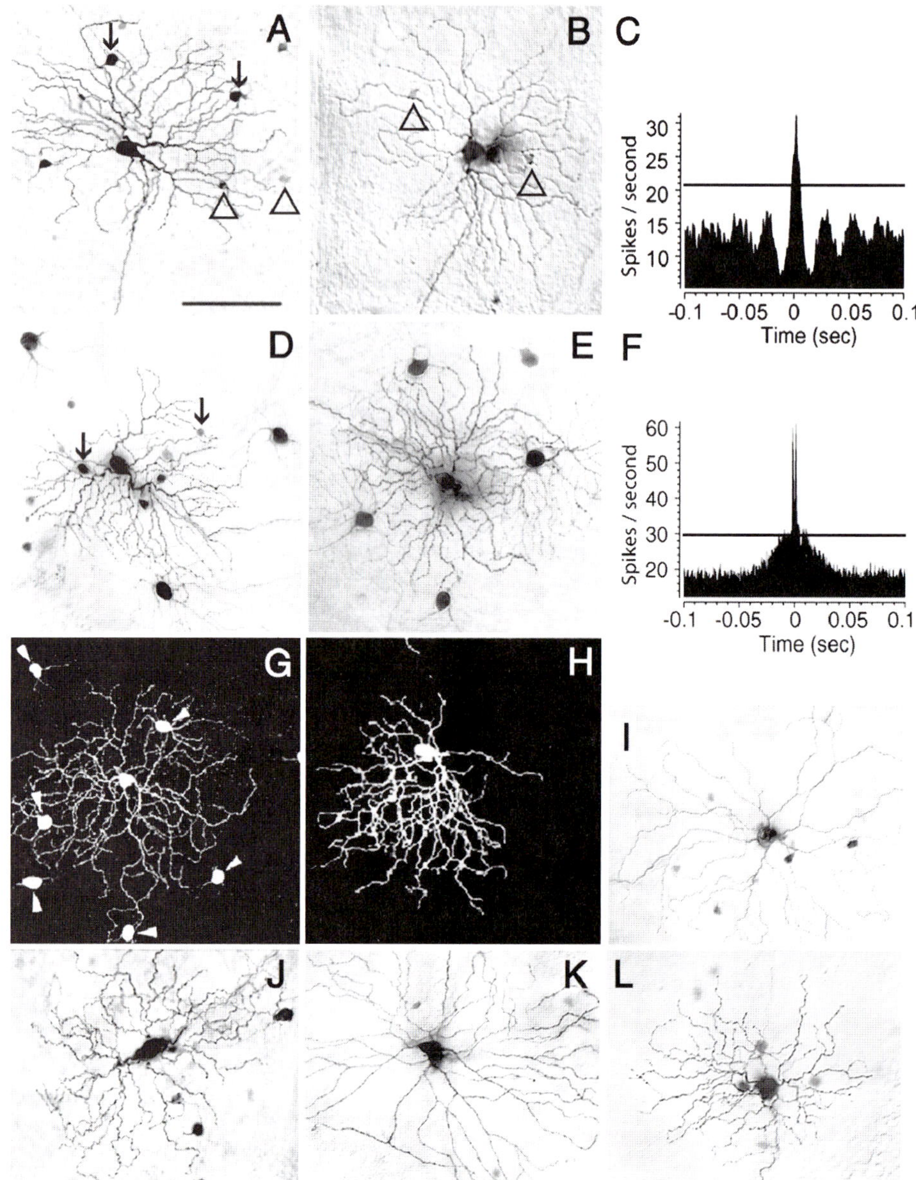

FIGURE 13.5 Tracer and electrical coupling of ganglion cells in the mouse retina. *A*, Photomicrograph of a Neurobiotin-labeled ON alpha ganglion cell in the wild-type mouse retina. This ON alpha cell is surrounded by a halo of tracer-coupled small (*open triangle*) and large, darkly labeled (*arrow*) amacrine cell somata. *B*, Neurobiotin-labeled ON alpha ganglion cell in the Cx36 KO mouse retina is tracer coupled only to small amacrine cells. *C*, Cross-correlogram of spontaneous spiking of a pair of neighboring ON alpha ganglion cells in the wild-type mouse retina shows a prominent central peak characteristic of unimodal spike synchrony. Line indicates 99% confidence limit. *D*, Photomicrograph of a Neurobiotin-labeled OFF alpha ganglion cell in the wild-type mouse retina. The OFF alpha cell is coupled both homologously to nearest neighbors and heterologously to two to three subtypes of amacrine cells (*arrow*). *E*, Neurobiotin-labeled OFF alpha ganglion cell in the Cx36 KO mouse retina reveals the loss of tracer coupling to amacrine cells. *F*, Cross-correlogram of a pair of OFF alpha ganglion cells in the wild-type retina shows two prominent peaks with short latency, which is a characteristic of bimodal spike correlation due to direct ganglion-to-ganglion cell coupling. *G*, Tracer coupling pattern of a Neurobiotin-labeled ON-OFF direction selective ganglion cell in the wild-type mouse retina. This cell displays homologous coupling to its nearest neighbor ganglion cells. *H*, Neurobiotin-labeled ON-OFF direction selective ganglion cell in the Cx45 KO retina shows no evidence of tracer coupling. *I–L*, Photomicrographs showing the tracer coupling pattern of a variety of ganglion cell subtypes injected with Neurobiotin. All these cells show heterologous coupling to amacrine cells. Scale bar = 100 μm for *A–H* and 150 μm for *I–L*. (*G* and *H*, Adapted from Schubert et al., 2005b, with permission.)

undiscovered connexins will likely be added to this list in the future. In a recent study, Dvoriantchikova et al. (2006) showed that pannexin 1 and 2 (Panx1, Panx2), two members of the pannexin protein family, are abundantly expressed by retinal neurons, including ganglion cells. This suggests that besides connexins, pannexin proteins may also constitute ganglion cell gap junctions in the mouse retina. The role of pannexins in retinal signal processing is unknown and will no doubt be an important aim of future research.

Functional role of ganglion cell coupling

Ganglion cells appear to couple in restricted groups, thereby preventing significant lateral spread of signals and maintaining spatial acuity. Thus, the gap junctions formed between ganglion cells appear to underlie local signal processing rather than global integration exemplified by the horizontal cells. It has been hypothesized that ganglion cell coupling underlies coherent firing of ganglion cell neighbors, ranging from broad correlations spanning tens of milliseconds to finely tuned spike synchrony with 1–3 ms latencies (Mastronarde, 1983; Meister et al., 1995; Brivanlou et al., 1998; DeVries, 1999; Hu and Bloomfield, 2003). Concerted firing accounts for up to one-half of retinal spike activity, suggesting that electrical coupling plays an important role in encoding visual information (Castelo-Branco et al., 1998; Schnitzer and Meister, 2003).

Direct ganglion cell to ganglion cell coupling is thought to mediate a fast (<2 ms) and reciprocal excitation that is reflected by prominent dual peaks in cross-correlograms of simultaneously recorded ganglion cell neighbors. This idea is supported by simultaneous recordings from homologously coupled OFF alpha ganglion cell pairs in the mouse retina, which produce bimodal, narrow spike correlations (figure 13.5*F*). In contrast, cross-correlograms of neighboring ON alpha ganglion cells, which are coupled only indirectly through amacrine cells, display a narrow, unimodal profile (figure 13.5*C*). This correlation profile for ON alpha cell neighbors likely reflects electrical synaptic inputs from common amacrine cells that give rise to synchronous spikes. These findings support the idea that homologous and heterologous coupling produce different types of correlated activity in neighboring ganglion cells (Brivanlou et al., 1998; DeVries, 1999; Hu and Bloomfield, 2003).

Finally, intercellular communication via gap junctions plays an important role in the development of neuronal circuits, including cell differentiation and pathfinding (Naus and Bani-Yaghoub, 1998). Ganglion cell gap junctions are thought to play a critical role in regulating the spontaneous activity, seen as spontaneous waves of depolarization, in developing retina that plays a role in refining retinal-thalamic and intraretinal connections (Sernagor et al., 2001; Grubb and Thompson, 2004). Bath application of gap junction blockers results in a reduction in the size and frequency of retinal waves (Singer et al., 2001; Syed et al., 2004). In a Cx36 KO mouse, Hansen et al. (2005) showed that Cx36 gap junctions play a critical role in suppressing ganglion cell firing between retinal waves during postnatal development. Thus, retinal gap junctions play an important role in the normal development of the visual system.

Conclusion

It is now abundantly clear that electrical coupling via gap junctions is ubiquitous in the vertebrate retina. Not only are gap junctions and their subunit connexin proteins widely expressed in both plexiform layers, but converging evidence suggests that they are expressed by most of the approximate 60 subtypes of retinal neurons. The finding that gap junctional conductances are affected by neuromodulators and changes in light adaptation indicates that electrical synaptic transmission forms a complex and dynamic mode of cellular communication. Although we are just beginning to elucidate the types of connexins (and pannexins) expressed in the retina, it is already clear that gap junctions play a wide variety of integrative functions, including (1) reducing the signal-to-noise ratio of the cellular responses of cones and amacrine cells, (2) synchronizing the spike activity of neighboring ganglion cells, (3) providing for interactions between the rod and cone pathways, (4) creating a secondary rod pathway, and (5) forming a syncytium of horizontal cells that signals ambient background illumination important for contrast signaling.

The retina is arguably the best model system in which to study the role of electrical synaptic transmission in the CNS. With the recent generation of mutant reporter and connexin KO models, the mouse has become the premier subject to study gap junctions in the retina. Future studies using cell-specific and inducible connexin KO mice models should be able to address the contribution of particular neuronal gap junctions to visual signaling. Determining the distribution and regulation of gap junction is an important challenge to understanding the functional roles of electrical coupling in the retina and their relationship to chemically mediated synaptic transmission. The mouse retina is expected to remain a vital resource in meeting this challenge.

REFERENCES

Bennett, M. V., and Zukin, R. S. (2004). Electrical coupling and neuronal synchronization in the mammalian brain. *Neuron* 41: 495–511.

Bloomfield, S. A., and Dacheux, R. F. (2001). Rod vision: Pathways and processing in the mammalian retina. *Prog. Retin. Eye Res.* 20:351–384.

Bloomfield, S. A., and Miller, R. F. (1982). A physiological and morphological study of the horizontal cell types of the rabbit retina. *J. Comp. Neurol.* 208:288–303.

Bloomfield, S. A., and Xin, D. (1997). A comparison of receptive-field and tracer-coupling size of amacrine and ganglion cells in the rabbit retina. *Vis. Neurosci.* 14:1153–1165.

Bloomfield, S. A., Xin, D., and Osborne, T. (1997). Light-induced modulation of coupling between AII amacrine cells in the rabbit retina. *Vis. Neurosci.* 14:565–576.

Bloomfield, S. A., Xin, D., and Persky, S. E. (1995). A comparison of receptive field and tracer coupling size of horizontal cells in the rabbit retina. *Vis. Neurosci.* 12:985–999.

Boycott, B. B., Peichl, L., and Wässle, H. (1978). Morphological types of horizontal cell in the retina of the domestic cat. *Proc. R. Soc. Lond. B Biol. Sci.* 203:229–245.

Brivanlou, I. H., Warland, D. K., and Meister, M. (1998). Mechanisms of concerted firing among retinal ganglion cells. *Neuron* 20:527–539.

Castelo-Branco, M., Neuenschwander, S., and Singer, W. (1998). Synchronization of visual responses between the cortex, lateral geniculate nucleus, and retina in the anesthetized cat. *J. Neurosci.* 18:6395–6410.

Deans, M. R., and Paul, D. L. (2001). Mouse horizontal cells do not express connexin26 or connexin36. *Cell Commun. Adhes.* 8:361–366.

Deans, M. R., Völgyi, B., Goodenough, D. A., Bloomfield, S. A., and Paul, D. L (2002). Connexin36 is essential for transmission of rod-mediated visual signals in the mammalian retina. *Neuron* 36:703–712.

Dedek, K., Schultz, K., Pieper, M., Dirks, P., Maxenier, S., Willecke, K., Weiler, R., and Janssen-Bienhold, U. (2006). Localization of heterotypic gap junctions composed of connexin45 and connexin36 in the rod pathway of the mouse retina. *Eur. J. Neurosci.* 24:1675–1686.

DeVries, S. H. (1999). Correlated firing in rabbit retinal ganglion cells. *J. Neurophysiol.* 81:908–920.

DeVries, S. H., and Baylor, D. A. (1995). An alternative pathway for signal flow from rod photoreceptors to ganglion cells in mammalian retina. *Proc. Natl. Acad. Sci. U.S.A.* 92:10658–10662.

DeVries, S. H., Qi, X., Smith, R., Makous, W., and Sterling, P. (2002). Electrical coupling between mammalian cones. *Curr. Biol.* 12(22):1900–1907.

DeVries, S. H., and Schwartz, E. A. (1992). Hemi-gap-junction channels in solitary horizontal cells of the catfish retina. *J. Physiol.* 445:201–230.

Dvoriantchikova, G., Ivanov, D., Panchin, Y., and Shestopalov, V. I. (2006). Expression of pannexin family of proteins in the retina. *FEBS Lett.* 580:2178–2182.

Feigenspan, A., Janssen-Bienhold, U., Hormuzdi, S., Monyer, H., Degen, J., Söhl, G., Willecke, K., Ammermuller, J., and Weiler, R. (2004). Expression of connexin36 in cone pedicles and OFF-cone bipolar cells of the mouse retina. *J. Neurosci.* 24:3325–3334.

Feigenspan, A., Teubner, B., Willecke, K., and Weiler, R. (2001). Expression of neuronal connexin36 in AII amacrine cells of the mammalian retina. *J. Neurosci.* 21:230–239.

Fisher, S. K., and Boycott, B. B. (1974). Synaptic connections made by horizontal cells within the outer plexiform layer of the retina of the cat and the rabbit. *Proc. R. Soc. Lond. B Biol. Sci.* 186:317–331.

Goodenough, D. A., and Revel, J. P. (1970). A fine structural analysis of intercellular junctions in the mouse liver. *J. Cell Biol.* 45:272–290.

Grubb, M. S., and Thompson, I. D. (2004). The influence of early experience on the development of sensory systems. *Curr. Opin. Neurobiol.* 14:503–512.

Guldenagel, M., Ammermuller, J., Feigenspan, A., Teubner, B., Degen, J., Söhl, G., Willecke, K., and Weiler, R. (2001). Visual transmission deficits in mice with targeted disruption of the gap junction gene connexin36. *J. Neurosci.* 21:6036–6044.

Hampson, E. C., Vaney, D. I., and Weiler, R. (1992). Dopaminergic modulation of gap junction permeability between amacrine cells in mammalian retina. *J. Neurosci.* 12:4911–4922.

Han, Y., and Massey, S. C. (2005). Electrical synapses in retinal ON cone bipolar cells: Subtype-specific expression of connexins. *Proc. Natl. Acad. Sci. U.S.A.* 102:13313–13318.

Hansen, K. A., Torborg, C. L., Elstrott, J., and Feller, M. B. (2005). Expression and function of the neuronal gap junction protein connexin 36 in developing mammalian retina. *J. Comp. Neurol.* 493:309–320.

He, S., Weiler, R., and Vaney, D. I. (2000). Endogenous dopaminergic regulation of horizontal cell coupling in the mammalian retina. *J. Comp. Neurol.* 418:33–40.

Hombach, S., Janssen-Bienhold, U., Sohl, G., Schubert, T., Bussow, H., Ott, T., Weiler, R., and Willecke, K. (2004). Functional expression of connexin57 in horizontal cells of the mouse retina. *Eur. J. Neurosci.* 19:2633–2640.

Hu, E. H., and Bloomfield, S. A. (2003). Gap junctional coupling underlies the short-latency spike synchrony of retinal alpha ganglion cells. *J. Neurosci.* 23:6768–6777.

Jeon, C. J., Strettoi, E., and Masland, R. H. (1998). The major cell populations of the mouse retina. *J. Neurosci.* 18:8936–8946.

Kamasawa, N., Furman, C. S., Davidson, K.G.V., Sampson, J. A., Magnie, A. R., Gebhardt, B. R., Kamasawa, M., Yasumura, T., Zumbrunnen, J. R., et al. (2006). Abundance and ultrastructural diversity of neuronal gap junctions in the OFF and ON sublaminae of the inner plexiform layer of rat and mouse retina. *Neuroscience* 142:1093–1117.

Kamermans, M., Kraaij, D., and Spekreijse, H. (2001). The dynamic characteristics of the feedback signal from horizontal cells to cones in the goldfish retina. *J. Physiol.* 534:489–500.

Kolb, H. (1974). The connections between horizontal cells and photoreceptors in the retina of the cat: Electron microscopy of Golgi preparations. *J. Comp. Neurol.* 155:1–14.

Kolb, H., and Jones, J. (1985). Electron microscopy of Golgi-impregnated photoreceptors reveals connections between red and green cones in the turtle retina. *J. Neurophysiol.* 54:304–317.

Lasater, E. M., and Dowling, J. E. (1985). Dopamine decreases conductance of the electrical junctions between cultured retinal horizontal cells. *Proc. Natl. Acad. Sci. U.S.A.* 82:3025–3029.

Lee, E. J., Han, J. W., Kim, H. J., Kim, I. B., Lee, M. Y., Oh, S. J., Chung, J. W., and Chun, M. H. (2003). The immunocytochemical localization of connexin 36 at rod and cone gap junctions in the guinea pig retina. *Eur. J. Neurosci.* 18:2925–2934.

Lin, B., Jakobs, T. C., and Masland, R. H. (2005). Different functional types of bipolar cells use different gap-junctional proteins. *J. Neurosci.* 25:6696–6701.

Massey, S. C., and Mills, S. L. (1996). A calbindin-immunoreactive cone bipolar cell type in the rabbit retina. *J. Comp. Neurol.* 366:15–33.

Mastronarde, D. N. (1983). Interactions between ganglion cells in cat retina. *J. Neurophysiol.* 49:350–365.

Maxeiner, S., Dedek, K., Janssen-Bienhold, U., Ammermuller, J., Brune, H., Kirsch, T., Pieper, M., Degen, J., Kruger, O., Willecke, K., and Weiler, R. (2005). Deletion of connexin45 in mouse retinal neurons disrupts the rod/cone signaling pathway between AII amacrine and ON cone bipolar cells and leads to impaired visual transmission. *J. Neurosci.* 25:566–576.

Meister, M., Legnado, L., and Baylor, D. A. (1995). Concerted signaling by retinal ganglion cells. *Science* 270:1207–1210.

Mills, S. L., and Massey, S. C. (1992). Morphology of bipolar cells labeled by DAPI in the rabbit retina. *J. Comp. Neurol.* 321:133–149.

Mills, S. L., and Massey, S. C. (1995). Differential properties of two gap junctional pathways made by AII amacrine cells. *Nature* 377:734–737.

Mills, S. L., and Massey, S. C. (2000). A series of biotinylated tracers distinguishes three types of gap junction in retina. *J. Neurosci.* 20:8629–8636.

Naka, K. I., and Nye, P. W. (1971). Role of horizontal cells in organization of the catfish retinal receptive field. *J. Neurophysiol.* 34:785–801.

Naka, K. I., and Rushton, W. A. (1967). The generation and spread of S-potentials in fish (Cyprinidae). *J. Physiol.* 192:437–461.

Naka, K. I., and Witkovsky, P. (1971). Dogfish ganglion cell discharge resulting from extrinsic polarization of the horizontal cells. *J. Physiol.* 223:449–460.

Naus, C. C., and Bani-Yaghoub, M. (1998). Gap junctional communication in the developing central nervous system. *Cell Biol. Int.* 22:751–763.

Nelson, R. (1977). Cat cones have rod input: A comparison of the response properties of cones and horizontal cell bodies in the retina of the cat. *J. Comp. Neurol.* 172:109–135.

Petrasch-Parwez, E., Habbes, H. W., Weickert, S., Lobbecke-Schumacher, M., Striedinger, K., Wieczorek, S., Dermietzel, R., and Epplen, J. T. (2004). Fine-structural analysis and connexin expression in the retina of a transgenic model of Huntington's disease. *J. Comp. Neurol.* 479:181–197.

Raviola, E., and Gilula, N. B. (1973). Gap junctions between photoreceptor cells in the vertebrate retina. *Proc. Natl. Acad. Sci. U.S.A.* 70:1677–1681.

Raviola, E., and Gilula, N. B. (1975). Intramembrane organization of specialized contacts in the outer plexiform layer of the retina: A freeze-fracture study in monkeys and rabbits. *J. Cell Biol.* 65:192–222.

Schneeweis, D. M., and Schnapf, J. L (1995). Photovoltage of rods and cones in the macaque retina. *Science* 268:1053–1056.

Schnitzer, M. J., and Meister, M. (2003). Multineuronal firing patterns in the signal from eye to brain. *Neuron* 37:499–511.

Schubert, T., Degen, J., Willecke, K., Hormuzdi, S. G., Monyer, H., and Weiler, R. (2005a). Connexin36 mediates gap junctional coupling of alpha-ganglion cells in mouse retina. *J. Comp. Neurol.* 485:191–201.

Schubert, T., Maxeiner, S., Kruger, O., Willecke, K., and Weiler, R. (2005b). Connexin45 mediates gap junctional coupling of bistratified ganglion cells in the mouse retina. *J. Comp. Neurol.* 490:29–39.

Sernagor, E., Eglen, S. J., and Wong, R. O. (2001). Development of retinal ganglion cell structure and function. *Prog. Retin. Eye Res.* 20:139–174.

Sharpe, L. T., and Stockman, A. (1999). Rod pathways: The importance of seeing nothing. *Trends Neurosci.* 22(11):497–504.

Shelley, J., Dedek, K., Schubert, T., Feigenspan, A., Schultz, K., Hombach, S., Willecke, K., and Weiler, R. (2006). Horizontal cell receptive fields are reduced in connexin57-deficient mice. *Eur. J. Neurosci.* 23(12):3176–3186.

Singer, J. H., Mirotznik, R. R., and Feller, M. B. (2001). Potentiation of L-type calcium channels reveals nonsynaptic mechanisms that correlate spontaneous activity in the developing mammalian retina. *J. Neurosci.* 21:8514–8522.

Smith, R. G., and Vardi, N. (1995). Simulation of the AII amacrine cell of mammalian retina: functional consequences of electrical coupling and regenerative membrane properties. *Vis. Neurosci.* 12:851–860.

Söhl, G., Maxeiner, S., and Willecke, K. (2005). Expression and functions of neuronal gap junctions. *Nat. Rev. Neurosci.* 6:191–200.

Söhl, G., and Willecke, K. (2003). An update on connexin genes and their nomenclature in mouse and man. *Cell Commun. Adhes.* 10:173–180.

Soucy, E., Wang, Y., Nirenberg, S., Nathans, J., and Meister, M. (1998). A novel signaling pathway from rod photoreceptors to ganglion cells in mammalian retina. *Neuron* 21: 481–493.

Strettoi, E., Dacheux, R. F., and Raviola, E. (1990). Synaptic connections of rod bipolar cells in the inner plexiform layer of the rabbit retina. *J. Comp. Neurol.* 295:449–466.

Strettoi, E., Raviola, E., and Dacheux, R. F. (1992). Synaptic connections of the narrow-field, bistratified rod amacrine cell (AII) in the rabbit retina. *J. Comp. Neurol.* 325:152–168.

Syed, M. M., Lee, S., He, S., and Zhou, Z. J. (2004). Stage-dependent dynamics and modulation of spontaneous waves in the developing rabbit retina. *J. Physiol.* 560:533–549.

Tomita, T. (1965). Electrophysiological study of the mechanisms subserving color coding in the fish retina. *Cold Spring Harb. Symp. Quant. Biol.* 30:559–566.

Tsukamoto, Y., Masarachia, P., Schein, S. J., and Sterling, P. (1992). Gap junctions between the pedicles of macaque foveal cones. *Vision Res.* 32:1809–1815.

Tsukamoto, Y., Morigiwa, K., Ueda, M., and Sterling, P. (2001). Microcircuits for night vision in mouse retina. *J. Neurosci.* 21:8616–8623.

Vaney, D. I. (1991). Many diverse types of retinal neurons show tracer coupling when injected with biocytin or neurobiotin. *Neurosci. Lett.* 125:187–190.

Vaney, D. I. (1994). Territorial organization of direction-selective ganglion cells in rabbit retina. *J. Neurosci.* (11 Pt. 1): 6301–6316.

Veruki, M. L., and Hartveit, E. (2002). Electrical synapses mediate signal transmission in the rod pathway of the mammalian retina. *J. Neurosci.* 22:10558–10566.

Völgyi, B., Abrams, J., Paul, D. L., and Bloomfield, S. A. (2005). Morphology and tracer coupling pattern of alpha ganglion cells in the mouse retina. *J. Comp. Neurol.* 492(1):66–77.

Völgyi, B., Deans, M. R., Paul, D. L., and Bloomfield, S. A. (2004). Convergence and segregation of the multiple rod pathways in mammalian retina. *J. Neurosci.* 24:11182–11192.

Witkovsky, P., and Dearry, A. (1991). Functional roles of dopamine in the vertebrate retina. *Prog. Ret. Res.* 11:247–292.

Xin, D., and Bloomfield, S. A. (1997). Tracer coupling pattern of amacrine and ganglion cells in the rabbit retina. *J. Comp. Neurol.* 383:512–528.

Xin, D., and Bloomfield, S. A. (1999a). Comparison of the responses of AII amacrine cells in the dark- and light-adapted rabbit retina. *Vis. Neurosci.* 16:653–665.

Xin, D., and Bloomfield, S. A. (1999b). Dark- and light-induced changes in coupling between horizontal cells in mammalian retina. *J. Comp. Neurol.* 405:75–87.

Yamada, E., and Ishikawa, T. (1965). The fine structure of the horizontal cells in some vertebrate retinae. *Cold Spring Harb. Symp. Quant. Biol.* 30:383–392.

14 Neurotransmission in the Mouse Retina

MAUREEN A. McCALL, NEAL S. PEACHEY, AND RONALD G. GREGG

Vision is initiated in rod and cone photoreceptors when light is transduced into an electrical signal. Much of our understanding of the general synaptic function of the retina has come from in vitro and in vivo studies of the salamander, cat, rabbit, and primate (Rodieck and Brening, 1983; Dowling, 1987). These elegant studies have provided a general framework of synaptic transmission (figure 14.1) that includes the vertical pathway of excitatory neurotransmission, beginning with photoreceptor (rod or cone) input to bipolar cells (BCs), followed by either a direct input from BCs to retinal ganglion cells (RGCs) or an indirect input to RGCs from BCs via an intermediary amacrine cell. In addition, lateral inhibitory pathways modulate the excitatory signaling in the vertical pathway. First, lateral inhibition occurs in the outer plexiform layer (OPL) via feedback from horizontal cells at the photoreceptor to BC synapse (Baylor et al., 1971; Shelley et al., 2006). In the inner plexiform layer (IPL), amacrine cells mediate lateral inhibition via feedback, feedforward, and serial inhibition (Cook and McReynolds, 1998; Werblin et al., 2001). Finally, there are other pathways that modulate retinal function, including dopaminergic control of light adaptation (Weiler et al., 2000), gap junctions (see chapter 13, this volume) and D-serine (Miller, 2004).

Because the morphological plan of the murine retina, described in chapter 12, is very similar to the structure of the retina in other mammalian species, it is likely that the basic function of the vertical and lateral pathways is also similar. Throughout this chapter, then, we compare the findings obtained in the murine model with those obtained in other mammalian and vertebrate models. With the advent of transgenic and knockout technology, the mouse has rapidly become an important model in which to explore the basic functional blueprint provided by earlier studies and begin to analyze the workings of the retina on a gene-by-gene basis.

This review focuses primarily on work conducted in murine mutants, both natural and induced, and in transgenics to elucidate the control of (1) excitatory synaptic transmission from the photoreceptors to the BCs in the OPL, (2) the depolarizing BC (DBC) signaling pathway, and (3) the control of feedback inhibition that shapes synaptic transmission from BCs to RGCs. The integration of these systems is manifested in the visual response properties of RGCs, which provide the basic interface between the visual environment and the rest of the CNS. Electrical communication among retinal neurons via gap junctions is a critical aspect of the modulation of synaptic transmission in the retina; because this topic is covered in chapter 13, it is not considered here.

Synaptic transmission in the outer retina

In the mouse retina, 97% of photoreceptors are rods and the remainder are cones. Although the mouse retina does not have a specialized area, such as the fovea, area centralis, or visual streak as in other mammals, there seem to be few other significant differences in the function of murine rods and cones. Rod photoreceptors are more sensitive and thus function under dark-adapted conditions and low light levels, and their responses saturate at higher light levels. Cone photoreceptors are less sensitive and function under light-adapted conditions. Rod and cone photoreceptor signaling is unique from almost every other neuron in the CNS. In the absence of light, the photoreceptors continuously release the excitatory neurotransmitter glutamate. A light stimulus results in hyperpolarization of the photoreceptor by a well-understood signal transduction cascade (for a review, see Calvert et al., 2006) that decreases intracellular cyclic guanosine monophosphate (cGMP) and closes a cGMP-gated cation channel on the photoreceptor outer segments. This causes the photoreceptor to hyperpolarize, which results in a decrease in the release of glutamate from its terminal in the OPL. Both rod and cone photoreceptors follow this general plan, although many of the molecules that function within the G protein cascades differ for each type of photoreceptor. Analysis of the molecular components of the phototransduction cascade has been aided by both their high molar concentrations and the large number of disease-causing mutations that have been identified (Chen, 2005). As for most neurons in the CNS, release of neurotransmitter from the photoreceptors is dependent on voltage-dependent calcium channels. However, unlike with most other neurons, the release of glutamate from the photoreceptors is graded,

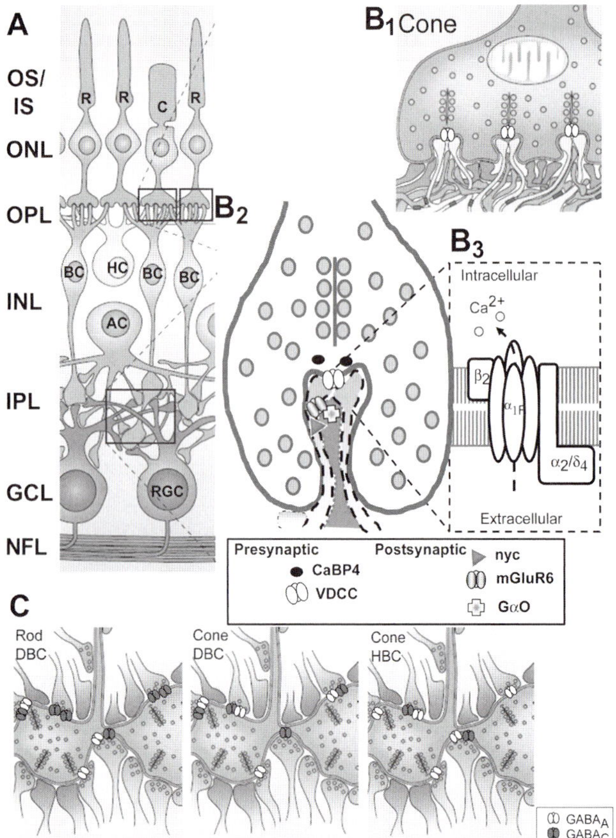

FIGURE 14.1 Schematic representation of the retinal circuit, showing the pattern of expression of the proteins that contribute to aspects of synaptic transmission discussed in this chapter. *A*, Overview of the retinal circuit. AC, amacrine cell; BC, bipolar cell; C, cone photoreceptor; GCL, ganglion cell layer; HC, horizontal cell; INL, inner nuclear layer; IPL, inner plexiform layer; NFL, nerve fiber layer; ONL, outer nuclear layer; OPL, outer plexiform layer; OS/IS outer and inner segments of the photoreceptors; R, rod photoreceptor; RGC, retinal ganglion cell. *B*, Detailed view of a cone pedicle (B_1) and a rod spherule (B_2) with their invaginating contacts from depolarizing bipolar cells and horizontal cells and their flat contacts from hyperpolarizing bipolar cells. Also included are most of the pre- and postsynaptic proteins expressed at this first synapse in the retina that are discussed in this chapter. Also shown is a detailed view of the hypothesized structure of a voltage-dependent calcium channel with the α_{1F} subunit forming the pore of this channel (B_3). CaBP4, calcium-binding protein 4; $G_{\alpha o}$, G protein αo; mGluR6, metabotropic glutamate receptor type 6; nyc, nyctalopin; VDCC, voltage-dependent Ca^{2+} channel. *C*, Detailed view of the axon terminals of bipolar cells in the inner plexiform layer. DBC, depolarizing bipolar cell; GABA, γ-aminobutyric acid; HBC, hyperpolarizing bipolar cell. (Adapted from Wässle, 2004, by permission of Macmillan Publishers Ltd.)

and this results in graded potentials in second-order neurons, the bipolar and horizontal cells.

In the dark, photoreceptors are relatively depolarized (resting potential of −40 mV; Schneeweis and Schnapf, 1999) and release glutamate continuously. This high rate of release is thought to be possible because of a unique synaptic specialization, the synaptic ribbon, present in both rod and cone terminals. This structure is thought to enable the continuous release of neurotransmitter by acting in a conveyer belt-like manner, shuttling synaptic vesicles from the readily releasable pool to the active zone. Synaptic ribbons also are present in BC axon terminals and in the terminals of the hair cells in the cochlea, which also utilize graded potentials and where synaptic release of glutamate is continuous.

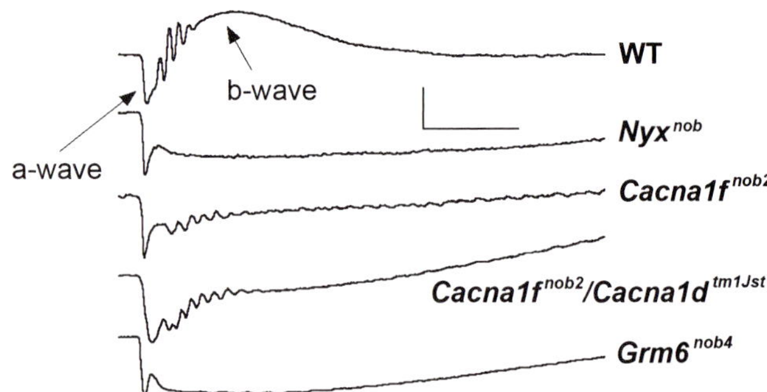

FIGURE 14.2 Dark-adapted ERGs from control and various pre- and postsynaptic mutants, with no b-wave (*nob*) phenotypes show some similarities and some differences. A C57Bl/6J (wild-type) mouse ERG response is shown at the top, and ERGs from various *nob* mutants are shown. The Nyx^{nob} mouse retina lacks expression of nyctalopin, a protein expressed on DBC dendrites. The $Cacna1f^{nob2}$ mouse retina lacks expression of the pore-forming voltage-dependent calcium channel subunit α_{1F}, expressed in photoreceptor terminals. The double mutant $Cacna1f^{nob2}/Cacna1d^{tm1Jst}$ lacks expression of both the α_{1F} and α_{1D} subunit of the voltage-dependent calcium channel, and its response is the same as that from $Cacna1f^{nob2}$. The $Grm6^{nob4}$ mouse mutant lacks expression of mGluR6 on DBC dendrites. All mutants have a normal a-wave and share the absence of a b-wave. It should be noted that there are subtle differences in the residual responses. Scale bar = 100 ms and 500 μV.

Mouse mutants of synaptic transmission in the outer retina

Photoreceptors make contact with two classes of BCs, hyperpolarizing bipolar cells (HBCs) and DBCs, which hyperpolarize or depolarize in response to reduced glutamate release (caused by a light stimulus), respectively. The activity of DBCs can be assessed noninvasively by the electroretinogram (ERG), a gross potential reflecting retinal activity to a light stimulus, recorded at the corneal surface. The wild-type (WT) murine ERG waveform, like that of most other vertebrates, has two major components relevant to synaptic transmission in the mouse retina, a- and b-waves (figure 14.2). The a-wave is the early negative-going wave that represents hyperpolarization of the photoreceptors in response to a light flash. Under dark-adapted conditions, this reflects the signal initiated in the rod photoreceptors, while under light-adapted conditions it reflects a cone photoreceptor–initiated response. The b-wave is derived from depolarization of DBCs, which may be rod or cone DBCs, depending on the adaptation condition of the retina (Robson and Frishman, 1998; Sharma et al., 2005). The ERG has been instrumental in identifying and characterizing spontaneous or genetically manipulated mice with defects in retinal signaling. In addition to being used to identify a host of mouse mutants with a-wave defects that have helped define the rod and cone opsin transduction cascades, the ERG has been used to identify mice that share another functional phenotype: a normal a-wave with an absent or greatly reduced b-wave in their dark- or light-adapted ERG. These mutants, collectively called *no b-wave*, or *nob*, have a human disease counterpart known as congenital stationary night blindness (Candille et al., 1999; Chang et al., 2006). The presence of a normal ERG a-wave indicates normal phototransduction and an absence of photoreceptor degeneration. The absent or diminished ERG b-wave indicates a defect in synaptic transmission between the photoreceptors and the DBCs.

The first spontaneous mouse mutant described with this functional phenotype was named *no b-wave* (*nob*; Pardue et al., 1998). Subsequent no b-wave mutants have been assigned the same nomenclature and numbered according to the chronology of their discovery (*nob, nob2, nob3, nob4*). Once the mutant genes were identified, and to enhance clarity, the official nomenclature now incorporates the gene name and the allele name (phenotype) for each mutant (see figure 14.1B_2 for the expression pattern of each protein, and table 14.1 for nomenclature). Because this ERG phenotype reflects a lack of synaptic activation of second-order DBCs by photoreceptors, mice with both presynaptic and postsynaptic mutations have been discovered. Mouse (and human) mutants with this functional phenotype fall into two groups: those with presynaptic mutations, involving genes expressed in photoreceptor terminals, and those with postsynaptic mutations, involving genes expressed in DBCs. Generally, mutations in postsynaptic genes have a more severe ERG phenotype and are referred to as complete congenital stationary night blindness. Presynaptic mutants retain a small ERG b-wave and are referred to as exhibiting incomplete congenital stationary night blindness. These mutant models have extended our understanding of the mechanisms that control neurotransmitter release from photoreceptors and the postsynaptic mechanisms that control BC depolarization. In the discussion that follows, we address what has been learned about synaptic transmission at the photoreceptor to BC synapse, within the DBC transduction cascade, and finally how these alterations affect the visual response properties of the RGCs in these models.

Presynaptic Mouse Mutants: Ca^{2+} and the Control of Neurotransmitter Release from Photoreceptors

Glutamate release from photoreceptors is mediated by Ca^{2+} influx through voltage-dependent calcium channels, which are heteromultimeric proteins (see figure 14.1B_3) consisting of an α_1 subunit that forms the pore of the Ca^{2+} channel and auxiliary β and $\alpha_2\delta$ subunits that modulate the Ca^{2+} current, regulate channel activation and inactivation, and, finally, control the proper assembly of the channel and its localization to the membrane (Catteral, 2000). Immunohistochemical data show that rod and cone photoreceptors express L-type voltage-dependent calcium channels, comprised of α_{1F} and α_{1D} subunits in cones and α_{1F} only in rods (Morgans et al., 2005). Although these two subunits result in channels with similar biophysical and pharmacological properties, their absence results in dramatically different functional outcomes.

Table 14.1

Nomenclature of mouse mutants discussed in this chapter

	Mutant Name	Gene Name	Protein Name	Official Mutant Name
Presynaptic mutants				
	nob2	*Cacna1f*	Ca_V1.4 (α_{1F} subunit of VDCCs)	*Cacna1f*^{nob2}
		Cacna1f	Ca_V 1.4 (α_{1F} subunit of VDCCs)	*Cacna1f*^{tm1Ntbh}
		Cacna1d	Ca_V 1.3 (α_{1D} subunit of VDCCs)	*Cacna1d*^{tm1Jst}
		Cacnb2	Ca_V 2.2 (β_2 subunit of VDCCs)	*Cacnb2*^{tm1Rgg}
		Cacna2d4	Ca_V 4.4 ($\alpha_2\delta$ subunit of VDCCs)	
		CaPB4	Calcium-binding protein 4	*Cabp4*^{tm1Kpal}
Postsynaptic mutants				
	nob	*Nyx*	Nyctalopin	*Nyx*^{nob}
		Gnao1	GαO	*Gnao1*^{tm1Lbi}
	nob4	*Grm6*	mGluR6	*Grm6*^{nob4}
		Grm6	mGluR6 (knockout)	*Grm6*^{tm1Nak}
		Gabrr1	GABA receptor C, ρ1 subunit	*Gabrr1*^{tm1Mmc}

Knockout and natural mutants of the α_{1F} subunit show a significantly reduced ERG b-wave under both light- and dark-adapted conditions, indicating that this subunit is utilized at both rod and cone photoreceptor terminals (Mansergh et al., 2005; Chang et al., 2006). The knockout of the α_{1D} subunit alone has little impact on the ERG b-wave (Wu et al., 2007). To investigate whether the residual light-adapted ERG b-wave in α_{1F} mutant mice might be due to the α_{1D} subunit, the ERG response in double mutants was characterized. The dark-adapted ERG of the α_{1F}/α_{1D} double mutant shows no significant difference from that of the single α_{1F} mutant (see figure 14.2). Therefore, the source of the residual ERG b-wave in α_{1F} mice is more complicated than initially anticipated and may involve other mechanisms, including voltage-dependent calcium channels with other α_1 subunits. In addition to mutations in α_1 subunits, loss of either the β_2 or α_2/δ_4 voltage-dependent calcium channel subunits also disrupts synaptic transmission (Ball et al., 2002; Wycisk et al., 2006). Further, the same phenotype and thus the same disruption in synaptic transmission in the OPL occur in mice with mutations in a component of the ribbon synapse, Bassoon (Dick et al., 2003), or molecules thought to modulate the voltage-dependent calcium channel CaBP4 (Haeseleer et al., 2004), and extracellular or intracellular matrix molecules (dystrophin: Pillers et al., 1999; *Rs1h*: Johnson et al., 2006) at the photoreceptor terminal.

In addition to the ERG phenotype, all these presynaptic mutants (with the exception of *Cacna1d*) share a morphological phenotype. The OPL thins and its synaptic architecture is disrupted. In all cases, the synaptic ribbons in the rod photoreceptors are disrupted, and the dendrites of horizontal cells and the rod BCs extend into the outer nuclear layer; in some cases ectopic synapses appear to form with photoreceptors (Dick et al., 2003; Chang et al., 2006; Bayley and Morgans, 2007).

Postsynaptic Mouse Mutants: Control of the Depolarizing Bipolar mGluR6 Signaling Cascade Synaptic transmission also requires detection of the changes in concentration of neurotransmitter in the synaptic cleft by the postsynaptic cells. Rod photoreceptors contact a single type of DBC (the rod DBC), while cones contact both DBCs and HBCs. The two classes of cone BCs can be distinguished by their response to the change in glutamate release following light activation of photoreceptors. HBCs use an ionotropic AMPA/kainate glutamate receptor that maintains electrical polarity (Saito and Kaneko, 1983, DeVries, 2000); for example, a hyperpolarization in the photoreceptor is matched by a hyperpolarization in HBCs. In contrast, DBCs employ a metabotropic glutamate receptor type 6 (mGluR6) mechanism (Nakajima et al., 1993), which switches the polarity of the response (from hyperpolarization in the photoreceptors to depolarization in these BCs) by opening a nonspecific cation conductance in response to the decrease in photoreceptor glutamate release (Slaughter and Miller, 1981).

Analysis of the molecular components involved in the DBC signal transduction cascade downstream of mGluR6 remains relatively incomplete (for a review, see Duvoisin et al., 2005). At this time, four mutant mouse models have been reported that disrupt signaling in DBCs. Two disrupt the mGluR itself (*Grm6*^{Tm1Nak}: Masu et al., 1995; *Grm6*^{nob4}: Pinto et al., 2007). Given their ERG phenotype, the other two, $G_{\alpha o}$ (*Gnao1*^{tm1Lbi}: Dhingra et al., 2000, 2002) and nyctalopin (*Nyx*^{nob}: Gregg et al., 2003), also must disrupt important components of the DBC signaling cascade. Again, ERG phenotypic screening has been crucial to the identification of two of these mutants (Gregg et al., 2003; Pinto et al., 2007) and to the characterization of the two knockout lines (Masu et al., 1995; Dhingra et al., 2000, 2002). All share the same ERG phenotype, a normal ERG a-wave, (photoreceptor response), and absence of the ERG b-wave (DBC) response (see figure 14.2). In fact, ERG characterization of the *Grm6*^{Tm1Nak} mouse verified that this receptor was responsible for the DBC component of the ERG b-wave (Masu et al., 1995). The absence of a b-wave in *Gnao1*^{tm1Lbi} (Valenzuela et al., 1997; Jiang et al., 1998; Dhingra et al., 2000, 2002), along with its postsynaptic expression in all DBCs, provided convincing evidence that this G protein subunit is a component of the DBC signal transduction cascade. Finally, in addition to its functional ERG phenotype, two other lines of evidence clearly place nyctalopin as an integral protein in DBC signaling. First, it is the only one of these models in which the absence of a DBC response to exogenous agonist (glutamate) administration has been verified (figure 14.3; Gregg et al., 2007). Second, a transgenic approach that expressed an EYFP-nyctalopin fusion protein only on the dendritic terminals of BCs produced a functional rescue of both the ERG b-wave (figure 14.4; Gregg et al., 2007) and other downstream visual (RGC) and anatomical defects (RGC axon terminals in the LGN) (Demas et al., 2006). While $G_{\alpha o}$ and nyctalopin are now established as elements critical to the function of the DBC signaling cascade, their exact roles and positions in this pathway remain a mystery, as does the identity of the nonspecific cation channel that is modulated in response to glutamate changes in the synaptic cleft.

In contrast to the mutant models of presynaptic neurotransmitter control described in the preceding section, retinal structure is normal at the light microscopic level in all four postsynaptic mutants (*Grm6*^{Tm1Nak}: Masu et al., 1995; Tagawa et al., 1999; *Grm6*^{nob4}: Pinto et al., 2007; *Gnao1*^{tm1Lbi}: Dhingra et al., 2000; and *Nyx*^{nob}: Pardue et al., 1998; Ball et al., 2003). In *Nyx*^{nob} and *Gnao1*^{tm1Lbi} mice, the only models studied at the electron microscopy level, both pre- and postsynaptic struc-

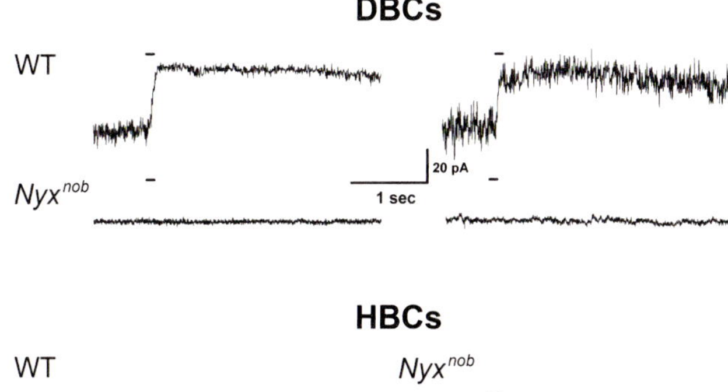

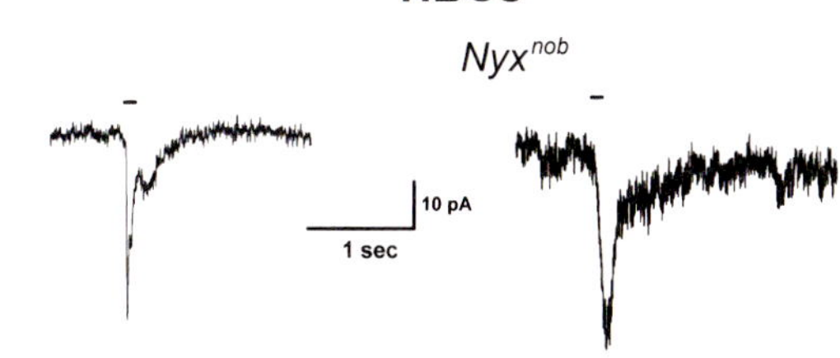

FIGURE 14.3 DBCs in Nyx^{nob} mouse retinal slices do not respond to exogenous application of the agonist glutamate. In WT mice, puffs of glutamate directed onto BC dendrites elicit robust outward currents in rod and cone DBCs and inward currents in HBCs. In Nyx^{nob} mice, HBC responses are identical to those in WT mice. In contrast, no response could be elicited in any DBC in Nyx^{nob} retina. The bar above each current trace indicates the glutamate puff duration (100 ms). (Adapted from Gregg et al., 2007.)

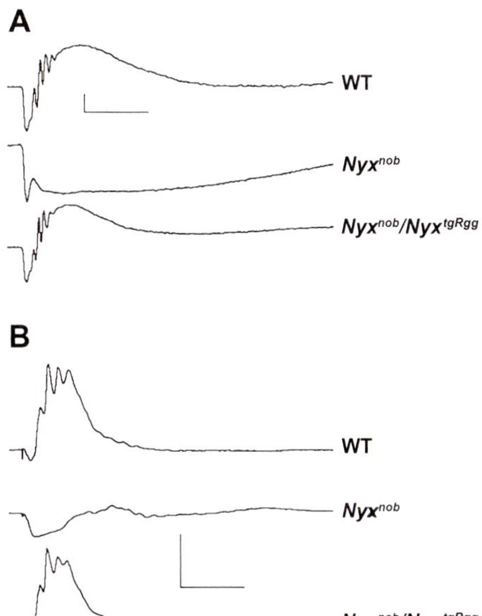

FIGURE 14.4 Expression of an EYFP: nyctalopin rescue transgene in BCs restores the b-wave component of the ERG in Nyx^{nob} mice. The transgene construct consisted of an 11-Kb fragment from the $GABA_C$ ρ1 gene, which drives expression of a murine nyctalopin cDNA with EYFP inserted after amino acid 19. *A*, Representative dark-adapted ERG waveforms of WT, Nyx^{nob}, and Nyx^{nob}/Nyx^{tgRgg} mice at a flash intensity of 1.4 log cd s/m^2. *B*, Light-adapted ERG waveforms of the same WT, Nyx^{nob}, and Nyx^{nob}/Nyx^{tg} mice evoked on a steady rod-adapting background (1.5 log cd/m^2) and with a flash intensity of 1.9 log cd s/m^2. (Adapted from Gregg et al., 2007.)

tures in the OPL are normal (Dhingra et al., 2000; Pardue et al., 2001). Finally, we know that nyctalopin expression is not required for expression of these other proteins, because its absence does not eliminate expression of either mGluR6 or $G_{\alpha o}$ (Ball et al., 2003).

Altered outer retina neurotransmission results in complex retinal ganglion cell phenotypes

The impact of these outer retinal defects on the retinal output has been explored by assessing the changes in the visual response properties of mutant RGCs relative to WT RGC function. These downstream effects represent the integration of the individual components of the retinal circuit by the RGCs. Both in vivo and in vitro studies have characterized the light-evoked responses of RGCs in *Cacna1f*^{nob2}, *Grm6*^{nob4}, and Nyx^{nob} mice. In vitro, RGC responses have been studied directly using multielectrode arrays (Demas et al., 2006; Renteria et al., 2006; Pinto et al., 2007) or indirectly analyzed by examining the visually evoked responses in the superior colliculus (SC), a structure that receives direct RGC synaptic input (Sugihara et al., 1997; Mansergh et al., 2005). In vivo, RGC responses have been evaluated using extracellular recording of the spiking activity of individual RGC axons. A broad generality can be made at this time: mutants with presynaptic defects have RGCs whose receptive fields (RFs) can be categorized as responding to either the onset (ON) or the offset (OFF) of a light stimulus. In contrast, mutants with postsynaptic defects that differentially affect the DBC signaling cascade lack normal ON RGC responses, although the effects on OFF RGC responses varies (Demas et al., 2006; Renteria et al., 2006; Pinto et al., 2007).

Retinal ganglion cell responses in mutants with outer plexiform layer presynaptic defects

RGCs responses in *Cacna1f*^{nob2} mice, which lack the voltage-dependent calcium channel α_{1F} subunit (Cav1.4), are surprisingly normal. At both light- and dark-adapted levels, *Cacna1f*^{nob2} RGCs have RFs with center-surround organization that can be classified as ON- or OFF-center (figure 14.5) (Chang et al., 2006). The most prominent defect observed under light-adapted conditions is a decrease in the spontaneous activity, along with a compression of the dynamic range of the ON-center *Cacna1f*^{nob2} RGCs compared to WT (Chang et al., 2006). The *Cacna1f*^{nob2} OFF-center RGCs are indistinguishable from WT OFF-center RGCs. Thus, there appears to be a specific deficit in the ON pathway in this mutant consistent with the reduction in its cone ERG b-wave (Sharma et al., 2005). Although the primary defect in visual processing occurs at the photoreceptor-to-BC synapse, *Cacna1f* is expressed in the inner retina, and therefore some changes at the level of the RGC could be due to downstream

A *Cacna1f nob2*

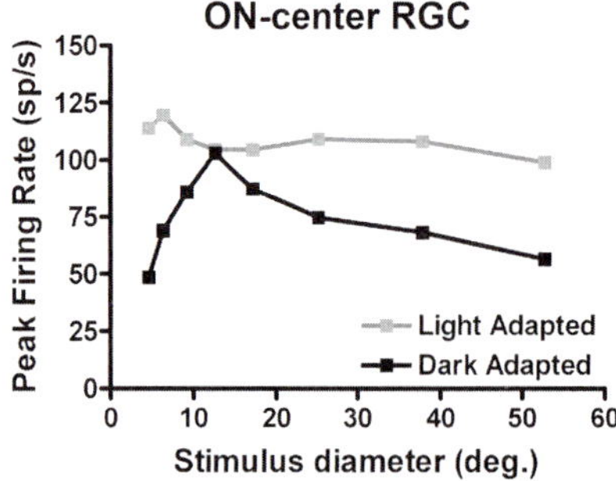

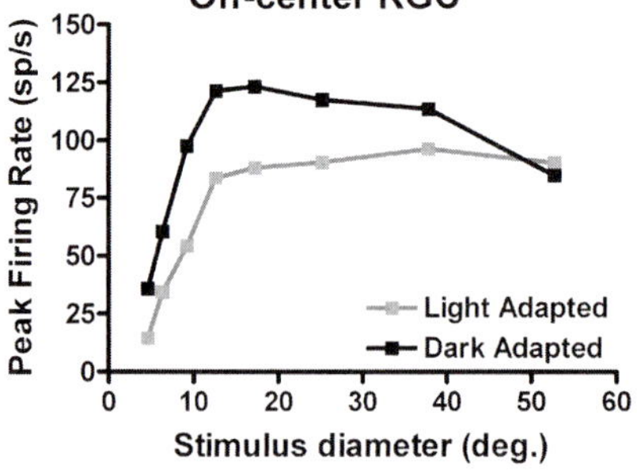

B WT

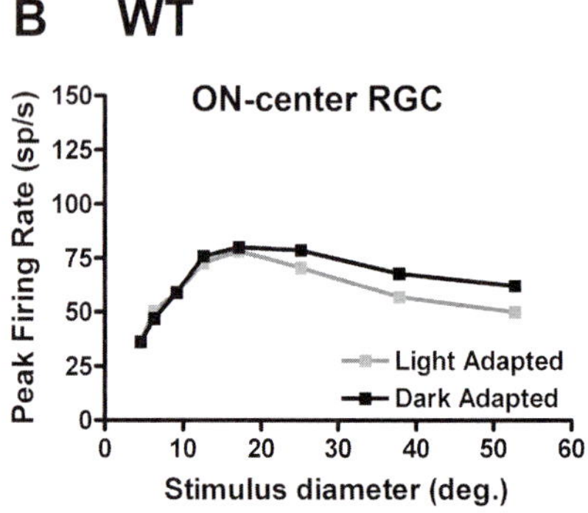

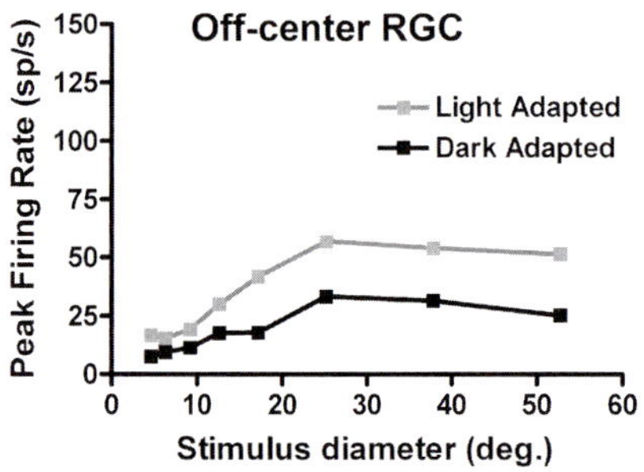

FIGURE 14.5 Visual responses of RGCs at light- and dark-adapted levels in *Cacna1f*^{nob2} RGCs show similar receptive field (RF) organization to WT controls. The RF organization of ON- (*left*) and OFF-center (*right*) RGCs in *Cacna1f*^{nob2} (*A*) and WT mice (*B*) was assessed with spots of standing contrast whose diameter varied from smaller than the RF center, to matching the RF center, to covering both the RF center and its antagonistic surround. An area response function (ARF) was generated for each RGC by plotting the cell's peak firing rate as a function of spot diameter. At both light-adapted (*gray traces*) and dark-adapted (*black traces*) levels, the representative curves show that RGC responses in the *Cacna1f*^{nob2} mice are as robust as in WT mice, and their RF organizations are similar.

alterations in IPL synaptic processing. In contrast to these effects, Mansergh et al. (2005) reported a loss of all visually evoked responses in the SC of the *Cacna1f*^{tmNtbh} knockout mouse, which implies there is no visually evoked activity in either ON or OFF RGCs. Although responses in the SC from *Cacna1f*^{nob2} have not been evaluated, a lack of visually evoked activity seems unlikely, given the robust RGC responses in this mutant (Chang et al., 2006). The reason for the differences in these two mutants with apparently identical genetic defects is unclear, as expression of the protein is eliminated in both (Mansergh et al., 2005; Chang et al., 2006). Although the mutations are on different genetic backgrounds (SV129 for the *Cacna1f*^{tmNtbh} knockout mouse and C57Bl/6J for the *Cacna1f*^{nob2} mouse), these phenotypic differences may correspond to the different clinical entities that have been associated with human *CACNA1F* mutations (congenital stationary night blindness type 2: Bech-Hansen et al., 1998; cone dystrophy: Jalkanen et al., 2006; Aland Island eye disease: Jalkanen et al., 2007).

Another mouse mutant that disrupts neurotransmitter release from photoreceptor terminals is knockout of the β_2 subunit of voltage-dependent calcium channels, *Cacnb2*^{tmRgg}. This mutant shares the ERG (Ball et al., 2003) and morphological (Gregg et al., 2008) phenotype characteristic of *Cacna1f*^{nob2} mice that lack normal release of glutamate from photoreceptors. Similar to what occurs in *Cacna1f*^{nob2}, RGCs in *Cacnb2*^{tmRgg} mice also can be classified as ON and OFF and have a well-defined center-surround RF organization. Again, OFF-center RGC responses are similar to those in WT animals. However, differences in RGC response properties in these two mutants appear at dark-adapted levels. Under these conditions, visual responses in *Cacnb2*^{tmRgg} RGCs are significantly reduced (M. A. McCall, unpublished observations) compared to *Cacna1f*^{nob2} and WT RGCs.

The subtlety of the changes in visual processing in the RGCs of these voltage-dependent calcium channel mutants strongly suggests that a scenario in which a single voltage-dependent calcium channel subunit combination controls synaptic transmission in rod versus cone photoreceptors is too simplistic. Instead, the differential effects on RF organization and visual responses of RGCs may reflect the presence of other subunits or the shuffling of subunits in the absence of expression of the primary subunit. There is support for this hypothesis from the characterization of Ca^{2+} currents in mouse BCs (Berntson et al., 2003). Alternatively, there could be no difference at the level of OPL, but rather alteration in the voltage-dependent calcium channels could occur in the inner retinal circuits (Pan, 2001; Cui et al., 2003; Ma and Pan, 2003), changing neurotransmitter release and synaptic transmission. What is needed now is a strategy in which the voltage-dependent calcium channels are expressed selectively in either the outer or the inner retina, but not both. For example, a transgenic rescue of each photoreceptor voltage-dependent calcium channel phenotype could provide insight into a definitive role for these subunits in outer versus inner retinal synaptic transmission.

Retinal ganglion cell responses in mouse mutants with postsynaptic defects in depolarizing bipolar cell signaling

With the exception of the *Nyx*^{nob} mouse, the analysis of BC responses has only used the ERG, and thus assessment of outer retinal synaptic function has been restricted to DBC signaling. All four mutants, *Grm6*^{nob4} and *Grm6*^{tm1Nak}, *Gnao1*^{tm1Lbi}, and *Nyx*^{nob}, share the same functional phenotype, a disruption in signaling that leads to DBC depolarization and b-wave generation. RGC visual response properties have been analyzed in both *Grm6* and *Nyx* mutants. The *Gnao1*^{tm1Lbi} mutant survives for only a few weeks after birth, complicating in vivo analyses. The RGC phenotype of the spontaneous mGluR6 mutant (*Grm6*^{nob4}) and the knockout (*Grm6*^{tm1Nak}) are similar and reflect the expected defect in synaptic transmission through the ON pathway (Renteria et al., 2006; Pinto et al., 2007). In both mutants there are spontaneously active RGCs that are not visually responsive, a result never found in WT retinas (Chang et al., 2006; Pinto et al., 2007). Visually responsive RGCs can be classified as ON, OFF, or ON/OFF relative to their response to the onset or offset of a full-field visual stimulus. In the few instances when an ON response could be identified in both *Grm6* mutants, its response onset was significantly delayed and its peak firing rate was significantly reduced compared to what is seen in WT animals. In both *Grm6* mutants, the characterizations via either multielectrode arrays in vitro (Renteria et al., 2006) or both multielectrode arrays in vitro and extracellular recording in vivo (Pinto et al., 2007) yielded similar results: OFF-center RGCs have RF center-surround organization similar to that of WT cells. The absence of signaling through the ON pathway in the context of normal function in the OFF pathway is consistent with a dysfunction of the mGluR6 receptor, which mediates signaling only in DBCs.

The *Nyx*^{nob} mouse has the same ERG phenotype as the *Grm6* mutants. In addition, *Nyx*^{nob} DBCs do not respond to exogenous application of agonist, but their HBCs do (see figure 14.3; Gregg et al., 2007). Thus, at the level of the BC, the functional phenotypes should be the same. However, the absence of nyctalopin produces a dramatically different effect on RGC response properties. Although the percentage of visually unresponsive *Nyx*^{nob} RGCs (Demas et al., 2006) is the same as in *Grm6*^{nob4} (Pinto et al., 2007), none of the *Nyx*^{nob} RGCs have classic center-surround RF organization (Vessey et al., 2005). Further, the spontaneous activity of the majority of *Nyx*^{nob} RGCs shows a rhythmic bursting at about 4 Hz (Demas et al., 2006), whereas spontaneous activity in both *Grm6*^{nob4} and WT RGCs is random (Pinto et al., 2007).

One hypothesis to account for this difference between *Grm6*^{nob4} and *Nyx*^{nob} RGCs is that nyctalopin is expressed in the IPL as well as in the OPL (Bayley and Morgans, 2007), whereas mGluR6 is expressed only in the OPL. However, transgenic expression of an EYFP nyctalopin fusion protein only on the tips of DBC dendrites of *Nyx*^{nob} mice restores not only the ERG b-wave but all spontaneous and visually evoked response properties of *Nyx*^{nob} RGCs to WT (Demas et al., 2006; Gregg et al., 2007). Thus, another mechanism must underlie these significant differences in downstream visual processing in the *Nyx*^{nob} mutant that ostensibly shares the same DBC functional phenotype as the *Grm6* mutants. If the axon terminals of *Nyx*^{nob} DBCs are in a constitutively more depolarized state than *Grm6*^{nob4} or *Grm6*^{tm1Nak} DBCs, this should alter the release properties of glutamate in the IPL. If this were the case, the mechanism might resemble the following scenario. In the dark in the WT retina, mGluR6 is activated by continuous glutamate release from the photoreceptors, and $G_{\alpha o}$ is free to modulate the unknown nonspecific cation channel, keeping it in a closed state and the DBC relatively hyperpolarized. Upon light stimulation, photoreceptor glutamate release is reduced, $G_{\alpha o}$ is sequestered as part of a tripartite G protein/mGluR6 complex, and the nonspecific cation channel opens, depolarizing the DBC. During the release of $G_{\alpha o}$ there is an exchange of GDP for GTP, but the exact nature of what controls the cation channel remains unknown. In *Grm6* mutants, the absence of mGluR6 expression should allow $G_{\alpha o}$ to be free to bind GTP and keep the cation channel in a constitutively closed state and the DBC relatively hyperpolarized, consistent with experimental observations (Nawy, 1999). If nyctalopin were required for the closure of the cation channel, then its absence in *Nyx*^{nob} mice would result in more depolarized DBCs. At this time, there is no empirical evidence for this scenario, and the differences between RGCs in *Nyx*^{nob} and the *Grm6* mutants await an understanding of the function of nyctalopin in this pathway.

Control of the synaptic output of bipolar cells by $GABA_C$R-mediated inhibition

Murine BCs have been divided into three functional classes, rod DBCs and cone DB or HBCs (for a review, see Sterling, 1995). Cone photoreceptors contact both cone DB and HBCs, which depolarize in response to increments and decrements of light intensity, respectively (Kolb and Famiglietti, 1974; Nelson et al., 1978, 1981). Cone BCs can be further divided into four types of HBC and five types of DBC, each distinguished by the morphology of their dendritic and axonal terminals, the IPL sublamina within which their axon terminals stratify, and, finally, by protein expression (Ghosh et al., 2004; Pignatelli and Strettoi, 2004). Rod photoreceptors contact a single type of rod DBC that depolarizes in response to a light increment (Bloomfield and Dacheux, 2001; but see Wu et al., 2004). Thus, visual information travels along these two sets of parallel pathways (reviewed by Wässle, 2004). One is segregated in terms of the light levels at which they function, with the rod pathway mediating visual function at low light levels and the cone pathway mediating vision at higher light levels. The second level of segregation occurs within the cone pathway, where cone photoreceptors signal to both DB and HBCs (Murakami et al., 1975). These functional pathways are thought to remain segregated, conveying information about the overall light level (rod and cone) and, within the cone pathway, information about intensity increments and decrements within the visual scene.

The differences in the kinetics of the photoreceptor output to rod and cone BCs have been characterized in other species and found to be temporally distinct. Two mechanisms cause these kinetic differences. First, there are distinct mechanisms of neurotransmitter release that cause synaptic transmission from cones to BCs to be faster than from rods to BCs. Second, there are distinct complements of postsynaptic glutamate receptors that enhance this temporal difference (Schnapf and Copenhagen, 1982; Ashmore and Copenhagen, 1983; Cadetti et al., 2005; Li and DeVries, 2006). While the differences in the kinetics of neurotransmitter release in murine rod and cone photoreceptors have not been thoroughly documented, their BCs utilize the same postsynaptic receptors, mGluR6 on rod and cone DBCs and AMPA/kainate receptors on cone HBCs (Nakanishi et al., 1998; Hack et al., 2001; Snellman and Nawy, 2004). Thus, the murine retina likely follows similar synaptic mechanisms in shaping photoreceptor-to-BC synaptic transmission.

Excitatory responses within the retina are shaped not only by synaptic release kinetics and the complement of postsynaptic glutamate receptors but also by inhibition mediated by GABA and glycine and their receptors (for a review, see Wässle, 2004). The role of inhibition in shaping excitatory transmission in the retina has been recognized for decades in a variety of species (Dowling, 1987); however, this is a developing area in the mouse, which is aided by our ability to eliminate specific receptor subunits using gene-targeting approaches. The presence of many GABA and glycine receptor subunits expressed in specific patterns within the IPL (Wässle et al., 1998; Haverkamp et al., 2004), as well as kinetic differences and sensitivities to agonists across these receptors, implies important functional differences. To date, the most thorough analyses have been undertaken for the role of the GABAc receptor ($GABA_C$R) in shaping both BC and RGC output, because of its restricted expression on BCs, the availability of relatively selective antagonists, and the production of a knockout mouse for the GABACρ1 subunit, which eliminates all $GABA_C$Rs in the retina (McCall et al., 2002), but see recent work of the Wässle lab (Ivanova et al., 2006; Majumdar et al., 2007; Weiss et al., 2008).

That BC outputs are shaped by presynaptic inhibitory input from GABAergic and glycinergic amacrine cells is well established in a number of species, including mouse (Lukasiewicz and Werblin, 1994; Pan and Lipton, 1995; Dong and Werblin, 1998; Euler and Masland, 2000). In the IPL, this is accomplished by activation of functionally distinct $GABA_A$, $GABA_C$, and glycine receptors on the axon terminals of the BCs (Euler and Wässle, 1998; Shields et al., 2000; Eggers and Lukasiewicz, 2006a, 2006b). Studies using exogenous application of agonists to reveal the types of receptors that mediate inhibitory currents suggest that $GABA_A$, $GABA_C$, and glycine receptor input varies with functional BC class (rod DBC, cone DBC or HBC) (Euler and Wässle, 1998; Shields et al., 2000; Ivanova et al., 2006; Eggers et al., 2007). Because the kinetics of each GABAergic and glycinergic receptor vary, there is the expectation that each provides a distinct modulation of BC output. Exogenous agonist application, however, cannot discriminate among differences in neurotransmitter release, receptor distribution, or circuitry interactions, each of which contributes to how much inhibition is activated from a given receptor when a light stimulus evokes inhibition. Thus, the combined use of stimulus control, receptor antagonists, and, when possible, knockout mice provides a more complete picture of the role of a particular receptor in synaptic transmission. Such an approach has been used to study the role of the $GABA_C$R in the control of the synaptic output of BCs and in the visual response properties of RGCs in the retina (McCall et al., 2002; Eggers and Lukasiewicz, 2006a, 2006b; Eggers et al., 2007).

$GABA_C$R-mediated inhibition was shown to be important in shaping BC output in several species using an arsenal of pharmacological agents (for a review, see Lukasiewicz et al., 2004). However, the availability of $GABA_CR^{tmMmc}$ knockout ($GABA_C$R) null mice has greatly extended these results in two ways. First, light stimulation has been used to induce inhibitory postsynaptic potentials in the BCs, and second, the absence of $GABA_CRs$ throughout the retina permits insight into its role in retinal circuitry both in vitro and in vivo. As with all knockout mice, one must establish that the observed effects of the knockout do not result from secondary effects. For example, is it possible that the absence of gene expression has developmental consequences? For this knockout model, the developmental consequences might include altered expression of other GABAR subunits or the formation of receptors with novel subunit composition, which could have altered kinetics. However, the $GABA_CR$ null mouse is an example of a well-behaved knockout. The likelihood of developmental alterations is relatively low because it normally is expressed relatively late in development, first detected around postnatal day 6 (Greka et al., 2000), near the time that rhodopsin is expressed and visual signals initiate activity in the retina. Elimination of the expression of the ρ1 subunit of the $GABA_CR$, also causes loss of retinal expression of the ρ2 and ρ3 subunits, so that formation of novel GABA receptors is unlikely (McCall et al., 2002).

These aspects have been confirmed functionally by demonstrating that no $GABA_CR$-mediated currents could be evoked by either exogenous agonist application (McCall et al., 2002; Eggers et al., 2007) or light stimulation (Eggers et al., 2007). Finally, the $GABA_AR$- and glycine receptor–mediated currents in $GABA_CR$ null BCs have similar kinetics and overall size as pharmacologically isolated currents in WT BCs (McCall et al., 2002; Eggers et al., 2007). Thus, this knockout fulfills all the necessary criteria to examine its role in synaptic transmission in the inner retina and its downstream effects on retinal processing at the level of the RGCs.

Comparisons of GABA- and light-evoked inhibitory currents in WT and $GABA_CR$ null mice have led to the following conclusions about the role of GABAergic and glycinergic inhibition in shaping the synaptic output of the three BC functional classes in the mouse retina. Glycine and $GABA_ARs$ shape the peak amplitude, while $GABA_CRs$ contribute to the time course of rod DBC inhibition (Eggers and Lukasiewicz, 2006a). Across the three functional BC classes, unique combinations of $GABA_C$, $GABA_A$, and glycine receptors contribute to inhibition. Specifically, large, slow, $GABA_C$ receptor-mediated inputs dominate rod DBC GABA- and light-evoked inhibitory postsynaptic currents (McCall et al., 2002; Eggers and Lukasiewicz, 2006a; Eggers et al., 2007). Slow $GABA_C$ and fast $GABA_A$ receptor-mediated inputs combine about equally and create inhibitory currents with shorter decays in cone DBCs relative to rod DBCs. Glycinergic inhibition is absent in cone DBCs and contributes relatively little, relative to GABAergic inhibition, in rod DBCs (Ivanova et al., 2006; Eggers et al., 2007). Glycinergic inhibition is most prominent relative to GABAergic input in the inhibitory responses of cone HBCs when the retina is dark-adapted, owing to inputs from the AII amacrine cell (Eggers et al., 2007). Under pharmacological conditions where the AII circuit is inactivated, which may mimic a light-adapted condition, inhibitory input to the cone HBCs is modified and comes directly through the cone pathway. Under these conditions $GABA_AR$ inhibition dominates, although a small contribution from $GABA_CRs$ is present. Thus, unique presynaptic receptor combinations mediate distinct forms of inhibition, which selectively modulate BC outputs across functional classes. This differential inhibitory input could work to enhance distinctions among these parallel retinal signals that are established by differences in the time course of their excitatory inputs that were discussed earlier.

$GABA_CR$-mediated feedback inhibition alters the visually and electrically evoked responses of ON-center retinal ganglion cells

Depolarization of BCs opens voltage-dependent calcium channels (Berntson et al., 2003; Awatramani et al., 2005), triggering the release of glutamate from their terminals in the IPL, which is translated into spiking activity in the third-order RGCs. Relative to the input of RGCs, $GABA_CR$ feedback inhibition onto the axon terminal of the BC is considered a form of presynaptic inhibition. Presynaptic inhibition has been shown in a number of systems in both invertebrates and vertebrates to be a critical factor that regulates neurotransmitter release probability (reviewed in MacDermott et al., 1999). In general, neurotransmitter release from a presynaptic neuron stimulates a postsynaptic inhibitory neuron, which feeds back and activates presynaptic inhibitory ionotropic receptors and induces a hyperpolarizing Cl^- current in the original output cell. This reduces Ca^{2+} influx, regulating neurotransmitter release (Dudel and Kuffler, 1961). In the retina, the presynaptic BC axon terminal releases glutamate, which provides an excitatory input to both the RGC and GABAergic amacrine cells. The $GABA_CR$ on the BC axon terminal detects a reciprocal input from the GABAergic amacrine cell and mediates feedback inhibition. To determine the role of this feedback inhibition in shaping the synaptic output of BCs, the visual response properties of RGCs in $GABA_CR$ null and WT mice were evaluated using both visually and electrically evoked stimuli. As described in this chapter, presynaptic inhibition mediated by $GABA_CRs$ differentially shapes inhibition among functional classes of BCs, and this would be expected to shape excitatory transmission between BCs and RGCs. Thus, under light-adapted conditions, ON-center RGCs, which receive direct input from cone DBCs, should be differentially affected compared to OFF-center RGCs when $GABA_CR$ null and WT responses are compared.

It has been observed that dynamic range and sensitivity differ between ON- and OFF-center RGCs (Chichilnisky and Kalmar, 2002; Zaghloul et al., 2003), but the synaptic mechanisms underlying these effects had not been explored. Differences in the visual response properties of $GABA_CR$ null and WT RGCs show that this feedback inhibition regulates the ability of the ON-center RGCs to encode light intensity increments and the dynamic range of their light-evoked responses (McCall et al., 2002; Sagdullaev et al., 2006). When the dynamic range was assessed using electrical stimulation of the OPL, a similar difference was noted. WT ON-center RGCs had a wider dynamic range than their counterparts in $GABA_CR$ null mice. This similarity strongly suggests that the changes observed result from $GABA_CR$-mediated control of synaptic transmission from BC to RGC. Consistent with the differential distribution of $GABA_CR$-mediated inhibition across functional BC classes, the visual response properties in OFF-center $GABA_CR$ null and WT RGCs are similar. This implies that $GABA_CR$ presynaptic inhibition regulates glutamate release from DBCs, but HBC output is not similarly controlled.

There is strong evidence that $GABA_CR$ input reduces glutamate release from DBCs. In the absence of $GABA_CR$ expression or in the WT retina when the BC circuit is driven by a very strong stimulus, glutamate release is enhanced, leading to spillover activation of perisynaptic NMDA receptors on ON-center RGCs (Sagdullaev et al., 2006). In addition, we have recently discovered that when stimuli of different luminance contrast are used to stimulate the ON-center cells, $GABA_CR$-mediated inhibition regulates surround inhibition, primarily when contrast is low (figure 14.6; Yarbrough et al., 2008). This difference is consistent with the same underlying mechanism regulating neurotransmitter release and spillover activation in encoding luminance contrast. The $GABA_CR$ regulation of neurotransmission at the BC-to-RGC synapse extends the dynamic range of the RGCs and enables this synapse to encode a wide range of light intensities and luminance contrasts.

The laboratory mouse is a relatively recent addition to the species used to characterize retinal circuitry. However, it is now clear that the morphology and much of the circuitry of the murine retina are similar to those in other species, including primates, even if mice lack a fovea or area of central retinal specialization. The power of forward and reverse genetics (Pinto and Enroth-Cugell, 2000), combined with gene targeting and transgenic and mutagenic approaches, is unique to the mouse and is greatly extending current knowledge regarding the role of specific molecules in visual function. In this chapter, we have highlighted just two areas where this approach has been fruitful, namely, to begin to analyze the role of signaling across the OPL and to understand the role of one inhibitory receptor in the IPL. These studies already have yielded surprises; no doubt, further surprises await us in the future.

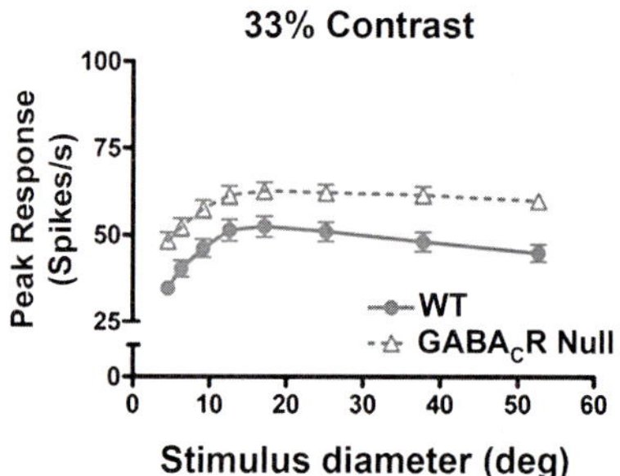

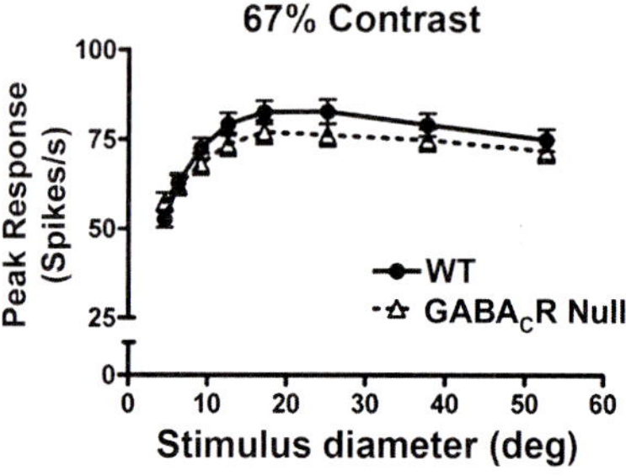

FIGURE 14.6 WT ON-center RGCs have smaller light-evoked responses throughout the RF than $GABA_CR$ null RGCs at low but not high luminance contrast. The RF organization of ON-center RGCs in WT and $GABA_CR$ null cells was assessed using spots of standing contrast (33% or 67%) and varying diameter on a $20 cd/m^2$ background. An ARF was generated for each RGC by plotting the cell's peak firing rate as a function of spot diameter. Average ARFs for WT and null mice at two different contrasts, 33% (*top*: WT, $n = 39$; null, $n = 44$) and 67% contrast (*bottom*: WT, $n = 35$; null, $n = 51$) show that, at low contrast, WT ON-center RGCs have significantly lower light-evoked responses than null cells across all spot sizes. (Repeated measures ANOVA for WT vs. null at 33%, genotype $P < 0.001$.) (Adapted from Yarbrough et al., 2008.)

ACKNOWLEDGMENTS Work was supported by NIH grant nos. EY014701 (MAMc), R24 EY15638 (NSP), and EY12354 (RGG) and by RPB awards to the Departments of Ophthalmology and Visual Science, University of Louisville, and the Department of Ophthalmology, Cleveland Clinic Lerner College of Medicine of Case Western Reserve University. The authors acknowledge the contributions of their laboratory staff and collaborators whose work is described in this review, in particular Drs. S. L. Ball, E. D. Eggers, M. T. Pardue, B. T. Sagdullaev, K. A. Vessey, and G. L. Yarbrough. The authors especially thank Dr. P. D. Lukasiewicz for his thoughtful comments on this chapter.

REFERENCES

ASHMORE, J. F., and COPENHAGEN, D. R. (1983). An analysis of transmission from cones to hyperpolarizing bipolar cells in the retina of the turtle. *J. Physiol.* 340:569–597.

AWATRAMANI, G. B., TURECEK, R., and TRUSSELL, L. O. (2005). Staggered development of GABAergic and glycinergic transmission in the MNTB. *J. Neurophysiol.* 93:819–828.

BALL, S. L., PARDUE, M. T., MCCALL, M. A., GREGG, R. G., and PEACHEY, N. S. (2003). Immunohistochemical analysis of the outer plexiform layer in the *nob* mouse shows no abnormalities. *Vis. Neurosci.* 20:267–272.

Ball, S. L., Powers, P. A., Shin, H.-S., Morgans, C. W., Peachey, N. S., and Gregg, R. G. (2002). Role of the β2 subunit of voltage-dependent calcium channels in the retinal outer plexiform layer. *Invest. Ophthalmol. Vis. Sci.* 43:1595–1603.

Bayley, P. R., and Morgans, C. W. (2007). Rod bipolar cells and horizontal cells form displaced synaptic contacts with rods in the outer nuclear layer of the *nob2* retina. *J. Comp Neurol.* 500:286–298.

Baylor, D. A., Fuortes, M. G. F., and O'Bryan, P. M. (1971). Receptive fields of cones in the retina of the turtle. *J. Physiol.* 214:265–294.

Bech-Hansen, N. T., Naylor, M. J., Maybaum, T. A., Pearce, W. G., Koop, B., Fishman, G. A., Mets, M., Musarella, M. A., and Boycott, K. M. (1998). Loss-of-function mutations in a calcium-channel alpha1-subunit gene in Xp11.23 cause incomplete x-linked congenital stationary night blindness. *Nat. Genet.* 19(3):264–267.

Berntson, A., Taylor, W. R., and Morgans, C. W. (2003). Molecular identity, synaptic localization, and physiology of calcium channels in retinal bipolar cells. *J. Neurosci. Res.* 71:146–151.

Bloomfield, S. A., and Dacheux, R. F. (2001). Rod vision: Pathways and processing in the mammalian retina. *Prog. Retin. Eye Res.* 20:351–384.

Cadetti, L., Tranchina, D., and Thoreson, W. B. (2005). A comparison of release kinetics and glutamate receptor properties in shaping rod-cone differences in EPSC kinetics in the salamander retina. *J. Physiol.* 569:773–788.

Calvert, P. D., Strissel, K. J., Schiesser, W. E., Pugh, E. N., Jr., and Arshavsky, V. Y. (2006). Light-driven translocation of signaling proteins in vertebrate photoreceptors. *Trends Cell Biol.* 16:560–568.

Candille, S. I., Pardue, M. T., McCall, M. A., Peachey, N. S., and Gregg, R. G. (1999). Localization of the mouse *nob* (*no b-wave*) gene to the centromeric region of the X chromosome. *Invest. Ophthalmol. Vis. Sci.* 40:2748–2751.

Catterall, W. A. (2000). Structure and regulation of voltage-gated Ca^{2+} channels. *Annu. Rev. Cell. Dev. Biol.* 16:521–555.

Chang, B., Heckenlively, J. R., Bayley, P. R., Brecha, N. C., Davisson, M. T., Hawes, N. L., Hirano, A. A., Hurd, R. E., Ikeda, A., et al. (2006). The *nob2* mouse, a null mutation in *Cacna1f*: Anatomical and functional abnormalities in the outer retina and their consequences on ganglion cell visual responses. *Vis. Neurosci.* 23:11–24.

Chen, C. K. (2005). The vertebrate phototransduction cascade: Amplification and termination mechanisms. *Rev. Physiol. Biochem. Pharmacol.* 154:101–121.

Chichilnisky, E. J., and Kalmar, R. S. (2002). Functional asymmetries in ON and OFF ganglion cells of primate retina. *J. Neurosci.* 22:2737–2747.

Cook, P. B., and McReynolds, J. S. (1998). Lateral inhibition in the inner retina is important for spatial tuning of ganglion cells. *Nat. Neurosci.* 1:714–719.

Cui, J., Ma, Y. P., Lipton, S. A., and Pan, Z. H. (2003). Glycine receptors and glycinergic synaptic input at the axon terminals of mammalian retinal rod bipolar cells. *J. Physiol.* 553:895–909.

Demas, J., Sagdullaev, B. T., Green, E., Jaubert-Miazza, L., McCall, M. A., Gregg, R. G., Wong, R. O., and Guido, W. (2006). Failure to maintain eye-specific segregation in *nob*, a mutant with abnormally patterned retinal activity. *Neuron* 50:247–259.

DeVries, S. H. (2000). Bipolar cells use kainate and AMPA receptors to filter visual information into separate channels. *Neuron* 28:847–856.

Dhingra, A., Jiang, M., Wang, T. L., Lyubarsky, A., Savchenko, A., Bar-Yehuda, T., Sterling, P., Birnbaumer, L., and Vardi, N. (2002). Light response of retinal ON bipolar cells requires a specific splice variant of Gαo. *J. Neurosci.* 22:4878–4884.

Dhingra, A., Lyubarsky, A., Jiang, M., Pugh, E. N., Jr., Birnbaumer, L., Sterling, P., and Vardi, N. (2000). The light response of ON bipolar neurons requires $G_{\alpha o}$. *J. Neurosci.* 20: 9053–9058.

Dick, O., tom Dieck, S., Altrock, W. D., Ammermuller, J., Weiler, R., Garner, C. C., Gundelfinger, E. D., and Brandstatter, J. H. (2003). The presynaptic active zone protein bassoon is essential for photoreceptor ribbon synapse formation in the retina. *Neuron* 37:775–786.

Dong, C. J., and Werblin, F. S. (1998). Temporal contrast enhancement via GABAC feedback at bipolar terminals in the tiger salamander retina. *J. Neurophysiol.* 79:2171–2180.

Dowling, J. E. (1987). *The retina: An approachable part of the brain.* Cambridge, MA: Belknap Press of Harvard University Press.

Dudel, J., and Kuffler, S. W. (1961). Presynaptic inhibition at the crayfish neuromuscular junction. *J. Physiol.* 155:543–562.

Duvoisin, R. M., Morgans, C. M., and Taylor, W. R. (2005). The mGluR6 receptors in the retina: Analysis of a unique G-protein signalling pathway. *Cell Sci. Rev.* 2(2):225–242.

Eggers, E. D., and Lukasiewicz, P. D. (2006a). GABA(A), GABA(C) and glycine receptor-mediated inhibition differentially affects light-evoked signalling from mouse retinal rod bipolar cells. *J. Physiol.* 572:215–225.

Eggers, E. D., and Lukasiewicz, P. D. (2006b). Receptor and transmitter release properties set the time course of retinal inhibition. *J. Neurosci.* 26:9413–9425.

Eggers, E. D., McCall, M. A., and Lukasiewicz, P. D. (2007). Presynaptic inhibition differentially shapes transmission in distinct circuits in the mouse retina. *J. Physiol.* 582:569–582.

Euler, T., and Masland, R. H. (2000). Light-evoked responses of bipolar cells in a mammalian retina. *J. Neurophysiol.* 83:1817–1829.

Euler, T., and Wässle, H. (1998). Different contributions of GABAA and GABAC receptors to rod and cone bipolar cells in a rat retinal slice preparation. *J. Neurophysiol.* 79:1384–1395.

Ghosh, K. K., Bujan, S., Haverkamp, S., Feigenspan, A., and Wässle, H. (2004). Types of bipolar cells in the mouse retina. *J. Comp. Neurol.* 469:70–82.

Gregg, R. G., Kamermans, M., Klooster, J., Lukasiewicz, P. D., Peachey, N. S. Vessey, K. A., and McCall, M. A. (2007). Nyctalopin expression in retinal bipolar cells restores visual function in mice with X-linked congenital stationary night blindness. *J. Neurophysiol.* 98:3023–3033.

Gregg, R. G., Mukhopadhyay, S., Candille, S. I., Ball, S. L., Pardue, M. T., McCall, M. A., and Peachey, N. S. (2003). Identification of the gene and the mutation responsible for the mouse *nob* phenotype. *Invest. Ophthalmol. Vis. Sci.* 44:378–384.

Gregg, R. G., Read, D. S., and McCall, M. A. (2008). VDCC β2 subunit is required for the development ribbon synapses in the outer plexiform layer in the mouse. Unpublished manuscript.

Greka, A., Lipton, S. A., and Zhang, D. (2000). Expression of GABAC receptor rho1 and rho2 subunits during development of the mouse retina. *Eur. J. Neurosci.* 12:3575–3582.

Hack, I., Frech, M., Dick, O., Peichl, L., and Brandstatter, J. H. (2001). Heterogeneous distribution of AMPA glutamate receptor subunits at the photoreceptor synapses of rodent retina. *Eur. J. Neurosci.* 13:15–24.

Haeseleer, F., Imanishi, Y., Maeda, T., Possin, D. E., Maeda, A., Lee, A., Rieke, F., and Palczewski, K. (2004). Essential role of Ca^{2+}-binding protein 4, a $Ca_V1.4$ channel regulator, in photoreceptor synaptic function. *Nat. Neurosci.* 7:1079–1087.

Haverkamp, S., Muller, U., Zeilhofer, H. U., Harvey, R. J., and Wässle, H. (2004). Diversity of glycine receptors in the mouse retina: localization of the α2 subunit. *J. Comp. Neurol.* 477:399–411.

Ivanova, E., Muller, U., and Wässle, H. (2006). Characterization of the glycinergic input to bipolar cells of the mouse retina. *Eur. J. Neurosci.* 23:350–364.

Jalkanen, R., Bech-Hansen, N. T., Tobias, R., Sankila, E. M., Mantyjarvi, M., Forsius, H., de la Chapelle, A., and Alitalo, T. (2007). A novel CACNA1F gene mutation causes Aland Island eye disease. *Invest. Ophthalmol. Vis. Sci.* 48:2498–2502.

Jalkanen, R., Mantyjarvi, M., Tobias, R., Isosomppi, J., Sankila, E. M., Alitalo, T., and Bech-Hansen, N. T. (2006). X linked cone-rod dystrophy, CORDX3, is caused by a mutation in the CACNA1F gene. *J. Med. Genet.* 43:699–704.

Jiang, M., Gold, M. S., Boulay, G., Spicher, K., Peyton, M., Brabet, P., Srinivasan, Y., Rudolph, U., Ellison, G., and Birnbaumer, L. (1998). Multiple neurological abnormalities in mice deficient in the G protein Go. *Proc. Natl. Acad. Sci. U.S.A.* 95:3269–3274.

Johnson, B. A., Ikeda, S., Pinto, L. H., and Ikeda, A. (2006). Reduced synaptic vesicle density and aberrant synaptic localization caused by a splice site mutation in the *Rs1h* gene. *Vis. Neurosci.* 23:887–898.

Kolb, H., and Famiglietti, E. V. (1974). Rod and cone pathways in the inner plexiform layer of cat retina. *Science* 186:47–49.

Li, W., and DeVries, S. H. (2006). Bipolar cell pathways for color and luminance vision in a dichromatic mammalian retina. *Nat. Neurosci.* 9:669–675.

Lukasiewicz, P. D., Eggers, E. D., Sagdullaev, B. T., and McCall, M. A. (2004). GABAC receptor-mediated inhibition in the retina. *Vision Res.* 44:3289–3296.

Lukasiewicz, P. D., and Werblin, F. S. (1994). A novel GABA receptor modulates synaptic transmission from bipolar to ganglion and amacrine cells in the tiger salamander retina. *J. Neurosci.* 14:1213–1223.

Ma, Y. P., and Pan, Z. H. (2003). Spontaneous regenerative activity in mammalian retinal bipolar cells: Roles of multiple subtypes of voltage-dependent Ca^{2+} channels. *Vis. Neurosci.* 20: 131–139.

MacDermott, A. B., Role, L. W., and Siegelbaum, S. A. (1999). Presynaptic ionotropic receptors and the control of transmitter release. *Annu. Rev. Neurosci.* 22:443–485.

Majumdar, S., Heinze, L., Haverkamp, S., Ivanova, E., and Wässle, H. (2007). Glycine receptors of A-type ganglion cells of the mouse retina. *Vis. Neurosci.* 24(4):471–487.

Mansergh, F., Orton, N. C., Vessey, J. P., Lalonde, M. R., Stell, W. K., Tremblay, F., Barnes, S., Rancourt, D. E., and Bech-Hansen, N. T. (2005). Mutation of the calcium channel gene *Cacna1f* disrupts calcium signaling, synaptic transmission and cellular organization in mouse retina. *Hum. Mol. Genet.* 14:3035–3046.

Masu, M., Iwakabe, H., Tagawa, Y., Miyoshi, T., Yamashita, J., Fukuda, Y., Sasaki, H., Hiroi, K., Nakamura, Y., et al. (1995). Specific deficit of the ON response in visual transmission by targeted disruption of the mGluR6 gene. *Cell* 80:757–765.

McCall, M. A., Lukasiewicz, P. D., Gregg, R. G., and Peachey, N. S. (2002). Elimination of the ρ1 subunit abolishes GABA(C) receptor expression and alters visual processing in the mouse retina. *J. Neurosci.* 22:4163–4174.

Miller, R. F. (2004). D-Serine as a glial modulator of nerve cells. *Glia* 47:275–283.

Morgans, C. W., Bayley, P. R., Oesch, N. W., Ren, G., Akileswaran, L., and Taylor, W. R. (2005). Photoreceptor calcium channels: Insight from night blindness. *Vis. Neurosci.* 22:561–568.

Murakami, M., Otsuka, T., and Shimazaki, H. (1975). Effects of aspartate and glutamate on the bipolar cells in the carp retina. *Vision Res.* 15:456–458.

Nakajima, Y., Iwakabe, H., Akazawa, C., Nawa, H., Shigemoto, R., Mizuno, N., and Nakanishi, S. (1993). Molecular characterization of a novel retinal metabotropic glutamate receptor mGluR6 with a high agonist selectivity for L-2-amino-4-phosphonobutyrate. *J. Biol. Chem.* 268:11868–11873.

Nakanishi, S., Nakajima, Y., Masu, M., Ueda, Y., Nakahara, K., Watanabe, D., Yamaguchi, S., Kawabata, S., and Okada, M. (1998). Glutamate receptors: Brain function and signal transduction. *Brain Res. Brain Res. Rev.* 26:230–235.

Nawy, S. (1999). The metabotropic receptor mGluR6 may signal through G(o), but not phosphodiesterase, in retinal bipolar cells. *J. Neurosci.* 19:2938–2944.

Nelson, R., Famiglietti, E. V., Jr., and Kolb, H. (1978). Intracellular staining reveals different levels of stratification for on- and off-center ganglion cells in cat retina. *J. Neurophysiol.* 41: 472–483.

Nelson, R., Kolb, H., Robinson, M. M., and Mariani, A. P. (1981). Neural circuitry of the cat retina: Cone pathways to ganglion cells. *Vision Res.* 21:1527–1536.

Pan, Z. H. (2001). Voltage-activated Ca^{2+} channels and ionotropic GABA receptors localized at axon terminals of mammalian retinal bipolar cells. *Vis. Neurosci.* 18:279–288.

Pan, Z. H., and Lipton, S. A. (1995). Multiple GABA receptor subtypes mediate inhibition of calcium influx at rat retinal bipolar cell terminals. *J. Neurosci.* 15:2668–2679.

Pardue, M. T., Ball, S. L., Mukhopadhyay, S., Candille, S. I., McCall, M. A., Gregg, R. G., and Peachey, N. S. (2001). *nob*: A mouse model of CSNB1. In R. E. Anderson, M. M. Lavail, and J. G. Hollyfield (Eds.), *New insights into retinal degenerative diseases*. New York: Kluwer Academic/Plenum Press.

Pardue, M. T., McCall, M. A., LaVail, M. M., Gregg, R. G., and Peachey, N. S. (1998). A naturally occurring mouse model of X-linked congenital stationary night blindness. *Invest. Ophthalmol. Vis. Sci.* 39:2443–2449.

Pignatelli, V., and Strettoi, E. (2004). Bipolar cells of the mouse retina: A gene gun, morphological study. *J. Comp. Neurol.* 476: 254–266.

Pillers, D. A., Weleber, R. G., Green, D. G., Rash, S. M., Dally, G. Y., Howard, P. L., Powers, M. R., Hood, D. C., Chapman, V. M., et al. (1999). Effects of dystrophin isoforms on signal transduction through neural retina: Genotype-phenotype analysis of Duchenne muscular dystrophy mouse mutants. *Mol. Genet. Metab.* 66:100–110.

Pinto, L. H., and Enroth-Cugell, C. (2000). Tests of the mouse visual system. *Mamm. Genome* 11:531–536.

Pinto, L. H., Vitaterna, M. H., Shimomura, K., Siepka, S. M., McDearmon, E. L., Balannik, V., Omura, C., Lumayag, S., Invergo, B. M., et al. (2007). Generation, identification and functional characterization of the *nob4* mutation of *Grm6* in the mouse. *Vis. Neurosci.* 24:111–123.

Renteria, R. C., Tian, N., Cang, J., Nakanishi, S., Stryker, M. P., and Copenhagen, D. R. (2006). Intrinsic ON responses of the retinal OFF pathway are suppressed by the ON pathway. *J. Neurosci.* 26:11857–11869.

Robson, J. G., and Frishman, L. J. (1998). Dissecting the dark-adapted electroretinogram. *Doc. Ophthalmol.* 95:187–215.

Rodieck, R. W., and Brening, R. K. (1983). Retinal ganglion cells: Properties, types genera, pathways and trans-species comparisons. *Brain Behav. Evol.* 23:121–164.

Sagdullaev, B. T., McCall, M. A., and Lukasiewicz, P. D. (2006). Presynaptic inhibition modulates spillover, creating distinct dynamic response ranges of sensory output. *Neuron* 50: 923–935.

Saito, T., and Kaneko, A. (1983). Ionic mechanisms underlying the responses of off-center bipolar cells in the carp retina. I. Studies on responses evoked by light. *J. Gen. Physiol.* 81:589–601.

Schnapf, J. L., and Copenhagen, D. R. (1982). Differences in the kinetics of rod and cone synaptic transmission. *Nature* 296: 862–864.

Schneeweis, D. M., and Schnapf, J. L. (1999). The photovoltage of macaque cone photoreceptors: Adaptation, noise, and kinetics. *J. Neurosci.* 19:1203–1216.

Sharma, S., Ball, S. L., and Peachey, N. S. (2005). Pharmacological studies of the mouse cone electroretinogram. *Vis. Neurosci.* 22:631–636.

Shelley, J., Dedek, K., Schubert, T., Feigenspan, A., Schultz, K., Hombach, S., Willecke, K., and Weiler, R. (2006). Horizontal cell receptive fields are reduced in connexin57-deficient mice. *Eur. J. Neurosci.* 23:3176–3186.

Shields, C. R., Tran, M. N., Wong, R. O., and Lukasiewicz, P. D. (2000). Distinct ionotropic GABA receptors mediate presynaptic and postsynaptic inhibition in retinal bipolar cells. *J. Neurosci.* 20:2673–2682.

Slaughter, M. M., and Miller, R. F. (1981). 2-amino-4-phosphonobutyric acid: A new pharmacological tool for retina research. *Science* 211:182–185.

Snellman, J., and Nawy, S. (2004). cGMP-dependent kinase regulates response sensitivity of the mouse on bipolar cell. *J. Neurosci.* 24:6621–6628.

Sterling, P. (1995). Vision: Tuning retinal circuits. *Nature* 377: 676–677.

Sugihara, H., Inoue, T., Nakanishi, S., and Fukuda, Y. (1997). A late ON response remains in visual response of the mGluR6-deficient mouse. *Neurosci. Lett.* 233:137–140.

Tagawa, Y., Sawai, H., Ueda, Y., Tauchi, M., and Nakanishi, S. (1999). Immunohistological studies of metabotropic glutamate receptor subtype 6–deficient mice show no abnormality of retinal cell organization and ganglion cell maturation. *J. Neurosci.* 19:2568–2579.

Valenzuela, D., Han, X., Mende, U., Fankhauser, C., Mashimo, H., Huang, P., Pfeffer, J., Neer, E. J., and Fishman, M. C. (1997). $G_{\alpha o}$ is necessary for muscarinic regulation of Ca^{2+} channels in mouse heart. *Proc. Natl. Acad. Sci. U.S.A.* 94:1727–1732.

Vessey, K. A., Sagdullaev, B. T., Gregg, R. G., and McCall, M. A. (2005). Retinal ganglion cell function is altered in two mouse models of congenital stationary night blindness. *Soc. Neurosci.* abstr. 977.21.

Wässle, H. (2004). Parallel processing in the mammalian retina. *Nat. Rev. Neurosci.* 5:747–757.

Wässle, H., Koulen, P., Brandstatter, J. H., Fletcher, E. L., and Becker, C. M. (1998). Glycine and GABA receptors in the mammalian retina. *Vision Res.* 38:1411–1430.

Weiler, R., Pottek, M., He, S., and Vaney, D. I. (2000). Modulation of coupling between retinal horizontal cells by retinoic acid and endogenous dopamine. *Brain Res. Brain Res. Rev.* 32:121–129.

Weiss, J., O'Sullivan, G. A., Heinze, L., Chen, H. X., Betz, H., and Wässle, H. (2008). Glycinergic input of small-field amacrine cells in the retinas of wildtype and glycine receptor deficient mice. *Mol. Cell Neurosci.* 37(1):40–55.

Werblin, F., Roska, B., and Balya, D. (2001). Parallel processing in the mammalian retina: Lateral and vertical interactions across stacked representations. *Prog. Brain Res.* 131:229–238.

Wu, J., Marmorstein, A. D., Striessnig, J., and Peachey, N. S. (2007). Voltage-dependent calcium channel $Ca_V1.3$ subunits regulate the light peak of the electroretinogram. *J. Neurophysiol.* 97:3731–3735.

Wu, S. M., Gao, F., and Pang, J. J. (2004). Synaptic circuitry mediating light-evoked signals in dark-adapted mouse retina. *Vision Res.* 44:3277–3288.

Wycisk, K. A., Budde, B., Feil, S., Skosyrski, S., Buzzi, F., Neidhardt, J., Glaus, E., Nurnberg, P., Ruether, K., and Berger, W. (2006). Structural and functional abnormalities of retinal ribbon synapses due to *Cacna2d4* mutation. *Invest. Ophthalmol. Vis. Sci.* 47:3523–3530.

Yarbrough, G. L., Sagdullaev, B. T., Vessey, K. A., and McCall, M. A. (2008). Contrast-dependent feedback inhibition contributes to spatial and temporal aspects of receptive field organization of retinal ganglion cells. Unpublished manuscript.

Zaghloul, K. A., Boahen, K., and Demb, J. B. (2003). Different circuits for ON and OFF retinal ganglion cells cause different contrast sensitivities. *J. Neurosci.* 23:2645–2654.

15 Morphological, Functional, and Developmental Properties of Mouse Retinal Ganglion Cells

JULIE L. COOMBS AND LEO M. CHALUPA

It is arguably the case that more is known about retinal ganglion cells (RGCs) in species commonly used in vision research, such as cat and monkey, than any other neurons in the CNS (Chalupa and Werner, 2004). In part, this reflects the paramount importance of vision in our lives, and the study of RGCs is vital to understanding how the visual system processes information. But it is also the case that RGCs have become important for understanding how neurons develop and form appropriate connections both over long (axonal pathfinding and target recognition in the brain) and short distances (formation of dendritic synapses and lamination in the inner plexiform layer, IPL). The advantages of the mouse model for addressing developmental issues are well recognized, yet our understanding of the morphological, functional, and developmental properties of mouse RGCs is still rudimentary. In recent years, however, a number of laboratories have begun making significant inroads with studies of mouse RGCs. In this chapter we summarize these recent advances and place them in an appropriate historical context.

Distinguishing retinal ganglion cell classes

A fundamental issue in the study of RGCs is defining the different cell classes constituting this population of neurons and categorizing each cell class in such a way that researchers in different laboratories can agree on their identity. The features distinguishing RGC classes are multiple and include morphological and functional properties, as well as their patterns of projections. In addition, the somata of a given cell class are presumed to be distributed across the retinal surface in nonrandom fashion with relatively little overlap of dendrites, to allow each RGC class to efficiently extract information from the entire visual field. Collectively, this has led to the important concept of parallel visual pathways or channels, which holds that different cell classes are specialized for processing and conveying different types of visual information to different retinorecipient targets.

In the mouse, we still lack basic information on the multiple criteria that have been used to distinguish among RGCs in some other species. Nevertheless, progress has been made on this front, particularly in the use of morphological criteria for differentiating among mouse RGC classes. In the past, studies of mouse RGCs relied on categorizations of these cells in other mammals to identify different cell types in the mouse; for instance, RGCs with large somata and dendritic fields were termed alpha cells, in reference to cells described in other species (see Peichl et al., 1987). A perusal of the published photomicrographs suggests, however, that the mouse RGCs identified as alpha are not the same cell types in the different studies that have used this designation (compare Pang et al., 2003, Lin et al., 2004, and Völgyi et al., 2005). There may indeed be alpha-equivalent RGCs in the mouse (Peichl et al., 1987), but a simple description of a large soma and dendritic field is inadequate for reproducible identification of these neurons.

In comparison to some other species, clear morphological distinctions among the majority of mouse RGCs are difficult to discern by eye. For this reason, distinguishing among different mouse RGCs requires painstaking morphometrics. But there is an advantage to studying mouse RGCs, besides the power of genetic manipulation: mouse RGCs show no discernible differences in size with retinal eccentricity. This uniformity across the retina simplifies the study and identification of different cell classes.

Morphological descriptions of RGCs have traditionally relied on the injection of individual cells with Lucifer yellow or other dyes, which is time-consuming, or the retrograde transport of dyes or particles injected into retinorecipient regions, a method that does not always reveal the full extent of dendrites (see Doi et al., 1995). Recently, new methods have been developed that make imaging of many isolated, completely labeled RGCs more straightforward. One such technique is diolistics, a modified gene gun method in which tiny particles (1–2 μm in diameter) coated with lipophilic dyes such as DiI are propelled into the tissue to be labeled using a gene gun (Gan et al., 2000). A subset of cells is hit by the particles, and the dye becomes incorporated into the membranes and diffuses throughout the perimeter of the cell, allowing fine cell structures such as spines to be readily visualized. Other workers have developed transgenic mice in which reporter genes, fluorescent proteins or alkaline phosphatase, are linked to genes expressed in RGCs (Feng et al., 2000; Badea et al., 2003). In particular, Feng et al. (2000) developed a number of mouse lines in which the expression of fluorescent proteins is linked to a regulator of the Thy-1 gene. Thy-1 is a protein found in RGCs whose function is unknown. Two of these mouse lines (M and H) have been used to visualize individual RGCs (Kong et al., 2005; Coombs et al., 2006). Other mice in which alkaline phosphatase expression is controlled by Cre-mediated recombination triggered by injections of 4-hydroxytamoxiphen have also been used successfully to visualize mouse RGCs (Badea et al., 2003; Badea and Nathans, 2004). These labeling methods, used alone (Sun et al., 2002) or in combination with new microscopy techniques and software that expedites morphological analysis, have prompted the erection of four proposed classification schemes for mouse RGCs (Badea and Nathans, 2004; Kong et al., 2005; Coombs et al., 2006). Each suggests a similar number of cell types, yet reconciling these four classifications remains problematic (e.g., figure 16 in Kong et al., 2005).

Sun et al. (2002) categorized mouse RGCs into different groups based mainly on qualitative criteria, as well as measurements of soma and dendritic field sizes. The resulting groupings showed a substantial degree of overlap, so in many cases, assigning a given cell to one group or another appears arbitrary. Badea and Nathans (2004) and Kong et al. (2005) used cluster analyses to sort out RGC types, but both studies relied primarily on only three cell traits in their analyses. Badea and Nathans (2004) used depth of dendritic stratification in the IPL (the location of both the topmost and the bottom-most dendrites) plus arbor area in their initial analysis, then relied on other parameters to sort out clusters that looked similar to each other. Kong et al. (2005) also used three measurements in their cluster analysis: dendritic stratification depth, arbor area, and dendrite density (dendrite length/arbor area). This approach was not able to distinguish as a separate group the melanopsin-expressing RGCs, which have a clearly distinctive morphology.

In an attempt to circumvent these problems, we used 14 different morphological measures to perform hierarchical cluster analyses (figure 15.1; mono- and bistratified cells were analyzed separately), using cells labeled with a melanopsin antibody as a control group to monitor the validity of the analysis (Coombs et al., 2006). Contrary to the assertion of others (e.g., Kong et al., 2005), we found that a larger number of parameters increased the power of the analysis rather than diminishing it. We also found that the analysis was more successful if we standardized each trait, by transforming the frequency distribution of each parameter to approximate a Gaussian curve and normalizing this curve to eliminate weighting due to differences in numerical scale. For example, without standardization, the dendritic field area (scale: 10^4 μm^2) would have much more sway over the final clustering outcome than the dendritic field diameter (scale: μm). The analysis resulted in 14 different clusters, with clusters 4 and 5 likely representing two RGC classes each (figures 15.2 and 15.3). The cells in this study were labeled in one of four different ways: with melanopsin antibody, by dioloistics, with Lucifer yellow, and by transgenic expression of YFP (H line). All the melanopsin-positive cells were clustered into a single group (cluster 6; x's in figure 15.1). The diolistically labeled cells were spread relatively evenly through the resulting clusters (though none appeared in cluster 6), but there were too few of the Lucifer yellow–

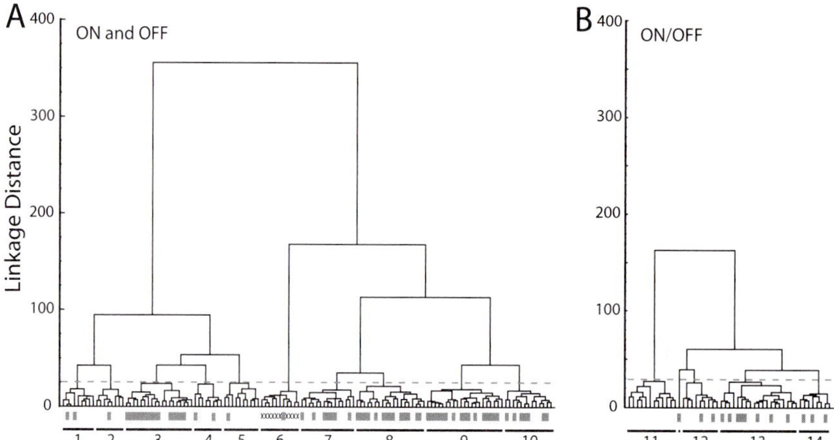

FIGURE 15.1 Cluster analysis trees. Linkage distance (*y*-axis) shows the relative similarity of cells (along *x*-axis) for monostratified (*A*) and bistratified cells (*B*). *Gray lines* indicate abrupt increases in linkage distance, thus demarking a cutoff point for defining distinct clusters. Cells linked together below the *gray lines* are defined as single cell types and given group numbers (shown under the trees). One cell forms its own cluster (* in *B*) and is not given a group name. YFP-expressing cells (*shaded boxes*) and melanopsin-positive cells (×) are shown below the *x*-axes. All other cells were labeled with DiI or Lucifer yellow.

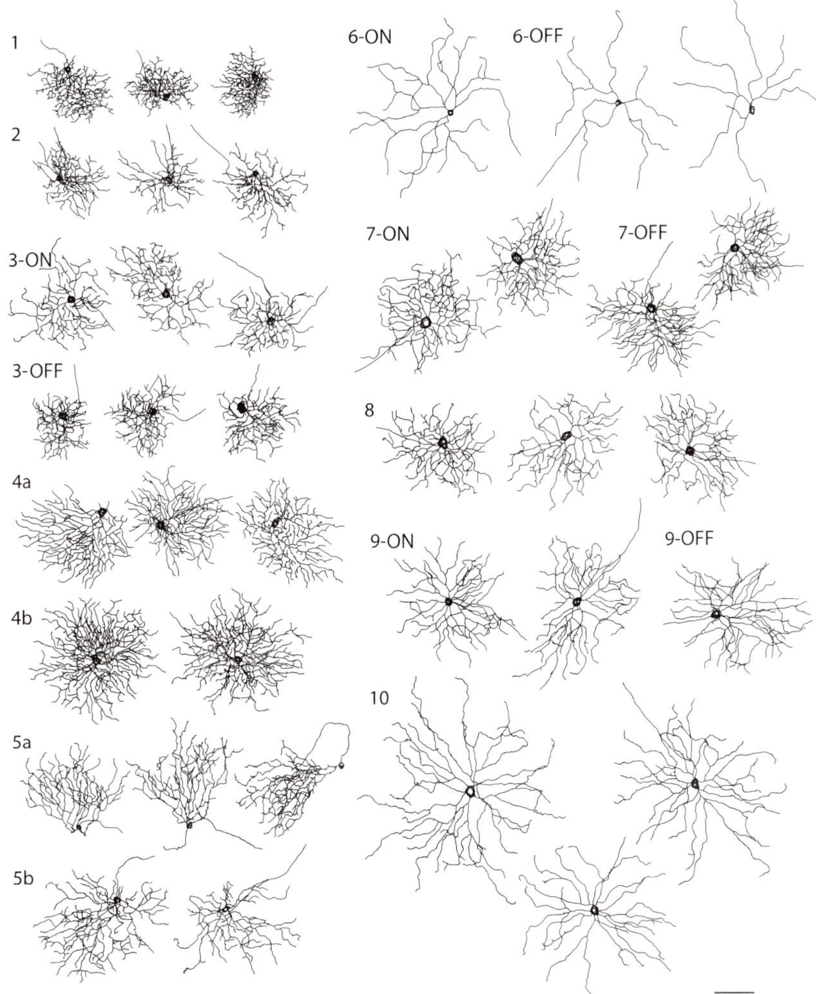

Figure 15.2 Tracings of cells from the monostratified cell clusters. Examples of ON and OFF cells are shown for groups M3, M6, M7, and M9. For groups M4 and M5, examples of two different morphologies (a and b) found in each cluster are shown. Scale bar = 100 μm.

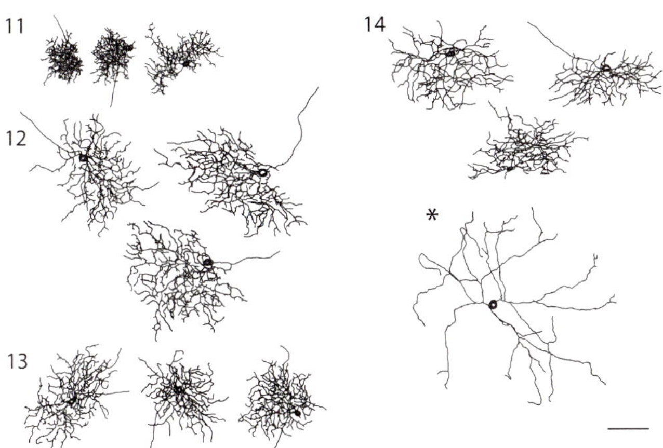

Figure 15.3 Tracings of cells from the bistratified cell clusters. *Asterisk* indicates a cell that was clustered by itself and thus was not given a group number. Scale bar = 100 μm.

filled cells to see any cluster trend for these. And though YFP-expressing cells were found in every cluster except cluster 11, they tended to be more heavily represented in 6 of the 14 clusters. This last observation suggests a bias for YFP to be expressed in specific RGC types in the H line of YFP-expressing mice (see figure 15.1, *shaded boxes* below *x*-axis).

Functional properties

The functional properties of mouse RGCs have been assessed by means of extracellular recordings from individual cells, multielectrode array recordings from multiple neurons, and whole-cell patch-clamp recordings. An early study by Stone and Pinto (1993) relied on extracellular recordings from individual neurons and reported that most mouse RGCs (90%) had concentric center-surround receptive fields (RFs), while the remaining 10% responded to both light onset and offset. Recently, three different response patterns were noted in alpha-like RGCs—an ON response to light onset and two types of OFF responses, transient or sustained, to light offset (Pang et al., 2003). A microelectrode array study reported four different response patterns to a simple step change in light: an increased firing rate to light onset, light offset, or to both onset and offset, and a decreased firing rate in response to light onset (Nirenberg and Meister, 1997). Moreover, these investigators noted that after the selective ablation of a population of amacrine cells situated in the ganglion cell layer (GCL), RGCs that normally responded to increases in light levels with transient responses showed sustained responses.

A recent multielectrode array recording study has suggested the presence of five different functional classes defined by a cluster analysis based on response latency, duration, relative size of ON and OFF responses, and the degree of nonlinearity of responses (Carcieri et al., 2003). It remains to be established how these functionally defined cell types relate to the 14 classes of mouse RGCs defined on the basis of morphological criteria.

A patch-clamp study of mouse RGCs defined these cells on the basis of their large sodium currents (Tian et al., 1998). Such cells showed synaptic events mediated by GABA and glutamate, with half of these also showing spontaneous synaptic events mediated by glycine. No cholinergic-mediated spontaneous synaptic events were noted. It remains to be established whether or not all classes of mouse RGCs express the same ionic conductances and show equivalent transmitter-mediated synaptic events.

Intrinsically photosensitive retinal ganglion cells

Mice without rods and cones in their retinas can still respond to light with normal pupillary reflexes and light-dependent photoentrainment. These responses were found to be mediated by cells in the inner rather than the outer retina, namely, by a class of intrinsically photosensitive RGCs (ipRGCs) that express melanopsin (Provencio et al., 1998, 2002; Hattar et al., 2002; Ruby et al., 2002; Berson, 2003; Panda et al., 2003). There is also intriguing evidence that ipRGCs may be involved in some aspects of visual processing as well (Barnard et al., 2006). They have dendrites in the inner or outer laminae (or both) of the IPL, and synapse on amacrine and bipolar cells in the ON lamina and only amacrine cells in the OFF lamina (Belenky et al., 2003). This suggests that the responses of ipRGCs to light in the inner retina may be modulated by inputs from rods and cones in the outer retina (Belenky et al., 2003). A recent study has indeed shown a direct influence of rods on ipRGCs (Doyle et al., 2006).

Projections of mouse retinal ganglion cells

There are two sets of targets in the mouse brain to which RGCs project axons, depending on whether the pathway is image forming or non-image forming (Provencio et al., 1998). Image-forming RGCs send axons to the lateral geniculate nucleus (LGN, both dorsal and ventral) and the superior colliculus (SC), with more than 70%, and possibly all, RGCs projecting to the SC (Hofbauer and Drager, 1985). Transgenic mouse lines linking expression of the GAP-lacZ protein to that of Brn-3b have been used to show that RGCs located in the dorsal half of the retina send axons to the lateral region of the SC and to the dorsal lateral geniculate nucleus (dLGN) and ventral lateral geniculate nucleus (vLGN), while RGCs in the ventral retina send axons to the medial region of the SC as well as the LGN (Zubair et al., 2002). Other studies have used a similar method to look at the axonal projections of ipRGCs. Although the bulk of RGCs send information to the visual centers in the brain, ipRGCs project to central circadian centers: the suprachiasmatic nucleus (SCN), intergeniculate leaflet of the thalamus, and the ventral lateral geniculate, as well as the olivary pretectal nucleus, which mediates pupil reflexes (Provencio et al., 1998; Hattar et al., 2002, 2006). Interestingly, a recent report has shown that these cells also project to brain nuclei involved in vision information processing, such as the dLG (Hattar et al., 2006).

Molecular markers for retinal ganglion cells

Ultimately, the definitive factor for differentiating among different classes of RGCs, as for all neurons in the CNS, will be some combination of genes and molecules that are uniquely expressed in all members of a given cell class. Presumably, their expression would account for the set of morphological and functional attributes that distinguish these cells from other cell classes. At present, we are a long way from attaining this long-term goal. Indeed, the ipRGCs that express melanopsin are the only cell class thus far identified on the basis of a molecular marker. Because these cells are molecularly identifiable based on their expression of this protein, a wealth of information has been obtained using genetic manipulations that tag reporter genes to the expression of melanopsin.

Specific markers for other RGCs have not been discovered, though there is information that junctional adhesion molecule-B (JAM-B) is expressed in the GCL of mice almost exclusively in asymmetric OFF RGCs (Kim et al., 2006). Antibodies against neurofilament H have been reported to label alpha-type cells in the mouse (Lin et al., 2004); however, a common antibody against this protein (SMI-32) has been shown to label more than one type of RGC in YFP-expressing mice (Coombs et al., 2006). Thy-1, a thymus protein, is found in all RGCs (Barnstable and Drager, 1984) and is often used to differentiate RGCs from other retinal cell types, but is not specific to any single type of RGC. Another widespread protein found in RGCs is islet-2, which is expressed in about a third of mouse RGCs; these neurons appear to all project to the opposite (or contralateral) side of the brain (Pak et al., 2004). Conversely, the transcription factor Zic2 is found only in the ventral/temporal (VT) part of the retina, where ipsilaterally projecting RGCs are located (Herrera et al., 2003).

Other possible markers for specific RGC types in the mouse include connexins 36 and 45, which are expressed by alpha-type and bistratified RGCs, respectively (Schubert et al., 2005a, 2005b; Völgyi et al., 2005). Connexin 36 (Cx36) is responsible for the formation of gap junctions between OFF alpha-type RGCs and amacrine cells. ON alpha-type cells show no tracer coupling with each other but do so with two amacrine cell types in the GCL. Some of this coupling is lost in Cx36 knockout mice. OFF alpha-type cells are tracer coupled with each other, in addition to some amacrine cell types. The homologous coupling remains intact in the Cx36 knockout, but the coupling of the OFF RGCs with amacrine cells is lost (Völgyi et al., 2005). As more molecular markers specific to different RGC types are found, it will be of interest to determine to what degree these can be related to the different cell classes differentiated on the basis of morphological and functional criteria.

Generation and differentiation of retinal ganglion cells

All retinal neurons are generated from the same ventricular cells in the developing mouse retina. Among the first retinal cells to be born from these progenitor cells are RGCs, starting around embryonic day 11 (E11; Young, 1985). Two distinct patterns of ganglion cell generation have been described, depending on the laterality of their projections. The vast majority of RGCs send axons to the opposite side of the brain (Drager and Olsen, 1980). These are born in a wave across the retinal surface, starting near the optic nerve head around E11, radiating outward, and ending at the retinal periphery, around E19–P0 (postnatal day zero; Drager, 1985). Conversely, RGCs with axons that project ipsilaterally (ca. 3% of RGCs in the GCL) originate in the VT crescent, though RGCs born in the VT crescent after E16.5 project contralaterally (Drager, 1985). A much larger percentage of the displaced RGCs (somata in the inner nuclear layer) send their axons ipsilaterally (ca. 30% vs. 3%).

RGC birth peaks around E13 (Drager, 1985), at a time when axons can be seen in the optic stalk (Hinds and Hinds, 1974). At P0, after all RGCs have been born, a large number of pyknotic cells become evident in the GCL, most of which are presumed RGCs. This cell death peaks around P3 and appears to radiate out from the optic nerve head region, ending around P11 in the peripheral retina (Young, 1984). Others have confirmed that most, if not all, RGC death occurs postnatally (Linden and Pinto, 1985; Pequignot et al., 2003; Farah and Easter, 2005). The incidence of cell death for RGCs generated earlier in development is somewhat higher than that for RGCs generated later in development. Farah and Easter (2005) reported that more than 48% of RGCs generated before E12.5 are eliminated by cell death, while about 30% of RGCs born after E15.5 succumb to this fate.

In mouse as in other animals, RGCs are the first cells to exit the mitotic cycle from a set of retinal progenitor cells (RGCs) that produce all neural cells in the retina. A host of molecular factors, both extrinsic and intrinsic, are emerging from studies dealing with the factors that control cell fate. Two secreted factors have been implicated in the early determination of mouse RGCs: sonic hedgehog (Shh; Wang et al., 2005) and growth and differentiation factor 11 (GDF11; Kim et al., 2005). Both molecules are expressed in central to peripheral waves across the retina starting around E12, just behind the leading edge of RGC birth, and have a negative effect on RGC production. The loss of either Shh or GDF11 increases the number of RGCs born, while an overproduction of either factor inhibits RGC birth (Kim et al., 2005; Wang et al., 2005). However, the mechanisms by which these two factors work are different. In the absence of Shh, RPCs tend to exit the cell cycle early, thus promoting an increase in RGC production (Wang et al., 2005). Moreover, RGCs appear to secrete Shh, thereby causing a cessation of further RGC production (Jensen and Wallace, 1997; Wang et al., 2005; in chick: Zhang and Yang, 2001). Mice transgenic for a null allele of GDF11 show normal cell proliferation but are unable to make the switch from producing RGCs to making other retinal cells. The number of RGCs is normal until about E17; after this time, when wild-type animals are showing a decrease in RGC production, these transgenic mice continue to generate RGCs (Kim et al., 2005).

A hierarchical suite of transcription factors appears to direct cell fate decisions during the course of RGC development. The homeobox gene *Pax6* directs optic vesicle formation and at a later stage is required for the maintenance of multipotency in mitotic retinal progenitor cells (Marquardt et al., 2001). Only amacrine cells are found in retinas of mice with *Pax6* conditionally knocked out (Marquadt et al., 2001). Starting at E10.5 and persisting through E15.5, a radial gradient of *Pax6* expression is seen across the mouse retina, with the weakest expression near the future optic nerve head (Marquardt et al., 2001; Baumer et al., 2002). The expression of subsequent transcription factors signals the commitment of retinal progenitor cells to specific retinal cell lineage fate. In the case of RGCs, the basic helix-loop-helix transcription factor Math5 (Atoh7) is expressed in postmitotic cells (Yang et al., 2003), just before the first RGCs are born (Brown et al., 1998). Math5 is expressed in a temporal wave, beginning near the future optic nerve at E11 and moving toward the retinal periphery in a pattern reminiscent of RGC births (Brown et al., 1998; Wang et al., 2001). In mice lacking Math5, the production of most RGCs is inhibited; however, about 20% of RGCs may still be found in adults, suggesting the presence of a Math5-independent RGC pathway (Brown et al., 2001; Wang et al., 2001). Moreover, Math5 is not sufficient to ensure a RGC fate, since it has also been found in other retinal cell types (Yang et al., 2003). Thus, other factors are required to commit these cells to an RGC fate (Mu et al., 2005).

Downstream of Math5 and first seen at E12, a POU domain transcription factor, POU4f2 (formerly Brn3b), is activated that promotes the expression of RGC phenotypic features such as axon elongation and pathfinding (Xiang et al., 1993; Erkman et al., 1996, 2000; Gan et al., 1996; Xiang, 1998; Brown et al., 2001; Wang et al., 2001; Yang et al., 2003). Even so, this transcription factor is not responsible for specification of RGC fate (Gan et al., 1999); thus there remains a missing link between Math5 and RGC determination. POU4f2 is first seen in postmitotic RGC precursors as they migrate from the neuroblast layer to the inner retina (Gan et al., 1996). The absence of POU4f2 expression causes an increase in the death of RGC precursors, leading to a loss of about 70% of RGCs from the mature retina (Xiang, 1998; Gan el al., 1999). In mice lacking the Wilms' tumor gene *Wt1*, no POU4f2 expression is seen, and the phenotype of the mice is similar to those lacking POU4f2 (Wagner et al., 2002). Two other POU domain transcription factors are found in RGCs in the mouse, POU4f1 and POU4f3 (formerly Brn3a and Brn3c). The three POU domain transcription factors have slightly different spatiotemporal expression patterns (Xiang et al., 1995, 1996; Erkman et al., 1996). All three play a role in RGC development, notably axon growth (Erkman et al., 1996; Xiang, 1998; Wang et al., 2002; Pan et al., 2005; Quina et al., 2005) and have the ability to substitute for one another when expressed in the appropriate time and place (Wang et al., 2002; Pan et al., 2005). At the same time, each may play a unique role in the development and differentiation of certain RGC properties; for instance, POU4f3 may control ipsilateral axon growth (Wang et al., 2002). Mice lacking two murine homologues of the *Drosophila* gene distal-less (*Dlx1* and *Dlx2*) also show a reduction in RGC number, acting upstream of the POU domain factors (de Melo et al., 2003, 2005).

Development of retinal ganglion cell morphological properties

Shortly after RGCs are born, they begin to extend axons into the optic nerve (Hinds and Hinds, 1974), and these reach the optic chiasm by E12–E13 (Godement et al., 1984, 1987; Zubair et al., 2002) and the dLGN and SC by E15–E16 (Godement et al., 1984; Edwards et al., 1986; Zubair et al., 2002). Within the retina, dendrites can be seen in the nascent IPL around the time of birth (E19 or P0). RGC dendrites grow and mature during the two postnatal weeks and appear morphologically mature by P20 (figure 15.4). As the dendritic trees extend and elaborate outward in the plane of the growing IPL, the orthogonal (or vertical) extent of these dendrites in the IPL remains relatively constant, even as the IPL itself widens. Thus, RGC dendrites stratify early in the postnatal development of the mouse retina (Coombs et al., 2007), though rearrangements of stratification pattern may occur at later stages (see Tian and Copenhagen, 2003).

The same morphological measurements used to distinguish among different RGC classes in the adult mouse have also been applied to RGCs on different postnatal days (Coombs et al., 2007). This effort revealed three different developmental trends. Five of the parameters showed little or no change. Five others increased steadily until around eye opening, after which these measures declined to reach adult-like values. And three other parameters showed little or no change early in postnatal development, then quickly increased to adult-like levels, showing an overall sigmoid shape in their growth pattern (figure 15.5). Thus, RGC dendritic growth appears to be regulated by different factors, all acting during the early postnatal period.

Development of retinal ganglion cell functional properties

The first synapses of RGCs are conventional, formed with amacrine cells, starting on P3 and ending around P20.

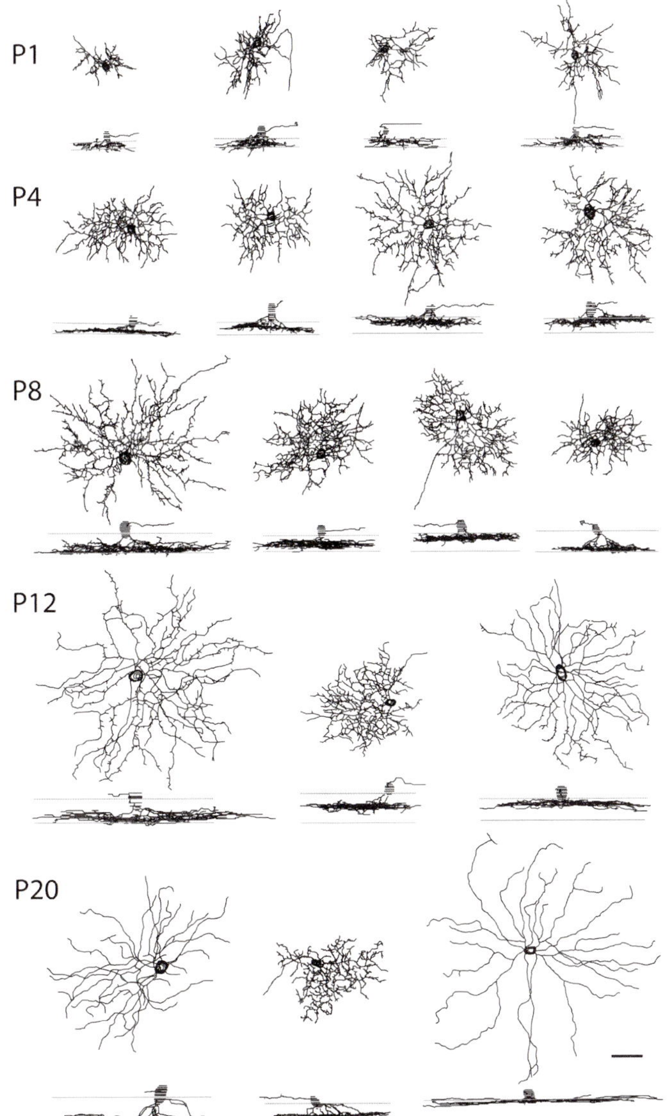

FIGURE 15.4 Tracings of immature RGCs, bird's-eye and side views (*top* and *bottom*, respectively, in each row). Five different ages are shown in rows from top to bottom: P1, P4, P8, P12, and P20. *Lines* in the side views represent the boundaries of the IPL, with the GCL on top and the INL on the bottom. Scale bar = 50 μm.

Ribbon synapses with bipolar cells are seen later in development, starting on P11, around the time of eye opening, and reaching a maximum density around P20 (Fisher, 1979). Correlated with this temporal sequence of synapse formation, waves of electrical and calcium activity move across the retina in large patches. The waves of activity seen between P1 and P10 are driven by cholinergic transmission, while subsequent waves are dependent on glutamate, correlating with the formation of synapses between RGCs and bipolar cells (Bansal et al., 2000). These waves of activity have been implicated in the refinement of RGC projection patterns (for reviews, see Torborg and Feller, 2005; see also chapter 28, this volume).

Spontaneous synaptic events are relatively infrequent before eye opening, with the number of such events recorded from RGCs increasing dramatically about 2 weeks after eye opening (Tian and Copenhagen, 2001). Using multielectrode array recordings, more than half of RGCs just before eye opening have been shown to respond to both On and Off changes in light. The incidence of ON/OFF-responsive cells decreases to the adult level of about 20% by 30 days after birth. This physiological change has been correlated with changes in the dendritic morphology occurring over the same time period. The percentage of the RGC population with both the physiological and anatomical properties of ON/OFF-responsive cells remains fixed if the

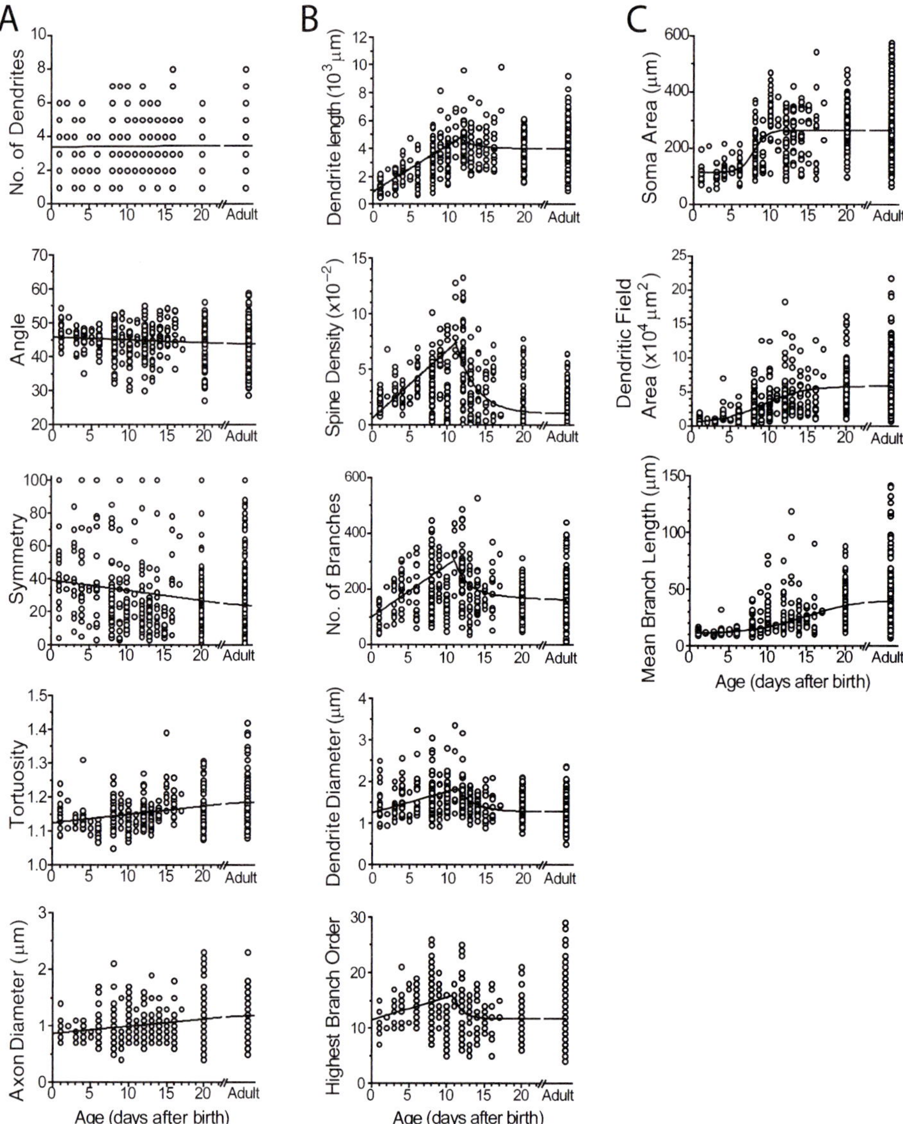

FIGURE 15.5 Thirteen different morphological measurements of developing mouse RGCs showed three main growth patterns. *A*, Little or no change was seen for five of the measurements. *Top to bottom*, number of dendrites, branch angle, symmetry (location of the soma in the dendritic field in bird's-eye view), tortuosity (the curviness of dendritic branches), and axon diameter. *B*, Five measurements showed a growth pattern characterized by linear growth, peaking around P11–P12, followed by decreases described by single exponential decays. *Top to bottom*, total dendrite length, spine density, number of branches, dendrite diameter, and the highest branch order for one dendrite. *C*, Three parameters followed a sigmoid growth pattern: little or no early change, fast change, followed by little or no change. *Top to bottom*, soma area, dendritic field area, and mean branch length. The changes in the means with age were fit by sigmoid curves (*black lines*). All fits were determined by the mean values at each age (*black lines* on each graph). The number of individual cells is the same in each graph, although some graphs appear to have fewer cells, owing to overlapping measurements.

mice are dark-reared (Tian and Copenhagen, 2003). A recent study from our laboratory, however, has shown that the percentage of bistratified cells (i.e., those with dendrites stratified in two distinct strata of the IPL) is relatively constant throughout postnatal development and equivalent to the incidence found at maturity (Coombs et al., 2007). Since the dendrites of many developing RGCs are stratified near the center of the IPL, it is possible that these could be innervated transiently by both ON and OFF bipolar cells, which would account for the apparent discrepancy between our morphological findings and the physiological results of Tian and Copenhagen (2003). However, these authors also reported a higher than normal percentage of RGCs with bistratified dendrites just before eye opening.

About 4 days after eye opening, the retinal waves that traverse the retina during development start to deteriorate, and by P21 they are gone. Unlike changes in the percentage of ON/OFF cells recorded in mouse retina, the loss of retinal waves is not dependent on visual experience, as they are lost over the normal time period when mice are dark-reared (Demas et al., 2003).

Early in development, before rods and cones are functional, ipRGCs can respond to light (Sekaran et al., 2005; Tu et al., 2005; Lupi et al., 2006). And though ipRGCs make up about 1% of the adult RGCs in the mouse, they account for more than 13% of ganglion cells on P0. Also, there are functional connections to the SCN at P0 in normal mice, but innervation of the SCN is not seen until P14 in mice lacking melanopsin (Sekaran et al., 2005). Multielectrode array recordings from early postnatal mouse retinas show three different physiological responses to light (in the absence of retinal waves), indicating three types of ipRGCs in these young retinas. Only two of these response types were also seen in the adult (Tu et al., 2005).

Concluding remarks

Mice are proving to be a remarkable resource for studies of RGCs in particular and the visual system in general. Though the visual capabilities of the mouse are relatively poor, increasingly sophisticated techniques for manipulating the mouse genome are already providing advances in our understanding of the visual system. Undoubtedly, we can look forward to more advances as more and more investigators become convinced of the utility of the mouse for their studies of the visual system.

REFERENCES

Badea, T. C., and Nathans, J. (2004). Quantitative analysis of neuronal morphologies in the mouse retina visualized by using a genetically directed reporter. *J. Comp. Neurol.* 480(4):331–351.

Badea, T. C., Wang, Y., and Nathans, J. (2003). A noninvasive genetic/pharmacologic strategy for visualizing cell morphology and clonal relationships in the mouse. *J. Neurosci.* 23(6): 2314–2322.

Bansal, A., Singer, J. H., Hwang, B. J., Xu, W., Beaudet, A., and Feller, M. B. (2000). Mice lacking specific nicotinic acetylcholine receptor subunits exhibit dramatically altered spontaneous activity patterns and reveal a limited role for retinal waves in forming ON and OFF circuits in the inner retina. *J. Neurosci.* 20(20):7672–7681.

Barnard, A. R., Hattar, S., Hankins, M. W., and Lucas, R. J. (2006). Melanopsin regulates visual processing in the mouse retina. *Curr. Biol.* 16(4):389–395.

Barnstable, C. J., and Drager, U. C. (1984). Thy-1 antigen: A ganglion cell specific marker in rodent retina. *Neuroscience* 11(4):847–855.

Baumer, N., Marquardt, T., Stoykova, A., Ashery-Padan, R., Chowdhury, K., and Gruss, P. (2002). *Pax6* is required for establishing naso-temporal and dorsal characteristics of the optic vesicle. *Development* 129(19):4535–4545.

Belenky, M. A., Smeraski, C. A., Provencio, I., Sollars, P. J., and Pickard, G. E. (2003). Melanopsin retinal ganglion cells receive bipolar and amacrine cell synapses. *J. Comp. Neurol.* 460(3):380–393.

Berson, D. M. (2003). Strange vision: ganglion cells as circadian photoreceptors. *Trends Neurosci.* 26(6):314–320.

Brown, N. L., Kanekar, S., Vetter, M. L., Tucker, P. K., Gemza, D. L., and Glaser, T. (1998). Math5 encodes a murine basic helix-loop-helix transcription factor expressed during early stages of retinal neurogenesis. *Development* 125(23):4821–4833.

Brown, N. L., Patel, S., Brzezinski, J., and Glaser, T. (2001). Math5 is required for retinal ganglion cell and optic nerve formation. *Development* 128(13):2497–2508.

Carcieri, S. M., Jacobs, A. L., and Nirenberg, S. (2003). Classification of retinal ganglion cells: A statistical approach. *J. Neurophysiol.* 90(3):1704–1713.

Chalupa, L. M., and Werner, J. S. (Eds.). (2004). *The visual neurosciences.* Cambridge, MA: MIT Press.

Coombs, J., van der List, D., and Chalupa, L. M. (2007). Morphological properties of mouse retinal ganglion cells during postnatal development. *J. Comp. Neurol.* 503(6):803–814.

Coombs, J., van der, List, D., Wang, G. Y., and Chalupa, L. M. (2006). Morphological properties of mouse retinal ganglion cells. *Neuroscience* 140(1):123–136.

Demas, J., Eglen, S. J., and Wong, R. O. (2003). Developmental loss of synchronous spontaneous activity in the mouse retina is independent of visual experience. *J. Neurosci.* 23(7):2851–2860.

de Melo, J., Du, G., Fonseca, M., Gillespie, L. A., Turk, W. J., Rubenstein, J. L., and Eisenstat, D. D. (2005). Dlx1 and Dlx2 function is necessary for terminal differentiation and survival of late-born retinal ganglion cells in the developing mouse retina. *Development* 132(2):311–322.

de Melo, J., Qiu, X., Du, G., Cristante, L., and Eisenstat, D. D. (2003). Dlx1, Dlx2, Pax6, Brn3b, and Chx10 homeobox gene expression defines the retinal ganglion and inner nuclear layers of the developing and adult mouse retina. *J. Comp. Neurol.* 461(2):187–204.

Doi, M., Uji, Y., and Yamamura, H. (1995). Morphological classification of retinal ganglion cells in mice. *J. Comp. Neurol.* 356:368–386.

Doyle, S. E., Castrucci, A. M., McCall, M., Provencio, I., and Menaker, M. (2006). Nonvisual light responses in the Rpe65 knockout mouse: Rod loss restores sensitivity to the melanopsin system. *Proc. Natl. Acad. Sci. U.S.A.* 103(27):10432–10437.

Drager, U. C. (1985). Birth dates of retinal ganglion cells giving rise to the crossed and uncrossed optic projections in the mouse. *Proc. R. Soc. Lond. B. Biol. Sci.* 224(1234):57–77.

Drager, U. C., and Olsen, J. F. (1980). Origins of crossed and uncrossed retinal projections in pigmented and albino mice. *J. Comp. Neurol.* 191(3):383–412.

Edwards, M. A., Schneider, G. E., and Caviness, V. S., Jr. (1986). Development of the crossed retinocollicular projection in the mouse. *J. Comp. Neurol.* 248(3):410–421.

Erkman, L., McEvilly, R. J., Luo, L., Ryan, A. K., Hooshmand, F., O'Connell, S. M., Keithley, E. M., Rapaport, D. H., Ryan, A. F., and Rosenfeld, M. G. (1996). Role of transcription factors Brn-3.1 and Brn-3.2 in auditory and visual system development. *Nature* 381(6583):603–606.

Erkman, L., Yates, P. A., McLaughlin, T., McEvilly, R. J., Whisenhunt, T., O'Connell, S. M., Krones, A. I., Kirby, M. A., Rapaport, D. H., et al. (2000). A POU domain transcription factor-dependent program regulates axon pathfinding in the vertebrate visual system. *Neuron* 28(3):779–792.

Farah, M. H., and Easter, S. S., Jr. (2005). Cell birth and death in the mouse retinal ganglion cell layer. *J. Comp. Neurol.* 489(1):120–134.

Feng, G., Mellow, R. H., Bernstein, M., Keller-Peck, C., Nguyen, Q. T., Wallace, M., Nerbonne, J. M., Lichtman, J. W., and Sanes, J. R. (2000). Imaging neuronal subsets in transgenic mice expressing multiple spectral variants of GFP. *Neuron* 28:41–51.

Fisher, L. J. (1979). Development of synaptic arrays in the inner plexiform layer of neonatal mouse retina. *J. Comp. Neurol.* 187(2):359–372.

Gan, L., Wang, S. W., Huang, Z., and Klein, W. H. (1999). POU domain factor Brn-3b is essential for retinal ganglion cell differentiation and survival but not for initial cell fate specification. *Dev. Biol.* 210(2):469–480.

Gan, L., Xiang, M., Zhou, L., Wagner, D. S., Klein, W. H., and Nathans, J. (1996). POU domain factor Brn-3b is required for the development of a large set of retinal ganglion cells. *Proc. Natl. Acad. Sci. U.S.A.* 93(9):3920–3925.

Gan, W. B., Grutzendler, J., Wong, W. T., Wong, R. O., and Lichtman, J. W. (2000). Multicolor "DiOlistic" labeling of the nervous system using lipophilic dye combinations. *Neuron* 27(2):219–225.

Godement, P., Salaun, J., and Imbert, M. (1984). Prenatal and postnatal development of retinogeniculate and retinocollicular projections in the mouse. *J. Comp. Neurol.* 230(4): 552–575.

Godement, P., Vanselow, J., Thanos, S., and Bonhoeffer, F. (1987). A study in developing visual systems with a new method of staining neurones and their processes in fixed tissue. *Development* 101(4):697–713.

Hattar, S., Kumar, M., Park, A., Tong, P., Tung, J., Yau, K. W., and Berson, D. M. (2006). Central projections of melanopsin-expressing retinal ganglion cells in the mouse. *J. Comp. Neurol.* 497(3):326–349.

Hattar, S., Liao, H. W., Takao, M., Berson, D. M., and Yau, K. W. (2002). Melanopsin-containing retinal ganglion cells: Architecture, projections, and intrinsic photosensitivity. *Science* 295(5557):1065–1070.

Herrera, E., Brown, L., Aruga, J., Rachel, R. A., Dolen, G., Mikoshiba, K., Brown, S., and Mason, C. A. (2003). Zic2 patterns binocular vision by specifying the uncrossed retinal projection. *Cell* 114(5):545–557.

Hinds, J. W., and Hinds, P. L. (1974). Early ganglion cell differentiation in the mouse retina: An electron microscopic analysis utilizing serial sections. *Dev. Biol.* 37:381–416.

Hofbauer, A., and Drager, U. C. (1985). Depth segregation of retinal ganglion cells projecting to mouse superior colliculus. *J. Comp. Neurol.* 234:465–474.

Jensen, A. M., and Wallace, V. A. (1997). Expression of Sonic hedgehog and its putative role as a precursor cell mitogen in the developing mouse retina. *Development* 124(2):363–371.

Kim, I., Yamagata, M., and Sanes, J. R. (2006). The cell adhesion molecule jam-b identifies a novel retinal ganglion cell subtype. *Soc. Neurosci.* abstract.

Kim, J., Wu, H. H., Lander, A. D., Lyons, K. M., Matzuk, M. M., and Calof, A. L. (2005). GDF11 controls the timing of progenitor cell competence in developing retina. *Science* 308(5730):1927–1930.

Kong, J. H., Fish, D. R., Rockhill, R. L., and Masland, R. H. (2005). Diversity of ganglion cells in the mouse retina: Unsupervised morphological classification and its limits. *J. Comp. Neurol.* 489(3):293–310.

Lin, B., Wang, S. W., and Masland, R. H. (2004). Retinal ganglion cell type, size, and spacing can be specified independent of homotypic dendritic contacts. *Neuron* 43(4):475–485.

Linden, R., and Pinto, L. H. (1985). Developmental genetics of the retina: Evidence that the pearl mutation in the mouse affects the time course of natural cell death in the ganglion cell layer. *Exp. Brain. Res.* 60(1):79–86.

Lupi, D., Sekaran, S., Jones, S. L., Hankins, M. W., and Foster, R. G. (2006). Light-evoked FOS induction within the suprachiasmatic nuclei (SCN) of melanopsin knockout (Opn4$^{-/-}$) mice: A developmental study. *Chronobiol. Int.* 23(1–2):167–179.

Marquardt, T., Ashery-Padan, R., Andrejewski, N., Scardigli, R., Guillemot, F., and Gruss, P. (2001). Pax6 is required for the multipotent state of retinal progenitor cells. *Cell* 105(1): 43–55.

Mu, X., Fu, X., Sun, H., Beremand, P. D., Thomas, T. L., and Klein, W. H. (2005). A gene network downstream of transcription factor Math5 regulates retinal progenitor cell competence and ganglion cell fate. *Dev. Biol.* 280(2):467–481.

Nirenberg, S., and Meister, M. (1997). The light response of retinal ganglion cells is truncated by a displaced amacrine circuit. *Neuron* 18(4):637–650.

Pak, W., Hindges, R., Lim, Y. S., Pfaff, S. L., and O'Leary, D. D. (2004). Magnitude of binocular vision controlled by islet-2 repression of a genetic program that specifies laterality of retinal axon pathfinding. *Cell* 119(4):567–578.

Pan, L., Yang, Z., Feng, L., and Gan, L. (2005). Functional equivalence of Brn3 POU-domain transcription factors in mouse retinal neurogenesis. *Development* 132(4):703–712.

Panda, S., Provencio, I., Tu, D. C., Pires, S. S., Rollag, M. D., Castrucci, A. M., Pletcher, M. T., Sato, T. K., Wiltshire, T., et al. (2003). Melanopsin is required for non-image-forming photic responses in blind mice. *Science* 301(5632): 525–527.

Pang, J. J., Gao, F., and Wu, S. M. (2003). Light-evoked excitatory and inhibitory synaptic inputs to ON and OFF alpha ganglion cells in the mouse retina. *J. Neurosci.* 23(14): 6063–6073.

Peichl, L., Ott, H., and Boycott, B. B. (1987). Alpha ganglion cells in mammalian retinae. *Proc. R. Soc. Lond. B. Biol. Sci.* 231(1263):169–197.

Pequignot, M. O., Provost, A. C., Salle, S., Taupin, P., Sainton, K. M., Marchant, D., Martinou, J. C., Ameisen, J. C., Jais, J. P., and Abitbol, M. (2003). Major role of BAX in apoptosis during retinal development and in establishment of a functional postnatal retina. *Dev. Dyn.* 228(2):231–238.

Provencio, I., Cooper, H. M., and Foster, R. G. (1998). Retinal projections in mice with inherited retinal degeneration: Implications for circadian photoentrainment. *J. Comp. Neurol.* 395(4): 417–439.

Provencio, I., Rollag, M. D., and Castrucci, A. M. (2002). Photoreceptive net in the mammalian retina: This mesh of cells may explain how some blind mice can still tell day from night. *Nature* 415(6871):493.

Quina, L. A., Pak, W., Lanier, J., Banwait, P., Gratwick, K., Liu, Y., Velasquez, T., O'Leary, D. D., Goulding, M., and Turner, E. E. (2005). Brn3a-expressing retinal ganglion cells project specifically to thalamocortical and collicular visual pathways. *J. Neurosci.* 25(50):11595–11604.

Ruby, N. F., Brennan, T. J., Xie, X., Cao, V., Franken, P., Heller, H. C., and O'Hara, B. F. (2002). Role of melanopsin in circadian responses to light. *Science* 298(5601):2211–2213.

Schubert, T., Degen, J., Willecke, K., Hormuzdi, S. G., Monyer, H., and Weiler, R. (2005a). Connexin36 mediates gap junctional coupling of alpha-ganglion cells in mouse retina. *J. Comp. Neurol.* 485(3):191–201.

Schubert, T., Maxeiner, S., Kruger, O., Willecke, K., and Weiler, R. (2005b). Connexin45 mediates gap junctional coupling of bistratified ganglion cells in the mouse retina. *J. Comp. Neurol.* 490(1):29–39.

Sekaran, S., Lupi, D., Jones, S. L., Sheely, C. J., Hattar, S., Yau, K. W., Lucas, R. J., Foster, R. G., and Hankins, M. W. (2005). Melanopsin-dependent photoreception provides earliest light detection in the mammalian retina. *Curr. Biol.* 15(12): 1099–1107.

Stone, C., and Pinto, L. H. (1993). Response properties of ganglion cells in the isolated mouse retina. *Vis. Neurosci.* 10(1):31–39.

Sun, W., Li, N., and He, S. (2002). Large-scale morphological survey of mouse retinal ganglion cells. *J. Comp. Neurol.* 451(2):115–126.

Tian, N., and Copenhagen, D. R. (2001). Visual deprivation alters development of synaptic function in inner retina after eye opening. *Neuron* 32(3):439–449.

Tian, N., and Copenhagen, D. R. (2003). Visual stimulation is required for refinement of ON and OFF pathways in postnatal retina. *Neuron* 39(1):85–96.

Tian, N., Hwang, T. N., and Copenhagen, D. R. (1998). Analysis of excitatory and inhibitory spontaneous synaptic activity in mouse retinal ganglion cells. *J. Neurophysiol.* 80(3):1327–1340.

Torborg, C. L., and Feller, M. B. (2005). Spontaneous patterned retinal activity and the refinement of retinal projections. *Prog. Neurobiol.* 76(4):213–235.

Tu, D. C., Zhang, D., Demas, J., Slutsky, E. B., Provencio, I., Holy, T. E., and Van Gelder, R. N. (2005). Physiologic diversity and development of intrinsically photosensitive retinal ganglion cells. *Neuron* 48(6):987–999.

Völgyi, B., Abrams, J., Paul, D. L., and Bloomfield, S. A. (2005). Morphology and tracer coupling pattern of alpha ganglion cells in the mouse retina. *J. Comp. Neurol.* 492(1):66–77.

Wagner, K. D., Wagner, N., Vidal, V. P., Schley, G., Wilhelm, D., Schedl, A., Englert, C., and Scholz, H. (2002). The Wilms' tumor gene Wt1 is required for normal development of the retina. *Embo. J.* 21(6):1398–1405.

Wang, S. W., Kim, B. S., Ding, K., Wang, H., Sun, D., Johnson, R. L., Klein, W. H., and Gan, L. (2001). Requirement for math5 in the development of retinal ganglion cells. *Genes Dev.* 15(1):24–29.

Wang, S. W., Mu, X., Bowers, W. J., Kim, D. S., Plas, D. J., Crair, M. C., Federoff, H. J., Gan, L., and Klein, W. H. (2002). Brn3b/Brn3c double knockout mice reveal an unsuspected role for Brn3c in retinal ganglion cell axon outgrowth. *Development* 129(2):467–477.

Wang, Y., Dakubo, G. D., Thurig, S., Mazerolle, C. J., and Wallace, V. A. (2005). Retinal ganglion cell-derived sonic hedgehog locally controls proliferation and the timing of RGC development in the embryonic mouse retina. *Development* 132(22): 5103–5113.

Xiang, M. (1998). Requirement for Brn-3b in early differentiation of postmitotic retinal ganglion cell precursors. *Dev. Biol.* 197(2):155–169.

Xiang, M., Zhou, L., Macke, J. P., Yoshioka, T., Hendry, S. H., Eddy, R. L., Shows, T. B., and Nathans, J. (1995). The Brn-3 family of POU-domain factors: Primary structure, binding specificity, and expression in subsets of retinal ganglion cells and somatosensory neurons. *J. Neurosci.* 15(7 Pt. 1):4762–4785.

Xiang, M., Zhou, L., and Nathans, J. (1996). Similarities and differences among inner retinal neurons revealed by the expression of reporter transgenes controlled by Brn-3a, Brn-3b, and Brn-3c promotor sequences. *Vis. Neurosci.* 13(5):955–962.

Xiang, M., Zhou, L., Peng, Y. W., Eddy, R. L., Shows, T. B., and Nathans, J. (1993). Brn-3b: A POU domain gene expressed in a subset of retinal ganglion cells. *Neuron* 11(4): 689–701.

Yang, Z., Ding, K., Pan, L., Deng, M., and Gan, L. (2003). Math5 determines the competence state of retinal ganglion cell progenitors. *Dev. Biol.* 264(1):240–254.

Young, R. W. (1984). Cell death during differentiation of the retina in the mouse. *J. Comp. Neurol.* 229(3):362–373.

Young, R. W. (1985). Cell differentiation in the retina of the mouse. *Anat. Rec.* 212:199–205.

Zhang, X. M., and Yang, X. J. (2001). Regulation of retinal ganglion cell production by Sonic hedgehog. *Development* 128(6): 943–957.

Zubair, M., Watanabe, E., Fukada, M., and Noda, M. (2002). Genetic labelling of specific axonal pathways in the mouse central nervous system. *Eur. J. Neurosci.* 15(5):807–814.

16 The Lamina Cribrosa Region and Optic Nerve of the Mouse

CHRISTIAN-ALBRECHT MAY

This chapter introduces structural and developmental aspects of the murine optic nerve. After an initial consideration of general morphological features, the first section describes the development of the optic nerve, with additional discussion of the optic nerve head region and myelinogenesis. The second section introduces the different cellular components of the optic nerve, namely, axons and glial cells (astrocytes, oligodendrocytes, microglia), while the third section focuses on connective tissue in the different optic nerve sections. The fourth section discusses the vascular supply of the murine optic nerve.

General morphological features

Four distinct sections of the optic nerve can be differentiated in the mouse orbit (figure 16.1): (1) The *optic nerve head*: efferent (axonal) processes of the retinal ganglion cells (RGCs) forming the nerve fiber layer of the retina accumulate toward the intraocular portion of the optic nerve. (2) The *lamina cribrosa region*: at the level of the choroid and sclera, the optic nerve fibers leave the eye. (3) The *unmyelinated portion*: the murine optic nerve first remains unmyelinated in the extraocular course. (4) The *myelinated portion*: in the posterior orbit, the optic nerve contains myelinated axons.

As part of the CNS, the extraocular portion of the optic nerve in the orbit is surrounded by three meningeal sheaths: (1) The pia mater covers the surface of the nerve and contains the small pial vessels. (2) A delicate arachnoid mater forms the subarachnoidal space containing cerebrospinal fluid. (3) The dura mater is the outermost sheath and merges anteriorly with the sclera.

Development

Next to the optic stalk, about 50–100 µm behind the eye, the first bundles of axons from the RGCs are seen on embryonic day 12.5 (E12.5) as a mixture of thin axons, thicker growth cones, and fine filopodial and foliopodial extensions (Colello and Guillery, 1992). Over the next 2 days, these bundles increase in size and number, and contain growth cones in all parts of the bundles. Toward the chiasm, the structure of the optic nerve pathway changes significantly: the growth cones become located predominantly close to the pial surface, and the deeper regions are filled by fine axons (Colello and Guillery, 1992). At the molecular level, the axon guidance molecule netrin-1 is necessary locally at the optic disc for proper pathfinding of the RGC axons (Deiner et al., 1997). The homebox gene *Vax1* and the sonic hedgehog protein seem to regulate the interaction between sprouting axons and optic nerve glia (astrocytes) deriving from the optic stalk (Bertuzzi et al., 1999; Wallace and Raff, 1999; Dakubo et al., 2003). At the level of the optic chiasm, *Vax1* and the paired homebox transcription factor Pax2 are required for proper formation of contralateral projections (Torres et al., 1996; Bertuzzi et al., 1999), while homebox gene *Vax2* is necessary for the formation of ipsilateral retinocollicular projections (Barbieri et al., 2002). Another crucial factor at the level of the optic chiasm is the growth-associated protein 43 (Strittmatter et al., 1995).

The optic nerve head/optic disc develops at the interface between the optic stalk and the retina. The initial step is the formation of the optic fissure on E10, which enables ganglion cell axons to exit the eye and mesenchymal cells to form hyaloid vessels. A crucial factor for this event seems to be the bone morphogenetic protein-7 (Bmp7), a factor known also to stimulate *Pax2* in an early phase of optic nerve head formation (Morcillo et al., 2006). *Pax2*, together with other homebox genes (e.g., *Vax2*), is necessary for guidance of the sprouting ganglion cell axons and for proper closure of the optic fissure (Torres et al., 1996; Otteson et al., 1998; Barbieri et al., 2002). Besides Bmp7, *Pax2* expression is also induced by other cytokines, among them Bmp4 and sonic hedgehog protein (Weston et al., 2003), but at a slightly later stage of the development. Closure of the optic fissure begins on E11 and is usually completed 2 days later (Hero, 1990; Ozeki et al., 2000). At birth (normally E21–E23), the optic nerve head is completely developed, showing a two- to three-fold increase in the number of axons, which falls to the adult value within 1 week (Sefton et al., 1985; Strom and Williams, 1998).

Myelinogenesis of the optic nerve axons begins by the end of the first week of postnatal life, starting selectively with the largest axons and in the direction of brain toward the eye (Bernstein et al., 1983; Dangata and Kaufman, 1997). At the

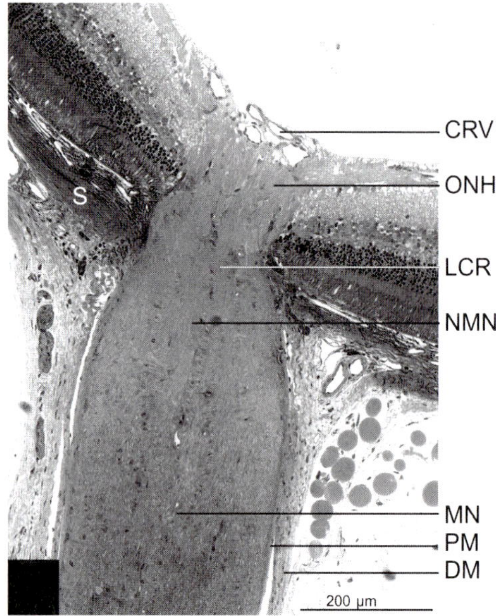

FIGURE 16.1 Optic nerve, sagittal section, showing four distinct sections: the optic nerve head (ONH), lamina cribrosa region (LCR), unmyelinated optic nerve (NMN), and myelinated optic nerve (MN). In the inner region of the optic nerve head several central retinal vessels (CRV) are visible. At the level of the sclera (S), no collagen bundles penetrate the optic nerve head; therefore, no lamina cribrosa is present. The extraocular optic nerve is surrounded by the pia mater (PM) and the dura mater (DM), separated by the subarachnoidal space.

end of the fifth week, about 73% of the fibers are myelinated, and by the 16th week virtually all axons enclose a myelin sheath (Dangata and Kaufman, 1997). The process of myelin sheath formation and differentiation continues even in adult animals, though on a very reduced scale. Quantification of optic nerve axons revealed that only about 1.2% of axons are unmyelinated in the optic nerve of the adult mouse (Honjin et al., 1977). Specific factors for oligodendrocyte morphogenesis and myelin formation in the optic nerve include the following: (1) for precursor cell numbers and cell spreading: brain-derived neurotrophic factor (Cellerino et al., 1997), gap junction proteins connexin 47 and connexin 32 (Menichella et al., 2003; Odermatt et al., 2003), laminin-2 (Chun et al., 2003), and Wiskott-Aldrich syndrome protein family verprolin homologous protein 1 (Kim et al., 2006); and (2) for axonal ensheathment and myelin compaction: myelin-associated glycoprotein (Biffiger et al., 2000), proteolipid protein (Thomson et al., 2005), and matrix metalloproteinases 9 and 12, which regulate insulin-like growth factor 1 (Larsen et al., 2006). Interestingly, myelination of the murine optic nerve stops 0.6–0.8 mm behind the eye globe. The precise mechanism is unknown, but potential molecular factors that might actively stop myelination at this level include tenascin C (Bartsch et al., 1994) and the polysialylated neural cell adhesion molecule (Charles et al., 2000).

Neuronal and glial tissue

The neuronal tissue in the optic nerve head and optic nerve consists of axons from the RGCs. Their number reveals profound variations in different mouse strains: in 60 inbred strains, the number of axons varies between 32,000 and 87,000, with distinct modes centered at 55,000 and 64,000 axons (Williams et al., 1996). The two most popular mouse strains represent the two modes, the lower (C57BL/6J) and the higher (Balb/cJ) mode, respectively. This difference is mainly due to a difference in RGC generation rather than apoptosis postpartum (Strom and Williams, 1998).

At birth, the unmyelinated axons have an average diameter of 0.4 μm (Strom and Williams, 1998). They are located next to each other without being separated by glial cell processes. In adult optic nerve sections, the myelinated nerve fibers (axons, including the myelin sheath) range in diameter from 0.3 to 4.2 μm, with a single peak at 0.7–0.9 μm. In the peripheral area of the murine optic nerve on cross section, the nerve fibers are relatively small and uniform in diameter, whereas the larger nerve fibers are mainly located in the central area (Honjin et al., 1977). In the optic nerve head, the axons remain unmyelinated and are clustered in bundles without glial separation of each single axon within the bundle. At the ultrastructural level the axons contain neurofilaments, neurotubuli, and mitochondria.

The presence and distribution of glial cells is different in the optic nerve head and the optic nerve: while the first contains only astrocytes, the latter contains astrocytes and oligodendrocytes. Microglia cells occur in both parts in rather small number (Wong et al., 1979; Lawson et al., 1994) and express MAC-1, but not Fc gamma II/III receptor, F4/80, or MAC-2 (Reichert and Rotshenker, 1996). Cell numbers of all three types of glial cells—astrocytes, oligodendrocytes, and microglia—show a distinct proportion to the number of axons: relating to 1,000 axons in a myelinated optic nerve cross section, one can detect 1.7–2.1 nuclei of oligodendrocytes, 0.9–1.2 nuclei of astrocytes, and 0.05–0.07 nuclei of microglia cells (adjusted from Burne et al., 1996).

Optic nerve astrocytes, stimulated by the ganglion cell axons to proliferate and differentiate (Burne and Raff, 1997), initially express vimentin (from E12 to E16) and then gradually change to their specific glial filament acidic protein (GFAP) expression. GFAP staining is first seen at the border of the nerve (beginning on E17) and spreads into the central optic nerve until birth. Astrocytes develop and express GFAP from the eye toward the optic tract (Bovolenta et al., 1987). In the mature myelinated optic nerve, astrocyte processes form multiple contacts with the nodes of Ranvier, blood vessels, and subpial glia limitans. They appear uniform, and there is no evidence for a specialized subpopulation of astrocytes in this part of the murine optic nerve (Butt et al., 1994).

In the optic nerve head, astrocytes also appear uniform ultrastructurally (May and Lütjen-Drecoll, 2002). However, at the level of the sclera, elongated astrocyte processes run transversally between the axon bundles, forming a meshlike frame and being extensively stuffed with intermediate glial filaments and cell organelles (Ding et al., 2002). Astrocytes are connected between each other by connexin 43, which is pronounced in the optic nerve head region (Yancey et al., 1992; May and Mittag, 2006).

The generation of oligodendrocytes and the myelin sheath was described earlier in the chapter. Mature oligodendrocytes of the murine optic nerve are characterized ultrastructurally by a dense nucleus and cytoplasm with sparse filaments (figure 16.2). Besides the production of myelin, optic nerve oligodendrocytes contain carbonic anhydrase II, presumably for local pH regulation (May and Lütjen-Drecoll, 2002; Ro and Carson, 2004).

Connective tissue

Although numerous species develop a lamina cribrosa at the level of the sclera, none of the different mouse strains analyzed shows any connective tissue bundles penetrating the optic nerve head in the unmyelinated portion (Tansley, 1956; Fujita et al., 2000; Morcos and Chan-Ling, 2000; May and Lütjen-Drecoll, 2002). At the level of the choroid and sclera, a smooth ring of densely packed collagen fibers separates the neuronal tissue. This ring is continuous with the pial connective tissue in the postbulbar portion of the nerve (figure 16.3), the bundles of collagen type I, III, and VI fibers arranged obliquely and longitudinally to the long axis of the nerve (May and Lütjen-Drecoll, 2002; May and Mittag, 2006). Toward the neuronal tissue of the optic nerve the collagen fibers of the sheath are connected to the basement membrane of the astrocyte processes surrounding the nerve. Occasionally, short, 5 μm extensions of the collagen sheath follow the basement membrane of the astrocyte processes, giving the internal surface of the ring a somewhat wavelike appearance. Elastic fibers are completely absent within the pial sheath, even at the level of the choroid (May and Lütjen-Drecoll, 2002). At the level of the sclera, the central retinal vessels enter the optic nerve and occupy about one-sixth of the ring.

In the murine optic nerve there are no connective tissue septa separating individual nerve fiber bundles from each other. Only some collagen fibers split from the pial connective tissue to follow the entering vessels into the myelinated part of the nerve.

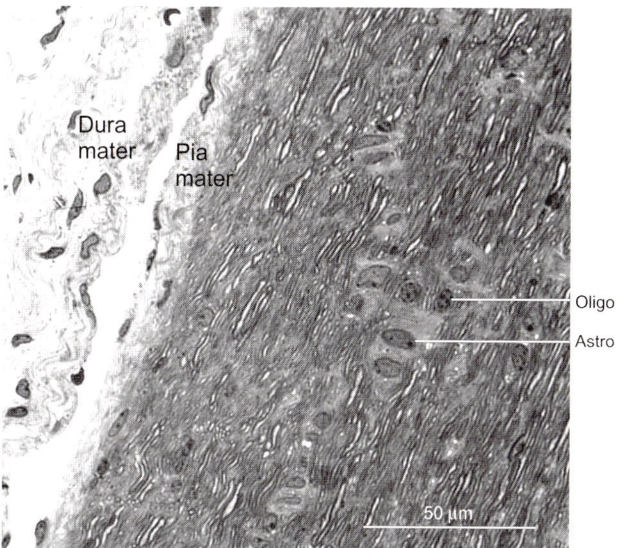

FIGURE 16.2 Myelinated portion of the optic nerve. Note the morphological differences between nuclei of astrocytes (Astro) and oligodendrocytes (Oligo).

Vascular supply

The central retinal artery (CRA) derives as a branch from the ophthalmic artery before ramifying into the posterior ciliary arteries. A triangular intra-arterial cushion is regularly present in the ophthalmic artery just before the

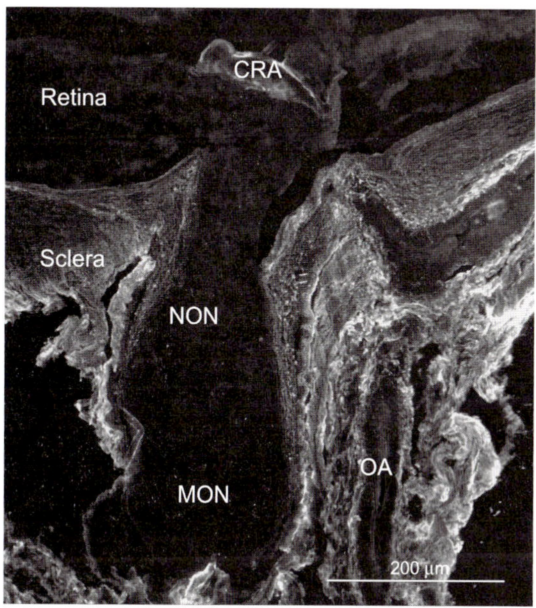

FIGURE 16.3 Optic nerve, sagittal section, immunostained with antibodies against collagen type III. Note the intense staining around the central retinal vessels (CRA), around the ophthalmic artery (OA), in the sclera, and around the optic nerve. No staining is present in the myelinated (MON) or unmyelinated (NON) portion of the optic nerve.

branching of the CRA. The cushion consists of smooth muscle cells and is covered by endothelial cells toward the lumen of the vessel. No nerve terminals are present in these protuberances. At the base of the cushion, the internal elastic lamina of the ophthalmic artery is interrupted, but fine elastic fibers within the cushion contact the internal elastic lamina (May and Lütjen-Drecoll, 2002). A similar cushion is also present in the rat ophthalmic artery (Lassmann et al., 1972), but does not exist in the human. The functional significance of this cushion is not clear, but it might modify blood flow in the entrance region of small branching vessels.

The CRA runs to the sclera and enters the optic nerve obliquely at the level of the sclera and choroid toward the center of the ONH (figure 16.4), where it branches further, forming the retinal arteries. The unmyelinated portion of the optic nerve is exclusively supplied by backward branches of the central retinal artery (May and Lütjen-Drecoll, 2002). These small vessels (two to three capillaries) are in direct contact with the neuronal tissue, showing a merged basement membrane of both endothelial cells and pericytes and astrocytes. The sheath of pericytes in this region is incomplete. The endothelial cells are connected by tight junctions supporting the blood–neural tissue barrier. The choroid does not contribute to the optic nerve head region blood supply in the mouse, and the arterial circle of Zinn and Haller is not present.

The myelinated portion of the optic nerve is supplied by capillaries deriving from pial vessels (May and Lütjen-Drecoll, 2002). These capillaries show a similar structure as in the unmyelinated portion, with two differences: the vessels are surrounded by a small connective tissue sheath separating the basement membrane from the vessel wall and the basement membrane of the astrocytes, and the endothelial cells do not show tight junctions, indicating a somewhat less potent blood barrier. Anastomoses between both capillary beds exist at the transit from the myelinated to the unmyelinated portion of the optic nerve.

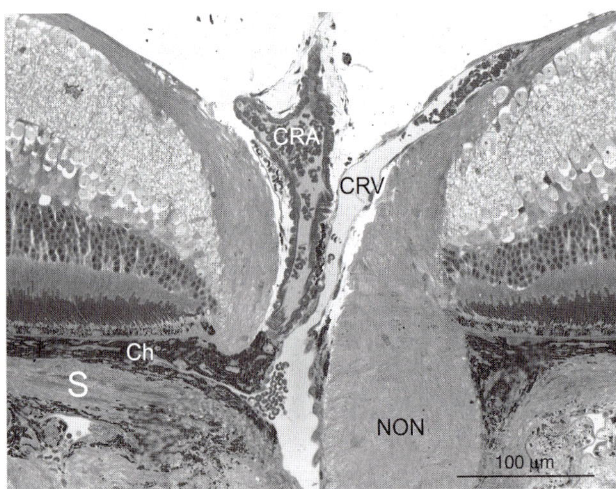

Figure 16.4 Sagittal section. The central retinal artery (CRA) and central retinal vein (CRV) enter the optic nerve obliquely at the level of the sclera (S) and choroid (Ch) toward the center of the optic nerve head. NON, unmyelinated portion of the optic nerve.

The central retinal vein runs closer to the optic nerve than the artery and is connected with the pial venous system. In contrast, the posterior ciliary veins draining blood from the posterior choroid continued to the orbital venous sinus (Pinkerton and Webber, 1964; Yamashita et al., 1980).

REFERENCES

Barbieri, A. M., Broccoli, V., Bovolenta, P., Alfano, G., Marchitiello, A., Mocchetti, C., Crippa, L., Bulfone, A., Marigo, V., et al. (2002). Vax2 inactivation in mouse determines alteration of the eye dorsal-ventral axis, misrouting of the optic fibres and eye coloboma. *Development* 129(3):805–813.

Bartsch, U., Faissner, A., Trotter, J., Dorries, U., Bartsch, S., Mohajeri, H., and Schachner, M. (1994). Tenascin demarcates the boundary between the myelinated and nonmyelinated part of retinal ganglion cell axons in the developing and adult mouse. *J. Neurosci.* 14(8):4756–4768.

Bartsch, U., Kirchhoff, F., and Schachner, M. (1989). Immunohistological localization of the adhesion molecules L1, N-CAM, and MAG in the developing and adult optic nerve of mice. *J. Comp. Neurol.* 284(3):451–462.

Bernstein, E., Tost, M., and Holzhausen, H. J. (1983). Myelinisierung des Nervus opticus bei der Albinomaus (the Agnes Bluhm Jena-Halle strain). *Klin. Monatsbl. Augenheilkd.* 183(4):265–269.

Bertuzzi, S., Hindges, R., Mui, S. H., O'Leary, D. D., and Lemke, G. (1999). The homeodomain protein vax1 is required for axon guidance and major tract formation in the developing forebrain. *Genes Dev.* 13(23):3092–3105.

Biffiger, K., Bartsch, S., Montag, D., Aguzzi, A., Schachner, M., and Bartsch, U. (2000). Severe hypomyelination of the murine CNS in the absence of myelin-associated glycoprotein and fyn tyrosine kinase. *J. Neurosci.* 20:7430–7437.

Bovolenta, P., Liem, R. K., and Mason, C. A. (1987). Glial filament protein expression in astroglia in the mouse visual pathway. *Brain Res.* 430(1):113–126.

Burne, J. F., and Raff, M. C. (1997). Retinal ganglion cell axons drive the proliferation of astrocytes in the developing rodent optic nerve. *Neuron* 18(2):223–230.

Burne, J. F., Staple, J. K., and Raff, M. C. (1996). Glial cells are increased proportionally in transgenic optic nerves with increased numbers of axons. *J. Neurosci.* 16(6):2064–2073.

Butt, A. M., Duncan, A., and Berry, M. (1994). Astrocyte associations with nodes of Ranvier: Ultrastructural analysis of HRP-filled astrocytes in the mouse optic nerve. *J. Neurocytol.* 23(8):486–499.

Cellerino, A., Carroll, P., Thoenen, H., and Barde, Y. A. (1997). Reduced size of retinal ganglion cell axons and hypomyelination in mice lacking brain-derived neurotrophic factor. *Mol. Cell Neurosci.* 9(5–6):397–408.

Charles, P., Hernandez, M. P., Stankoff, B., Aigrot, M. S., Colin, C., Rougon, G., Zalc, B., and Lubetzki, C. (2000). Negative regulation of central nervous system myelination by polysialylated-neural cell adhesion molecule. *Proc. Natl. Acad. Sci. U.S.A.* 97(13):7585–7590.

Chun, S. J., Rasband, M. N., Sidman, R. L., Habib, A. A., and Vartanian, T. (2003). Integrin-linked kinase is required for laminin-2-induced oligodendrocyte cell spreading and CNS myelination. *J. Cell Biol.* 163(2):397–408.

Colello, R. J., and Guillery, R. W. (1992). Observations on the early development of the optic nerve and tract of the mouse. *J. Comp. Neurol.* 317(4):357–378.

Dakubo, G. D., Wang, Y. P., Mazerolle, C., Campsall, K., McMahon, A. P., and Wallace, V. A. (2003). Retinal ganglion cell-derived sonic hedgehog signaling is required for optic disc and stalk neuroepithelial cell development. *Development* 130(13): 2967–2980.

Dangata, Y. Y., and Kaufman, M. H. (1997). Myelinogenesis in the optic nerve of (C57BL × CBA) F1 hybrid mice: A morphometric analysis. *Eur. J. Morphol.* 35(1):3–17.

Deiner, M. S., Kennedy, T. E., Fazeli, A., Serafini, T., Tessier-Lavigne, M., and Sretavan, D. W. (1997). Netrin-1 and DCC mediate axon guidance locally at the optic disc: loss of function leads to optic nerve hypoplasia. *Neuron* 19(3):575–589.

Ding, L., Yamada, K., Takayama, C., and Inoue, Y. (2002). Development of astrocytes in the lamina cribrosa sclerae of the mouse optic nerve, with special reference to myelin formation. *Okajimas Folia Anat. Jpn.* 79(5):143–157.

Fujita, Y., Imagawa, T., and Uehara, M. (2000). Comparative study of the lamina cribrosa and the pial septa in the vertebrate optic nerve and their relationship to the myelinated axons. *Tissue Cell* 32:293–301.

Hero, I. (1990). Optic fissure closure in the normal cinnamon mouse. An ultrastructural study. *Invest. Ophthalmol. Vis. Sci.* 31(1): 197–216.

Honjin, R., Sakato, S., and Yamashita, T. (1977). Electron microscopy of the mouse optic nerve: A quantitative study of the total optic nerve fibers. *Arch. Histol. Jpn.* 40(4):321–332.

Kim, H. J., DiBernardo, A. B., Sloane, J. A., Rasband, M. N., Solomon, D., Kosaras, B., Kwak, S. P., and Vartanian, T. K. (2006). WAVE1 is required for oligodendrocyte morphogenesis and normal CNS myelination. *J. Neurosci.* 26(21):5849–5859.

Larsen, P. H., DaSilva, A. G., Conant, K., and Yong, V. W. (2006). Myelin formation during development of the CNS is delayed in matrix metalloproteinase-9 and -12 null mice. *J. Neurosci.* 26(8):2207–2214.

Lassmann, H., Pamperl, H., and Stockinger, G. (1972). Intimapolster der Arteria ophthalmica der Ratte in morphologisch-funktioneller Sicht. *Z. Mikrosk. Anat. Forsch.* 85:139–148.

Lawson, L. J., Frost, L., Risbridger, J., Fearn, S., and Perry, V. H. (1994). Quantification of the mononuclear phagocyte response to Wallerian degeneration of the optic nerve. *J. Neurocytol.* 23(12):729–744.

May, C. A., and Lütjen-Drecoll, E. (2002). Morphology of the murine optic nerve. *Invest. Ophthalmol. Vis. Sci.* 43:2206–2212.

May, C. A., and Mittag, T. (2006). Optic nerve degeneration in the DBA/2NNia mouse: Is the lamina cribrosa important in the development of glaucomatous optic neuropathy? *Acta Neuropathol.* 111:158–167.

Menichella, D. M., Goodenough, D. A., Sirkowski, E., Scherer, S. S., and Paul, D. L. (2003). Connexins are critical for normal myelination in the CNS. *J. Neurosci.* 23(13):5963–5973.

Morcillo, J., Martinez-Morales, J. R., Trousse, F., Fermin, Y., Sowden, J. C., and Bovolenta, P. (2006). Proper patterning of the optic fissure requires the sequential activity of BMP7 and SHH. *Development* 133(16):3179–3190.

Morcos, Y., and Chan-Ling, T. (2000). Concentration of astrocytic filaments at the retinal optic nerve junction is coincident with the absence of intra-retinal myelination: Comparative and developmental evidence. *J. Neurocytol.* 29:665–678.

Odermatt, B., Wellershaus, K., Wallraff, A., Seifert, G., Degen, J., Euwens, C., Fuss, B., Bussow, H., Schilling, K., et al. (2003). Connexin 47 (Cx47)-deficient mice with enhanced green fluorescent protein reporter gene reveal predominant oligodendrocytic expression of Cx47 and display vacuolized myelin in the CNS. *J. Neurosci.* 23(11):4549–4559.

Otteson, D. C., Shelden, E., Jones, J. M., Kameoka, J., and Hitchcock, P. F. (1998). Pax2 expression and retinal morphogenesis in the normal and Krd mouse. *Dev. Biol.* 193(2):209–224.

Ozeki, H., Ogura, Y., Hirabayashi, Y., and Shimada, S. (2000). Apoptosis is associated with formation and persistence of the embryonic fissure. *Curr. Eye Res.* 20(5):367–372.

Pinkerton, W., and Webber, M. (1964). A method of injecting small laboratory animals by the ophthalmic plexus route. *Proc. Soc. Exp. Biol. Med.* 116:959–961.

Reichert, F., and Rotshenker, S. (1996). Deficient activation of microglia during optic nerve degeneration. *J. Neuroimmunol.* 70 (2):153–161.

Ro, H. A., and Carson, J. H. (2004). pH microdomains in oligodendrocytes. *J. Biol. Chem.* 279(35):37115–37123.

Sefton, A. J., Horsburgh, G. M., and Lam, K. (1985). The development of the optic nerve in rodents. *Aust. N.Z. J. Ophthalmol.* 13(2):135–145.

Strittmatter, S. M., Fankhauser, C., Huang, P. L., Mashimo, H., and Fishman, M. C. (1995). Neuronal pathfinding is abnormal in mice lacking the neuronal growth cone protein GAP-43. *Cell* 80(3):445–452.

Strom, R. C., and Williams, R. W. (1998). Cell production and cell death in the generation of variation in neuron number. *J. Neurosci.* 18(23):9948–9953.

Tansley, K. (1956). Comparison of the lamina cribrosa in mammalian species with good and with indifferent vision. *Br. J. Ophthalmol.* 40:178–182.

Thomson, C. E., Vouyiouklis, D. A., Barrie, J. A., Wease, K. N., and Montague, P. (2005). Plp gene regulation in the developing murine optic nerve: Correlation with oligodendroglial process alignment along the axons. *Dev. Neurosci.* 27(1):27–36.

Torres, M., Gomez-Pardo, E., and Gruss, P. (1996). Pax2 contributes to inner ear patterning and optic nerve trajectory. *Development* 122(11):3381–3391.

Wallace, V. A., and Raff, M. C. (1999). A role for Sonic hedgehog in axon-to-astrocyte signalling in the rodent optic nerve. *Development* 126(13):2901–2909.

Weston, C. R., Wong, A., Hall, J. P., Goad, M. E., Flavell, R. A., and Davis, R. J. (2003). JNK initiates a cytokine cascade that causes Pax2 expression and closure of the optic fissure. *Genes Dev.* 17(10):1271–1280.

Williams, R. W., Strom, R. C., Rice, D. S., and Goldowitz, D. (1996). Genetic and environmental control of variation in retinal ganglion cell number in mice. *J. Neurosci.* 16:7193–7205.

Wong, S. L., Ip, P. P., and Yew, D. T. (1979). Comparative ultrastructural study of the optic nerves and visual cortices of young (2.5 months) and old (17 months) mice. *Acta Anat. (Basel)* 105(4):426–430.

Yamashita, T., Takahashi, A., and Honjin, R. (1980). Spatial aspect of the mouse orbital venous sinus. *Okajimas Folia Anat. Jpn.* 56(6):329–336.

Yancey, S. B., Biswal, S., and Revel, J. P. (1992). Spatial and temporal patterns of distribution of the gap junction protein connexin43 during mouse gastrulation and organogenesis. *Development* 114(1):203–212.

17 Photoentrainment of the Circadian Oscillator

SATCHIDANANDA PANDA

Circadian rhythms are near-24-hour oscillations in behavior and physiology found in most living organisms that enable the orchestration of endogenous processes to the appropriate time of day. An endogenous timekeeping mechanism or oscillator generates and maintains these rhythms. Thus, a property of circadian oscillations is their sustenance under constant environmental conditions in the absence of any timing cue. Interestingly, most free-running circadian pacemakers oscillate with a periodicity different from that of Earth's rotation. Therefore, the oscillator requires daily adjustment to maintain a constant phase relationship with geophysical time. Furthermore, the phase of the oscillator must be adjusted to seasonal day-length variations. Of all the potential environmental factors that fluctuate daily and can serve as an input, light is the predominant *Zeitgeiber* (time giver) or entrainment stimulus for the clock. Therefore, under natural conditions, the daily rhythms in behavior and physiology result from the interactions of the endogenous circadian clock and the ambient light-dark cycle.

The photopigments and the cell types that play dominant roles in entrainment of the mammalian circadian oscillator have recently become known. A small subset of retinal ganglion cells (RGCs) express a novel photopigment, melanopsin, and are intrinsically photosensitive (mRGCs or ipRGCs). These RGCs make direct synaptic contact with the hypothalamic brain center harboring a master circadian oscillator. Mouse behavior and genetics have played a major role in our understanding of how mRGCs mediate entrainment of the master oscillator to the ambient lighting conditions.

The mouse as a model system for human circadian function

A wide range of human behaviors and functions, such as maintenance of core body temperature, heart function, muscle tone, alertness, eating and drinking, insulin sensitivity, the synthesis and release of several hormones, and the sleep/wake cycle, exhibit robust circadian fluctuations (Cauter, 2000), which underscores the importance of proper circadian regulation to human health and function. For example, transient desynchronization of circadian rhythms from local physical time, as occurs during jet lag, leads to productivity loss, while chronic desynchronization, caused by shift work, can contribute to several pathological conditions, including sleep disorders, seasonal affective disorder, metabolic syndromes, and even cancer (reviewed in Waterhouse and DeCoursey, 2004). Furthermore, various nonprimate animal species exhibit seasonal breeding behavior that arises from the interaction of the circadian oscillator and seasonal day lengths (Goldman, 2001). These pervasive effects of circadian rhythms on mammalian health and disease have been a major impetus to investigating the molecular bases of the circadian system.

Remarkably, both the circadian oscillation of different behaviors and functions and the molecular mechanisms that underlie the circadian system appear to be conserved from mice to humans (Panda, Hogenesch, et al., 2002), such that mutations that cause circadian oscillator disorders in humans have similar effects in mice (Xu et al., 2007). The circadian system is largely modular in organization and function. For simplicity, it is presumed to consist of three modules: (1) the entrainment or light input, (2) the core oscillator, and (3) the outputs. Anatomically, the master circadian oscillator in mammals is located in the hypothalamic suprachiasmatic nucleus (SCN), which receives direct retinal input and, through both synaptic and diffusible signals, orchestrates rhythmic output behavior and functions in distant brain regions and peripheral organs (Reppert and Weaver, 2002).

In general, owing to their physical size, large rodents such as hamsters and rats have traditionally been used to examine the neuroanatomy of the mammalian circadian system. However, with the strength of murine genetics and the availability of genetic techniques to label and track different cell types, mice have increasingly become the model organism of choice for the study of the circadian system.

Circadian behaviors in mice

The most obvious output of the circadian oscillator in animals is the daily rhythm of activity and rest. Thus, long-term (i.e., across days), continuous measurement of general activity under controlled lighting conditions is a widely used approach in analyzing the circadian oscillator. Although general activity may be measured by infrared beam-break systems, the wheel-running assay is a robust readout of temporal activity, because rodents limit their wheel-running activity to night and rest during the day. In a typical assay, mice are individually housed in special cages equipped with a running wheel whose rotation is computer monitored (Siepka and Takahashi, 2005). Under a normal 12-hour light, 12-hour dark (LD) lighting regimen, mice of the widely used C57Bl/6J strain start their wheel-running activity at dark onset and are active throughout the night. Such a tight, 24-hour activity rhythm arises from photoentrainment of the circadian clock to the imposed LD cycle and from the light-induced suppression of activity, or negative masking, that occurs in mice (Mrosovsky, 1999). Because negative masking may be confused with bona fide circadian entrainment, it is important to be able to distinguish between them. This is best accomplished by administering a discrete period of light to the animals during the dark phase. In mice, this action results in the immediate cessation of wheel-running behavior and the onset of an inactive state for the duration of the light pulse. In other words, light negatively masks or inhibits the activity of nocturnal animals, and the phenomenon is called negative masking.

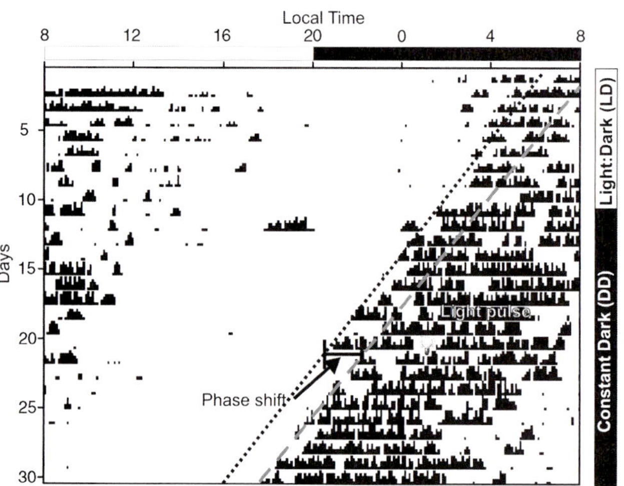

Figure 17.1 Circadian photoentrainment in mice. Wheel-running activity record of a mouse shows daily activity entrainment to an imposed light-dark cycle, free running under constant darkness, and the activity phase-shifting effect of a single light pulse. Each *horizontal line* shows the temporal activity pattern over one geophysical day. The mouse was entrained to LD cycle for 10 days and subsequently released into constant darkness. On day 20, the animal received a 30-minute light pulse approximately 4 hours after activity onset. Phase shift (if any) in response to the light pulse is usually determined by calculating the time difference (on the day of light pulse) between two extrapolated regression lines fitting daily activity onsets before and after the light pulse.

The effect of light in adjusting the phase of the oscillator is best assessed in mice held under constant darkness. Mice are first entrained to a LD cycle for up to 2 weeks and then released into constant darkness (DD). Under DD, the time of activity onset is no longer determined by the time of dark onset but by the phase of the clock. The time difference between activity onset on the first day of DD and dark onset during the prior entrainment period is referred to as the phase angle of entrainment and reflects the true phase of entrainment. Although mice of wild-type C57Bl/6J background have a phase angle of almost zero, other strains exhibit a significant phase angle of entrainment, which might arise from abnormal phototransduction mechanism, core circadian clock function, or masking. During the subsequent days under DD, with no scheduled lighting or other timing cues, the temporal activity is said to "free run" entirely under the control of the circadian clock (figure 17.1). The temporal activity pattern still exhibits tight circadian control, so that the activity is mostly consolidated to the "subjective night" time. C57Bl/6J mice typically exhibit a DD free-running period length of about 23.5 hours, which truly reflects the daily rhythm in individual SCN neural activity and the rhythm of the molecular oscillator (Welsh et al., 1995; Yoo et al., 2004). Because the DD period length is slightly different from that of the geophysical day, the temporal activity is no longer expressed with reference to the local time. Instead, the temporal measures are referenced as the endogenous circadian time (CT), where the free-running period length is normalized to 24 hours. In this convention, the daily activity onset is referenced as CT12, so that the subjective day spans from CT0 to CT12 and the subjective night extends from CT12 to CT24 or CT0. A pulse of light administered during the subjective night causes a shift in the phase of the clock, so that the wheel-running activity onset of the mouse shifts during the subsequent days. Such a light-induced phase shift in the circadian activity rhythm is a widely used approach when measuring the interaction between light input and the circadian oscillator. This interaction is also assessed by measuring the free-running period length under constant light. After entrainment to the LD cycle, the mice are released into constant light (LL). Constant light has a period-lengthening effect in mice, such that the free-running LL period length is longer than 24 hours. In combination, these assays form a powerful set of tools for distinguishing between perturbations of the circadian clock and perturbations of the photoentrainment mechanism. For instance, mice with mutations in the core clock components exhibit a DD period length that is different from that of littermate controls, while photoentrainment mutations typically produce no change in DD period length but a significant change in the phase angle of entrainment, light-induced phase shift, or LL period length.

Other adaptive photic responses

While the interaction between the day-night cycle and the circadian oscillator helps organisms adapt to daily fluctuation in ambient light, several other adaptive responses are also directly modulated by light. For example, some circadian outputs are directly regulated by light. As mentioned earlier, general activity in mice is suppressed by light. Similarly, melatonin synthesis and release by the pineal gland is both clock-regulated and strongly light-suppressed. These effects of light are independent of photoentrainment of the clock and are observed within minutes of light exposure. Finally, a much faster photoadaptive response is constriction of the pupil diameter in response to increased light intensity, which helps the outer retina photoreceptors adapt to environmental changes in irradiance. These adaptive responses, along with circadian photoentrainment, can persist in the absence of image-forming visual responses and are commonly referred to as nonvisual, non-image-forming or adaptive light responses (Van Gelder, 2001). These responses exhibit similar action spectra as photoentrainment and are valuable to the elucidation of the molecular basis of the latter.

Circadian photosensitivity

Photoentrainment in mice and humans is entirely mediated by retinal photoreceptors. When rodents are subjected to experimental bilateral enucleation, their circadian oscillator is rendered unresponsive to light and, as a consequence, free runs even under constant light conditions (Yamazaki et al., 1999). Despite the dependence on retinal photoreceptors, the sensitivity of circadian photoentrainment is quite distinct from that of patterned vision. The administration of discrete light pulses of varying intensities, wavelengths, and duration at different circadian time to rodents held under constant darkness has been extensively used to study features of circadian photosensitivity (Takahashi et al., 1984). Intriguingly, the phase-shifting effect of light exhibits strong circadian modulation, such that a bright light pulse administered during the subjective day produces no or only small phase shifts, while the same light pulse administered during the subjective evening causes significant phase delays, and during subjective late night causes phase advances (Pittendrigh, 1981). Although the molecular mechanism of such circadian gating of entrainment in mammals remains unclear, it highlights a novel mechanism for integrating both time and light information in appropriate resetting of the phase of the oscillator.

The threshold sensitivity of circadian photoentrainment is significantly higher than that of patterned vision, which protects the clock from photic noise in nature. For example, a brief light pulse of several seconds, as occurs during lightning, or a low-intensity light, such as moonlight, rarely causes a phase shift of the circadian clock. Circadian entrainment also exhibits characteristic features of spectral integration over time (Takahashi et al., 1984). Light pulses of defined wavelengths and intensities have been used to generate irradiance response curves and action spectra. The action spectrum of photoentrainment fits an opsin nomogram with a peak sensitivity around 480–500 nm (Takahashi et al., 1984; Yoshimura and Ebihara, 1996). Comparable action spectra are also observed for the pupillary light reflex (PLR) in mice (Lucas et al., 2001) and pineal melatonin suppression in human (Brainard et al., 2001; Thapan et al., 2001). Circadian photoentrainment, PLR, negative masking (light suppression of activity), and photic suppression of pineal melatonin synthesis remain intact in mice with outer retina degeneration (Keeler, 1927; Foster et al., 1991; Mrosovsky et al., 1999). Furthermore, in these mice, the sensitivity of circadian phase shift, as well as the phase angle of entrainment, does not show any significant difference from those of normal mice. This suggests that non-rod, non-cone photopigments play a dominant role in circadian photoentrainment (Foster et al., 1991).

Neuroanatomy of the circadian photoentrainment pathway

The circadian system in mammals, including mice, is hierarchical in nature, with a master circadian oscillator resident in the 10,000–20,000 neurons of the paired SCN coordinating tissue autonomous oscillators in the rest of the body. The SCN neurons in turn are entrained to the ambient light-dark cycle via a direct synaptic projection to a small subset of RGCs that constitute what is known as the retinohypothalamic tract (RHT) (Abrahamson and Moore, 2001). This basic organization of the SCN and RHT is well conserved among mammals, with some minor variations. In most mammals, the axon termini of RHT neurons are restricted to the ventral portion of the SCN, whereas in mice they extend more dorsally (Cassone et al., 1988). Such neuroanatomical organization implies that only a small fraction of all SCN neurons receive direct retinal input, and therefore intercellular communication among SCN neurons is important to achieve complete resetting of the master oscillator.

The evolutionary conservation of direct projection of the RHT to the SCN and the observation that functionally active mRGCs make synaptic connections to the SCN during prenatal life in mice raise the possibility that tonic light input and/or interaction with the neurons of the RHT may influence the ontogeny and function of the master circadian oscillator of the SCN. In support of this, anophthalmic mice or mice experimentally enucleated immediately after birth have an aberrant SCN morphology (Silver, 1977; Holtzman et al., 1989; Nagai et al., 1992). In these mice, the SCN either is reduced in size or is unilateral. Consistently, these anophthalmic mice exhibit no circadian photoresponse, but intriguingly, their DD period length is significantly lengthened compared with that of the normal mice. These results had earlier suggested a role of functional light input to the SCN in the development of normal circadian system. However, results from other genetic models with specific disruption of RGCs showed little effect of ocular light input on SCN oscillator development and endogenous function. *Math5*-null mutants (*Math5*$^{-/-}$) have been useful in addressing this question. The *Math5* gene encodes a basic helix-loop-helix (bHLH) class of transcription factor that plays a key role in RGC differentiation. *Math5*$^{-/-}$ mice lack fully differentiated RGCs and a functional optic tract. Circadian behavioral assessment from two different laboratories conclusively established that RGCs are necessary and sufficient for circadian photoentrainment (Wee et al., 2002; Brzezinski et al., 2005); however, the effect of this mutation on the endogenous circadian oscillator appears to be strain specific. On a C57Bl/6J.129S1/SvIMJ mixed background, the mutation leads to almost 90% reduction in the number of RGCs, including mRGCs, and the mice exhibit a free-running period length that is significantly longer than that of wild-type littermates (Wee et al., 2002). However, the same mutation on a C57Bl/6J background does not affect the endogenous pace of the oscillator, which indicates that the SCN oscillator can develop normally in the absence of any signal input from the retina (Brzezinski et al., 2005). This view is further supported by the observation of normal circadian function but lack of entrainment in mice lacking both rod/cone and melanopsin function (Hattar et al., 2003; Panda et al., 2003). In summary, the RHT plays a major role in circadian photoentrainment of the SCN oscillator. However, light signaling from the retina is not necessary for normal development of the SCN or for its endogenous circadian rhythm.

Other circadian and light-regulated responses, such as pineal melatonin rhythm and negative masking, involve more complex neuronal connections. A multisynaptic connection from the SCN to the pineal gland that traverses the paraventricular nucleus (PVN), spinal cord, and superior cervical ganglion (SCG) mediates both SCN and light regulation of pineal melatonin synthesis and release (Larsen et al., 1998; Teclemariam-Mesbah et al., 1999). The neuroanatomic circuit regulating negative masking is less clear. The SCN is dispensable for negative masking, and several brain regions, including hypothalamic and visual centers, modulate negative masking (Edelstein and Mrosovsky, 2001; Redlin et al., 2003).

Melanopsin-expressing retinal ganglion cells play a key role in circadian photoentrainment

The existence of a novel inner retina photopigment with a dominant role in entraining the SCN oscillator via the RHT has long been suggested from the observations that mice with outer retinal degeneration have an intact circadian photosensitivity and that a small subset of RGCs make direct synaptic connections to the SCN. The search for this novel photopigment led to the discovery of melanopsin (Provencio et al., 1998, 2000, 2002). The majority of the SCN-projecting RGCs express melanopsin and are intrinsically photosensitive. Mice deficient in melanopsin (*Opn4*$^{-/-}$) entrain their circadian activity rhythm to an imposed light-dark cycle, yet the magnitude of circadian phase shift in response to discrete light pulses of varying intensities is significantly attenuated. Such a reduced circadian photosensitivity is also evident in their period length when placed in LL, which is significantly shorter than that of their littermate wild-type controls (Panda, Sata, et al., 2002; Ruby et al., 2002). Furthermore, the negative masking response is also attenuated in the *Opn4*$^{-/-}$ mice. When exposed to prolonged illumination during subjective night, wild-type (WT) and *Opn4*$^{-/-}$ mice stop activity immediately after light onset. While the activity of wild-type mice remains suppressed for the entire length of the light pulse, the *Opn4*$^{-/-}$ mice gradually become more active (Mrosovsky and Hattar, 2003). In addition, *Opn4*$^{-/-}$ mice exhibit reduced PLR at high light intensity, while at low to medium intensity light their responses are indistinguishable from those of their wild-type littermates (Lucas et al., 2003). The reduced photosensitivity phenotypes in *Opn4*$^{-/-}$ mice correlates with the loss of intrinsic photosensitivity of the SCN-projecting RGCs, whose number, overall morphology, and projections remain intact (Lucas et al., 2003), while the residual photosensitivity in the *Opn4*$^{-/-}$ mice is mediated by rod/cone photoreceptors. Indeed, mice deficient in both rod/cone and melanopsin function fail to entrain to the imposed light-dark cycles and exhibit no masking, and their pupils remain completely open even under high-intensity light. Irrespective of the light environment, the circadian activity rhythm in these mice always free runs with a period length similar to the DD period length of wild-type mice (Hattar et al., 2003; Panda et al., 2003). Such a phenotype further highlights the modular nature of the circadian system, in which the cellular development and function of the core oscillator are independent of any mechanisms responsible for mediating light input.

The behavioral and cellular phenotypes of rod/cone- and melanopsin-deficient mice bear several implications for circadian photoentrainment and other adaptive photoresponses. The complete loss of ocular photosensitivity in rod/cone- and melanopsin-deficient mice highlights the necessity and sufficiency of these photopigment systems for all ocular photoresponses. These genetic analyses also unraveled an important role for rod/cone photoreceptors in circadian photoentrainment, which may account for the residual entrainment of *Opn4*$^{-/-}$ mice to the imposed LD cycle. Further genetic analysis may elucidate the relative contribution of rods or any of the specific cones to circadian photoentrainment. However, the neuroanatomical basis of signal integration from rod/cone and melanopsin photopigment remains unclear. It is highly likely that the mRGCs that remain intact in *Opn4*$^{-/-}$ mice also transmit the rod/cone-initiated photic signal to target brain regions, including the SCN. The rod/cone response may also be transmitted to the SCN via non-mRGCs, some of which directly project to the SCN, and some which make indirect connections to the SCN via the IGL or the OPN (Hannibal and Fahrenkrug, 2004; Hattar et al., 2006). In either case, the molecular bases of signal integration from inner and outer retina photopigments remain undiscovered. Finally, the high threshold sensitivity of circadian phase shift in *Opn4*$^{-/-}$ mice (Panda, Sato, et al., 2002; Ruby et al., 2002) suggests that this property of circadian photoentrainment is independent of the threshold sensitivity of the photopigments and may be encoded in the signal transduction pathway or in the oscillator itself.

Intrinsically photosensitive retinal ganglion cells

As mentioned earlier, the majority of the SCN-projecting RGCs express melanopsin and are intrinsically photosensitive (Berson et al., 2002; Hattar et al., 2002). The photoresponses of the ipRGCs is distinct from that of the outer retina photoreceptors. Their responses are characterized by long latencies approaching almost 1 minute, with a depolarizing current exhibiting fast action potentials sustained for the duration of the light pulse, relatively slow turn-off rates, and resistance to bleaching. The photoresponse in ipRGCs is resistant to synaptic blockade and persists in physically isolated cells, thus conclusively establishing the intrinsic nature of the photosensitivity. The action spectrum of the ipRGC photoresponse shows peak sensitivity around 480 nm, which is distinct from the peak sensitivity of rod/cone photoreceptors in rodents.

The sustained depolarizing current of the ipRGCs faithfully reflects the light intensity, which sets them apart from other RGCs. No other mammalian RGCs can encode ambient light level in this way. Although the ipRGCs were characterized in detail only recently, they may have been described as a luminance unit almost three decades earlier (Barlow and Levick, 1969). Their rare occurrence, accounting for about 1% of the total number of RGCs in adult rodent retina, might have been a major reason for the lack of their detection and characterization in the intervening years.

ipRGC Morphology, Ontogeny, and Functional Diversity The unique efferent projections of the ipRGCs, coupled with the power of retinal multielectrode array recording and the availability of genetic resources and specific antibodies identifying these cells, have catalyzed their cellular and functional characterization. Direct projection of a majority of the ipRGCs to the SCN allows retrograde labeling of these cells by injecting fluorescent dyes into the SCN (Berson et al., 2002; Hattar et al., 2002). Furthermore, specific staining of these cells and axons in a mouse strain carrying a functional *lacZ* gene in the melanopsin locus (Hattar et al., 2002), as well as the fortuitous tropism of adenoassociated virus-2 serotype (Gooley et al., 2003), has facilitated the comprehensive characterization of mRGC cell distribution and their brain targets. High-quality anti-melanopsin antibodies (Provencio et al., 2002) have also been instrumental in immunohistological and ultrastructural characterization of these cells in the inner retina.

In the mouse CNS, melanopsin expression is extremely restricted, present only in 1%–3% of RGCs. The cell bodies of mRGCs are almost uniformly distributed throughout the retina, with occasional crowding along the periphery. Most of the cell bodies reside in the ganglion cell layer; however, approximately 5% of the cell bodies are found in the inner border of the inner nuclear layer. All melanopsin-expressing cells send their axons to the optic nerve, thus establishing that all melanopsin-expressing cells are RGCs (Hannibal et al., 2002; Hattar et al., 2002, 2006). Melanopsin protein is almost uniformly distributed throughout the plasma membrane of the dendrites, cell bodies, and axons of RGCs (Provencio et al., 2002). Such spatial distribution of melanopsin is distinct from vertebrate rod/cone and invertebrate image-forming opsins, which are densely packed in defined membrane ultrastructures. The dendrites of mRGCs arborize heavily and overlap in the synapse-rich inner plexiform layer (IPL), thus creating what appears to be a photoreceptive dendritic net covering the entire retina (figure 17.2*A*). The dendritic field of individual ipRGCs is relatively large and can approach 500 μM or 15°, which closely matches the calculated receptive field of SCN neurons. Ultrastructural studies have indicated that the melanopsin immunoreactive dendrites in the ON sublayer of the IPL make synaptic contact with both bipolar and amacrine terminals, while those in the OFF sublayer receive only amacrine terminals (Belenky et al., 2003).

As is evident from the reduced number of the mRGCs in *Math5*$^{-/-}$ mice, it is clear that the development of mRGCs is also controlled by the bHLH protein Math5. RGC differentiation begins early in the mouse retina, around embryonic day 11.5, and is almost complete by the first week after birth (P7; reviewed in Mu and Klein, 2004). The mRGCs are also detected by immunostaining starting at E12.5, and at P0, each murine eye contains almost 200 ipRGCs/mm^2 that are fully functional and transmit light information to the SCN (Tarttelin et al., 2003; Sekaran et al. 2005; Tu et al., 2005). The number of melanopsin-positive RGCs in murine retina declines dramatically after birth during a period when bipolar, amacrine, and outer retina photoreceptor cells are differentiated. By P14, when the mouse eyes are open and rods and cones are functioning, almost 75% of the melanopsin-expressing RGCs are lost, leaving approximately 700–1,000 melanopsin-positive cells in each adult mouse retina. This decline in ipRGC population, along with changes in the physiological diversity among them, has been more thoroughly examined by multielectrode array recording. This approach has enabled the simultaneous recording of the photoresponses of sufficiently large numbers of ipRGCs and has led to the accurate measurements of their sensitivity, onset speed, and offset kinetics. In young, P8 mice, three distinct types of ipRGCs are observed: slow onset (>12 s), sensitive (irradiance yielding half-maximal response or log IR50 < 12.85), fast off (type I); slow onset, insensitive, slow off (type II); and rapid onset, sensitive, and very slow off (type III). The majority (ca. 75%) of the ipRGCs in P8 mice are type I, which are almost undetectable in adult retina (Tu et al., 2005). The functional significance of the observed physiological diversity among ipRGCs is currently unclear. The subtypes may differ in projections to the target brain regions controlling various adaptive responses. Identification of molecular marker to tag or specifically perturb ipRGC subtypes may help elucidate their functional significance.

A

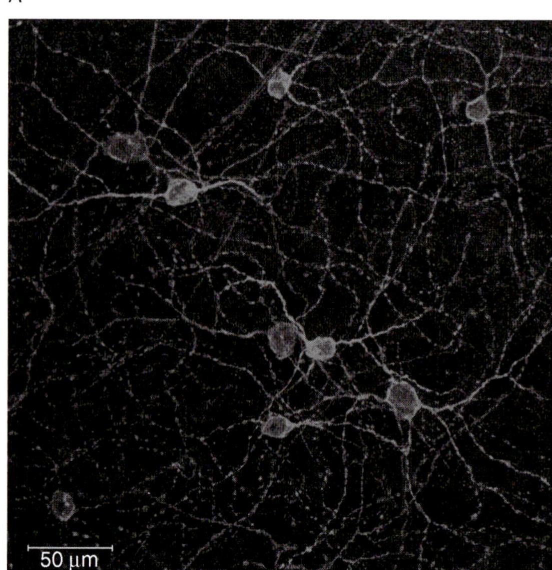

B

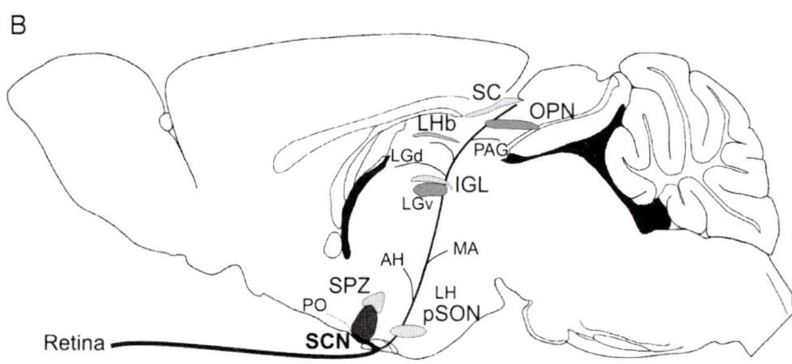

Figure 17.2 Morphology and projections of mRGCs in mouse. *A*, Retina flat mount stained with a polyclonal antimouse melanopsin antibody showing specific staining of dendrites, somata, and axons of a small subset of retinal ganglion cells. *B*, Schematic drawing showing direct axonal projections of mRGCs to several brain regions. (Results from Hattar et al., 2006, are redrawn here.) Brain regions receiving significant projections are represented in large, bold letters. AH, anterior hypothalamic nucleus; IGL, intergeniculate leaflet; LGd, lateral geniculate nucleus, dorsal division; LGv, lateral geniculate nucleus, ventral division; LH, lateral hypothalamus; LHb, lateral habenula; MA, median amygdaloid nucleus; OPN, olivary pretectal nucleus; PAG, periaqueductal gray; PO, preoptic; pSON, perisupraoptic nucleus; SC, superior colliculus; SCN, suprachiasmatic nucleus; SPZ, subparaventricular zone. See color plate 6.

Target brain regions innervated by mRGCs

The projections of the mRGCs differ significantly from those of the rest of the RGCs (figure 17.2*B*). In the optic nerve the axons of the mRGCs are almost uniformly distributed up to the optic chiasm, beyond which the fibers run mostly contralaterally and are clustered along the dorsal surface of the optic tract (Gooley et al., 2003; Hannibal and Fahrenkrug, 2004; Hattar et al., 2006). The SCN, resident above the optic chiasm, is the most densely innervated brain target of the mRGCs. An almost equal number of crossed and uncrossed fibers innervate the SCN. The nerve terminals are distributed throughout the SCN, and some extend dorsally to reach the ventral subparaventricular zone (vSPZ). Sparse projections also reach the lateral preoptic nucleus (LPO), ventrolateral preoptic nucleus (VLPO), medial preoptic nucleus (MPO), and supraoptic nucleus (SON). Direct mRGC innervations of these hypothalamic targets may form a basis for the well-characterized photic modulation of sleep, body temperature, and neuroendocrine outputs. Beyond the hypothalamus, most of the mRGCs projections are contralateral, and their major brain target areas include the intergeniculate leaflet (IGL) and olivary pretectal nucleus (OPN), both of which are also reciprocally connected to the SCN. The direct projection to the OPN forms the basis for the mRGC regulation of PLR. A small but detectable number of melanopsin-negative RGCs also send direct projections to the SCN. Additionally, nonmelanopsin RGC projections to the OPN and IGL may suggest potential non-mRGC regulation of circadian photoentrainment (Gooley et al., 2003; Hannibal and Fahrenkrug, 2004; Hattar et al., 2006).

While the majority of the mRGCs project to brain regions implicated in non-image-forming photoresponses, involvement of mRGCs in visual processes cannot be ruled out. Sparse projections to the lateral geniculate, which forms the primary relay center to the visual cortex, and projections to OPN and superior colliculus, which sends projections to the visual thalamus, may suggest a potential role of mRGCs in visual processing. Furthermore, in the RGC layer, the ipRGCs maintain gap junction connections with other retinal cell types (Sekaran et al., 2003), raising the possibility that they may directly influence other intraretinal functions, including rod/cone initiated signaling events. In support of this, cone ERG of mice has been shown to be modulated in *Opn4*$^{-/-}$ mice (Barnard et al., 2006).

The melanopsin photopigment

The mouse melanopsin gene spans 7.8 kb on chromosome 14 and encodes a protein of 521 amino acids (aa). The predicted seven transmembrane region (amino acids 72–350) shows sequence homology with opsins and contains a lysine residue in the seventh transmembrane region that may serve as the binding site for a retinal-based chromophore (Provencio et al., 2000). Targeted mutation of this site abolishes photoactivation of melanopsin (Newman et al., 2003; Kumbalasiri et al., 2007). Phylogenetic comparisons of this region show higher sequence similarity to rhodopsins from invertebrates than to those from vertebrates (Provencio et al., 2000). Specifically, the cytoplasmic regions of the opsin segment show sequence features suggestive of potential activation of the $G_{\alpha q}$ class of G proteins instead of transducin (Nayak et al., 2007). However, unlike mouse rhodopsin (full length 348 aa) or *Drosophila* rhodopsin-1 (373 aa), the mouse melanopsin contains an unusually long C-terminal sequence (351–521 aa) with no sequence similarity to any other known protein. This C-terminal region contains multiple putative phosphorylation sites and may serve as a target region for several regulatory proteins.

Melanopsin Phototransduction Mechanism The scarcity of melanopsin-expressing cells in the mouse has prevented a systematic characterization of its signaling properties. The ipRGCs exhibit light-evoked transient increases in intracellular calcium levels (Sekaran et al., 2003) and a depolarizing membrane current that bears characteristic features of nonselective cation channels, like those of the Trp class (Warren et al., 2003). Successful heterologous expression of functional melanopsin in cultured cell lines and in *Xenopus* oocytes has shed light on the potential phototransduction mechanism in ipRGCs. In both cultured cells and oocytes, photoactivated mouse melanopsin signals through $G_{\alpha q}/G_{\alpha 11}$, and phosphoinositide signaling pathways to trigger the release of intracellular calcium store (Panda et al., 2005; Qiu et al., 2005). When coexpressed with the TrpC class of ion channels, it can also trigger light-induced opening of Trp channels, leading to membrane depolarization. The photocurrent in these melanopsin-expressing cells exhibits a peak sensitivity at about 480 nm, which is similar to that of ipRGC and circadian phase shift. The heterologous expression experiments have also suggested that melanopsin, like *Drosophila* Rh1 opsin, may possess an intrinsic photoisomerase activity to photoconvert *all-trans* retinal photoproduct to its 11-*cis* isomer (Melyan et al., 2005; Panda et al., 2005).

Despite the successful demonstration of potential phototransduction mechanism in a heterologous system, the steps from photoactivation to membrane channel opening in the ipRGCs remain unclear. Both $G_{\alpha q}$ and $G_{\alpha 11}$ G proteins are almost ubiquitously expressed and can functionally compensate for each other's loss. To further complicate the analysis, mammalian melanopsin has also been shown to signal through the $G_{\alpha i/o}$ class of G protein (Newman et al., 2003; Melyan et al., 2005), and melanopsin may likely activate promiscuous G proteins such as $G_{\alpha 14}$ and $G_{\alpha 16}$. Genetic analysis of the subsequent candidate steps, such as PLC and Trp channels, also suffers from a similar problem of functional redundancy among family members. Generation of ipRGC specific loss-of-function mutants may be a promising option to conclusively establish the melanopsin phototransduction pathway.

The biochemical characterization of melanopsin photopigment has been achieved with some success. Melanopsin purified from COS cells and reconstituted with 11-*cis* retinal can activate a G protein (Newman et al., 2003). However, the peak absorption spectrum of the purified melanopsin is significantly different from the peak action spectra of photoresponses of ipRGCs, and also different from the photoresponses of cells heterologously expressing mouse melanopsin. This disparity highlights the potential differences between the expression system and the chemical environment.

The nature of the native chromophore used by melanopsin in ipRGCs is currently unknown. Heterologously expressed melanopsin can use *all-trans* retinal and several *cis*-isomers of retinaldehyde, which implies that melanopsin photopigment can photoisomerize its chromophore and that the photosensitivity of ipRGCs may be independent of the RPE retinoid cycle. Consistently, mice carrying loss-of-function mutations in key components of the retinoid cycle still exhibit some, if reduced, circadian photosensitivity and PLR (Fu et al., 2005; Doyle et al., 2006; Tu et al., 2006). Although these mice can entrain to an imposed LD cycle, the discrete light pulse–induced phase shift during free running in DD is retained only at high light intensities. The ipRGC responses in *Rpe65*$^{-/-}$ mice as measured by microelectrode arrays remain normal. Yet both the number of melanopsin-expressing RGCs and dendritic staining for melanopsin are reduced. The diminished behavioral photosensitivity these mice display, as well as the weak melanopsin immunostaining seen in their retina, can be rescued by abolishing rod function (*Rpe65*$^{-/-}$;*rdta*) (Doyle et al., 2006), which demonstrates that disruption of retinoid cycle in the RPE can indirectly influence the function of the ipRGCs. Intriguingly, double mutant mice (*Rpe65*$^{-/-}$;*Opn4*$^{-/-}$) with no functional RPE65 and melanopsin are largely diurnal under bright light/dark condition, while triple mutants (*Rpe65*$^{-/-}$;*rdta*;*Opn4*$^{-/-}$) show no photoresponses. The temporal niche switching in *Rpe65*$^{-/-}$;*Opn4*$^{-/-}$ mice shows how interaction between the photic input pathway from the retina and the circadian oscillator can contribute to establishing diurnal or nocturnal behavior in animals.

Molecular basis of circadian photoentrainment

Our knowledge of the core molecular mechanism of circadian oscillation, the neurotransmitters of the RHT and their mode of action, has provided a framework for understanding the molecular bases of circadian photoentrainment (figure 17.3). In mammals, the core mechanism of circadian oscillator is composed of interlocked transcription-translation negative feedback loops. In a simplified model, the positive transcription factors Bmal1, Clock, and NPAS2 heterodimerize and drive transcription of the *Period* and *Cryptochrome* genes (*Per1*, *Per2*, *Per3*, *Cry1*, *Cry2*), whose protein products repress their own transcription. The transcriptional inhibitors are eventually degraded, relieving repression and allowing the start of another round of transcription; this ultimately produces oscillating levels of *Per* and *Cry* gene products (Reppert and Weaver, 2002). The phase of *Per1* or *Per2* gene product roughly correlates with the phase of the behavioral rhythm. A discrete light pulse administered to mice in constant darkness causes transient induction of *Per1* and *Per2* transcripts and a concomitant change in the phase of their oscillations. This molecular event may underlie the change in phase of the behavioral rhythm (Yan and Silver, 2004).

Nonetheless, the components and signaling events that begin from light detection in the retina and progress to the acute induction of *Per* genes in the SCN are yet to be fully elucidated. It is thought that light-induced RGC membrane depolarization releases the neurotransmitters glutamate and PACAP, both of which are stored in the SCN-projecting RGCs, from their axon terminals in the SCN (Hannibal et al., 2000). Glutamate acts through ionotropic glutamate receptors in the SCN neurons (Ding et al., 1994). In addition, SCN neurons also express at least two receptors that can bind to PACAP: Pac1 receptor (Pac1r) and VPAC2 receptor (Vpac2r). The signaling events downstream of glutamate or PACAP receptors ultimately converge and include increases in cytosolic calcium, phosphorylation of CREB at serine 133, histone modification, and phospho-CREB-mediated transient induction of *Per1* or *Per2* gene products leading to a change in the phase of the molecular oscillator (reviewed in Meijer and Schwartz, 2003). In support of this model, mice that lack PACAP or Pac1 receptor exhibit an attenuated phase shift in response to light (Hannibal et al., 2001; Colwell et al., 2004). Vpac2r is also a receptor for vasoactive intestinal peptide (VIP) which is significantly expressed in the SCN. Signaling via Vpac2r is presumed to synchronize or entrain the individual cellular oscillators with each other. As a consequence, Vpac2r-deficient mice exhibit a more severe circadian dysfunction and are generally arrhythmic (Harmar et al., 2002; Maywood et al., 2006).

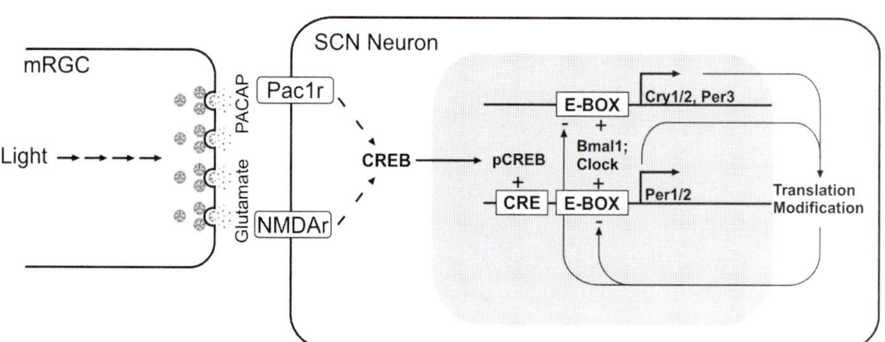

FIGURE 17.3 Model depicting major steps during photoentrainment of the SCN oscillator. Light received by the rod/cone and mRGCs ultimately causes depolarization of mRGCs and release of glutamate and PACAP from their axon termini in the SCN. These neurotransmitters activate their cognate receptors in the SCN neurons and ultimately trigger CREB phosphorylation, binding of pCREB to *cis*-acting CRE site and transcriptional induction of *Per1* and *Per2* genes. An increased level of Per1/Per2 proteins resets the phase of the oscillator. Under constant conditions, a negative feedback loop maintains oscillation of *Per* gene products. Transcriptional activators Clock and BMAL1 drive *Per* and *Cry* gene transcription by binding to *cis*-acting E-box. *Per* and *Cry* gene products are translated, phosphorylated, and translocated into the nucleus, where they inhibit Clock/BMAL1 function.

The linear model of circadian photoentrainment in its current format is too simplistic, because it does not take into account some signal integration steps. First, it is unknown whether rod and cone input is exclusively transmitted via mRGCs. If an alternate pathway, such as direct projection of non-mRGCs to the SCN or indirect projections via the IGL and OPN, contributes significantly to photoentrainment, the neurotransmitters and receptors transmitting light information through these pathways are not clearly known. Furthermore, it is known that several nonphotic cues also modulate the phase of the SCN oscillator. The molecular bases of integration of the photic and nonphotic entraining cues are just beginning to be understood.

Other mouse models for circadian photoentrainment

Mouse genetic studies have suggested that several additional genes may participate in circadian photoentrainment, although the causal genes and the mechanism are unknown. For instance, the mechanism of participation of cryptochromes in mammalian circadian photoentrainment is still unclear. Although cryptochromes from plants and flies have been demonstrated to be functional photopigments (Cashmore, 2003), the mammalian cryptochromes are best described as transcriptional repressors (Griffin et al., 1999; Kume et al., 1999), and evidence for direct light-dependent function, as has been demonstrated in plants and flies, is still lacking. Cryptochrome-deficient mice (*Cry1*$^{-/-}$;*Cry2*$^{-/-}$) lack a functional circadian oscillator, which prevents the evaluation of their role in circadian photoentrainment. However, other surrogate roles in negative masking and pupillary light reflex suggest some role in these processes. As mentioned earlier, *rd* mice entrain to LD cycle and free run with a wild-type period length under DD (Foster et al., 1991), and *Cry1*$^{-/-}$;*Cry2*$^{-/-}$ mice entrain (negative masking) to the LD cycle but are arrhythmic under DD (van der Horst et al. 1999). On the other hand, triple mutant *rd*; *Cry1*$^{-/-}$;*Cry2*$^{-/-}$ mice exhibit no negative masking, and their locomotor activity is arrhythmic under both LD and DD conditions, thus suggesting a role of cryptochromes in photic control of activity (Selby et al., 2000). Similarly, the triple mutants exhibit significantly lower photosensitivity in pupil constriction than either *rd* or *Cry1*$^{-/-}$;*Cry2*$^{-/-}$ mice (Van Gelder et al., 2003). Despite these observations, extensive expression of *Cry1* and *Cry2* in the retina, SCN, and other brain regions, and lack of tissue-specific loss-of-function mutants makes it difficult to assess whether their function in the photoreceptive cells, in downstream cells, or in brain regions regulating masking or pupillary light reflex underlies the observed deficits.

Quantitative trait analyses in mice have implicated several loci regulating the phase angle of entrainment or masking response (Shimomura et al., 2001; Panda et al., 2003). The genetic intervals for these loci are relatively large, spanning several megabases. None of these chromosomal regions harbors any known photopigment or light-signaling component. Some of these loci modulate the phase angle of entrainment (Shimomura et al., 2001). A different locus modifying melanopsin function does not affect general entrainment when the LD cycle is shifted by several hours, but it significantly attenuates masking, resulting in increased activity during the light period (Panda et al., 2003). Finally, a wild species of mouse, *Peromyscus californicus* (de Groot and Rusak, 2002), exhibits normal masking but impaired photoentrainment. Cloning and characterization of the relevant genes in these mouse lines is expected to offer new tools to understand the interplay between masking and circadian photoentrainment.

Summary

The identification of mRGCs and the demonstration that melanopsin is a functional photopigment have precipitated systematic studies of circadian photoentrainment. The rarity of mRGCs still poses a major challenge for the cellular and molecular understanding of photoentrainment. Although possible mechanisms of melanopsin phototransduction have been demonstrated in several heterologous expression systems, the exact mechanism, its preferred chromophore, and the effecter channels in ipRGCs are still unknown. Methods to isolate, culture, and extract RNA or protein materials from ipRGCs will have a profound impact on the systematic analysis of the photosensitivity of ipRGCs by verifying expression of candidate signaling molecules and channels in these cells.

Understanding the molecular properties of the melanopsin photopigment will still heavily depend on heterologous expression. Despite sharing sequence similarity with a group of fast-acting GPCRs, the slow photosensitivity of the ipRGCs and of cells that heterologously express melanopsin raises questions about the biophysical basis of slow activation of melanopsin photocurrent. It is unknown whether the slow kinetics reflects a property of the photopigment or of the signaling cascade.

Genetic analyses have shown that rod and cone photoreceptors also play a significant role in photoentrainment. Identifying the specific (if any) rod or cone photopigment that can largely compensate for the loss of melanopsin will also be a major finding. Furthermore, it is yet to be tested whether the photopotentiation effect on melanopsin function shown in cultured cells (Melyan et al., 2005) is also evident in the whole animal. Overall progress in understanding the mammalian photoentrainment mechanism has the potential to improve therapy for sleep and mood disorders.

REFERENCES

Abrahamson, E. E., and Moore, R. Y. (2001). Suprachiasmatic nucleus in the mouse: retinal innervation, intrinsic organization and efferent projections. *Brain Res.* 916(1–2):172–191.

Barlow, H. B., and Levick, W. R. (1969). Changes in the maintained discharge with adaptation level in the cat retina. *J. Physiol.* 202(3):699–718.

Barnard, A. R., Hattar, S., Hankins, M. W., and Lucas, R. J. (2006). Melanopsin regulates visual processing in the mouse retina. *Curr. Biol.* 16(4):389–395.

Belenky, M. A., Smeraski, C. A., Provencio, I., Sollars, P. J., and Pickard, G. E. (2003). Melanopsin retinal ganglion cells receive bipolar and amacrine cell synapses. *J. Comp. Neurol.* 460(3):380–393.

Berson, D. M., Dunn, F. A., and Takao, M. (2002). Phototransduction by retinal ganglion cells that set the circadian clock. *Science* 295(5557):1070–1073.

Brainard, G. C., Hanifin, J. P., Greeson, J. M., Byrne, B., Glickman, G., Gerner, E., and Rollag, M. D. (2001). Action spectrum for melatonin regulation in humans: Evidence for a novel circadian photoreceptor. *J. Neurosci.* 21(16):6405–6412.

Brzezinski, J. A. T., Brown, N. L., Tanikawa, A., Bush, R. A., Sieving, P. A., Vitaterna, M. H., Takahashi, J. S., and Glaser, T. (2005). Loss of circadian photoentrainment and abnormal retinal electrophysiology in Math5 mutant mice. *Invest. Ophthalmol. Vis. Sci.* 46(7):2540–2551.

Cashmore, A. R. (2003). Cryptochromes: Enabling plants and animals to determine circadian time. *Cell* 114(5):537–543.

Cassone, V. M., Speh, J. C., Card, J. P., and Moore, R. Y. (1988). Comparative anatomy of the mammalian hypothalamic suprachiasmatic nucleus. *J. Biol. Rhythms* 3(1):71–91.

Cauter, E. V. (2000). Endocrine rhythms. In K. L. Becker (Ed.), *Principles and practice of endocrinology and metabolism* (pp. 57–67). Philadelphia: Lippincott Williams and Wilkins.

Colwell, C. S., Michel, S., Itri, J., Rodriguez, W., Tam, J., Lelievre, V., Hu, Z., and Waschek, J. A. (2004). Selective deficits in the circadian light response in mice lacking PACAP. *Am. J. Physiol. Regul. Integr. Comp. Physiol.* 287(5):R1194–R1201.

de Groot, M. H., and Rusak, B. (2002). Entrainment impaired, masking spared: An apparent genetic abnormality that prevents circadian rhythm entrainment to 24-h lighting cycles in California mice. *Neurosci. Lett.* 327(3):203–207.

Ding, J. M., Chen, D., Weber, E. T., Faiman, L. E., Rea, M. A., and Gillette, M. U. (1994). Resetting the biological clock: Mediation of nocturnal circadian shifts by glutamate and NO. *Science* 266(5191):1713–1717.

Doyle, S. E., Castrucci, A. M., McCall, M., Provencio, I., and Menaker, M. (2006). Nonvisual light responses in the Rpe65 knockout mouse: Rod loss restores sensitivity to the melanopsin system. *Proc. Natl. Acad. Sci. U.S.A.* 103(27):10432–10437.

Edelstein, K., and Mrosovsky, N. (2001). Behavioral responses to light in mice with dorsal lateral geniculate lesions. *Brain Res.* 918(1–2):107–112.

Foster, R. G., Provencio, I., Hudson, D., Fiske, S., De Grip, W., and Menaker, M. (1991). Circadian photoreception in the retinally degenerate mouse (rd/rd). *J. Comp. Physiol. A* 169(1): 39–50.

Fu, Y., Zhong, H., Wang, M. H., Luo, D. G., Liao, H. W., Maeda, H., Hattar, S., Frishman, L. J., and Yau, K. W. (2005). Intrinsically photosensitive retinal ganglion cells detect light with a vitamin A-based photopigment, melanopsin. *Proc. Natl. Acad. Sci. U.S.A.* 102(29):10339–10344.

Goldman, B. D. (2001). Mammalian photoperiodic system: formal properties and neuroendocrine mechanisms of photoperiodic time measurement. *J. Biol. Rhythms* 16(4):283–301.

Gooley, J. J., Lu, J., Fischer, D., and Saper, C. B. (2003). A broad role for melanopsin in nonvisual photoreception. *J. Neurosci.* 23(18):7093–7106.

Griffin, E. A., Jr., Staknis, D., and Weitz, C. J. (1999). Light-independent role of CRY1 and CRY2 in the mammalian circadian clock. *Science* 286(5440):768–771.

Hannibal, J., and Fahrenkrug, J. (2004). Target areas innervated by PACAP-immunoreactive retinal ganglion cells. *Cell Tissue Res.* 316(1):99–113.

Hannibal, J., Hindersson, P., Knudsen, S. M., Georg, B., and Fahrenkrug, J. (2002). The photopigment melanopsin is exclusively present in pituitary adenylate cyclase-activating polypeptide-containing retinal ganglion cells of the retinohypothalamic tract. *J. Neurosci.* 22(1):RC191.

Hannibal, J., Jamen, F., Nielsen, H. S., Journot, L., Brabet, P., and Fahrenkrug, J. (2001). Dissociation between light-induced phase shift of the circadian rhythm and clock gene expression in mice lacking the pituitary adenylate cyclase activating polypeptide type 1 receptor. *J. Neurosci.* 21(13): 4883–4890.

Hannibal, J., Moller, M., Ottersen, O. P., and Fahrenkrug, J. (2000). PACAP and glutamate are co-stored in the retinohypothalamic tract. *J. Comp. Neurol.* 418(2):147–155.

Harmar, A. J., Marston, H. M., Shen, S., Spratt, C., West, K. M., Sheward, W. J., Morrison, C. F., Dorin, J. R., Piggins, H. D., et al. (2002). The VPAC(2) receptor is essential for circadian function in the mouse suprachiasmatic nuclei. *Cell* 109(4): 497–508.

Hattar, S., Kumar, M., Park, A., Tong, P., Tung, J., Yau, K. W., and Berson, D. M. (2006). Central projections of melanopsin-expressing retinal ganglion cells in the mouse. *J. Comp. Neurol.* 497(3):326–349.

Hattar, S., Liao, H. W., Takao, M., Berson, D. M., and Yau, K. W. (2002). Melanopsin-containing retinal ganglion cells: architecture, projections, and intrinsic photosensitivity. *Science* 295(5557):1065–1070.

Hattar, S., Lucas, R. J., Mrosovsky, N., Thompson, S., Douglas, R. H., Hankins, M. W., Lem, J., Biel, M., Hofmann, F., Foster, R. G., and Yau, K. W. (2003). Melanopsin and rod-cone photoreceptive systems account for all major accessory visual functions in mice. *Nature* 424(6944):76–81.

Holtzman, R. L., Malach, R., and Gozes, I. (1989). Disruption of the optic pathway during development affects vasoactive intestinal peptide mRNA expression. *New Biologist* 1(2):215–221.

Keeler, C. E. (1927). Iris movements in blind mice. *Am. J. Physiol.* 81(1):107–112.

Kumbalasiri, T., Rollag, M. D., Isoldi, M., de Lauro Castrucci, A. M., and Provencio, I. (2007). Melanopsin triggers the release of internal calcium stores in response to light. *Photochem. Photobiol.* 83(2):273–279.

Kume, K., Zylka, M. J., Sriram, S., Shearman, L. P., Weaver, D. R., Jin, X., Maywood, E. S., Hastings, M. H., and Reppert, S. M. (1999). mCRY1 and mCRY2 are essential components of the negative limb of the circadian clock feedback loop. *Cell* 98(2):193–205.

Larsen, P. J., Enquist, L. W., and Card, J. P. (1998). Characterization of the multisynaptic neuronal control of the rat pineal gland using viral transneuronal tracing. *Eur. J. Neurosci.* 10(1):128–145.

Lucas, R. J., Douglas, R. H., and Foster, R. G. (2001). Characterization of an ocular photopigment capable of driving pupillary constriction in mice. *Nat. Neurosci.* 4(6):621–626.

Lucas, R. J., Hattar, S., Takao, M., Berson, D. M., Foster, R. G., and Yau, K. W. (2003). Diminished pupillary light reflex at high irradiances in melanopsin-knockout mice. *Science* 299(5604):245–247.

Maywood, E. S., Reddy, A. B., Wong, G. K., O'Neill, J. S., O'Brien, J. A., McMahon, D. G., Harmar, A. J., Okamura, H., and Hastings, M. H. (2006). Synchronization and maintenance of timekeeping in suprachiasmatic circadian clock cells by neuropeptidergic signaling. *Curr. Biol.* 16(6):599–605.

Meijer, J. H., and Schwartz, W. J. (2003). In search of the pathways for light-induced pacemaker resetting in the suprachiasmatic nucleus. *J. Biol. Rhythms* 18(3):235–249.

Melyan, Z., Tarttelin, E. E., Bellingham, J., Lucas, R. J., and Hankins, M. W. (2005). Addition of human melanopsin renders mammalian cells photoresponsive. *Nature* 433(7027):741–745.

Mrosovsky, N. (1999). Masking: history, definitions, and measurement. *Chronobiol. Int.* 16(4):415–429.

Mrosovsky, N., Foster, R. G., and Salmon, P. A. (1999). Thresholds for masking responses to light in three strains of retinally degenerate mice. *J. Comp. Physiol. A* 184(4):423–428.

Mrosovsky, N., and Hattar, S. (2003). Impaired masking responses to light in melanopsin-knockout mice. *Chronobiol. Int.* 20(6):989–999.

Mu, X., and Klein, W. H. (2004). A gene regulatory hierarchy for retinal ganglion cell specification and differentiation. *Semin. Cell Dev. Biol.* 15(1):115–123.

Nagai, N., Nagai, K., and Nakagawa, H. (1992). Effect of orbital enucleation on glucose homeostasis and morphology of the suprachiasmatic nucleus. *Brain Res.* 589(2):243–252.

Nayak, S. K., Jegla, T., and Panda, S. (2007). Role of a novel photopigment, melanopsin, in behavioral adaptation to light. *Cell. Mol. Life Sci.* 64(2):144–154.

Newman, L. A., Walker, M. T., Brown, R. L., Cronin, T. W., and Robinson, P. R. (2003). Melanopsin forms a functional short-wavelength photopigment. *Biochemistry* 42(44):12734–12738.

Panda, S., Hogenesch, J. B., and Kay, S. A. (2002). Circadian rhythms from flies to human. *Nature* 417(6886):329–335.

Panda, S., Nayak, S. K., Campo, B., Walker, J. R., Hogenesch, J. B., and Jegla, T. (2005). Illumination of the melanopsin signaling pathway. *Science* 307(5709):600–604.

Panda, S., Provencio, I., Tu, D. C., Pires, S. S., Rollag, M. D., Castrucci, A. M., Pletcher, M. T., Sato, T. K., Wiltshire, T., et al. (2003). Melanopsin is required for non-image-forming photic responses in blind mice. *Science* 301(5632):525–527.

Panda, S., Sato, T. K., Castrucci, A. M., Rollag, M. D., DeGrip, W. J., Hogenesch, J. B., Provencio, I., and Kay, S. (2002). Melanopsin (Opn4) requirement for normal light-induced circadian phase shifting. *Science* 298(5601):2213–2216.

Pittendrigh, P. S. (1981). Circadian systems: Entrainment. In J. Aschoff (Ed.), *Handbook of behavioral neurobiology* (pp. 95–124). New York: Plenum Press.

Provencio, I., Jiang, G., De Grip, W. J., Hayes, W. P., and Rollag, M. D. (1998). Melanopsin: An opsin in melanophores, brain, and eye. *Proc. Natl. Acad. Sci. U.S.A.* 95(1):340–345.

Provencio, I., Rodriguez, I. R., Jiang, G., Hayes, W. P., Moreira, E. F., and Rollag, M. D. (2000). A novel human opsin in the inner retina. *J. Neurosci.* 20(2):600–605.

Provencio, I., Rollag, M. D., and Castrucci, A. M. (2002). Photoreceptive net in the mammalian retina: This mesh of cells may explain how some blind mice can still tell day from night. *Nature* 415(6871):493.

Qiu, X., Kumbalasiri, T., Carlson, S. M., Wong, K. Y., Krishna, V., Provencio, I., and Berson, D. M. (2005). Induction of photosensitivity by heterologous expression of melanopsin. *Nature* 433(7027): 745–749.

Redlin, U., Cooper, H. M., and Mrosovsky, N. (2003). Increased masking response to light after ablation of the visual cortex in mice. *Brain Res.* 965(1–2):1–8.

Reppert, S. M., and Weaver, D. R. (2002). Coordination of circadian timing in mammals. *Nature* 418(6901):935–941.

Ruby, N. F., Brennan, T. J., Xie, X., Cao, V., Franken, P., Heller, H. C., and O'Hara, B. F. (2002). Role of melanopsin in circadian responses to light. *Science* 298(5601):2211–2213.

Sekaran, S., Foster, R. G., Lucas, R. J., and Hankins, M. W. (2003). Calcium imaging reveals a network of intrinsically light-sensitive inner-retinal neurons. *Curr. Biol.* 13(15):1290–1298.

Sekaran, S., Lupi, D., Jones, S. L., Sheely, C. J., Hattar, S., Yau, K. W., Lucas, R. J., Foster, R. G., and Hankins, M. W. (2005). Melanopsin-dependent photoreception provides earliest light detection in the mammalian retina. *Curr. Biol.* 15(12):1099–1107.

Selby, C. P., Thompson, C., Schmitz, T. M., Van Gelder, R. N., and Sancar, A. (2000). Functional redundancy of cryptochromes and classical photoreceptors for nonvisual ocular photoreception in mice. *Proc. Natl. Acad. Sci. U.S.A.* 97(26):14697–14702.

Shimomura, K., Low-Zeddies, S. S., King, D. P., Steeves, T. D., Whiteley, A., Kushla, J., Zemenides, P. D., Lin, A., Vitaterna, M. H., et al. (2001). Genome-wide epistatic interaction analysis reveals complex genetic determinants of circadian behavior in mice. *Genome Res.* 11(6):959–980.

Siepka, S. M., and Takahashi, J. S. (2005). Methods to record circadian rhythm wheel running activity in mice. *Methods Enzymol.* 393:230–239.

Silver, J. (1977). Abnormal development of the suprachiasmatic nuclei of the hypothalamus in a strain of genetically anophthalmic mice. *J. Comp. Neurol.* 176(4):589–606.

Takahashi, J. S., DeCoursey, P. J., Bauman, L., and Menaker, M. (1984). Spectral sensitivity of a novel photoreceptive system mediating entrainment of mammalian circadian rhythms. *Nature* 308(5955):186–188.

Tarttelin, E. E., Bellingham, J., Bibb, L. C., Foster, R. G., Hankins, M. W., Gregory-Evans, K., Gregory-Evans, C. Y., Wells, D. J., and Lucas, R. J. (2003). Expression of opsin genes early in ocular development of humans and mice. *Exp. Eye Res.* 76(3):393–396.

Teclemariam-Mesbah, R., Ter Horst, G. J., Postema, F., Wortel, J., and Buijs, R. M. (1999). Anatomical demonstration of the suprachiasmatic nucleus-pineal pathway. *J. Comp. Neurol.* 406(2):171–182.

Thapan, K., Arendt, J., and Skene, D. J. (2001). An action spectrum for melatonin suppression: evidence for a novel non-rod, non-cone photoreceptor system in humans. *J. Physiol.* 535(Pt. 1):261–267.

Tu, D. C., Owens, L. A., Anderson, L., Golczak, M., Doyle, S. E., McCall, M., Menaker, M., Palczewski, K., and Van Gelder, R. N. (2006). Inner retinal photoreception independent of the visual retinoid cycle. *Proc. Natl. Acad. Sci. U.S.A.* 103(27):10426–10431.

Tu, D. C., Zhang, D., Demas, J., Slutsky, E. B., Provencio, I., Holy, T. E., and Van Gelder, R. N. (2005). Physiologic diversity and development of intrinsically photosensitive retinal ganglion cells. *Neuron* 48(6):987–999.

van der Horst, G. T., Muijtjens, M., Kobayashi, K., Takano, R., Kanno, S., Takao, M., de Wit, J., Verkerk, A., Eker, A. P., et al. (1999). Mammalian Cry1 and Cry2 are essential for maintenance of circadian rhythms. *Nature* 398(6728):627–630.

Van Gelder, R. N. (2001). Non-visual ocular photoreception. *Ophthalmic Genet.* 22(4):195–205.

Van Gelder, R. N., Wee, R., Lee, J. A., and Tu, D. C. (2003). Reduced pupillary light responses in mice lacking cryptochromes. *Science* 299(5604):222.

Warren, E. J., Allen, C. N., Brown, R. L., and Robinson, D. W. (2003). Intrinsic light responses of retinal ganglion cells projecting to the circadian system. *Eur. J. Neurosci.* 17(9):1727–1735.

Waterhouse, J. M., and DeCoursey, P. J. (2004). The relevance of circadian rhythms for human welfare. In J. C. Dunlap, J. J. Loros, and P. J. DeLaney (Eds.), *Chronobiology: Biological timekeeping* (pp. 325–358). Sunderland, MA: Sinauer.

Wee, R., Castrucci, A. M., Provencio, I., Gan, L., and Van Gelder, R. N. (2002). Loss of photic entrainment and altered free-running circadian rhythms in math5^{-}/$^{-}$ mice. *J. Neurosci.* 22(23):10427–10433.

Welsh, D. K., Logothetis, D. E., Meister, M., and Reppert, S. M. (1995). Individual neurons dissociated from rat suprachiasmatic nucleus express independently phased circadian firing rhythms. *Neuron* 14(4):697–706.

Xu, Y., Toh, K. L., Jones, C. R., Shin, J. Y., Fu, Y. H., and Ptacek, L. J. (2007). Modeling of a human circadian mutation yields insights into *Clock* regulation by PER2. *Cell* 128(1): 59–70.

Yamazaki, S., Goto, M., and Menaker, M. (1999). No evidence for extraocular photoreceptors in the circadian system of the Syrian hamster. *J. Biol. Rhythms* 14(3):197–201.

Yan, L., and Silver, R. (2004). Resetting the brain clock: Time course and localization of mPER1 and mPER2 protein expression in suprachiasmatic nuclei during phase shifts. *Eur. J. Neurosci.* 19(4):1105–1109.

Yoo, S. H., Yamazaki, S., Lowrey, P. L., Shimomura, K., Ko, C. H., Buhr, E. D., Siepka, S. M., Hong, H. K., Oh, W. J., et al. (2004). PERIOD2::LUCIFERASE real-time reporting of circadian dynamics reveals persistent circadian oscillations in mouse peripheral tissues. *Proc. Natl. Acad. Sci. U.S.A.* 101(15): 5339–5346.

Yoshimura, T., and Ebihara, S. (1996). Spectral sensitivity of photoreceptors mediating phase-shifts of circadian rhythms in retinally degenerate CBA/J (rd/rd) and normal CBA/N (+/+) mice. *J. Comp. Physiol. A* 178(6):797–802.

18 Physiology of the Mouse Dorsal Lateral Geniculate Nucleus

MATTHEW S. GRUBB

The dorsal lateral geniculate nucleus (dLGN) plays a key role in the mouse brain's processing of the visual world. Positioned in the flow of information from eye to cortex, its most fundamental job is to provide the neocortex with visual input. It does this not only by passing on the results of processing achieved in the retina but also by introducing more complexity and flexibility into the visual signal—the dLGN is not a passive relay, and reshapes retinal information in important ways. Studying the physiology of this important processing station, then, is key to understanding higher vision. Indeed, it is impossible to understand cortical visual physiology without first knowing the properties of its major driving input. This need for information about geniculate physiology is even more marked in the mouse, since mutation-induced changes in cortical visual function can only be safely interpreted if we know their effects on dLGN function, too (e.g., Rossi et al., 2001; Grubb et al., 2003). To use the mouse to understand higher visual processing, then, we need to understand the physiology of the mouse dLGN. It is a vital link in our knowledge of how the mouse visual system functions.

There is another good reason to study mouse dLGN physiology: the dLGN is the best understood nucleus of the thalamus and has long been used as a model for thalamic function as a whole. This means that questions of mouse dLGN physiology and function are intimately bound up with basic issues of how the thalamus works. We know the thalamus acts as a relay, and appears to change its relayed information in subtle ways, but how exactly? The dLGN is considered a first-order thalamic relay, receiving driving inputs from subcortical structures and sending them on to cortex (e.g., Sherman and Guillery, 2003). As such, it is in a minority within the thalamus, with most nuclei being higher order and subserving communication between different areas within cortex. However, the dLGN is still a good model for general thalamic physiology: almost all of its basic intrinsic and circuit-level function is mirrored in the known properties of other thalamic nuclei (e.g., Sherman, 2005). Furthermore, in any search for a mouse model of primate thalamic function, the dLGN is by far the best candidate. Like all thalamic nuclei in primates, but unlike all other thalamic nuclei in mice, the mouse dLGN contains both glutamatergic relay cells and GABAergic local interneurons (Arcelli et al., 1997). Studying mouse dLGN physiology, therefore, is useful not only when one is trying to understanding mouse vision. It also provides important information about general thalamic function.

This chapter describes our current knowledge of mouse dLGN physiology, from the level of intrinsic cell physiology up to the visual response properties of mouse dLGN neurons. Well aware that many of the most insightful visual and cellular physiology studies of the dLGN were performed in other species, I try to be comparative as much as possible; in many cases it is a matter of showing that the mouse dLGN is just like, or slightly different from, other cases we already know well. However, this situation should change in the future. The availability of powerful genetic manipulations in the mouse should make the mouse dLGN a leading site for studies relating visual and thalamic physiology to the action of individual proteins, and indeed this is already starting to happen. So, whereas carnivore and primate physiology currently informs and shapes our knowledge of the mouse dLGN, the flow of information should soon be headed at least partly in the opposite direction. In this spirit, throughout this chapter I highlight some areas in which the mouse dLGN could lead the way in our understanding of both thalamic and visual physiology.

Intrinsic physiology of mouse dLGN neurons

Understanding the visual role of the mouse dLGN requires basic knowledge about the intrinsic physiological properties of its neurons. Any visual computation taking place in the nucleus will, after all, fundamentally depend on changes in the ionic currents flowing into and out of mouse dLGN cells. Indeed, many of the intrinsic features of mouse dLGN neurons are rather specialized for thalamic functioning. This section describes the basic ionic currents possessed by mouse dLGN cells, concentrating on thalamocortical relay cells, where almost all of our knowledge is based. The species focus in this field has largely been on other rodents (guinea pig, rat) and carnivores (cat, ferret), but we are beginning to develop a good picture of how mice compare. Indeed, genetic manipulations are becoming increasingly useful for studying the molecular bases of intrinsic geniculate physiological properties. The good news is that the main features of intrinsic thalamic physiology seem extremely well conserved, both across individual thalamic nuclei within a given species and across different species and even different phyla (Llinas and Steriade, 2006), so that what we know about the mouse dLGN largely applies to other animals, and vice versa.

Sodium Currents Like most neurons in the brain, those in the mouse dLGN possess a fast transient sodium current ($I_{Na,t}$), which activates and then inactivates rapidly at depolarized membrane potentials (e.g., MacLeod et al., 1997; Jaubert-Miazza et al., 2005; figure 18.1). This current underlies the firing of rapid action potentials, which among other functions sends visual information out of the dLGN toward cortex.

Calcium Currents The presence of a particular calcium current, I_T, is a hallmark of thalamocortical relay cells (TCs) and underlies some of their most important physiological functions. The current, like the transient sodium current underlying action potentials, is activated and then inactivated at depolarized membrane potentials, although I_T kinetics are much slower, and I_T needs less depolarization to activate (it is a low-threshold calcium current). The main effect of I_T is to produce low-threshold calcium spikes (LTSs), which depolarize membrane voltage to levels at which $I_{Na,t}$ is activated, resulting in a burst of sodium spikes riding on a slower calcium LTS (Jahnsen and Llinas, 1984; see figure 18.1). This firing pattern (burst mode) is very different from that produced by depolarization in the absence of I_T activation, which produces trains of action potentials with much longer interspike intervals (tonic mode). It is this distinction between burst and tonic TC activity that may be crucial in determining the geniculate relay of visual information at any given point in time.

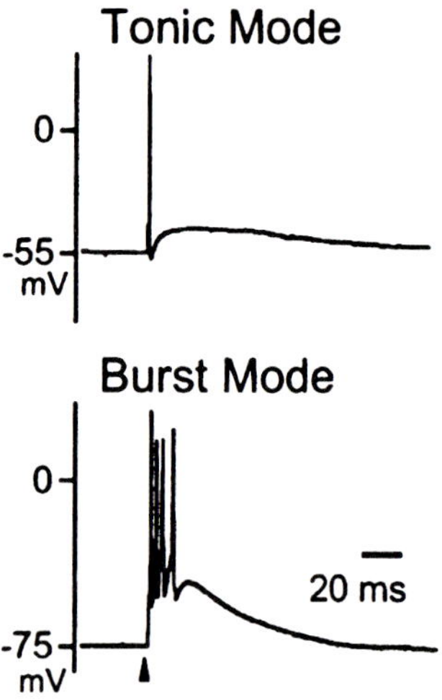

Figure 18.1 Burst and tonic firing modes in a mouse dLGN neuron. The figure shows thalamocortical cell responses in current clamp following stimulation of RGC axons in the optic tract (*arrowhead*). *Top*, When the cell is relatively depolarized, at −55 mV, RGC stimulation produces an EPSP accompanied by a single sodium spike. *Bottom*, When the cell is relatively hyperpolarized, at −75 mV, RGC stimulation produces an EPSP accompanied by a low-threshold calcium spike. A burst of sodium action potentials rides the crest of this LTS. (From Blitz and Regehr, 2003.) Scale bar applies to both traces.

The slow nature of I_T kinetics has important implications for the circumstances in which it is activated. Once inactivated at depolarized membrane potentials (a process that takes ca. 100 ms), the cell membrane must undergo hyperpolarization for about 100 ms or more before I_T channels become deinactivated and ready for re-use. This means that control of IT is achieved through slow-acting modulation that can alter membrane voltage for periods of 100 ms or more. In this way modulatory metabotropic neurotransmission can regulate I_T activity, and thus TC firing mode, in ways that fast ionotropic neurotransmission cannot.

I_T has been identified in all TCs in all species studied to date (Sherman and Guillery, 2003), and the mouse is no exception (MacLeod et al., 1997; Blitz and Regehr, 2003; Jaubert-Miazza et al., 2005; Meuth et al., 2006a, 2006b). Possible functional implications of burst versus tonic firing modes, and the modulation of these two response states in the mouse dLGN, are discussed in detail in the pages that follow.

Mouse dLGN cells also have other, less well-studied calcium currents. High-threshold calcium spikes through $I_{L/N}$ currents, crucial to fully explaining TC cell responses under depolarization (Rhodes and Llinas, 2005), have been identified in the mouse dLGN (MacLeod et al., 1997), while “plateau” potentials arising through activation of L-type calcium channels have also been described in a mouse dLGN preparation, although these figured predominantly in immature developmental stages (Jaubert-Miazza et al., 2005).

Potassium Currents A wide range of potassium currents shapes the subthreshold and action potential firing capabilities of all central neurons, including mouse TCs. The rectifying current I_K, which is activated at highly depolarized membrane voltages and which helps, among other functions, the repolarization following sodium spikes (McCormick, 2003), has been clearly identified in mouse TCs in vitro (MacLeod et al., 1997; Jaubert-Miazza et al., 2005). Mouse dLGN cells also possess a slow afterhyperpolarization potassium current (I_{AHP}; Jaubert-Miazza et al., 2005), which can act as a brake on repetitive sodium spike firing (McCormick, 2003). In addition, mouse TCs are known to possess the I_A potassium current (MacLeod et al., 1997), which activates and inactivates rapidly on membrane depolarization and can therefore slow or delay the firing of both sodium- and calcium-based spikes (Huguenard and McCormick, 1992). Finally, a leak potassium current $I_{K,leak}$, which contributes to the resting membrane potential of TCs, has been well described in the mouse dLGN; in fact, genetic manipulations in murine models have proved crucial in understanding the particular TASK channels that underlie this current (Meuth et al., 2006a).

Hyperpolarization-Activated Currents I_h is a mixed cation current that activates at hyperpolarized membrane potentials and acts to depolarize the cell. Its presence in TCs has been well described because of the role it can play, in conjunction with I_T, in setting up intrinsic slow oscillations in thalamic neurons. LTSs produced by I_T activation wane once I_T is inactivated, producing a membrane hyperpolarization that can activate I_h, thus depolarizing the cell again and providing enough activation for another I_T-based LTS (e.g., Huguenard and McCormick, 1992; McCormick and Bal, 1997). I_h is certainly present in mouse dLGN cells (Meuth et al., 2006a), where, along with potassium leak currents, it plays a key role in setting resting membrane potential levels. The presence or absence of slow oscillations produced from the combined actions of I_h and I_T, however, has not been directly addressed in the mouse geniculate.

Oscillations in the Mouse dLGN? As described earlier, particular combinations of membrane currents possessed by thalamic cells can produce oscillatory activity. Important oscillations are also set up in the dLGN by interactions between TCs and cells in other brain areas, including cortex and the thalamic reticular nucleus (TRN; McCormick and Bal, 1997). These oscillations are prevalent in the naturally sleeping or anesthetized brain, and thalamic/dLGN cells are known to be a vital part of the circuits producing normal and pathological network oscillations (e.g., Llinas and Steriade, 2006). Indeed, one vital function of the dLGN may be to regulate the flow of visual information during different states of alertness by altering rhythmic activity patterns. However, the seminal work describing these oscillations has occurred exclusively in non-mouse mammalian models, and although the mouse dLGN appears to have all the intrinsic currents, cells, and circuits necessary to oscillate, it is unclear whether it has the same network behavior. There has been one report of slow, approximately 1 Hz oscillations in extracellularly recorded mouse dLGN spikes in vitro (Zhu et al., 2006), but we need to build on these initial data before we can use the full power of the mouse model to understand the basis, and maybe even the functional implications, of these oscillations in health and disease.

Overall, then, mouse dLGN cells are model examples of thalamic units, with no great differences across species. There are gaps left to fill in our knowledge, of course, not least concerning oscillatory activity. It is also unclear whether mouse dLGN cells have other important currents—including I_{K2} and $I_{Na,p}$—that have been identified in the TCs of other species (e.g., Jahnsen and Llinas, 1984; Huguenard and McCormick, 1992). Furthermore, it is important to note that our knowledge of intrinsic mouse dLGN physiology comes almost entirely from TC recordings, and although we know there are important differences between TCs and local interneurons in terms of intrinsic capabilities in other species (e.g., McCormick and Bal, 1997; Llinas and Steriade, 2006), nothing is known about these differences in mice. This knowledge would be particularly useful insofar as the dLGN is the only thalamic nucleus in the mouse to possess GABAergic interneurons (Arcelli, et al., 1997). Nevertheless, as the case of resting membrane potential shows (Meuth et al., 2006a, 2006b), using the mouse dLGN as a model for these intrinsic properties has great value, allowing molecular-level understanding of crucial electrophysiological features.

Relaying the retinal signal

The intrinsic properties of mouse dLGN cells combine with the input received by the nucleus from various sources to produce the dLGN's output—sodium spikes transmitted to visual cortex. And although the majority of synapses received by TCs come from nonretinal sources, the roughly 7% of synapses that derive from the eye (Sherman, 2005) dominate the visual physiology of the dLGN—they are "driving" inputs. At least in part, then, the mouse dLGN serves to relay visual information from the eye to cortex. How it does so and the consequences for the visual response properties of mouse dLGN neurons are described in this section.

Retinogeniculate Inputs and Spatial Information In vitro recordings have shown that mouse TCs receive input from very few (one to three) individual retinal ganglion cell (RGC) fibers, and that these inputs always arise from the same eye (Chen and Regehr, 2000; Jaubert-Miazza et al., 2005; figure 18.2). Insofar as these inputs are also strong, with high release probability (Chen and Regehr, 2000; Reichova and Sherman, 2004; Kielland et al., 2006), one might expect the spatial visual response properties of mouse dLGN neurons to reflect very closely those of their individual RGC inputs. This is certainly the case in other species (Hubel and Wiesel, 1961; Usrey et al., 1999), and is true in the mouse, where dLGN cells all respond to visual stimulation through one eye only (Metin et al., 1983; Grubb et al., 2003), and share many important spatial properties with their RGC input. In particular, the receptive fields (RFs) of most mouse dLGN cells, like those in other mammalian species (e.g., Hubel and Wiesel, 1961; Wiesel and Hubel, 1966), are

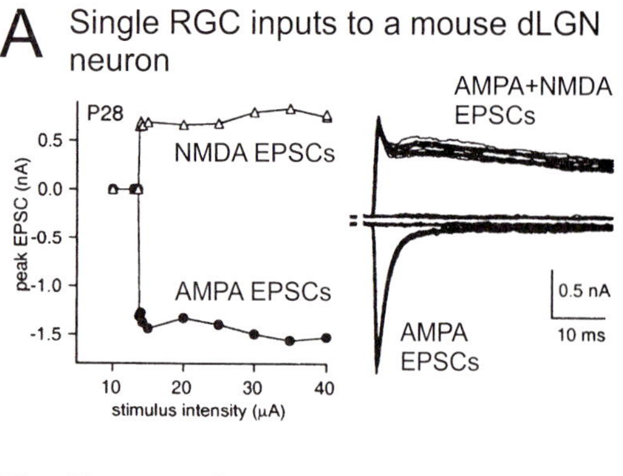

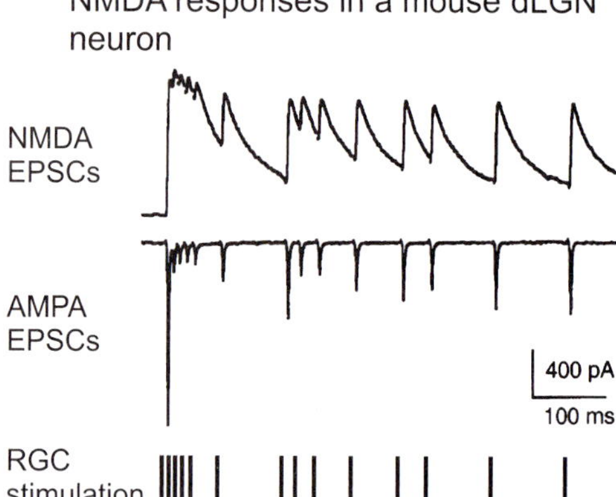

FIGURE 18.2 Features of retinogeniculate inputs in the mouse. *A*, Mature mouse dLGN neurons receive input from one or few RGCs. *Left plot* shows retinogeniculate EPSC amplitude, for both NMDA events (*open triangles*) and for AMPA events (*filled circles*), as a function of increasing RGC stimulation amplitude. *Right plot* shows whole-cell-recorded EPSC traces at +40 mV (AMPA + NMDA; *top*) and −70 mV (AMPA only; *bottom*) after RGC stimulation of varying amplitude. Both plots show clearly that increasing the number of stimulated RGC fibers produces an all-or-nothing step in postsynaptic response size, consistent with a single presynaptic RGC input to the recorded cell. *B*, AMPA and NMDA events in mouse dLGN neurons differ in the temporal patterns produced by RGC inputs. Plots show NMDA EPSCs (*top*; +40 mV in NBQX) and AMPA EPSCs (*middle*; −70 mV in CPP) in a mouse thalamocortical neuron during stimulation of RGC inputs with a pattern mimicking a mouse RGC's response to a flash of light (*bottom*). Notice the large diminution in AMPA current produced by high-frequency RGC inputs, in contrast to the sustained level of NMDA activation in such circumstances. Scale bar applies to both top and middle traces. (*A*, Modified from Chen and Regehr, 2000. *B*, Modified from Chen et al., 2002.)

circular, concentric, and center-surround in organization (figure 18.3). They can be ON- or OFF-center, so responding best to either a light spot on a dark background (ON-center) or a dark spot on a light background (OFF-center; Grubb and Thompson, 2003). The mouse retina contains cells of this type too (e.g., Balkema and Pinto, 1982; Tian and Copenhagen, 2003), although the question of whether particular types of mouse RGC project only to dLGN neurons with the same RF type (see Usrey et al., 1999) has yet to be definitively examined. It is also important to note that center-surround RFs are very probably not the only RF type present in either mouse retina or dLGN (they represented ca. 60% of a dLGN sample; Grubb and Thompson, 2003); for the moment, they simply represent the population we know the most about. However, given the physiology of the retinogeniculate projection, one would also expect the RF features of other mouse RGC types to be mapped fairly faithfully onto their geniculate targets. This is probably the case in cats and in primates, where some W-type or koniocellular (K) dLGN neurons, respectively, possess non-center-surround RFs (e.g., Sur and Sherman, 1982; Xu et al., 2001).

Not only are there similarities in RF structure between the mouse retina and dLGN, there is also great similarity in RF size. RF center diameter in mouse RGCs is about 5–10° (Balkema and Pinto, 1982), while the mean value in mouse dLGN, calculated from spatial frequency (SF) tuning curves, is about 6° (Grubb and Thompson, 2003). Center size largely predicts a cell's spatial acuity, reflected in its SF cutoff frequencies, and there the similarities continue: the average mouse dLGN cell can resolve an SF of 0.18 c/deg, and maximum acuity values in the nucleus are about 0.5 c/deg. In comparison, mouse RGCs have SF cutoffs of around 0.2 c/deg, while the ERG response of the retina as a whole has a spatial acuity (reflective of that of its best-performing units) of about 0.6 c/deg. It should be apparent from this discussion that, comparatively, mouse vision at the thalamic level is extremely poor in terms of spatial acuity: macaque dLGN RF centers are normally less than 1° in diameter, for example, leading to an acuity of about 40 c/deg (e.g., Merigan et al., 1991; figure 18.4). However, this poor performance cannot be blamed on the mouse dLGN. It is simply making the most of the low-resolution information it receives from the retina.

The spatial signal relayed by dLGN cells can depend on the particular type of cell that is doing the relaying. In primates, three main classes of geniculate cell have been identified—parvocellular (P), magnocellular (M), and koniocellular (K)—based on a multitude of distinguishing biochemical, anatomical, and physiological characteristics. In terms of spatial response characteristics, P cells have smaller RFs than M cells, which in turn have smaller RFs than K cells (e.g., Xu et al., 2002). Most RFs in all classes, however, are center-surround in organization and summate spatial influences linearly across their RFs (e.g., Xu et al., 2001). These features, at least for P and M cells, are likely to stem directly from the response properties of different classes of primate RGC (Callaway, 2005). Similarly, the cat dLGN also contains cell populations that differ in their spatial response characteristics. X cells have smaller RFs than Y cells, which in turn have smaller RFs than W cells (e.g., Sur

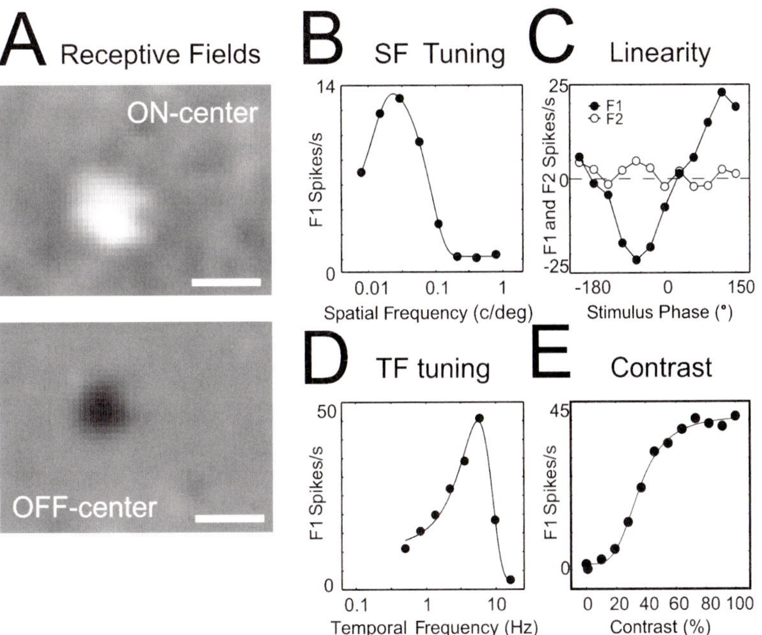

Figure 18.3 Representative visual response properties of mouse dLGN neurons. *A*, Mouse dLGN cell receptive fields (RFs), mapped from responses to localized flashed black-and-white square stimuli. The resultant circular, concentric RFs are typical of most mouse dLGN cells and are either ON-center (*top*) or OFF-center (*bottom*). *B*, Spatial frequency (SF) tuning. Cell response magnitude is plotted against the SF of drifting sinusoidal grating stimuli. Like this cell, most mouse dLGN neurons prefer SFs of about 0.02 c/deg, and have SF cutoffs of about 0.2 c/deg. *C*, Linearity of spatial summation. Cell response amplitude at both the first (F1) and second (F2) harmonics of the stimulus is plotted against the phase of stationary, counterphased sinusoidal gratings. Two null positions, where the F1 response is zero, along with small F2 responses are indicative of linear spatial summation; almost all mouse dLGN cells displayed this type of behavior. *D*, Temporal frequency (TF) tuning, assessed with drifting sinusoidal gratings. Like this cell, most mouse neurons have bandpass TF tuning curves and prefer TFs of about 4 Hz. *E*, Contrast response properties, also assessed using drifting sinusoidal grating stimuli. Mouse neurons, like this one, showed sigmoidal increases in response amplitude with increasing stimulus contrast, and usually had half-maximal responses (c_{50}) at around 30%. Plots in different panels reflect the responses of different mouse dLGN cells. (Modified from Grubb and Thompson, 2003.)

and Sherman, 1982). Most cells in all groups have center-surround RF organization, but the linearity of summation differs among the different classes: X cells are linear, Y cells display nonlinear doubling responses at high SFs, and the W cell population shows examples of both types of behavior (Sur and Sherman, 1982). Again, these differences are likely to arise directly from the spatial properties of the retinal input: X and Y cells in particular are known to receive strong inputs only from the corresponding RGC type (Usrey et al., 1999). Evidence for different functional cell classes in the mouse dLGN, however, is lacking (Grubb and Thompson, 2003). RF sizes in our sample did not segregate into distinct groups, whereas almost all mouse dLGN cells displayed linear spatial summation. This latter finding was surprising, given that both linear and nonlinear summation have been observed in mouse RGCs (Balkema and Pinto, 1982). However, it is possible that "Y-like" mouse RGCs project to nongeniculate targets, or that they project (weakly) to postsynaptic targets that display X-like properties (see Usrey et al., 1999). It also should be stressed that, although we found no evidence for "parallel processing" of visual information in the mouse dLGN cells we recorded, these data were based on the approximately 60% of cells that had clear center-surround RFs. The remaining 40% of cells, perhaps with more complex RFs, may then relay rather different, parallel information.

Retinogeniculate Inputs and Temporal Information

The processing of temporal information across the retinogeniculate synapse has been particularly well described in the mouse. RGCs are glutamatergic, and the signal they transmit to TCs is received exclusively (Chen and Regehr, 2000; Reichova and Sherman, 2004) by two types of ionotropic glutamate receptor with very different temporal properties: AMPA receptors (AMPARs), which display very rapid kinetics, and NMDA receptors (NMDARs), which operate on a far slower time scale (e.g., Chen and Regehr, 2000, 2003). Additional important differences, apart from the NMDAR's famous voltage dependency, are that AMPARs desensitize rapidly on glutamatergic stimulation, while NMDARs, with their higher affinity for the neurotransmitter, can saturate under repetitive stimulation. Both of these

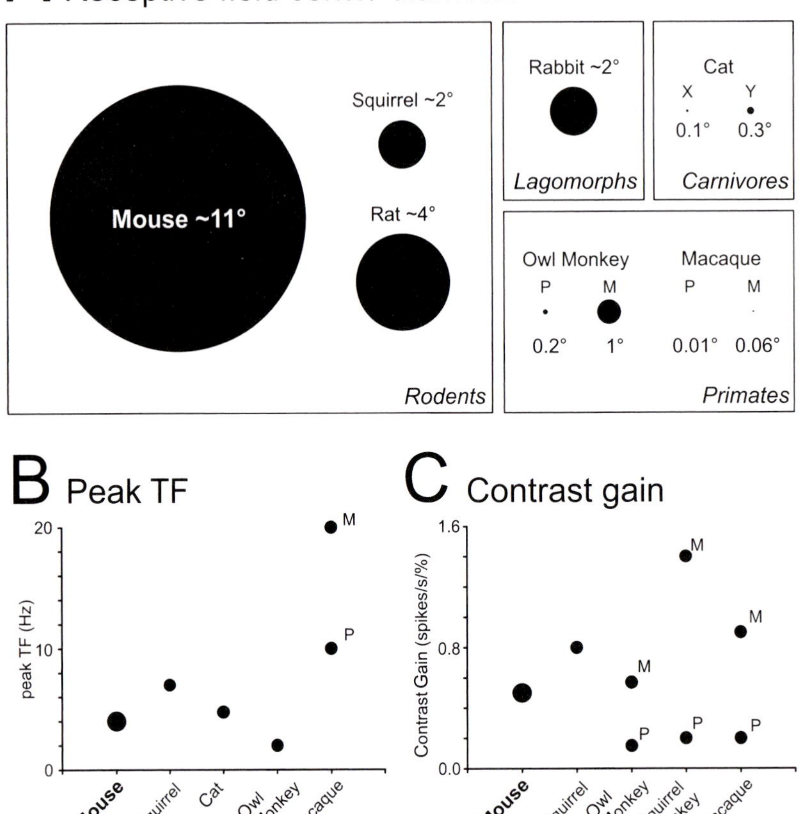

Figure 18.4 Cross-species comparison of dLGN visual response properties. *A*, In the spatial domain, mouse RF center diameters are by far the largest of any mammalian species studied, conferring low spatial acuity on the visual system as a whole. *B*, In the temporal domain, however, mouse peak temporal frequency (TF) compares favorably with that of other mammals, aside from macaque. *C*, In terms of contrast gain, cells in the mouse dLGN tend to fall midway between the performance of parvocellular (P) and magnocellular (M) primate dLGN neurons. For the sake of simplicity, only selected species and cell classes are shown, and separate cell classes are shown for a given species only when they differ largely from each other. (Mouse data from Grubb and Thompson, 2003; all other RF diameter data from table 1 in Van Hooser et al., 2005. Squirrel data from Van Hooser et al., 2003; cat data from Mukherjee and Kaplan, 1995; TF owl monkey data from Xu et al., 2001; TF macaque data from Derrington and Lennie, 1984; contrast squirrel monkey and owl monkey data from Usrey and Reid, 2000; contrast macaque data from Levitt et al., 2001.)

phenomena lead to reduced responses at high RGC firing frequencies (Chen and Regehr, 2003). However, the slow nature of NMDAR responses can counteract the effects of saturation, allowing high-frequency firing to lead to summation of NMDA currents, whereas similar firing reduces the contribution made by rapid-kinetic AMPARs (Blitz and Regehr, 2003, see figure 18.2). The upshot is that AMPARs relay single RGC spikes more precisely, but NMDARs are required to allow TC responses to high-frequency RGC activity. TCs can follow RGC action potential trains precisely (so long as they are in tonic mode), but the precise effect of a given RGC firing pattern on TC activity will depend on the relative numbers of AMPARs and NMDARs at the retinogeniculate synapse (Blitz and Regehr, 2003).

A prediction based on this information, and given the strong, unitary nature of the retinogeniculate connection, would be that the visual temporal properties of mouse dLGN cells would depend both on the temporal properties of their driving RGC input and on the mixture of ionotropic glutamate receptors present at their synapses. We know that mouse dLGN cells respond best to sinusoidal grating stimuli with temporal frequencies of about 4 Hz (Grubb and Thompson, 2003), but unfortunately, we have very little information about the temporal visual response properties of mouse RGCs. Similarly, since the responses of RGCs generally increase monotonically with increases in visual stimulus contrast (e.g., Kaplan and Shapley, 1986), one might expect the contrast response characteristics of mouse dLGN cells to also depend on RGC tuning and AMPAR-NMDAR distributions. Higher NMDAR ratios could be needed to be able to signal increases in the highest stimulus contrasts, reflected in higher RGC firing rates, but higher

AMPA ratios might allow changes in lower contrast to be reflected more faithfully in TC firing patterns. Again, although the contrast response properties are well described for mouse dLGN neurons (mean gain ca. 0.5 spikes/s/%, mean c_{50} ca. 33%; Grubb and Thompson, 2003), we lack the appropriate RGC data for comparison. Perhaps if future studies reveal large differences between RGCs and TCs in these phenomena, AMPAR-NMDAR distributions could be the reason. Indeed, it could be extremely interesting to look at mice carrying kinetics-altering mutations in AMPAR/NMDAR subunits (e.g., Lu et al., 2006)—would this lead to geniculate abnormalities in temporal or contrast visual response properties? This would be one situation in which the mouse dLGN would be a perfect model to combine the strengths of both in vitro and in vivo electrophysiological approaches. Indeed, the strength of the mouse dLGN as such a model is clear from the quantitative data noted: although mouse dLGN performs extremely poorly in the spatial domain, its performance is rather good in the temporal and contrast domains (see figure 18.4). Preferred temporal frequency may be much lower (ca. 4 Hz) in mouse than in macaque (ca. 10–16 Hz; Derrington and Lennie, 1984), but the mouse compares favorably with the cat (ca. 5 Hz; Mukherjee and Kaplan, 1995) and other primates (owl monkey: ca. 2 Hz, Xu et al., 2001; galago: ca. 2–4 Hz, Norton et al., 1988) in this respect. In terms of contrast responses, mouse dLGN values fall between those reported for primate M and P dLGN cells (Levitt et al., 2001; Usrey and Reid, 2000). So, even though the mouse visual thalamus operates at very low spatial resolution, it still provides cortex with good temporal and contrast information.

Reshaping the retinal signal

The previous section showed that retinal input to the mouse dLGN determines many of its most important physiological features. In particular, mouse dLGN cells resemble their RGC inputs extremely closely in terms of visual spatial processing. However, although one role of the mouse dLGN is undoubtedly to relay information from retina to cortex, the huge number of non-RGC synapses impinging on TCs (e.g., Sherman, 2005) suggests that this is certainly not all the mouse dLGN is doing. In fact, there are numerous ways in which modulatory input to the geniculate can alter the visual information passing through the structure. This subtle modulation of the visual signal, compared with the drastic changes in visual RF structure as vision is processed through both retina and cortex, is a unique feature of the dLGN within the visual system (Sherman, 2005). One can even view the mouse dLGN's main role as providing a subtle reshaping of the retinal signal based on its owner's current state and environmental demands.

Presynaptic Modulation of Retinal Input Before visual information arrives postsynaptically in the dLGN, it can be controlled by the effects of modulating inputs onto RGC terminals. These effects have been well described in the mouse and appear to be inhibitory: GABA acting through metabotropic $GABA_B$ receptors decreases the otherwise strong release probability at retinogeniculate terminals, while serotonin, operating through 5-HT_1 receptors, also inhibits transmitter release (Chen and Regehr, 2003). This latter effect has been shown specifically to improve the signal-to-noise ratio for high-frequency RGC inputs (Seeburg et al., 2004). Another opportunity for the mouse to lead our knowledge in this field: retina-specific genetic manipulations of either of these regulatory channels could prove extremely useful in determining the importance of such presynaptic modulation in visual or thalamic function.

Local Geniculate Inhibition As noted earlier, the dLGN is special in the mouse thalamus, but normal when compared with all primate thalamic nuclei, for containing a population of GABAergic interneurons (Arcelli et al., 1997). The effect of these cells can be seen following electrical stimulation of the optic tract in an in vitro preparation and depends on the particular circuitry of the cell being studied. "Locked" IPSCs (Blitz and Regehr, 2005) can be seen with very short and consistent latencies following glutamatergic EPSCs, and likely reflect feed-forward inhibition: a single RGC monosynaptically contacts both a TC and a local inhibitory neuron, with the latter then contacting the same TC (figure 18.5). This could occur in specialized synaptic structures known as triads, where the terminal of a RGC, the dendrite of a TC, and the dendrite of a geniculate interneuron are all closely opposed and synaptically interconnected (Rafols and Valverde, 1973; Sherman and Guillery, 2003). What is the role of this locked inhibition? Probably to sharpen a TC's temporal response to retinal input, especially that carried through AMPARs (Blitz and Regehr, 2005). "Nonlocked" inhibition (Blitz and Regehr, 2005) is also seen after optic tract stimulation, occurring at variable latencies, and probably reflecting input to TCs from inhibitory cells that are not presynaptically connected to the same RGCs (see figure 18.5). The unlocked inhibition likely serves to increase surround inhibition within the dLGN. If inhibitory cells are driven by inputs from the region surrounding a TC's RF center, and if they share same center type (ON/OFF) as that TC cell, their action would increase the contrast of visual information sent to cortex.

In fact, this is one transformation of the visual signal that is well characterized over the retinogeniculate pathway—surround inhibition is much stronger in dLGN cells than in the RGCs that feed them (Hubel and Wiesel, 1961; Usrey et al., 1999), and this difference depends on local geniculate inhibitory activity (Norton et al., 1989). It also appears to be

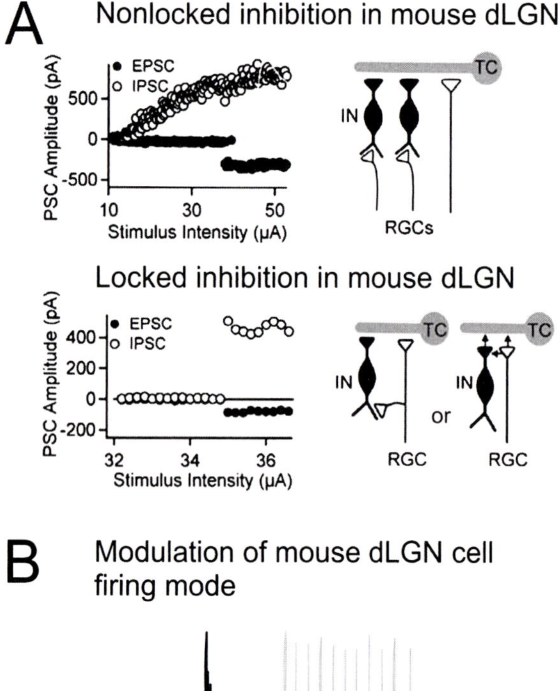

FIGURE 18.5 Reshaping the retinal signal in the mouse dLGN. *A*, Nonlocked and locked inhibition produced by RGC stimulation. *Left plots* show the amplitude of EPSCs (*solid circles*) and IPSCs (*open circles*) produced as the stimulation of RGC fibers in the optic tract becomes stronger. In both cases, the all-or-nothing increase in EPSC magnitude signifies a single-input retinogeniculate connection (see figure 18.2). In nonlocked inhibition (*top*), IPSCs increase gradually in strength. This is consistent with the recruitment of RGC fibers other than those that contacted the recorded cell; these fibers then project to inhibitory dLGN neurons that *do* contact the recorded neuron (*right*). In locked inhibition (*bottom*), the IPSCs also show an all-or-nothing jump in response amplitude with increased stimulation strength. This is consistent with the inhibition depending on activation of the same RGC fiber that provides excitation to the recorded cell (*right*). IN, interneuron. *B*, Switching TC response mode through modulatory neurotransmission. In control conditions (*black trace*), the response of a mouse dLGN cell is recorded in current clamp from a holding potential of −73 mV. A depolarizing current injection then results in an LTS accompanied by burst mode firing. Without any alteration in the holding current, application of muscarine then depolarizes the cell to −58 mV, and subsequent current injection leads to a train of spikes in tonic mode. (*A*, Modified from Blitz and Regehr, 2005. *B*, From Meuth et al., 2006a.)

the case in the mouse. Although strong surround inhibition was seen in almost all mouse dLGN cells studied (only 12 of 92 were low-pass for SF-varying stimuli; Grubb and Thompson, 2003), such effects were rarely seen in mouse RGCs (Stone and Pinto, 1993; but it should be noted that the retinal recordings were carried out in vitro, while those from the dLGN were in vivo). Interestingly, if this is an effect of local inhibition in the mouse dLGN, it does not depend on the topographical organization of the nucleus. In mice lacking the β2 subunit of the nicotinic acetylcholine (ACh) receptor, the retinotopic organization of the dLGN is disrupted (Grubb et al., 2003), but RF surrounds are entirely normal (Grubb and Thompson, 2004). We hope that other genetic manipulations could offer the chance in the near future to study the effects of GABAergic inhibition on visual thalamic processing.

MODULATING INTRINSIC TC PHYSIOLOGY Other modulatory influences come from outside the dLGN and act on the intrinsic conductances of TCs. A huge number of glutamatergic feedback projections impinge on dLGN TCs from visual cortex, where the effects of each individual synapse are weak, with low release probability (Reichova and Sherman, 2004). However, in addition to the AMPARs and NMDARs that act at the glutamatergic retinogeniculate synapse, strong synergistic activation of inputs from mouse cortex can also activate metabotropic glutamate receptors (mGluRs), producing a slow depolarization of the TC membrane (Reichova and Sherman, 2004).

Many other extrinsic inputs to mouse dLGN TCs also act to produce slow changes in membrane potential. Studies in the mouse have shown that the easiest way to alter TC membrane voltage is probably through changes in the opening of K_{leak} and I_h channels—the two interact to largely determine resting membrane potential (Meuth et al., 2006b). Indeed, ACh acting through metabotropic muscarinic receptors (mAChRs) in the mouse dLGN produces a slow TC depolarization by closing K_{leak} channels (Meuth et al., 2006a). In contrast, activation of β-adrenergic receptors or $GABA_B$ receptors (from interneurons in the TRN, and maybe from local interneurons, too) have depolarizing and hyperpolarizing effects, respectively, on mouse TC membrane voltage through cAMP-controlled modulation of I_h (Frere and Luthi, 2004). It remains to be shown whether the multitude of other slow modulatory effects on TC membrane potential, as have been described in other species (see, e.g., McCormick and Bal, 1997), also occur in the mouse, where once again, the application of genetic interventions might prove crucial in explaining their underlying molecular mechanisms (e.g., Meuth et al., 2006a, 2006b).

The common and most important feature of all of these modulatory mechanisms is that their effects on TC membrane potential are slow. The importance of this becomes obvious when considering the properties of I_T. Both inactivation and deinactivation of I_T are slow processes. It takes approximately 100 ms for I_T to inactivate at depolarized potentials, and approximately 100 ms for it to become deinactivated at hyperpolarized voltages (Jahnsen and Llinas,

1984). The kinds of depolarization or hyperpolarization produced by ionotropic receptors or by depolarizing action potentials, then, although having huge effects on mouse dLGN response properties, will not affect TC response mode. In contrast, the slow hyperpolarizations and depolarizations produced by the mouse dLGN's modulatory input are ideal for regulating I_T, and thus the burst versus tonic response mode of the nucleus's relay neurons. Indeed, to give just one example from the mouse, ACh shifts TCs from burst (I_T-activated) to tonic (I_T-inactivated) mode through the slow depolarizing influence of closed K_{leak} channels brought about by mAChR activation (Meuth et al., 2006a; see figure 18.5). The final effect of dLGN modulation, then, is often to switch TC response mode from burst to tonic mode, or vice versa.

This effect is extremely important in transitions from sleeping to waking states. Bursting predominates in the former, but with the transition from slow-wave sleep to wakefulness, modulatory inputs from the brainstem produce a slow depolarization of TCs that inactivates I_T, decreasing burst firing and promoting the tonic responses that dominate the waking state (McCarley et al., 1983; McCormick and Bal, 1997; Llinas and Steriade, 2006). But could modulatory influences, and thus the firing mode of mouse TCs, also play a role in the way visual information is coded?

Burst and Tonic Mode Contributions to Visual Processing Because rhythmic bursting is most prominent during slow-wave sleep (McCarley et al., 1983; Weyand et al., 2001), and because during sleep the responsiveness of dLGN neurons to RF stimulation is decreased (Livingstone and Hubel, 1981), it might appear that burst firing in TCs is unimportant as a carrier of visual information. However, experiments carried out mainly in the cat have uncovered the possibility that burst and tonic responses carry specific types of visual information. Intracellular recordings in cat dLGN showed that burst responses driven by I_T activation can occur during visual stimulation (Lu et al., 1992), and also showed that burst spikes could be accurately identified purely on the basis of temporal patterns in spike firing. The latter finding has allowed less technically demanding extracellular recordings to confirm that bursting, like tonic firing, can occur in the dLGN in awake behaving animals (Guido and Weyand, 1995; Weyand et al., 2001), and to show in anesthetized animals that the visual response properties of the two firing modes can be very different. Among other differences, burst spikes in the cat follow temporal changes in visual stimuli less faithfully (Guido et al., 1992; Lu et al., 1992), offer better stimulus detection (Guido et al., 1995), are more tightly tuned for TF (Mukherjee and Kaplan, 1995), and have more reliable timing (Guido and Sherman, 1998) than their tonic counterparts. Changes in firing mode in mouse thalamic relay cells brought about by modulatory influences on I_T might therefore affect the information relayed by those cells to cortex.

We recently explored whether burst and tonic firing might also be able to encode different forms of visual information in the mouse dLGN (Grubb and Thompson, 2005). As expected given the cross-species homology of I_T and firing modes described in vitro, we found that the criteria developed to identify burst spikes in cat dLGN also identified distinct groups of spikes in the mouse—the criteria successfully classified *preexisting* temporal patterns of neuronal firing (figure 18.6). Comparing burst and tonic spikes classified in this way across a range of quantitative visual response parameters revealed that both firing modes were identical in terms of the spatial information they could encode. RF characteristics, the linearity of spatial summation, and SF tuning were all identical in burst versus tonic firing (Grubb and Thompson, 2005). Indeed, RF center and surround sizes were also shown to be identical in cat dLGN (Alitto et al., 2005). However, the two firing modes in the mouse dLGN did differ significantly in the temporal domain. Just as in the cat, bursts are more phase advanced, more rectified, have sharper TF tuning, and prefer lower TFs (Grubb and Thompson, 2005). We also demonstrated that contrast-response curves are more steplike for burst responses, a feature that may arise, at least in part, from the all-or-none nature of the I_T-driven LTS (see Zhan et al., 1999). Finally, just as in the cat, we found in the mouse dLGN that higher levels of bursting are associated with better stimulus detection (see figure 18.6), and that burst spikes offer more reliable information about stimulus onset (Grubb and Thompson, 2005).

This all suggests not only that the cat and mouse dLGN may be extremely functionally similar but also the possibility that burst and tonic firing in the mouse dLGN could signal (subtly) different types of visual information. Why might this be important? It may not be. It is a distinct possibility that the response properties of burst versus tonic firing are epiphenomena arising from mechanisms that evolved to switch cortex on and off during sleeping and waking states (e.g., Llinas and Steriade, 2006). However, another hypothesis of thalamic function (e.g., Sherman, 2001) suggests that bursting may function as a wake-up call for cortex: occurring at the start of a stimulus, and possessing good capability for stimulus detection, bursts could signal to cortex that that stimulus has occurred, and that it started a certain time ago. Bursts could also send a great deal of information about the stimulus (especially in the spatial domain), information that cortex can start to process before more detailed tonic spike-driven information arrives. It remains to be shown whether burst firing during stimulus presentation produces better behavioral detection of that stimulus (see Ruiz et al., 2006). However, the observation that the burst-tonic distinction occurs in the mouse dLGN and that it appears to have many

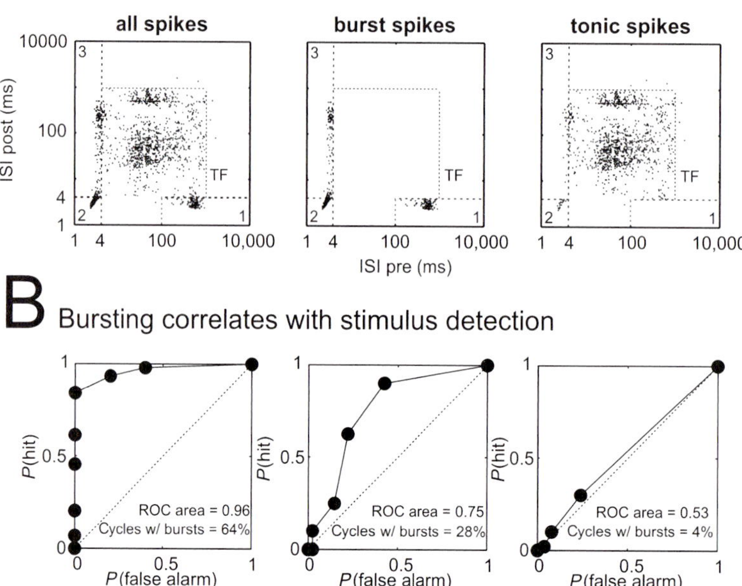

FIGURE 18.6 Burst and tonic firing in the visual responses of mouse dLGN cells. *A*, Identifying burst and tonic spikes in extracellularly recorded dLGN cell responses. Criteria based on spike timing, taken from intracellular recordings in vivo (Lu et al., 1992), were used to categorize events: bursts were preceded by >100 ms of silence and consisted of ≥2 spikes separated by interspike intervals (ISIs) of <4 ms. Spikes fired by a single mouse dLGN cell to a sinusoidal grating stimulus are plotted here based on their preceding and following ISIs, and it is clear that the criteria segregate *preexisting* patterns of spiking behavior. Spikes in box 1 are the first spikes in bursts, those in box 2 are mainly the middle spikes of bursts, and those in box 3 are mainly the last spikes in bursts. All other spikes form part of tonic firing. TF, stimulus temporal frequency. *B*, Bursting correlates positively with stimulus detection ability. The receiver operating characteristic (ROC) curves here take responses fired by a single cell to a drifting sinusoidal grating stimulus and, for a given spike count, plot the probability *P(hit)* of attaining this count during stimulus presentation versus the probability *P(false alarm)* of attaining this count during an equal period of spontaneous activity. The area under the resulting curve (ROC area) then provides a nonparametric measure of the cell's ability to distinguish visual from nonvisual stimulation. This ability correlates positively with the burstiness of a mouse dLGN cell: the ROC area increases as the percentage of stimulus cycles with bursts increases. (From Grubb and Thompson, 2005.)

functional similarities to that in other mammals leaves open the possibility for some interesting genetic experiments. What happens to mouse vision, for example, when the calcium channel underlying I_T is knocked out in the thalamus (Kim et al., 2001)? At the geniculate level, given the subtle coding differences noted earlier, maybe no drastic effects would be observed, but at the cortical or behavioral level, what would be the consequence of dLGN cells that were always in tonic mode? If the knockout could be more specific—perhaps to TCs or interneurons only—we could start to strip down the functional role of I_T even further. And even if there are no visual functional differences between burst and tonic firing, an I_T knockout would be the ideal model to show this. Other fun manipulations also spring to mind. How about mutating the HCN channels underlying I_h (e.g., Meuth et al., 2006b) to specifically control rhythmic bursting in an intact preparation? Or producing mutations in any of the modulatory neurotransmitter receptors that affect TC firing mode? The easiest way to look for causality in the functional role of properties produced by a single molecule may well be to delete that molecule and see what happens. And, for the moment, those experiments are easiest by far in the mouse.

Conclusion

Currently, a good outline of mouse dLGN physiology exists. Neurons in the structure possess all the major intrinsic physiological features of thalamic cells, and knowledge of how these features can be modulated to produce changes in firing rate or firing mode is advancing nicely. We know a great deal about the spatial and temporal features of retinogeniculate input and are able to relate this information (at least indirectly) to the fundamental quantitative visual response properties of mouse dLGN cells. Finally, the features of the two major thalamic firing modes, burst and tonic, and their possible contributions to visual processing have started to be investigated in the structure.

However, much remains to be uncovered. The areas in which our understanding of geniculate function is far ahead in other species have been highlighted where appropriate in this chapter, but that still leaves a long list of things the physiologist might like to know about the mouse dLGN. Simply in terms of visual response properties, we know nothing about chromatic responses in the mouse dLGN, the responses of mouse dLGN neurons to natural scene stimuli, the effects of contextual influences on mouse dLGN RF properties, the coding possible in populations of mouse dLGN cells, or how any or all of these properties relate to the mouse's visual behavior. In terms of circuitry, our knowledge of the oscillatory properties of mouse dLGN cells and networks is hugely lacking. It is also difficult to fully understand the functions of the mouse dLGN when we have so little quantitative data on the visual properties of both its retinal input and of its cortical target neurons, and no information at all about physiology in a major provider of thalamic inhibition, the TRN. No nucleus is an island.

The potential benefits of obtaining this information are huge. With the advent of more and more sophisticated techniques for controlling gene expression in a spatially and temporally regulated manner (Lewandowski, 2001; Aronoff and Petersen, 2006), the mouse dLGN offers a good model of both visual processing and thalamic function in which we can investigate the effects of single molecules on physiological phenomena. The hope is that in the near future, studies of wild-type and mutant mouse dLGN physiology will lead us closer to an understanding of what the visual thalamus actually does.

ACKNOWLEDGMENTS I thank Murray Sherman and Ian Thompson for their helpful comments.

REFERENCES

Alitto, H. J., Weyand, T. G., and Usrey, W. M. (2005). Distinct properties of stimulus-evoked bursts in the lateral geniculate nucleus. *J. Neurosci.* 25:514–523.

Aronoff, R., and Petersen, C. C. (2006). Controlled and localized genetic manipulation in the brain. *J. Cell. Mol. Med.* 10: 333–352.

Arcelli, P., Frassoni, C., Regondi, M. C., De Biasi, S., and Spreafico, R. (1997). GABAergic neurons in mammalian thalamus: A marker of thalamic complexity? *Brain Res. Bull.* 42:27–37.

Balkema, G. W., Jr., and Pinto, L. H. (1982). Electrophysiology of retinal ganglion cells in the mouse: A study of a normally pigmented mouse and a congenic hypopigmentation mutant, pearl. *J. Neurophysiol.* 48:968–980.

Blitz, D. M., and Regehr, W. G. (2003). Retinogeniculate synaptic properties controlling spike number and timing in relay neurons. *J. Neurophysiol.* 90:2438–2450.

Blitz, D. M., and Regehr, W. G. (2005). Timing and specificity of feed-forward inhibition within the LGN. *Neuron* 45:917–928.

Callaway, E. M. (2005). Structure and function of parallel pathways in the primate early visual system. *J. Physiol.* 566: 13–19.

Chen, C., Blitz, D. M., and Regehr, W, G. (2002). Contributions of receptor desensitization and saturation to plasticity at the retinogeniculate synapse. *Neuron* 33:779–788.

Chen, C., and Regehr, W. G. (2000). Developmental remodeling of the retinogeniculate synapse. *Neuron* 28:955–966.

Chen, C., and Regehr, W. G. (2003). Presynaptic modulation of the retinogeniculate synapse. *J. Neurosci.* 23:3130–3135.

Derrington, A. M., and Lennie, P. (1984). Spatial and temporal contrast sensitivities of neurons in lateral geniculate nucleus of macaque. *J. Physiol.* 357:219–240.

Frere, S. G., and Luthi, A. (2004). Pacemaker channels in mouse thalamocortical neurons are regulated by distinct pathways of cAMP synthesis. *J. Physiol.* 554:111–125.

Grubb, M. S., Rossi, F. M., Changeux, J. P., and Thompson, I. D. (2003). Abnormal functional organization in the dorsal lateral geniculate nucleus of mice lacking the β2 subunit of the nicotinic acetylcholine receptor. *Neuron* 40:1161–1172.

Grubb, M. S., and Thompson, I. D. (2003). Quantitative characterization of visual response properties in the mouse dorsal lateral geniculate nucleus. *J. Neurophysiol.* 90:3594–3607.

Grubb, M. S., and Thompson, I. D. (2004). Visual response properties in the dorsal lateral geniculate nucleus of mice lacking the beta2 subunit of the nicotinic acetylcholine receptor. *J. Neurosci.* 24:8459–8469.

Grubb, M. S., and Thompson, I. D. (2005). Visual response properties of burst and tonic firing in the mouse dorsal lateral geniculate nucleus. *J. Neurophysiol.* 93:3224–3247.

Guido, W., Lu, S. M., and Sherman, S. M. (1992). Relative contributions of burst and tonic responses to the receptive field properties of lateral geniculate neurons in the cat. *J. Neurophysiol.* 68:2199–2211.

Guido, W., Lu, S. M., Vaughan, J. W., Godwin, D. W., and Sherman, S. M. (1995). Receiver operating characteristic (ROC) analysis of neurons in the cat's lateral geniculate nucleus during tonic and burst response mode. *Vis. Neurosci.* 12:723–741.

Guido, W., and Sherman, S. M. (1998). Response latencies of cells in the cat's lateral geniculate nucleus are less variable during burst than tonic firing. *Vis. Neurosci.* 15:231–237.

Guido, W., and Weyand, T. (1995). Burst responses in thalamic relay cells of the awake behaving cat. *J. Neurophysiol.* 74: 1782–1786.

Hubel, D. H., and Wiesel, T. N. (1961). Integrative action in the cat's lateral geniculate body. *J. Physiol.* 155:385–398.

Huguenard, J. R., and McCormick, D. A. (1992). Simulation of the currents involved in rhythmic oscillations in thalamic relay neurons. *J. Neurophysiol.* 68:1373–1383.

Jahnsen, H., and Llinas, R. (1984). Electrophysiological properties of guinea-pig thalamic neurons: An in vitro study. *J. Physiol.* 349:205–226.

Jaubert-Miazza, L., Green, E., Lo, F. S., Bui, K., Mills, J., and Guido, W. (2005). Structural and functional composition of the developing retinogeniculate pathway in the mouse. *Vis. Neurosci.* 22:661–676.

Kaplan, E., and Shapley, R. M. (1986). The primate retina contains two types of ganglion cells, with high and low contrast sensitivity. *Proc. Natl. Acad. Sci. U.S.A.* 83:2755–2757.

Kielland, A., Erisir, A., Walaas, S. I., and Heggelund, P. (2006). Synapsin utilization differs among functional classes of synapses on thalamocortical cells. *J. Neurosci.* 26:5786–5793.

Kim, D., Song, I., Keum, S., Lee, T., Jeong, M. J., Kim, S. S., McEnery, M. W., and Shin, H. S. (2001). Lack of the burst firing of thalamocortical relay neurons and resistance to absence seizures in mice lacking alpha(1G) T-type Ca(2+) channels. *Neuron* 31:35–45.

Levitt, J. B., Schumer, R. A., Sherman, S. M., Spear, P. D., and Movshon, J. A. (2001). Visual response properties of neurons in the LGN of normally reared and visually deprived macaque monkeys. *J. Neurophysiol.* 85:2111–2129.

Lewandoski, M. (2001). Conditional control of gene expression in the mouse. *Nat. Rev. Genet.* 2:743–755.

Livingstone, M. S., and Hubel, D. H. (1981). Effects of sleep and arousal on the processing of visual information in the cat. *Nature* 291:554–561.

Llinas, R. R., and Steriade, M. (2006). Bursting of thalamic neurons and states of vigilance. *J. Neurophysiol.* 95:3297–3308.

Lu, C., Fu, Z., Karavanov, I., Yasuda, R. P., Wolfe, B. B., Buonanno, A., and Vicini, S. (2006). NMDA receptor subtypes at autaptic synapses of cerebellar granule neurons. *J. Neurophysiol.* 96:2282–2294.

Lu, S. M., Guido, W., and Sherman, S. M. (1992). Effects of membrane voltage on receptive field properties of lateral geniculate neurons in the cat: Contributions of the low-threshold Ca^{2+} conductance. *J. Neurophysiol.* 68:2185–2198.

MacLeod, N., Turner, C., and Edgar, J. (1997). Properties of developing lateral geniculate neurones in the mouse. *Int. J. Dev. Neurosci.* 15:205–224.

McCarley, R. W., Benoit, O., and Barrionuevo, G. (1983). Lateral geniculate nucleus unitary discharge in sleep and waking: State- and rate-specific aspects. *J. Neurophysiol.* 50:798–818.

McCormick, D. A. (2003). Membrane properties and neurotransmitter actions. In G. M. Shepherd (Ed.), *The synaptic organization of the brain.* New York: Oxford University Press.

McCormick, D. A., and Bal, T. (1997). Sleep and arousal: Thalamocortical mechanisms. *Annu. Rev. Neurosci.* 20:185–215.

Merigan, W. H., Katz, L. M., and Maunsell, J. H. (1991). The effects of parvocellular lateral geniculate lesions on the acuity and contrast sensitivity of macaque monkeys. *J. Neurosci.* 11:994–1001.

Metin, C., Godement, P., Saillour, P., and Imbert, M. (1983). [Physiological and anatomical study of the retinogeniculate projections in the mouse]. *C.R. Seances Acad. Sci. III* 296:157–162.

Meuth, S. G., Aller, M. I., Munsch, T., Schuhmacher, T., Seidenbecher, T., Meuth, P., Kleinschnitz, C., Pape, H. C., Wiendl, H., et al. (2006a). The contribution of TWIK-related acid-sensitive K^+-containing channels to the function of dorsal lateral geniculate thalamocortical relay neurons. *Mol. Pharmacol.* 69:1468–1476.

Meuth, S. G., Kanyshkova, T., Meuth, P., Landgraf, P., Munsch, T., Ludwig, A., Hofmann, F., Pape, H. C., and Budde, T. (2006b). Membrane resting potential of thalamocortical relay neurons is shaped by the interaction among TASK3 and HCN2 channels. *J. Neurophysiol.* 96:1517–1529.

Mukherjee, P., and Kaplan, E. (1995). Dynamics of neurons in the cat lateral geniculate nucleus: In vivo electrophysiology and computational modeling. *J. Neurophysiol.* 74:1222–1243.

Norton, T. T., Casagrande, V. A., Irvin, G. E., Sesma, M. A., and Petry, H. M. (1988). Contrast-sensitivity functions of W-, X-, and Y-like relay cells in the lateral geniculate nucleus of bush baby, *Galago crassicaudatus*. *J. Neurophysiol.* 59:1639–1656.

Norton, T. T., Holdefer, R. N., and Godwin, D. W. (1989). Effects of bicuculline on receptive field center sensitivity of relay cells in lateral geniculate nucleus. *Brain Res.* 488:348–352.

Rafols, J. A., and Valverde, F. (1973). The structure of the dorsal lateral geniculate nucleus in the mouse: A Golgi and electron microscopic study. *J. Comp. Neurol.* 150:303–332.

Reichova, I., and Sherman, S. M. (2004). Somatosensory corticothalamic projections: Distinguishing drivers from modulators. *J. Neurophysiol.* 92:2185–2197.

Rhodes, P. A., and Llinas, R. (2005). A model of thalamocortical relay cells. *J. Physiol.* 565:765–781.

Rossi, F. M., Pizzorusso, T., Porciatti, V., Marubio, L. M., Maffei, L., and Changeux, J. P. (2001). Requirement of the nicotinic acetylcholine receptor beta 2 subunit for the anatomical and functional development of the visual system. *Proc. Natl. Acad. Sci. U.S.A.* 98:6453–6458.

Ruiz, O., Royal, D., Sary, G., Chen, X., Schall, J. D., and Casagrande, V. A. (2006). Low-threshold Ca^{2+}-associated bursts are rare events in the LGN of the awake behaving monkey. *J. Neurophysiol.* 95:3401–3413.

Seeburg, D. P., Liu, X., and Chen, C. (2004). Frequency-dependent modulation of retinogeniculate transmission by serotonin. *J. Neurosci.* 24:10950–10962.

Sherman, S. M. (2001). Tonic and burst firing: dual modes of thalamocortical relay. *Trends Neurosci.* 24:122–126.

Sherman, S. M. (2005). Thalamic relays and cortical functioning. *Prog. Brain. Res.* 149:107–126.

Sherman, S. M., and Guillery, R. W. (2003). Thalamus. In G. M. Shepherd (Ed.), *The synaptic organization of the brain.* New York: Oxford University Press.

Stone, C., and Pinto, L. H. (1993). Response properties of ganglion cells in the isolated mouse retina. *Vis. Neurosci.* 10:31–39.

Sur, M., and Sherman, S. M. (1982). Linear and nonlinear W-cells in C-laminae of the cat's lateral geniculate nucleus. *J. Neurophysiol.* 47:869–884.

Tian, N., and Copenhagen, D. R. (2003). Visual stimulation is required for refinement of ON and OFF pathways in postnatal retina. *Neuron* 39:85–96.

Usrey, W. M., and Reid, R. C. (2000). Visual physiology of the lateral geniculate nucleus in two species of New World monkey: *Saimiri sciureus* and *Aotus trivirgatis*. *J. Physiol.* 523(Pt 3):755–769.

Usrey, W. M., Reppas, J. B., and Reid, R. C. (1999). Specificity and strength of retinogeniculate connections. *J. Neurophysiol.* 82:3527–3540.

Van Hooser, S. D., Heimel, J. A., and Nelson, S. B. (2003). Receptive field properties and laminar organization of lateral geniculate nucleus in the gray squirrel (*Sciurus carolinensis*). *J. Neurophysiol.* 90:3398–3418.

Van Hooser, S. D., Heimel, J. A., and Nelson, S. B. (2005). Functional cell classes and functional architecture in the early visual system of a highly visual rodent. *Prog. Brain Res.* 149:127–145.

Weyand, T. G., Boudreaux, M., and Guido, W. (2001). Burst and tonic response modes in thalamic neurons during sleep and wakefulness. *J. Neurophysiol.* 85:1107–1118.

Wiesel, T. N., and Hubel, D. H. (1966). Spatial and chromatic interactions in the lateral geniculate body of the rhesus monkey. *J. Neurophysiol.* 29:1115–1156.

Xu, X., Bonds, A. B., and Casagrande, V. A. (2002). Modeling receptive-field structure of koniocellular, magnocellular, and parvocellular LGN cells in the owl monkey (*Aotus trivigatus*). *Vis. Neurosci.* 19:703–711.

Xu, X., Ichida, J. M., Allison, J. D., Boyd, J. D., Bonds, A. B., and Va, V. A. (2001). A comparison of koniocellular, magnocellular and parvocellular receptive field properties in the lateral geniculate nucleus of the owl monkey (*Aotus trivirgatus*). *J. Physiol.* 531:203–218.

Zhan, X. J., Cox, C. L., Rinzel, J., and Sherman, S. M. (1999). Current clamp and modeling studies of low-threshold calcium spikes in cells of the cat's lateral geniculate nucleus. *J. Neurophysiol.* 81:2360–2373.

Zhu, L., Blethyn, K. L., Cope, D. W., Tsomaia, V., Crunelli, V., and Hughes, S. W. (2006). Nucleus- and species-specific properties of the slow (<1 Hz) sleep oscillation in thalamocortical neurons. *Neuroscience* 141:621–636.

19 Superior Colliculus and Saccade Generation in Mice

TOMOYA SAKATANI AND TADASHI ISA

When animals orient to objects of particular interest in their immediate environment, combined movements of the eyes, head, trunk, and limbs are induced. If movements of the head, trunk, and limbs are then restrained, isolated eye movement can be investigated as a component of such orienting movements. It is under this condition of restraint that saccadic eye movements are studied in cats, monkeys, and humans (Sparks, 1999).

In general, saccadic eye movement is a rapid shift of eye position to capture an object in the visual environment. Studying saccadic eye movements as a way to understand the neural mechanisms underlying control of accurate movements has several advantages. First, the muscular mechanics of the oculomotor control system are relatively simple when compared with limb movement controllers. Therefore, quantification of movements is relatively easy; the parameter to calculate is the angle of eyeball direction. Second, electrical stimulation of part of the underlying neural circuits can mimic naturally evoked movements. Finally, much is now known about the properties of identified neuronal elements of the related circuits. The neuronal circuitries underlying the generation of saccades have been intensively studied, especially in cats and monkeys (Wurtz and Goldberg, 1989; Moschovakis et al., 1996; Scudder et al., 2002; Sparks, 2002). Moreover, numerous theoretical models have been proposed to explain the saccadic system (Girard and Berthoz, 2005).

Several kinds of studies have been pursued in mice to investigate slow eye movements such as the vestibular-ocular reflex (VOR) and optokinetic responses and their adaptive control mechanism (De Zeeuw et al., 1998; Katoh et al., 1998; Blazquez et al., 2004; Stahl, 2004). In contrast to these slow eye movement systems and, despite some previous reports (Mitchiner et al., 1976; Balkema et al., 1984; Grusser-Cornehls and Bohm, 1988), quantitative and systematic analyses of saccades have not been carried out in mice. The mouse is an ideal experimental model animal in which to study the molecular mechanism of saccade control. However, saccades have not been thought to be important in mice, because mice have a poor fovea and are lateral-eyed, and they are thought to use mainly head movements for orientation.

We have recently developed a PC-based high-speed video-oculography system to perform online analysis of eye movements of mice with high temporal resolution. Using this system, we are able to investigate the ocular component of orienting movements that are saccade-like rapid eye movements (SLREMs), and we have conducted quantitative and systematic analyses of SLREMs in head-fixed mice (Sakatani and Isa, 2004, 2007). Our results suggest that mice have neural circuits for the generation of REMs that share common mechanisms with those in other animal species. Because the behavioral meaning of REMs in mice under natural conditions is still unclear, we use the term SLREM rather than saccade in this chapter, emphasizing our focus on the kinematics of these eye movements.

Saccades are controlled by large-scale neural networks distributed widely over many brain areas, including the brainstem, basal ganglia, frontal and parietal cortex, and cerebellum, and these circuits have not been studied in mice or rats. Among the various components of these networks, the superior colliculus (SC) is presumed to be a pivotal brainstem structure for determination of saccade vectors. We have recently found that electrical stimulation of the SC induce SLREMs in mice.

In addition, over the past decade considerable progress was made in understanding signal processing in local circuits of the mammalian SC by applying whole-cell patch-clamp recording and intracellular labeling techniques in the rodent slice preparation (for reviews, see Isa, 2002; Isa et al., 2003; Helms et al., 2004; Isa and Sparks, 2006).

In this chapter, we introduce recent research conducted by our group on the neural system for the control of orienting movements in rodents and discuss structure-function relationships of the related neural circuits, mainly focusing on the SC.

Saccade-like rapid eye movements in mice

Measurement of Rapid Eye Movements Although the existence of SLREMs has been reported in mice (Mitchiner et al., 1976; Balkema et al., 1984; Grusser-Cornehls and Bohm, 1988), no previous work has focused on quantitative measurements of REMs in this species except for the fast phase of the VOR (Stahl, 2004). It is difficult to measure REMs stably and continuously in such small animals. Our recent development of a PC-based high-speed video-oculography technique enabled us to perform online analysis of spontaneously evoked SLREMs in mice in a quantitative manner (Sakatani and Isa, 2004).

Figure 19.1 shows schematically the procedures used to measure eye movements in mice. Movements of the right eye are monitored with a high-speed CCD camera (CS3720, Toshiba TELI Corp., Tokyo) at a sampling rate of 240 frames/s placed at an angle of 60° laterally from the body axis and 30° down from the horizontal plane (figure 19.1*A*). The awake animal is placed in a stereotaxic apparatus with the body loosely restrained on a soft rubber sheet, so that the legs hang in the air, not touching anything else. The animal's head is fixed painlessly to the platform with a brass rod attached to a manipulator (figure 19.1*B*).

Captured images of the eyes are processed online using custom software that detects the center of the pupil by fitting a circular function to the pupil boundary and tracks the eye position online (figure 19.1*C*). Subsequently, pupillary displacement in the two-dimensional video plane is geometrically converted to angular rotation of the eyeball by estimating its rotation center based on the anatomical eyeball model (figure 19.1*D*). Detailed procedures can be found in the original publication by Sakatani and Isa (2004).

Spontaneous SLREMs in Mice Eye movement trajectories were successfully recorded and analyzed in C57BL/6JjmsSlc mice in a quantitative manner using the high-speed video-oculography technique (figure 19.1*E*). Naturally evoked, spontaneous SLREMs were observed in a dimly lit (<100 lux), sound-attenuated box (figure 19.1*F*). *Arrowheads* in the figure indicate the occurrence of SLREMs.

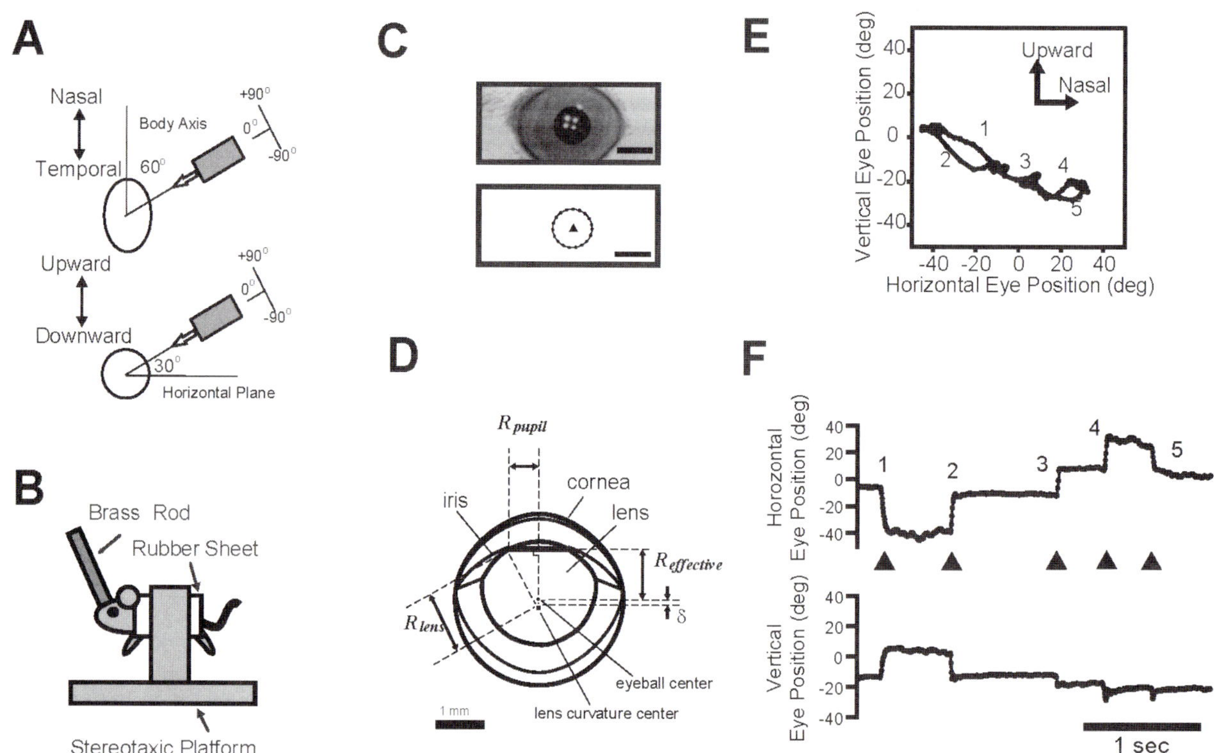

Figure 19.1 Spontaneously evoked saccade-like rapid eye movements (SLREMs). *A*, Top-view (*top*) and back-view (*bottom*) diagrams of the video coordinate system. The optical axis of the camera is shown as a *white arrow*. The movements of the right eye were monitored with a high-speed (240 frames/s) video camera. A CCD camera (shaded box) was set at an angle of 60° right with regard to the body axis and 30° down against the horizontal plane. *B*, A mouse was loosely restrained with a rubber sheet and the head was fixed with a brass rod and a pedestal. *C*, Image processing software detected a boundary of the pupil (*dotted circle in bottom panel*) and its center (▲) online from a captured frame image (*top panel*). Angular eye positions were then calculated based on an anatomical eyeball model (Sakatani and Isa, 2004). *D*, Anatomy of the eyeball in the mouse. The effective rotation radius ($R_{effective}$) is calculated from the pupil radius (R_{pupil}: obtained from a video image) and lens radius (R_{lens}: 1.25 mm). The radius is 1.6 mm and δ is 0.1 mm in this model. *E*, Eye trajectories in the *x-y* plane. Each number represents the corresponding SLREM shown in *F*. *F*, Horizontal (*top*) and vertical (*bottom*) eye positions. SLREMs were observed at the time indicated by *arrowheads* (*top*).

Male C57BL/6jmsSlc mice (n = 7) spontaneously made SLREMs at a nearly constant rate under the recording condition. On average, spontaneous SLREMs in all animals in the head-fixed condition occurred at a frequency of 7.5 ± 4.7/min (n = 7) with a median amplitude of 14.3 ± 2.1°, mainly in the horizontal direction (88%; −45 ~ +45° and +135 ~ +225° in polar coordinates). The observed maximal eye deviation from the central position ranged from 66.7° to 99.6° in the horizontal plane and from 39.8° to 59.8° in the vertical plane. The observed maximum oculomotor range in the horizontal direction in the mouse is relatively wider than in the cat (50°: Guitton et al., 1980) or rabbit (30°: Collewijn, 1970) and is close to the oculomotor range in humans (110°: Guitton and Volle, 1987).

The eye often returned toward the central position by a centripetal saccade or drifted back slowly toward the center of the orbit after the SLREM. Thus, SLREMs usually occurred from the center of the orbit.

To investigate the effect of auditory and visual stimuli on triggering SLREMs, an attempt was made to check the ability of these stimuli to induce SLREMs. Although mice responded with SLREMs when presented with a novel stimulus (sound or light), they tended to become habituated to these stimuli quickly, and then they became almost unresponsive to these sound or visual stimuli.

The kinematics of SLREM can be defined on the basis of velocity-amplitude characteristics (Bahill et al., 1975). Figure 19.2*A* shows velocity profiles of SLREMs with four different amplitudes in a single animal.

The peak velocity of the SLREM relative to its amplitude increased in mice in a way similar to that seen in other mammals, such as humans, monkeys, and cats. Even though there is a similar tendency among these mammals, mice exhibited some unique characteristics. The peak velocity did not saturate, at least in the range of observation (2–50°). The velocity profile of SLREMs with different amplitudes exhibited a characteristic appearance. Figure 19.2*B* shows an example of the relationship between amplitude and peak velocity in a single animal. This relationship exhibited a nearly linear correlation (correlation coefficient 0.92 in the nasal direction and 0.92 in the temporal direction) and could be well fitted by linear regression. The peak velocity increased almost linearly with a slope of 52.2 deg/s-deg in the nasal direction and 34.7 deg/s-deg in the temporal direction. The amplitude and peak velocity of SLREMs were found to be linearly correlated in all seven animals tested (correlation coefficient 0.91 ± 0.03 in the nasal direction and 0.85 ± 0.07 in the temporal direction), with a mean slope of 51.3 ± 3.9 deg/s-deg in the nasal direction and 31.7 ± 3.2 deg/s-deg in the temporal direction. These values are much higher than those recorded in other mammals, such as human: 20 deg/s-deg (Boghen et al., 1974), monkey: 40 deg/s-deg (Fuchs, 1967), cat: 10 deg/s-deg (Evinger and Fuchs, 1978), rabbit: 13 deg/s-deg (Collewijn, 1970), and rat: 20–40 deg/s-deg (Fuller, 1985; Hikosaka and Sakamoto, 1987).

These results suggest that the mouse may have neural circuits for the generation of REM that share some common properties with those in cats, monkeys, and humans. However, there might also be some different properties related to the control of SLREM duration, which should be a subject of future studies.

The difference between the nasal and temporal directions was significant (Tukey's test: $P < 0.01$). In humans, the kinematics of centrifugal saccadic eye movements differ from those of centripetal saccades (Pelisson and Prablanc, 1988). In a recent study on the VOR in mice, Stahl (2004) also noted that abducting fast phases of nystagmus tended to be slower than adducting fast phase.

Electrically Induced SLREMs in Mice The SC is comprised of several layers. The dorsal three layers—the stratum zonale (SZ), the stratum griseum superficiale (SGS), and the stratum opticum (SO)—are designated the superficial layers and receive visual input either directly from the retina or indirectly from the visual cortex. The next two layers, the stratum griseum intermediale (SGI) and the stratum album intermediale (SAI), ventral to the superficial layers are designated intermediate layers, and the ventralmost two layers, the stratum griseum profundum (SGP) and the stratum album profundum (SAP), are designated deep layers. The intermediate and deep layers send descending outputs to the brainstem reticular formation and spinal cord. In monkeys, it is well known that a population of neurons in the intermediate and deep layers exhibits high-frequency burst discharges starting about 20 ms prior to contraversive saccades (Schiller and Stryker, 1972; Wurtz and Goldberg, 1972) and that repetitive electrical stimulation of these layers evokes saccades (Robinson, 1972). To clarify whether the SC controls SLREM in mice, we tested the effects of repetitive electrical stimulation of the SC in awake, head-fixed mice.

Electrical stimulation of the intermediate layer of the SC can induce eye movements closely resembling spontaneously evoked SLREMs in awake, head-fixed mice (figure 19.3). As shown in figure 19.3*A*, SLREMs were induced above a certain threshold stimulus intensity (biphasic current, 333 Hz, 180 ms duration, 0.1 ms negative and 0.1 ms positive pulse duration, 20 μA in this case) of stimulation. Increasing the stimulus current beyond the threshold shortened latencies of the induced SLREMs from 96 ms to 42 ms (from the onset of stimulation), whereas the amplitude of the eye movements remained constant at higher stimulus intensities. The average latency was 59.8 ± 22.3 ms, and the latency was never shorter than 16.7 ms. As exemplified in figure 19.3*B*, the threshold stimulus intensity to induce the SLREM was systematically examined at different depths in the SC. Threshold current

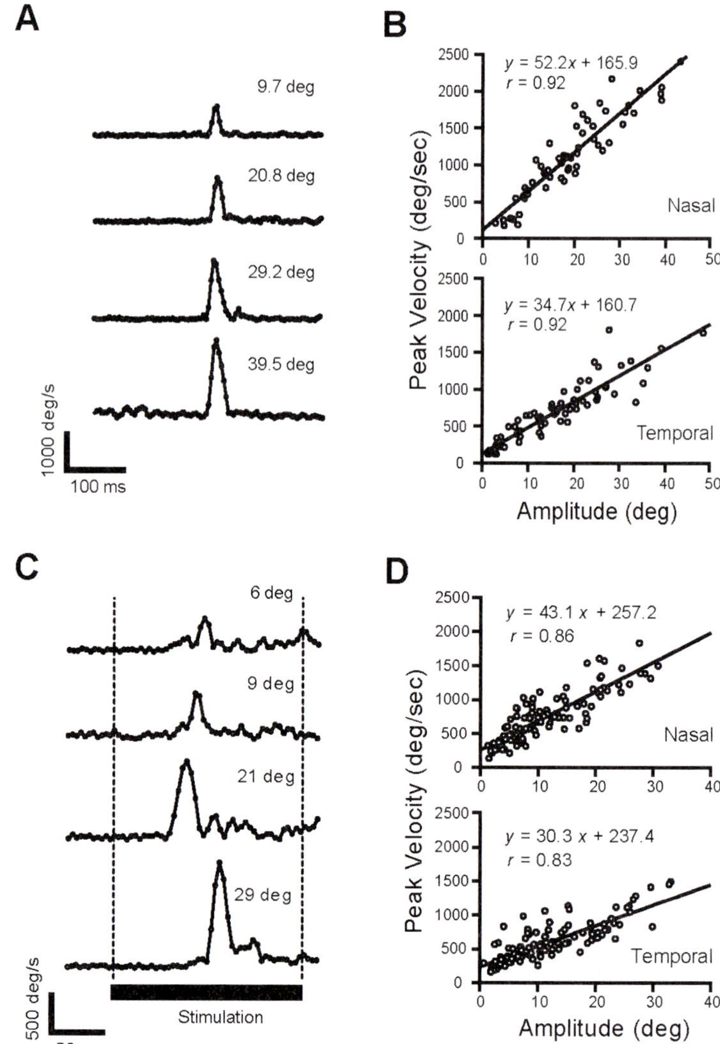

FIGURE 19.2 Peak velocity versus amplitude relationships of spontaneously evoked and electrically induced SLREMs. *A*, Examples of velocity profiles of spontaneously evoked SLREMs of different size and velocity. Each velocity trace is aligned with the onset of SLREM determined by a velocity threshold above 100 deg/s. The amplitude of spontaneous SLREMs is 9.7°, 20.8°, 29.2°, and 39.5° (*top to bottom*). The peak velocity is 2,222, 1,685, 1,284, and 851 deg/s, respectively. *B*, Example of the peak velocity versus amplitude plot in a single animal. *Solid line* indicates the linear regression line. *C*, Velocity profile of electrically induced SLREMs. The amplitude of the SLREM is 6°, 9°, 21°, and 29° (*top to bottom*). Note that the velocity curve has a nearly bell-shaped profile. A second peak observed for 21° movements reflects overshoot. *D*, Relationship between the peak velocity and amplitude of the electrically induced SLREM. The entire data set pooled across 31 sites in 7 animals is plotted in the nasal direction (*top*, $n = 106$) and temporal direction (*bottom*, $n = 121$) separately. Each data point represents the value of peak velocity in an individual stimulation trial. A linear regression line is superimposed (*solid line*).

intensities were lower in the intermediate and deep layers. The threshold was often lower than 10 μA in these layers. This suggests that the cell bodies or axons of projection neurons responsible for induction of SLREMs are located in the intermediate and deep layers of the SC in mice as in other species.

We examined the motor representation of various rostrocaudal and mediolateral locations in the SC (figure 19.3*C* and *D*) at the depth of the intermediate layer. The trajectories of eye movements evoked at different sites in a single mouse SC are shown in figure 19.3*D*. Since the left SC was stimulated and movements of the right eye were recorded, an ipsiversive SLREM means movement in the nasal direction, while a contraversive movement means temporal movement in this figure. From most stimulation sites in the SC, SLREMs were evoked in the contraversive (temporal) direction. The amplitude of evoked REMs became larger when more caudal sites were stimulated and smaller at more rostral sites, showing a similar motor representation pattern to that in other mammals. These results suggest that mice are equipped with saccade generator circuits downstream of the SC. On the other hand, nasal (ipsiversive) SLREMs could be induced

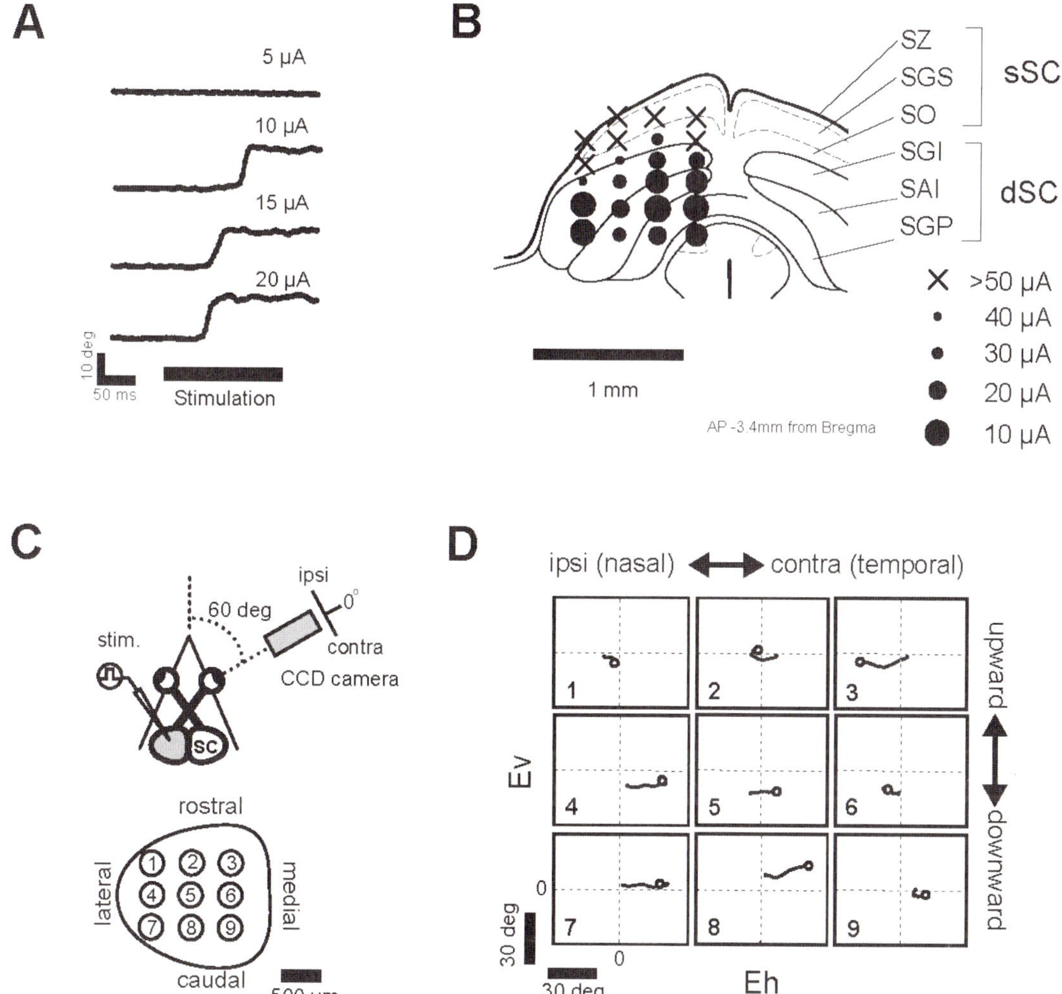

Figure 19.3 SLREMs induced by stimulation of the superior colliculus (SC). *A*, Eye position traces of an electrically induced REM in response to different current intensities of SC stimulation. The threshold current (T) to evoke the eye movements was 20 μA at the site of electrical stimulation (b). Stimulation was applied at 333 Hz for 180 ms duration as indicated by the *thick black line* along the time axis (individual pulse width was 0.2 ms). *Top to bottom*, 0.5 × T, 1.0 × T, 1.5 × T, and 2.0 × T, respectively. *B*, Threshold current intensities to induce SLREMs at various points in the SC in a single animal are presented on a coronal section. The threshold current intensities are represented by the size of the symbol. dSC, deeper layers of the SC; SAI, stratum album intermediale; SGI, stratum griseum intermediale; SGP, stratum griseum profundum; SGS, stratum griseum superficiale; SO, stratum opticum; sSC, superficial layers of the SC; SZ, stratum zonale. *C*, Schematic drawing of the experimental arrangement (*top*) and dorsal view of the left SC, showing the stimulation sites (*bottom*). *Circled numbers* indicate penetrations of the stimulation electrode plotted on the dorsal view of the left SC. *D*, Examples of eye movements evoked at different sites in a mouse SC. The stimulation sites are indicated with numbers corresponding to those in *C*. *Open circles* indicate terminal points of the movements. *Dotted lines* indicate the horizontal and vertical midline determined arbitrarily as shown in *C*.

from the rostromedial portion (stimulation sites 3 and 6). In this region, the visual representation of the superficial layer is the same as that of the visual field with the opposite SC (Dräger and Hubel, 1975). Therefore, this region represents the ipsilateral visual field. Thus, in mice, the SC on one side likely controls both contraversive and ipsiversive SLREMs, in agreement with the overlying retinotopic map in the superficial layer (Dräger and Hubel, 1975).

The velocity profile of the electrically induced SLREMs had a somewhat bell-shaped curve, which was reported as a typical feature of SLREMs in other mammals (see Wurtz and Goldberg, 1989) (see figure 19.2*C*). Larger eye movements often tended to overshoot, resulting in the second peak of the velocity profile (see figure 19.2*C*). For SLREMs with larger amplitude, the peak velocity was higher than that associated with smaller SLREMs. This relationship was clearly demonstrated in the pooled data from a single animal (nine tracks) in figure 19.2*D*. Also, the peak velocities of SLREMs differed depending on the direction of the SLREM. The relationship between the peak velocity and the amplitude of SLREMs induced by the electrical stimulation was well fitted by the linear regression line (for temporal SLREMs: slope = 43.1, $r = 0.86$; for nasal SLREMs: slope = 30.3, $r = 0.83$), which was similar to that of the spontaneous SLREMs (see figure 19.2*B*), although values of the electrically induced SLREMs are lower than those of the spontaneously evoked SLREMs.

All these results indicate that SLREMs in mice share common properties with those previously described in cats and monkeys, a finding suggesting the existence of similar saccade generator circuits downstream of the mouse SC.

Local circuits of the rodent superior colliculus

Cellular Properties A 1974 study by Langer and Lund used Golgi staining to reveal the cytoarchitecture of local circuits in the SC superficial layers. This study showed that the local circuit in the superficial layers involves five neuron types: narrow-field vertical cells, wide-field vertical cells, piriform or stellate cells, horizontal cells, and marginal cells (figure 19.4). Among these, wide-field vertical cells are the major projection neurons connected to the deeper layers of the SC (Mooney et al., 1988b) and to the lateral posterior nucleus of the pulvinar (Lane et al., 1993). Their dendritic arbors extend widely into a horizontally wide area of the superficial layer. In addition, narrow-field vertical and marginal cells are also projection neurons targeted to the SC deeper layers and the parabigeminal nucleus. Subsequent immunohistochemical studies suggested that horizontal, stellate, and piriform cells are GABA-ergic, based on the morphology of soma and proximal dendrites (Mize, 1992). Compared with neurons in the superficial layers, the morphological properties of neurons in the intermediate layer are more heterogeneous and less distinct. They are classified into multipolar, pyramidal, fusiform, horizontal, and wide-field vertical cells (Norita, 1980; Ma et al., 1990).

The electrophysiological properties of SC neurons are very heterogeneous. Based on the firing pattern in response to the depolarizing current step, they are classified into regular spiking, late spiking, burst spiking, fast spiking, and rapid adaptation types (Saito and Isa, 1999). The regular spiking type constitutes the majority of the neurons both in the superficial (50%; Isa and Saito, 2001) and intermediate layer (50%; Saito and Isa, 1999). Surprisingly, no clear correlation has so far been observed between the electrophysiological properties and somatodendritic morphology of neurons, except the expression of large and fast hyperpolarization-activated current (Ih) in wide-field vertical cells. These neurons exclusively express Ih of large amplitude and fast activation time course (Lo et al., 1998; Saito and Isa, 1999).

Among a variety of SC neurons, the morphological and electrophysiological properties of deeper layer neurons projecting to the contralateral paramedian pontine reticular formation (PPRF) were studied by whole-cell patch-clamp recordings from cells that had been retrogradely labeled with dextran-conjugated Texas red injected into the PPRF a few days before the experiments (Sooksawate, Saito, et al., 2005). Among the 112 identified projection neurons in the SGI, regular, burst, late, and fast spiking and rapid inactivation types accounted for 73%, 12%, 11%, 0%, and 4%, respectively. Among the 76 projection neurons that were successfully stained with biocytin, multipolar, fusiform, pyramidal, horizontal, and round-shaped cells accounted for 66%, 13%, 8%, 11%, and 3%, respectively. Thus, multipolar and regular spiking neurons made up the largest population of SGI neurons projecting to the contralateral PPRF.

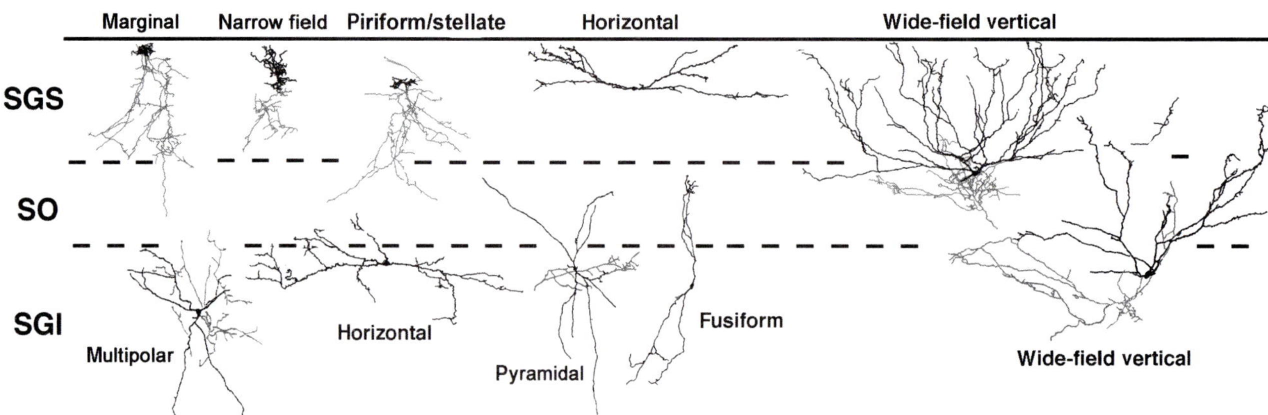

Figure 19.4 Morphological properties of neurons in the mammalian SC. Five major subclasses of neurons in the superficial layer (marginal cell, narrow-field vertical cells, piriform/stellate cells, horizontal cells, and wide-field vertical cells) and five major subclasses of neurons in the intermediate layer (multipolar cells, horizontal cells, pyramidal cells, fusiform cells, and wide-field vertical cells) are illustrated. Somata and dendrites are shown in black and axons in gray. SGI, stratum griseum intermediale; SGS, stratum griseum superficiale; SO, stratum opticum. (Modified from Isa and Saito, 2001.)

GABAERGIC CIRCUITS Recently, we studied the electrophysiological and morphological properties of GABAergic neurons in GAD67 (*Gad1*)-GFP knock-in mice (Endo et al., 2003, 2005; Sooksawate, Isa, et al., 2005), in which GABAergic neurons are labeled with fluorescence of green fluorescent protein (GFP) (Tamamaki et al., 2003).

The superficial layers contain a very high density of GABAergic neurons. Mize (1992) noted that about 45% of neurons in the SGS are GABAergic. In the GAD67 (*Gad1*)-GFP knock-in mice, all the recorded GABAergic neurons revealed the morphology of horizontal cells, which issued relatively long dendritic trees (Endo et al., 2003). They exhibited the firing pattern of regular spiking (18 of 65, 28%), burst spiking (14 of 65, 22%), or fast spiking (18 of 65, 28%) patterns. They are likely to be involved in lateral inhibition of visual responses in the SGS. So far we have not been able to stain the cells with piriform or stellate cell-type morphology, which were proposed to be GABAergic in the immunohistochemical study by Mize (1992), among the neurons with GFP fluorescence in the GAD67 (*Gad1*)-GFP knock-in mice. The reason may be that neurons of this subclass exhibit weak GFP expression in this mouse genotype.

We analyzed the electrophysiological and/or morphological properties of 231 GABAergic neurons in the SGI of the GAD67 (*Gad1*)-GFP mice (Sooksawate, Isa, et al., 2005). In the electrophysiological analysis, a majority of these cells exhibited either fast spiking (135 of 231, 58%) or burst spiking (67 of 231, 29%) properties. Based on the axonal trajectories, the GABAergic cells that were successfully stained by intracellular labeling ($n = 115$) were classified as (1) intralaminar local interneurons (19 cells), (2) intralaminar horizontal neurons (19 cells), (3) interlaminar interneurons (38 cells), (4) commissural neurons (5 cells), or (5) extrinsic projection neurons (34 cells). The axodendritic morphology of individual subclasses of neurons suggests they may provide recurrent inhibition or lateral inhibition. Detailed information on the input-output relationship of each cell type is required to determine the function of individual subtypes of GABAergic neurons.

INTERLAMINAR CONNECTIONS As described earlier in the chapter, the visual topography of the superficial layer and the distribution of SLREM vectors in the deeper layers showed good coincidence. This is a similar to what is seen in cats and monkeys, but in these animal species, the connection between the superficial and deeper layers had long been a subject of debate (Edwards, 1980; Mays and Sparks, 1980; Mooney et al., 1988a; Moschovakis et al., 1988; Behan and Appell, 1992).

In the late 1990s, the existence of the interlaminar connection was investigated in detail by using electrophysiological techniques in combination with intracellular staining techniques in slice preparations of the rodent SC (Lee et al., 1997; Isa et al., 1998). In this section, we summarize the observations obtained in slice studies.

Figure 19.5*A* summarizes the design of our experiments in slices obtained from rats ages 17–22 days, roughly 1 week after eye opening. Stimulating electrodes were placed in the SGS and in the optic tract (OT) near the lateral border of the optic layer (SO), where the OT comprises a bundle of fibers. Electrical pulses delivered through the OT electrode induced EPSPs with long and fluctuating onset latencies, presumably of di- or oligosynaptic origin, in SGI neurons following stimulation of the OT (figure 19.5*B* and *C*). These responses were markedly enhanced by application of $GABA_A$ receptor antagonists such as bicuculline (see figure 19.5*C*) or SR95531; the bursting spike discharges evoked in the SGI cells were superimposed on large clusters of EPSPs, which could last longer than 1 s, even when single brief electrical pulses were delivered through the OT electrode. The longlasting depolarization and bursting spike discharges were evoked in an all-or-none fashion at threshold stimulus intensities (see figure 19.5*C*). Stimulation of the SGS induced monosynaptic EPSPs in SGI neurons, which were again amplified into bursting spike discharges superimposed on the longlasting depolarization following application of bicuculline (figure 19.5*D*). These results confirm the existence of an excitatory pathway from the OT to SGI neurons, presumably mediated by SGS or SO neurons, as previously demonstrated by Lee et al. (1997) in SC slices from the tree shrew. These observations in slice preparations were confirmed in in vivo experiments. The bursting responses evoked in SGI neurons by OT stimulation were observed following blockade of $GABA_A$ receptor-mediated synaptic transmission in anesthetized rats (Katsuta and Isa, 2003) and more recently in anesthetized monkeys (N. Nikitin, R. Kato, and T. Isa, unpublished observations).

Thus, the existence of the interlaminar connection has been demonstrated, and signal transmission through the pathway is enhanced by disinhibition from $GABA_A$ receptor-mediated inhibition. It has been argued that the interlaminar connection is likely used for "express saccades," which are executed with extremely short reaction times (see Isa, 2002; Isa et al., 2003; Helms et al., 2004; Isa and Sparks, 2006) in monkeys. The function of this interlaminar connection remains elusive in rodents.

The results of the present experiments were confirmed in mice.

MECHANISM OF BURST GENERATION Saccade-related activities in the deeper layers of the SC have been intensively investigated in nonhuman primates. Under conditions in which the subject can anticipate the forthcoming target location, a gradual increase in activity is observed in a subpopulation of deeper layer neurons ("prelude" or

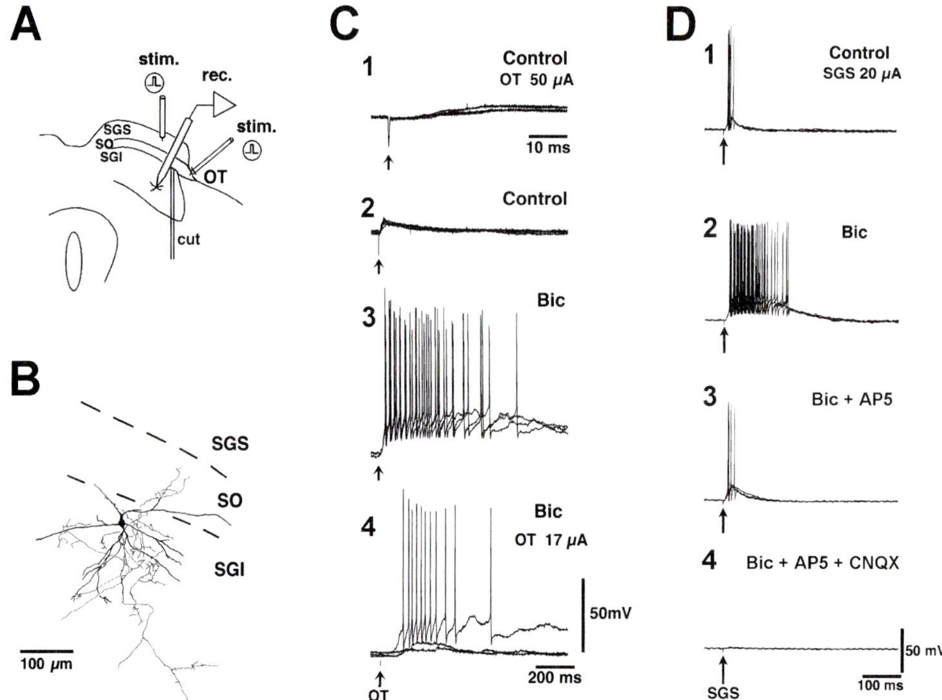

FIGURE 19.5 Interlaminar connection in the rodent SC. *A*, Experimental setup of in vitro slice experiments. Stimulating electrodes are placed in the bundle of the optic tract, at the most lateral portion of the optic layer (SO), or in the superficial gray layer (SGS). Whole-cell recordings were made from neurons in the intermediate gray layer (SGI). *B*, The morphology of the recorded neuron, stained with biocytin. Dendrites are drawn as *thick lines*. The axon and its collaterals are drawn as *thin lines*. C_1 shows the synaptic responses of this neuron to the OT stimulation (50 μA) in the control solution. C_2 and C_3 show the effects of application of 10 μM Bic (C_2, control; C_3, after application of Bic). C_4 shows the synaptic responses to the critical stimulus strength (17 μA) for induction of longlasting responses with the application of 10 μM Bic. *D*, Effect of SGS stimulation on another SGI neuron. Shown is the effect of 10 μM Bic on the EPSP (compare D_1 and D_2) and of the additional application of 50 μM APV (D_3) or 50 μM APV plus 10 μM CNQX (D_4). (Modified from Isa et al., 1998.)

"buildup" activity), and the sudden change from low-level activity to high-frequency bursts is thought to trigger the initiation of saccades. The timing of the high-frequency burst of collicular neurons is tightly coupled to saccade onset, leading the movement by 18–20 ms (Sparks et al., 2000). Accordingly, clarifying the cellular or circuit mechanism of burst generation in the SC deeper layer neurons should facilitate understanding of the neural mechanism underlying the saccade initiation. In vitro slice preparations of the SC that have been separated from other brain structures can be a powerful tool in this regard. The bursting responses of neurons may arise via several alternative mechanisms related to either the intrinsic membrane properties of individual neurons or the structure of the circuit.

As a first step in exploring this issue, it was essential to know the intrinsic membrane properties of individual identified tectofugal cells. We found that most of the crossed tectoreticular SGI cells identified by retrograde labeling with a fluorescent tracer exhibited regular spiking properties and a quasi-linear f-I relationship (Sooksawate, Saito, et al., 2005). In contrast, as shown in figure 19.5*C*, the bursts emitted by SGI neurons in response to stimulation of the SGS in the presence of bicuculline were suppressed by application of 50 μM APV, an NMDA-type glutamate receptor antagonist, and thus the bursts depended on activation of NMDA-type glutamate receptors. It is well known that NMDA receptors have a J-shaped current-voltage relationship. Due to Mg^{2+} block, the NMDA-type glutamate receptors admit inward currents only when the cell is sufficiently depolarized. Once the membrane potential exceeds the value necessary for activation of the NMDA receptor, a regenerative process ensues and further enhances their depolarization. This nonlinear activation of NMDA receptors can account for the all-or-none character of the bursts emitted by SGI neurons.

Presaccadic neurons of the primate SC are known to have recurrent collaterals that ramify in the neighborhood of the parent somata (Moschovakis et al., 1988). To further investigate whether a local circuit including these neurons may support their longlasting depolarization and bursting activity, we obtained simultaneous dual whole-cell patch-clamp recordings from pairs of adjacent SGI neurons in rats (Saito and Isa, 2003, 2004, 2005). Figure 19.6*A* illustrates an

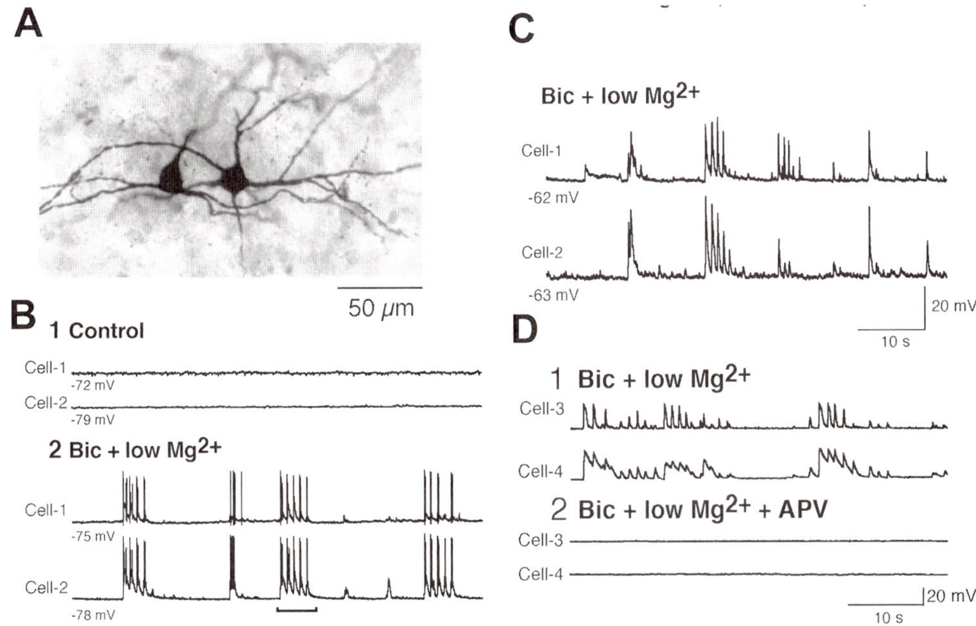

FIGURE 19.6 Simultaneous recordings from a pair of SGI neurons in an SC slice. *A*, Photomicrograph of a pair of recorded SGI neurons (injected with biocytin intracellularly). *B*, Spontaneous membrane potentials in control solution (*1*) and in the presence of 10 μM bicuculline (Bic) and low (0.1 mM) Mg^{2+} (*2*). *C*, Spontaneous membrane potentials recorded simultaneously from a pair of SGI neurons (cell-1 and cell-2) in the presence of 10 μM Bic and low (0.1 mM) Mg^{2+}. The intracellular solution contained 5 mM QX-314. *D*, Effect of 50 μM APV on the synchronous depolarization.

example obtained from a pair of neurons horizontally separated by less than 100 μm. When we applied 10 μM bicuculline (or SR95531) to block $GABA_A$ receptors and reduced the extracellular concentration of Mg^{2+} from 1.0 mM to 0.1 mM to enhance the NMDA receptor-mediated responses, the SGI neurons exhibited bursting spike activity superimposed on repetitive, spontaneous, depolarizing potentials (figure 19.6*B*). Interestingly, the spontaneous depolarization and the bursting spike activity occurred almost simultaneously in both neurons. Since the spiking discharges of two adjacent presaccadic burst neurons are synchronous, synchronization of SC neuron discharges could underlie the generation of their presaccadic bursts in vivo. Such synchronous depolarization could be observed when spikes were blocked by intracellular application of QX-314 (figure 19.6*C*), which suggested common input to the neuron pair. We further found that activation of NMDA-type glutamate receptors is essential for such synchronous depolarization to occur, since it was completely abolished by APV (figure 19.6*D*). These results suggest that a recurrent excitatory network would generate synchronous bursting responses in the SC deeper layer neurons via NMDA receptor-dependent synaptic transmission. The experiments were conducted in rats; however, later studies confirmed the results in mice.

ACTION OF NEUROMODULATORS It has been reported that the SC receives innervation from several neuromodulator systems, such as cholinergic, serotonergic, and purinergic systems (Binns, 1999). These neuromodulator systems may modulate the signal processing in the SC local circuits in a context-dependent manner. Among these, the actions of cholinergic inputs are becoming clear.

The superficial layer of the SC (sSC) receives cholinergic innervation from the parabigeminal nucleus (Graybiel, 1978a; Sherk, 1979; Hall et al., 1989). The cholinergic action on the sSC was examined by testing the current responses induced by acetylcholine (ACh) in the GAD67 (*Gad1*)-GFP knock-in mouse (Endo et al., 2005). Brief air pressure application of 1 mM ACh elicited nicotinic inward current responses in both GABAergic and non-GABAergic neurons. The inward current responses in the GABAergic neurons were highly sensitive to a selective antagonist for α3β2 (Gabra3/Gabrb2 subunits)- and α6β2 (Gabra6/Gabrb2 subunits)-containing receptors, α-conotoxin MII (αCtxMII). A subset of these neurons exhibited a faster α-bungarotoxin-sensitive inward current component, indicating the expression of α7 (Chrna7)-containing nicotinic ACh receptors (nAChRs). We also found that activation of presynaptic nAChRs induced release of GABA, which elicited a burst of miniature inhibitory postsynaptic currents mediated by $GABA_A$ receptors in non-GABAergic neurons. This ACh-induced GABA release was mediated mainly by αCtxMII-sensitive nAChRs and resulted from the activation of voltage-dependent calcium channels. Morphological analysis of the recorded neurons revealed that recorded GFP-positive neurons were interneurons and GFP-negative neurons include projection neurons. These findings suggest that nAChRs are involved in the regulation of GABAergic inhibition, especially enhancement of contrast of visual responses by facilitation of lateral inhibition in the sSC.

On the other hand, the SGI receives cholinergic innervation mainly from the pedunculopontine and laterodorsal tegmental nuclei of the midbrain (PPTN and LDTN; Graybiel, 1978b; Illing and Graybiel, 1985; Beninato and Spencer, 1986; Hall et al., 1989). The effect of bath application of carbachol, an agonist of both nicotinic and muscarinic ACh receptors, has been analyzed in 246 randomly sampled SGI neurons (Sooksawate and Isa, 2006). It has been clarified that carbachol application induces postsynaptic responses with various combination of nicotinic inward, muscarinic inward, and muscarinic outward currents. Pharmacological analysis clarified that nicotinic inward currents are mainly mediated by the $\alpha 4\beta 2$ (Gabra4/Gabrb2 subunits) subtype of nicotinic receptors, and muscarinic inward currents are mainly mediated by M3 (*Chrm3*)-type and muscarinic outward currents by M2 (*Chrm2*)-type muscarinic receptors. Among these, projection neurons of the SGI, which were identified by their axonal trajectories, mainly exhibit combination of nicotinic inward + muscarinic inward + muscarinic outward currents (15 of 28), or nicotinic inward + muscarinic inward currents (9 of 28). Thus, the major action of the cholinergic inputs on SGI output neurons would be excitatory.

On the other hand, cholinergic inputs suppress GABAergic synaptic transmission in the SGI with presynaptic mechanisms, mediated by M1 (*Chrm1*)- and M3 (*Chrm3*)-type muscarinic receptors (Li et al., 2004). Both of these results suggest that cholinergic inputs to the SGI mainly facilitate the generation of output command from the SGI. Thus, cholinergic inputs to the sSC and SGI originate from different sources and exhibit different roles in modulation of sensorimotor processing in the SC.

Conclusion

High-speed video-oculography system has made it possible to analyze SLREMs in head-fixed mice. We found that mice exhibit spontaneous SLREMs with kinematic properties similar to those seen in cats, monkeys, and humans. In addition, electrical stimulation of the deeper layer of the SC induces SLREMs. Investigation of SLREMs in genetically engineered mice should allow us to study the molecular mechanisms underlying the operation of saccade generator circuits.

For this purpose, an in-depth understanding of the structure of the saccade control systems is required. Considerable knowledge is emerging on the structure and the way signals are processed in local circuits of the SC, including their modulation by the neuromodulator system. Further understanding of the saccade control system as a whole, including the downstream circuits of the SC located in the brainstem reticular formation and upstream structures in the cerebral cortex and basal ganglia, will facilitate a multiscale analysis of saccade control, from molecular control to neural circuits to the final behavioral motor output.

REFERENCES

Bahill, A. T., Clark, M. R., and Stark, L. (1975). The main sequence, a tool for studying human eye movements. *Math. Biosci.* 24:191–204.

Balkema, G. W., Mangini, N. J., Pinto, L. H., and Vanable, J. W., Jr. (1984). Visually evoked eye movements in mouse mutants and inbred strains: A screening report. *Invest. Ophthalmol. Vis. Sci.* 25:795–800.

Behan, M., and Appell, P. P. (1992). Intrinsic circuitry in the cat superior colliculus: Projections from the superficial layers. *J. Comp. Neurol.* 315:230–243.

Beninato, M., and Spencer, R. F. (1986). A cholinergic projection to the rat superior colliculus demonstrated by retrograde transport of horseradish peroxidase and choline acetyltransferase immunohistochemistry. *J. Comp. Neurol.* 253:525–538.

Binns, K. E. (1999). The synaptic pharmacology underlying sensory processing in the superior colliculus. *Prog. Neurobiol.* 59:129–159.

Blazquez, P. M., Hirata, Y., and Highstein, S. M. (2004). The vestibulo-ocular reflex as a model system for motor learning: What is the role of the cerebellum? *Cerebellum* 3:188–192.

Boghen, D., Troost, B. T., Daroff, R. B., Dell'Osso, L. F., and Birkett, J. E. (1974). Velocity characteristics of normal human saccades. *Invest. Ophthalmol.* 13:619–623.

Collewijn, H. (1970). The normal range of horizontal eye movements in the rabbit. *Exp. Neurol.* 28:132–143.

De Zeeuw, C. I., Hansel, C., Bian, F., Koekkoek, S. K., van Alphen, A. M., Linden, D. J., and Oberdick, J. (1998). Expression of a protein kinase C inhibitor in Purkinje cells blocks cerebellar LTD and adaptation of the vestibulo-ocular reflex. *Neuron* 20:495–508.

Dräger, U. C., and Hubel, D. H. (1975). Responses to visual stimulation and relationship between visual, auditory, and somatosensory inputs in mouse superior colliculus. *J. Neurophysiol.* 38:690–713.

Edwards, S. B. (1980). The deep cell layers of the superior colliculus: Their reticular characteristics and structural organization. In A. Hobson and M. Brazier (Eds.), *The reticular formation revisited* (pp. 193–209). New York: Raven Press.

Endo, T., Yanagawa, Y., Obata, T., and Isa, T. (2003). Characteristics of GABAergic neurons in the superficial superior colliculus in mice. *Neurosci. Lett.* 346:81–84.

Endo, T., Yanagawa, Y., Obata, K., and Isa, T. (2005). Nicotinic acetylcholine receptor subtypes involved in facilitation of GABAergic inhibition in mouse superficial superior colliculus. *J. Neurophysiol.* 94:3893–3902.

Evinger, C., and Fuchs, A. F. (1978). Saccadic, smooth pursuit, and optokinetic eye movements of the trained cat. *J. Physiol.* 285:209–229.

Fuchs, A. F. (1967). Saccadic and smooth pursuit eye movements in the monkey. *J. Physiol.* 191:609–631.

FULLER, J. H. (1985). Eye and head movements in the pigmented rat. *Vision Res.* 25:1121–1128.

GIRARD, B., and BERTHOZ, A. (2005). From brainstem to cortex: Computational models of saccade generation circuitry. *Prog. Neurobiol.* 77:215–251.

GLIMCHER, P. W., and SPARKS, D. L. (1992). Movement selection in advance of action in the superior colliculus. *Nature* 355: 542–545.

GRAYBIEL, A. M. (1978a). A satellite system of the superior colliculus: The parabigeminal nucleus and its projections to the superficial collicular layers. *Brain Res.* 145:365–374.

GRAYBIEL, A. M. (1978b). A stereometric pattern of distribution of acetylthiocholinesterase in the deep layers of the superior colliculus. *Nature* 272:539–541.

GRUSSER-CORNEHLS, U., and BOHM, P. (1988). Horizontal optokinetic ocular nystagmus in wild-type ($B6CBA^{+/+}$) and weaver mutant mice. *Exp. Brain Res.* 72:29–36.

GUITTON, D., CROMMELINCK, M., and ROUCOUX, A. (1980). Stimulation of the superior colliculus in the alert cat. I. Eye movements and neck EMG activity evoked when the head is restrained. *Exp. Brain Res.* 39:63–73.

GUITTON, D., and VOLLE, M. (1987). Gaze control in humans: Eye-head coordination during orienting movements to targets within and beyond the oculomotor range. *J. Neurophysiol.* 58:427–459.

HALL, W. C., FITZPATRICK, D., KLATT, L. L., and RACZKOWSKI, D. (1989). Cholinergic innervation of the superior colliculus in the cat. *J. Comp. Neurol.* 287:495–514.

HELMS, M. C., OZEN, G., and HALL, W. C. (2004). Organization of the intermediate gray layer of the superior colliculus. I. Intrinsic vertical connections. *J. Neurophysiol.* 91:1706–1715.

HIKOSAKA, O., and SAKAMOTO, M. (1987). Dynamic characteristics of saccadic eye movements in the albino rat. *Neurosci. Res.* 4: 304–308.

HILBIG, H., and SCHIERWAGEN, A. (1994). Interlayer neurones in the rat superior colliculus: A tracer study using DiI/Di-ASP. *Neuroreport* 5:477–480.

ILLING, R. B., and GRAYBIEL, A. M. (1985). Convergence of afferents from frontal cortex and substantia nigra onto acetylcholinesterase-rich patches of the cat's superior colliculus. *Neuroscience* 14:455–482.

ISA, T. (2002). Intrinsic processing in the mammalian superior colliculus. *Curr. Opin. Neurobiol.* 12:668–677.

ISA, T., ENDO, T., and SAITO, Y. (1998). The visuo-motor pathway in the local circuit of the rat superior colliculus. *J. Neurosci.* 15:8496–8504.

ISA, T., KOBAYASHI, Y., and SAITO, Y. (2003). Dynamic modulation of signal transmission in the local circuit of mammalian superior colliculus. In W. C. Hall and A. K. Moschovakis (Eds.), *The superior colliculus: New approaches for studying sensorimotor integration* (pp. 159–171). Boca Raton, FL: CRC Press.

ISA, T., and SAITO, Y. (2001). The direct visuo-motor pathway in mammalian superior colliculus: Novel perspective on the interlaminar connection. *Neurosci. Res.* 41:107–113.

ISA, T., and SPARKS, D. (2006). Microcircuit of the superior colliculus: A neuronal machine that determines timing and endpoint of saccadic eye movements. Paper presented at the 93rd Dahlem Workshop on Microcircuits: The Interface Between Neurons and Global Brain Function, pp. 1–34.

KATOH, A., KITAZAWA, H., ITOHARA, S., and NAGAO, S. (1998). Dynamic characteristics and adaptability of mouse vestibulo-ocular and optokinetic response eye movements and the role of the flocculo-olivary system revealed by chemical lesions. *Proc. Natl. Acad. Sci. U.S.A.* 95:7705–7710.

KATSUTA, H., and ISA, T. (2003). Release from $GABA_A$ receptor-mediated inhibition unmasks interlaminar connection within superior colliculus in anesthetized adult rats. *Neurosci. Res.* 46: 73–83.

LANE, R. D., BENNETT-CLARKE, C. A., ALLAN, D. M., and MOONEY, R. D. (1993). Immunochemical heterogeneity in the tecto-LP pathway of the rat. *J. Comp. Neurol.* 333:210–222.

LANGER, T. P., and LUND, R. D. (1974). The upper layers of the superior colliculus of the rat: A Golgi study. *J. Comp. Neurol.* 158:418–435.

LI, F., ENDO, T., and ISA, T. (2004). Presynaptic muscarinic acetylcholine receptors suppress GABAergic synaptic transmission in the intermediate grey layer of mouse superior colliculus. *Eur. J. Neurosci.* 20:2079–2088.

LEE, P. H., HELMS, M. C., AUGUSTINE, G. J., and HALL, W. C. (1997). Role of intrinsic synaptic circuitry in collicular sensorimotor integration. *Proc. Natl. Acad. Sci. U.S.A.* 94:13299–13304.

LO, F. S., CORK, R. J., and MIZE, R. R. (1998). Physiological properties of neurons in the optic layer of the rat's superior colliculus. *J. Neurophysiol.* 80:331–343.

MA, T. P., CHENG, H. W., CZECH, J. A., and RAFOLS, J. A. (1990). Intermediate and deep layers of the macaque superior colliculus: A Golgi study. *J. Comp. Neurol.* 295:92–110.

MAYS, L. E., and SPARKS, D. L. (1980). Dissociation of visual and saccade-related responses in superior colliculus. *J. Neurophysiol.* 43:207–232.

MITCHINER, J. C., PINTO, L. H., and VANABLE, J. W., JR. (1976). Visually evoked eye movements in the mouse (*Mus musculus*). *Vision Res.* 16:1169–1171.

MIZE, R. R. (1992). The organization of GABAergic neurons in the mammalian superior colliculus. *Prog. Brain Res.* 90:219–248.

MOONEY, R. D., NIKOLETSEAS, M. M., HESS, P. R., ALLEN, Z., LEWIN, A. C., and RHOADES, R. W. (1988a). The projection from the superficial to the deep layers of the superior colliculus: An intracellular horseradish peroxidase injection study in the hamster. *J. Neurosci.* 8:1384–1399.

MOONEY, R. D., NIKOLETSEAS, M. M., RUIZ, S. A., and RHOADES, R. W. (1988b). Receptive-field properties and morphological characteristics of the superior collicular neurons that project to the lateral posterior and dorsal lateral geniculate nuclei in the hamster. *J. Neurophysiol.* 59:1333–1351.

MOSCHOVAKIS, A. K., KARABELAS, A. B., and HIGHSTEIN, S. M. (1988). Structure-function relationships in the primate superior colliculus. II. Morphological identity of presaccadic neurons. *J. Neurophysiol.* 60:263–302.

MOSCHOVAKIS, A. K., SCUDDER, C. A., and HIGHSTEIN, S. M. (1996). The microscopic anatomy and physiology of the mammalian saccadic system. *Prog. Neurobiol.* 50:133–254.

NORITA, M. (1980). Neurons and synaptic patterns in the deep layers of the superior colliculus of the cat: A Golgi and electron microscopic study. *J. Comp. Neurol.* 190:29–48.

PELISSON, D., and PRABLANC, C. (1988). Kinematics of centrifugal and centripetal saccadic eye movements in man. *Vision Res.* 28:87–94.

PETTIT, D. L., HELMS, M. C., AUGUSTINE, G. J., and HALL, W. C. (1999). Local excitatory circuits in the intermediate gray layer of the superior colliculus. *J. Neurophysiol.* 81:1424–1427.

ROBINSON, D. A. (1972). Eye movements evoked by collicular stimulation in the alert monkey. *Vision Res.* 12:1795–1808.

SAITO, Y., and ISA, T. (1999). Electrophysiological and morphological properties of neurons in the rat superior colliculus. I. Neurons in the intermediate layer. *J. Neurophysiol.* 82:754–767.

Saito, Y., and Isa, T. (2003). Local excitatory network and NMDA receptor activation generate a synchronous and bursting command from the superior colliculus. *J. Neurosci.* 23:5854–5864.

Saito, Y., and Isa, T. (2004). Laminar specific distribution of lateral excitatory connections in the rat superior colliculus. *J. Neurophysiol.* 92:3500–3510.

Saito, Y., and Isa, T. (2005). Organization of interlaminar interactions in the rat superior colliculus. *J. Neurophysiol.* 93:2898–2907.

Sakatani, T., and Isa, T. (2004). PC-based high-speed video-oculography for measuring rapid eye movements in mice. *Neurosci. Res.* 49:123–131.

Sakatani, T., and Isa, T. (2007). Quantitative analysis of spontaneous saccade-like rapid eye movements in C57BL/6 mice. *Neurosci. Res.* 58:324–331.

Schiller, P. H., and Stryker, M. (1972). Single-unit recording and stimulation in superior colliculus of the alert rhesus monkey. *J. Neurophysiol.* 35:915–924.

Scudder, C. A., Kaneko, C. S., and Fuchs, A. F. (2002). The brainstem burst generator for saccadic eye movements: A modern synthesis. *Exp. Brain Res.* 142:439–462.

Sherk, H. (1979). A comparison of visual-response properties in cat's parabigeminal nucleus and superior colliculus. *J. Neurophysiol.* 42:1640–1655.

Sooksawate, T., Saito, Y., and Isa, T. (2005). Electrophysiological and morphological properties of identified crossed tecto-reticular neurons in the rat superior colliculus. *Neurosci. Res.* 52:174–184.

Sooksawate, T., and Isa, T. (2006). Properties of cholinergic responses in neurons in the intermediate grey layer of rat superior colliculus. *Eur. J. Neurosci.* 24:3096–3108.

Sooksawate, T., Isa, K., Obata, K., Yanagawa, Y., and Isa, T. (2005). Electrophysiological and morphological properties of GABAergic neurons in the intermediate gray layer of superior colliculus in GAD67-GFP knock-in mice. Presented at the annual meeting of the Society for Neuroscience, abstr. 167.8.

Sparks, D. (1999). Conceptual issues related to the role of the superior colliculus in the control of gaze. *Curr. Opin. Neurobiol.* 9:698–707.

Sparks, D. (2002). The brainstem control of saccadic eye movements. *Nat. Rev. Neurosci.* 3:952–964.

Sparks, D., Rohrer, W. H., and Zhang, Y. (2000). The role of the superior colliculus in saccade initiation: A study of express saccades and the gap effect. *Vision Res.* 40:2763–2777.

Stahl, J. S. (2004). Eye movements of the murine P/Q calcium channel mutant rocker, and the impact of aging. *J. Neurophysiol.* 91:2066–2078.

Tamamaki, N., Yanagawa, Y., Tomioka, R., Miyazaki, J. I., Obata, K., and Kaneko, T. (2003). Green fluorescent protein expression and colocalization with calretinin, parvalbumin, and somatostatin in the GAD67-GFP knock-in mouse. *J. Comp. Neurol.* 467:60–79.

van Alphen, A. M., Stahl, J. S., and De Zeeuw, C. I. (2001). The dynamic characteristics of the mouse horizontal vestibulo-ocular and optokinetic response. *Brain Res.* 890:296–305.

Wurtz, R. H., and Goldberg, M. E. (1972). Activity of superior colliculus in behaving monkey. III. Cells discharging before eye movements. *J. Neurophysiol.* 35:575–586.

Wurtz, R., and Goldberg, M. (1989). *The neurobiology of saccadic eye movements.* New York: Elsevier.

20 Interconnections of Visual Cortical Areas in the Mouse

ANDREAS BURKHALTER AND QUANXIN WANG

Visual cortical functions are impaired in many disorders that affect children. For example, in autism spectrum disorders, individuals have a predisposition to see local stimulus features but have difficulty grouping these features to recognize global shapes (Dakin and Frith, 2005). In Williams syndrome, individuals suffer from a visuospatial construction deficit that makes it difficult for them to put together even the simplest of puzzles (Meyer-Lindenberg et al., 2004). Both of these disorders are linked to a variety of gene mutations (Polleux and Lauder, 2004; Eckert et al., 2006; Grice and Buxbaum, 2006) and are associated with structural abnormalities that reduce the connectivity of the parietal cortex, which belongs to the dorsal cortical processing stream (Van Essen et al., 2006; Just et al., 2007). To develop an understanding of the mechanisms that underlie these structural malformations, there is growing interest in using a mouse model in which the expression of specific genes can be manipulated and the effects on the visual cortical network can be studied (Eckert et al., 2006). To interpret these effects, it is important to understand the connectivity in wild-type mice and to ask whether the mouse is a good model of the primate visual cortex.

Investigation of the connectivity of mouse visual cortex was pioneered in the 1970s by Vernon Caviness, Ursula Dräger, and Alan Pearlman, and to this day, our understanding of mouse visual cortical connectivity is dominated by their contributions. After the publication of their classic papers, however, research focused more on the cortical anatomy of rats and squirrels than on mice, with a corresponding lag in understanding the connectivity of mouse visual cortex. This chapter considers primarily studies in mice, to collect the research and establish a clear picture of what is known today.

Area map of mouse visual cortex

Cytoarchitectonic Fields It is widely accepted that the brain operations responsible for perception and cognitive processing of visual information occur in an interconnected network of functionally specialized cortical areas. Knowing where these areas are, how they are connected and what they do is therefore key to understanding how the network processes visual information. In the tradition of Brodmann's work on the structural diversity of cortical areas (Garey, 2006), early studies of mouse cerebral cortex identified areas based on variations in cell size, cell density, and lamination (Isenschmid, 1911; De Vries, 1912; Rose, 1912; Fortuyn, 1914). Using such cytoarchitectonic features, Rose (1929) distinguished an astonishingly large number of 55 fields, and speculated that they may be linked by 1,458 possible connections. In Rose's 1929 map, occipital cortex was dominated by a large elliptical region, which, owing to its thick granular layer, became known as striate area. Many years later this area was shown to undergo structural changes after enucleation (Valverde, 1968). This discovery was followed by labeling the structure by transneuronal transport of ^{3}H-proline from the eye (Dräger, 1974), which identified the area as primary visual cortex (i.e., striate cortex, V1).

The first hint that visual cortex extends beyond the striate area came from a lesion study that revealed degenerating connections to the surrounding medial and lateral extrastriate cortex (Valverde and Estéban, 1968). A short time later, studies showed that these cortical regions contain visuotopic maps and demonstrated that receptive fields (RFs) in mouse striate and extrastriate cortex are tuned to moving oriented light bars (Dräger, 1975; Métin et al., 1988). The topographic organization of Dräger's (1975) area 18a adjacent to lateral V1 resembled area 18 in cat and area V2 in hedgehog and gray squirrel (Hubel and Wiesel, 1965; Kaas et al., 1970; Hall et al., 1971). Area 18 on the medial side of mouse V1 (Dräger, 1975) resembled the prostriate area (Sanides and Hoffman, 1969) or the visually responsive splenial cortex in cats (Kalia and Whitteridge, 1973). Based on these similarities, Caviness (1975) reinterpreted Rose's (1929) map and proposed that, similar to what is seen in rat (Krieg, 1946), mouse V1 is adjoined laterally by area 18a and medially by area 18b (figure 20.1*A*). In more recent maps, however, considerable uncertainty persists about the shape, size, and boundaries of areas 18a and 18b (Caviness, 1975; Caviness and Frost, 1980; Frost and Caviness, 1980) and how these areas relate to the cytoarchitectonically defined visual areas V2L, V2ML, V2MM, and TeA depicted in the most widely used atlas, by Paxinos and Franklin (2001) (figure 20.1*B*).

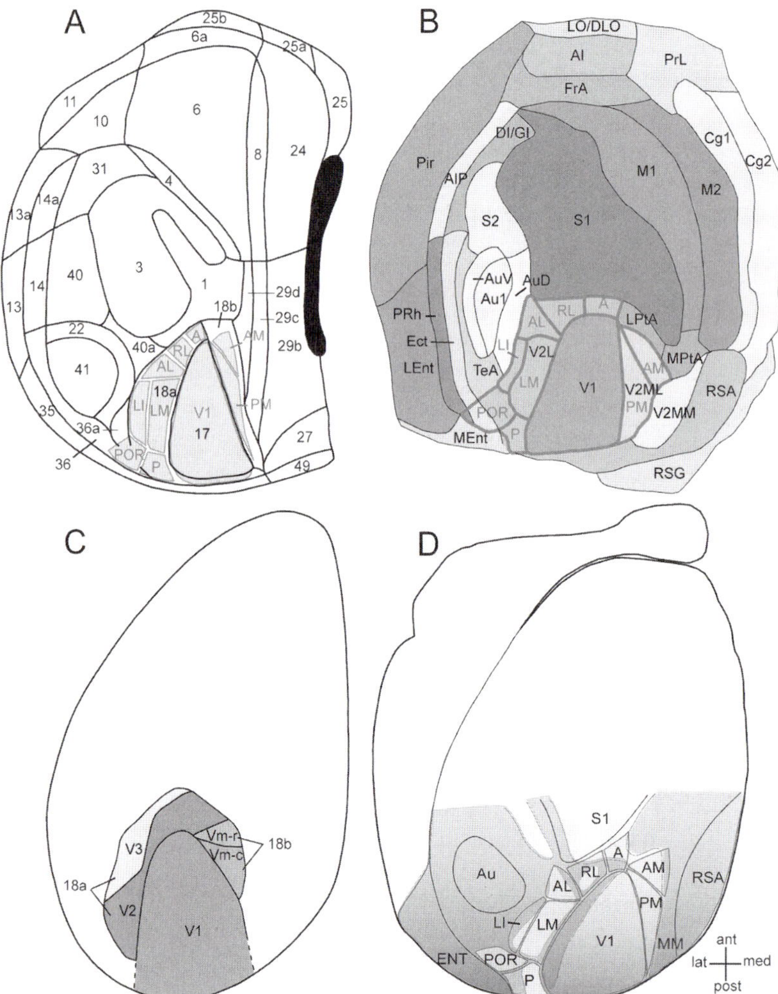

FIGURE 20.1 Different maps of mouse visual cortex. *A*, Flat map of cytoarchitectonic areas (*black outlines*) in the left hemisphere of mouse cerebral cortex published by Caviness and Frost (1980). *Red shaded regions* represent schematic outlines of visuotopically organized areas, identified by Wang and Burkhalter (2006). Note that areas 18a and 18b contain multiple visuotopic areas. *B*, Flat map of cytoarchitectonic areas of the left mouse cerebral cortex constructed by David C. Van Essen by unfolding coronal sections taken from the atlas of Paxinos and Franklin (2001). *Red outlines* represent schematic borders of visuotopically defined areas identified by Wang and Burkhalter (2007). Note that areas V2L and V2ML contain multiple visuotopically organized areas. *C*, Visuotopic organization of the left mouse visual cortex derived by mapping of receptive fields, published by Wagor et al. (1980). In this map, cytoarchitectonic area 18a contains areas V2 and V3 and cytoarchitectonic area 18b contains the rostral and caudal medial visual areas, Vm-r and Vm-c. *D*, Area map of left mouse visual cortex derived by topographic mapping of V1 connections and receptive field mapping (Wang and Burkhalter, 2007). *Blue shading* represents the distribution of callosal connections in superficial layers. See color plate 7.

TOPOGRAPHICALLY DEFINED AREAS Studies in monkey have shown that only a minority of areas can be identified based on cytoarchitectonic features. In fact, even within the original borders of Brodmann's area 18, visuotopic mapping has revealed as many as four complete topographic representations of the visual field that are considered discrete visual areas (Van Essen, 1979; Van Essen and Maunsell, 1981). To study whether cytoarchitectonic areas correspond to visuotopically defined areas, Wagor et al. (1980) recorded RFs in mouse visual cortex and showed that area 18a contains two complete visuotopic maps, V2 and V3, that flank V1 on the lateral side (figure 20.1*C*). On the medial side of V1, Wagor et al. (1980) found a rostral and a caudal visual area, Vm-r and Vm-c, both of which were contained within area 18b (see figure 20.1*C*). Using intrinsic optical signal imaging, Kalatsky and Stryker (2003) confirmed that mouse V1 is adjoined laterally by a single area, V2. In addition, they showed that V2 is adjoined laterally by area V3, and that V3 shares its lateral border with area V4. On the medial side of V1, they found only a single area, V5. Although Kalatsky and Stryker (2003) suggest that their optical map resembles the map of Wagor et al. (1980), it is important to note this has not been demonstrated directly. Using a similar optical imaging approach, Schuett et al. (2002) found a completely different map, in which mouse V1 is adjoined on the lateral side not by a single area V2 but by the lateromedial area, LM, and the anterolateral area, AL. These conflicting maps prompted Wang and Burkhalter (2007) to revisit the issue by using a combination of axonal tracing of V1 connections, RF mapping, and referencing projection and recording sites to fixed callosal landmarks and myeloarchitectonic boundaries. The tracing experiments revealed a total of 15 V1 projection fields, nine of which contained a complete representation of the visual field and can therefore be considered distinct areas (Felleman and Van Essen, 1991). Based on similar studies in rat visual cortex (Olavarria and Montero, 1984; Montero, 1993) we have designated these fields posterior (P), lateromedial (LM), anterolateral (AL), rostrolateral (RL), anterior (A), posteromedial (PM), anteromedial (AM), laterointermediate (LI), and postrhinal (POR) areas (figure 20.2*A*, *B*, and *D*). Each of these areas has a characteristic location relative to the fixed pattern of callosal connections (figure 20.2*C*), but the callosally connected regions do not necessarily correspond to areal boundaries (see figure 20.2*B* and *C*). Some of these locations (e.g., LM, AL, LI, P, AM) correspond to projection sites that were previously identified by tracing connections of mouse V1 with ^{3}H-proline (Olavarria and Montero, 1989). On the medial side of V1, Wang and Burkhalter's (2007) connection map strongly resembles the RF map of Wagor et al. (1980) (see figure 20.1*C* and *D*). However, unlike Wagor et al. (1980), who found a single area V2 on the lateral side of V1, Wang and Burkhalter (2007) found that lateral V1 is adjoined by five distinct areas, P, LM, AL, RL, and A. One explanation for these differences is that Wang and Burkhalter's (2007) map was constructed by high-resolution mapping in single animals and the referencing of projection and recording sites against fixed callosal and myeloarchitectonic landmarks. In contrast, Wagor et al. (1980) faced the challenging task of constructing maps by pooling recording sites across animals with a dearth of fixed anatomical references. As a result, Wagor et al. (1980) overlooked the reversal of the elevation map at the LM/AL border and the polarity change of the azimuthal map at the vertical meridian representation that coincides with the AL/RL border (see figure10*A* and *B* of Wang and Burkhalter, 2007). In addition, Wagor et al. (1980) mistook the horizontal meridians of LM and RL as a single split horizontal meridian representation at the V2/V3 border. Thus, the string of areas on the lateral side of V1 resembles more closely the complex organization found in rat (Montero, 1993) than the simple organization found in many rodent and nonrodent species, in which lateral V1 is adjoined by a single area V2 (Rosa and Krubitzer, 1999). However, unlike in rat (Thomas and Espinoza, 1987; Montero, 1993), Wang and Burkhalter

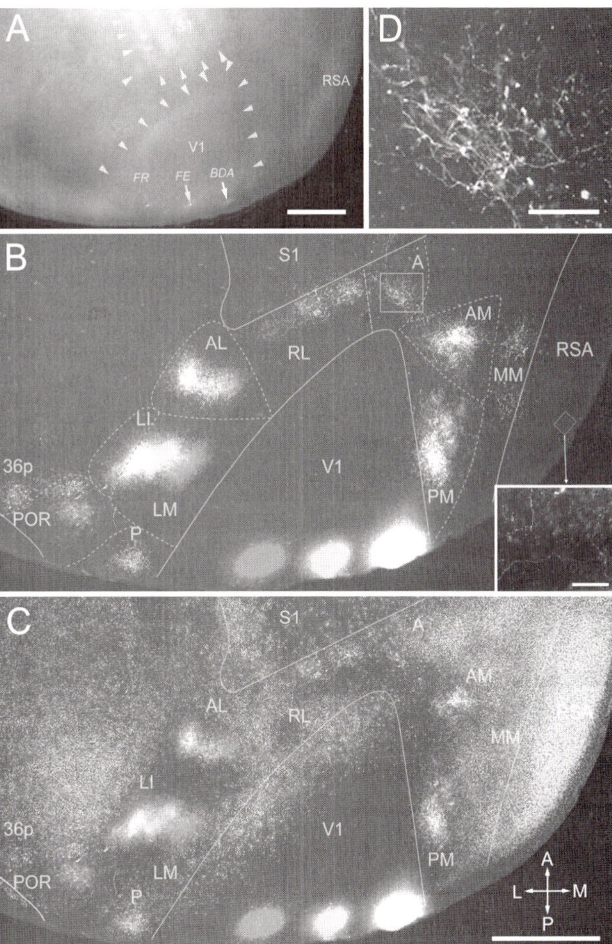

Figure 20.2 Topographic maps of V1 connections in mouse visual cortex. Representation of azimuth in extrastriate visual cortex is shown in horizontal sections of left occipital cortex. The maps were generated by making three simultaneous injections of fluororuby (FR, red), fluoroemerald (FE, green), and biotinylated dextran amine (BDA, yellow) into V1, followed by triple-anterograde tracing of intracortical connections. *A*, Darkfield image showing heavy myelination in primary visual cortex (V1) and the barrel field of primary somatosensory cortex (S1). *Arrowheads* indicate myeloarchitectonic borders. *Arrows* indicate injection sites in V1. *B*, Fluorescently labeled axonal connections after injections of FR, FE, and BDA at different nasotemporal locations (azimuth) of the upper visual field representation in V1. *Dashed lines* indicate areal borders, which were determined by mapping inputs from the perimeter of V1. *Solid lines* indicate myeloarchitectonic borders. *C*, Overlay of BDA-labeled axonal projections shown in *B* and bisbenzimide-labeled callosally projecting neurons (blue). *D*, Higher magnification image of axonal labeling shown in area A (inset in *B*). A, anterior; L, lateral; M, medial; P, posterior. Scale bar = 1 mm (*A*–*C*), 0.1 mm (*B*, *inset*), and 0.3 mm (*D*). See color plate 8.

(2007) found that in mouse, the vertical meridian is represented only at the V1/LM border, suggesting that LM is homologous to V2 (Van Essen, 1979). Thus, in respect to V1 and LM, mouse visual cortex is simple. But, unlike the simple extrastriate cortex of primates, in which V1 is surrounded by a single area, V2, containing multiple compartments with distinct connections and RF properties embedded in a single global visuotopic map (Roe and Ts'o, 1995), V1 in mice is adjoined by multiple areas, each of which contains a map of the entire visual field. This organization exhibits the hallmark feature of a complex extrastriate cortex and supports the hypothesis that in ancestral mammals, V1 was surrounded by multiple areas that gave rise to homologous areas in distantly related species (Rosa and Krubitzer, 1999).

Relationship between Cytoarchitectonic Areas and Topographic Maps To determine the shape and size of extrastriate visual areas, Wang and Burkhalter (2007) traced the connections from the perimeter of V1. The borders of the nine visuotopically organized areas are shown in the flat map illustrated in figure 20.1*D*. The overlay of the topographic map with the cytoarchitectonic map of Caviness and Frost (1980) shows that in medial extrastriate cortex, PM and AM overlap with area 18b, whereas in lateral extrastriate cortex, P, LM, AL, LI, RL, and A overlap with areas 18a and 36a, which may correspond to POR (see figure 20.1*A*). The overlay of Wang and Burkhalter's (2007) map with the cytoarchitectonic map of Paxinos and Franklin (2001) shows that V2ML in medial extrastriate cortex overlaps with PM and AM (see figure 20.1*B*). In lateral extrastriate cortex, V2L coincides with P, LM, LI, AL, RL, A, and POR, which encroaches on ectorhinal cortex (see figure 20.1*B*).

Connections of mouse visual cortex

Subcortical Inputs In the mouse, at least 12 different morphological types of retinal ganglion cells (RGCs) have been identified that convey image-forming and non-image-forming visual information from the eye to a variety of subcortical structures, including the dorsal lateral geniculate nucleus (dLGN) and the superior colliculus (SC) (Godement et al., 1984; Sun et al., 2002; Badea and Nathans, 2004; Hattar et al., 2006). Based on morphological criteria, 11–14 different types of RGC have been identified in the mouse retina (Kong et al., 2005; Coombs et al., 2006). The image-forming RGCs have been classified into three to five distinct groups with short- and long-latency responses (Carcieri et al., 2003; Pang et al., 2003). Short-latency neurons are further classified as ON- and OFF-center cells, and ON neurons are subdivided into separate groups with transient and sustained response properties (Carcieri et al., 2003). But, unlike recordings in the isolated retina (Stone and Pinto, 1993), in vivo studies have found that linear and nonlinear spatial summation properties of RGC RFs lie on a continuum with various degrees of nonlinearities, and there is no evidence for distinct classes of cells with linear (X-like) and nonlinear (Y-like) RFs (Carcieri et al., 2003). This differs from mouse and squirrel dLGN, in which most RFs show linear spatial summation properties and resemble monkey magnocellular dLGN neurons (Usrey and Reid, 2000; Grubb and Thompson, 2003; Van Hooser et al., 2003). Although there is no evidence for distinct linear and nonlinear channels, ON-center dLGN cells are more sensitive to contrast than OFF-center cells, suggesting that geniculocortical inputs are carried through parallel high-contrast-gain ON and low-contrast-gain OFF channels (Grubb and Thompson, 2003).

Neurons of the dLGN send axons to the visual cortex, where they terminate in layers 1, 3, 4, and the layer 5/6 border of V1 (Frost and Caviness, 1980; Simmons et al., 1982). Individual axonal arbors have different laminar distributions, terminal densities, and fields of innervation, which in layer 4 are 50–1,700 μm in diameter (Antonini et al., 1999). Descending outputs from V1 to the dLGN originate from layer 6 (Simmons et al., 1982; Brumberg et al., 2003), whereas layer 5 cells send output to the SC (Kozloski et al., 2001).

About 90% of retinal inputs project to the opposite hemisphere (Dräger and Olson, 1980). Cortical inputs from the contralateral dLGN are distributed across the entire primary visual area, whereas inputs from the same side terminate in the lateral half of V1, which corresponds to the binocular zone (Dräger, 1974; Antonini et al., 1999; Kalatsky and Stryker, 2003).

Connections within V1 Most connections within V1 are local but account for only 3.5% of the total length of 4 km of axons contained within 1 mm^3 of cortex (Braitenberg and Schüz, 1991; Schüz et al., 2006). Studies in the adult mouse somatosensory cortex suggest that approximately 85% of these axons are excitatory and 15% are inhibitory (DeFelipe et al., 1997). Although in mouse visual cortex, isolated examples of spiny stellate cells have been described that project from layer 4 to layer 2/3 (Valverde, 1968, 1976), interlaminar connections of pyramidal neurons have only been studied systematically in somatosensory cortex. In mouse S1, Larsen and Callaway (2006) found that layer 2/3 pyramidal cells either project to both layers 5 and 6 or make connections to layers 4, 5, and 6. Further, Larsen and Callaway (2006) identified three types of layer 5 pyramidal cells with distinct dendritic arbors that all send axonal projections to layers 2/3 and 6. An even greater diversity of pyramidal cell types was observed in layer 5 of V1, but whether these cells have different connections is not known (Tsiola et al., 2003). Corticogeniculate layer 6 neurons, however, are known to send recurrent axon collaterals to layer 4 (Brumberg et al., 2003). Taken together, this sketchy evidence suggests that V1 contains a columnar network that links chains of neurons, which act as conduits for the propagation of ascending and descending sequences of spontaneous neuronal firing that have been observed with calcium indicator dyes in slices of mouse visual cortex (Ikegaya et al., 2004).

The horizontal connections within layers 2/3, 5, and 6 of V1 are anisotropic and are longer in rostrocaudal axis than in mediolateral axis (Q. Wang and A. Burkhalter, unpublished observations). This phenomenon is location dependent and more prominent in the upper than the lower visual field representation. Within this oval region, the distribution of terminals is uniform and resembles the nonpatchy horizontal connections within V1 of the gray squirrel (Van Hooser et al., 2006). This differs from earlier claims of patchy horizontal connections within rat V1 (Rumberger et al., 2001). However, it is quite possible that individual cells or very small clusters make patchy intrinsic connections, as has been shown in rat visual cortex (Burkhalter and Charles, 1990).

Connections between Different Cortical Areas Little is known about interareal connections of mouse visual cortex. Early studies using ^{3}H-proline as tracer found that V1 projects to as many as nine discrete projection fields (Olavarria et al., 1982; Olavarria and Montero, 1989). Using high-resolution pathway tracing with dextran dyes to label axon terminal fields in combination with bisbenzimide retrograde labeling of fixed callosal landmarks, we have found that mouse V1 projects to 15 fields (Wang and Burkhalter, 2007). These targets are best visualized in flat mounts of the injected cortical hemisphere. In the example shown in figure 20.2*A*, we injected three different dyes—fluororuby (red), fluoroemerald (green), and biotinylated dextran amine (BDA, yellow)—at different azimuths of the upper visual field representation in V1 (Wang and Burkhalter, 2007). Groups of nonoverlapping red/green and yellow projection patches were found in nine topographically organized extrastriate areas (i.e., LM, AL, RL, A, PM, AM, LI, P, and POR). In addition, we found projection fields in which the red, green, and yellow patches largely overlapped (see figure 20.2*B–D*). These nonvisuotopically organized fields include area 36p, the lateral entorhinal area (LEA), the face representation of area S1, the mediomedial area (MM), which overlaps with V2MM of Paxinos and Franklin (2001), the primary cingulate cortex (Cg1), and the retrosplenial agranular area (RSA). These results show that the connections of mouse V1 are more extensive than previously demonstrated (Olavarria and Montero, 1989), and that similar to what is seen in rat, V1 provides direct inputs to somatosensory cortex, the frontal eye field, and retrosplenial, perirhinal, and entorhinal cortex (Miller and Vogt, 1984; Coogan and Burkhalter, 1993).

There is only a single study on the connections of mouse extrastriate visual cortex, demonstrating that areas V1, 18a, and 18b are reciprocally connected (Simmons et al., 1982). Our area map (see figure 20.1*D*) (Wang and Burkhalter, 2007) and the overlay with the map of Caviness and Frost (1980) (see figure 20.1*A*), however, suggest that the cytoarchitectonic areas 18a and 18b contain more than a single visuotopic map (see figure 20.1*A*). We have therefore sought to determine whether areas LM and AL, both of which are contained within area 18a, have distinct connections. Tracing the connections of area LM with BDA shows that this V2-like area has strong projections to areas V1, AL, RL, LI, P, POR, 36p, AM, and PM, and weaker projections to the rostral temporal area (TeAr), LEA, the dorsal auditory belt (AuD), retrosplenial cortex (RSA), and the frontal eye field (Cg1, not shown) (figure 20.3). These connections closely resemble those of rat LM (Coogan and Burkhalter, 1993) and show similarities to the projections labeled by tracer injections into the rat posterior lateral extrastriate cortex, which is strongly connected with the parahippocampal cortex and the amygdala (McDonald and Mascagni, 1996; Burwell and Amaral, 1998).

Tracer injections into area AL revealed a set of connections that differ from those of LM. The AL connections shown in figure 20.4 include strong projections to V1, LM, RL, LI, AM, PM, AuD, S1, the lateral parietal cortex (PL), area A of the posterior parietal cortex, the transition zone between cingulate and retrosplenial cortex (Cg/RS), Cg1, and the dorsal orbitofrontal area (DLO), and weak inputs to area P, POR, TeAr, 36p, and LEA. In the rat, similar connections were observed after injections into AL and rostral lateral extrastriate cortex, which, unlike posterior lateral cortex, is only very weakly connected with the amygdala (Coogan and Burkhalter, 1993; McDonald and Mascagni, 1996).

From these results it is evident that LM and AL share many targets. However, the projection strengths in these shared targets are not the same. For example, LM projects more strongly to area P, area LI, and 36p, whereas AL provides stronger inputs to AuD and A. An even stronger preference of LM for ventral targets is evident in the input to POR, which has very sparse connections with AL. In contrast, the strong preference of AL for dorsal targets is seen in the projections to PL, area Cg/RS, and DLO, which do not receive input from LM. These differences suggest that the projections of LM and AL contribute to distinct but intertwined visual processing streams (Wang and Burkhalter, 2003, 2004, 2005). In mice, the ventral stream appears to originate from LM and flows into parahippocampal (i.e., area POR) and perirhinal cortex (i.e., area 36p). Single-unit recordings have shown that LM neurons carry high spatial frequency information (Gao et al., 2006), which may be used by POR neurons to detect changes in the visual environment (Burwell and Hafeman, 2003). Lesion studies further suggest that the detected signals are used further downstream in

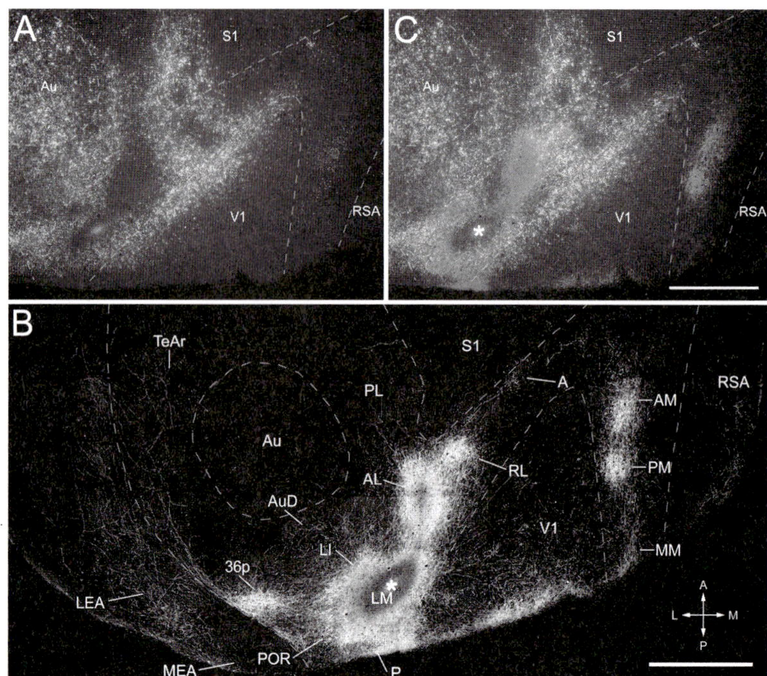

FIGURE 20.3 Intracortical connections of the extrastriate lateromedial area (LM) in mouse visual cortex, shown in tangential sections through the flattened posterior cerebral cortex. *A*, Fluorescence image showing the distribution of retrogradely labeled callosal connections. *Dashed lines* represent the myeloarchitectonic borders of V1, S1, and RSA. *B*, Darkfield image of biotinylated dextran amine (BDA)–labeled axonal connections of area LM. *Asterisk* indicates the injection site. Note the strong connections to areas POR and 36p. *C*, Superimposition of BDA-labeled LM connections (gold) with callosal connections (blue somata). A, anterior; L, lateral; M, medial; P, posterior. Scale bar = 1 mm in all images. See color plate 9.

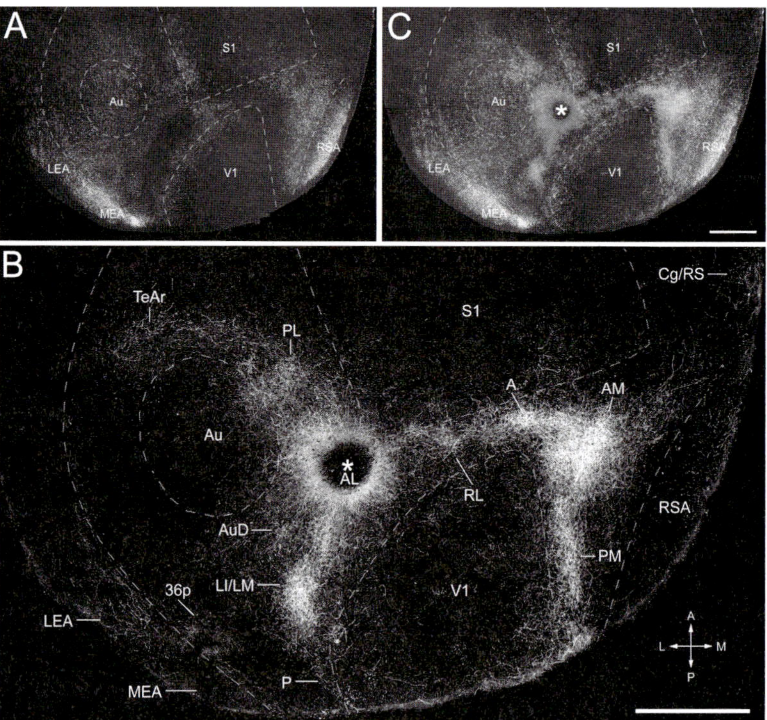

FIGURE 20.4 Intracortical connections of the extrastriate lateromedial area (AL) in mouse visual cortex, shown in tangential sections through the flattened posterior cerebral cortex. *A*, Fluorescence image showing the distribution of retrogradely labeled callosal connections. *Dashed lines* represent the myeloarchitectonic borders of V1, S1, and RSA. *B*, Darkfield image of biotinylated dextran amine (BDA)–labeled axonal connections of area AL. *Asterisk* indicates injection site. Note the strong connections to areas PL, A, and Cg/RS. *C*, Superimposition of BDA-labeled LM connections (gold) with callosal connections (blue somata). A, anterior; L, lateral; M, medial; P, posterior. Scale bar = 1 mm in all images. See color plate 10.

perirhinal cortex to make visual discriminations and for object recognition (Prusky et al., 2004; Davies et al., 2007). Thus, the ventral stream may play a role in navigation that relies on the dynamic recognition and identification of landmarks along routes. In contrast, AL sends low-frequency information about rapidly changing, fast-moving objects (Gao et al., 2006) to polymodal areas in posterior and lateral parietal cortex, which in rat represent tactile and auditory stimuli (Toldi et al., 1986; Brett-Green et al., 2003). This information may be used further downstream in retrosplenial cortex and the frontal eye field to direct eye, head, and body movements (Neafsey, 1990; Taube, 1998). Thus, areas of the dorsal stream may process visual motion-related cues that may be employed for navigation and the construction of reference frames used for the generation of head direction cells and hippocampal place cells (Save et al., 2005).

Areal Hierarchy Most interareal connections in mouse visual cortex originate from layers 2/3 and 5 pyramidal neurons (Simmons et al., 1982). Feedforward projections from V1 to higher visual areas such as LM, AM, and S1 (viewed from the perspective of the visual system) were shown to terminate principally in layers 2/3–6 (Olavarria and Montero, 1989; Yamashita et al., 2003; Dong et al., 2004a; figure 20.5*A*). In contrast, feedback projections from the higher visual area, LM, terminate in layers 1, 2/3, 5, and 6 of V1 and exclude layer 4 (Yamashita et al., 2003; Dong et al., 2004a, 2004b) (figure 20.5*B*). These laminar connection patterns are reminiscent of those found in rat visual cortex, in which feedforward and feedback circuits interconnect areas to a hierarchical network (Coogan and Burkhalter, 1993). Although the reconstruction of the structure of the areal hierarchy of mouse visual cortex is incomplete, multiunit recordings in different visual areas have shown significant areal differences in RF size (i.e., V1 < LM < POR < AL < P < LI < PM < AM < RL < A < MM; Wang and Burkhalter, 2007), suggesting that the structural hierarchy correlates with a functional hierarchy. The present anatomical evidence suggests that the neocortical hierarchy has at least four levels, including V1, LM/AL, POR/36p, and LEA.

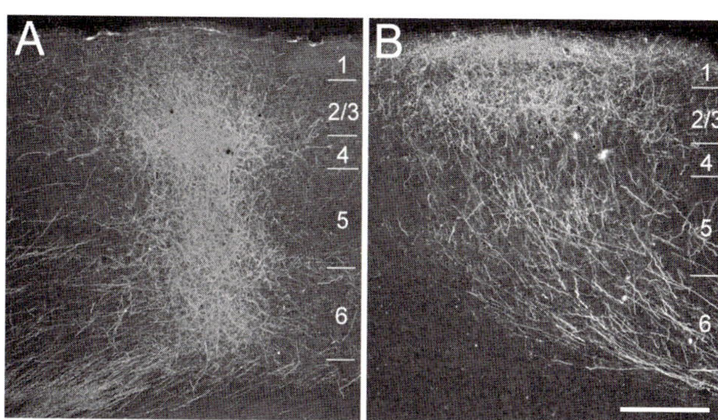

Figure 20.5 Laminar organization of inter-areal feedforward and feedback connections in mouse visual cortex labeled by anterograde tracing with BDA. *A*, Coronal section showing feedforward axons that originate from the lower area V1 and terminate in the higher extrastriate area LM. The projection column includes layers 2/3 to 6, and inputs to layer 1 are sparse. *B*, Coronal section showing feedback axons that originate from area LM and terminate in V1. The projections to layer 1, 2/3, and 5 are dense, whereas inputs to layer 4 are sparse. Scale bar = 0.2 mm. See color plate 11.

Conclusion

The presence of 10 complete orderly maps of the visual field strongly suggests that mouse visual cortex contains at least 10 distinct visual areas. Thus, the arealization of mouse visual cortex rivals the complexity of that in prosimian monkeys (Striedter, 2006). Unlike in many other rodent and nonrodent mammals, however, lateral primary visual cortex in mice is adjoined by multiple distinct areas, not by a single area V2 containing repeating structurally and functionally distinct modules (Rosa and Krubitzer, 1999). Only one of these areas, LM, shares the vertical meridian representation with V1 and can therefore be considered homologous to V2. Thus, according to the complex cortex hypothesis, the remaining visuotopically organized areas can be considered homologous to extrastriate areas in other mammalian lineages (Rosa and Krubitzer, 1999). Unlike primate V2, however, LM, including all the other visual areas, contains maps that are topologically equivalent to V1. The reason for this mapping format may be that the mouse brain is small and there is little pressure to minimize the length of connections between homotopic locations of different maps (Allman and Kaas, 1974). Similar rules may apply to intra-areal connections and may explain the absence of patchy horizontal connections within mouse V1 (Chklovskii and Koulakov, 2004).

Geniculocortical inputs are conveyed in a high-contrast-gain ON channel and a low-contrast-gain OFF channel, both of which have linear spatial summation properties and resemble the magnocellular geniculocortical pathway in primates. In cortex, the distinction between high- and low-contrast pathways is lost. However, high spatial frequency/low temporal frequency information is preferentially represented in area LM, whereas AL neurons are selective for fast-moving, low spatial frequency/high temporal frequency stimuli. Interestingly, the outputs of LM are strongly biased toward ventral cortex, whereas AL projects more strongly to dorsal areas. These connections are reminiscent of the "where" and "what" streams in primates (Ungerleider and Pasternak, 2004) and suggest that similar streams exist in mouse visual cortex.

Lower and higher visual areas are interconnected by feedforward and feedback circuits, which are identified by their distinct laminar termination patterns. On the basis of these anatomical features, the few areas that have been studied so far can be ordered in a hierarchy that has at least 4 levels, with V1 at the bottom and entorhinal cortex at the top. By comparison, in macaque monkey there are 11 levels between V1 and entorhinal cortex (Felleman and Van Essen, 1991). But the lower number of levels found in mouse neocortex may not be surprising, given that the difference between the smallest and largest RFs in monkey is approximately 50 times greater than in mouse (Gao et al., 2006; Wang and Burkhalter, 2007). Thus, the shorter chain of command in mouse visual cortex suggests that the visual world is represented over a much narrower spatial scale than in primates. Although the mouse visual cortex is clearly very different from that in primates, both species share a basic common plan of organization, suggesting that mouse visual cortex is a good model for studies of arealization, hierarchical networks, interareal synaptic processing, and how visual inputs are used to construct an environment-independent spatial coordinate system.

ACKNOWLEDGMENTS Work was supported by grant nos. EY-05935 and EY-016184 from the U.S. National Institutes of Health, grant no. HFSP123/200-B, and funding from the McDonnell Center for Studies of Higher Brain Function. We thank David C. Van Essen for the flat map of cytoarchitectonic areas shown in figure 20.1*B*.

REFERENCES

Allman, J. M., and Kaas, J. H. (1974). The organization of the second visual area (VII) in the owl monkey: A second order transformation of the visual hemifield. *Brain Res.* 76:247–265.

Antonini, A., Fagolini, M., and Stryker, M. P. (1999). Anatomical correlates of functional plasticity in mouse visual cortex. *J. Neurosci.* 19:4388–4406.

Badea, T. C., and Nathans, J. (2004). Quantitative analysis of neuronal morphologies in the mouse retina visualized by using a genetically directed reporter. *J. Comp. Neurol.* 480:331–351.

Braitenberg, V., and Schüz, A. (1991). *Anatomy of the cortex: Statistics and geometry*. Berlin: Springer-Verlag.

Brett-Green, B., Fifková, E., Larue, D. T., Winer, J. A., and Barth, D. S. (2003). A multisensory zone in rat parietotemporal cortex: Intra- and extracellular physiology and thalamocortical connections. *J. Comp. Neurol.* 460:223–237.

Brumberg, J. C., Hamzei-Sichani, F., and Yuste, R. (2003). Morphological and physiological characterization of layer VI corticofugal neurons of mouse primary visual cortex. *J. Neurophysiol.* 89:2854–2867.

Burkhalter, A., and Charles, V. (1990). Organization of local axon collaterals of efferent projection neurons in rat visual cortex. *J. Comp. Neurol.* 302:920–934.

Burwell, R. D., and Amaral, D. G. (1998). Cortical afferents of the perirhinal, postrhinal, and entorhinal cortices of the rat. *J. Comp. Neurol.* 398:179–205.

Burwell, R. D., and Hafeman, D. M. (2003). Positional firing properties of postrhinal cortex neurons. *Neuroscience* 119:577–588.

Carcieri, S. M, Jacobs, A. L., and Nirenberg, S. (2003). Classification of retinal ganglion cells: A statistical approach. *J. Neurophysiol.* 90:1704–1713.

Caviness, V. S. (1975). Architectonic map of neocortex of the normal mouse. *J. Comp. Neurol.* 164:247–263.

Caviness, V. S., and Frost, D. O. (1980). Tangential organization of thalamic projections to the neocortex in the mouse. *J. Comp. Neurol.* 194:335–367.

Chklovskii, D. B., and Koulakov, A. A. (2004). Maps in the brain: What can we learn from them? *Annu. Rev. Neurosci.* 27: 369–392.

Coogan, T. A., and Burkhalter, A. (1993). Hierarchical organization of areas in rat visual cortex. *J. Neurosci.* 13:3749–3772.

Coombs, J., Van Der List, D., Wang, G.-Y., and Chalupa, J. M. (2006). Morphological properties of mouse retinal ganglion cells. *Neuroscience* 140:123–136.

Dakin, S., and Frith, U. (2005). Vagaries of visual perception in autism. *Neuron* 48:497–507.

Davies, M., Machin, P. E., Sanderson, D. J., Pearce, J. M., and Aggleton, J. P. (2007). Neurotoxic lesions of the rat perirhinal and postrhinal cortices and their impact on biconditional visual discrimination tasks. *Behav. Brain Res.* 176:274–283.

DeFelipe, J., Marco, P., Fairen, A., and Jones, E. G. (1997). Inhibitory synaptogenesis in mouse somatosensory cortex. *Cereb. Cortex* 7:619–634.

De Vries, I. (1912). Über die Zytoarchitektonik der Grosshirnrinde der Maus und über die Beziehungen der einzelnen Zellschichten zum Corpus Callosum auf Grund von experimentellen Läsionen. *Folia Neurobiol. (Haarlem)* 6:289–322.

Dong, H., Shao, Z., Nerbonne, J. M., and Burkhalter, A. (2004a). Differential depression of inhibitory synaptic responses in feedforward and feedback circuits between different areas of mouse visual cortex. *J. Comp. Neurol.* 475:361–373.

Dong, H., Wang, Q., Valkova, K., Gonchar, Y., and Burkhalter, A. (2004b). Experience-dependent development of feedforward and feedback circuits between lower and higher areas of mouse visual cortex. *Vision Res.* 44:3389–3400.

Dräger, U. C. (1974). Autoradiography of tritiated proline and fucose transported transneuronally from the eye to the visual cortex in pigmented and albino mice. *Brain Res.* 82:284–292.

Dräger, U. C. (1975). Receptive fields of single cells and topography in mouse visual cortex. *J. Comp Neurol.* 160:269–290.

Dräger, U. C., and Olson, J. F. (1980). Origins of crossed and uncrossed retinal projections in pigmented and albino mice. *J. Comp. Neurol.* 191:383–412.

Eckert, M. A., Galaburda, A. M., Mills, D. L., Belluggi, U., Korenberg, J. R., and Reiss, A. L. (2006). The neurobiology of Williams syndrome: Cascading influences of visual system impairment? *Cell. Mol. Life Sci.* 63:1867–1875.

Felleman, D. J., and Van Essen, D. C. (1991). Distributed hierarchical processing in the primate cerebral cortex. *Cereb. Cortex* 1:1–47.

Fortuyn, A. (1914). Cortical cell-lamination of the hemispheres of some rodents. *Arch. Neurol. Psychiatry* 17:215–247.

Frost, D. O., and Caviness, V. S. (1980). Radial organization of thalamic projections of the neocortex in the mouse. *J. Comp. Neurol.* 194:369–393.

Gao, E., DeAngelis, G. C., and Burkhalter, A. (2006). Specialized areas for shape and motion analysis in mouse visual cortex. *Soc. Neurosci. Abstr.* 641.6.

Garey, L. J. (2006). *Brodmann's localization in the cerebral cortex*. New York: Springer-Verlag.

Godement, P., Salaün, J., and Imbert, M. (1984). Prenatal and postnatal development of retinogeniculate and retinocollicular projections in the mouse. *J. Comp. Neurol.* 230:552–575.

Grice, D. E., and Buxbaum, J. D. (2006). The genetics of autism spectrum disorders. *Neuromolecular Med.* 8:451–460.

Grubb, M. S., and Thompson, I. D. (2003). Quantitative characterization of visual response properties in the mouse dorsal lateral geniculate nucleus. *J. Neurophysiol.* 90:3594–3607.

Hall, W. C., Kaas, J. H., and Diamond, I. T. (1971). Cortical visual areas in the grey squirrel (*Sciurus carolensis*): A correlation between cortical evoked potential maps and architectonic subdivisions. *J. Neurophysiol.* 34:43–452.

Hattar, S., Kumar, M., Park, A., Tong, P., Tung, J., Yau, K. W., and Berson, D. M. (2006). Central projections of melanopsin-expressing retinal ganglion cells in the mouse. *J. Comp. Neurol.* 497:326–349.

Hubel, D. H., and Wiesel, T. N. (1965). Receptive fields and functional architecture in two nonstriate visual areas (18 and 19) of the cat. *J. Neurophysiol.* 28:229–289.

Ikegaya, Y., Aaron, G., Cossart, R., Aronov, D., Lampl, I., Ferster, D., and Yuste, R. (2004). Synfire chains and cortical songs: Temporal modules of cortical activity. *Science* 304: 559–564.

Isenschmid, R. (1911). Zur Kenntnis der Grosshirnrinde der Maus. *Abhandl. Königl. Preuss. Akad. Wiss.* 3:1–46.

Just, M. A., Cherkassky, V. L., Keller, T. A., Kana, R. K., and Minshew, N. J. (2007). Functional and anatomical cortical underconnectivity in autism: Evidence from fMRI study of an executive function and task and corpus callosum optometry. *Cereb. Cortex* 17:951–961.

Kaas, J., Hall, W. C., and Diamond, I. T. (1970). Cortical visual areas I and II in the hedgehog: Relation between evoked potential maps and architectonic subdivisions. *J. Neurophysiol.* 33: 595–615.

Kalatsky, V. A., and Stryker, M. P. (2003). New paradigm for optical imaging: Temporally encoded maps of intrinsic signal. *Neuron* 38:529–545.

Kalia, M., and Whitteridge, D. (1973). The visual areas in the splenial sulcus of the cat. *J. Physiol.* 232:275–283.

Kong, J.-H., Fish, D. R., Rockhill, R. J., and Masland, R. H. (2005). Diversity of ganglion cells in the mouse retina: Unsupervised morphological classification and its limits. *J. Comp. Neurol.* 489:293–310.

Kozloski, J., Hamzei-Sichani, F., and Yuste, R. (2001). Stereotyped position of local synaptic targets in neocortex. *Science* 292:868–872.

Krieg, W. J. S. (1946). Connections of the cerebral cortex. *J. Comp. Neurol.* 84:278–323.

Larsen, D. D., and Callaway, E. M. (2006). Development of layer-specific axonal arborizations in mouse primary somatosensory cortex. *J. Comp. Neurol.* 494:398–414.

McDonald, A. J., and Mascagni, F. (1996). Cortico-cortical and cortico-amygdaloid projections of the rat occipital cortex: A *Phaseolus vulgaris* leucoagglutinin study. *Neuroscience* 71:37–54.

Métin, C., Godement, P., and Imbert, M. (1988). The primary visual cortex in the mouse: Receptive field properties and functional organization. *Exp. Brain Res.* 69:594–612.

Meyer-Lindenberg, A., Kohn, P., Mervis, C. B., Kippenhan, J. S., Olsen, R. K., Morris, C. A., and Berman, K. F. (2004). Neural basis of genetically determined visuospatial construction deficit in Williams syndrome. *Neuron* 43:623–631.

Miller, M. W., and Vogt, B. A. (1984). Direct connections of rat visual cortex with sensory, motor, and association cortices. *J. Comp. Neurol.* 226:184–202.

Montero, V. M. (1993). Retinotopy of cortical connections between the striate cortex and extrastriate visual areas in the rat. *Exp. Brain Res.* 94:1–15.

Neafsey, E. J. (1990). The complete ratunculus: Output organization of layer V of the cerebral cortex. In B. Kolb and R. C. Tees (Eds.), *The cerebral cortex of the rat* (pp. 197–212). Cambridge, MA: MIT Press.

Olavarria, J., Mignano, L. R., and Van Sluyters, R. C. (1982). Pattern of extrastriate visual areas connecting reciprocally with striate cortex in mouse. *Exp. Neurol.* 78:775–779.

Olavarria, J., and Montero, V. M. (1984). Relation of callosal and striate-extrastriate cortical connections in the rat: Morphological definition of extrastriate visual areas. *Exp. Brain Res.* 54:240–252.

Olavarria, J., and Montero, M. V. (1989). Organization of visual cortex in the mouse revealed by correlating callosal and striate-extrastriate connections. *Vis. Neurosci.* 3:59–69.

Pang, J. J., Gao, F., and Wu, S. M. (2003). Light-evoked excitatory and inhibitory synaptic inputs to ON and OFF alpha ganglion cells in the mouse retina. *J. Neurosci.* 23:6063–6073.

Paxinos, G., and Franklin, K. B. J. (2001). *The mouse brain in stereotaxic coordinates.* New York: Academic Press.

Polleux, F., and Lauder, J. M. (2004). Toward a developmental neurobiology of autism. *Ment. Retard. Dev. Dis. Res. Rev.* 10: 303–317.

Prusky, G. T., Douglas, R. M., Nelson, L., Shabanpoor, A., and Sutherland, R. J. (2004). Visual memory task for rats reveals an essential role for hippocampus and perirhinal cortex. *Proc. Natl. Acad. Sci. U.S.A.* 101:5064–5068.

Roe, A. W. and Ts'o, D. Y. (1995). Visual topography in primate V2: Multiple representations across functional stripes. *J. Neurosci.* 15:3689–3715.

Rosa, M. G. P., and Krubitzer, L. A. (1999). The evolution of visual cortex: Where is V2? *Trends Neurosci.* 22:242–248.

Rose, M. (1912). Histologische Lokalisation der Grosshirnrinde bei kleinen Säugetieren (Rodentia, Insectivora, Chiroptera). *J. Psychol. Neurol.* 19:119–479.

Rose, M. (1929). Cytoarchitektonischer Atlas der Grosshirnrinde der Maus. *J. Psychol. Neurol.* 40:1–32.

Rumberger, A., Tyler, C. J., and Lund, J. S. (2001). Intra- and inter-areal connections between the primary visual cortex V1 and the areas immediately surrounding V1 in the rat. *Neuroscience* 102:35–52.

Sanides, F., and Hoffman, J. (1969). Cyto- and myeloarchitecture of the visual cortex of the cat and the surrounding integration cortices. *J. Hirnforsch.* 11:79–104.

Save, E., Paz-Villagran, V., Alexinsky, T., and Poucet, B. (2005). Functional interaction between the associative parietal cortex and hippocampal place cell firing in the rat. *J. Eur. Neurosci.* 21:522–530.

Schuett, S., Bonhoffer, T., and Hübener, M. (2002). Mapping retinotopic structure in mouse visual cortex with optical imaging. *J. Neurosci.* 22:6549–6559.

Schüz, A., Chaimov, D., Liewald, D., and Dortenman, M. (2006). Quantitative aspects of cortical connections: A tracer study in the mouse. *Cereb. Cortex* 16:1474–1486.

Simmons, P. A., Lemmon, V., and Pearlman, A. L. (1982). Afferent and efferent connections of the striate and extrastriate visual cortex of the normal and reeler mouse. *J. Comp. Neurol.* 211: 295–308.

Stone, C., and Pinto, L. H. (1993). Response properties of retinal ganglion cells in the isolated mouse retina. *Vis. Neurosci.* 10: 31–39.

Striedter, G. F. (2006). *Principles of brain evolution.* Sunderland, MA: Sinauer.

Sun, W., Li, N., and He, S. (2002). Large-scale morphological survey of mouse retinal ganglion cells. *J. Comp. Neurol.* 451: 115–126.

Taube, J. S. (1998). Head direction cells and the neurophysiological basis for a sense of direction. *Prog. Neurobiol.* 55:225–256.

Thomas, H. C., and Espinoza, S. G. (1987). Relationship between interhemispheric cortical connections and visual areas in hooded rats. *Brain Res.* 417:214–224.

Toldi, J., Fehér, O., and Wolf, J. R. (1986). Sensory interactive zones in the rat cerebral cortex. *Neuroscience* 18:461–465.

Tsiola, A., Hamzei-Sichani, F., Peterlin, Z., and Yuste, R. (2003). Quantitative morphologic classification of layer 5 neurons from mouse primary visual cortex. *J. Comp. Neurol.* 461:415–428.

Ungerleider, L. G., and Pasternak, T. (2004). Ventral and dorsal cortical processing streams. In L. M. Chalupa and J. S. Werner (Eds.), *The visual neurosciences* (pp. 541–562). Cambridge, MA: MIT Press.

Usrey, W. M., and Reid, R. C. (2000). Visual physiology and the lateral geniculate nucleus in two species of New World monkey: *Saimiri sciureus* and *Aotus trivirgatus*. *J. Physiol.* 523.3:755–769.

Valverde, F. (1968). Structural changes in the area striate of the mouse after enucleation. *Exp. Brain Res.* 5:274–292.

Valverde, F. (1976). Aspects of cortical organization related to the geometry of neurons with intra-cortical axons. *J. Neurocytol.* 5:509–529.

Valverde, F., and Estéban, E. (1968). Peristriate cortex of mouse: Location and the effects of enucleation on the number of dendritic spines. *Brain Res.* 9:145–148.

Van Essen, D. C. (1979). Visual areas of the mammalian cerebral cortex. *Annu. Rev. Neurosci.* 2:227–263.

Van Essen, D. C., Dierker, D., Snyder, A. Z., Raichle, M. E., Reiss, A. L., and Korenberg, J. (2006). Symmetry of cortical folding abnormalities in Williams syndrome revealed by surface-based analyses. *J. Neurosci.* 26:5470–5483.

Van Essen, D. C., and Maunsell, J. H. R. (1981). The middle temporal visual area in the macaque: Myeloarchitecture, connections, functional properties and topographic organization. *J. Comp Neurol.* 199:293–326.

Van Hooser, S. D., Heimel, J. A., Chung., S., and Nelson, S. B. (2006). Lack of patchy horizontal connectivity in primary visual cortex of a mammal without orientation maps. *J Neurosci.* 26:7680–7692.

Van Hooser, S. D., Heimel, J. A., and Nelson, S. B. (2003). Receptive field properties and laminar organization of lateral geniculate nucleus in the gray squirrel (*Sciurus carolensis*). *J. Neurophysiol.* 90:3398–3418.

Wagor, E., Mangini, N. J., and Pearlman, A. L. (1980). Retinotopic organization of striate and extrastriate visual cortex in the mouse. *J. Comp. Neurol.* 193:187–202.

Wang, Q., and Burkhalter, A. (2003). Anatomical evidence for different processing streams in mouse visual cortex. *Soc. Neurosci. Abstr.* 701.3.

Wang, Q., and Burkhalter, A. (2004). Dorsal and ventral streams for processing of visual information in mouse cerebral cortex. *Soc. Neurosci. Abstr.* 300.5.

Wang, Q., and Burkhalter, A. (2005). Separate output streams from V1 to higher areas of mouse visual cortex. *Soc. Neurosci. Abstr.* 854.1.

Wang, Q., and Burkhalter, A. (2007). Area map of mouse visual cortex. *J. Comp. Neurol.* 502(3):339–357.

Yamashita, A., Valkova., K., Gonchar., Y., and Burkhalter, A. (2003). Rearrangement of synaptic connections with inhibitory neurons in developing mouse visual cortex. *J. Comp. Neurol.* 464:426–437.

IV DEVELOPMENT OF THE MOUSE EYE

21 Chronology of Development of the Mouse Visual System: Comparisons with Human Development

BARBARA L. FINLAY AND BARBARA CLANCY

In this first era of genomic analysis of neural systems, the emphasis falls on what genes code, where particular genes are expressed, and what kinds of disorders appear when genes are mutated, absent, or misapplied. Less emphasis is placed on when and for how long genes are expressed, and less still on the control that coordinates the expression of ensembles of genes that construct developing sensory systems and brains. Control of the timing and duration of gene expression is certainly the major way in which vertebrate eyes differ from each other, because vertebrate eyes are quite conservative in their cell types, neurotransmitters, neuromodulators, and general structure (Rodieck, 1973; Arendt, 2003), with variation in opsins the notable exception (Shyue et al., 1995). The most significant differences in vertebrate eyes are in size, in the ratios of numbers of cell types, and in the arrangement of these cells. These differences suggest that alterations in the control of genes expressed, rather than the nature of the genes expressed, is the principal source of variation in evolution. Understanding the class of variations in developmental timing that can give rise to functional eyes should be a focus of genomic work as well. How the components of the eye are caused to scale gracefully and integrate with each other gives us a different way of approaching the genome than the more static version presented by the study of a single species.

The conservation of the constitutive elements of the eye, and of the visual system in general, is thus good and bad news for the mouse model. Because of the conservation, mechanistic comparability in most domains will be good. On the other hand, permissible and pathological variations in the duration and timing of gene expression are difficult to distinguish or characterize in an animal with such a relatively brief gestation period (ca. 18.5 days). The qualitative trait locus method of correlating variations in parameters such as brain size or gestational length with regions of the genome (e.g., Zhou and Williams, 1999) is a first step toward integrating intra- and interspecies variation with pathological variation. In addition, some natural variations in rapidly and slowly developing mice chimeras could be used to investigate basic questions about overarching control of rates of neurodevelopment (Williams and Goldowitz, 1992).

Understanding the chronology of development has an empirical aspect and a theoretical aspect. In this chapter, we first describe the chronology of development of the mouse visual system in relation to that in humans and monkeys, using a comprehensive model we and our colleagues have developed. This model capitalizes on the essential conservation of developmental timing in mammals for interspecies comparison and for interpolating missing data accurately in those cases where the data have not been or cannot be determined empirically (neurogenesis data, for example, require invasive techniques). This database is intended as a resource for the optimal developmental placement of any observation or experiment, as well as for investigating the control of developmental timing per se. We point out areas of greatest similarity between mice, other experimental animals, and humans that suggest the most reliable prediction, and also point out areas of difference that would make the mouse model less reliable. Finally, we suggest areas of investigation that would be particularly interesting to pursue in light of mouse and human similarities and differences in chronology.

Timetable of mouse development

Table 21.1 lists the observed and computed times of various visual developmental events in mouse, human, and rhesus macaque, all given in postconception (PC) days, where the day of conception is designated day zero. This table is excerpted from a much more extensive database that includes 102 events in early development (principally neurogenesis, tract formation, and structure innervation) from all sensory

Table 21.1

Observed and computed (predicted) times of visual developmental events in mouse, human, and rhesus macaque (PC days)

Structure	Event	Mouse		Human		Monkey	
		Pred.	Obs.	Pred.	Obs.	Pred.	Obs.
Retina	*Ganglion cell—start*	*10*	*10.5*	*38.1*		*30.8*	*30*
Cortex	Subplate—start	10.1	10	48.2		38.7	39.5
SC	Superficial SC—start	10.7	10.5	41.9		33.8	30
LGN	dLGN—start	10.8	10.5	43		34.6	36
Cortex	Subplate—peak	10.9	11	54.5		43.6	43
Cortex	Cortical layer VI—start	11.4	11	57.9		46.3	45
LGN	vLGN—peak	11.7	11.5	47.9		38.4	
Optic nerve	Axons in optic stalk	11.7	12.3	48.2	51	38.7	
Connectivity	Internal capsule appears	11.7		60.8	63	48.5	40
LGN	dLGN—peak	12	12	50		40.1	43
Optic nerve	Optic axons at chiasm	12.2	13	50.9		40.8	36
Retina	*Horizontal cells—peak*	*12.4*		*52.4*		*42*	*40*
SC	SC—peak	12.7	13	53.9		43.1	41
LGN	dLGN—end	12.8	12.5	54.4		43.5	43
Cortex	Cortical layer V—start	12.8	12	68.6		54.6	58.5
Retina	*Ganglion cells—peak*	*12.9*	*13*	*55.6*		*44.4*	*43*
Cortex	Subplate—end	12.9	12	69.8		55.6	48
Cortex	Layer VI—peak	13	12.5	70.3		56	53
Optic nerve	Axons reach dLGN and SC	13.7	14.5	59.8		47.7	
Optic nerve	Axons invade visual centers	14.2	15.5	63.2	60	50.4	
SC	Superficial SC—end	14.2	14	62.8		50.1	56
Cortex	Layer V—peak	14.2	13	79.7		63.3	70
Cortex	Lamina VI—end	14.4	13	80.8		64.2	65
Cortex	Lamina IV—start	14.4	15	81.2		64.5	70
Retina	*Cones—peak*	*14.8*	*14*	*66.3*		*52.8*	*56*
Retina	*Amacrine cells—peak*	*15.3*	*15*	*69.3*		*55.2*	*56*
Cortex	Layer II/III—start	15.2		87.4		69.4	85.5
Cortex	Layer V—end	15.3	14	87.8		69.7	75
Cortex	Layer IV—peak	15.5	17	89.3		70.9	80
Retina	*Ganglion cells—end*	*15.8*	*18.5*	*72.4*		*57.6*	*57*
Connectivity	Corpus callosum appears	15.9	17	92.6	87.5	73.4	
Connectivity	LGN axons in subplate	16.2		94.7		75.1	78
Connectivity	Cortical axons reach dLGN	16.3		95.9		76	67
Cortex	Layer II/III—peak	16.9	15	100.4		79.6	90
Cortex	Layer IV—end	17.1	17	101.7		80.5	85
Optic nerve	Axonal number—peak	17.2		80.9		64.3	69
Cortex	Layer II/III—end	18.3		110.6		87.5	100
Connectivity	Cortical axons in dLGN	18.4		111.5		88.2	81.5
Connectivity	LGN axons in layer IV	21.1		132.3		104.5	91
SC	Superficial—start lamination	21.2		104.7		82.9	86
Retina	*Rods—peak of neurogenesis*	*21.6*	*19*	*106.9*		*84.6*	*85*
Connectivity	Cortical axons in SC	22.5		143.2		113.1	96
Retina	*Onset of retinal waves*	*20.6*		*101.3*		*80.2*	
Retina	*Bipolar cells—peak*	*23*		*115.6*		*91.4*	*85*
Optic nerve	Rapid axonal loss ends	24.3		123.1		97.3	110
LGN/SC	Ipsi-, contralateral segregation	24.5	25.5	124.4	175	98.3	87
Eye opening	Eye opening	29.7	30	155.4	158	122.6	123

Note: Table lists model-derived values (Pred.) versus empirical observations (Obs.) for the postconceptional day of occurrence of various developmental events in the laboratory mouse, human, and rhesus macaque. Retinal events are in italic type for easier identification.
LGN, lateral geniculate nucleus; SC, superior colliculus.

systems and brain regions, and 10 species (also hamster, rat, rabbit, spiny mouse, guinea pig, ferret, and cat). The complete database (www.translatingtime.net) describes the sources in more detail and allows calculation of the desired developmental windows in the species listed; it also gives the confidence intervals for each value calculated (Clancy et al., 2007). Predicted developmental times are derived through a general linear model incorporating all the data sources listed on the Web site; a sample calculation on the site is shown in figure 21.1. This model was first derived for a more limited set of developmental events (principally neurogenesis) and a more limited set of species to query about a systematic function to transform the schedule of developmental events of one species into the developmental schedule of another (Finlay and Darlington, 1995; Finlay et al., 1998, 2001). It proved possible to do so with high accuracy, and in subsequent versions the model was expanded to include marsupial mammals and more classes of developmental events (Darlington et al., 1999), to account for the particular deviations of primates in the timing of cortical versus limbic developmental events (Clancy et al., 1999), and finally, to include more species, including humans (Clancy et al., 2001). These citations, as well as the Web site, give the references to the source empirical data; the majority of sources for the mouse data included here come from the laboratories of Angevine, Sidman, Caviness, and their collaborators, and the monkey data come from Rakic and collaborators.

The model predicts PC dates transformed to the mathematical term Y as $Y = \ln$ (PC days − 4.34). The form of the equation, containing a natural logarithm modified by a constant, is the empirically determined best-fitting function for this data. The biological significance of the constant (4.34) is probably that the function fits best with its zero located after early germinal events (blastulation, differentiation of basic germinal layers) common to all eutherian mammals have occurred, averaging 4.34 days. The biological account of why a logarithmic function best fits the relation between developmental schedules is not so clear (in contrast to, for example, the inaccurate multiplicative rule of thumb that is used to transform dog years to human years). The greater separation, in absolute days, of late events in slow-developing species compared with separation of the same events in more rapidly developing species is the feature of the data reflected in the log function.

Each neural event in the database is assigned an event score (with later events having higher scores), and each species is assigned a species score (with slower-developing species having higher scores) consistent with the general linear model described previously (Darlington, 1990; Finlay and Darlington, 1995). Then Y is modeled as the sum of three terms: the event score, the species score, and a primate interaction term where appropriate. The primate interaction factor accounts for the fact that limbic and cortical components of rodent and human brains mature at different rates with respect to the rest of the brain (Clancy et al., 1999). This third factor adds 0.248683 to the estimated Y score of every primate cortical event and subtracts 0.079280 from the estimated Y score of every primate limbic event. This general linear model has been fitted simultaneously to all cells with data, but it also generates estimates for cells with no empirical data (figure 21.2).

Technical and qualitative evaluation of the model's predictions

Utilizing a regression model to formulate predictions is unusual in developmental neurobiology, and we spend some time here describing considerations at several levels that

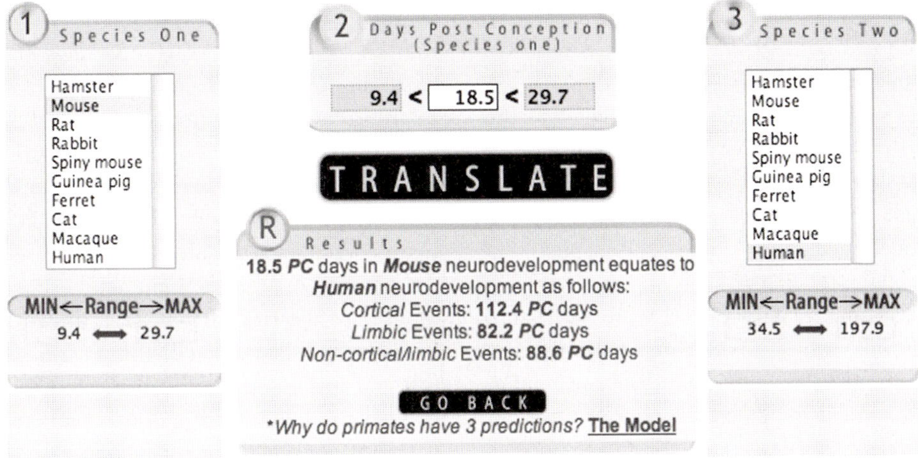

FIGURE 21.1 Representative Web page (www.translatingtime.net) depicting a "translation" from mouse on the day of birth to human neurodevelopmental time. The model predicts that neural events that occur in the mouse brain on the day of birth (14.5 days post-conception, PC) translate into PC112 in human cortical development, PC82 in human limbic system development, and PC88 for noncortical, nonlimbic neural events.

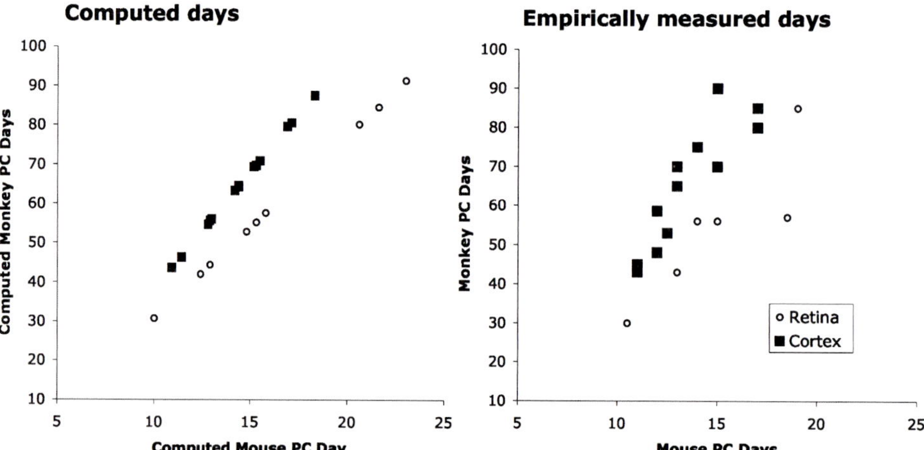

FIGURE 21.2 These graphs contrast the overall function relating the PC day of a number of developmental events in the mouse (x-axis) to the monkey (y-axis). Plot at *left* shows the generalized relationship determined from a much larger sample of neuroembryological events and species; plot at right shows the empirical measures made for the visual system of mice and monkeys, using data drawn from table 21.1. There are fewer measured than computed events because the generalized function computes a value for all desired events, not just the ones measured empirically for these two species. A further contrast is made in both graphs concerning the different scaling of the cortex (*black squares*) versus the retina (*white circles*) between primates and rodents.

should guide the use of this model in empirical applications. Fitting any mathematical model involves three steps: (1) selecting the variables to include in the model, together with the general way they will be combined (e.g., additively, multiplicatively), (2) estimating the specific numerical values to be used in the model, and (3) testing the fit of data to model. We are convinced that we have the correct overall form for the model based on the high correlation (0.990223) between observed values and the model's predictions, this based on the extended data set (Clancy et al., 2007). We should also mention that exhaustive investigation of potential additional factors (by species hierarchies, by grouping of functional systems such as visual or auditory, or grouping by location, such as midbrain or spinal cord) produce no further improvements in predictability. Even though the correlations are high, however, the specific numerical values predicted by the model do not exactly match the available empirical data, particularly for the human data (see table 21.1 and figure 21.2). Based on the assumption just mentioned, how do we understand the model's accuracy?

SAFETY IN NUMBERS Empirical investigators are aware that their observations can be subject to individual variation and observational error, and this is especially true for human developmental data, where specimens are rather rare and often subject to errors in birth dating. For this particular database, intralaboratory differences in the interpretation of such events as "first retinal axons in LGN" are an additional source of concern. However, when numerous error-plagued figures are averaged, the average is likely to be more accurate than the individual figures. The same is true for statistical models of the type described here. Since the estimates generated by the model are each based on all the observations used to build the model, errors can average out, making the model's estimates more accurate than the individual observations on which the model was based.

An illustrative example of the bootstrap effect can be seen in simple regression. Suppose a regression has been derived in a sample of 200 mice, predicting an animal's weight from its age in days, for ages running from one to 100 days. To estimate the average weight of a mouse at 50 days, one could use the regression model (entering age = 50) or one could average the weights of the one or two mice in the sample that happened to be exactly 50 days of age when studied. Assuming a linear relation, the regression model is likely to give a far more accurate estimate of the value of interest than an average of one or two weights. The same argument applies to more complex regression models, such as the one described in this chapter (Clancy et al., 2001). The difference between model predictions and empirical observations for retinal and cortical developmental events in monkey versus mouse are shown in figure 21.2, drawn directly from table 21.1. (It should be noted that the range of empirical observations for this comparison is truncated because there is not a complete matching range of observations).

Because of the difficulty encountered when working with humans, published human data appear to contain about twice as much error as figures for other species, as measured by the fit of human data to the model described here (Clancy et al., 2001). Thus the model is particularly useful for estimating neural dates in humans, not because the model estimates dates for humans better than for other species (it does not) but because the alternatives may be so much worse. Insofar as each predicted event is based not simply on data available for that particular species but on data available for all species, the model is less restricted than might be expected from the limited—or even inaccurate—data set pertaining to humans. Although we are confident the predictions and comparisons for the neural events that are included in our database are of value, we also caution against overeager interpretations until more data become available.

Production of the cortex: Timetable differs in primates

In figure 21.2, the events associated with corticogenesis and maturation (*black squares*) are contrasted with events associate with the retina (*open circles*), with the timing of mouse events plotted against the same events in rhesus macaque. This figure demonstrates that at any given developmental day, events that occur at the same time in the retina and cortex of the mouse occur at a corresponding time in the retina but later in the cortex in the monkey. This effect is specific to the primates of this database (human and rhesus macaque), not simply any animal with a brain larger than a mouse's. So, for example, the peak of cone generation and the start of generation of pyramidal cells destined for layers II/III of the cortex both happen on PC14 in the mouse but separate in the monkey to occur between PC53 for the retina event and PC69 for the cortical event. All noncortical events (with the exception of the limbic system, not shown here) scale with the retina, which has been selected for illustrative purposes only for figure 21.2. For example, to take another subcortical event that happens at about the same time in the mouse, the end of generation of the superficial layers of the superior colliculus occurs on PC14 in the mouse and PC50 in the monkey. Therefore, to set up appropriate comparisons in experiments, the different scales of the cortex compared to the rest of the brain in primates must be attended to.

This timing difference correlates with an allometric difference in overall brain organization of rodents versus primates, one that has been described in detail numerous times: in rodents and insectivores, relatively more neural mass is allocated to olfactory bulb, olfactory cortex, and entorhinal, subicular, and hippocampal cortices, as well as other basal forebrain structures (the classic limbic system), while in primates relatively more mass is allocated to the neocortex (Jerison, 1973; Gould, 1975; Stephan et al., 1988). We have argued that not only is the difference in developmental timing correlated with the varying size of brain components, it is the direct cause of it, using the shorthand of "late equals large" (Finlay et al., 2001; Reep et al., 2007). In the monkey, the "birthdays" of neurons destined for limbic structures occur comparatively earlier than they would in rodents, which corresponds to precursor cells becoming postmitotic and removing themselves from the precursor pool, thus depleting it. By contrast, the birthdays of cells destined for cortex are comparatively later in primates, allowing their precursor pools to proliferate exponentially for a longer time and thus become disproportionately large.

This timing distinction may have some consequences for the organization of innervation between structures, including guidance molecules and trophic support. A debate existed for some time, for example, about whether there was a "waiting period" for thalamocortical axons in the subplate region or whether thalamocortical fibers directly invaded the cortical plate on arrival (Miller et al., 1990; Catalano et al., 1991; Ghosh and Shatz, 1992). The debate may have been caused directly by this species difference, since the studies that suggested direct innervation were done in rodents, while those suggesting a "waiting period" were done in the cat. Carnivores' cortices scale in the direction of primates' (Reep et al., 2007), and the measured times of cat corticogenesis systematically occur later than their predicted times, though the trend is not distinct enough to justify a "carnivore" factor.

What mice cannot model in human developmental timing

A notable feature of the development of the monkey and human retina that is deliberately absent from table 21.1 is the presence of distinct gradients of neurogenesis and other aspects of maturation within single cell classes, such as retinal ganglion cells (RGCs), or the sublaminae of layer IV of cortex (Rakic, 1974; Rapaport et al., 1992, 1996). In the retina, for example, a distinct gradient of neurogenesis from the center to the periphery of the retina is observed in every mammal studied. Most pronounced is the offset of neurogenesis—the peak of rod neurogenesis in the retina center—in monkey is PC70, but for the very periphery it is PC120 (Rapaport et al., 1996). This allows the extracellular environment of groups of precursor cells to be systematically biased by their spatial location, which is employed to advantage to produce regional differences in the retina. Though the "clock" of cell specification appears to proceed in a rather uniform manner across the retina surface in the well-established order of ganglion cells, cones, amacrine cells, rod, and rod bipolar cells (figure 21.3), the early provision and cessation of precursor cells for specification in the central retina produces an abundance of RGCs and cones and fewer rods, with the opposite the case in the peripheral retina (Cepko et al., 1996; Finlay et al., 2005b). The short distances and time available in the mouse retina appear to produce only the shallowest gradients of cell classes across the retinal surface, while in the monkey, the pronounced gradients produce no rods in the central retina (the eventual

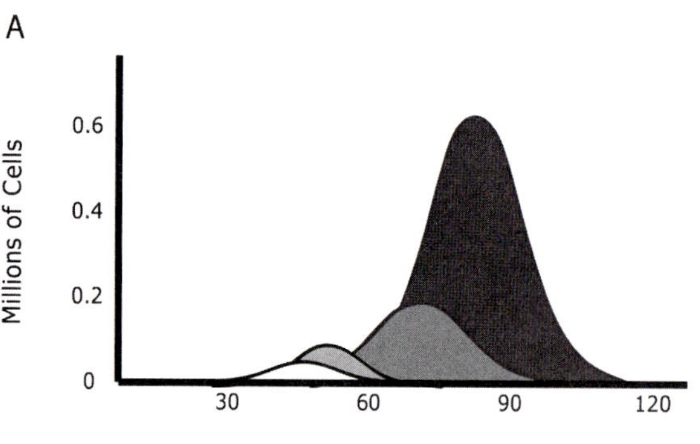

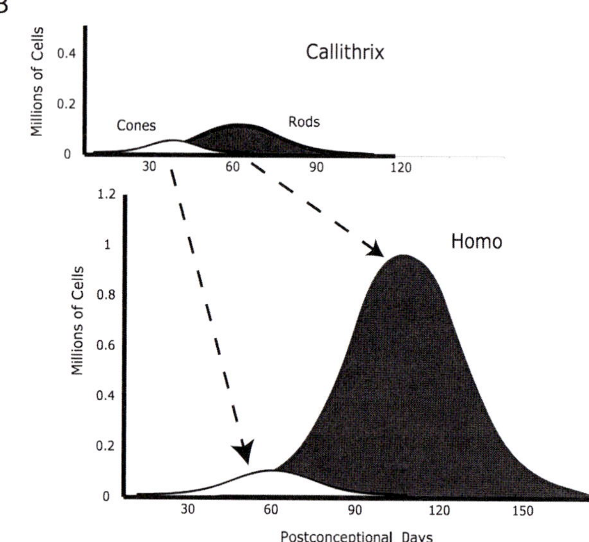

FIGURE 21.3 *A*, Schematized order of production of retinal ganglion cells, cones, bipolar cells, and rods in the retina of rhesus macaque. For the two types of neurons omitted from this map, horizontal cells virtually overlap cones; amacrine cells lead bipolars slightly. The abscissa shows the postconceptional day of terminal cell division, the ordinate the percentage of each cell class produced on that day. *B*, Schematic demonstrating how extension of the period of retina neurogenesis may disproportionately increase the number of later-generated cell groups, in this case rods, by allowing a disproportionate increase in the precursor pool from which later cell groups are drawn.

site of the fovea) and an abundance of rods with virtually no cones in the very periphery. It is possible that the extension of the gradient producing the retina in primates that resulted in a small rod-free region might serve as the initial signaling event to locate the fovea, and that secondary events, such as the compaction of cone outer segments and displacement of cell bodies, might be instigated by this time-based morphological singularity (Finlay et al., 2005b). Insofar as these unusual cell complements might be the features permissive of the production of the notable primate specialization of the fovea and whatever new features of genetic specialization that come linked to it, there can be no real mouse homologue, as the fovea is linked to a feature of retinal chronology that mice simply do not have.

The layers of the cortex are a comparable case: every mammal studied exhibits the well-known inside-out gradient of corticogenesis (Rakic, 1974). In mice, however, the overlapping nature of the layer gradients and the small numbers of cells produced would make lamination in cortical layer IV unobservable, though possibly the features that give rise to lamination in a larger structure might be distributed through it (Sidman and Angevine, 1962). In passing, while much has been made of cortical "uniformity" across species (Rockel et al., 1980), it simply is not so. As the cortex gets larger overall, it also increases in column depth somewhat, and the increase in number is most pronounced in the upper cortical layers, 4 and 2/3. In the animals with the smallest extent of neocortex, layer 4, as distinguished by the presence of spiny stellate cells (Valverde, 1990), may be entirely absent, with thalamocortical axons terminating on the basal dendrites of layer 3 pyramidal cells.

The variability of mouse strains

The often deliberately inbred, "unselected" nature of the various mouse strains raises concern about how representative the mouse is of general mammalian brain organization. And there is some cause for concern: for example, in an allometric study of the relative sizes of subcortical components of the auditory system in a wide range of mammals, the mouse was a notable outlier, along with the little brown bat and the mountain beaver, even though there is no reason to suspect any unusual functionality of the auditory system in the mouse (Glendenning and Masterton, 1998). We have been collecting data on strain variability in the relative sizes of brain parts and comparing examples of individual mouse strains (11 individuals) with individual wild and domesticated pigs (24 individuals) and wild and domesticated minks (12 individuals) (Finlay et al., 2005a, analyzing data from Kruska, 1988, and from the Mouse Brain Library, www.mbl.org). When we examined the factorial structure of the size of brain components in this unusual collection of animals, data from four of 49 individuals fell outside the 90% confidence interval, and of those four, three were mice, each of a different strain. Although this study is preliminary, and the majority of the mouse strains used fell into the range of normal variability, it suggests that in planning future studies it would not be a wasted effort to pay close attention to the normality of the structure to be studied in whichever mouse strain is chosen.

What evolutionary variability suggests we should look for in mouse models of the developing visual system

The studies of comparative brain allometry and timing described so far highlight questions of the relative sizes of structures and the problems that arise from scaling animals over a variety of sizes, and these questions have been addressed in the mouse genome literature. Williams and colleagues have done multiple studies employing natural variation in brain and eye size in mouse strains to highlight regions of the genome involved in control of retinal, visual system, and overall brain size (Williams et al., 1996, 1998; Strom and Williams, 1998; Zhou and Williams, 1999; Airey et al., 2001; Seecharan et al., 2003). Several studies have examined mutations and deletions in mice that have caused the development of abnormally large cortices (Chenn and Walsh, 2002; Kingsbury et al., 2003). Researchers studying the control of cortex size in rodents naturally speculate that the mutations they see might be involved in the production of the "unusually developed" human cortex. Is this a possibility? We are entering an entirely unexplored field when we ask what the relationship is among evolutionary variability, variability between individual species members, "natural" pathology of the kind found in human development that we would like to remediate, and the induced pathologies we might see as a result of mutations and deletions of the mouse genome. We might caricature two types of views of the genome, one in which each feature of the visual system, each cell type in the retina, each connection decision, each instruction for cellular growth, has its own committed and relatively encapsulated genomic machinery. This is in contrast to a second view, in which all features of cell morphology, connectivity, and function are overlapping and contingent, where all the action is in the control genes to set very general parameters of size and timing. We would expect very different relationships among evolutionary variation, individual variation, naturally occurring pathology, and induced pathology, depending on the view of the genome we hold.

We present two pieces of evidence that the emerging features of conserved developmental timing are employed to advantage for the scaling of visual system structures. Both suggest that individual variability and phylogenetic variability are tightly linked at the level of control genes (Finlay et al., 2005b), and both are based on the fundamental evolutionary scaling concept that late equals large. In other words, if the schedule of cytogenesis or neurogenesis is extended to make a larger eye, brain, or visual system, those groups of cells exiting cytogenesis last will have a longer time to experience the exponential growth of precursor doubling and will become disproportionately large compared with cell groups exiting early. The most obvious example of this phenomenon is the size of the spinal cord relative to cortex between small- and large-brained mammals. Similarly, if the time of precursor cell differentiation is pushed early or late, as previously described for the cortex and limbic system, the associated structure will become smaller or larger accordingly. The overwhelming evidence in the case of the brains of eutherian mammals is that in order to become larger, brains are made for a longer time, not generated at a faster rate (Darlington et al., 1999).

Scaling the eye and the cortex

The eyes of diurnal primates are large absolutely compared with those of most mammals and scale allometrically with body size (Ross, 2000), ranging from around 10 mm in diameter in the smallest monkeys to around 30 mm in various anthropoid apes and humans (Heesy and Ross, 2001). Scaling an organ (made of cells of constrained size) that has several geometrical features under different constraints is an interesting construction puzzle—not all parts of the eye may scale the same and retain function. The overall conformation of the optics of the eye scale up linearly. For example, the eye of the rat and the eye of the mouse, appropriately scaled, are superimposable (Remtulla and Hallet, 1985). Within the eye, however, retinal thickness may not vary much, owing to the constraints of perfusion and light passage, and stays close to a thickness of approximately 200 μm.

Numbers of rods and cones must scale at different slopes with eye size in order to hold constant their particular functions. If an eye becomes twice as large in diameter, no change in the number of cones is necessary to retain the same visual acuity: since the retina is flooded with photons in diurnal vision, a single cone will have no difficulty encountering a photon in the visual angle it represents, regardless of the angle the cone itself subtends. More cones could be added to improve acuity, but we are discussing here what is required to maintain equivalent, not improved, function over different eye sizes.

The same solution will not work for rods. At low light levels and low photon numbers, a single rod located in a larger absolute retinal angle will fail to detect most photons, even allowing for biologically plausible increases in the size of a single rod. Rods must tile the surface of the retina to maintain sensitivity, increasing in number approximately as the square of change in retinal diameter. The observed scaling of rods and cones in diurnal primates conforms closely to this functional necessity: where cones increase in number by less than a factor of 2 between marmosets (*Callithrix jacchus*) and humans, rods increase by more than a factor of 10 (Finlay et al., 2005b).

How is this consistent, within- and across-species scaling executed in the schedule of neurogenesis of the retina? Although the precise kinetics remain to be worked out, the schedule of neurogenesis in the retina is arranged such that extension of the period of embryogenesis automatically produces the desired differential scaling. Such is the case for the relative timing of cone and rod neurogenesis in the retina, as modeled for marmoset versus human (see figure 21.3). Those cell types that must change in number exponentially with eye diameter, rods and their attendant bipolar cells are differentiated last, and those that need not change are produced first. Those potential ancestors with the opposite order of neurogenesis in the retina that might have had a selective advantage at a larger body size but that unfortunately became blind in the dark as a result presumably would enjoy less reproductive success.

This obligatory, coordinated scaling of retinal cell classes to match functional requirements has direct consequences for the kind of genetic control we might look for. For example, a researcher noticing the markedly large number of rods in the human retina might be tempted to look for the genetic specification events that produce the greater number. We argue that there is no such effect, except for the genetic event that causes the overall extension of neurogenesis for the entire brain, because the change in the relative numbers of rods and cones in larger eyes comes directly out of the kinetics of cell division and the longer period of neurogenesis required for larger retinas.

The enlarged size of the human cortex has a similar explanation. It has been shown repeatedly that the size of the cortex and the size of its subcomponents, such as primary visual cortex, or frontal cortex in humans, are precisely the size they should be with respect to overall brain size (visual cortex: Frahm et al., 1984; Kaskan et al., 2005; frontal cortex: Hofman, 1989; Jerison, 1997; Semendeferi et al., 2002). We argue that this phenomenon has exactly the same late-equals-large explanation given for the rods and cones in the retina, and that the apparently disproportionate size of the human cortex similarly falls directly out of cell cycle kinetics and an extended period of neurogenesis, given first a larger allocation of precursor cells to the cortex in all primates. Therefore, mutations in mice that cause unusual proliferation of the cortex through alterations in the rate of proliferation or changes in the amount of early cell death, though very interesting, would be unlikely to have anything to do with the particular size of the human cortex. Mutations in genes that alter cortex size may well be involved in the normal regulation of cortex size in mice and humans, but they would be unlikely to be essentially different in their regulation.

Future directions

Change in the duration of embryogenesis is one of the principal ways that animals differ from each other: it simply takes more cell divisions, and thus more time, to make a larger brain or body. Given the notable size differences both within species and between species, the filter of evolution appears to have positioned the order of cytogenesis with respect to nonlinearity of the kinetics of cytogenesis. This permits graceful scaling, as we have discussed for rods and cones in the retina, and for the cortex, and probably for any number of other functional systems. But what sets the overall duration of neurogenesis, and the developmental clock overall? Are there chronology mutants in mice that complete cytogenesis in abnormally short or long times? If so, what covaries with this property, and what controls it? These aspects of cell cycle regulation, yet to be identified, are fundamental to our understanding of both development and evolution.

ACKNOWLEDGMENTS Work was supported by grant nos. IBN-0138113, P20 RR-16460, and P20 RR-16460 (the IDeA Networks of Biomedical Research Excellence Program of the National Center for Research Resources), National Institutes of Health. We thank Richard Darlington for his central role in the original studies on which this chapter depends.

REFERENCES

Airey, D. C., Lu, L., and Williams, R. W. (2001). Genetic control of the mouse cerebellum: Identification of quantitative trait loci modulating size and architecture. *J. Neurosci.* 21:5099–5109.

Arendt, D. (2003). Evolution of eyes and photoreceptor cell types. *Int. J. Dev. Biol.* 47:563–571.

Catalano, S. M., Robertson, R. T., and Killackey, H. P. (1991). Early ingrowth of thalamocortical afferents to the neocortex of the prenatal rat. *Proc. Natl. Acad. Sci. U.S.A.* 88:2999–3003.

Cepko, C. L., Austin, C. P., Yang, X. J., and Alexiades, M. (1996). Cell fate determination in the vertebrate retina. *Proc. Natl. Acad. Sci. U.S.A.* 93:589–595.

Chenn, A., and Walsh, C. A. (2002). Regulation of cerebral cortical size by control of cell cycle exit in neural precursors. *Science* 297:365–369.

Clancy, B., Darlington, R. B., and Finlay, B. L. (1999). The course of human events: Predicting the timing of primate neural development. *Dev. Sci.* 3:57–66.

Clancy, B., Darlington, R. B., and Finlay, B. L. (2001). Translating developmental time across mammalian species. *Neuroscience* 105:7–17.

Clancy, B., Kersh, B., Hyde, J., Anand K. J. S., Darlington, R. B., and Finlay, B. L. (2007). Web-based method for translating neurodevelopment from laboratory species to humans. *Neuroinformatics* 5:79–94.

Darlington, R. B. (1990). *Regression and linear models.* New York: McGraw-Hill.

Darlington, R. B., Dunlop, S. A., and Finlay, B. L. (1999). Neural development in metatherian and eutherian mammals: Variation and constraint. *J. Comp. Neurol.* 411:359–368.

Finlay, B. L., and Darlington, R. B. (1995). Linked regularities in the development and evolution of mammalian brains. *Science* 268:1578–1584.

Finlay, B. L., Darlington, R. B., and Nicastro, N. (2001). Developmental structure in brain evolution. *Behav. Brain Sci.* 24: 263–307.

Finlay, B. L., Hersman, M. N., and Darlington, R. B. (1998). Patterns of vertebrate neurogenesis and the paths of vertebrate evolution. *Brain Behav. Evol.* 52:232–242.

Finlay, B. L., Hinz, F., and Darlington, R. D. (2005a). The relationship of individual variability to phylogenetic variability in the evolution of brain component structure. *Brain Behav. Evol.* 58:112.

Finlay, B. L., Silveira, L. C. L., and Reichenbach, A. (2005b). Comparative aspects of visual system development. In J. Kremers (Ed.), *The structure, function and evolution of the primate visual system* (pp. 37–72). New York: John Wiley and Sons.

Frahm, H. K., Stephan, H., and Baron, G. (1984). Comparisons of brain structure volumes in Insectivora and Primates: V. Area striata. *J. Hirnforsch.* 25:537–557.

Ghosh, A., and Shatz, C. J. (1992). Involvement of subplate neurons in the formation of ocular dominance columns. *Science* 255:1441–1443.

Glendenning, K. K., and Masterton, R. B. (1998). Comparative morphometry of mammalian central auditory systems: Variation in nuclei and form of the ascending system. *Brain Behav. Evol.* 51:59–89.

Gould, S. J. (1975). Allometry in primates, with emphasis on scaling and the evolution of the brain. In P. Andrews and J. A. H. van Couvering (Eds.), *Approaches to primate paleobiology* (p. 244–292). Basel: S. Karger.

Heesy, C. P., and Ross, C. F. (2001). Evolution of activity patterns and chromatic vision in primates: Morphometrics, genetics and cladistics. *J. Hum. Evol.* 40:111–149.

Hofman, M. A. (1989). On the evolution and geometry of the brain in mammals. *Prog. Neurobiol.* 32:137–158.

Jerison, H. J. (1973). *Evolution of the brain and intelligence.* New York: Academic Press.

Jerison, H. J. (1997). Evolution of prefrontal cortex. In N. A. Krasnegor, G. R. Lyon, and P. S. Goldman-Rakic (Eds.), *Development of the prefrontal cortex: Evolution, neurobiology and behavior* (pp. 9–26). Baltimore: Paul H. Brooks.

Kaskan, P., Franco, C., Yamada, E., Silveira, L. C. L., Darlington, R., and Finlay, B. L. (2005). Peripheral variability and central constancy in mammalian visual system evolution. *Proc. R. Soc. Lond. B. Biol. Sci.* 272:91–100.

Kingsbury, M. A., Rehen, S. K., Contos, J. J. A., Higgins, C. M., and Chun, J. (2003). Nonproliferative effects of lysophosphatidic acid enhance cortical growth and folding. *Nat. Neurosci.* 6:1292–1299.

Kruska, D. (1988). Mammalian domestication and its effect on brain structure and behavior. In H. J. Jerison, and I. Jerison (Eds.), *Intelligence and evolutionary biology.* Berlin: Springer-Verlag.

Miller, B., Chou, L., and Finlay, B. L. (1993). The early development of thalamocortical and corticothalamic projections. *J. Comp. Neurol.* 335:16–41.

Rakic, P. (1974). Neurons in the rhesus monkey visual cortex: Systematic relation between time of origin and eventual disposition. *Science* 183:425–427.

Rapaport, D. H., Fletcher, J. T., LaVail, M. M., and Rakic, P. (1992). Genesis of neurons in the retinal ganglion cell layer of the monkey. *J. Comp. Neurol.* 322:577–588.

Rapaport, D. H., Rakic, P., and LaVail, M. M. (1996). Spatiotemporal gradients of cell genesis in the primate retina. *Perspect. Dev. Neurobiol.* 3:147.

Reep, R., Darlington, R. B., and Finlay, B. L. (2007). The limbic system in mammalian brain evolution. *Brain Behav. Evol.* 70: 57–70.

Remtulla, S., and Hallet, P. E. (1985). A schematic eye for the mouse and comparisons with the rat. *Vision Res.* 25: 21–31.

Rockel, A. J., Hiorns, R. W., and Powell, T. P. S. (1980). Basic uniformity in the structure of the cerebral cortex. *Brain* 103: 221–243.

Rodieck, R. W. (1973). *The vertebrate retina: Principles of structure and function.* San Francisco: W. H. Freeman.

Ross, C. F. (2000). Into the light: The origin of Anthropoidea. *Annu. Rev. Anthropol.* 29:147–194.

Seecharan, D. J., Kulkarni, A. L., Lu, L., Rosen, G. D., and Williams, R. W. (2003). Genetic control of interconnected neuronal populations in the mouse primary visual system. *J. Neurosci.* 23:11178–11188.

Semendeferi, K., Lu, A., Schenker, N., and Damasio, H. (2002). Humans and great apes share a large frontal cortex. *Nat. Neurosci.* 5:272–276.

Shyue, S. K., Hewettemmett, D., Sperling, H. G., Hunt, D. M., Bowmaker, J. K., Mollon, J. D., and Li, W. H. (1995). Adaptive evolution of color vision genes in higher primates. *Science* 269: 1265–1267.

Sidman, R. L., and Angevine, J. B. (1962). Autoradiographic analysis of time of origin of nuclear versus cortical components of the mouse telencephalon. *Anat. Rec.* 142:327.

Stephan, H., Baron, G., and Frahm, H. D. (1988). Comparative size of brain and brain components. In *Comparative primate biology* (pp. 1–38). New York: Alan R. Liss.

Strom, R. C., and Williams, R. W. (1998). Cell production and cell death in the generation of variation in neuron number. *J. Neurosci.* 18:9948–9953.

Valverde, F. (1990). Aspects of phylogenetic variability in neocortical intrinsic organization. In B. L. Finlay, C. Innocenti, and H. Scheich (Eds.), *The neocortex: Ontogeny and phylogeny* (pp. 87–102). New York: Plenum Press.

Williams, R. W., and Goldowitz, D. (1992). Structure of clonal and polyclonal cell arrays in the chimeric mouse retina. *Proc. Natl. Acad. Sci. U. S. A.* 89:1184–1188.

Williams, R. W., Strom, R. C., and Goldowitz, D. (1998). Natural variation in neuron number in mice is linked to a major quantitative trait locus on Chr 11. *J. Neurosci.* 18:138–146.

Williams, R. W., Strom, R. C., Rice, D. S., and Goldowitz, D. (1996). Genetic and environmental control of variation in retinal ganglion cell number in mice. *J. Neurosci.* 16:7193–7205.

Zhou, G., and Williams, R. W. (1999). Eye1 and Eye2: Gene loci that modulate eye size, lens weight, and retinal area in the mouse. *Invest. Ophthalmol. Vis. Sci.* 40:817–825.

22 Developmental Studies of the Mouse Lens: Past, Present, and Future

MICHAEL L. ROBINSON

The basic structure and development of all vertebrate lenses are similar. Particularly striking is the similarity of the genetic pathways dictating the formation of vertebrate lenses. In reviewing what has been learned in the mouse, it is important to recall how and why the mouse lens emerged as the premier model for understanding lens development and function. The lens holds a special place historically in the rise of experimental embryology, and many features of the lens ensure that it will remain the gem of developmental biology for years to come.

Basic structure and development of the vertebrate lens

The vertebrate lens is a most unusual tissue. It is both clear, like glass, and entirely cellular in composition. The mature lens contains no blood supply or nervous input and depends solely on diffusion for nutrients and oxygen. Vertebrate lenses are entirely derived from a sheet of surface ectoderm cells known as the presumptive lens ectoderm (PLE). The PLE overlies an evagination of the embryonic forebrain known as the optic vesicle (OV). In the mouse embryo, the OV and PLE come in close contact approximately 9 days after fertilization (E9), and this apposition is soon followed by a thickening of a portion of the PLE into a lens placode (figure 22.1). The lens placode is the first morphological evidence of lens induction. Soon after the formation of the lens placode, the placode and OV undergo a simultaneous invagination, forming the lens pit and optic cup, respectively. The lens pit forms at E10 in the mouse embryo. The lens pit subsequently closes (at approximately E11 in the mouse), forming an initially hollow lens vesicle between the optic cup on the posterior side and the overlying anterior surface ectoderm that will eventually differentiate into the corneal epithelium.

All vertebrate lenses consist of only two basic cell types, lens epithelial cells and lens fiber cells. Lens epithelial cells consist of a single layer of cells that lines the anterior hemisphere of the lens, facing the cornea. The fiber cells make up the remainder of the lens mass. Fiber cells can be subdivided into primary fiber cells and secondary fiber cells. Primary fiber cells are the fiber cells produced by differentiation of the cells originally lining the posterior half of the lens vesicle, while secondary fiber cells result from continuous differentiation of lens epithelial cells at the lens equator. In the mouse, primary fiber cells entirely fill the lumen of the lens vesicle by elongating toward the apical surface of the epithelium between E12 and E13. The lens continues to grow in size throughout the vertebrate life span through continuous lens epithelial cell proliferation and differentiation of secondary fiber cells. The structure of the lens is also stereotypical in that the oldest lens cells are found in the center of the lens (composed of primary fiber cells produced during embryonic development), with progressively younger lens fiber cells being found in a central-to-peripheral gradient. In vertebrates, the lens is enclosed within a modified basement membrane known as the lens capsule that is composed largely of type IV collagen. Enclosure within the capsule effectively seals the lens away from direct physical contact with other cell types, meaning that no cells enter or leave the intact lens except through proliferation or apoptosis. Lens fiber cells do not turn over and must continue to function for the lifetime of the organism to ensure clear sight. Mature lens fiber cells, like mature mammalian erythrocytes, are devoid of intracellular membrane-bound organelles, including nuclei. Also, like erythrocytes, lens fiber cells accumulate cell-type-specific proteins (crystallins) and undergo extensive structural changes in the cell membrane. Unlike erythrocytes, which act as individual units of oxygen transport, lens fiber cells function in a closely packed aggregate and are interconnected by gap junctions, forming an electrically coupled syncytium. All these unusual features represent engineering modifications that allow light to pass through the lens unobstructed by light-scattering particles within the cell.

The lens plays a very important role in the eye. While the lens is responsible for nearly all the focusing activity in fishes, in terrestrial vertebrates the cornea provides most of the refractive power of the eye, and the cornea and lens

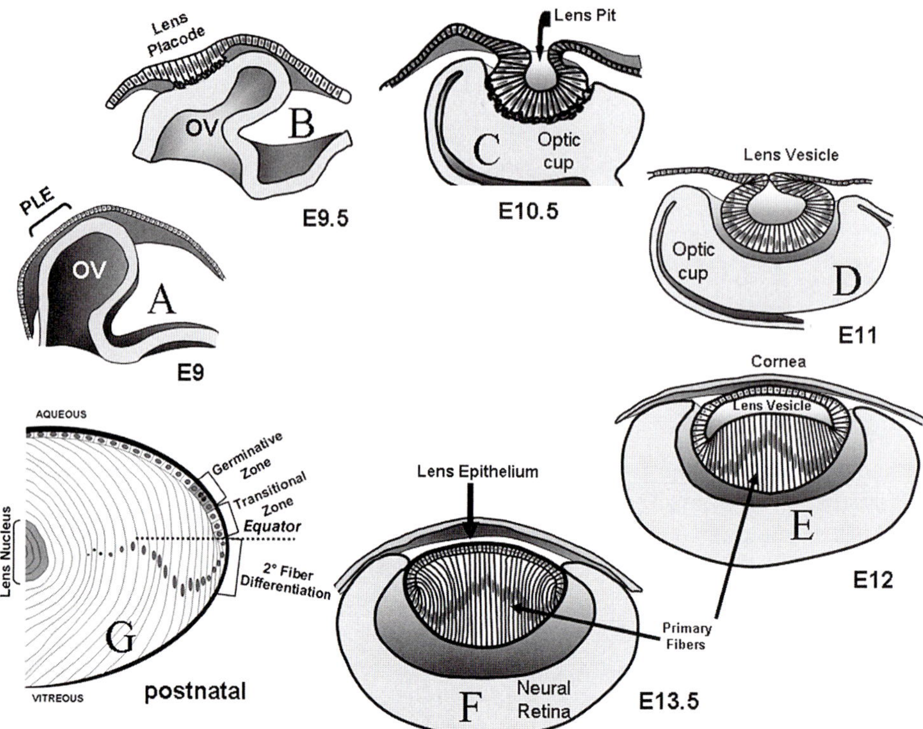

Figure 22.1 Morphological stages of lens development from the presumptive lens ectoderm (PLE) and optic vesicle (OV) at E9 (*A*) through the postnatal stage (*G*). (Adapted from Lovicu and McAvoy, 2005.)

collaborate to focus a clear image onto the retina. In terrestrial vertebrates, the lens is responsible for accommodation for near or far vision. This is accomplished by muscular activity outside the lens either to move the lens forward and backward or to change the shape of the lens within the eye (reviewed in Robinson and Lovicu, 2004). Perhaps more important than the functional role of the lens in the adult animal is the instructive role the lens plays in the overall development of other structures in the eye. The lens is the major determinant of the overall size of the vertebrate eye, and a small lens (microphakia) always results in a small eye (microphthalmia). In addition to dictating ocular size, the lens is absolutely required for the development of the anterior chamber and the neural crest–derived structures of the anterior segment, including the corneal stroma, corneal endothelium, iris stroma, and the trabecular meshwork (Beebe and Coats, 2000). The precise molecular signals sent by the lens to these developing structures are unknown.

History of lens research: The rise of experimental embryology

Although interest in the lens and its development predates the twentieth century (reviewed in Robinson and Lovicu, 2004), lens research has remained at the forefront of developmental biology since the classic experiments of Hans Spemann (1901). In these studies, Spemann demonstrated that the OV was required for the subsequent formation of the lens from the overlying PLE in the frog, *Rana fusca*. This finding was the first description of the concept of embryonic induction. In addition to revealing a fundamental concept of developmental biology, these experiments were also the first to introduce microsurgery as an embryological tool (reviewed in Okada, 2000). Spemann's discovery of embryonic lens induction spawned numerous subsequent investigations of lens development by Spemann and others, some of which demonstrated that the OV was not universally required for vertebrate lens induction (King, 1905; Lewis, 1904; Mencl, 1903; Spemann, 1907). These species-specific differences in the importance of the OV in the process of lens development have been addressed in more recently developed models, which have demonstrated that the OV is simply the last in a stepwise series of embryonic tissues responsible for inducing vertebrate lens formation (reviewed in Fisher and Grainger, 2004).

Nonmurine model systems dominated lens research throughout much of the twentieth century. Spemann's initial discovery of lens induction in frogs, coupled with the accessibility and rapid development of tadpoles, fostered the popularity of this model system for embryonic studies. The discovery of lens regeneration in select species of salamanders and fishes (reviewed in Okada, 2000, 2004) also led to productive investigations of lens development in these species. The developing chick also provided an excellent model for experimental studies on lens development. Chick embryos have large eyes and, like amphibian embryos, are amenable to surgical manipulation during development. This property was exploited by Alfred and Jane Coulombre in classic lens reversal experiments which revealed that the polarity of the lens (with the lens epithelium normally facing the cornea) is dependent on extrinsic factors within the eye (Coulombre and Coulombre, 1963). In contrast to chicks and tadpoles, mammalian embryos develop within a largely inaccessible uterine environment, making experimental manipulations more difficult. These difficulties are compounded in the mouse, as the developing eye is extremely small.

History of lens research: Enter the mighty mouse

Rodents have the advantage of being easy and inexpensive to breed in captivity, with short generation times and multiple animals per litter. Less than a decade after Hans Spemann's initial experiments on lens induction in frogs, early mouse geneticists began creating the first inbred mice (reviewed in Morse, 1978). These animals, largely descendants of mice domesticated centuries ago by Asian and European mouse fanciers, were initially created to investigate cancer (Paigen, 2003a) but have subsequently served as keystone species for investigating all aspects of mammalian biology. Inbred mice, according to the 1989 International Committee on Standardized Nomenclature for Mice, are the result of at least 20 generations of brother-sister mating (Silver, 1995). This level of inbreeding theoretically results in genetic homozygosity for 98.7% of the genome (Green, 1981). In essence, this means that all animals in a given inbred strain are basically genetically identical. All of the common, commercially available inbred strains have been inbred many more than 20 generations, dictating that any heterozygosity within an inbred strain is the result of mutations arising since the initial creation of the strain. From the beginning, it was the power of mouse genetics that provided the most potent experimental benefit to this unassuming rodent.

Although the mouse lens did not start out as the most popular developmental system for investigations of lens development, it was not entirely ignored even in these early years. In 1938, Herman Chase obtained a strain of anophthalmic (having no eyes) mice from Clarence Cook Little (founder of the Jackson Laboratory in Bar Harbor, Maine). Chase continued inbreeding these mice, forming the strain now known as ZRDCT. Chase published a number of papers on these mice, the first of which described the ocular morphology of developing mutant embryos (Chase and Chase, 1941). The key morphological feature of these mice was an OV that was smaller than normal and that failed, in most cases, to make good contact with the overlying PLE. About 90% of mice in the ZRDCT strain are anophthalmic, and the remainder are microphthalmic (having very small eyes). Chase also investigated the genetics of the ZRDCT strain by making crosses with other inbred mouse strains. These crosses confirmed that the anophthalmic trait was recessive, as all F_1 progeny from crosses involving one ZRDCT parent had normal eyes. Subsequent crossing suggested that the anophthalmic trait was not the result of a single mutant gene but, more likely, the combination of a major genetic determinant, designated ey1, and a small number of additional modifying genetic characters (Chase, 1942). In later experiments, Chase hypothesized that most of the ZRDCT anophthalmic phenotype was the result of homozygosity for ey1 and a major modifier that he designated ey2 (Chase, 1944). Therefore, anophthalmia in the ZRDCT mice represented an early example of a complex genetic trait in mammals.

The ZRDCT mice are highlighted here for a number of reasons. First, these studies were among the first, if not the first, published works exploiting both the embryology and genetics of mice to study eye development. Second, these mice demonstrate that although the PLE undergoes inductive influences prior to encountering the OV (reviewed in Fisher and Grainger, 2004), physical contact between the OV and the surface ectoderm is indeed important for normal development of the mouse lens and eye. Third, the ZRDCT strain still exists nearly 70 years after Clarence Little first noticed their anophthalmic ancestors, and these mice continue to inspire scientific investigation. The ey1 mutation was identified by positional cloning as a point mutation in an alternative start codon for the *Rx/rax* homeobox transcription factor (Tucker et al., 2001), but the identity of the ey2 modifier gene(s) remains unknown. *Rx/rax* is expressed in the OV but is not expressed in the PLE or the lens, so the effects of the ey1 mutation on lens development are indirect. Mice homozygous for null (loss of function) mutations in *Rx/rax* fail to form OVs and are also anophthalmic (Mathers et al., 1997), and homozygous mutations in the human *Rx/rax* orthologue are associated with human anophthalmia (Voronina et al., 2004). In many ways, the ZRDCT mice studies pointed the way toward the power of mouse genetics to elucidate problems of eye development.

There were other, nongenetic, studies of mouse eye development that were notable in these early years. As early as 1948, Ida Mann showed that mouse lens epithelial cells were capable of elongating in vitro (Mann, 1948) preceding similar findings by others in chicks (Philpott and Coulombre, 1965) and amphibians (McDevitt and Yamada, 1969). Muthukkaruppan performed tissue recombination experiments using E9 mouse embryos to explore the presumed requirement of the OV to induce formation of the mammalian lens (Muthukkaruppan, 1965). He found that both a lens and a retina could form in vitro from explanted mouse

OV with surrounding mesenchyme and PLE. In these experiments, lenses (as judged by the morphological appearance of elongated fiber cells) were not able to form from isolated PLE, from isolated OV, or from PLE cultured in association with various sources of embryonic mesenchyme. Muthukkaruppan was able to achieve lens formation from the PLE in association with optic cup tissue from E10 embryos or from E13 neural retina, but not from E13 spinal cord, demonstrating that lens-inductive influence was not present in all embryonic neural tissue. Furthermore, the lens-inductive influence of the optic cup or neural retina was able to pass through a Millipore filter (Muthukkaruppan, 1965).

Yujiro Yamamoto used lenses from 6- to 8-day-old mouse pups to perform lens transplantation experiments into the eyes of adult mice (Yamamoto, 1976). Yamamoto found that when a normal lens was placed into a normal adult eye with the normal orientation (epithelial cells facing the cornea), lens growth continued and the lens remained transparent for more than 5 months. As in experiments performed more than a decade earlier in chicks (Coulombre and Coulombre, 1963), mouse lenses transplanted into mouse eyes in reverse orientation (epithelial cells facing the retina) underwent a reorientation. In other words, the lens epithelium facing the retina elongated into fiber cells, and a new monolayer of epithelium formed over the original posterior surface of the lens facing the cornea. Yamamoto found that the reformation of the lens epithelium on the posterior surface of the reversed lens (facing the cornea) did not depend on the recipient mouse having an intact neural retina, but that the neural retina was necessary for the differentiation of fibers of the original lens epithelium in the reversed donor lens or for the continued lens growth in the correctly oriented donor lens (Yamamoto, 1976).

Perhaps the first morphological descriptions of normal mouse eye and lens development were provided by Paul Leonhard Kessler in 1877, and these were followed by Rugh in 1968 and beautiful photographic views of mouse eye development by Pei and Rhodin in 1970, and more recently by Kaufmann in 1992. Other morphological processes such as fiber cell denucleation (Kuwabara and Imaizumi, 1974; Vrensen et al., 1991) have been covered in the mouse lens using transmission electron microscopy, and excellent scanning electron micrographs of mouse eye and lens development by Kathleen Sulik can be found online (www.med.unc.edu/embryo_images).

One essential component of lens development and growth is lens cell proliferation. Cell proliferation in the lens is confined to the lens epithelium, and some of the finest early characterization of the normal mouse lens epithelium was carried out by Nancy Rafferty using adult CF_1 strain outbred (nongenetically identical) mice (Rafferty, 1972; Rafferty and Rafferty, 1981). Rafferty used ^{3}H-thymidine labeling to characterize cell cycle kinetics in the mouse lens epithelium. These studies estimated that the mouse lens epithelium consisted of 44,000 cells that could be subdivided based on position and rate of proliferation. This estimate included approximately 3,600 cells of the most peripheral cells, where nuclei line up into what are called meridional rows. These cells are currently characterized as very young fiber cells. Rafferty also observed a slowly cycling subpopulation of approximately 5,000 cells in the periphery of the lens epithelium whose divisions would ultimately fuel the production of secondary fiber cells at the rate of 207 cells per day (Rafferty and Rafferty, 1981). This zone is now referred to at the germinative zone (figure 22.1*G*). An adjacent zone approximately seven cell diameters thick and consisting of approximately 9,000 epithelial cells that were no longer incorporating ^{3}H-thymidine but had not yet begun to line up in meridional rows was also denoted by the Raffertys. This zone of post-mitotic epithelial cells is now referred to as the transitional zone (see figure 22.1*G*), as these are epithelial cells in transition to becoming secondary fiber cells. Although these studies were not the first to recognize that different subpopulations of lens epithelial cells with different proliferative potentials exist in vertebrate lenses, they were benchmarks in the specific characterization of the mouse lens epithelium and served as a framework by which later molecular studies of mouse lens cell proliferation could proceed.

The relationship of mouse and human lenses

Mice, like humans, are mammals and therefore share a closer genetic relationship with humans than with other nonmammalian vertebrates such as amphibians or chickens. In fact, humans are genetically closer to mice than to cats, dogs, cows, pigs, or many other familiar nonprimate mammals (Reyes et al., 2004). Insofar as cataracts remain the number one cause of human blindness worldwide (Resnikoff et al., 2004), the study of lens development in an animal model closely related to humans has obvious potential medical benefit. That said, mice are not simply small, furry humans, and there are fundamental differences between the mouse and human lens. The mouse lens is much rounder and takes up a larger percentage of the eye volume than does the flatter human lens. The mouse and human lens also differ in the arrangement and type of lens sutures (reviewed in Kuszak and Costello, 2004). Lens sutures are formed when differentiating fiber cells lose contact with the basement membrane and associate with the ends of other differentiating fiber cells. This process explains why older, more mature fiber cells are found deep within the lens, while the youngest fiber cells remain in contact with the lens capsule at the surface. Mouse lenses have Y-suture lenses and primates have star suture lenses. Suture patterns, and the overall geometry of individual fiber cells, also dictate the accommodating power of the lens, with human lenses having significant accommodation power, versus the negligible accommodating power of the mouse lens (Kuszak et al., 2006).

There are several biochemical differences between mouse and human lenses as well. Among these are differences in the composition of lens membrane lipids. Human lens cell membranes contain large amounts of dihydrosphingomyelin, a lipid virtually absent from mouse lens membranes, and mouse lens membranes have far more phosphatidylcholine than the membranes of human lenses (R. Truscott, pers. comm.). These differences in murine and human lenses are more apparent in their mature forms than during embryonic development, and there is strong reason to suspect that nearly all the genetic pathways dictating mouse and human lens development are similar.

Beware: Not all mice are created equal

The existence of inbred mice is one of the great strengths of working with the mouse system. Each inbred strain can be thought of as a pool of identical individuals from a genetic standpoint. At the same time, different inbred strains represent different pools of genetically identical individuals. It is prudent to be aware of the possible complications inherent to the interpretation of phenotypes arising in a particular strain of inbred mice. Other chapters in this book alert readers to the common *Pde6b*^{rd1} mutation leading to rapid postnatal retina degeneration in many inbred mouse strains. Lurking in the eyes of several "normal" inbred mouse strains are mutations and polymorphisms that have an impact on lens development as well. Among the more recently identified of these is a null mutation in the *Bfsp2* gene encoding the lens fiber cell–specific beaded filament protein, CP49. This *Bfsp2* mutation is shared by several inbred strains, including 129X1/SvJ, 129S1/SvImJ, 129S4/SvJae, 129S2/SvPas, C3H, CBA, 101 and FVB/N (Alizadeh et al., 2004; Sandilands et al., 2004; Simirskii et al., 2006). As a result, the lenses of these mice lack intermediate beaded filaments. Although the overall development of the lenses from *Bfsp2* mutant mice appears normal, beaded filament loss leads to increased light scattering in the lens and alterations in other optical properties as well (reviewed in Perng and Quinlan, 2005). FVB/N and 129 are the most commonly used inbred strains for the production of transgenic and knockout mice, respectively. Therefore, it is not unlikely that mice derived from genetic engineering approaches carry *Bfsp2* mutations.

Inbred mice derived from the C57 Black strains (most notably C57BL/6 and C57BL/10) are inherently prone to develop microphthalmia and/or anophthalmia. This was first noted in the experiments of Herman Chase, who used C57 Black mice as a control strain in comparisons with the ZRDCT anophthalmic strain (Chase, 1942; Chase and Chase, 1941). The frequency of spontaneous microphthalmia or anophthalmia in C57BL mice has been reported to be as low as 4.4% (N = 2,200; Chase, 1942) to as high as 9.6% (N = 2,709; Kalter, 1968). For reasons that remain unclear, eye defects are more common in females than in males and, when unilateral, are more commonly seen in the right eye than in the left (Chase, 1942; Kalter, 1968). There is also evidence that environmental factors influence the frequency of eye defects in C57BL mice (Pierro and Spiggle, 1969), and C57BL/6 mice are particularly susceptible (compared to C3H, CF-1, and CD-1 strains) to ocular defects resulting from teratogenic insults such as alcohol (Cook et al., 1987). The apparently stochastic appearance of ocular defects within genetically identical C57BL mice suggests an inherent genetic deficiency of eye development universally present in the strain. Like the eye defects present in the ZRDCT strain (although seen at a much higher frequency), eye defects in C57BL mice are most likely a complex genetic trait consisting of multiple genetic loci.

There are two main hypotheses as to the mechanistic nature of C57BL ocular defects. The first derived from observations that C57BL OVs, like those of the ZRDCT strain, are smaller than normal and make less than optimal contact with the PLE, resulting in a smaller lens (Cook and Sulik, 1986; Harch et al., 1978). The second hypothesis is that the defects in C57BL mice are intrinsic to problems within the PLE or the lens cells derived from the PLE (LoCascio et al., 1987; Robinson et al., 1993). This hypothesis descends from the analysis of ocular tissues derived from chimeric mice made from the aggregation of preimplantation embryos from C57BL/6 mice and DBA/2 or A/J strain mice. Chimeras made with C57BL/6 embryos demonstrated a uniform and dramatic underrepresentation of C57BL/6 cells in the lens relative to the overall chimeric contribution of C57BL/6 cells to other ocular and nonocular tissues. Notably, the OV-derived chimeric retinas tended to have a C57BL/6 contribution reflective of the overall C57BL/6 chimeric contribution. Even those supporting the lens-intrinsic hypothesis noted consistent morphological differences in the early stages of lens development between C57BL/6 and control (DBA/2 and A/J) embryos resulting in a universally smaller initial lens pit and vesicle (Robinson et al., 1993). The fact that most C57BL/6 mice do not exhibit frank postnatal microphthalmia suggests that size deficiencies present early in lens development can largely be compensated for, presumably by increased proliferation. It is interesting to note, however, that adult C57BL/6 mice were recently shown to exhibit a lens axial thickness significantly ($P < 0.001$) smaller than that of DBA/2 (Puk et al., 2006). Unfortunately, the molecular nature of C57BL/6 ocular deficiencies remains unknown. Perhaps with the application of current molecular genetic tools the answer will be forthcoming. In any case, C57BL/6 is among the most commonly used inbred mouse strains, and it is frequently used as a "normal" control strain. It is also common practice to breed mutations created in 129 strain-derived embryonic stem (ES) cells onto a C57BL/6 genetic background. Therefore, it is important for those interested in ocular development to realize the C57BL/6 mice do carry a genetic predisposition to ocular abnormalities.

Molecular biology of the lens: Developing the tools

The first half of this chapter described the historical context in which developmental studies on the mouse lens arose. It was only with the advent of molecular techniques and, most important, the ability to experimentally manipulate the mouse genome that the mouse truly became the keystone for mechanistic understanding of vertebrate lens development. It is appropriate here to briefly discuss lens crystallins. The literature on lens crystallins is rich and enormous, far greater than can be adequately discussed here.

Lens biochemists first isolated and characterized crystallin proteins from nonmurine sources, and resultant antibodies to these proteins gave lens biologists the tools to follow development in tissue sections. Despite their critical functional role in maintaining lens clarity, lens crystallins are likely not major regulators of lens development. Crystallins have, however, been used extensively as molecular markers of lens differentiation, and eventually any genetic pathway leading to lens differentiation will ultimately regulate crystallin gene expression. Pioneering work on the regulation of crystallin gene expression made the first transgenic studies on lens development possible. Crystallins are the most abundant water-soluble proteins in the lens, and their high concentrations are necessary to maintain lens transparency. The mammalian lens contains α-, β-, and γ-crystallins. In the mouse there are multiple genes encoding each crystallin subclass: *αA-, αB-, βA3/A1-, βA2-, βA3-, βB1-, βB2-, βB3-, γA-, γB-, γC-, γD-, γE-, γF-,* and *γS-crystallin* (reviewed in Duncan et al., 2004). The developmental expression of the three different mammalian crystallin classes was first shown by John McAvoy with immunocytochemical studies in the rat (McAvoy, 1978). McAvoy showed that α-crystallins were expressed in lens epithelial cells and lens fiber cells, while β- and γ-crystallins were restricted to lens fiber cells. McAvoy also demonstrated that β-crystallin expression precedes γ-crystallin expression in the fiber differentiation pathway. This expression pattern was later seen by others in the mouse. The first crystallin genes expressed during mouse development are the α-crystallins (Zwaan, 1983), with αB-crystallin initiating expression at the lens placode stage and αA-crystallin appearing at the lens pit stage (Haynes et al., 1996; Robinson and Overbeek, 1996). Both α-crystallin genes are expressed in lens epithelial cells and lens fiber cells, but *αA-crystallin* is expressed at significantly higher levels in lens fiber cells. β- and γ-crystallins have been and continue to be used as markers of lens fiber cell differentiation. This is not inappropriate, as the expression of *γ-crystallin* transcripts in the rodent embryo does not initiate until after fiber cell differentiation commences (Goring et al., 1992; Van Leen et al., 1987), and antibodies to β-crystallins do not detect these proteins in the embryonic mouse lens epithelium (Carper et al., 1986). Recently, however, βB1- and γS-crystallin proteins were found to be reasonably abundant in normal postnatal rat lens epithelium, and transcripts for *βA2-* and *γS-crystallins* are induced in lens epithelial cells cultured in nondifferentiating media, demonstrating that these particular crystallins are not exclusive to lens fiber cells (Wang et al., 2004).

The mouse *αA-crystallin* gene was the first crystallin promoter to be cloned and analyzed in detail (King and Piatigorsky, 1983). These analyses began by fusing 5′ flanking regions of the *αA-crystallin* gene to a *chloramphenicol acetyl transferase* (*CAT*) reporter gene. Two methods were initially used to evaluate the αA/CAT constructs. The first was to transfect the αA/CAT construct into primary explants of chick lens epithelia and then to analyze the explant for expression of the *CAT* reporter gene. The constructs containing 364 nucleotides upstream and 46 nucleotides downstream of the transcription initiation site (−364/+45) of the mouse were capable of driving CAT expression in explanted chick lens epithelia but were not capable of promoting CAT expression in chick fibroblasts. In contrast, a shorter, −87/+45 construct was not capable of eliciting CAT expression in either chick lens epithelia or fibroblasts (Chepelinsky et al., 1985). These experiments first demonstrated that sequences between −87 and −364 of the mouse *αA-crystallin* gene contained sufficient information to drive the expression of a heterologous gene (CAT) in a tissue-specific way, and that chicken regulatory proteins were able to interpret the instructions encoded in mouse noncoding DNA. Similar previous experiments by Kondoh and colleagues demonstrated that a genomic clone for *δ-crystallin* (a crystallin not normally expressed in the mammalian lens), containing 2 kb of upstream noncoding sequence, was able to direct δ-crystallin synthesis following microinjection into cultured mouse lens epithelial cells but not into nonlens cells (Kondoh et al., 1983). These experiments showed that the regulatory sequences directing gene expression to the lens exhibit amazing functional conservation despite millions of years of evolution separating chickens from mice.

Lens research enters the transgenic era

The second method used to investigate the regulatory activity of the αA-crystallin gene 5′-flanking region was to inject the αA/CAT constructs into pronuclear stage mouse zygotes to create transgenic mice. The −364/+45 αA/CAT construct exhibited lens-specific CAT expression in the resultant transgenic mice, and expression was detected as early as E12.5 in the mouse embryo (Overbeek et al., 1985). At the time, this was very new technology. The first transgenic mice ever made were published in 1980 and 1981 (reviewed in Paigen, 2003b). The αA/CAT transgenic mice published in 1985 were the first transgenic mice produced in which transgene expression was directed specifically to the visual system (Overbeek et al., 1985). For the first time in the history of lens research it was possible to ectopically express virtually any gene in the developing lens.

The αA/CAT transgenic mice opened a virtual floodgate to lens transgenic experiments. Many of these were designed to directly test various promoter constructs for their lens activity and specificity in vivo. Transgenic mice were soon being made with the murine −759/+45 γF-crystallin promoter, in which transgene expression was directed specifically to central lens fiber cells (Goring et al., 1987), and a δ-crystallin genomic clone containing a 2.5 kb promoter that directed δ-crystallin expression to both the lens and the brain (Kondoh et al., 1987). Transgenic studies proved to be the gold standard for functional activity of lens promoter regions in vivo. Over the years, several different promoter constructs have directed transgene expression to the mouse lens with varying degrees of lens specificity. Among these are various crystallin promoters from a variety of species (reviewed in Duncan et al., 2004), as well as the chicken vimentin (Capetanaki et al., 1989) and human keratin 14 (Nguyen et al., 2002) promoters and elements of the murine *Pax6* promoter (Ashery-Padan et al., 2000; Williams et al., 1998). These promoters have proven to be valuable tools for lens developmental biologists.

A common misconception, even among lens biologists, is that the overexpression or ectopic expression of any gene in the lens will cause a cataract. While the expression of many genes in the lens does lead to cataract, this is not universally true. In fact, a number of different transgenes have been expressed ubiquitously, as well as in the lens specifically, without causing lens cataracts. The first lens transgenic mice produced with the αA/CAT construct did not develop cataracts (Overbeek et al., 1985).

Other lens transgenic experiments were designed to ectopically express ectopic proteins in the lens to alter normal lens development. Lenses are not prone to the development of tumors in any vertebrate species, but transgenic mice expressing the SV40 T-antigen readily formed lens tumors (Mahon et al., 1987). These lens tumor–bearing mice spawned numerous productive investigations of cell cycle regulation and apoptosis in which the transgenic mouse lens was used as a model system (reviewed in Griep and Zhang, 2004). Other early ectopic lens expression experiments directed toxin genes to the lens to achieve lens-specific cell ablation (Breitman et al., 1987; Landel et al., 1988). Specific loss of lens cells in these mice uniformly led to microphthalmia, demonstrating that eye size in mice is directly dependent on lens size during development.

In addition to the ectopic expression of viral proteins, reporter genes, and toxin genes, the lens was used to express a wide variety of growth factors. Some of these growth factors were expressed endogenously by the lens and others were not normally expressed by the lens at all. Often these experiments were designed to influence either the development of the lens or the development of tissues in the eye surrounding the lens. Growth factors and cytokines expressed in the lens of transgenic mice include transforming growth factor-alpha (TGF-α; Decsi et al., 1994; Reneker et al., 1995, 2000), epidermal growth factor (EGF; Reneker et al., 2000), TGF-β (Flugel-Koch et al., 2002; Srinivasan et al., 1998; Zhao and Overbeek, 2001), bone morphogenic protein 7 (BMP7; Hung et al., 2002), vascular endothelial growth factor (VEGF; Ash and Overbeek, 2000), insulin-like growth factor-I (IGF-I; Shirke et al., 2001), platelet-derived growth factor (PDGF; Reneker and Overbeek, 1996), neurotrophin-3 (NT3; Robinson, 2008), insulin (Reneker et al., 2004), optineurin (Kroeber et al., 2006), interleukin-1β (IL-1β; Vinores et al., 2003), leukocyte inhibitory factor (LIF; Graham et al., 2005), and several different fetal growth factors (reviewed in Robinson, 2006). In addition, a number of different growth factor receptor genes (wild-type, constitutively active and dominant negative) have been expressed in the lens. These have contributed significantly to our understanding of the regulation of lens development, particularly in the regulation of lens fiber differentiation (reviewed in Lovicu and McAvoy, 2005). Although transgenic-mediated overexpression provided insights into lens development, they were limited. It was often difficult to determine if lens phenotypes in transgenic mice were the result of a fundamental interference with a specific normal developmental process or if overexpression of proteins in the lens resulted in nonspecific, ectopic effects.

Customizing the mouse genome to study lens development

The advent of homologous gene targeting in mouse ES cells quickly made it possible to delete or alter genes in the mouse genome at will. This was the technology that firmly cemented the mouse at the forefront of understanding lens development. Today, the mouse remains the only vertebrate in which targeted germline genetic alterations are routine. Genes in which null mutations are introduced by gene targeting are often referred to as knockout mice. Not all targeted mutations are knockouts, however. Targeted mutations can lead to hypomorphic (partial function) or dominant negative alleles. Sometimes gene targeting is used to replace the coding sequence of one gene with another to create a "knock-in" mouse. Targeted mutations in many different mouse genes, sometimes unexpectedly, led to problems with eye development. The opposite also proved true.

Amazingly, lens development in mice with null mutations in genes encoding major lens proteins such as αA-crystallin (Brady et al., 1997), αB-crystallin (Brady et al., 2001), CP49 (Alizadeh et al., 2002), or filensin (Alizadeh et al., 2003) was largely normal, at least in the sense that the lenses were formed and were initially free from cataract.

The lens complementation system

Perhaps the most challenging aspects of using gene targeting approaches to study lens development is that many genes important for lens development are also essential for the development of other organ systems. In this case, lens phenotypes in a particular knockout mouse may be secondary to developmental deficiencies in another tissue. Even worse, many homozygous knockout mice die prior to the lens placode stage, complicating the use of these knockouts to study lens development. One way to address this issue is with the use of chimeras, in which wild-type cells can often compensate for the early lethality that may be present in an uncompensated homozygous knockout. Nanette Liegéois and colleagues devised a lens complementation system using embryos homozygous for the mouse *aphakia* (*ak*) mutation for precisely this purpose (Liegéois et al., 1996). The *ak* mutation consists of deletions in the promoter region of the *Pitx3* transcription factor, and *ak* homozygotes are unable to form lenses (reviewed in Graw and Loster, 2003). Injection of wild-type ES cells into homozygous *ak* blastocysts rescues lens development in the chimeras, and the resulting lenses are entirely derived from the ES cell component (Liegéois et al., 1996). The lens complementation strategy was recently used to determine if *Fgfr1* played an essential role in mouse lens development. *Fgfr1* homozygous knockouts die shortly after gastrulation, well before morphological signs of lens development (Deng et al., 1994; Yamaguchi et al., 1994). Chimeras made from *Fgfr1* null ES cells and *ak*/*ak* embryos exhibited normally formed lenses entirely lacking *Fgfr1*, demonstrating that *Fgfr1* was not required for normal lens development (Zhao et al., 2006). The use of the *aphakia* lens complementation strategy has at least two complications. First, lack of lens development in a chimera might be indirect and the result of problems with mutant ES cell migration or differentiation prior to lens induction. Second, lens development does initiate in *ak* mutants, and early lens structures such as the lens placode, lens pit, and lens vesicle, are likely to consist of a mixture of cells rather than strictly being derived from the ES cell component.

Conditional gene alterations using Cre recombinase

The manipulation of gene expression, both temporally and in a tissue-specific manner, is the most powerful way to exploit genetics to gain developmental insight. Fortunately, lens biologists have several tools at their disposal to do this, and new and better tools are doubtless forthcoming. Today, the most widely used system for temporal control of genome manipulation in the mouse is the Cre-loxP system, derived from P1 bacteriophage (reviewed in Branda and Dymecki, 2004). In essence, genomic DNA flanked by directly oriented 34 bp loxP sites can be deleted, in the presence of Cre recombinase, in vivo. Gene targeting constructs can be designed to insert loxP sites on each end of a gene, or within introns surrounding essential exons within that gene to preserve gene function in the targeted allele. The loxP-flanked gene or exons can then be deleted at will by controlling the temporal and spatial expression of Cre recombinase. The mouse lens was the first tissue in which tissue-specific DNA deletion using Cre recombinase was demonstrated in vivo (Lakso et al., 1992).

There are several different transgenic strains with patterns of Cre expression potentially useful for lens developmental studies. *Rx-Cre* transgenic mice, where Cre expression is under the regulatory control of a 4 kb medaka fish Rx3 promoter fragment, express Cre in the entire OV prior to lens placode formation, making these mice useful for evaluating the roles of OV-expressed genes on the subsequent induction and differentiation of the lens (Swindell et al., 2006). Within the lens, several different transgenic lines have been used to delete loxP-flanked genes (figure 22.2). The earliest acting of these are directed by genomic sequences from the murine *Pax6* gene. The Le-Cre transgenic line exploits a 6.5 kb genomic fragment that includes the P0 promoter from the mouse *Pax6* gene to drive Cre expression (Ashery-Padan et al., 2000). In Le-Cre mice, Cre expression initiates in the *Pax6*-expressing head ectoderm, including all the cells of the PLE at 9.0. Conditional (*loxP*-flanked) gene deletion in these mice takes place in virtually all of the ocular tissues derived from the surface ectoderm, including the lens, corneal epithelium, conjunctiva epithelium, and portions of the eyelid. The Le-Cre mice also experience conditional gene deletion in cells of the developing endocrine pancreas and in the olfactory epithelium (see figure 22.1). The Pax6(Lens)-Cre line is similar to Le-Cre except that it only includes the 340 bp *Pax6* ectoderm enhancer fused to the P0 promoter and exhibits a more eye-specific expression pattern (Yoshimoto et al., 2005). MLR10 transgenic mice express Cre under the control of a murine *αA-crystallin* promoter modified by the insertion of a Pax6 consensus binding site (Zhao et al., 2004). In MLR10 mice, Cre expression initiates at the lens pit/vesicle stage (E10.5) and effectively deletes many loxP-flanked sequences in the majority of lens epithe-

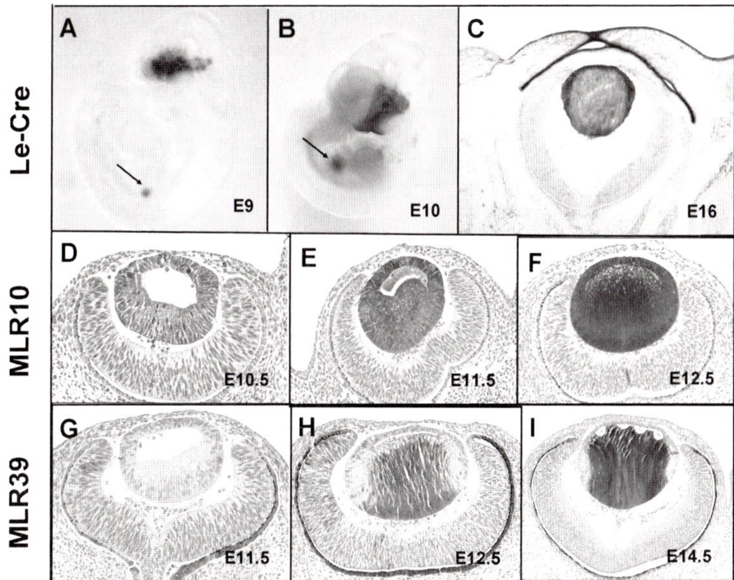

FIGURE 22.2 Cre expression patterns in three different transgenic strains: Le-Cre (*A–C*), MLR10 (*D–F*), and MLR39 (*G–I*). Cre expression in whole-mount (*A* and *B*) or tissue sections (*C–I*) is indicated by blue (*B* and *D–I*) or purple (*A* and *C*) staining following histochemical detection of a Cre-activated reporter allele. *Arrows* in *A* and *B* indicate Cre expression in the developing pancreas of Le-Cre mice. Developmental time points are indicated. See color plate 12. (Adapted from Ashery-Padan et al., 2000, and Zhao et al., 2004.)

lial cells and lens fiber cells. The lens is the only site of ocular Cre expression in MLR10 mice. MLR39 transgenic mice express Cre from the α*A-crystallin* promoter, initiating in the lens fiber cells at approximately E12.5. Although Cre expression can also be seen in the developing retina pigment epithelium, within the lens, Cre expression in MLR39 mice is largely fiber cell specific (Zhao et al., 2004). Although the endogenous α*A-crystallin* gene is expressed in both lens epithelial cells and lens fiber cells, the −364/+45 αA-crystallin promoter (most commonly used in transgenic mice) efficiently directs gene expression only to lens fiber cells. It is now clear that the α*A-crystallin* gene contains several regulatory elements missing in the −364/+45 αA-crystallin promoter (Yang et al., 2006).

The different Cre-expressing mouse strains allow genes to be deleted in the lens at distinct developmental time points. This makes the evaluation of gene function at multiple stages of lens development and differentiation possible (see figure 22.2). For studies of lens induction, it may be valuable to delete genes in the presumptive lens prior to the initiation of *Pax6* expression in the PLE. One potentially useful mouse strain for this purpose is the AP2α-Cre strain (Macatee et al., 2003), where Cre expression initiates in the head surface ectoderm at the 10 somite stage (E8.5). Mouse strains also exist in which Cre expression can be induced in a global fashion following induction with a drug such as tamoxifen (Hayashi and McMahon, 2002). These tools, and better ones sure to follow, permit exquisite manipulation of specific gene expression during lens development. With any conditional gene deletion strategy it is important to determine precisely when and where Cre is expressed and to assess the efficiency with which the loxP-flanked DNA of interest is deleted within the particular Cre driver strain chosen. This information is essential to interpreting the results of conditional gene deletion experiments.

Mouse lens induction

Perhaps no stage of mouse lens development has been more clearly elucidated from a molecular perspective than that of lens induction. Mouse lens induction is the subject of a recent review article by Richard Lang, who has contributed much to the current understanding of this subject (Lang, 2004). At the heart of lens induction in mice (and likely all vertebrates) is the transcription factor Pax6. *Pax6* expression is absolutely required for eye formation in *Drosophila* as well as in vertebrates. Ectopic expression of *Pax6* is also sufficient to induce the formation of ectopic eyes in both *Drosophila* and *Xenopus*, demonstrating that Pax6 exhibits a conserved and critical role in metazoan eye development. Mutations in *Pax6* are responsible for the dominant *small eye* (*Sey*) series of allelic mutations in mice and aniridia (as well as other ocular anomalies) in humans. *Pax6* expression in the mouse PLE can be divided into two distinct phases (figure 22.3). The first phase of *Pax6* expression ($Pax6^{pre\text{-}placode}$) covers a large region of the head surface ectoderm that subsequently (after the

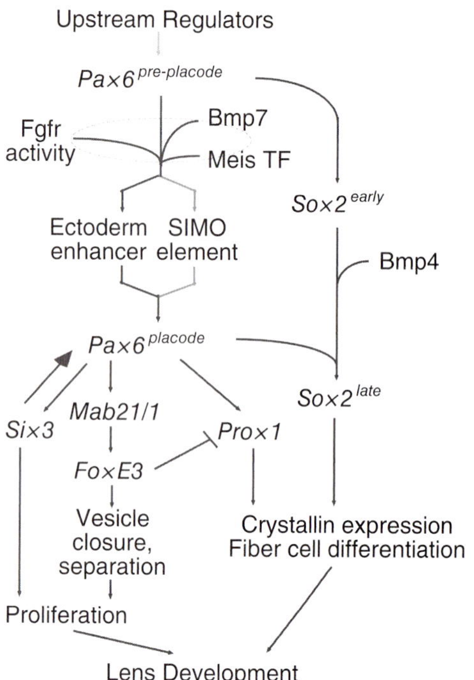

FIGURE 22.3 A model for the genetic pathways regulating lens induction. (Reprinted with permission from Lang, 2004.)

PLE comes in close contact with the OV) becomes restricted in the second phase (Pax6^{placode}) to a region including and immediately surrounding the lens placode. The second phase of *Pax6* expression is dependent on functional Pax6 protein being produced in the first phase, indicating that Pax6 regulates its own expression (Grindley et al., 1995). Although there are many regulatory elements controlling *Pax6* gene expression, two have been analyzed in detail with respect to their ability to regulate the Pax6^{placode} phase of *Pax6* expression. These elements are the *Pax6* ectoderm enhancer, upstream of the P0 promoter, and the SIMO element, approximately 140 kb downstream from *Pax6* (reviewed in Lang, 2004).

Inhibition of Fgf receptor (Fgfr) signaling (either by a chemical Fgfr inhibitor or by expression of a dominant negative Fgfr transgene) reduces the level of Pax6 in the mouse lens placode. Lenses that subsequently form under Fgfr inhibition are abnormally small, with reduced rates of cell proliferation. Heterozygous loss of *Bmp7* exacerbated the reduction of Pax6^{placode} expression in combination with Fgfr inhibition, suggesting a genetic cooperation of the Bmp and Fgfr signaling pathways in regulating *Pax6* expression during lens induction (Faber et al., 2001). Mice homozygous for null mutations in either *Bmp7* or *Bmp4* most often fail to induce a lens. Although *Bmp4* is not expressed in the PLE, and its loss does not reduce Pax6^{placode} expression, it is expressed in the OV and required for the upregulation of the transcription factor Sox2 (Furuta and Hogan, 1998). *Bmp7* is expressed in the PLE, and while there is phenotypic variability in lens defects resulting from *Bmp7* loss (Dudley et al., 1995; Luo et al., 1995), Bmp7 deficiency often results in the loss of Pax6^{placode} expression (Wawersik et al., 1999). Pax6^{placode} expression is also regulated by Meis transcription factors, at least in part, through binding sites identified in the *Pax6* ectoderm enhancer (Zhang et al., 2002).

Vertebrate lens development also depends on members of the Sox family of HMG box transcription factors. *Sox2* expression in the mouse PLE follows that of *Pax6* and is dependent on BMP4. Pax6 and Sox2 proteins physically interact to control δ-crystallin gene expression in the chick lens (Kamachi et al., 2001). Recent evidence also suggests that Sox2 may cooperate with Oct-1 in mice to activate the *Pax6* promoter through binding sites in the ectoderm enhancer (Donner et al., 2007). Null mutations in *Sox2* cause early embryonic lethality and mice with *Sox2* specifically deleted in the PLE have not been reported (Avilion et al., 2003). Gene-targeting mutations have determined a specific requirement for Sox1 for fiber cell elongation and γ-crystallin expression (Nishiguchi et al., 1998).

The regulation of Pax6$^{pre\text{-}placode}$ expression is less clear. There is evidence suggesting that vertebrate sensory and neurogenic placodes arise from a common preplacodal region (PPR) near the edge of the neural plate that expresses transcription factors from the Six (from *Drosophila, sine oculis*), Eya (from *Drosophila*, eyes absent), and Dach (from *Drosophila*, dachshund) families (reviewed in Donner et al., 2006; Schlosser, 2006). *Pax6* is subsequently expressed in the portion of the PPR fated to become the lens. Although the direct relationship of *Six/Eye/Dach* expression and Pax6$^{pre\text{-}placode}$ expression is not firmly established in mouse lens induction, there is experimental evidence that Six3 may be required. First, *Six3* expression may precede *Pax6* expression in the PLE, and deletion of loxP-flanked exons of *Six3* at E8.5 reduces Pax6$^{pre\text{-}placode}$ expression. Furthermore, Six3 binds both the *Pax6* ectoderm enhancer and the SIMO element in vitro and in vivo, transactivates a reporter construct consisting of the *Pax6* ectoderm enhancer fused to luciferase in cultured cells, and expands the *Pax6* expression domain of chick embryo head ectoderm following in ovo electroporation (Liu et al., 2006). Pax6^{placode} expression is required for the upregulation of *Six3* expression in the lens placode, and a *Six3* transgene under the regulatory control of the αA-crystallin promoter upregulates *Pax6* expression, leading to a rescue of *Pax6* heterozygous deficiency in the lens (Goudreau et al., 2002). Evidence suggests that Pax6 and Six3 are each able to regulate the expression of the other, and this reciprocal regulatory relationship is also seen in *eyeless* and *sin oculis*, the *Drosophila* orthologues of these genes.

Additional evidence for the role of Fgfr signaling in early lens development comes from recent analysis of mice lacking

Ndst1. Ndst1 is a member of a family of enzymes responsible for the synthesis of heparan sulfate required for heparan sulfate proteoglycan (HSPG) formation. HSPGs have been shown to participate in several different signal transduction pathways during development (reviewed in Lin, 2004), including the Wnt, Bmp, and Fgf pathways. Mice with targeted deletions in *Ndst1* have ocular defects ranging from microphthalmia to anophthalmia resulting from a small lens placode invagination and reduced proliferation in the resultant lens (Pan et al., 2006). Despite the ability of HSPGs to participate in several different signaling pathways, the early lens in Ndst1 knockout mice is specifically compromised in Fgfr signaling and exhibits dramatic reductions in the level of phosphorylated (active) Erk in the lens (Pan et al., 2006). Targeted mutations in *Frs2α* phosphorylation sites, specifically linking Fgfr signaling to Erk activation, also led to defective lens induction (Gotoh et al., 2004).

AP2α is widely expressed in the embryonic head ectoderm, and its expression is not dependent on Pax6. Targeted mutations in *AP2α* lead to numerous craniofacial malformations, including abnormal lens development. Furthermore, *Pax6* expression in lens tissue present in *AP2α* null mice is reduced relative to that in wild-type lenses, suggesting that AP2α may play a role in *Pax6* gene regulation (West-Mays et al., 1999).

Several genes regulating lens development appear to be downstream from Pax6 in the lens induction pathway. Another gene that is upregulated in lens placode is *Mab21l1*, named after the *C. elegans* gene *mab-21* required for ray identity specification. Mice lacking *Mab21l1* exhibit severe microphthalmia, at least in part because of lowered proliferation in cells comprising the lens placode and early lens vesicle. Mab21l1 deficiency in lens cells is cell autonomous, as *Mab21l1* homozygous mutant cells are specifically underrepresented in the lenses of chimeric mice. *Pax6* expression is not altered in Mab21l1-deficient embryos, but *Mab21l1* expression is lost in the absence of Pax6 (Yamada et al., 2003). Although Mab21l1-deficient lens cells are able express transcripts for differentiation-specific crystallins, *Foxe3* expression within the lens is dramatically reduced.

Foxe3 is a winged-helix transcription factor that is normally expressed in the PLE prior to placode formation, and *Foxe3* expression becomes restricted to the lens epithelial cells as development progresses. A mutation in *Foxe3* is responsible for the spontaneously occurring *dysgenetic lens* (*dyl*) allele in mice (Blixt et al., 2000). Foxe3-deficient lenses display numerous developmental anomalies. Primary fiber cell differentiation, as assessed by the expression of differentiation-specific crystallins, does take place in the absence of Foxe3, but proliferation in the lens epithelium is severely reduced (Blixt et al., 2000; Medina-Martinez et al., 2005). Epithelial cells in Foxe3 mutants also display characteristics consistent with premature differentiation and undergo high rates of apoptosis (Blixt et al., 2000). *Foxe3*-deficient lens vesicles also fail to separate from the surface ectoderm, leading to a persistent lens stalk. In the eye, *Foxe3* is not expressed in the absence of Pax6 (Brownell et al., 2000), and *Foxe3* expression is reduced in *Sey* heterozygotes (Blixt et al., 2007). Foxe3 deficiency also leads to abnormal differentiation of the neural crest–derived structures of the anterior segment, including the corneal endothelium, iris, and trabecular meshwork. This is not particularly surprising, as many mutations interfering with early lens development affect these tissues (Beebe and Coats, 2000). More surprising is the finding of subtle abnormalities in these anterior segment tissues in *Foxe3* heterozygous mutants, where morphological lens development appears normal (Blixt et al., 2007). Within the eye, Foxe3 is not expressed outside the lens. Therefore, Foxe3 may be involved in the signaling from the lens responsible for the organization of neural crest cells into ocular structures of the anterior segment.

Foxe3 expression is also lost in the absence of Sip1, a Smad-binding homeodomain transcription factor (Yoshimoto et al., 2005). *Sip1* is normally expressed in the lens placode and after lens formation; *Sip1* is expressed in the lens epithelium and at the equator where secondary fiber differentiation occurs. Sip1 acts cooperatively with Smad8 to activate the *Foxe3* promoter in transfection assays, but the promoter element responsible for this activation does not confer lens specificity in transgenic mice (Yoshimoto et al., 2005). Conditional deletion of *Sip1* in the lens placode leads to lens cell apoptosis and failure of the lens to separate from the surface ectoderm, features common to *Sey* heterozygotes and Foxe3-deficient mice. In addition, the loss of Sip1 inhibits lens fiber differentiation. Sip1-deficient fiber cells express low levels of β-crystallins, fail to fully elongate, and do not express γ-crystallins (Yoshimoto et al., 2005). *Sip1* expression is not affected by Foxe3 loss, but the dependence of *Sip1* expression in the lens placode on Pax6 is unknown.

In addition to factors that promote lens induction, there are also factors that appear to act to inhibit lens induction in the head ectoderm. Conditional deletion of β-*catenin* in the PLE leads to ectopic appearance of lentoid bodies expressing β-crystallins and Prox1 in the surface ectoderm located nasally relative to the normal lens (Smith et al., 2005). β-catenin is an essential component of the canonical Wnt signaling pathway, and analysis of canonical Wnt signaling reporter mice suggests that this pathway is not active in the ectoderm that will form the lens but is active in adjacent ectoderm that will normally form the conjunctival epithelium and nasal epidermis (Miller et al., 2006; Smith et al., 2005). Furthermore, ectopic activation of canonical Wnt signaling in the developing lens inhibits lens formation (Miller et al., 2006; Smith et al., 2005). This evidence suggests that the normal role for Wnt signaling in the early lens is to suppress lens formation in *Pax6*-expressing head ectoderm outside the lens. Canonical Wnt signaling may play an important role in the lens during later (post E12.5) development as the loss of another essential component of this pathway, Lrp6, leads to discontinuities in the lens epithelium (Stump et al., 2003).

Lens fiber differentiation

Shortly after the lens pit invaginates with the optic cup, the cells at the bottom of the pit begin elongating and primary fiber cell differentiation commences. The subject of fiber cell differentiation is discussed in several recent reviews (Bassnett and Beebe, 2004; Beebe et al., 2004; Boros et al., 2006; Lovicu and McAvoy, 2005; Menko and Walker, 2004; Rao and Maddala, 2006; Robinson, 2006) and so is discussed only briefly here. Many of the same molecules important for lens induction, namely Bmps and Fgfs, are thought to be essential for the process of lens fiber differentiation. The endpoints of fiber cell differentiation are elongation, cell cycle exit, expression of fiber cell–specific proteins (e.g., CP49, filensin, connexin46, aquaporin0, β-crystallins, γ-crystallins), and ultimately loss of subcellular organelles.

Homozygosity for targeted mutations in the genes encoding the transcription factors *c-Maf* (Kawauchi et al., 1999; Kim et al., 1999; Ring et al., 2000), *Sox1* (Nishiguchi et al., 1998), and *Prox1* (Wigle et al., 1999) all result in failed lens fiber cell elongation. The loss of any of these three transcription factors also compromises the expression of differentiation-specific crystallin expression. Expression of αA- as well as all the β- and γ-crystallins is severely compromised in *c-Maf* knockout mice, consistent with the observation of Maf-binding sites in many crystallin gene promoters (reviewed in Cvekl et al., 2004; Reza and Yasuda, 2004a; Reza and Yasuda, 2004b). It must be noted however, that secondary fiber cells do not form in *c-Maf* knockout mice, and several of the γ-crystallin genes are not expressed in primary fiber cells. The expression of other fiber cell proteins such as CP49, filensin, and aquaporin0 is also reduced in *c-Maf* knockout mice, but these genes may not be directly regulated by c-Maf (DePianto et al., 2003). *Sox1* loss results in a loss of γ-crystallin expression but is not needed for the expression of *αA-*, *αB-* and *βA3/A1-crystallin* (Nishiguchi et al., 1998). *Prox1* knockout mice demonstrated a specific loss in *γB-* and *γD-crystallin* expression, but it is not known if this is a direct or an indirect effect of *Prox1* loss. The regulatory relationships of c-Maf, Sox1 and Prox1 are unclear. *Sox1* and *Prox1* are expressed normally in the absence of c-Maf (Ring et al., 2000), suggesting that these regulatory proteins may be involved in parallel rather than linear pathways of crystallin regulation.

Cell cycle withdrawal in differentiating lens fiber cells ultimately depends on Rb hypophosphorylation. This is largely achieved in lens cells through the regulation of cyclin-dependent kinase inhibitors $p27^{Kip1}$ and $p57^{Kip2}$ (reviewed in Griep and Zhang, 2004). Notably, the expression of $p57^{Kip2}$ dramatically increases as fiber cells begin to differentiate. This increase in $p57^{Kip2}$ expression is lost in the absence of *Prox1*, and Prox1-deficient lens cells remain in the cell cycle (Wigle et al., 1999). *Prox1* is expressed in the lens placode and its expression depends on Pax6 (Ashery-Padan et al., 2000). *Prox1* is expressed in the lens epithelium and is upregulated on fiber cell differentiation (Wigle et al., 1999). Prox1 protein also undergoes a change in subcellular localization from a primarily cytoplasmic location to a nuclear location as lens fiber cells differentiate (Duncan et al., 2002). Loss of Foxe3 function leads to an upregulation of *Prox1* in the mouse lens epithelium, consistent with a role for Foxe3 and Prox1 in promoting and inhibiting lens epithelial cell proliferation, respectively.

The loss of subcellular organelles marks the final stage of lens fiber cell differentiation. Organelle loss during fiber differentiation is coordinated and takes place over a relatively short period of time, forming an organelle-free zone in the center of the mature lens. Many have compared the breakdown of nuclei and mitochondria in the lens to apoptosis (reviewed in Bassnett, 2002). While some lens epithelial cell apoptosis normally takes place in the lens epithelium, excessive apoptosis leads to pathology (reviewed in Yan et al., 2006). Caspases, largely responsible for cellular proteolysis during apoptosis, were considered likely mediators of organelle breakdown during lens fiber cell differentiation. These observations were based on the finding that caspase substrates were cleaved during lens organelle breakdown (Bassnett and Mataic, 1997; Ishizaki et al., 1998; Wride et al., 1999). Examination of knockout mice in which each of the so-called executioner caspases was deleted called this presumption into question. No abnormalities in fiber cell organelle loss were noted in mice deficient in caspase-3, caspase-6, caspase-7 or mice doubly deficient in caspase-3 and caspase-6 (Zandy et al., 2005). In contrast, recent evidence suggests that the ubiquitin-proteasome pathway mediates mitochondrial degradation in maturing lens fiber cells and is responsible for VEIDase activity (normally attributed to caspase-6) in lens extracts (Zandy and Bassnett, 2007).

Conclusion

There are many important aspects of mouse lens development, and many important scientific contributions are beyond the scope of this chapter. To cover lens development comprehensively would take far more than a chapter. The goal of this review is rather to inspire those with an interest in lens development with an introduction to the rich history of mouse lens research and with the virtually limitless current possibilities to analyze the molecular mechanisms of lens development through the power of mouse genetics. The use of Cre recombinase for conditional gene deletion in the lens is already becoming commonplace, and other molecular tools, including Flp and ϕC31, promise to expand the ability to fine-tune manipulation of the mouse genome for inducible, tissue-specific gene manipulation (reviewed in Branda and Dymecki, 2004). Breakthroughs are forthcoming in nearly all aspects of lens development research. Although many of the key molecules, particularly transcription factors, for lens development are now known, the precise regulatory relationship of these molecules is often still unclear. For example, the genetic hierarchy of *Six3*, *Pax6*, and *Sox2* in mouse lens development is still an area of debate. The genes responsible for ocular defects in C57BL/6 mice remain unknown, as well as the precise Fgf ligands that influence lens development. The nature of the molecular communication between the lens and the neural crest cells remains a mystery. These are but a few of the thousands of questions that are yet to be answered. With the current and future ability to exploit the mouse genome to map and manipulate genes, these answers await only the talent, time, imagination, and resources required from those willing to uncover them.

ACKNOWLEDGMENTS Work was supported by grant no. EY012995 from the National Eye Institute. The author thanks members of the Robinson laboratory for proofreading the manuscript, and Frank Lovicu, Richard Lang, and Ruth Ashery-Padan for providing high-resolution images for use in figure construction.

REFERENCES

Alizadeh, A., Clark, J., Seeberger, T., Hess, J., Blankenship, T., and FitzGerald, P. G. (2003). Targeted deletion of the lens fiber cell-specific intermediate filament protein filensin. *Invest. Ophthalmol. Vis. Sci.* 44:5252–5258.

Alizadeh, A., Clark, J., Seeberger, T., Hess, J., Blankenship, T., and FitzGerald, P. G. (2004). Characterization of a mutation in the lens-specific CP49 in the 129 strain of mouse. *Invest. Ophthalmol. Vis. Sci.* 45:884–891.

Alizadeh, A., Clark, J. I., Seeberger, T., Hess, J., Blankenship, T., Spicer, A., and FitzGerald, P. G. (2002). Targeted genomic deletion of the lens-specific intermediate filament protein CP49. *Invest. Ophthalmol. Vis. Sci.* 43:3722–3727.

Ash, J. D., and Overbeek, P. A. (2000). Lens-specific VEGF-A expression induces angioblast migration and proliferation and stimulates angiogenic remodeling. *Dev. Biol.* 223:383–398.

Ashery-Padan, R., Marquardt, T., Zhou, X., and Gruss, P. (2000). Pax6 activity in the lens primordium is required for lens formation and for correct placement of a single retina in the eye. *Genes Dev.* 14:2701–2711.

Avilion, A. A., Nicolis, S. K., Pevny, L. H., Perez, L., Vivian, N., and Lovell-Badge, R. (2003). Multipotent cell lineages in early mouse development depend on SOX2 function. *Genes Dev.* 17:126–140.

Bassnett, S. (2002). Lens organelle degradation. *Exp. Eye Res.* 74: 1–6.

Bassnett, S., and Beebe, D. (2004). Lens fiber differentiation. In F. J. Lovicu and M. L. Robinson (Eds.), *Development of the ocular lens* (pp. 214–244). New York: Cambridge University Press.

Bassnett, S., and Mataic, D. (1997). Chromatin degradation in differentiating fiber cells of the eye lens. *J. Cell Biol.* 137:37–49.

Beebe, D., and Coats, J. M. (2000). The lens organizes the anterior segment: Specification of neural crest cell differentiation in the avian eye. *Dev. Biol.* 220:424–431.

Beebe, D., Garcia, C., Wang, X., Rajagopal, R., Feldmeier, M., Kim, J. Y., Chytil, A., Moses, H., Ashery-Padan, R., and Rauchman, M. (2004). Contributions by members of the TGFbeta superfamily to lens development. *Int. J. Dev. Biol.* 48:845–856.

Blixt, A., Landgren, H., Johansson, B. R., and Carlsson, P. (2007). *Foxe3* is required for morphogenesis and differentiation of the anterior segment of the eye and is sensitive to *Pax6* gene dosage. *Dev. Biol.* 302(1):218–219.

Blixt, A., Mahlapuu, M., Aitola, M., Pelto-Huikko, M., Enerback, S., and Carlsson, P. (2000). A forkhead gene, *FoxE3*, is essential for lens epithelial proliferation and closure of the lens vesicle. *Genes Dev.* 14:245–254.

Boros, J., Newitt, P., Wang, Q., McAvoy, J. W., and Lovicu, F. J. (2006). Sef and Sprouty expression in the developing ocular lens: Implications for regulating lens cell proliferation and differentiation. *Semin. Cell Dev. Biol.* 17:741–752.

Brady, J. P., Garland, D., Duglas-Tabor, Y., Robison, W. G., Jr., Groome, A., and Wawrousek, E. F. (1997). Targeted disruption of the mouse alpha A-crystallin gene induces cataract and cytoplasmic inclusion bodies containing the small heat shock protein alpha B-crystallin. *Proc. Natl. Acad. Sci. U.S.A.* 94:884–889.

Brady, J. P., Garland, D. L., Green, D. E., Tamm, E. R., Giblin, F. J., and Wawrousek, E. F. (2001). AlphaB-crystallin in lens development and muscle integrity: A gene knockout approach. *Invest. Ophthalmol. Vis. Sci.* 42:2924–2934.

Branda, C. S., and Dymecki, S. M. (2004). Talking about a revolution: The impact of site-specific recombinases on genetic analyses in mice. *Dev. Cell* 6:7–28.

Breitman, M. L., Clapoff, S., Rossant, J., Tsui, L., Glode, L. M., Maxwell, I. H., and Bernstein, A. (1987). Genetic ablation: Targeted expression of a toxin gene causes microphthalmia in transgenic mice. *Science* 238:1563–1565.

Brownell, I., Dirksen, M., and Jamrich, M. (2000). Forkhead Foxe3 maps to the dysgenetic lens locus and is critical in lens development and differentiation. *Genesis* 27:81–93.

Capetanaki, Y., Starnes, S., and Smith, S. (1989). Expression of the chicken vimentin gene in transgenic mice: Efficient assembly of the avian protein into the cytoskeleton. *Proc. Natl. Acad. Sci. U.S.A.* 86:4882–4886.

Carper, D., Smith-Gill, S. J., and Kinoshita, J. H. (1986). Immunocytochemical localization of the 27K beta-crystallin polypeptide in the mouse lens during development using a specific monoclonal antibody: Implications for cataract formation in the Philly mouse. *Dev. Biol.* 113:104–109.

Chase, H. B. (1942). Studies on an anophthalmic strain of mice. III. Results of crosses with other strains. *Genetics* 27:339–348.

Chase, H. B. (1944). Studies on an anophthalmic strain of mice. IV. A second major gene for anophthalmia. *Genetics* 29: 264–269.

Chase, H. B., and Chase, E. B. (1941). Studies of an anophthalmic strain of mice. I. Embryology of the eye region. *J. Morph.* 68:279–301.

Chepelinsky, A. B., King, C. R., Zelenka, P. S., and Piatigorsky, J. (1985). Lens-specific expression of the chloramphenicol acetyltransferase gene promoted by 5′ flanking sequences of the murine alpha A-crystallin gene in explanted chicken lens epithelia. *Proc. Natl. Acad. Sci. U.S.A.* 82:2334–2338.

Cook, C. S., Nowotny, A. Z., and Sulik, K. K. (1987). Fetal alcohol syndrome: Eye malformations in a mouse model. *Arch. Ophthalmol.* 105:1576–1581.

Cook, C. S., and Sulik, K. K. (1986). Sequential scanning electron microscopic analyses of normal and spontaneously occurring abnormal ocular development in C57Bl/6J mice. *Scan. Electron Microsc.* (pt. 3):1215–1227.

Coulombre, J. L., and Coulombre, A. J. (1963). Lens development: Fiber elongation and lens orientation. *Science* 142: 1489–1490.

Cvekl, A., Yang, Y., Chauhan, B. K., and Cveklova, K. (2004). Regulation of gene expression by Pax6 in ocular cells: A case of tissue-preferred expression of crystallins in lens. *Int. J. Dev. Biol.* 48:829–844.

Decsi, A., Peiffer, R. L., Qiu, T., Lee, D. C., Friday, J. T., and Bautch, V. L. (1994). Lens expression of TGF alpha in transgenic mice produces two distinct eye pathologies in the absence of tumors. *Oncogene* 9:1965–1975.

Deng, C. X., Wynshaw-Boris, A., Shen, M. M., Daugherty, C., Ornitz, D. M., and Leder, P. (1994). Murine FGFR-1 is required for early postimplantation growth and axial organization. *Genes Dev.* 8:3045–3057.

DePianto, D. J., Blankenship, T. N., Hess, J. F., and FitzGerald, P. G. (2003). Analysis of non-crystallin lens fiber cell gene expression in *c-Maf−/−* mice. *Mol. Vis.* 9:288–294.

Donner, A. L., Episkopou, V., and Maas, R. L. (2007). Sox2 and Pou2f1 interact to control lens and olfactory placode development. *Dev. Biol.* 303:784–799.

Donner, A. L., Lachke, S. A., and Maas, R. L. (2006). Lens induction in vertebrates: Variations on a conserved theme of signaling events. *Semin. Cell Dev. Biol.* 17:676–685.

Dudley, A. T., Lyons, K. M., and Robertson, E. J. (1995). A requirement for bone morphogenetic protein-7 during development of the mammalian kidney and eye. *Genes Dev.* 9:2795–2807.

Duncan, M. K., Cui, W., Oh, D. J., and Tomarev, S. I. (2002). Prox1 is differentially localized during lens development. *Mech. Dev.* 112:195–198.

Duncan, M. K., Cvekl, A., Kantorow, M., and Piatigorsky, J. (2004). Lens crystallins. In F. J. Lovicu and M. L. Robinson (Eds.), *Development of the ocular lens* (pp. 119–150). New York: Cambridge University Press.

Faber, S. C., Dimanlig, P., Makarenkova, H. P., Shirke, S., Ko, K., and Lang, R. A. (2001). Fgf receptor signaling plays a role in lens induction. *Development* 128:4425–4438.

Fisher, M., and Grainger, R. M. (2004). Lens induction and determination. In F. J. Lovicu and M. L. Robinson (Eds.), *Development of the ocular lens* (pp. 27–47). New York: Cambridge University Press.

Flugel-Koch, C., Ohlmann, A., Piatigorsky, J., and Tamm, E. R. (2002). Disruption of anterior segment development by TGF-beta1 overexpression in the eyes of transgenic mice. *Dev. Dyn.* 225:111–125.

Furuta, Y., and Hogan, B. L. (1998). BMP4 is essential for lens induction in the mouse embryo. *Genes Dev.* 12:3764–3775.

Goring, D. R., Breitman, M. L., and Tsui, L. C. (1992). Temporal regulation of six crystallin transcripts during mouse lens development. *Exp. Eye Res.* 54:785–795.

Goring, D. R., Rossant, J., Clapoff, S., Breitman, M. L., and Tsui, L. C. (1987). In situ detection of beta-galactosidase in lenses of transgenic mice with a gamma-crystallin/lacZ gene. *Science* 235:456–458.

Gotoh, N., Ito, M., Yamamoto, S., Yoshino, I., Song, N., Wang, Y., Lax, I., Schlessinger, J., Shibuya, M., and Lang, R. A. (2004). Tyrosine phosphorylation sites on FRS2alpha responsible for Shp2 recruitment are critical for induction of lens and retina. *Proc. Natl. Acad. Sci. U.S.A.* 101:17144–17149.

Goudreau, G., Petrou, P., Reneker, L. W., Graw, J., Loster, J., and Gruss, P. (2002). Mutually regulated expression of *Pax6* and *Six3* and its implications for the *Pax6* haploinsufficient lens phenotype. *Proc. Natl. Acad. Sci. U.S.A.* 99:8719–8724.

Graham, D. R., Overbeek, P. A., and Ash, J. D. (2005). Leukemia inhibitory factor blocks expression of Crx and Nrl transcription factors to inhibit photoreceptor differentiation. *Invest. Ophthalmol. Vis. Sci.* 46:2601–2610.

Graw, J., and Loster, J. (2003). Developmental genetics in ophthalmology. *Ophthalmic Genet.* 24:1–33.

Green, E. L. (1981). Genetics and probability in animal breeding experiments. New York: Oxford University Press.

Griep, A. E., and Zhang, P. (2004). Lens cell proliferation: The cell cycle. In F. J. Lovicu and M. L. Robinson (Eds.), *Development of the ocular lens* (pp. 191–213). New York: Cambridge University Press.

Grindley, J. C., Davidson, D. R., and Hill, R. E. (1995). The role of *Pax-6* in eye and nasal development. *Development* 121:1433–1442.

Harch, C., Chase, H. B., and Gonsalves, N. I. (1978). Studies on an anophthalmic strain of mice. VI. Lens and cup interaction. *Dev. Biol.* 63:352–357.

Hayashi, S., and McMahon, A. P. (2002). Efficient recombination in diverse tissues by a tamoxifen-inducible form of Cre: A tool for temporally regulated gene activation/inactivation in the mouse. *Dev. Biol.* 244:305–318.

Haynes, J. I., Duncan, M. K., and Piatigorsky, J. (1996). Spatial and temporal activity of the alpha B-crystallin/small heat shock protein gene promoter in transgenic mice. *Dev. Dyn.* 207:75–88.

Hung, F. C., Zhao, S., Chen, Q., and Overbeek, P. A. (2002). Retinal ablation and altered lens differentiation induced by ocular overexpression of BMP7. *Vision Res.* 42:427–438.

Ishizaki, Y., Jacobson, M. D., and Raff, M. C. (1998). A role for caspases in lens fiber differentiation. *J. Cell Biol.* 140:153–158.

Kalter, H. (1968). Sporadic congenital malformations of newborn inbred mice. *Teratology* 1:193–199.

Kamachi, Y., Uchikawa, M., Tanouchi, A., Sekido, R., and Kondoh, H. (2001). Pax6 and SOX2 form a co-DNA-binding partner complex that regulates initiation of lens development. *Genes Dev.* 15:1272–1286.

Kaufman, M. H. (1992). *The atlas of mouse development.* New York: Academic Press.

Kawauchi, S., Takahashi, S., Nakajima, O., Ogino, H., Morita, M., Nishizawa, M., Yasuda, K., and Yamamoto, M. (1999). Regulation of lens fiber cell differentiation by transcription factor c-Maf. *J. Biol. Chem.* 274:19254–19260.

Kessler, P. L. (1877). *Zur Entwickelung des Auges der Wirberthiere.* Leipzig: Vogel.

Kim, J. I., Li, T., Ho, I. C., Grusby, M. J., and Glimcher, L. H. (1999). Requirement for the c-Maf transcription factor in crystallin gene regulation and lens development. *Proc. Natl. Acad. Sci. U.S.A.* 96:3781–3785.

King, C., and Piatigorsky, J. (1983). Alternative RNA splicing of the murine αA-crystallin gene: protein-coding information within an intron. *Cell* 32:707–712.

King, H. (1905). Experimental studies on the eye of the frog embryo. *Arch. Entw. Mech.* 19:85–107.

Kondoh, H., Katoh, K., Takahashi, Y., Fujisawa, H., Yokoyama, M., Kimura, S., Katsuki, M., Saito, M., Nomura, T., Hiramoto, Y., et al. (1987). Specific expression of the chicken delta-crystallin gene in the lens and the pyramidal neurons of the piriform cortex in transgenic mice. *Dev. Biol.* 120:177–185.

Kondoh, H., Yasuda, K., and Okada, T. S. (1983). Tissue-specific expression of a cloned chick delta-crystallin gene in mouse cells. *Nature* 301:440–442.

Kroeber, M., Ohlmann, A., Russell, P., and Tamm, E. R. (2006). Transgenic studies on the role of optineurin in the mouse eye. *Exp. Eye Res.* 82:1075–1085.

Kuszak, J. R., and Costello, M. J. (2004). The structure of the vertebrate lens. In F. J. Lovicu and M. L. Robinson (Eds.), *Development of the ocular lens* (pp. 71–118). New York: Cambridge University Press.

Kuszak, J. R., Mazurkiewicz, M., Jison, L., Madurski, A., Ngando, A., and Zoltoski, R. K. (2006). Quantitative analysis of animal model lens anatomy: Accommodative range is related to fiber structure and organization. *Vet. Ophthalmol.* 9:266–280.

Kuwabara, T., and Imaizumi, M. (1974). Denucleation process of the lens. *Invest. Ophthalmol.* 13:973–981.

Lakso, M., Sauer, B., Mosinger, B., Jr., Lee, E. J., Manning, R. W., Yu, S. H., Mulder, K. L., and Westphal, H. (1992). Targeted oncogene activation by site-specific recombination in transgenic mice. *Proc. Natl. Acad. Sci. U.S.A.* 89:6232–6236.

Landel, C. P., Zhao, J., Bok, D., and Evans, G. A. (1988). Lens-specific expression of recombinant ricin induces developmental defects in the eyes of transgenic mice. *Genes Dev.* 2:1168–1178.

Lang, R. A. (2004). Pathways regulating lens induction in the mouse. *Int. J. Dev. Biol.* 48:783–791.

LaVail, M. M., Overbeek P. A., Ash, J. D., and Robinson, M. L. (2008). [Sustained delivery of NT3 by lens fiber cells results in hypertrophy and hypermyelination of peripheral nerves entering the eye without influencing lens development.] Unpublished data.

Lewis, W. (1904). Experimental studies on the development of the eye in amphibia. I. On the origin of the lens. *Rana palustris. Am. J. Anat.* 3:505–536.

Liegéois, N. J., Horner, J. W., and DePinho, R. A. (1996). Lens complementation system for the genetic analysis of growth, differentiation, and apoptosis in vivo. *Proc. Natl. Acad. Sci. U.S.A.* 93:1303–1307.

Lin, X. (2004). Functions of heparan sulfate proteoglycans in cell signaling during development. *Development* 131:6009–6021.

Liu, W., Lagutin, O. V., Mende, M., Streit, A., and Oliver, G. (2006). Six3 activation of *Pax6* expression is essential for mammalian lens induction and specification. *Embo. J.* 25:5383–5395.

LoCascio, N. J., LoCascio, J. A. III, and Dewey, M. J. (1987). Cellular competition in the development of ocular tissues in allophenic mice. *Dev. Biol.* 124:291–294.

Lovicu, F. J., and McAvoy, J. W. (2005). Growth factor regulation of lens development. *Dev. Biol.* 280:1–14.

Luo, G., Hofmann, C., Bronckers, A. L., Sohocki, M., Bradley, A., and Karsenty, G. (1995). BMP-7 is an inducer of nephrogenesis, and is also required for eye development and skeletal patterning. *Genes Dev.* 9:2808–2820.

Macatee, T. L., Hammond, B. P., Arenkiel, B. R., Francis, L., Frank, D. U., and Moon, A. M. (2003). Ablation of specific expression domains reveals discrete functions of ectoderm- and endoderm-derived FGF8 during cardiovascular and pharyngeal development. *Development* 130:6361–6374.

Mahon, K. A., Chepelinsky, A. B., Khillan, J. S., Overbeek, P. A., Piatigorsky, J., and Westphal, H. (1987). Oncogenesis of the lens in transgenic mice. *Science* 235:1622–1628.

Mann, I. (1948). Tissue culture of mouse lens epithelium. *Br. J. Ophthalmol.* 32:591–596.

Mathers, P. H., Grinberg, A., Mahon, K. A., and Jamrich, M. (1997). The Rx homeobox gene is essential for vertebrate eye development. *Nature* 387:603–607.

McAvoy, J. W. (1978). Cell division, cell elongation and distribution of alpha-, beta- and gamma-crystallins in the rat lens. *J. Embryol. Exp. Morphol.* 44:149–165.

McDevitt, D. S., and Yamada, T. (1969). Acquisition of antigenic specificity by amphibian lens epithelial cells in culture. *Am. Zool.* 9:1130–1131.

Medina-Martinez, O., Brownell, I., Amaya-Manzanares, F., Hu, Q., Behringer, R. R., and Jamrich, M. (2005). Severe defects in proliferation and differentiation of lens cells in Foxe3 null mice. *Mol. Cell Biol.* 25:8854–8863.

Mencl, E. (1903). Ein Fall von Beiderseitiger Augenlinsenaußbildung während der Abwesenheit von Augenblasen. *Arch. Entw. Mech.* 16:328–339.

Menko, A. S., and Walker, J. L. (2004). Role of matrix and cell adhesion molecules in lens differentiation. In F. J. Lovicu and M. L. Robinson (Eds.), *Development of the ocular lens* (pp. 245–289). New York: Cambridge University Press.

Miller, L. A., Smith, A. N., Taketo, M. M., and Lang, R. A. (2006). Optic cup and facial patterning defects in ocular ectoderm beta-catenin gain-of-function mice. *BMC Dev. Biol.* 6:14.

Morse, H. C. I. (1978). *Origins of inbred mice.* New York: Academic Press.

Muthukkaruppan, V. (1965). Inductive tissue interaction in the development of the mouse lens in vitro. *J. Exp. Zool.* 159:269–288.

Nguyen, M. M., Potter, S. J., and Griep, A. E. (2002). Deregulated cell cycle control in lens epithelial cells by expression of inhibitors of tumor suppressor function. *Mech. Dev.* 112:101–113.

Nishiguchi, S., Wood, H., Kondoh, H., Lovell-Badge, R., and Episkopou, V. (1998). Sox1 directly regulates the gamma-crystallin genes and is essential for lens development in mice. *Genes Dev.* 12:776–781.

Okada, T. S. (2000). Lens studies continue to provide landmarks of embryology (developmental biology). *J. Biosci.* 25:133–141.

Okada, T. S. (2004). From embryonic induction to cell lineages: Revisiting old problems for modern study. *Int. J. Dev. Biol.* 48:739–742.

Overbeek, P. A., Chepelinsky, A. B., Khillan, J. S., Piatigorsky, J., and Westphal, H. (1985). Lens-specific expression and developmental regulation of the bacterial chloramphenicol acetyltransferase gene driven by the murine alpha A-crystallin promoter in transgenic mice. *Proc. Natl. Acad. Sci. U.S.A.* 82:7815–7819.

Paigen, K. (2003a). One hundred years of mouse genetics: An intellectual history. I. The classical period (1902–1980). *Genetics* 163:1–7.

Paigen, K. (2003b). One hundred years of mouse genetics: An intellectual history. II. The molecular revolution (1981–2002). *Genetics* 163:1227–1235.

Pan, Y., Woodbury, A., Esko, J. D., Grobe, K., and Zhang, X. (2006). Heparan sulfate biosynthetic gene *Ndst1* is required for FGF signaling in early lens development. *Development* 133:4933–4944.

Pei, Y. F., and Rhodin, J. A. (1970). The prenatal development of the mouse eye. *Anat. Rec.* 168:105–125.

Perng, M. D., and Quinlan, R. A. (2005). Seeing is believing! The optical properties of the eye lens are dependent upon a functional intermediate filament cytoskeleton. *Exp. Cell Res.* 305: 1–9.

Philpott, G. W., and Coulombre, A. J. (1965). Lens development. I. The differentiation of embryonic chick lens epithelial cells in vitro and in vivo. *Exp. Cell Res.* 38:635–644.

Pierro, L. J., and Spiggle, J. (1969). Congenital eye defects in the mouse. II. The influence of litter size, litter spacing, and suckling of offspring on risk of eye defects in C57BL mice. *Teratology* 2:337–343.

Puk, O., Dalke, C., Favor, J., de Angelis, M. H., and Graw, J. (2006). Variations of eye size parameters among different strains of mice. *Mamm. Genome* 17:851–857.

Rafferty, N. S. (1972). The cytoarchitecture of normal mouse lens epithelium. *Anat. Rec.* 173:225–228.

Rafferty, N. S., and Rafferty, K. A., Jr. (1981). Cell population kinetics of the mouse lens epithelium. *J. Cell Physiol.* 107: 309–315.

Rao, P. V., and Maddala, R. (2006). The role of the lens actin cytoskeleton in fiber cell elongation and differentiation. *Semin. Cell Dev. Biol.* 17:698–711.

Reneker, L. W., Chen, Q., Bloch, A., Xie, L., Schuster, G., and Overbeek, P. A. (2004). Chick delta1-crystallin enhancer influences mouse alphaA-crystallin promoter activity in transgenic mice. *Invest. Ophthalmol. Vis. Sci.* 45:4083–4090.

Reneker, L. W., and Overbeek, P. A. (1996). Lens-specific expression of PDGF-A alters lens growth and development. *Dev. Biol.* 180:1–12.

Reneker, L. W., Silversides, D. W., Patel, K., and Overbeek, P. A. (1995). TGFα can act as a chemoattractant to perioptic mesenchymal cells in developing mouse eyes. *Development* 121: 1669–1680.

Reneker, L. W., Silversides, D. W., Xu, L., and Overbeek, P. A. (2000). Formation of corneal endothelium is essential for anterior segment development: A transgenic mouse model of anterior segment dysgenesis. *Development* 127:533–542.

Resnikoff, S., Pascolini, D., Etya'ale, D., Kocur, I., Pararajasegaram, R., Pokharel, G. P., and Mariotti, S. P. (2004). Global data on visual impairment in the year 2002. *Bull. WHO* 82:844–851.

Reyes, A., Gissi, C., Catzeflis, F., Nevo, E., Pesole, G., and Saccone, C. (2004). Congruent mammalian trees from mitochondrial and nuclear genes using Bayesian methods. *Mol. Biol. Evol.* 21:397–403.

Reza, H. M., and Yasuda, K. (2004a). Lens differentiation and crystallin regulation: A chick model. *Int. J. Dev. Biol.* 48:805–817.

Reza, H. M., and Yasuda, K. (2004b). Roles of Maf family proteins in lens development. *Dev. Dyn.* 229:440–448.

Ring, B. Z., Cordes, S. P., Overbeek, P. A., and Barsh, G. S. (2000). Regulation of mouse lens fiber cell development and differentiation by the Maf gene. *Development* 127:307–317.

Robinson, M. L. (2006). An essential role for FGF receptor signaling in lens development. *Semin. Cell Dev. Biol.* 17:726–740.

Robinson, M. L., Holmgren, A., and Dewey, M. J. (1993). Genetic control of ocular morphogenesis: Defective lens development associated with ocular anomalies in C57BL/6 mice. *Exp. Eye Res.* 56:7–16.

Robinson, M. L., and Lovicu, F. J. (2004). The lens: Historical and comparative perspectives. In F. J. Lovicu and M. L. Robinson (Eds.), *Development of the ocular lens* (pp. 3–26). New York: Cambridge University Press.

Robinson, M. L., and Overbeek, P. A. (1996). Differential expression of alpha A- and alpha B-crystallin during murine ocular development. *Invest. Ophthalmol. Vis. Sci.* 37:2276–2284.

Rugh, R. (1968). *The mouse: Its reproduction and development.* Minneapolis, MN: Burgess Publishing Co.

Sandilands, A., Wang, X., Hutcheson, A. M., James, J., Prescott, A. R., Wegener, A., Pekny, M., Gong, X., and Quinlan, R. A. (2004). Bfsp2 mutation found in mouse 129 strains causes the loss of CP49′ and induces vimentin-dependent changes in the lens fibre cell cytoskeleton. *Exp. Eye Res.* 78:875–889.

Schlosser, G. (2006). Induction and specification of cranial placodes. *Dev. Biol.* 294:303–351.

Shirke, S., Faber, S. C., Hallem, E., Makarenkova, H. P., Robinson, M. L., Overbeek, P. A., and Lang, R. A. (2001). Misexpression of IGF-I in the mouse lens expands the transitional zone and perturbs lens polarization. *Mech. Dev.* 101: 167–174.

Silver, L. M. (1995). *Mouse genetics: Concepts and applications.* New York: Oxford University Press.

Simirskii, V. N., Lee, R. S., Wawrousek, E. F., and Duncan, M. K. (2006). Inbred FVB/N mice are mutant at the cp49/Bfsp2 locus and lack beaded filament proteins in the lens. *Invest. Ophthalmol. Vis. Sci.* 47:4931–4934.

Smith, A. N., Miller, L. A., Song, N., Taketo, M. M., and Lang, R. A. (2005). The duality of beta-catenin function: a requirement in lens morphogenesis and signaling suppression of lens fate in periocular ectoderm. *Dev. Biol.* 285:477–489.

Spemann, H. (1901). Über Correlationen in der Entwicklung des Auges. *Anat. Anz.* 15:61–79.

Spemann, H. (1907). Neue Tatsächen zum Linsenproblem. *Zool. Anz.* 31:379–386.

Srinivasan, Y., Lovicu, F. J., and Overbeek, P. A. (1998). Lens-specific expression of transforming growth factor beta1 in transgenic mice causes anterior subcapsular cataracts. *J. Clin. Invest.* 101:625–634.

Stump, R. J., Ang, S., Chen, Y., von Bahr, T., Lovicu, F. J., Pinson, K., de Iongh, R. U., Yamaguchi, T. P., Sassoon, D. A., and McAvoy, J. W. (2003). A role for Wnt/beta-catenin signaling in lens epithelial differentiation. *Dev. Biol.* 259:48–61.

Swindell, E. C., Bailey, T. J., Loosli, F., Liu, C., Amaya-Manzanares, F., Mahon, K. A., Wittbrodt, J., and Jamrich, M. (2006). Rx-Cre, a tool for inactivation of gene expression in the developing retina. *Genesis* 44:361–363.

Tucker, P., Laemle, L., Munson, A., Kanekar, S., Oliver, E. R., Brown, N., Schlecht, H., Vetter, M., and Glaser, T. (2001). The eyeless mouse mutation (ey1) removes an alternative start codon from the Rx/rax homeobox gene. *Genesis* 31:43–53.

Van Leen, R. W., Breuer, M. L., Lubsen, N. H., and Schoenmakers, J. G. (1987). Developmental expression of crystallin genes: In situ hybridization reveals a differential localization of specific mRNAs. *Dev. Biol.* 123:338–345.

Vinores, S. A., Xiao, W. H., Zimmerman, R., Whitcup, S. M., and Wawrousek, E. F. (2003). Upregulation of vascular endothelial growth factor (VEGF) in the retinas of transgenic mice overexpressing interleukin-1beta (IL-1beta) in the lens and mice undergoing retinal degeneration. *Histol. Histopathol.* 18:797–810.

Voronina, V. A., Kozhemyakina, E. A., O'Kernick, C. M., Kahn, N. D., Wenger, S. L., Linberg, J. V., Schneider, A. S., and Mathers, P. H. (2004). Mutations in the human RAX homeobox gene in a patient with anophthalmia and sclerocornea. *Hum. Mol. Genet.* 13:315–322.

Vrensen, G. F., Graw, J., and De Wolf, A. (1991). Nuclear breakdown during terminal differentiation of primary lens fibres in mice: A transmission electron microscopic study. *Exp. Eye Res.* 52:647–659.

Wang, X., Garcia, C. M., Shui, Y. B., and Beebe, D. C. (2004). Expression and regulation of alpha-, beta-, and gamma-crystallins in mammalian lens epithelial cells. *Invest. Ophthalmol. Vis. Sci.* 45:3608–3619.

Wawersik, S., Purcell, P., Rauchman, M., Dudley, A. T., Robertson, E. J., and Maas, R. (1999). BMP7 acts in murine lens placode development. *Dev. Biol.* 207:176–188.

West-Mays, J. A., Zhang, J., Nottoli, T., Hagopian-Donaldson, S., Libby, D., Strissel, K. J., and Williams, T. (1999). AP-2alpha transcription factor is required for early morphogenesis of the lens vesicle. *Dev. Biol.* 206:46–62.

Wigle, J. T., Chowdhury, K., Gruss, P., and Oliver, G. (1999). Prox1 function is crucial for mouse lens-fibre elongation. *Nat. Genet.* 21:318–322.

Williams, S. C., Altmann, C. R., Chow, R. L., Hemmati-Brivanlou, A., and Lang, R. A. (1998). A highly conserved lens transcriptional control element from the *Pax-6* gene. *Mech. Dev.* 73:225–229.

Wride, M. A., Parker, E., and Sanders, E. J. (1999). Members of the bcl-2 and caspase families regulate nuclear degeneration during chick lens fibre differentiation. *Dev. Biol.* 213:142–156.

Yamada, R., Mizutani-Koseki, Y., Hasegawa, T., Osumi, N., Koseki, H., and Takahashi, N. (2003). Cell-autonomous involvement of Mab21l1 is essential for lens placode development. *Development* 130:1759–1770.

Yamaguchi, T. P., Harpal, K., Henkemeyer, M., and Rossant, J. (1994). *fgfr-1* is required for embryonic growth and mesodermal patterning during mouse gastrulation. *Genes Dev.* 8:3032–3044.

Yamamoto, Y. (1976). Growth of lens and ocular environment: Role of neural retina in the growth of mouse lens as revealed by an implantation experiment. *Dev. Growth Differ.* 18:273–278.

Yan, Q., Liu, J. P., and Li, D. W. (2006). Apoptosis in lens development and pathology. *Differentiation* 74:195–211.

Yang, Y., Stopka, T., Golestaneh, N., Wang, Y., Wu, K., Li, A., Chauhan, B. K., Gao, C. Y., Cveklova, K., Duncan, M. K., et al. (2006). Regulation of alphaA-crystallin via *Pax6*, c-Maf, CREB and a broad domain of lens-specific chromatin. *Embo J.* 25:2107–2118.

Yoshimoto, A., Saigou, Y., Higashi, Y., and Kondoh, H. (2005). Regulation of ocular lens development by Smad-interacting protein 1 involving Foxe3 activation. *Development* 132:4437–4448.

Zandy, A. J., and Bassnett, S. (2007). Proteolytic mechanisms underlying mitochondrial degradation in the ocular lens. *Invest. Ophthalmol. Vis. Sci.* 48:293–302.

Zandy, A. J., Lakhani, S., Zheng, T., Flavell, R. A., and Bassnett, S. (2005). Role of the executioner caspases during lens development. *J. Biol. Chem.* 280:30263–30272.

Zhang, X., Friedman, A., Heaney, S., Purcell, P., and Maas, R. L. (2002). Meis homeoproteins directly regulate *Pax6* during vertebrate lens morphogenesis. *Genes Dev.* 16:2097–2107.

Zhao, H., Yang, Y., Partanen, J., Ciruna, B. G., Rossant, J., and Robinson, M. L. (2006). Fibroblast growth factor receptor 1 (Fgfr1) is not essential for lens fiber differentiation in mice. *Mol. Vis.* 12:15–25.

Zhao, H., Yang, Y., Rizo, C. M., Overbeek, P. A., and Robinson, M. L. (2004). Insertion of a *Pax6* consensus binding site into the alphaA-crystallin promoter acts as a lens epithelial cell enhancer in transgenic mice. *Invest. Ophthalmol. Vis. Sci.* 45:1930–1939.

Zhao, S., and Overbeek, P. A. (2001). Elevated TGFbeta signaling inhibits ocular vascular development. *Dev. Biol.* 237:45–53.

Zwaan, J. (1983). The appearance of α-crystallin in relation to cell cycle phase in the embryonic mouse lens. *Dev. Biol.* 96:173–181.

23 Development of the Retinal Vasculature and the Effects of High Oxygen (Retinopathy of Prematurity)

MICHAEL R. POWERS

Retinopathy of prematurity (ROP) was initially described and characterized in the 1940s and early 1950s in premature infants and continues to be a leading cause of blindness in children (Ashton, 1968; Recchia and Capone, 2004). Pathological retinal neovascularization and retinal detachment characterize the severe forms of the disease. Infants born at 24–25 weeks' gestation are now surviving and are at highest risk for developing ROP (Recchia and Capone, 2004).

The mouse retina is an ideal model in which to study the pathogenesis of ROP because the retinal vessels develop and mature during the first 3 weeks of life, and the mouse retinal vasculature at birth is similar to that of a 25-week gestation infant (Connolly et al., 1988). Over the past two decades, the normal vascular development in the mouse retina and the effects of oxygen-induced injury have been extensively characterized. The mouse is now the most commonly used animal model in which to study retinal angiogenesis, both in normal development of the retina and in models of oxygen-induced retinopathy (OIR; Madan and Penn, 2003). A literature search of the past 10 years shows that approximately 250 publications referenced the mouse model of OIR. This review highlights many of the murine studies that have contributed to our current understanding of normal retinal vascular development and the pathogenesis of oxygen-induced neovascularization in the immature retina.

Development of the mouse retinal vasculature

The mouse retina is an ideal structure in which to study normal vascular development because it develops after birth and can be easily monitored using retinal flat-mount preparations. Early studies used selective lectin binding and immunohistochemistry to label and visualize the developing retinal vessels in mice (Connolly et al., 1988). Initially, the vessels enter the inner retina from the optic nerve head shortly after birth. The superficial vessels continue to grow and remodel in radial fashion, reaching the retinal periphery at postnatal day 7 (P7) (figure 23.1*A*). Between P7 and P8, branching sprouts from the superficial vascular network grow into the deeper layers of the retina (figure 23.1*B*), completing the deep vascular network in the outer plexiform layer (OPL) by approximately P12 (figure 23.1*C*). The superficial network consists of arteries, veins, and capillaries, while the deep network of vessels is not remodeled beyond a plexus of capillaries. An intermediate vascular network at the inner edge of the inner nuclear layer (INL) is also formed and remodeled during the third week after birth and completed at approximately P18–P20 (Dorrell and Friedlander, 2006). In addition, the mouse retinal vascular networks exhibit vessel remodeling as late as P45 (Connolly et al., 1988). Retinal endothelial cells (ECs) interact with retinal astrocytes and Müller cells to form the blood-retinal barrier (Janzer and Raff, 1987; Tout et al., 1993). Mature retinal ECs are also covered, almost in a 1:1 ratio, by pericytes (Armulik et al., 2005). The retinal capillary networks supply oxygen and nutrients to the inner retina, while the outer nuclear layer (ONL; photoreceptors) receives oxygen from the choroidal circulation.

Vessel formation can occur by a process called vasculogenesis, whereby vascular precursor cells (angioblasts) proliferate and coalesce into a primitive vascular network, or by the process of angiogenesis, the sprouting of new vessels from preexisting vessels (Risau, 1997). Currently there is disagreement in the literature over which mechanism gives rise to the superficial vascular network in the retina (Gariano and Gardner, 2005; Saint-Geniez and D'Amore, 2004). Studies on human and canine retinas have suggested that angioblasts are present in the developing retina and participate in retinal neovascularization (Lutty et al., 2006b). In contrast, recent studies in the mouse retina have suggested that the superficial vascular network is formed by angiogenesis (Dorrell et al., 2002; Fruttiger, 2002; Gerhardt et al., 2003). However, there is general agreement among investigators

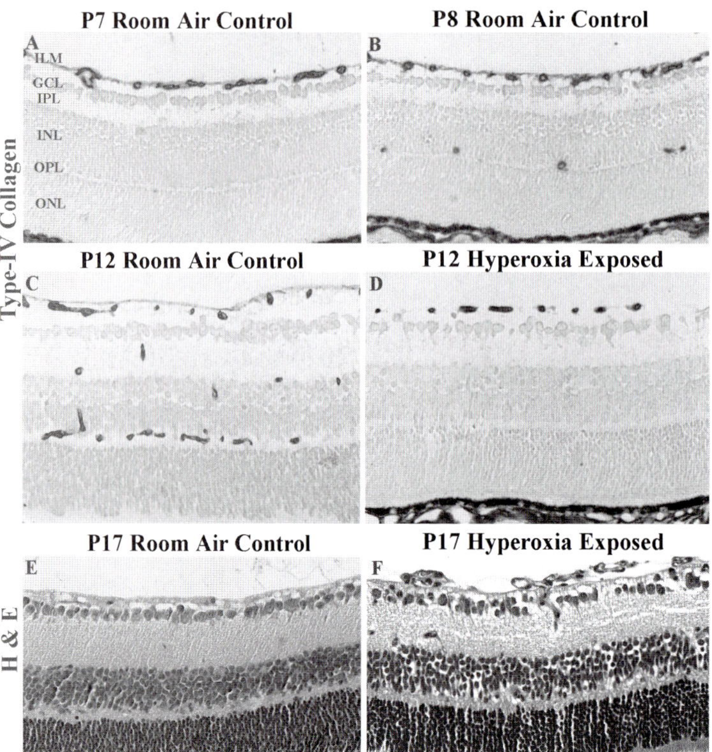

Figure 23.1 Type IV collagen-stained retinal cross sections with the mouse retinal vessels labeled. *A*, P7 retinas show positive staining in the superficial vascular network. *B*, Staining on P8 demonstrates the onset of formation of the deep vascular network. *C*, Normal vascular development is seen on P12 with the completion of the deep network and the onset of the intermediate plexus. *D*, Vascular obliteration in the OIR model is evident on P12. *E*, Hematoxylin-eosin staining on P17 demonstrates normal development of the retina, compared with the neovascularization seen in the OIR model (*F*). *E*, eosin; *H*, hematoxylin; GCL, ganglion cell layer; ILM, inner limiting membrane; INL, inner nuclear layer; IPL, inner plexiform layer; ONL, outer nuclear layer; OPL, outer plexiform layer. Original magnification ×400.

that the deep vascular network, as well as pathological retinal neovascularization, occurs via angiogenesis.

A major advance in understanding retinal vascularization and pathological retinal neovascularization came from early studies that associated retinal hypoxia with the expression of vascular endothelial growth factor-A (VEGF-A), a potent hypoxia-induced angiogenic factor (Pierce et al., 1995). In brief, astrocytes peripheral to the leading edge of the developing superficial vascular network express VEGF-A in response to relative hypoxia, thereby stimulating the proliferation and migration of the immature vessels from the central retina to the periphery. Subsequently, with neuronal activation in the maturing retina, a second wave of VEGF-A expression occurs by Müller cells located in the INL, leading to the formation of the deep vascular network.

Despite the apparent differences between species in the development of the superficial network (vasculogenesis versus angiogenesis), studies of the developing mouse vasculature have been invaluable in advancing our understanding of retinal vascular development (Gariano, 2003). Studies using mice have taken advantage of the wealth of transgenic and gene deletion strains available to investigators. In addition, the postnatal development of the mouse retina permits the directed use of specific agonists or antagonists to delineate specific developmental pathways. Recent studies have focused on the cellular and molecular mechanisms that regulate vessel formation and the pattern of the retinal vascular system. These studies have included examining the interactions of ECs with glial and mural cells, the role of specific VEGF-A isoforms and other growth factors, the role of novel guidance molecules, and the contribution of progenitor cells in vessel formation (Carmeliet and Tessier-Lavigne, 2005; Dorrell and Friedlander, 2006; Gariano and Gardner, 2005).

A variety of growth factor peptides have been localized and evaluated during normal mouse retinal vascular development since the initial VEGF studies were conducted. We review some of these studies in this chapter, but we also discuss additional growth factors and their receptors in the context of interactions with glial and mural cells. Placental growth factor (PGF) is a member of the VEGF family and activates Flt-1 (VEGFR-1). PGF has been localized to large vessels and capillaries in the superficial network of the P9 mouse retina. PGF does not bind to KDR (VEGFR-2) and therefore does not stimulate angiogenesis directly, but it may play a regulatory role by binding to VEGF-A and limiting the activation of KDR (Feeney et al., 2003). Angiopoietin2 (Angpt2) is a pleiotrophic cytokine that, in the absence of VEGF-A, causes vessel regression via induction of EC apoptosis, but in the presence of VEGF-A stimulates vessel sprouting (for a review, see Jain, 2003). Angpt2 appears to sensitize the deep vascular capillaries to VEGF-A-mediated proliferation (Oshima et al., 2004). Tumor necrosis factor (TNF) receptor–deficient mice display a delay in the development of the deep vascular network. Development of the deep network in these mice does not start until P10, and the animals continue to exhibit a reduced number of deep intraretinal vessels compared with controls at P21 (Ilg et al., 2005). Hence, the proliferation of retinal ECs in the deep vascular network may be under the control of TNF, Angpt2, and VEGF-A.

In contrast to alterations in the deep vascular network, two recent reports have linked specific growth factors with the failed development of the superficial vascular network. Near complete inhibition of normal vascular development in mouse retina has been demonstrated both in mice with transgenic overexpression of leukemia inhibitory factor (LIF) and in transgenic mice overexpressing a truncated fibroblast growth factor receptor-1 (FGFR-1) (Rousseau et al., 2003; Ash et al., 2005). These two studies indicate that both LIF and FGFs are essential molecules for normal retinal vascularization. However, when the antiangiogenic factor pigment epithelium–derived factor (PEDF, *Serpinf1*) is overexpressed in the postnatal mouse retina, the vascular networks develop normally, indicating that PEDF does not appear to play a significant role in normal retinal vascularization (Wong et al., 2004).

Two groups have recently examined the vascular pattern and guidance of retinal vessels in the mouse in elegant in vivo studies (Dorrell et al., 2002; Gerhardt et al., 2003). Prior studies have characterized the migration of retinal astrocytes from the optic nerve between embryonic day (E) 18 and 19 and the association of astrocytes with the postnatal development of blood vessels in the superficial network (Zhang and Stone, 1997). This astrocyte influx into the retina and subsequent proliferation is mediated by the expression of platelet-derived growth factor-A (PDGF-A) from retinal ganglion cells, which binds to platelet-derived growth factor receptor-alpha (PDGFR-α) expressed on retinal astrocytes (Fruttiger et al., 1996). Friedlander and colleagues have extended these findings through the use of glial fibrillary acidic protein-green fluorescent protein (GFAP-GFP) transgenic mice, whole-mount immunohistochemistry, and multiphoton confocal microscopy. GFAP-GFP mice allow visualization of GFAP monomers, a marker for more immature astrocytes, through the detection of GFP. In contrast to earlier reports, GFAP-GFP-positive cells (astrocytes) are nearing the retinal periphery at birth, revealing a nearly complete astrocytic network. ECs in the superficial layer are always associated with underlying astrocytes, with ECs exhibiting filopodia-like projections. The fingerlike projections are observed at the leading edge of the superficial network, at points of vessel interconnections, and at branch points heading toward the deep vascular network. Betsholtz and colleagues further characterized the role that VEGF plays in regulating the filopodial extensions at the tips of these vessel sprouts (see Gerhardt et al., 2003). The long filopodia are restricted to a single, highly polarized EC that expresses KDR. These "tip cells" do not proliferate but migrate over the astrocyte's template in response to VEGF-A expressed by astrocytes that are just ahead of the growing vascular network. The "stalk" cells, just posterior to the tip cells, also respond to VEGF-A and are the major site of EC proliferation in the growing vascular plexus.

Local gradients of VEGF-A isoforms have also been shown to play a critical role in normal vessel growth and branching (Gerhardt et al., 2003; Stalmans et al., 2002). The $VEGF_{120}$ isoform is diffusible, while $VEGF_{188}$ is heparin bound to the matrix, and $VEGF_{164}$ demonstrates intermediate properties. Thus, $VEGF_{120}$ acts over a longer distance, while $VEGF_{188}$ action is restricted to a short range. Transgenic mice have been created to express a single VEGF isoform to examine the role of isoforms in retinal vascular development (Stalmans et al., 2002). $VEGF_{120}$ mice ($VEGF_{164,188}$ null) fail to provide the normal gradient of VEGF-A isoforms along the growing vasculature, thereby lacking the proper signals to the tip cell filopodia, resulting in reduced vessel branching. In contrast, $VEGF_{188}$ mice ($VEGF_{120,164}$ null) have excessive matrix-bound VEGF-A expression, resulting in extensive branching of multiple small vessels, as well as the lack of arteriolar specification. $VEGF_{164}$ mice have normal vascular branching, providing enough diffusible VEGF-A to stimulate EC proliferation and enough matrix-bound VEGF-A to provide spatial information and guidance to the growing retinal vessels along the astrocyte template (for a review, see Carmeliet and Tessier-Lavigne, 2005). It is presumed that in wild-type mice, all three forms of VEGF-A contribute to retinal vascular development to some extent; however, $VEGF_{164}$ is required for pathological neovascularization (Saint-Geniez and D'Amore, 2004).

In addition to VEGF-A, the cell surface adhesion molecule cadherin 4 (Cdh4) is localized temporally and spatially at sites of retinal vascularization, specifically at the sites of endothelial filopodia (Dorrell et al., 2002). Retinas treated with an anti-cadherin 4 antibody exhibit stunted vessels, failure of ECs to follow the astrocyte template, and subsequent invasion of vessels from the deep network into the normally avascular photoreceptor region. This suggests that cadherin 4 provides guidance cues to the developing vessels.

Recently, several axon guidance molecules have been implicated in endothelial tip cell guidance and vascular network formation. It appears that the developing vascular system has adopted several molecules that guide neural network formation and axonal growth cone migration, which resembles vascular tip cell migration. These molecules include the netrins, semaphorins, slits, and ephrins and their receptors (Carmeliet and Tessier-Lavigne, 2005; Dorrell and Friedlander, 2006). Specifically, Sema3E-PlexinD1 and Netrin-1-UNC5B interactions have been characterized to provide repulsive signals to the endothelial tip cells during mouse vascular development.

Ephrin ligands and Eph receptors have been the most extensively studied guidance molecules in regard to the formation of vascular and neural networks. The Eph receptor family is the largest group of receptor tyrosine kinases (RTK) known to date, currently made up of 15 receptors that engage nine ephrin ligands. Ephrin ligands contain an extracellular and transmembrane domain. However, ephrin ligands of the A class lack a cytoplasmic tail, while ephrin ligands of the B class contain a cytoplasmic domain, which can initiate an intracellular signaling cascade on interaction with an Eph receptor. Several of the ephrin ligands and ephrin receptors have been implicated in adult angiogenesis, while both ephrin-B2 (EFNB2) and ephrin receptor-B4 (EPhB4) have emerged as key regulators of vascular development. Ephrin-B2 ligand and EphB4 receptor identify arterial and venous ECs, respectively, helping define molecular boundaries between arteries and veins, arresting EC migration at the arterial-venous interface. Both *Efnb2* and *Ephb4* are essential for vascular development, and targeted disruptions of these genes results in embryonic lethality due to defects in arteries and veins and failure to properly remodel vascular networks. EphrinB2 and EPhB4 have recently been localized to the developing retinal vasculature in the mouse retina, and examination of the superficial vascular network allows one to follow the establishment of arteries, veins, and capillaries. Uemura et al (2006) characterized *Efnb2* and *Ephb4* expression in the retinal vessels by detecting *LacZ* expression in retinas from mutant mice heterozygous for each gene. At P2, most of the vascular sprouts around the optic nerve express *Ephb4*, indicating venous origin. However, between P3 and P4, *Efnb2* is expressed in the arteries and associated capillaries, while *Ephb4* expression becomes restricted to veins. Other investigators have also detected *Ephb4* expression in retinal veins as well as in some of the capillaries by in situ hybridization, indicating that the retinal capillaries may have both arterial and venous origins (Saint-Geniez et al., 2003). Retinal mRNA expression of *Efnb2* has been shown to be constitutively expressed in the developing mouse retina, while expression of *Ephb4* was modestly reduced between P12 and P17 (Zamora et al., 2005).

Of interest, oxygen levels can regulate *Ephb2* expression in retinal ECs in the developing retina (Claxton and Fruttiger, 2005). Mice raised in 10% oxygen from birth exhibit reduced capillary-free zones around retinal arteries on P6, and concurrently, *Efnb2* expression was absent from the arteries. Increasing the oxygen exposure to 60% at birth resulted in widening of the capillary-free zone around arteries but did not alter the expression of *Efnb2*. Mice exposed to hypoxic conditions develop a retinal vascular network that exhibits an abnormal double superficial capillary network and unusual spacing between arteries and veins. Despite the lack of *Efnb2* expression in response to hypoxia, the arterial ECs do not express vein-specific markers, indicating the arteries do not convert to veins, and oxygen levels do not directly determine cell fate. However, it appears that arterial ECs require a threshold of oxygen to express *Efnb2*, and its absence results in an abnormal spatial organization of the developing retinal vasculature, perhaps from inability to develop proper boundaries between arteries and veins.

Pericytes are mural cells that colocalize with retinal vessels. These cells are distributed evenly throughout the developing vascular network but always lag slightly behind the leading edge of the vessel sprout (Fruttiger, 2002). Pericytes, which express PDGFR-β, proliferate and migrate in response to the PDGF-B, which is expressed by the EC tip cells. The major role of pericytes is to provide stability to the nascent vessel. Pericytes encircle the vessel with long cytoplasmic extensions, making focal contacts with ECs via junctional complexes located at sites where the shared basement membrane is absent (Armulik et al., 2005). The critical role of PDGF-B in EC-pericyte interactions was confirmed in endothelium-specific *Pdgf-b* knockout mice. In this strain, pericyte recruitment is altered, resulting in a diabetic-like retinopathy (Enge et al., 2002). Transforming growth factor-beta$_1$ (TGF-β_1, *Tgfb1*) expressed by EC is also important for pericyte differentiation and function. There are numerous studies of gene deletion of TGF-β ligands, TGF-β receptors, binding proteins, and other downstream signaling molecules, resulting in cardiovascular defects and vascular malformations (Armulik et al., 2005). Recent coculture studies have shown that mesenchymal cells can express VEGF-A as they differentiate into pericytes in response to TGF-β, while in vivo studies have confirmed that capillary-associated pericytes express VEGF-A in the developing mouse retinal vasculature (Darland et al., 2003). These findings suggest that astrocytes and pericytes are sources for VEGF-A and both cell types are important for vessel stabilization.

Pericyte-derived angiopoietin-1 (Angpt1) also contributes to vessel stabilization by activating the TEK receptor on vascular ECs, mediating maturation and quiescence of the retinal microvessels (Jain, 2003). Angpt1 null mice die in midgestation and exhibit microvascular defects of altered pericyte coverage. In the absence of pericytes, exogenous Angpt1 helps restore vessel integrity in the developing mouse retina, reducing edema and hemorrhage (Armulik et al., 2005).

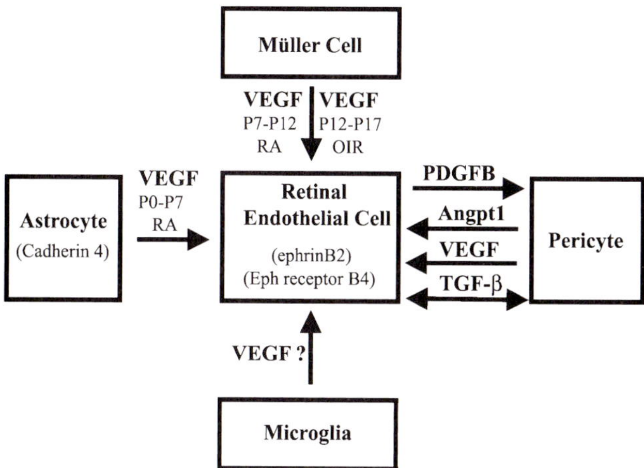

FIGURE 23.2 Schematic summary of cytokine interactions between endothelial cells and resident cells during postnatal retinal vascular development.

Figure 23.2 is a schematic summary of cytokine interactions between ECs and resident cells during retinal vasculature development, which are subject to alteration by high oxygen exposure.

Bone marrow–derived hematopoietic stem cells (HSCs) can differentiate into nonhematopoietic (Lin^-) lineages, function as endothelial progenitor cells (EPCs), and participate in retinal neovascularization (Grant et al., 2002). In the neonatal mouse retina, EPCs can target retinal astrocytes and incorporate into the developing vasculature (Otani et al., 2002). Alternatively, when a subset of Lin^- HSC cells ($CD44^{hi}$) are intravitreally injected into eyes of neonatal mice, the $CD44^{hi}$ cells differentiate into microglia and promote revascularization of the central retina, as well as reduce neovascular tuft formation in the mouse model of OIR. These studies suggest there is a subpopulation of Lin^- HSCs that participates in normal vascular development and pathological retinal neovascularization. The use of cell-based therapies certainly needs further investigation, but they hold promise for future approaches to the treatment of ischemic retinopathies and retinal degenerative diseases.

Historical perspective: Mouse model of retinopathy of prematurity

The association between high levels of supplemental oxygen and ROP was characterized by several investigators in the early 1950s (Ashton, 1968; Madan and Penn, 2003). These studies recognized the obliteration of developing retinal vessels from hyperoxia and subsequent pathological retinal neovascularization on returning to room air. Concurrently with these clinical observations, several groups were also investigating the effect of hyperoxia on the mouse retina (for a review, see Ashton, 1968; Madan and Penn, 2003). These studies entailed using 100% oxygen for variable lengths of time, with the exposure initiated at birth or shortly after birth. The studies demonstrated obliteration of vascular development in newborn mice from hyperoxia exposure. Furthermore, when these mice recovered in room air, preretinal neovascularization was also observed around the optic disc. When older mice were exposed to hyperoxia, neovascularization was observed in the peripheral retina. In addition to the retinal changes observed, marked dilation and proliferation of hyaloid vessels were noted.

The early studies of oxygen toxicity to developing mouse retina were reviewed and repeated by Ashton in the late 1960s to directly compare the mouse studies with the kitten and rat models of oxygen-induced retinopathy (Ashton, 1968). Ashton confirmed that if the mouse retina is exposed to hyperoxia before 5 days of age, a severe hyaloidopathy is the major pathology observed, with a mild retinal neovascularization confined to the disc region. However, when a P5 mouse was exposed to 80%–90% oxygen for 4 days, a star-shaped pattern of vaso-obliteration was observed, but in contrast to earlier studies, Ashton did not observe abnormal retinal neovascularization when the animals were returned to room air (Ashton, 1968). Gole et al. in 1990 suggested that the mouse is a suitable model of OIR, based on their ultrastructural findings of vitreous vessels, and suggested that histological cross sections could be used to grade preretinal neovascularization in future studies. Hence, the early studies using the mouse as a model of OIR were inconsistent and lacked reproducible quantification, and the animals developed a severe hyaloidopathy.

Contemporary perspective: Mouse model of oxygen-induced retinopathy

CHARACTERIZATION OF MODEL Smith and colleagues in the early 1990s developed and characterized a consistent and reproducible model of OIR in neonatal mice (Smith et al., 1994). This model continues to be used today to investigate the pathogenesis and molecular mechanisms of the proliferative retinopathies (ROP, diabetic retinopathy). To develop the model, Smith et al. examined the effect of initiating the hyperoxia exposure from P0 (birth) to P7, while varying the oxygen concentrations between 50% and 95%. Eventually, P7 mice (C57BL/6J) were chosen in order to balance the oxygen-induced injury of the developing retinal vasculature with the regression of the hyaloid vasculature. This aided in avoiding the hyaloidopathy that was observed by earlier investigators. In addition, a 75% oxygen exposure protocol was chosen because it yielded a reproducible pathological preretinal neovascularization without the maternal or pup mortality that was associated with higher oxygen exposures. Neonatal mice (P7) were exposed to 75% oxygen for 5 days and then returned to room air on P12.

Mouse eyes were evaluated daily to assess the neovascular response from P12 until P44. Exposure of adult mice (P24) to 75% oxygen for 5 days did not result in vaso-obliteration or retinal neovascularization, confirming that developing vessels, but not mature retinal vessels, were sensitive to oxygen toxicity. A recent study also determined that mice exhibit a mature vascular response to hyperoxia by P15, by failing to exhibit a vaso-obliteration response (Gu et al., 2002).

Two different techniques were used to assess and quantify the vascular response. The first method used high-molecular-weight (HMW) fluorescein-labeled dextrans that were perfused through the left ventricle just prior to sacrifice, allowing visualization of the entire retinal vasculature with fluorescence microscopy. This technique had the advantage over the previously used India ink or low-molecular-weight fluorescein-labeled dextran perfusion in that the HMW dextrans filled the entire vasculature without leaking. As suggested by Gole et al., the second method used to evaluate retinal neovascularization was to examine histological cross sections of the retinas. Two to four sections on each side of the optic nerve, 30–90 μm apart, were evaluated from each sectioned eye. Preretinal vascular cell nuclei that extended into the vitreous beyond the inner limiting membrane (ILM) were counted from each cross section to quantify neovascularization. Cross sections that included the optic nerve were excluded to avoid counting regressing hyaloid vessels. GFAP was also immunolocalized in the retinal sections to examine whether astrocytes and Müller cells contributed to retinal response in OIR.

After 24 hours of hyperoxia, the central retina exhibited a nonreversible central vasoconstriction. After 5 days of hyperoxia exposure (P12), the central retina displayed a severe hypoperfusion with apparent vaso-obliteration of both the superficial network capillaries and deep vascular network (see figure 23.1*D*). Subsequent studies did confirm obliteration of the central superficial vascular capillaries at P12; however, in contrast to the superficial network, the entire deep vascular network failed to develop both centrally and peripherally in response to hyperoxia (Banin et al., 2006; Davies et al., 2003). This observation is consistent with the fact that the superficial network is almost complete at P7, but the deep network starts to develop between P7 and P8 (Dorrell et al., 2002; Fruttiger, 2002). Hence, normal retinal vascular development was altered by hyperoxia, with vaso-obliteration of superficial capillaries in the central retina and inhibition of the deep network capillaries in both the central and peripheral retina. After 5 days in hyperoxia and 2 days in room air (P14), the retinas continued to display a lack of central retinal capillaries; however, the arteries and veins now had a dilated and tortuous appearance.

At P17 and P21, preretinal neovascular tufts were appreciated at the transition zone between the nonperfused central retina and the perfused peripheral retina in both the fluorescein-dextran-perfused retinal flat mounts and the retinal cross sections (see figure 23.1*F*). The neovascular tuft response occurred in 100% of the mice and was similar in both male and female mice (Smith et al., 1994). The retinal neovascularization that is observed in ROP also occurred at the transition zone between the vascular and avascular retina. However, in contrast to mice, in humans the avascular zone is located at the periphery of the retina and often exhibits a well-defined mesenchymal ridge. The neovascular tufts in the mice were noted to gradually regress after P21 and were absent after approximately P24–P26. In the initial studies by Smith et al., intense GFAP immunostaining was exhibited by astrocytes along the superficial layer of vessels, as well as in Müller cell processes beneath the areas of preretinal neovascularization. GFAP expression is increased in a variety of retinal injuries, and it appears to be a marker for intraretinal injury in this model. Despite the overall increased GFAP expression in the retina, the neovascular tufts were negative for GFAP, indicating that despite their activation, astrocytes and Müller cells are not physically associated with the tufts.

The extent of retinal neovascularization in the mouse model of OIR is also strain dependent because of differential expression of angiogenic factors (Chan et al., 2005). The mouse strain used to characterize the OIR model, C57BL/6J, is relatively resistant to angiogenic stimuli when compared with the 129/SvImJ strain (Chan et al., 2005; Rohan et al., 2000). Therefore it is essential to understand the genetic background of mice when evaluating the angiogenesis response in the OIR model. Investigators must ensure the use of proper genetic controls when comparing the effects of gene deletion (commonly made in 129 mice) or gene overexpression. The effect of genetic diversity on angiogenesis has been recently characterized and reviewed (Rogers and D'Amato, 2006).

Two recent studies have attempted to explain the selective vulnerability of central retinal vessels in mice to hyperoxia as opposed to the peripheral retina observed in humans (Claxton and Fruttiger, 2003; Shih et al., 2003a). One hypothesis is that the hyperoxia results in a larger capillary-free zone around arteries emanating from the optic nerve head (including the regressing hyaloid) with an associated downregulation of astrocyte-derived VEGF-A. A reduction in VEGF-A would result in additional vascular regression in the central retina. The second hypothesis is that the pericytes that are located in the central neonatal mouse retina fail to express TGF-β, with a secondary failure to induce expression of FLT1 on their associated EC. Protection of capillaries from oxygen-induced injury is mediated by VEGF-A binding to FLT1 (Shih et al., 2003b). Of interest, the pericytes at the leading edge of the superficial network express TGF-β at P5, which correlates with the area of the mouse superficial network that is resistant to hyperoxia. In addition, TGF-β-expressing pericytes are localized to all vessels in P15 retinas (resistant to oxygen-induced injury, as noted earlier). Hence, these studies suggest that the sensitivity of the neonatal vessels to hyperoxia-induced injury is related to reduced VEGF-A ligand and FLT1 expression in the central immature retina. The human hyaloid vasculature exhibits more regression prior to birth, even in the 25-week premature infant; therefore, excessive hyperoxia may not be present in the central retina compared with the periphery. Human studies examining the pericyte expression of TGF-β in the immature retina are lacking. Figure 23.3 is timeline of retinal vessel formation in normal development and in OIR in the mouse.

The mouse model of OIR continues to be further characterized, and additional methods of quantification have been developed. Higgins et al. (1999) developed a retinopathy scoring system using features from scoring systems used in kittens and humans. This scoring system grades blood vessel growth, blood vessel tufts, extraretinal neovascularization, central vasoconstriction, retinal hemorrhage, and blood vessel tortuosity as evaluated with HMW fluorescein-labeled dextran-perfused retinal flat mounts. This quantitative scoring system was validated by the quantification of preretinal neovascular nuclei as described by Smith et al. This scoring system has the advantage of evaluating several features of retinopathy that might be differentially altered by genetic manipulation or other therapeutic interventions but requires very consistent fluorescein perfusion and well-trained scorers. Mice with OIR were recently evaluated with three-dimensional in vivo imaging to assess the retinal vasculature in a living animal (Ritter et al., 2005). Imaging at P18 confirmed the presence of pathological neovascularization, as well as vascular leakage, a feature of the model not well appreciated when using HMW-fluorescein dextran perfusions, since they are designed not to leak out of the vasculature. This technique of imaging can provide new insights into retinal neovascularization that are not available when fixed tissues are used. However, improvements in optics and microscopy are likely required before investigators can routinely employ this methodology.

Banin et al. have developed a new, complementary methodology of quantification for the mouse model of OIR that can provide a detailed time course of the vaso-obliteration and retinal neovascularization (Banin et al., 2006). Isolectin *Griffonia simplicifolia* (isolectin GS)-stained retinal flat mounts were analyzed using confocal microscopy and image analysis software. To measure the area of vaso-obliteration in the retina, the border of the avascular retina was traced using the "freehand" selection tool from Photoshop. To measure neovascularization, the vascular tufts were traced using the "magic wand" tool. The total areas were measured in pixels and then converted to square micrometers. Dextranperfused retinas were also stained with the isolectin GS, with the vascular tufts being more clearly visualized with isolectin GS and therefore used for quantification. In contrast, both the dextran-perfused and isolectin GS–stained retinas delineated the avascular regions in a comparable fashion. This neovascular tuft quantification method correlated well with results obtained by counting preretinal neovascular tufts in tissue sections. The data analysis revealed good correlation between both eyes from each animal with regard to the extent of vaso-obliteration and vascular tuft formation. This allows one eye to be used for intraocular treatment while the other eye is used as a control, with a predictable and consistent response. The data analysis also revealed that vaso-obliteration significantly recovers by P16 and is nearly resolved on P21, while the neovascularization peaks on P17, with a gradual regression until P22. Figure 23.4 shows a retinal flat mount from a P17 oxygen-injured animal with preretinal neovascularization. The sample has been stained with isolectin GS and digitally imaged using a conventional fluorescence microscope in the author's laboratory.

Studies of VEGF, Growth Factors, and Cytokines The mouse model of OIR has played an important role in defining the contribution of VEGF-A to the pathogenesis of pathological retinal neovascularization and its link to the human diseases of ROP and diabetic retinopathy (Lutty et al., 2006a; Saint-Geniez and D'Amore, 2004). Smith and colleagues initially investigated the expression and regulation of VEGF-A in the mouse retina using the model (Pierce et al., 1995, 1996). During the hyperoxia phase (P7–P12), VEGF-A expression was downregulated within 6 hours and remained reduced after 5 days (P12). After animals were returned to room air on P12, VEGF-A expression was significantly increased compared with that seen in room air controls within 12 hours and remained elevated through P17, the peak of retinal neovascularization. VEGF-A expression was localized to Müller cell processes and their end-feet along the inner retina. Intravitreal injection of

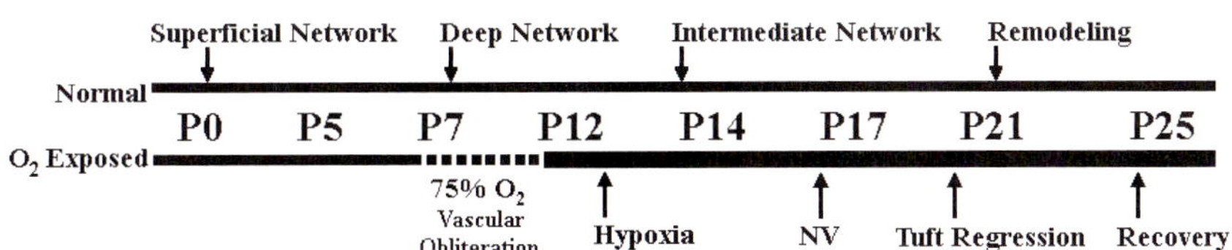

Figure 23.3 Timeline of normal vascular development and oxygen-induced retinopathy in the mouse retina. NV, neovascularization.

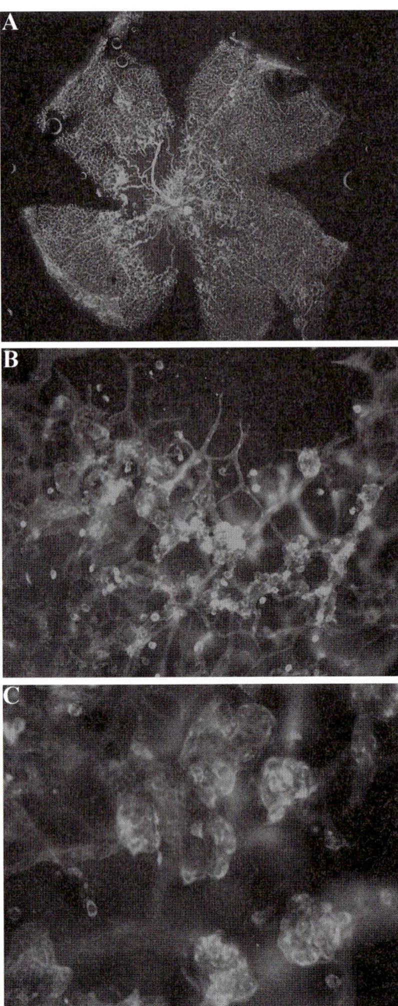

FIGURE 23.4 Visualization of vessels in P17 retinal flat-mount preparations stained with GS-lectin from a mouse model of OIR. *A*, Low-power (magnification ×25) image of the retina shows areas of central vaso-obliteration, as well as neovascular tufts. *B*, Higher magnification (×200) shows neovascular tuft formation at the transition zone between vascular and central avascular retina. *C*, At even greater magnification (×400), multiple neovascular tufts are evident. See color plate 13.

recombinant VEGF-A on P7 reduced the extent of vaso-obliteration typically observed in the model.

These early findings shed light on the interactions between VEGF-A and the retinal vasculature: (1) VEGF-A is down-regulated in response to hyperoxia, (2) reduced VEGF-A expression is associated with vaso-obliteration, and (3) over-production of VEGF-A in avascular (relative hypoxic) regions of the retina results in abnormal retinal neovascularization. Subsequent studies have experimentally determined that the avascular areas of the mouse retina are indeed hypoxic, and that a transcription factor that stimulates *Vegfa* expression, hypoxia inducible factor-1α (HIF-1α), is increased in the mouse model of OIR, with a temporal and spatial correlation with VEGF-A expression (P12.5–P17) (Ozaki et al., 1999; West et al., 2005). The central role that VEGF-A plays in proliferative retinopathies was further confirmed by the suppression of retinal neovascularization with intravitreal injection (P12 and P14) of a soluble VEGF receptor (ca. 42% reduction) and antisense oligodeoxynucleotides targeting *Vegfa* (ca. 50% reduction) (Aiello et al., 1995; Robinson et al., 1996). The fact the specific inhibitors did not completely block the pathological neovascularization suggests that additional angiogenic factors are involved or the inhibitors did not penetrate into the intraretinal locations of VEGF-A.

Several additional studies have used the mouse model of OIR to demonstrate a major role for VEGF-A in ischemic retinopathies, with potential translation of VEGF-A inhibition to human disease (Al-Shabrawey et al., 2005; Deng et al., 2005; Shen et al., 2006). For example, reduction of VEGF-A expression and retinal neovascularization has been achieved after treatment with virus-mediated expression of small VEGF peptides, inhibition of NAD(P)H oxidase, or siRNA targeting of Flt-1. Insulin-like growth factor-I (IGF-I) also modulates VEGF-A function during angiogenesis and is an additional target for inhibition of retinal neovascularization (Smith et al., 1999). Mice treated with an IGF-I receptor antagonist exhibited a reduction in neovascularization by 53% compared to control. The IGF-I receptor antagonist did not alter levels of VEGF-A or VEGF receptors but rather modulated VEGF-A-mediated intracellular signaling pathways. IGF-I has also been linked to ROP in infants (Hellstrom et al., 2003).

As previously discussed, the angiopoietin/Tek system is critical for normal retinal vasculature development, playing a role in the EC–mural cell interactions. In postnatal angiogenesis, Angpt2 is also specifically upregulated in microvascular ECs by hypoxia in vitro and in the mouse model of OIR in vivo, and localizes to neovascular tufts in P17 mice. The coexpression of Angpt2 and VEGF-A in response to hypoxia is required for retinal neovascularization to occur (Hackett et al., 2000). In the mouse model of OIR, retinal neovascularization was suppressed by 23% by the intraocular injection of a soluble Tek (sTek-Fc). However, when the sTek-Fc was combined with a soluble Flt1 (sFlt-1-Fc), neovascularization was inhibited by 50% compared to control. In the absence of VEGF-A, Angpt2 will induce vascular regression of nascent vessels but have no effect on more mature vessels (Campochiaro, 2006). This finding implies that Angpt2 has the potential to be a therapeutic antiangiogenic agent if used in combination with a specific VEGF-A antagonist.

Briefly, two cytokines that have been implicated in human proliferative retinopathy, erythropoietin and interleukin-8, are also increased during the phase of retinal neovascularization in the mouse model of OIR (Powers et al., 2005; Watanabe et al., 2005). Expression of retinal erythropoietin mRNA is increased dramatically on P17 compared to control, and intraocular injection of a soluble erythropoietin receptor reduces the neovascularization when evaluated on P19. The chemokine KC, a mouse homologue of interleukin-8, is markedly increased on P17 and P21 compared to control, immunolocalizes to the Müller cell processes, and is induced by interleukin-1.

As outlined in this section, multiple angiogenic factors contribute to neovascularization in the immature retina. For clinical use, inhibitors of retinal neovascularization will likely need to be administered in combined fashion, and they should affect only pathological vessels, not the normal pattern of retinal vascular development.

Endothelial Cell Apoptosis and Oxygen-Induced Retinopathy It is now recognized that there is a critical link between angiogenesis and apoptosis (Folkman, 2003). After ECs are incorporated into new vessels, they continue to depend on angiogenic factors (survival factors) to block apoptotic pathways while simultaneously stimulating intracellular survival pathways. Alon et al. (1995) correlated downregulation of VEGF-A by hyperoxia with the apoptosis of retinal ECs in a rat model of OIR, implicating VEGF-A as an EC survival factor. Thus, during the phase of hyperoxia exposure, growth factor withdrawal results in EC apoptosis and contributes to the subsequent vaso-obliteration. Survival factor withdrawal has since been characterized to activate the mitochondrial pathway of apoptosis, although specific intracellular apoptotic pathways need to be delineated during vaso-obliteration in the mouse model of OIR.

In addition to growth factor withdrawal, proliferating ECs upregulate the death receptor Fas on their cell surface, making immature vessels vulnerable to regression via FasL-induced apoptosis (Stuart et al., 2003). In a variety of mouse models, the Fas/FasL pathway has been shown to play an important role in retinal vessel regression during normal vascular development and neovascular tuft regression (Barreiro et al., 2003; Davies et al., 2003; Ishida et al., 2003b). Two independent groups utilized FasL-defective mice (*Gld*) in the mouse model of OIR and observed a significant increase (ca. 50%) in preretinal neovascularization on P17 (Barreiro et al., 2003; Davies et al., 2003). The *gld* mice also exhibited a significantly reduced number of apoptotic EC (ca. 50%) in the neovascular tufts as compared to control mice at P17. These findings suggest that Fas/FasL-mediated apoptosis helps to regulate the extent of pathological neovascularization observed in the mouse model of OIR. However, other apoptotic mediators also likely contribute to the delicate balance between angiogenic and antiangiogenic factors, because even in the *Gld* mice the tufts eventually regressed by P26. Another observation from these studies was that normal vascular development (in room air controls) and vaso-obliteration were not altered in the *Gld* mice on P8 or P12 compared to C57BL/6 controls. Additional studies are needed to further define the apoptosis pathways that regulate development of the retinal vasculature and their role in hyperoxia-induced EC death.

Mice deficient in Bcl-2 (an intracellular apoptosis inhibitor) exhibited significantly (70%) reduced neovascularization compared to controls during OIR despite the characteristic increase in VEGF-A expression on P15 (Wang et al., 2005). Bcl-2 inhibits apoptosis in ECs and is normally upregulated by VEGF-A to stabilize new vessel formation. Wang et al. (2005) found that VEGF-A is unable to counterbalance the endogenous pro-apoptotic factors, owing to lack of functional Bcl-2; thus, the balance is tipped toward vascular regression and not vascular proliferation. Endostatin, a cleavage product of collagen XVIII and endogenous antiangiogenic factor, inhibits angiogenesis by inducing EC apoptosis through the downregulation of Bcl-2 and VEGF-A (Dhanabal et al., 1999; Zhang et al., 2006). Retinal neovascularization on P17 is nearly completely inhibited by exogenous intraocular injection of endostatin on P12 in the mouse model of OIR. The inhibition of NV was also associated with a 3.5-fold reduction in retinal VEGF-A expression, downregulating an antiapoptotic factor (VEGF-A), again tipping the balance toward vascular regression. Thrombospondin 1 (Thbs1) is an endogenous inhibitor of angiogenesis and induces EC apoptosis through the upregulation of FasL (Quesada et al., 2005). Overexpression of ocular thrombospondin-1 in transgenic mice results in significant inhibition of retinal neovascularization on P17 in the mouse model of OIR. These studies highlight the potential novel approaches in developing antiangiogenic therapies, through the modulation of apoptosis pathways with specific agonists or antagonists, or by enhancing endogenous antiangiogenic factors. During the phase of vaso-obliteration, prevention of EC apoptosis should prove an invaluable approach to treating ischemic retinopathies. For example, thrombospondin-1-deficient mice (decreased apoptosis) are less sensitive to hyperoxia-mediated vessel obliteration (Wang et al., 2003). If vaso-obliteration can be minimized, there should be less hypoxia during the room air recovery phase, less VEGF-A expression, and ultimately less retinal neovascularization.

Role of Microglia and Leukocytes in the Mouse Model of OIR Microglia (myeloid-derived) and leukocytes have the potential to play many different roles in the process of angiogenesis and vascular regression, depending on the temporal and spatial biological context. For example, macrophages can produce many angiogenic growth factors, but they are also capable of expressing several antiangiogenic/pro-apoptotic factors. Infiltrating leukocytes (lymphocytes) have been observed to contribute to vaso-obliteration via a FasL-dependent pathway in P7 mice that had been exposed to 80% oxygen for 2 days. However, this study did not evaluate the impact of leukocytes during the period of neovascularization (Ishida et al., 2003b).

Two recent studies explored the contribution of endogenous retinal microglia to the development of the retinal vasculature and the retinal response to oxygen-induced injury (Checchin et al., 2006; Ritter et al., 2006). The depletion of microglia during vascular development resulted in reduced vascular density, while mice exposed to 75% oxygen from P7 to P12 exhibited a marked loss of microglia in the central retina, correlating with the regions of vaso-obliteration. Mice strains that are more resistant to oxygen-induced vaso-obliteration and that have a quicker vascular recovery also have a greater number of microglial cells in the central retina. These studies imply that microglia promote the survival of nascent vessels in the immature retina.

Macrophages/microglia also colocalize to the neovascular tufts in the OIR model, as determined by the mouse macrophage marker F4/80 (Banin et al., 2006; Davies et al., 2006). The contribution of retinal microglial cells cannot be excluded because F4/80 specifically labels both macrophages and microglia. The monocyte/macrophage chemokine, monocyte chemoattractant protein-1 (MCP-1, CCL2), is also significantly elevated on P14–P17, indicating that many of the F4/80-positive cells observed in the neovascular tufts are likely blood-borne macrophages recruited to the retina (Davies et al., 2006). Retinal sections also revealed that microglial cells exhibit an activated morphology and are localized to the inner retina/neovascular tufts by P17. Quantification of F4/80-positive cells from P12–P21 indicated the monocytes/macrophages infiltrate into the retina after P14, peaking on P21 (a fivefold increase), with continued localization to the neovascular tufts. In a rat model of OIR, depletion of monocytes led to a suppression of retinal neovascularization, suggesting an angiogenic role for infiltrating monocytes/macrophages, while blocking lymphocytes increased the neovascularization (Ishida et al., 2003a). In the mouse model of OIR, the number of macrophages peaks at a time when the neovascular tufts are beginning to regress (after P17). Activated macrophages are quite capable of inducing EC apoptosis, a finding that may suggest that macrophages could contribute to vascular tuft regression in the mouse model of OIR (Lobov et al., 2005). This concept does not exclude an angiogenic function during an earlier phase of disease injury (Checchin et al., 2006; Ritter et al., 2006). Studies in MCP-1-deficient mice demonstrated reduced infiltration of F4/80 cells into the retina, reduced apoptosis in the neovascular tufts, and increased retinal neovascularization on P21 and P24 compared to controls (Davies and Powers, 2005).

Miscellaneous Molecules in the Mouse Model of OIR More than 250 publications referenced the mouse model of OIR within the past decade. The details of many of these studies could not be outlined here. A plethora of molecules have been evaluated to determine whether they contribute to the pathogenesis of pathological retinal neovascularization. A short list of the types of molecules examined in these studies includes TNF, integrins, matrix metalloproteinases and their inhibitors, nitric oxide and nitric oxide synthase, cyclooxygenases, angiotensin-converting enzyme, and several transcription factors. Many of these contributions have been recently reviewed (Das and McGuire, 2003; Lutty et al., 2006a; Saint-Geniez and D'Amore, 2004).

Summary

Basic scientific studies are critical if we are to advance our understanding of normal retinal vascular development and the response of developing retinal vessels to oxygen-induced injury. As noted by Patz, "The mouse model of OIR has become the gold standard for research on retinal angiogenesis" (cited in Lutty et al., 2006a). Studies in mice have created a fundamental understanding of blood vessel guidance, the role of VEGF-A isoforms in both normal and pathological retinal neovascularization, the critical interactions of retinal ECs and mural cells, and the role of apoptosis in balancing angiogenic and antiangiogenic factors. The results of these studies have also translated to human clinical trials, such as the application of a specific VEGF inhibitor to the $VEGF_{165}$ isoform, in order to selectively treat pathological retinal neovascularization without altering normal vessels (Lutty et al., 2006a). Future studies of angiogenesis in the mouse retina should lead to new targets for selective therapies in human proliferative retinopathies.

acknowledgments I thank Michael Davies for his dedicated assistance, and David Zamora for critically reading the manuscript. Work was supported by grant no. EY011548 from the National Eye Institute, Fight For Sight, the Collins Medical Trust, and Research to Prevent Blindness.

REFERENCES

Aiello, L. P., Pierce, E. A., Foley, E. D., Takagi, H., Chen, H., Riddle, L., Ferrara, N., King, G. L., and Smith, L. E. (1995). Suppression of retinal neovascularization in vivo by inhibition of vascular endothelial growth factor (VEGF) using soluble VEGF-receptor chimeric proteins. *Proc. Natl. Acad. Sci. U.S.A.* 92(23):10457–10461.

Alon, T., Hemo, I., Itin, A., Pe'er, J., Stone, J., and Keshet, E. (1995). Vascular endothelial growth factor acts as a survival factor for newly formed retinal vessels and has implications for retinopathy of prematurity. *Nat. Med.* 1(10):1024–1028.

Al-Shabrawey, M., Bartoli, M., El-Remessy, A. B., Platt, D. H., Matragoon, S., Behzadian, M. A., Caldwell, R. W., and Caldwell, R. B. (2005). Inhibition of NAD(P)H oxidase activity blocks vascular endothelial growth factor overexpression and neovascularization during ischemic retinopathy. *Am. J. Pathol.* 167(2):599–607.

Armulik, A., Abramsson, A., and Betsholtz, C. (2005). Endothelial/pericyte interactions. *Circ. Res.* 97(6):512–523.

Ash, J., McLeod, D. S., and Lutty, G. A. (2005). Transgenic expression of leukemia inhibitory factor (LIF) blocks normal vascular development but not pathological neovascularization in the eye. *Mol. Vis.* 11:298–308.

Ashton, N. (1968). Donders Lecture, 1967. Some aspects of the comparative pathology of oxygen toxicity in the retina. *Br. J. Ophthalmol.* 52(7):505–531.

Banin, E., Dorrell, M. I., Aguilar, E., Ritter, M. R., Aderman, C. M., Smith, A. C., Friedlander, J., and Friedlander, M. (2006). T2-TrpRS inhibits preretinal neovascularization and enhances physiological vascular regrowth in OIR as assessed by a new method of quantification. *Invest. Ophthalmol. Vis. Sci.* 47(5):2125–2134.

Barreiro, R., Schadlu, R., Herndon, J., Kaplan, H. J., and Ferguson, T. A. (2003). The role of Fas-FasL in the development and treatment of ischemic retinopathy. *Invest. Ophthalmol. Vis. Sci.* 44(3):1282–1286.

Campochiaro, P. A. (2006). Ocular versus extraocular neovascularization: Mirror images or vague resemblances. *Invest. Ophthalmol. Vis. Sci.* 47(2):462–474.

Carmeliet, P., and Tessier-Lavigne, M. (2005). Common mechanisms of nerve and blood vessel wiring. *Nature* 436(7048):193–200.

Chan, C. K., Pham, L. N., Zhou, J., Spee, C., Ryan, S. J., and Hinton, D. R. (2005). Differential expression of pro- and antiangiogenic factors in mouse strain–dependent hypoxia-induced retinal neovascularization. *Lab. Invest.* 85(6):721–733.

Checchin, D., Sennlaub, F., Levavasseur, E., Leduc, M., and Chemtob, S. (2006). Potential role of microglia in retinal blood vessel formation. *Invest. Ophthalmol. Vis. Sci.* 47(8):3595–3602.

Claxton, S., and Fruttiger, M. (2003). Role of arteries in oxygen induced vaso-obliteration. *Exp. Eye Res.* 77(3):305–311.

Claxton, S., and Fruttiger, M. (2005). Oxygen modifies artery differentiation and network morphogenesis in the retinal vasculature. *Dev. Dyn.* 233(3):822–828.

Connolly, S. E., Hores, T. A., Smith, L. E., and D'Amore, P. A. (1988). Characterization of vascular development in the mouse retina. *Microvasc. Res.* 36(3):275–290.

Darland, D. C., Massingham, L. J., Smith, S. R., Piek, E., Saint-Geniez, M., and D'Amore, P. A. (2003). Pericyte production of cell-associated VEGF is differentiation-dependent and is associated with endothelial survival. *Dev. Biol.* 264(1):275–288.

Das, A., and McGuire, P. G. (2003). Retinal and choroidal angiogenesis: Pathophysiology and strategies for inhibition. *Prog. Retin. Eye Res.* 22(6):721–748.

Davies, M. H., Eubanks, J. P., and Powers, M. R. (2003). Increased retinal neovascularization in Fas ligand–deficient mice. *Invest. Ophthalmol. Vis. Sci.* 44(7):3202–3210.

Davies, M. H., Eubanks, J. P., and Powers, M. R. (2006). Microglia and macrophages are increased in response to ischemia-induced retinopathy in the mouse retina. *Mol. Vis.* 12:467–477.

Davies, M. H., and Powers, M. R. (2005). MCP-1 deficient mice exhibit a prolonged neovascular response in a mouse model of oxygen-induced retinopathy. IOVS; ARVO E-Abstract 4185.

Deng, W. T., Yan, Z., Dinculescu, A., Pang, J., Teusner, J. T., Cortez, N. G., Berns, K. I., and Hauswirth, W. W. (2005). Adeno-associated virus-mediated expression of vascular endothelial growth factor peptides inhibits retinal neovascularization in a mouse model of oxygen-induced retinopathy. *Hum. Gene Ther.* 16(11):1247–1254.

Dhanabal, M., Ramchandran, R., Waterman, M. J., Lu, H., Knebelmann, B., Segal, M., and Sukhatme, V. P. (1999). Endostatin induces endothelial cell apoptosis. *J. Biol. Chem.* 274(17):1721–1726.

Dorrell, M. I., Aguilar, E., and Friedlander, M. (2002). Retinal vascular development is mediated by endothelial filopodia, a preexisting astrocytic template and specific R-cadherin adhesion. *Invest. Ophthalmol. Vis. Sci.* 43(11):3500–3510.

Dorrell, M. I., and Friedlander, M. (2006). Mechanisms of endothelial cell guidance and vascular patterning in the developing mouse retina. *Prog. Retin. Eye Res.* 25(3):277–295.

Enge, M., Bjarnegard, M., Gerhardt, H., Gustafsson, E., Kalen, M., Asker, N., Hammes, H. P., Shani, M., Fassler, R., and Betsholtz, C. (2002). Endothelium-specific platelet-derived growth factor-B ablation mimics diabetic retinopathy. *Embo J.* 21(16):4307–4316.

Feeney, S. A., Simpson, D. A., Gardiner, T. A., Boyle, C., Jamison, P., and Stitt, A. W. (2003). Role of vascular endothelial growth factor and placental growth factors during retinal vascular development and hyaloid regression. *Invest. Ophthalmol. Vis. Sci.* 44(2):839–847.

Folkman, J. (2003). Angiogenesis and apoptosis. *Semin. Cancer Biol.* 13(2):159–167.

Fruttiger, M. (2002). Development of the mouse retinal vasculature: Angiogenesis versus vasculogenesis. *Invest. Ophthalmol. Vis. Sci.* 43(2):522–527.

Fruttiger, M., Calver, A. R., Kruger, W. H., Mudhar, H. S., Michalovich, D., Takakura, N., S. Nishikawa, S., and Richardson, W. D. (1996). PDGF mediates a neuron-astrocyte interaction in the developing retina. *Neuron* 17(6):1117–1131.

Gariano, R. F. (2003). Cellular mechanisms in retinal vascular development. *Prog. Retin. Eye Res.* 22(3):295–306.

Gariano, R. F., and Gardner, T. W. (2005). Retinal angiogenesis in development and disease. *Nature* 438(7070):960–966.

Gerhardt, H., Golding, M., Fruttiger, M., Ruhrberg, C., Lundkvist, A., Abramsson, A., Jeltsch, M., Mitchell, C., Alitalo, K., et al. (2003). VEGF guides angiogenic sprouting utilizing endothelial tip cell filopodia. *J. Cell Biol.* 161(6):1163–1177.

Gole, G. A., Browning, J., and Elts, S. M. (1990). The mouse model of oxygen-induced retinopathy: A suitable animal model for angiogenesis research. *Doc. Ophthalmol.* 74(3):163–169.

Grant, M. B., May, W. S., Caballero, S., Brown, G. A., Guthrie, S. M., Mames, R. N., Byrne, B. J., Vaught, T., Spoerri, P. E., et al. (2002). Adult hematopoietic stem cells provide functional hemangioblast activity during retinal neovascularization. *Nat. Med.* 8(6):607–612.

Gu, X., Samuel, S., El-Shabrawey, M., Caldwell, R. B., Bartoli, M., Marcus, D. M., and Brooks, S. E. (2002). Effects of sustained hyperoxia on revascularization in experimental retinopathy of prematurity. *Invest. Ophthalmol. Vis. Sci.* 43(2):496–502.

Hackett, S. F., Ozaki, H., Strauss, R. W., Wahlin, K., Suri, C., Maisonpierre, P., Yancopoulos, G., and Campochiaro, P. A. (2000). Angiopoietin 2 expression in the retina: Upregulation during physiologic and pathologic neovascularization. *J. Cell Physiol.* 184(3):275–284.

Hellstrom, A., Engstrom, E., Hard, A. L., Albertsson-Wikland, K., Carlsson, B., Niklasson, A., Lofqvist, C., Svensson, E., Holm, S., Ewald, U., et al. (2003). Postnatal serum insulin-like growth factor I deficiency is associated with retinopathy of prematurity and other complications of premature birth. *Pediatrics* 112(5):1016–1020.

Higgins, R. D., Yu, K., Sanders, R. J., Nandgaonkar, B. N., Rotschild, T., and Rifkin, D. B. (1999). Diltiazem reduces retinal neovascularization in a mouse model of oxygen-induced retinopathy. *Curr. Eye Res.* 18(1):20–27.

Ilg, R. C., Davies, M. H., and Powers, M. R. (2005). Altered retinal neovascularization in TNF receptor-deficient mice. *Curr. Eye Res.* 30(11):1003–1113.

Ishida, S., Usui, T., Yamashiro, K., Kaji, Y., Amano, S., Ogura, Y., Hida, T., Oguchi, Y., Ambati, J., et al. (2003a). VEGF164-mediated inflammation is required for pathological, but not physiological, ischemia-induced retinal neovascularization. *J. Exp. Med.* 198(3):483–489.

Ishida, S., Yamashiro, K., Usui, T., Kaji, Y., Ogura, Y., Hida, T., Honda, Y., Oguchi, Y., and Adamis, A. P. (2003b). Leukocytes mediate retinal vascular remodeling during development and vaso-obliteration in disease. *Nat. Med.* 9(6):781–788.

Jain, R. K. (2003). Molecular regulation of vessel maturation. *Nat. Med.* 9(6):685–693.

Janzer, R. C., and Raff, M. C. (1987). Astrocytes induce blood-brain barrier properties in endothelial cells. *Nature* 325(6101):253–257.

Lobov, I. B., Rao, S., Carroll, T. J., Vallance, J. E., Ito, M., Ondr, J. K., Kurup, S., Glass, D. A., Patel, M. S., Shu, W., et al. (2005). WNT7b mediates macrophage-induced programmed cell death in patterning of the vasculature. *Nature* 437(7057):417–421.

Lutty, G. A., Chan-Ling, T., Phelps, D. L., Adamis, A. P., Berns, K. I., Chan, C. K., Cole, C. H., D'Amore, P. A., Das, A., et al. (2006a). Proceedings of the Third International Symposium on Retinopathy of Prematurity: An update on ROP from the lab to the nursery (November 2003, Anaheim, California). *Mol. Vis.* 12:532–580.

Lutty, G. A., Merges, C., Grebe, R., Prow, T., and McLeod, D. S. (2006b). Canine retinal angioblasts are multipotent. *Exp. Eye Res.* 83(1):183–193.

Madan, A., and Penn, J. S. (2003). Animal models of oxygen-induced retinopathy. *Front. Biosci.* 8:d1030–d1043.

Oshima, Y., Deering, T., Oshima, S., Nambu, H., Reddy, P. S., Kaleko, M., Connelly, S., Hackett, S. F., and Campochiaro, P. A. (2004). Angiopoietin-2 enhances retinal vessel sensitivity to vascular endothelial growth factor. *J. Cell Physiol.* 199(3):412–417.

Otani, A., Kinder, K., Ewalt, K., Otero, F. J., Schimmel, P., and Friedlander, M. (2002). Bone marrow-derived stem cells target retinal astrocytes and can promote or inhibit retinal angiogenesis. *Nat. Med.* 8(9):1004–1010.

Ozaki, H., Yu, A. Y., Della, N., Ozaki, K., Luna, J. D., Yamada, H., Hackett, S. F., Okamoto, N., Zack, D. J., et al. (1999). Hypoxia inducible factor-1alpha is increased in ischemic retina: Temporal and spatial correlation with VEGF expression. *Invest. Ophthalmol. Vis. Sci.* 40(1):182–189.

Pierce, E. A., Avery, R. L., Foley, E. D., Aiello, L. P., and Smith, L. E. (1995). Vascular endothelial growth factor/vascular permeability factor expression in a mouse model of retinal neovascularization. *Proc. Natl. Acad. Sci. U.S.A.* 92(3):905–909.

Pierce, E. A., Foley, E. D., and Smith, L. E. (1996). Regulation of vascular endothelial growth factor by oxygen in a model of retinopathy of prematurity. *Arch. Ophthalmol.* 114(10):1219–1228.

Powers, M. R., Davies, M. H., and Eubanks, J. P. (2005). Increased expression of chemokine KC, an interleukin-8 homologue, in a model of oxygen-induced retinopathy. *Curr. Eye Res.* 30(4):299–2307.

Quesada, A. J., Nelius, T., Yap, R., Zaichuk, T. A., Alfranca, A., Filleur, S., Volpert, O. V., and Redondo, J. M. (2005). In vivo upregulation of CD95 and CD95L causes synergistic inhibition of angiogenesis by TSP1 peptide and metronomic doxorubicin treatment. *Cell Death Differ.* 12(6):649–658.

Recchia, F. M., and Capone, A., Jr. (2004). Contemporary understanding and management of retinopathy of prematurity. *Retina* 24(2):283–292.

Risau, W. (1997). Mechanisms of angiogenesis. *Nature* 386(6626):671–674.

Ritter, M. R., Aguilar, E., Banin, E., Scheppke, L., Uusitalo-Jarvinen, H., and Friedlander, M. (2005). Three-dimensional in vivo imaging of the mouse intraocular vasculature during development and disease. *Invest. Ophthalmol. Vis. Sci.* 46(9):3021–3026.

Ritter, M. R., Banin, E., Moreno, S. K., Aguilar, E., Dorrell, M. I., and Friedlander, M. (2006). Myeloid progenitors differentiate into microglia and promote vascular repair in a model of ischemic retinopathy. *J. Clin. Invest.* 116(12):3266–3276.

Robinson, G. S., Pierce, E. A., Rook, S. L., Foley, E., Webb, R., and Smith, L. E. (1996). Oligodeoxynucleotides inhibit retinal neovascularization in a murine model of proliferative retinopathy. *Proc. Natl. Acad. Sci. U.S.A.* 93(10):4851–4856.

Rogers, M. S., and D'Amato, R. J. (2006). The effect of genetic diversity on angiogenesis. *Exp. Cell Res.* 312(5):561–574.

Rohan, R. M., Fernandez, A., Udagawa, T., Yuan, J., and D'Amato, R. J. (2000). Genetic heterogeneity of angiogenesis in mice. *FASEB J.* 14(7):871–876.

Rousseau, B., Larrieu-Lahargue, F., Bikfalvi, A., and Javerzat, S. (2003). Involvement of fibroblast growth factors in choroidal angiogenesis and retinal vascularization. *Exp. Eye Res.* 77(2):147–156.

Saint-Geniez, M., Argence, C. B., Knibiehler, B., and Audigier, Y. (2003). The *msr/apj* gene encoding the apelin receptor is an early and specific marker of the venous phenotype in the retinal vasculature. *Gene Expr. Patterns* 3(4):467–472.

Saint-Geniez, M., and D'Amore, P. A. (2004). Development and pathology of the hyaloid, choroidal and retinal vasculature. *Int. J. Dev. Biol.* 48(8–9):1045–1058.

Shen, J., Samul, R., Silva, R. L., Akiyama, H., Liu, H., Saishin, Y., Hackett, S. F., Zinnen, S., Kossen, K., et al. (2006). Suppression of ocular neovascularization with siRNA targeting VEGF receptor 1. *Gene Ther.* 13(3):225–234.

Shih, S. C., Ju, M., Liu, N., Mo, J. R., Ney, J. J., and Smith, L. E. (2003a). Transforming growth factor beta1 induction of vascular endothelial growth factor receptor 1: mechanism of pericyte-induced vascular survival in vivo. *Proc. Natl. Acad. Sci. U.S.A.* 100(26):15859–15864.

Shih, S. C., Ju, M., Liu, N., and Smith, L. E. (2003b). Selective stimulation of VEGFR-1 prevents oxygen-induced retinal vascular degeneration in retinopathy of prematurity. *J. Clin. Invest.* 112(1):50–57.

Smith, L. E., Shen, W., Perruzzi, C., Soker, S., Kinose, F., Xu, X., Robinson, G., Driver, S., Bischoff, J., et al. (1999). Regulation of vascular endothelial growth factor-dependent retinal neovascularization by insulin-like growth factor-1 receptor. *Nat. Med.* 5(12):1390–1395.

Smith, L. E., Wesolowski, E., McLellan, A., Kostyk, S. K., D'Amato, R., Sullivan, R., and D'Amore, P. A. (1994). Oxygen-induced retinopathy in the mouse. *Invest. Ophthalmol. Vis. Sci.* 35(1):101–111.

Stalmans, I. Y., Ng, S., Rohan, R., Fruttiger, M., Bouche, A., Yuce, A., Fujisawa, H., Hermans, B., Shani, M., et al. (2002). Arteriolar and venular patterning in retinas of mice selectively expressing VEGF isoforms. *J. Clin. Invest.* 109(3):327–336.

Stuart, P. M., Pan, F., Plambeck, S., and Ferguson, T. A. (2003). FasL-Fas interactions regulate neovascularization in the cornea. *Invest. Ophthalmol. Vis. Sci.* 44(1):93–98.

Tout, S., Chan-Ling, T., Hollander, H., and Stone, J. (1993). The role of Müller cells in the formation of the blood-retinal barrier. *Neuroscience* 55(1):291–301.

Uemura, A., Kusuhara, S., Katsuta, H., and Nishikawa, S. (2006). Angiogenesis in the mouse retina: A model system for experimental manipulation. *Exp. Cell Res.* 312(5):676–683.

Wang, S., Sorenson, C. M., and Sheibani, N. (2005). Attenuation of retinal vascular development and neovascularization during oxygen-induced ischemic retinopathy in *Bcl-2−/−* mice. *Dev. Biol.* 279(1):205–219.

Wang, S., Wu, Z., Sorenson, C. M., Lawler, J., and Sheibani, N. (2003). Thrombospondin-1-deficient mice exhibit increased vascular density during retinal vascular development and are less sensitive to hyperoxia-mediated vessel obliteration. *Dev. Dyn.* 228(4):630–642.

Watanabe, D., Suzuma, K., Matsui, S., Kurimoto, M., Kiryu, J., Kita, M., Suzuma, I., Ohashi, H., Ojima, T., et al. (2005). Erythropoietin as a retinal angiogenic factor in proliferative diabetic retinopathy. *N. Engl. J. Med.* 353(8):782–792.

West, H., Richardson, W. D., and Fruttiger, M. (2005). Stabilization of the retinal vascular network by reciprocal feedback between blood vessels and astrocytes. *Development* 132(8):1855–1862.

Wong, W. T., Rex, T. S., Auricchio, A., Maguire, A. M., Chung, D., Tang, W., and Bennett, J. (2004). Effect of over-expression of pigment epithelium-derived factor (PEDF) on developing retinal vasculature in the mouse. *Mol. Vis.* 10:837–844.

Zamora, D. O., Davies, M. H., Planck, S. R., Rosenbaum, J. T., and Powers, M. R. (2005). Soluble forms of ephrinB2 and EphB4 reduce retinal neovascularization in a model of proliferative retinopathy. *Invest. Ophthalmol. Vis. Sci.* 46(6):2175–2182.

Zhang, M., Yang, Y., Yan, M., and Zhang, J. (2006). Downregulation of vascular endothelial growth factor and integrinbeta3 by endostatin in a mouse model of retinal neovascularization. *Exp. Eye Res.* 82(1):74–80.

Zhang, Y., and Stone, J. (1997). Role of astrocytes in the control of developing retinal vessels. *Invest. Ophthalmol. Vis. Sci.* 38(9):1653–1666.

24 Specification, Histogenesis, and Photoreceptor Development in the Mouse Retina

DEEPAK LAMBA, BRANDEN NELSON, MIKE O. KARL, AND THOMAS A. REH

The eye has long been an excellent model for studies of nervous system development. Many principles of developmental biology, such as embryonic induction, thymidine birth dating, and cell fate and lineage analysis, were first analyzed in the retina. This felicitous situation has arisen in part because of its laminated structure, its well-defined cell types, and the wealth of studies characterizing retinal cell biology, physiology, and histology. In this review, we focus primarily on studies carried out in mice and on the critical contributions of molecular genetic experiments. There has been a virtual explosion of information about the development of the eye in the last 10 to 15 years, only a small part of which we can address here. Three areas that have received the most attention in studies of the mouse retina are (1) early eye development, (2) cell fate determination, and (3) photoreceptor development. We have not reviewed studies on the regulation of proliferation in the retinal progenitors, since Michael Dyer reviews this work in the context of retinoblastoma in chapter 25.

Genes that control early eye development: Eye field transcription factors

The presumptive eye field is specified prior to the development of the optic pits in the diencephalon. This eye field specification in the neural plate is caused by a group of transcription factors expressed in this region called eye field transcription factors (EFTFs). The first of the EFTFs to be identified was *Pax6* or *eyeless*. It belongs to the family of paired homeodomain genes and has been highly conserved from nematodes (*C. elegans*; Chisholm and Horvitz, 1995) and *Drosophila* (Quiring et al., 1994) to humans (Glaser et al., 1992; Jordan et al., 1992), especially in the region of its DNA-binding domains, the paired box and homeobox. *Pax6* is expressed in the anterior neural plate at the end of gastrulation and is then restricted to the optic vesicle and lens ectoderm. Its expression persists throughout eye development in retinal progenitor cells (RPCs), and it is ultimately expressed by ganglion, horizontal, and amacrine cells in the mature retina (Grindley et al., 1995; de Melo et al., 2003). Small eye (Sey) mutations in mouse were linked to the *Pax6* gene by Robert Hill and his colleagues (1991). Animals mutant in both alleles of the *Pax6* gene ($Sey^{-/-}$) have almost no eye development (anophthalmia); the homozygous mutants can be identified as early as embryonic day (E) 9.5 by the absence of optic vesicles and lens placode at E9.75 (Grindley et al., 1995), and all subsequent steps of optic development are arrested. The gene dosage of *Pax6* is also critical: heterozygous Sey mice show a small eye phenotype, whereas overexpression of *Pax6* also results in a small eye phenotype (Schedl et al., 1996). In addition to being required for eye development, *Pax6* is also sufficient for eye formation; *Pax6* mRNA injected into 16–32-cell-stage *Xenopus* embryos caused the resultant tadpoles to grow multiple ectopic eyes in their head region (Chow et al., 1999), and ectopic expression of eyeless, the *Drosophila Pax6* homologue, is sufficient to initiate eye formation in many regions of the fly, even the leg.

In addition to Pax6, several other transcription factors are critical for eye development. Rx *(Rax)* is expressed early in the presumptive eye field and, like *Pax6*, belongs to the family of paired homeodomain genes. The expression of Rx begins in areas that will give rise to the ventral forebrain and optic vesicles at approximately E7.5. Once the optic vesicles form, Rx expression is restricted to the ventral diencephalon and the optic vesicles and eventually to the developing retina (Furukawa et al., 1997a). Rx is not as well conserved as *Pax6*; it is absent in planaria eye cells and *Drosophila* eye imaginal discs (Eggert et al., 1998; Salo et al., 2002). Like *Pax6*, homozygous null mutations of the *Rx* gene in mouse result in anophthalmia (Mathers et al., 1997). Eye defects can be seen as early as E9; there is a defect in the formation of the optic sulci. $Rx^{-/-}$ mice do not express other EFTFs, like *Pax6* and *Six3* (see later), in the optic region, indicating that Rx may have a role in inducing these genes (Zhang et al., 2000). Overexpression of Rx in embryonic *Xenopus* or zebrafish results in hyperproliferation of the neural retina and retinal pigment epithelium, as well as the formation of ectopic retinal tissue (Mathers et al., 1997; Andreazzoli et al., 1999; Chuang et al., 1999).

Some of the other EFTFs are members of the Six (sine oculis) homeodomain family of genes, characterized by a six domain and a six-type homeodomain. This family of genes was originally identified by their homology to the *Drosophila* sine oculis (so) gene, which is required for eye development in flies. One of the members of this family, Six3, appears in the region of the presumptive eye field close to E7.5 (Oliver et al., 1995; Bovolenta et al., 1998; Loosli et al., 1998; Lagutin et al., 2001). Targeted disruption of the *Six3* gene in mice results in a lack of anterior head structures, including eyes (Lagutin et al., 2003), and mutations of *Six3* in humans cause holoprosencephaly, a severe malformation of the brain. *Six3* inactivation in medaka fishes also results in anophthalmia and forebrain agenesis (Carl et al., 2002), whereas misexpression of *Six3* in medaka fishes results in multiple eyelike structures (Kobayashi et al., 1998; Loosli et al., 1999). In mice, ectopic expression of *Six3* under the control of the *Pax2* promoter element induces the formation of ectopic optic vesicles in the midbrain and hindbrain. *Optx2* (*Six6, Six9*) also belongs to the Six homeodomain family of genes and is expressed in the optic vesicles beginning at E8.5 in mice (Toy et al., 1998; Jean et al., 1999; Lopez-Rios et al., 1999; Toy and Sundin, 1999). Misexpression of *Optx2* in *Xenopus* embryos results in a large expansion of the retinal domain, as well as hyperproliferation (Zuber et al., 1999; Bernie et al., 2000).

Not all of the EFTFs fall into the Pax or Six family of genes. *Lhx2* is an EFTF belonging to the family of Lim-homeobox genes, with a LIM-type homeodomain and two zinc finger-like domains. It is expressed in the optic vesicles as early as E8.5 (Xu et al., 1993; Porter et al., 1997). In *Lhx2* null mutants, eye formation stalls at the optic vesicle stage, and the optic cup and lens do not form or fail to develop (Porter et al., 1997). *Lhx2*-knockout mice have a normal pattern of Pax6 expression in the optic vesicle, placing *Lhx2* downstream of *Pax6*. ET (*Tbx2,Tbx3,Tbx5*) is a member of another family of developmental regulator transcription factors, the T-domain proteins. It has been shown to be expressed in early vertebrate eye field induction, and its expression is subsequently restricted to the dorsal retina (Li et al., 1997).

There has been considerable debate in the literature as to which of the various EFTFs is the primary one, or "master regulator." Among the known EFTFs already described, Rx is expressed earliest in the presumptive eye field, followed shortly by Pax6, Six3, and ET. In Rx mutant mice, Pax6, Six3, and other EFTFs are not specifically upregulated in the optic region, though the initial expression of Pax6 and Six3 is unaffected. In *Pax6* null mice, Rx is induced in the optic vesicle, suggesting *Pax6* is downstream of *Rx*. However, *Pax6* may still have a role in inducing or upregulating *Rx*, since ectopic Pax6 can induce retinal tissue that expresses Rx. Similarly, overexpression of either Pax6 or Six3 results in expression of the other in the ectopic eye tissue that forms, suggesting that these genes also induce and cross-regulate one another. To better understand the hierarchy and regulation of the EFTFs, Harris and colleagues injected various combinations of EFTFs into *Xenopus* embryos and analyzed their role in eye field induction and the expression of the other EFTFs that had been left out of the mix (Zuber et al., 2003). They then injected Otx2, ET, Pax6, Six3, Rx, and Optx2 RNAs simultaneously (or with one factor at a time left out) into a single blastomere of the two-cell-stage *Xenopus* embryo. Of all the combinations, absence of Pax6 from the mix resulted in least induction of ectopic tissue, while absence of Optx2 least affected ectopic tissue induction. Also, injection of ET alone resulted in strong Rx induction, while Rx mRNA injection had no effect on ET expression. The authors thus postulated that ET lies at the front of the EFTF circuit inducing Rx, which then activates a cross-regulatory network involving Pax6, Six3, Lhx2, and Optx2.

The EFTFs have also been shown to interact directly with each other. Coimmunoprecipitation experiments following cotransfection showed the existence of complexes between the homeodomain of Pax6 and the paired-like domain of Rx in vivo (Mikkola et al., 2001). Similarly, GST pulldown assays revealed that the homeodomains of Six3 and Lhx2 can bind to Pax6 and enhance Pax6-mediated transactivation (Mikkola et al., 2001). Taken together, the data suggest that the master regulation of eye development relates to a complex set of factors rather than a single factor.

Although we know much about the EFTFs and early eye development, we know relatively little about the extracellular signaling molecules that regulate them. Recently, investigators have looked into the role of Wnt signaling in the initiation and regulation of the eye fields (Rasmussen et al., 2001; Cavodeassi et al., 2005). Wnt signaling can be divided into a canonical, β-catenin-dependent pathway and a noncanonical, β-catenin-independent pathway, and ligands and receptors for both pathways are expressed at the site of the prospective eye field. Wnt1 and Wnt8b activate the canonical Wnt-β-catenin pathway and cause a reduction in the eye fields when overexpressed in *Xenopus* embryos by suppressing Rx and Six3 expression. On the other hand, Wnt11 activates the noncanonical pathway and results in larger eyes in *Xenopus* when overexpressed (Cavodeassi et al., 2005). Overexpression of the Wnt receptor frizzled-3 (Fz3 [*Fzd3*]) in *Xenopus* results in formation of multiple ectopic eyes: Fz3 is believed to preferentially activate the noncanonical Wnt pathway (Rasmussen et al., 2001). Wnt4 is also required for *Xenopus* eye formation, and likely acts via Fz3 to induce EAF2 (*Eaf2*), which in turn regulates Rx expression in

Xenopus (Maurus et al., 2005). Loss of EAF2 function results in loss of eyes, while loss of Wnt4 function is rescued by EAF2 misexpression.

Antagonizing both Wnt and bone morphogenic protein (BMP) signaling also seems important for eye development. Dickkopf1 (Dkk1) is a potent antagonist of canonical Wnt signaling, and mice carrying null deletions of Dkk1 lose all cranial structures anterior to the midbrain, including the eyes (Mukhopadhyay et al., 2001). Noggin (*Nog*), a known inhibitor of BMP signaling, is believed to play an important role in neural induction and eye field formation (Lamb et al., 1993; Zuber et al., 2003). In animal cap assays, noggin causes increased expression of many EFTFs, including Pax6, Six3, Rx, Lhx2, and Optx2 (Zuber et al., 2003). In mice, Dkk1 and noggin pathways synergize to induce head formation during gastrulation by dually antagonizing Wnt and BMP signaling, acting as a head organizer (del Barco Barrantes et al., 2003): loss of one copy each of Dkk1 and noggin also results in total loss of the anterior head. Insulin-like growth factors (IGF-I [*Igf1*]) are believed to play an important role in head and eye formation (Pera et al., 2001) and achieve this by inhibition of canonical Wnt signaling (Richard-Parpaillon et al., 2002) via kermit2 (*Gipc1*), which is both an IGF receptor– and frizzled receptor–interacting protein (Wu et al., 2006). After the initial formation of the eye field, sonic hedgehog (Shh) signaling from the midline splits the eye field to form two eyes (Chiang et al., 1996). Shh has been shown to repress Pax6 expression via Vax2 (*Vax2*), a homeodomain transcription factor (Li et al., 1997; Kim and Lemke, 2006). Loss of Shh in the midline results in cyclopia, the development of a single midline eye (Chiang et al., 1996). Thus, a balance largely between Wnt and BMP signaling activation and inhibition by localized extracellular signaling centers is crucial in regulating eye field induction and morphogenesis during early stages of development.

Even less is known about intrinsic factors regulating EFTF activity. CCCTC binding factor (CTCF [*Ctcf*]), a transcriptional regulator, has recently been shown to control Pax6 transcription by interacting with a repressor element located in the 5′-flanking region upstream of the Pax6 P0 promoter. Overexpression of CTCF results in the small-eye phenotype by suppressing Pax6 gene transcription (Li et al., 2004). Members of the TALE family of homeobox proteins (Meis1, Meis2 [*Mrg1*], Prep1 [*Pknox1*]) have recently been implicated in regulation of Pax6 expression. Loss of Meis1/2 homeobox activity in the prospective lens ectoderm represses Pax6 expression and subsequent lens placodal development (Zhang et al., 2002). Meis1 and Prep1 are also expressed in the retina (Zhang et al., 2002; Ferretti et al., 2006). Loss of Prep1 activity concomitantly leads to loss of Meis1 and Pbx1/2 (TALE activation partners) expression, resulting in decreased Pax6 expression (Ferretti et al., 2006). Although these studies are beginning to reveal regulatory inputs for EFTFs (Pax6 in particular), the molecular mechanisms linking extrinsic and intrinsic pathways directly to EFTFs remain obscure.

One other recently emerging signaling pathway with roles in specification of neural tissues is the Notch pathway. Classically, the Notch intercellular inhibitory signaling system is composed of interactions between a Notch-ligand (Delta/Jagged [*Jag1*]) expressed on one cell, which binds and activates a Notch receptor in neighboring cells to inhibit their cellular differentiation in a process termed lateral inhibition. Yet several recent studies suggest that certain components of the Notch signaling system may contribute to earlier tissue specification and induction events. Overexpression of a constitutively active Notch internal cytoplasmic domain (NICD) in *Xenopus* embryos induced expression of Pax6 and the formation of ectopic eyes (Onuma et al., 2002). Mouse genetic studies of Notch pathway components also suggest an early role for some in eye development. Hes1, a key component of the Notch signal transduction pathway, is expressed at E8.5 in the anterior neural plate and subsequent stages of optic cup formation (Lee et al., 2005). Loss of Hes1 alone results in microphthalmia (Tomita et al., 1996a), but the combined loss of Hes1 and Pax6 seems to totally prevent optic cup formation, although Rx expression is not affected (Lee et al., 2005). Loss of Hes5, another component of the Notch pathway, reduces Müller glia cell number without any obvious microphthalmia (Hojo et al., 2000), but the combined loss of Hes1 and Hes5 results in failure of optic cup formation (Hatakeyama et al., 2004). The likely ligand for the Notch pathway at these early stages of eye development is Jagged1, which is expressed in the early optic cup and becomes restricted to the peripheral retina later (Lindsell et al., 1996; Bao and Cepko, 1997).

The preceding analysis highlights how the eye field is defined though the expression of a set of transcription factors that are constrained to this domain by multiple signaling factors. Less well defined are the transcriptional targets of the EFTFs. In other words, how does this set of genes make an eye? The overexpression studies described earlier have implicated many of these factors in the regulation of mitotic proliferation: for example, Six6/Optx2 overexpression causes hyperproliferation of the cells in the eye field. Since the Six genes appear to act primarily as transcriptional repressors, Six6/Optx2 regulation of cell proliferation is mediated at least in part by its repression (together with Dach1) of expression of the cyclin-dependent kinase inhibitors p27kip1 (*Cdkn1b*), p19Ink4d (*Cdkn2d*), and p57kip2 (*Cdkn1c*) (Li et al., 2002). Targeted deletion of Six6 leads to an upregulation of Cdki expression and a premature cell cycle exit for retinal neurons, leading to a reduction in the RPC pool and an overall reduction in eye size. In addition to a transcriptional mechanism, a recent study has implicated another type of protein, geminin (*Gmnn*), in the cell cycle–regulatory activity of Six3 (Del Bene et al., 2004). Geminin is a key cell cycle inhibitor that acts to sequester and inhibit Cdt1, part of the prereplication complex. Six3 binds to geminin directly, thereby reducing the sequestration of Cdt1 and promoting mitotic proliferation. Several direct targets of Pax6 have also been identified in the retina, including Optimedin (*Olfm3*), a protein involved in cell-cell adhesion and cell-matrix attachment (Grinchuk et al., 2005); Necab (*Efcbp1*), a Ca^{2+}-binding protein (Bernier et al., 2001), and delta-catenin (*Ctnnd1*), a component of adherens junctions (Duparc et al., 2006). These studies highlight the variety of mechanisms that will most likely be found to be involved in eye growth as we learn more about the targets of the EFTFs.

Cell fate in the retina: Transcription factors and signaling molecules

The retina is built by the sequential production of different types of retinal cells. RGCs are the first to be generated, and the other cell classes are then produced in a regular sequence that was first described using the ^{3}H-thymidine "birth dating" technique (Sidman et al., 1961). Thymidine birth dating analysis has been carried out in the retina in many different animals, and the sequence of cell generation is remarkably conserved among vertebrates. Overall, the cell classes can be divided into two phases of generation. In the first phase, ganglion cells, cones, and horizontal cells are generated. In the second phase of histogenesis, rod photoreceptors, bipolar cells, and Müller glial cells are produced. Amacrine cells are primarily generated in the later phase, but many amacrine cells become postmitotic at the same time as ganglion cells, so these cells do not fall as neatly into one or the other phase (for a review, see Robinson and Dreher, 1990; Reh and Cagan, 1994). A key feature of the progenitor cells that are responsible for the production of all the retinal neurons and Müller glia is that they are multipotent: there is not a different progenitor for each cell type. Two methods were developed for tracing the lineage of individual RPCs: (1) retroviral infection of progenitors with a virus containing a reporter gene and (2) direct injection of progenitors with an intracellular dye. Both types of methods yielded the same results (Holt et al., 1988; Turner et al., 1990): the retina has a common progenitor that can make all the different cell types, through sequential cell divisions.

The sequential development of the different retinal cell types has led several investigators to propose that the production of one cell class induces the progenitor cells to make the next cell type in the sequence. Such a model would be analogous to the way in which the R8 photoreceptor of *Drosophila is* required for the sequential induction of the other photoreceptors in ommatidia (Cagan, 1993; Reh and Cagan, 1994). For example, RGCs being generated first by the progenitor cells, might secrete a substance that prevents additional cells from differentiating into this fate and at the same time instructs the progenitor cells to begin making the next cell type, the horizontal cells; the horizontal cells would then secrete a factor that instructs the progenitor cells to make cones, and so on until all the retinal cell types had been generated. Despite the seeming simplicity of this model and its clear applicability to the recruitment of the different types of photoreceptors to the ommatidial clusters in the *Drosophila* eye, it has been difficult to show that sequential cell inductions are required for the generation of the vertebrate retinal cell classes. Elimination of ganglion cells, the first cell type to be generated, does not appear to drastically affect the development of the other retinal cells, as would have been predicted from a sequential cell induction model (Brown et al., 1998).

Several years ago, we found that forcing RPCs to differentiate prematurely led to their adoption of early generated fates, whereas inducing the differentiation of RPCs later in development caused them to adopt late fates (Reh and Kljavin, 1989; Taylor and Reh, 1990; Reh, 1992). This led us to propose that RPCs have an intrinsic "clock" that changes their competence over developmental time (Reh and Cagan, 1994). A similar mechanism appears to be responsible for generating different types of neurons in systems as diverse as the cerebral cortex (McConnell and Kaznowski, 1991) and the *Drosophila* CNS (Pearson and Doe, 2004). In this model, RPCs change throughout development as to the cell types they are competent to give rise to. First is the RGC. The progenitor cells then shift their competence so they are more likely to produce horizontal cells, then cone photoreceptors, and so on. A cascade of transcription factors might be responsible, with the first one setting in motion the mechanism for the production of the second, which acts to produce a third transcription factor, and so on. This model begs the question, what are the transcription factors that define the identities of the different retinal cell types? There is now a considerable amount of information about various transcription factors and their expression patterns in the retina (for a review, see Akagi et al., 2004). These transcription factors fall primarily into two basic types: (1) homeodomain and (2) proneural basic helix-loop-helix (bHLH). Knockout and overexpression of these factors have been carried out in the developing retina to try to gain insight into the role of these factors in neurogenesis and cell fate.

Many of the EFTFs already mentioned are also expressed in RPCs and in specific types of mature retinal neurons. For example, Pax6 is expressed in RPCs throughout the stages of histogenesis, and is maintained in amacrine cells, some ganglion cells, and horizontal cells (Hitchcock et al., 1996; Belecky-Adams et al., 1997; Hirsch and Harris, 1997).

Chx10, another member of the paired homeodomain class of transcription factors, is also expressed in RPCs and then later in bipolar cells (Burmeister et al., 1996; Belecky-Adams et al., 1997; de Melo et al., 2003; Green et al., 2003). Six6/Optx2 is expressed in progenitors and all retinal neurons (Toy and Sundin, 1999). Prox1, a divergent homeodomain protein, is expressed in RPCs and horizontal cells (Belecky-Adams et al., 1997; Dyer et al., 2003). The expression of these homeodomain transcription factors in both progenitors and specific types of retinal neurons led to the hypothesis that specific types of homeodomain transcription factors specify individual types of retinal neurons. An early example consistent with this idea came from studies of Chx10. As noted earlier, Chx10 is expressed in RPCs and then remains expressed in bipolar cells. Loss-of-function mutations of Chx10 lead to a reduction in progenitor proliferation and ultimately to a specific defect in bipolar cell development (Burmeister et al., 1996). The loss of bipolar cells is due not to the reduction in proliferation (Green et al., 2003) but rather to a repression of the rod photoreceptor program in these cells (Livne-Bar et al., 2006). However, this model does not fit with a retinal-specific deletion of Pax6 (Marquardt et al., 2001). Although Pax6 is expressed in progenitors and then primarily in amacrine cells in the mature retina, loss of Pax6 resulted in a retina that was comprised almost entirely of amacrine cells (Marquardt et al., 2001). Thus, the roles these transcription factors play are likely to be more complex than simply "specifying" a cell type. The identification of some of their direct targets will most likely provide great insight into this issue.

The other major class of transcription factors that has been implicated in cell fate during retinal development consists of the "proneural" bHLH transcription factors. In situ localization studies have demonstrated that Mash1 (*Ascl1*; Jasoni et al., 1994; Jasoni and Reh, 1996; Marquardt et al., 2001) and Ngn2 (*Neurog2*; Marquardt et al., 2001) are expressed in the progenitor cells, while many others are expressed in various types of postmitotic cells. Neurod1 is expressed in photoreceptors (Yan and Wang, 1998; Morrow et al., 1999; Inoue et al., 2002; Pennesi et al., 2003) and amacrine cells. Math3 (*Neurod4*) is expressed in amacrine cells (Inoue et al., 2002). Math5 (*Atoh7*) is expressed in ganglion cells (Kanekar et al., 1997; Brown et al., 1998), and bHLHb4 (*Bhlhb4*) and bHLHb5 (*Bhlhb5*) are expressed in bipolar cells (Bramblett et al., 2004; Feng et al., 2006). The cell-type-specific expression of these factors has also led to the idea that they are important in establishing the identities of the various types of retinal neurons (Jasoni et al., 1994; Tomita et al., 1996b; Akagi et al., 2004).

Loss-of-function studies have been carried out for most members of the bHLH gene family to gain insight into their function in retinal development. In some cases the results of knockout studies have shown a requirement for a specific member of this family in the genesis of a specific cell type. Homozygous deletion of Math5 leads to nearly complete ganglion cell loss (Brown et al., 1998), targeted deletion of bHLHb4 causes the death of most bipolar cells (Bramblett et al., 2004), and mice with Ptf1a knocked out lack most amacrine cells and horizontal cells (Fujitani et al., 2006). However, in other cases, targeted deletion of single members of this class has not demonstrated a simple relationship between the expression of a particular bHLH gene and the development of a specific cell type. Kageyama's laboratory has therefore studied double and triple knockouts of these genes to determine whether they have redundant functions in retinal development (Inoue et al., 2002; Akagi et al., 2004). Some of these double-knockout experiments have led to clear phenotypes. For example, loss of both NeuroD1 and Math3 results in a severe reduction in the number of amacrine cells (Inoue et al., 2002). However, many of the triple deletion combinations do not show simple phenotypes (Akagi et al., 2004). Even more surprising, one triple deletion (*Mash1*, *NeuroD1*, and *Math3*) results in a partial rescue of one of the double deletions (*NeuroD1* and *Math3*), restoring amacrine cells to near normal numbers. Although an early study of *Mash1* knockout mice led to the conclusion that this gene was required specifically for bipolar cell development (Tomita et al., 1996b), recent analysis of the double- and triple-knockout mice revealed that this phenotype is observed in every combination (Akagi et al., 2004), including those that do not remove *Mash1*, and so this phenotype may be due to an overall reduction in late-generated cell types as the progenitor pool is lost from a lack of Notch signaling. The studies of bHLH transcription factors and retinal development thus parallel those of homeodomain transcription factors: some of the results support a relatively simple model, others do not. Nevertheless, a molecular picture of cell fate is beginning to take shape for at least some of the cell types, such as the RGCs, and many of the transcriptional targets are being identified (Skowronska-Krawczyk et al., 2004; Mu et al., 2005).

To adequately review the literature of signaling molecules and retinal cell fate would require considerably more space than this brief review allows; however, several recent studies of the function of the Notch pathway in the regulation of retinogenesis deserve mention, since we understand most about the interactions of this pathway with underlying transcriptional regulation of the proneural bHLH factors. Retinogenesis in the mouse begins after optic cup stage (ca. E10–E11) and lasts to approximately postnatal day 10 (P10). The Notch signaling pathway functions in part to prevent progenitor cells from differentiating over a long developmental period in which all of the various cell types are born (Austin et al., 1995; Bao and Cepko, 1997; Dorsky et al., 1997; Henrique et al., 1997; Furukawa et al., 2000; Silva et al., 2003; Jadhav et al., 2006; Nelson et al., 2006;

Yaron et al., 2006). Mutations in Notch1 lead to early embryonic lethality, preventing analysis of Notch's role in retinogenesis. Two recent studies analyzed a Notch1 floxed allele using RPC-specific Cre drivers to conditionally knock out Notch1 (Notch1 CKO): Chx10-Cre (Jadhav et al., 2006) and Pax6-Cre (Yaron et al., 2006). Notch1 CKO eyes are smaller, RPC proliferation is reduced, and cone photoreceptor differentiation is increased early (Yaron et al., 2006; Jadhav et al., 2006), while rod photoreceptor differentiation is increased and Müller glial cell differentiation is decreased later (Jadhav et al., 2006). Similar results are observed in mice with deletion of the gene coding for Hes1, a key component of the Notch signal transduction pathway (Tomita et al., 1996a): the mice have more rod, horizontal, amacrine, and ganglion cells, with fewer Müller glial and bipolar cells. Deletion of another member of this gene family, Hes5, does not have as dramatic effects on retinal development (the retinas have ca. 35% fewer Müller glia [Hojo et al., 2000]), suggesting there is compensation between Hes5 and Hes1. Complementary gain-of-function studies in mice and chick are consistent with the analysis of the mutants: activated Notch suppresses neural differentiation and either maintains progenitors in an undifferentiated state or promotes their differentiation into Müller glia (Austin et al., 1995; Bao and Cepko, 1997; Dorsky et al., 1997; Henrique et al., 1997). Pharmacological inactivation of the γ-secretase complex, which is necessary for activation of all Notch1–4 homologues, recapitulates virtually all aspects of the genetic phenotypes discussed earlier but allows more precise temporal regulation (Nelson et al., 2006). Addition of a γ-secretase inhibitor causes rapid downregulation of Notch activity and the concomitant differentiation of age-appropriate cell types and a reduction in the development of Müller glia (Nelson et al., 2006).

Photoreceptor development

The development of photoreceptors has received a great deal of attention as a specific model for studies of cell fate during retinal neurogenesis. This is due in part to the availability of specific markers for these cells because of their distinctive biochemistry and gene expression profile. Early studies focused on the rod photoreceptors, although recently we have learned a great deal about the genes that control cone subtype in the mouse.

Studies in rat retinal cultures demonstrated that cell interactions (Watanabe and Raff, 1988; Reh, 1992) are important in the differentiation of rod photoreceptors, as assayed by rhodopsin expression. Some candidates for the signaling molecules responsible for promoting opsin expression in developing rods include retinoic acid (Kelley et al., 1994; Wallace and Jensen, 1999), taurine (Altshuler et al., 1993; Young and Cepko, 2004; Young et al., 2006), S-laminin (Hunter et al., 1992), Shh (Levine et al., 1997), activin (Davis et al., 2000), and VEGF (Yourey et al., 2000). In addition, EGF, LIF, and CNTF antagonize opsin expression in primary cultures of developing rat or mouse retina (Anchan et al., 1991; Lillien and Cepko, 1992; Neophytou et al., 1997; Kirsch et al., 1998), likely mediated by STAT3 (Ozawa et al., 2004; Rhee et al., 2004). It appears that immature rods go through a phase in their differentiation program in which they are very sensitive to the inhibition of rhodopsin expression via these signaling molecules, though recent data suggest that this mechanism of rhodopsin regulation persists to adulthood (Wen et al., 2006). The molecular details by which these signaling factors control opsin expression are not yet clear in most cases, though recent data indicate that some of these factors may affect the expression or function of one or more of the photoreceptor-specific transcription factors.

In conjunction with the aforementioned signaling factors, photoreceptor development is controlled by several different types of transcription factors. The homeodomain transcription factor *Otx2* is an early factor that biases RPCs to become photoreceptors: conditional deletion of Otx2 leads to loss of photoreceptors; retroviral gene transfer of Otx2 into RPCs promotes the photoreceptor fate (Nishida et al., 2003). Otx2 also activates transcription of the cone-rod homeobox gene (*Crx*) (Furukawa et al., 1997b), which is also required for the expression of photoreceptor-specific genes, including the opsins. A third transcription factor expressed in photoreceptors is NeuroD1. While overexpression studies have shown a role for this bHLH transcription factor in promoting photoreceptor development (Moore et al., 2002; Ma et al., 2004), and it is expressed in both rods and cones early in their development, rods and cones appear to be generated in normal numbers in mice with homozygous deletion of NeuroD1 (Pennesi et al., 2003).

In the next stage of photoreceptor development, the Otx2/Crx/NeuroD1-expressing photoreceptors develop as either rods or cones, depending on their expression of at least two other transcription factors, Nrl and Nr2e3. Nrl (neural leucine zipper1; Swaroop et al., 1992) is a member of the Maf family of transcriptional activators (Friedman et al., 2004), which is expressed only in rods in the developing retina. Nrl binds to and activates the rhodopsin promoter (Kumar et al., 1996; Rehemtulla et al., 1996) and is required for rod photoreceptor development; deletion of this gene results in all the rods developing instead as s-opsin-expressing cones (Mears et al., 2001; Daniele et al., 2005). Rod photoreceptor development also requires another transcription factor, Nr2e3, a member of the nuclear hormone receptor family of transcription factors. This gene was first identified as important in rod development by the demonstration that mutations in Nr2e3 result in enhanced S cone syndrome in humans (Haigh et al., 2003) and a similar phenotype in mice (Haider et al., 2001). Like Nrl, retinas from mice deficient in *Nr2e3* develop either excess cones or cone-like "hybrid" photoreceptors at the expense of rods (Haider et al., 2001; Chen et al., 2005; Corbo and Cepko, 2005). Nr2e3 also acts as a transcriptional activator of rhodopsin and other rod-specific genes, likely in a complex with Nrl and Crx (Chen et al., 2005). Nrl is likely to be upstream of Nr2e3, since deletion of Nrl leads to a loss of Nr2e3, but not the reverse. Interestingly, Nrl and Nr2e3 have some distinct functions, since replacement of Nrl with Nr2e3 results in activation of some, but not all, of the rod-specific gene profile (Cheng et al., 2006). Remarkably, Nr2e3 is a strong repressor of the cone fate, since expression of Nr2e3 under the control of the s-opsin promoter causes the developing cones to switch their fate and develop as rodlike cells (Cheng et al., 2006).

Ultimately we would like to know how the signaling factors regulate the transcription factors, and vice versa. However, at this time there is still relatively little information on this point. LIF inhibits rod development in part through the inhibition of Crx and Nrl expression (Graham et al., 2005), while retinoic acid, one of the factors that promotes rod differentiation during development, promotes expression of Nrl through a retinoic acid response element in its promoter (Khanna et al., 2006). One of the other factors that regulate rod development, taurine, appears to act through the glycine receptor (Altshuler et al., 1993; Young and Cepko et al., 2004). In the developing retina, taurine-synthesizing enzymes and transporters are expressed (Pasantes-Morales and Cruz, 1985; Lombardini, 1991) and taurine expression is upregulated during differentiation (Lake and Malik, 1987). The effects of taurine on photoreceptor development can be blocked by antagonists to either glycine or GABA receptors (Altshuler et al., 1993; Thio et al., 2003). It appears that taurine acts on postmitotic cells, altering their opsin expression (Wallace and Jensen, 1999). Glycine receptor α2 (GlyRα2 [*Glra2*]) is expressed in the prospective layer of RPCs and photoreceptor precursors in mice at P0 (Young and Cepko, 2004). Misexpression of GlyRα2 leads to an increase in photoreceptor development and a decrease in Müller glia, suggesting a change in cell fate (Young and Cepko, 2004). Moreover, using an siRNA loss-of-function approach, Young and Cepko (2004) inhibited GlyRα2 and found that photoreceptor development was reduced. However, mice with a targeted deletion of GlyRα2 do not have a gross morphological retinal phenotype (Young et al., 2006), and the number of rods apparently is normal. Moreover, transgenic mice with a taurine transporter deletion have lower taurine levels, but not fewer photoreceptors (Heller-Stilb et al., 2002). Therefore, although taurine is sufficient to promote rod photoreceptor development, it may be that some of its function can be replaced by redundant factors.

Although we know relatively little about the relationships between the signaling factors and the transcriptional regulators of rod photoreceptor development, we are beginning to understand these relationships in the development of cone photoreceptors. Like most mammals, mice have two opsin proteins that respond maximally to different wavelengths: s-opsin to short wavelengths and m-opsin to longer wavelengths. In mice there is an opposing gradient of m- and s-opsin such that m-opsin expression is highest in dorsal cones and s-opsin predominates in the ventral retina. Cone photoreceptors are generated in the early stages of retinal histogenesis, and the presumptive postmitotic cones express Crx, NeuroD1, and Otx2, and instead of Nrl or Nr2e3, they express two cone-specific transcription factors: thyroid hormone receptor-β_2 (*TRβ2* [*Thrb2*]) and RXR-γ (*RXRγ* [*Rxrg*]). These two factors, members of the nuclear hormone receptor family, are critical for the developmental "choice" of which of the two cone opsin genes to express in developing cone photoreceptors (Ng et al., 2001). *TRβ2* null mice show a profound disruption in the cone opsin gradient. These mice fail to express m-opsin (*Opn1mw*) in any cones, indicating that *TRβ2* is necessary for m-opsin expression. Additionally, *all* cones in *TRβ2* null mice express s-opsin (*Opn1sw*), which indicates that *TRβ2* is also necessary to repress s-opsin. Mice with a mutation in the ligand-binding domain of TR-β show the same defects as the *TRβ2*$^{-/-}$ mice, indicating that binding of endogenous TH to the TR-β receptor is required, both for the inhibition of s-opsin and for the activation of m-opsin in vivo. TRs often regulate transcription as heterodimers with RXRs. RXR-γ is expressed in developing cone photoreceptors in both mice and humans (Roberts et al., 2005). Mice deficient in RX*Rγ* express s-opsin in every cone, resulting in a loss of normal cone opsin patterning (Roberts et al., 2005). Thus, it is likely that heterodimers of *RXRγ* and *TRβ2* normally establish the pattern of s-opsin expression by inhibiting it in many of the dorsal retinal cones. Interestingly, both *RXRγ* and *TRβ2* are transiently downregulated at s-opsin onset (Roberts et al., 2005, 2006), suggesting that this downregulation is necessary for the timing of s-opsin expression in both mice and humans. However, neither of the two RXR genes expressed in developing cone photoreceptors, *RXRγ* or *RXRβ*-, is required to activate m-opsin expression (Roberts et al., 2005, 2006). Thus, an RXR-γ:TR-β_2 heterodimer regulates s-opsin, while a TR-β_2:TR-β_2 homodimer appears to regulate m-opsin expression. Both *RXRγ* and *TRβ2* are regulated by ligands; are these ligands important in cone development? Both T_3 and T_4 are present in the developing retina, and both are more highly localized to the dorsal retina at the time of m-opsin onset, P10 (Roberts et al., 2006). Exogenous T_3 administration inhibits s-opsin when experimentally elevated at the time of s-opsin onset but activates m-opsin when animals are treated at the time of m-opsin onset (Roberts et al., 2006).

These studies have led to the following model of photoreceptor development. Cones are generated in mice from multipotent progenitors beginning at E10.5, and rods begin to be generated a few days later. Shortly after withdrawal from the cell cycle, both rods and cones express photoreceptor-specific transcription factors such as NeuroD1, Crx, and Otx2. Nrl and Nr2e3 are expressed in the cells fated to become rods, and these repress cone genes while activating the rod-specific genetic program. Those cells fated to become cones, however, express TRβ2 and RXRγ. These two transcription factors repress s-opsin expression in a T3-dependent manner. Both genes are then downregulated around P0 in the cones that will turn on s-opsin but remain high in the cells that will go on to express m-opsin. Later in retinal development (P10), T3 and the TRβ2 receptor are necessary to activate m-opsin expression, and the level of m-opsin expression reflects the level of T3 and T4 in the retina at that time. *RXRγ*:*TRβ2* heterodimers repress s-opsin expression, while m-opsin is regulated by either a *TRβ2* homodimer or *TRβ2* with an unknown heterodimeric partner.

Conclusion

Our understanding of eye development has grown tremendously over the past 20 years. Although many of the basic phenomena of eye development can now be at least partly explained by their underlying molecular mechanisms, there are still fundamental gaps in our understanding. We hope that this review has highlighted some of these gaps, and may thereby stimulate research in these areas. One thing is certain, however: the beauty and complexity of the eye and retina will continue to fascinate and challenge new generations of developmental biologists.

REFERENCES

Akagi, T., Inoue, T., Miyoshi, G., Bessho, Y., Takahashi, M., Lee, J. E., Guillemot, F., and Kageyama, R. (2004). Requirement of multiple basic helix-loop-helix genes for retinal neuronal subtype specification. *J. Biol. Chem.* 279:28492–28498.

Altshuler, D., Lo Turco, J. J., Rush, J., and Cepko, C. (1993). Taurine promotes the differentiation of a vertebrate retinal cell type in vitro. *Development* 119:1317–1328.

Anchan, R. M., Reh, T. A., Angello, J., Balliet, A., and Walker, M. (1991). EGF and TGF-alpha stimulate retinal neuroepithelial cell proliferation in vitro. *Neuron* 6:923–936.

Andreazzoli, M., Gestri, G., Angeloni, D., Menna, E., and Barsacchi, G. (1999). Role of Xrx1 in *Xenopus* eye and anterior brain development. *Development* 126:2451–2460.

Austin, C. P., Feldman, D. E., Ida, J. A., Jr., and Cepko, C. L. (1995). Vertebrate retinal ganglion cells are selected from competent progenitors by the action of Notch. *Development* 121: 3637–3650.

Bao, Z. Z., and Cepko, C. L. (1997). The expression and function of Notch pathway genes in the developing rat eye. *J. Neurosci.* 17:1425–1434.

Belecky-Adams, T., Tomarev, S., Li, H. S., Ploder, L., McInnes, R. R., Sundin, O., and Adler, R. (1997). *Pax-6*, *Prox 1*, and *Chx10* homeobox gene expression correlates with phenotypic fate of retinal precursor cells. *Invest. Ophthalmol. Vis. Sci.* 38: 1293–1303.

Bernier, G., Panitz, F., Zhou, X., Hollemann, T., Gruss, P., and Pieler, T. (2000). Expanded retina territory by midbrain transformation upon overexpression of *Six6* (*Optx2*) in *Xenopus* embryos. *Mech. Dev.* 93:59–69.

Bernier, G., Vukovich, W., Neidhardt, L., Herrmann, B. G., and Gruss, P. (2001). Isolation and characterization of a downstream target of *Pax6* in the mammalian retinal primordium. *Development* 128:3987–3994.

Bovolenta, P., Mallamaci, A., Puelles, L., and Boncinelli, E. (1998). Expression pattern of *cSix3*, a member of the Six/sine oculis family of transcription factors. *Mech. Dev.* 70:201–203.

Bramblett, D. E., Pennesi, M. E., Wu, S. M., and Tsai, M. J. (2004). The transcription factor Bhlhb4 is required for rod bipolar cell maturation. *Neuron* 43:779–793.

Brown, N. L., Kanekar, S., Vetter, M. L., Tucker, P. K., Gemza, D. L., and Glaser, T. (1998). *Math5* encodes a murine basic helix-loop-helix transcription factor expressed during early stages of retinal neurogenesis. *Development* 125:4821–4833.

Burmeister, M., Novak, J., Liang, M. Y., Basu, S., Ploder, L., Hawes, N. L., Vidgen, D., Hoover, F., Goldman, D., et al. (1996). Ocular retardation mouse caused by *Chx10* homeobox null allele: Impaired retinal progenitor proliferation and bipolar cell differentiation. *Nat. Genet.* 12:376–384.

Cagan, R. (1993). Cell fate specification in the developing *Drosophila* retina. *Development* Suppl. 19–28.

Carl, M., Loosli, F., and Wittbrodt, J. (2002). Six3 inactivation reveals its essential role for the formation and patterning of the vertebrate eye. *Development* 129:4057–4063.

Cavodeassi, F., Carreira-Barbosa, F., Young, R. M., Concha, M. L., Allende, M. L., Houart, C., Tada, M., and Wilson, S. W. (2005). Early stages of zebrafish eye formation require the coordinated activity of *Wnt11*, *Fz5*, and the *Wnt*/beta-catenin pathway. *Neuron* 47:43–56.

Chen, J., Rattner, A., and Nathans, J. (2005). The rod photoreceptor-specific nuclear receptor Nr2e3 represses transcription of multiple cone-specific genes. *J. Neurosci.* 25:118–129.

Cheng, H., Aleman, T. S., Cideciyan, A. V., Khanna, R., Jacobson, S. G., and Swaroop, A. (2006). In vivo function of the orphan nuclear receptor NR2E3 in establishing photoreceptor identity during mammalian retinal development. *Hum. Mol. Genet.* 15:2588–2602.

Chiang, C., Litingtung, Y., Lee, E., Young, K. E., Corden, J. L., Westpha, H., and Beachy, P. A. (1996). Cyclopia and defective axial patterning in mice lacking Sonic hedgehog gene function. *Nature* 383:407–413.

Chisholm, A. D., and Horvitz, H. R. (1995). Patterning of the *Caenorhabditis elegans* head region by the Pax-6 family member vab-3. *Nature* 377:52–55.

Chow, R. L., Altmann, C. R., Lang, R. A., and Hemmati-Brivanlou, A. (1999). *Pax6* induces ectopic eyes in a vertebrate. *Development* 126:4213–4222.

Chuang, J. C., Mathers, P. H., and Raymond, P. A. (1999). Expression of three Rx homeobox genes in embryonic and adult zebrafish. *Mech. Dev.* 84:195–198.

Corbo, J. C., and Cepko, C. L. (2005). A hybrid photoreceptor expressing both rod and cone genes in a mouse model of enhanced S-cone syndrome. *PLoS Genet.* 1:e11.

Daniele, L. L., Lillo, C., Lyubarsky, A. L., Nikonov, S. S., Philp, N., Mears, A. J., Swaroop, A., Williams, D. S., and Pugh, E. N., Jr. (2005). Cone-like morphological, molecular, and electrophysiological features of the photoreceptors of the Nrl knockout mouse. *Invest. Ophthalmol. Vis. Sci.* 46:2156–2167.

Davis, A. A., Matzuk, M. M., and Reh, T. A. (2000). Activin A promotes progenitor differentiation into photoreceptors in rodent retina. *Mol. Cell. Neurosci.* 15:11–21.

del Barco Barrantes, I., Davidson, G., Grone, H. J., Westphal, H., and Niehrs, C. (2003). Dkk1 and noggin cooperate in mammalian head induction. *Genes Dev.* 217:2239–2244.

Del Bene, F., Tessmar-Raible, K., and Wittbrodt, J. (2004). Direct interaction of geminin and Six3 in eye development. *Nature* 427:745–749.

de Melo, J., Qiu, X., Du, G., Cristante, L., and Eisenstat, D. D. (2003). *Dlx1*, *Dlx2*, *Pax6*, *Brn3b*, and *Chx10* homeobox gene expression defines the retinal ganglion and inner nuclear layers of the developing and adult mouse retina. *J. Comp. Neurol.* 461:187–204.

Dorsky, R. I., Chang, W. S., Rapaport, D. H., and Harris, W. A. (1997). Regulation of neuronal diversity in the *Xenopus* retina by delta signalling. *Nature* 385:67–70.

Duparc, R. H., Boutemmine, D., Champagne, M. P., Tetreault, N., and Bernier, G. (2006). Pax6 is required for delta-catenin/neurojugin expression during retinal, cerebellar and cortical development in mice. *Dev. Biol.* 300:647–655.

Dyer, M. A., Livesey, F. J., Cepko, C. L., and Oliver, G. (2003). Prox1 function controls progenitor cell proliferation and horizontal cell genesis in the mammalian retina. *Nat. Genet.* 34:53–58.

Eggert, T., Hauck, B., Hildebrandt, N., Gehring, W. J., and Walldorf, U. (1998). Isolation of a *Drosophila* homolog of the vertebrate homeobox gene Rx and its possible role in brain and eye development. *Proc. Natl. Acad. Sci. U.S.A.* 95:2343–2348.

Feng, L., Xie, X., Joshi, P. S., Yang, Z., Shibasaki, K., Chow, R. L., and Gan, L. (2006). Requirement for Bhlhb5 in the specification of amacrine and cone bipolar subtypes in mouse retina. *Development* 133:4815–4825.

Ferretti, E., Villaescusa, J. C., Di Rosa, P., Fernandez-Diaz, L. C., Longobardi, E., Mazzieri, R., Miccio, A., Micali, N., Selleri, L., et al. (2006). Hypomorphic mutation of the TALE gene *Prep1* (pKnox1) causes a major reduction of Pbx and Meis proteins and a pleiotropic embryonic phenotype. *Mol. Cell Biol.* 26:5650–5662.

Friedman, J. S., Khanna, H., Swain, P. K., Denicola, R., Cheng, H., Mitton, K. P., Weber, C. H., Hicks, D., and Swaroop, A. (2004). The minimal transactivation domain of the basic motif-leucine zipper transcription factor NRL interacts with TATA-binding protein. *J. Biol. Chem.* 279:47233–47241.

Fujitani, Y., Fujitani, S., Luo, H., Qiu, F., Burlison, J., Long, Q., Kawaguchi, Y., Edlund, H., MacDonald, R. J., Furukawa, T., et al. (2006). Ptf1a determines horizontal and amacrine cell fates during mouse retinal development. *Development* 133:4439–4450.

Furukawa, T., Kozak, C. A., and Cepko, C. L. (1997a). *Rax*, a novel paired-type homeobox gene, shows expression in the anterior neural fold and developing retina. *Proc. Natl. Acad. Sci. U.S.A.* 94:3088–3093.

Furukawa, T., Morrow, E. M., and Cepko, C. L. (1997b). *Crx*, a novel *otx*-like homeobox gene, shows photoreceptor-specific expression and regulates photoreceptor differentiation. *Cell* 91: 531–541.

Furukawa, T., Mukherjee, S., Bao, Z. Z., Morrow, E. M., and Cepko, C. L. (2000). rax, Hes1, and notch1 promote the formation of Müller glia by postnatal retinal progenitor cells. *Neuron* 26:383–394.

Glaser, T., Walton, D. S., and Maas, R. L. (1992). Genomic structure, evolutionary conservation and aniridia mutations in the human *PAX6* gene. *Nat. Genet.* 2:232–239.

Graham, D. R., Overbeek, P. A., and Ash, J. D. (2005). Leukemia inhibitory factor blocks expression of Crx and Nrl transcription factors to inhibit photoreceptor differentiation. *Invest. Ophthalmol. Vis. Sci.* 46:2601–2610.

Green, E. S., Stubbs, J. L., and Levine, E. M. (2003). Genetic rescue of cell number in a mouse model of microphthalmia: interactions between Chx10 and G1-phase cell cycle regulators. *Development* 130:539–552.

Grinchuk, O., Kozmik, Z., Wu, X., and Tomarev, S. (2005). The Optimedin gene is a downstream target of Pax6. *J. Biol. Chem.* 280:35228–35237.

Grindley, J. C., Davidson, D. R., and Hill, R. E. (1995). The role of Pax-6 in eye and nasal development. *Development* 121: 1433–1442.

Haider, N. B., Naggert, J. K., and Nishina, P. M. (2001). Excess cone cell proliferation due to lack of a functional NR2E3 causes retinal dysplasia and degeneration in rd7/rd7 mice. *Hum. Mol. Genet.* 10:1619–1626.

Haigh, J. J., Morelli, P. I., Gerhardt, H., Haigh, K., Tsien, J., Damert, A., Miquerol, L., Muhlner, U., Klein, R., et al. (2003). Cortical and retinal defects caused by dosage-dependent reductions in VEGF-A paracrine signaling. *Dev. Biol.* 262:225–241.

Hatakeyama, J., Bessho, Y., Katoh, K., Ookawara, S., Fujioka, M., Guillemot, F., and Kageyama, R. (2004). *Hes* genes regulate size, shape and histogenesis of the nervous system by control of the timing of neural stem cell differentiation. *Development* 131:5539–5550.

Heller-Stilb, B., van Roeyen, C., Rascher, K., Hartwig, H. G., Huth, A., Seeliger, M. W., Warskulat, U., and Häussinger, D. (2002). Disruption of the taurine transporter gene (taut) leads to retinal degeneration in mice. *FASEB J.* 16: 231–233.

Henrique, D., Hirsinger, E., Adam, J., Le Roux, I., Pourquié, O., Ish-Horowicz, D., and Lewis, J. (1997). Maintenance of neuroepithelial progenitor cells by Delta-Notch signalling in the embryonic chick retina. *Curr. Biol.* 7:661–670.

Hill, R. E., Favor, J., Hogan, B. L., Ton, C. C., Saunders, G. F., Hanson, I. M., Prosser, J., Jordan, T., Hastie, N. D., and van Heyningen V. (1991). Mouse small eye results from mutations in a paired-like homeobox-containing gene. *Nature* 354: 522–525.

Hirsch, N., and Harris, W. A. (1997). *Xenopus Pax-6* and retinal development. *J. Neurobiol.* 32:45–61.

Hitchcock, P. F., Macdonald, R. E., VanDeRyt, J. T., and Wilson, S. W. (1996). Antibodies against Pax6 immunostain amacrine and ganglion cells and neuronal progenitors, but not rod precursors, in the normal and regenerating retina of the goldfish. *J. Neurobiol.* 29:399–413.

Hojo, M., Ohtsuka, T., Hashimoto, N., Gradwohl, G., Guillemot, F., and Kageyama, R. (2000). Glial cell fate specification modulated by the bHLH gene Hes5 in mouse retina. *Development* 127:2515–2522.

Holt, C. E., Bertsch, T. W., Ellis, H. M., and Harris, W. A. (1988). Cellular determination in the *Xenopus* retina is independent of lineage and birth date. *Neuron* 1:15–26.

Hunter, D. D., Murphy, M. D., Olsson, C. V., and Brunken, W. J. (1992). S-laminin expression in adult and developing retinae: A potential cue for photoreceptor morphogenesis. *Neuron* 8:399–413.

Inoue, T., Hojo, M., Bessho, Y., Tano, Y., Lee, J. E., and Kageyama, R. (2002). Math3 and NeuroD regulate amacrine cell fate specification in the retina. *Development* 129:831–842.

Jadhav, A. P., Mason, H. A., and Cepko, C. L. (2006). Notch 1 inhibits photoreceptor production in the developing mammalian retina. *Development* 133:913–923.

Jasoni, C. L., and Reh, T. A. (1996). Temporal and spatial pattern of MASH-1 expression in the developing rat retina demonstrates progenitor cell heterogeneity. *J. Comp. Neurol.* 369:319–327.

Jasoni, C. L., Walker, M. B., Morris, M. D., and Reh, T. A. (1994). A chicken achaete-scute homolog (CASH-1) is expressed in a temporally and spatially discrete manner in the developing nervous system. *Development* 120:769–783.

Jean, D., Bernier, G., and Gruss, P. (1999). Six6 (Optx2) is a novel murine Six3-related homeobox gene that demarcates the presumptive pituitary/hypothalamic axis and the ventral optic stalk. *Mech. Dev.* 84:31–40.

Jordan, T., Hanson, I., Zaletayev, D., Hodgson, S., Prosser, J., Seawright, A., Hastie, N., and van Heyningen, V. (1992). The human *PAX6* gene is mutated in two patients with aniridia. *Nat. Genet.* 1:328–332.

Kanekar, S., Perron, M., Dorsky, R., Harris, W. A., Jan, L. Y., Jan, Y. N., and Vetter, M. L. (1997). *Xath5* participates in a network of bHLH genes in the developing *Xenopus* retina. *Neuron* 19:981–994.

Kelley, M. W., Turner, J. K., and Reh, T. A. (1994). Retinoic acid promotes differentiation of photoreceptors in vitro. *Development* 120:2091–2102.

Khanna, H., Akimoto, M., Siffroi-Fernandez, S., Friedman, J. S., Hicks, D., and Swaroop, A. (2006). Retinoic acid regulates the expression of photoreceptor transcription factor NRL. *J. Biol. Chem.* 281:27327–27334.

Kim, J. W., and Lemke, G. (2006). Hedgehog-regulated localization of Vax2 controls eye development. *Genes Dev.* 20:2833–2847.

Kirsch, M., Schulz-Key, S., Wiese, A., Fuhrmann, S., and Hofmann, H. (1998). Ciliary neurotrophic factor blocks rod photoreceptor differentiation from postmitotic precursor cells in vitro. *Cell Tissue Res.* 291:207–216.

Kobayashi, M., Toyama, R., Takeda, H., Dawid, I. B., and Kawakami, K. (1998). Overexpression of the forebrain-specific homeobox gene six3 induces rostral forebrain enlargement in zebrafish. *Development* 125:2973–2982.

Kumar, R., Chen, S., Scheurer, D., Wang, Q. L., Duh, E., Sung, C. H., Rehemtulla, A., Swaroop, A., Adler, R., and Zack, D. J. (1996). The bZIP transcription factor Nrl stimulates rhodopsin promoter activity in primary retinal cell cultures. *J. Biol. Chem.* 271:29612–29618.

Lagutin, O., Zhu, C. C., Furuta, Y., Rowitch, D. H., McMahon, A. P., and Oliver, G. (2001). Six3 promotes the formation of ectopic optic vesicle-like structures in mouse embryos. *Dev. Dyn.* 221:342–349.

Lagutin, O. V., Zhu, C. C., Kobayashi, D., Topczewski, J., Shimamura, K., Puelles, L., Russell, H. R., McKinnon, P. J., et al. (2003). Six3 repression of Wnt signaling in the anterior neuroectoderm is essential for vertebrate forebrain development. *Genes Dev.* 17:368–379.

Lake, N., and Malik, N. (1987). Retinal morphology in rats treated with a taurine transport antagonist. *Exp. Eye Res.* 44:331–346.

Lamb, T. M., Knecht, A. K., Smith, W. C., Stachel, S. E., Economides, A. N., Stahl, N., Yancopolous, G. D., and Harland, R. M. (1993). Neural induction by the secreted polypeptide noggin. *Science* 262:713–718.

Lee, H. Y., Wroblewski, E., Philips, G. T., Stair, C. N., Conley, K., Reedy, M., Mastick, G. S., and Brown, N. L. (2005). Multiple requirements for Hes 1 during early eye formation. *Dev. Biol.* 284:464–478.

Levine, E. M., Roelink, H., Turner, J., and Reh, T. A. (1997). Sonic hedgehog promotes rod photoreceptor differentiation in mammalian retinal cells in vitro. *J. Neurosci.* 17:6277–6288.

Li, H., Tierney, C., Wen, L., Wu, J. Y., and Rao, Y. (1997). A single morphogenetic field gives rise to two retina primordia under the influence of the prechordal plate. *Development* 124: 603–615.

Li, T., Lu, Z., and Lu, L. (2004). Regulation of eye development by transcription control of CCCTC binding factor (CTCF). *J. Biol. Chem.* 279:27575–27583.

Li, X., Perissi, V., Liu, F., Rose, D. W., and Rosenfeld, M. G. (2002). Tissue-specific regulation of retinal and pituitary precursor cell proliferation. *Science* 297:1180–1183.

Lillien, L., and Cepko, C. (1992). Control of proliferation in the retina: Temporal changes in responsiveness to FGF and TGF alpha. *Development* 115:253–266.

Lindsell, C. E., Boulter, J., diSibio, G., Gossler, A., and Weinmaster, G. (1996). Expression patterns of Jagged, Delta1, Notch1, Notch2, and Notch3 genes identify ligand-receptor pairs that may function in neural development. *Mol. Cell Neurosci.* 8:14–27.

Livne-Bar, I., Pacal, M., Cheung, M. C., Hankin, M., Trogadis, J., Chen, D., Dorval, K. M., and Bremner, R. (2006). Chx10 is required to block photoreceptor differentiation but is dispensable for progenitor proliferation in the postnatal retina. *Proc. Natl. Acad. Sci. U.S.A.* 103:4988–4993.

Lombardini, J. B. (1991). Taurine: Retinal function. *Brain Res. Brain Res. Rev.* 16:151–169.

Loosli, F., Koster, R. W., Carl, M., Krone, A., and Wittbrodt, J. (1998). Six3, a medaka homologue of the *Drosophila* homeobox gene sine oculis is expressed in the anterior embryonic shield and the developing eye. *Mech. Dev.* 74:159–164.

Loosli, F., Winkler, S., and Wittbrodt, J. (1999). Six3 overexpression initiates the formation of ectopic retina. *Genes Dev.* 13:649–654.

Lopez-Rios, J., Gallardo, M. E., Rodriguez de Cordoba, S., and Bovolenta, P. (1999). Six9 (Optx2), a new member of the six gene family of transcription factors, is expressed at early stages of vertebrate ocular and pituitary development. *Mech. Dev.* 83:155–159.

Ma, W., Yan, R. T., Xie, W., and Wang, S. Z. (2004). A role of Math5 in inducing neuroD and the photoreceptor pathway. *J. Neurosci.* 24:7150–7158.

Marquardt, T., Ashery-Padan, R., Andrejewski, N., Scardigli, R., Guillemot, F., and Gruss, P. (2001). Pax6 is required for the multipotent state of retinal progenitor cells. *Cell* 105:43–55.

Mathers, P. H., Grinberg, A., Mahon, K. A., and Jamrich, M. (1997). The Rx homeobox gene is essential for vertebrate eye development. *Nature* 387:603–607.

Maurus, D., Heligon, C., Burger-Schwarzler, A., Brandli, A. W., and Kuhl, M. (2005). Noncanonical Wnt-4 signaling and

EAF2 are required for eye development in *Xenopus laevis. EMBO J.* 24:1181–1191.

McConnell, S. K., and Kaznowski, C. E. (1991). Cell cycle dependence of laminar determination in developing neocortex. *Science* 254:282–285.

Mears, A. J., Kondo, M., Swain, P. K., Takada, Y., Bush, R. A., Saunders, T. L., Sieving, P. A., and Swaroop, A. (2001). Nrl is required for rod photoreceptor development. *Nat. Genet.* 29: 447–452.

Mikkola, I., Bruun, J. A., Holm, T., and Johansen, T. (2001). Superactivation of Pax6-mediated transactivation from paired domain-binding sites by DNA-independent recruitment of different homeodomain proteins. *J. Biol. Chem.* 276:4109–4118.

Moore, K. B., Schneider, M. L., and Vetter, M. L. (2002). Posttranslational mechanisms control the timing of bHLH function and regulate retinal cell fate. *Neuron* 34:183–195.

Morrow, E. M., Furukawa, T., Lee, J. E., and Cepko, C. L. (1999). NeuroD regulates multiple functions in the developing neural retina in rodent. *Development* 126:23–36.

Mu, X., Fu, X., Sun, H., Beremand, P. D., Thomas, T. L., and Klein, W. H. (2005). A gene network downstream of transcription factor Math5 regulates retinal progenitor cell competence and ganglion cell fate. *Dev. Biol.* 2280:467–481.

Mukhopadhyay, M., Shtrom, S., Rodriguez-Esteban, C., Chen, L., Tsukui, T., Gomer, L., Dorward, D. W., Glinka, A., Grinberg, A., et al. (2001). Dickkopf1 is required for embryonic head induction and limb morphogenesis in the mouse. *Dev. Cell* 1:423–434.

Nelson, B. R., Gumuscu, B., Hartman, B. H., and Reh, T. A. (2006). Notch activity is downregulated just prior to retinal ganglion cell differentiation. *Dev. Neurosci.* 28:128–141.

Neophytou, C., Vernallis, A. B., Smith, A., and Raff, M. C. (1997). Müller-cell-derived leukaemia inhibitory factor arrests rod photoreceptor differentiation at a postmitotic pre-rod stage of development. *Development* 124:2345–2354.

Ng, L., Hurley, J. B., Dierks, B., Srinivas, M., Saltó, C., Vennström, B., Reh, T. A., and Forrest, D. (2001). A thyroid hormone receptor that is required for the development of green cone photoreceptors. *Nat. Genet.* 27:94–98.

Nishida, A., Furukawa, A., Koike, C., Tano, Y., Aizawa, S., Matsuo, I., and Furukawa, T. (2003). Otx2 homeobox gene controls retinal photoreceptor cell fate and pineal gland development. *Nat. Neurosci.* 6:1255–1263.

Oliver, G., Mailhos, A., Wehr, R., Copeland, N. G., Jenkins, N. A., and Gruss, P. (1995). Six3, a murine homologue of the sine oculis gene, demarcates the most anterior border of the developing neural plate and is expressed during eye development. *Development* 121:4045–4055.

Onuma, Y., Takahashi, S., Asashima, M., Kurata, S., and Gehring, W. J. (2002). Conservation of Pax 6 function and upstream activation by Notch signaling in eye development of frogs and flies. *Proc. Natl. Acad. Sci. U.S.A.* 99:2020–2025.

Ozawa, Y., Nakao, K., Shimazaki, T., Takeda, J., Akira, S., Ishihara, K., Hirano, T., Oguchi, Y., and Okano, H. (2004). Downregulation of STAT3 activation is required for presumptive rod photoreceptor cells to differentiate in the postnatal retina. *Mol. Cell Neurosci.* 26:258–270.

Pasantes-Morales, H., and Cruz, C. (1985). Taurine: A physiological stabilizer of photoreceptor membranes. *Prog. Clin. Biol. Res.* 179:371–381.

Pearson, B. J., and Doe, C. Q. (2004). Specification of temporal identity in the developing nervous system. *Annu. Rev. Cell. Dev. Biol.* 20:619–647.

Pennesi, M. E., Cho, J. H., Yang, Z., Wu, S. H., Zhang, J., Wu, S. M., and Tsai, M. J. (2003). BETA2/NeuroD1 null mice: A new model for transcription factor-dependent photoreceptor degeneration. *J. Neurosci.* 23:453–461.

Pera, E. M., Wessely, O., Li, S. Y., and De Robertis, E. M. (2001). Neural and head induction by insulin-like growth factor signals. *Dev. Cell* 1:655–665.

Porter, F. D., Drago, J., Xu, Y., Cheema, S. S., Wassif, C., Huang, S. P., Lee, E., Grinberg, A., Massalas, J. S., et al. (1997). Lhx2, a LIM homeobox gene, is required for eye, forebrain, and definitive erythrocyte development. *Development* 124: 2935–2944.

Quiring, R., Walldorf, U., Kloter, U., and Gehring, W. J. (1994). Homology of the eyeless gene of *Drosophila* to the small eye gene in mice and aniridia in humans. *Science* 265:785–789.

Rasmussen, J. T., Deardorff, M. A., Tan, C., Rao, M. S., Klein, P. S., and Vetter, M. L. (2001). Regulation of eye development by frizzled signaling in *Xenopus. Proc. Natl. Acad. Sci. U.S.A.* 98: 3861–3866.

Reh, T. A. (1992). Cellular interactions determine neuronal phenotypes in rodent retinal cultures. *J. Neurobiol.* 23:1067–1083.

Reh, T. A., and Cagan, R. L. (1994). Intrinsic and extrinsic signals in the developing vertebrate and fly eyes: Viewing vertebrate and invertebrate eyes in the same light. *Perspect. Dev. Neurobiol.* 2: 183–190.

Reh, T. A., and Kljavin, I. J. (1989). Age of differentiation determines rat retinal germinal cell phenotype: Induction of differentiation by dissociation. *J. Neurosci.* 9:4179–4189.

Rehemtulla, A., Warwar, R., Kumar, R., Ji, X., Zack, D. J., and Swaroop, A. (1996). The basic motif-leucine zipper transcription factor Nrl can positively regulate rhodopsin gene expression. *Proc. Natl. Acad. Sci. U.S.A.* 93:191–195.

Rhee, K. D., Goureau, O., Chen, S., and Yang, X. J. (2004). Cytokine-induced activation of signal transducer and activator of transcription in photoreceptor precursors regulates rod differentiation in the developing mouse retina. *J. Neurosci.* 24: 9779–9788.

Richard-Parpaillon, L., Heligon, C., Chesnel, F., Boujard, D., and Philpott, A. (2002). The IGF pathway regulates head formation by inhibiting Wnt signaling in *Xenopus. Dev. Biol.* 244: 407–417.

Roberts, M. R., Hendrickson, A., McGuire, C. R., and Reh, T. A. (2005). Retinoid X receptor (gamma) is necessary to establish the s-opsin gradient in cone photoreceptors of the developing mouse retina. *Invest. Ophthalmol. Vis. Sci.* 46:2897–2904.

Roberts, M. R., Srinivas, M., Forrest, D., Morreale de Escobar, G., and Reh, T. A. (2006). Making the gradient: Thyroid hormone regulates cone opsin expression in the developing mouse retina. *Proc. Natl. Acad. Sci. U.S.A.* 103:6218–6223.

Robinson, S. R., and Dreher, B. (1990). The visual pathways of eutherian mammals and marsupials develop according to a common timetable. *Brain Behav. Evol.* 36:177–195.

Salo, E., Pineda, D., Marsal, M., Gonzalez, J., Gremigni, V., and Batistoni, R. (2002). Genetic network of the eye in Platyhelminthes: Expression and functional analysis of some players during planarian regeneration. *Gene* 287:67–74.

Schedl, A., Ross, A., Lee, M., Engelkamp, D., Rashbass, P., van Heyningen, V., and Hastie, N. D. (1996). Influence of PAX6 gene dosage on development: Overexpression causes severe eye abnormalities. *Cell* 86:71–82.

Sidman, R. L., Mottla, P. A., and Feder, N. (1961). Improved polyester wax embedding for histology. *Stain Technol.* 36: 279–284.

Silva, A. O., Ercole, C. E., and McLoon, S. C. (2003). Regulation of ganglion cell production by Notch signaling during retinal development. *J. Neurobiol.* 54:511–524.

Skowronska-Krawczyk, D., Ballivet, M., Dynlacht, B. D., and Matter, J. M. (2004). Highly specific interactions between bHLH transcription factors and chromatin during retina development. *Development* 131:4447–4454.

Swaroop, A., Xu, J. Z., Pawar, H., Jackson, A., Skolnick, C., and Agarwal, N. (1992). A conserved retina-specific gene encodes a basic motif/leucine zipper domain. *Proc. Natl. Acad. Sci. U.S.A.* 89:266–270.

Taylor, M., and Reh, T. A. (1990). Induction of differentiation of rat retinal, germinal, neuroepithelial cells by dbcAMP. *J. Neurobiol.* 21:470–481.

Thio, L. L., Shanmugam, A., Isenberg, K., and Yamada, K. (2003). Benzodiazepines block alpha2-containing inhibitory glycine receptors in embryonic mouse hippocampal neurons. *J. Neurophysiol.* 90:89–99.

Tomita, K., Ishibashi, M., Nakahara, K., Ang, S. L., Nakanishi, S., Guillemot, F., and Kageyama, R. (1996a). Mammalian hairy and Enhancer of split homolog 1 regulates differentiation of retinal neurons and is essential for eye morphogenesis. *Neuron* 16:723–734.

Tomita, K., Nakanishi, S., Guillemot, F., and Kageyama, R. (1996b). Mash1 promotes neuronal differentiation in the retina. *Genes Cells* 1:765–774.

Toy, J., and Sundin, O. H. (1999). Expression of the optx2 homeobox gene during mouse development. *Mech. Dev.* 83:183–186.

Toy, J., Yang, J. M., Leppert, G. S., and Sundin, O. H. (1998). The optx2 homeobox gene is expressed in early precursors of the eye and activates retina-specific genes. *Proc. Natl. Acad. Sci. U.S.A.* 95:10643–10648.

Turner, D. L., Snyder, E. Y., and Cepko, C. L. (1990). Lineage-independent determination of cell type in the embryonic mouse retina. *Neuron* 4:833–845.

Wallace, V. A., and Jensen, A. M. (1999). IBMX, taurine and 9-cis retinoic acid all act to accelerate rhodopsin expression in postmitotic cells. *Exp. Eye Res.* 69:617–627.

Watanabe, T., and Raff, M. C. (1998). Retinal astrocytes are immigrants from the optic nerve. *Nature* 332:834–837.

Wen, R., Song, Y., Kjellstrom, S., Tanikawa, A., Liu, Y., Li, Y., Zhao, L., Bush, R. A., Laties, A. M., and Sieving, P. A. (2006). Regulation of rod phototransduction machinery by ciliary neurotrophic factor. *J. Neurosci.* 26:13523–13530.

Wu, J., O'Donnell, M., Gitler, A. D., Klein, P. S. (2006). Kermit 2/XGIPC, an IGF1 receptor interacting protein, is required for IGF signaling in *Xenopus* eye development. *Development* 133:3651–3660.

Xu, Y., Baldassare, M., Fisher, P., Rathbun, G., Oltz, E. M., Yancopoulos, G. D., Jessell, T. M., and Alt, F. W. (1993). LH-2: A LIM/homeodomain gene expressed in developing lymphocytes and neural cells. *Proc. Natl. Acad. Sci. U.S.A.* 90:227–231.

Yan, R. T., and Wang, S. Z. (1998). neuroD induces photoreceptor cell overproduction in vivo and de novo generation in vitro. *J. Neurobiol.* 36:485–496.

Yaron, O., Farhy, C., Marquardt, T., Applebury, M., and Ashery-Padan, R. (2006). Notch1 functions to suppress cone-photoreceptor fate specification in the developing mouse retina. *Development* 133:1367–1378.

Young, T. L., and Cepko, C. L. (2004). A role for ligand-gated ion channels in rod photoreceptor development. *Neuron* 41:867–879.

Young-Pearse, T. L., Ivic, L., Kriegstein, A. R., and Cepko, C. L. (2006). Characterization of mice with targeted deletion of glycine receptor alpha 2. *Mol. Cell Biol.* 26:5728–5734.

Yourey, P. A., Gohari, S., Su, J. L., and Alderson, R. F. (2000). Vascular endothelial cell growth factors promote the in vitro development of rat photoreceptor cells. *J. Neurosci.* 20:6781–6788.

Zhang, L., Mathers, P. H., and Jamrich, M. (2000). Function of Rx, but not Pax6, is essential for the formation of retinal progenitor cells in mice. *Genesis* 28:135–142.

Zhang, X., Friedman, A., Heaney, S., Purcell, P., and Maas, R. L. (2002). Meis homeoproteins directly regulate Pax6 during vertebrate lens morphogenesis. *Genes Dev.* 16:2097–2107.

Zuber, M. E., Gestri, G., Viczian, A. S., Barsacchi, G., and Harris, W. A. (2003). Specification of the vertebrate eye by a network of eye field transcription factors. *Development* 130:5155–5167.

Zuber, M. E., Perron, M., Philpott, A., Bang, A., and Harris, W. A. (1999). Giant eyes in *Xenopus laevis* by overexpression of XOptx2. *Cell* 98:341–352.

25 Rb and the Control of Retinal Development

MICHAEL A. DYER

The decision to exit the cell cycle during retinal development must be carefully coordinated with intrinsic changes in retinal progenitor competence to ensure that the correct proportion of each cell type is generated. The Rb family of proteins—Rb, p107, and p130—are at the heart of the cell cycle machinery that executes the decision to exit the cell cycle in retinal progenitor cells (RPCs). The individual Rb family members are expressed in a dynamic pattern during retinogenesis, and genetic studies have revealed that intrinsic genetic compensation and redundancy helps to prevent deregulated proliferation when individual family members are absent. Interestingly, the expression of the Rb family during retinal development and their compensatory mechanisms are different in mouse and human retinas. These differences are important because they provide an explanation for the unique susceptibility of humans to retinoblastoma following *RB1* gene inactivation. Beyond its role in RPC proliferation, Rb is also required for rod photoreceptor development in mice. This role is unique to Rb and illustrates how a single protein can contribute to the coordination of cell cycle exit and cell fate specification in the developing retina. More recent studies have extended these data by using mice with mosaic inactivation of *Rb* in their developing retina to study synaptogenesis between rods, bipolar cells, and horizontal cells. These examples highlight how studying tumor suppressor genes in the developing retina can contribute to our understanding of RPC proliferation, retinoblastoma formation, neuronal cell fate specification, and synaptogenesis.

The regulation of proliferation during development is often associated with the regulation of tissue size. In the developing retina, defects in proliferation can result in microphthalmia, retinal degeneration, and partial or complete loss of vision (Burmeister et al., 1996; Ma et al., 1998). Alternatively, ectopic proliferation during retinal development can lead to retinoblastoma, which is fatal if left untreated and often results in compromised vision when treatment is successful (Dyer, 2004; Dyer et al., 2005; Dyer and Harbour, 2006). Beyond the regulation of tissue size, the decision to exit the cell cycle must also be precisely coordinated with intrinsic changes in RPC competence to ensure that each neuronal cell type is generated in the correct proportion (Dyer and Cepko, 2001a). Because retinal neurons are believed to process visual information as functional clusters (Jeon et al., 1998), generation of the correct proportion of each neuronal cell type is critical for normal visual signal processing. Precisely how the decision to exit the cell cycle is coordinated with the changing competence of RPCs remains a significant challenge in the field of retinal development today (Donovan and Dyer, 2005).

Efforts to better understand the regulation of RPC proliferation during development have benefited from advances in our understanding of the regulation of changes in RPC competence (Cepko et al., 1996) and of the proteins that regulate cell cycle progression (Dyer and Cepko, 2001c). Over the past decade, several laboratories have focused on the intrinsic factors that regulate RPC proliferation during development. These studies have focused on the cell cycle proteins themselves, including cyclin D1, p27, p57, Rb, p107, and p130 (Ma et al., 1998; Dyer and Cepko, 2000a, 2000b, 2001a, 2001b, 2001c; Donovan and Dyer, 2004; Zhang et al., 2004a, 2004b; Donovan et al., 2006; Johnson et al., 2006; Laurie et al., 2006; Sun et al., 2006), and the transcription factors that regulate proliferation in RPCs, such as Prox1, Chx10, and Six3 (Zhu et al., 2002; Dyer, 2003; Dyer et al., 2003). In addition to intrinsic regulators of RPC proliferation, extrinsic factors such as sonic hedgehog (Dakubo et al., 2003) and glutamate (Martins et al., 2006) provide mitogenic cues in the developing retina. Therefore, both proliferation and cell fate specification are regulated by carefully orchestrated signaling cascades between extrinsic and intrinsic factors. However, unlike the aforementioned studies on RPC competence, less is known about how signals from growth factors are balanced by the intrinsic ability of RPCs to respond to those cues. For example, how are postmitotic cells kept from reentering the cell cycle? Newly born cells are often adjacent to proliferating RPCs, and it is not known why they no longer respond to the surrounding growth factors that drive their neighboring RPCs to proliferate. As a first step toward improving our understanding of these issues, we must understand better how each of the intrinsic factors regulates RPC proliferation, and then explore how the intrinsic programs are coordinated with extrinsic signals.

There are three major reasons for studying the coordination of cell cycle exit with cell fate specification. First, we hope to learn how the ratios of different cell types are generated during retinogenesis from multipotent RPCs. A better understanding of this process is needed to develop cell-based therapies for retinal degeneration involving retinal stem cells (Tropepe et al., 2000; Coles et al., 2004) or RPCs (MacLaren et al., 2006). Second, a thorough understanding of intrinsic genetic compensation and redundancy has facilitated the development of the first knockout mouse models of retinoblastoma (Chen et al., 2004; MacPherson et al., 2004; Zhang et al., 2004b). These and other preclinical models have been used to test new therapies for the treatment of retinoblastoma in clinical trials (Laurie et al., 2005, 2006). Third, studies on cell cycle proteins have led to some unexpected insights into processes not traditionally associated with proliferation control, such as photoreceptor development and synaptogenesis (Johnson et al., 2006). In the absence of Rb, rod photoreceptors fail to form, and this has allowed researchers to study the response of their synaptic partners (bipolar cells and horizontal cells) in the absence of rod inputs. These different lines of inquiry demonstrate how genetic, molecular, cellular, and neuroanatomical studies of tumor suppressor knockout mice can contribute to our understanding of retinal development and disease.

Intrinsic genetic compensation and redundancy

For most researchers using mouse genetics to study retinal development and disease, separating the cell-autonomous and non-cell-autonomous roles of a given gene is of fundamental importance for interpreting the retinal phenotype. Once the cell-autonomous and non-cell-autonomous effects of genetic changes have been elucidated, intrinsic genetic compensation and redundancy must also be addressed (figure 25.1). This is of particular importance for the cell cycle genes in the developing retina, because most genetic changes in this pathway lead to some form of compensation or there is redundant gene expression (discussed in Dyer and Cepko, 2001c). Intrinsic genetic redundancy occurs in a cell that expresses two or more gene family members that have overlapping functions. As a result, inactivation of more than one gene is required to see changes in proliferation, apoptosis, or differentiation. In this example, the different gene

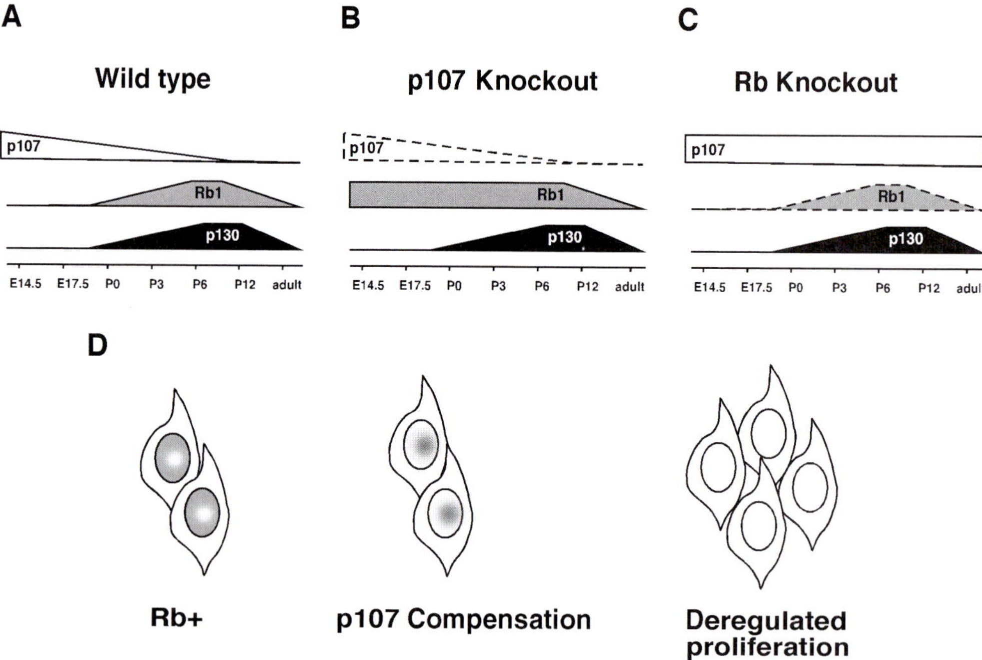

FIGURE 25.1 Intrinsic genetic redundancy and compensation among the Rb family of proteins. *A*, The Rb family members (Rb, p107, and p130) are expressed in a dynamic pattern during mouse retinal development. Shown is a summary of expression data from real-time RT-PCR, in situ hybridization, immunofluorescence, and immunoblotting: p107 is expressed at high levels during embryonic retinal development in the proliferating retinal progenitor cells (RPCs). Rb is expressed in postnatal RPCs and newly postmitotic neurons and glia. In the adult retina, virtually all cell types express Rb, and p130 is expressed in the inner nuclear layer and ganglion cell layer redundantly. *B*, In the absence of p107, Rb is upregulated in embryonic RPCs to prevent deregulated proliferation and retinoblastoma. *C*, In the absence of Rb, p107 is upregulated in postnatal RPCs to prevent deregulated proliferation and retinoblastoma. *D*, Intrinsic genetic compensation is distinct from redundancy. In the case of postnatal RPCs, they normally express Rb and little p107. However, when Rb is absent, the cells sense this imbalance and upregulate p107 in a compensatory manner to prevent deregulated proliferation. Only when both Rb and p107 are inactivated does retinoblastoma form.

family members do not necessarily have the same molecular function or partners, but they can effect the same eventual outcome in a given cell at a particular time during development.

Intrinsic genetic compensation can occur in a number of different ways when the expression of one gene family member is lost. For example, another gene family member that was not previously expressed may become upregulated (see figure 25.1). Alternatively, compensation may occur through unrelated proteins that lead to the induction of downstream events by an alternative pathway (discussed in Dyer and Cepko, 2001c).

In the developing mouse retina, p107 is expressed in embryonic RPCs and Rb is expressed in postnatal RPCs (Donovan et al., 2006). When Rb is deleted, p107 compensation prevents deregulated proliferation of postnatal RPCs, and when p107 is deleted, Rb compensation prevents deregulated proliferation of embryonic RPCs (Zhang et al., 2004a; Dyer and Bremner, 2005; Donovan et al., 2006). The p107 promoter has E2F binding sites, and there is evidence to suggest that induction of *p107* in the absence of *Rb* is mediated through these regulatory elements (Aslanian et al., 2004). Specifically, when *Rb* is present, it binds E2F/DP at the *p107* promoter and prevents its transcription. When *Rb* is deleted, repression is lost and the *p107* gene is upregulated in a compensatory manner. It is not known how *Rb* compensation is induced in the embryonic retina when *p107* is deleted. The functional significance of *p107* compensation was revealed when both *Rb* and *p107* were deleted in the developing mouse retina. Retinoblastoma does not form in *Rb*-deficient or *p107*-deficient retinas. However, when both *Rb* and *p107* are deleted, retinoblastoma forms (Robanus-Maandag et al., 1998; Chen et al., 2004; MacPherson et al., 2004; Zhang et al., 2004a), which indicates that inactivation of these two family members is sufficient to initiate tumorigenesis.

There is no compensation by p130 when either Rb or p107 are deleted. However, *Rb* and *p130* are redundantly expressed in the inner nuclear layer (INL) of the developing mouse retina (Donovan et al., 2006). It is possible that redundant expression of *Rb* and *p130* in these cells may prevent tumorigenesis because *Rb;p130*-deficient mice develop retinoblastoma (MacPherson et al., 2004). It will be interesting to test whether *p107* is upregulated in a compensatory manner in the developing INL cells of *Rb;p130*-deficient retinas and whether *p107* compensation is sufficient for normal development of INL neurons and glia in these mice.

Species-specific differences in Rb family compensation

Children who inherit a defective copy of the *RB1* gene have an increased susceptibility to develop retinoblastoma through inactivation of the remaining wild-type allele (Knudson, 1971; Friend et al., 1986). In contrast, mice with one defective copy of the *Rb* gene have normal retinas and never develop retinoblastoma (Clarke et al., 1992; Jacks et al., 1992; Lees et al., 1992). As mentioned earlier, mice with both copies of the *Rb* gene inactivated in the developing retina also fail to develop retinoblastoma (Robanus-Maandag et al., 1998).

The first clue to this species-specific difference in the susceptibility to retinoblastoma came from chimeric mouse studies using *Rb;p107*-deficient embryonic stem (ES) cells (Robanus-Maandag et al., 1998). Chimeric mice made by mixing *Rb;p107*-deficient and wild-type ES cells developed retinoblastoma (Robanus-Maandag et al., 1998). Analysis of the expression of the Rb family during retinal development and their redundant and compensatory roles provided the key mechanistic insight into these data and the mouse retinoblastoma paradox. *Rb*-deficient and *p107*-deficient mice do not develop retinoblastoma because of reciprocal compensation by other family members in the developing retina (Donovan et al., 2006). However, simultaneous inactivation of both genes results in deregulated proliferation and retinoblastoma (Chen et al., 2004; MacPherson et al., 2004; Zhang et al., 2004a).

The expression of the Rb protein family during human retinal development is different from that reported for mice (Donovan et al., 2006). There is very little if any p107 expression in the developing human retina, and RB1 is the primary family member expressed throughout retinogenesis (Donovan et al., 2006). To test whether *p107* can compensate for loss of *RB1* in human retinas, the *RB1* gene was inactivated in human fetal week 14 retinas by square wave electroporation of a plasmid expressing an *RB1* siRNA (Donovan et al., 2006). There was no increase in p107 expression following *RB1* gene inactivation in human fetal RPCs using this experimental approach (Donovan et al., 2006). Therefore, it is possible that the difference between mouse and human susceptibility to retinoblastoma following *RB1* gene inactivation can be explained by these differences in p107 expression and compensation.

The role of Rb in rod development

In addition to the role of *Rb* as a tumor suppressor, it regulates rod photoreceptor development in mice (Donovan and Dyer, 2004; MacPherson et al., 2004; Zhang et al., 2004a; MacPherson and Dyer, 2007). Because traditional *Rb*-knockout mice die in utero, for these studies *Rb* was inactivated by mating Rb^{Lox} mice (Marino et al., 2000) with the *Chx10-Cre* transgenic mouse line (Rowan and Cepko, 2004), which targets Cre recombinase to RPCs and bipolar cells. In the *Chx10-Cre*;$Rb^{Lox/-}$ retina, Cre is expressed in a mosaic pattern (Donovan and Dyer, 2004; Rowan and

Cepko, 2004) such that the *Rb*-deficient retina is chimeric, that is, apical-basal stripes of retina in which *Rb* has been inactivated are flanked by wild-type stripes of retina (Donovan and Dyer, 2004; Rowan and Cepko, 2004; Zhang et al., 2004a). This model provides an internal control with which to differentiate direct, cell-autonomous effects and non-cell-autonomous effects within a single retina. The genetic mosaic feature of the *Chx10-Cre;Rb*$^{Lox/-}$ retinas has suggested that Rb is cell autonomous for rod development (Zhang et al., 2004a). These data are consistent with data from cultured retinas from Rb-deficient E13.5 embryos, as well as *Mox-Cre;Rb*$^{Lox/Lox}$ mice (Zhang et al., 2004a). As further evidence of a cell-autonomous role of Rb in rod development, lineage analysis using a replication-incompetent retrovirus that expresses Cre-recombinase and alkaline phosphatase (LIA-Cre) showed that rod photoreceptors fail to form in the absence of Rb (Zhang et al., 2004a). Subsequent studies using square wave electroporation to acutely inactivate Rb in the developing retina with a plasmid expressing Cre-recombinase confirmed the finding from the retroviral lineage studies (Donovan et al., 2006). Interestingly, p107 cannot take the place of Rb in rod development in the mouse retina (Zhang et al., 2004a, 2004b; Donovan et al., 2006). This shows that some roles for the Rb family, such as proliferation control, are overlapping for Rb and p107, but other roles, such as rod development, are not.

An alternative to the hypothesis that Rb regulates rod development in the mouse retina is that Rb is required to keep newly postmitotic rod photoreceptors from reentering the cell cycle. According to this alternative hypothesis, when Rb is deleted, rods are formed normally but reenter the cell cycle and undergo apoptosis, leading to retinal degeneration. In support of this hypothesis, it has been shown previously that ectopic expression of cyclin D1 or other oncogenes in rod photoreceptors leads to ectopic cell cycle exit and cell death (Howes et al., 1994; Skapek et al., 2001). However, it is unlikely that this is the primary mechanism of photoreceptor cell loss in *Rb*-deficient retinas. The reason is that there is limited ectopic proliferation of Rb-deficient ONL cells during the period of rod commitment and differentiation, and this cannot account for their death (Zhang et al., 1993; Donovan et al., 2006). Moreover, this does not account for the presence of immature cells that express RPC markers and have morphological features of RPCs in the ONL of *Chx10-Cre;Rb*$^{Lox/Lox}$ and *Pax6-Cre;Rb*$^{Lox/Lox}$ retinas (Donovan and Dyer, 2004; Donovan et al., 2006; Johnson et al., 2006). It is more plausible that rods fail to mature properly in the absence of Rb and the presence of immature cells in the ONL leads to neuronal stress and cell death of neighboring rod photoreceptors. Of course, a combination of the two models is also a reasonable possibility, as discussed later in the chapter.

One important consideration that has come from these and other genetic studies is the timing of *Rb* inactivation during rod genesis. Previous analysis of *IRBP-Cre;Rb*$^{Lox/Lox}$ mice revealed that rods developed normally when Rb was inactivated in cells already committed to the rod fate (Vooijs et al., 2002). These data, combined with the data from *Chx10-Cre;Rb*$^{Lox/Lox}$, *Pax6-Cre;Rb*$^{Lox/Lox}$, and *Nestin-Cre;Rb*$^{Lox/Lox}$ mice (Chen et al., 2004; MacPherson et al., 2004; Zhang et al., 2004a), suggest that Rb is required during the early stages of rod development but once they commit to the rod fate, Rb is no longer required. The LIA-Cre lineage studies are consistent with these data. Specifically, when LIA-Cre is injected into the eyes of newborn mice, the retrovirus integrates into the genome of proliferating RPCs. However, at P0, most RPCs are undergoing terminal cell cycle exit or one to two rounds of cell division. Studies in mouse embryonic fibroblasts have shown that it takes 36–48 hours for LIA-Cre to recombine two copies of a floxed gene (Schweers and Dyer, 2005). Therefore, LIA-Cre inactivates *Rb*^{Lox} around the time that cells are exiting the cell cycle and committing to the rod fate, and, depending on the number of rounds of cell division following retroviral integration, some cells may inactivate *Rb* after they have committed to the rod fate. The prediction based on these data is that some clones would contain normal rods and some clones would contain cells that failed to commit to the rod fate because of the timing of Rb inactivation. This is exactly what has been reported (Zhang et al., 2004a; Donovan et al., 2006). Similarly, if the retroviral injection is performed 12–24 hours later, the prediction is that the proportion of normal rods in clones would be increased over that seen following injection on P0. Preliminary studies suggest this is also true.

Another consideration is the selection of the reporter gene used in the retroviral lineage studies. The advantage of alkaline phosphatase in LIA-Cre is that the enzyme reporter gene provides excellent sensitivity because of the enzymatic amplification of the signal. Moreover, alkaline phosphatase is membrane associated, so it provides exquisite detail on the morphology of the infected cells using light microscopy and transmission electron microscopy (TEM) (Zhang et al., 2004a; Donovan et al., 2006; Johnson et al., 2006). In contrast, green fluorescent protein (GFP) is not suitable for most retroviral lineage studies. The reason is that the expression of GFP is often too low for the fluorescence to be directly detected. Some researchers rely on immunofluorescent detection of GFP from replication-incompetent retroviruses expressing GFP, but these approaches suffer from similar limitations in reporter gene detection. Of particular importance is the reduction in reporter gene expression from retroviruses when genes are ectopically expressed or when cells fail to develop normally. For example, when Rb is inactivated in *Rb*$^{Lox/Lox}$ retinas in vivo with the use of LIA-Cre, the Rb-deficient cells that fail to develop into rods express lower levels of the reporter gene than do their normal rod counterparts or control littermates. When a GFP-reporter gene is used instead of alkaline phosphatase in $Rb^{Lox/Lox}$ mice, the Rb-deficient cells that fail to develop as rods are below the level of detection, leading to a very different interpretation of the data. These examples demonstrate how important it is to use multiple independent approaches to elucidate the role of cell cycle proteins such as Rb in the developing retina, and the importance of using well-characterized genetic tools.

Caution must also be taken when distinguishing the cell-autonomous and non-cell-autonomous roles of Rb in rod development. Even though there is considerable evidence that Rb plays a cell-autonomous role in regulating rod development, this does not eliminate the possibility of a non-cell-autonomous role for Rb in rod maturation or survival. Indeed, rod photoreceptors are very sensitive to their microenvironment, and it is reasonable to propose that the failure of some Rb-deficient cells to differentiate into rods may have a profound effect on their normal neighboring cells that retain their Rb locus. Consistent with this hypothesis, all the genetic studies using conditional inactivation of Rb during retinal development have reported extensive rod photoreceptor degeneration in addition to the failure of rods to differentiate normally (Chen et al., 2004; MacPherson et al., 2004; Zhang et al., 2004a). These non-cell-autonomous effects on normal Rb+ rods can make the interpretation of studies directed toward elucidating the cell-autonomous role of Rb difficult, especially if the analysis is performed at late stages of development. Moreover, broad inactivation of the *Rb* gene in the developing retina using *Pax6-Cre* or *Nestin-Cre* can amplify these non-cell-autonomous effects and further complicate data interpretation. To minimize these effects, comprehensive analysis of several early developmental stages is required, as well as a Cre transgenic line that has a mosaic pattern of expression, such as *Chx10-Cre* (figure 25.2).

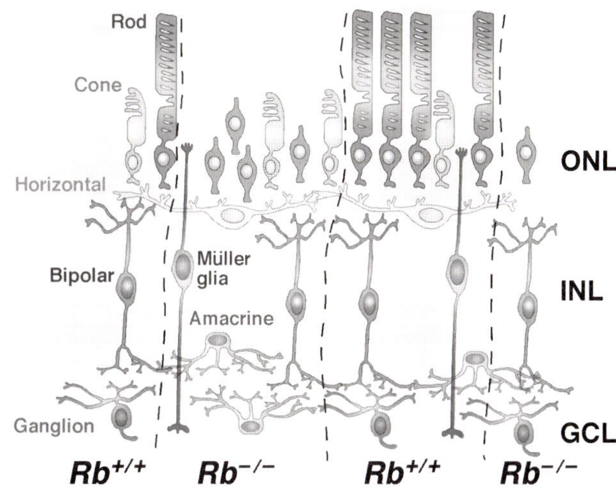

FIGURE 25.2 Mosaic Rb inactivation in the *Chx10-Cre;Rb*$^{Lox/Lox}$ retina. A key question that must be addressed to distinguish between primary and secondary effects of gene inactivation is whether the changes are cell autonomous or non-cell autonomous. Specifically, is the change caused by loss of that gene in the cell (i.e., a cell-autonomous effect), or is it caused by the loss of that gene in a neighboring cell (i.e., non-cell-autonomous effect)? If the effect is cell autonomous, then changes in that cell are more likely to reflect a primary role of that gene in that cell. On the other hand, if the effect is non-cell autonomous, then changes are more likely to be a secondary effect. Traditionally, these effects have been distinguished by genetic mosaic analysis. Mosaic patches of genetically altered cells are generated on a background of normal tissue. By analyzing the cells at the boundaries of mutant and wild-type mosaic patches and comparing their phenotypes with those of cells surrounded by mutant cells, one can distinguish between cell-autonomous and non-cell-autonomous effects. For example, if loss of a gene leads to a particular cellular phenotype, and if mosaic analysis shows that this phenotype is reverted when mutant cells contact wild-type cells, then the phenotype is probably non-cell autonomous. A key feature of performing genetic mosaic analysis is labeling the mutant cells and wild-type cells unambiguously. For synaptogenesis studies this is particularly important. The *Chx10-Cre;Rb*$^{Lox/Lox}$ mice are ideal for such studies because there are alternating stripes of cells that are wild type and Rb-deficient. GCL, ganglion cell layer; INL, inner nuclear layer; ONL, outer nuclear layer.

In addition, genetic mosaic analysis is required at the level of individual cells. To achieve this, it is possible to perform EM analysis of lead citrate–stained *Chx10-Cre;Rb*$^{Lox/Lox}$*;Z/AP* retinas. The *Z/AP* transgene expresses alkaline phosphatase in every cell that expressed Cre at some time during its development (Lobe et al., 1999). Lead citrate staining of samples processed for TEM facilitates the detection of AP-expressing cells and provides enough resolution to study individual processes and synapses (Gustincich et al., 1997; Johnson et al., 2006).

Bipolar cells are also affected in the *Rb*-deficient retinas. Analysis of early-stage retinas lacking Rb showed no defect in bipolar cell development, yet there was some reduction in later stages of development (Zhang et al., 2004a). This suggests that Rb does not play a role in bipolar cell formation but may be important for their survival. Further evidence came from TEM analysis of *Chx10-Cre;Rb*$^{Lox/Lox}$ retinas stained with lead citrate (Johnson et al., 2006). In addition to Cre, the *Chx10* promoter also drives alkaline phosphatase expression in a subset of bipolar cells of mature *Chx10-Cre;Rb*$^{Lox/Lox}$ retinas. These studies have shown that some bipolar cells can develop normally in the absence of Rb and form functional synapses with rods and horizontal cells (Johnson et al., 2006). It remains a formal possibility that a subtype of bipolar cells that do not express *Chx10* are susceptible to dying in the absence of Rb.

Nonetheless, despite these important considerations in interpreting genetic data on the role of Rb in retinal development, there is now broad consensus in the field that Rb is required for rod development. Indeed, independent laboratories using distinct genetic approaches have all shown that Rb is required for rod photoreceptor development (reviewed in MacPherson and Dyer, 2007). Current efforts are focused on elucidating the mechanism underlying the regulation of rod development by Rb.

The first clue regarding the mechanism for the regulation of rod development by Rb came from studies on p107 compensation in the mouse retina. As mentioned earlier, p107 can compensate for Rb loss in RPCs, but it cannot take the place of Rb in differentiating rod photoreceptors. The other Rb family member, p130, does not compensate for loss of Rb, p107, or the combination of the two (Donovan et al., 2006). It has been well established that different Rb family members bind to different E2F/DP heterodimers, and the first evidence pertaining to specific targets of Rb in rod development came from analysis of an exon-specific Rb knock-in allele (*Rb*^{654}) with a single amino acid substitution at position 654 of the mouse Rb protein (Sun et al., 2006). The Rb^{654} mutant protein has reduced binding to E2F1 and E2F3, and rods fail to form in *Chx10-Cre;Rb*$^{654/Lox}$ retinas (Sun et al., 2006). This suggests that Rb regulates rod development through E2F1 or E2F3, or both. Specifically, it has been proposed that there is a putative rod repressor gene that is regulated by Rb/E2F1 and/or Rb/E2F3 (figure 25.3) (Sun et al., 2006). The prediction from this model is that *Rb;E2F1*-deficient retinas will have normal rod development, and preliminary data have confirmed this hypothesis.

Another possible mechanism for the regulation of rod development by Rb is through the genes that are important for early rod development, such as *Nrl*, *Crx*, and *Nr2e3* (Furukawa et al., 1997; Haider et al., 2001; Mears et al., 2001). The evidence for this has come from preliminary studies showing that these genes are downregulated in Rb-deficient retinas at all stages of development. Preliminary chromatin immunoprecipitation experiments have shown that Rb can bind to the promoters of these genes (Chen and Dyer, 2008), suggesting that Rb may modulate the rod commitment and differentiation pathway more directly. It will be important to perform genetic epistasis analysis to determine if Rb lies functionally upstream of *Nrl*, *Crx*, and *Nr2e3* and to confirm Rb protein binding at the promoters of these genes.

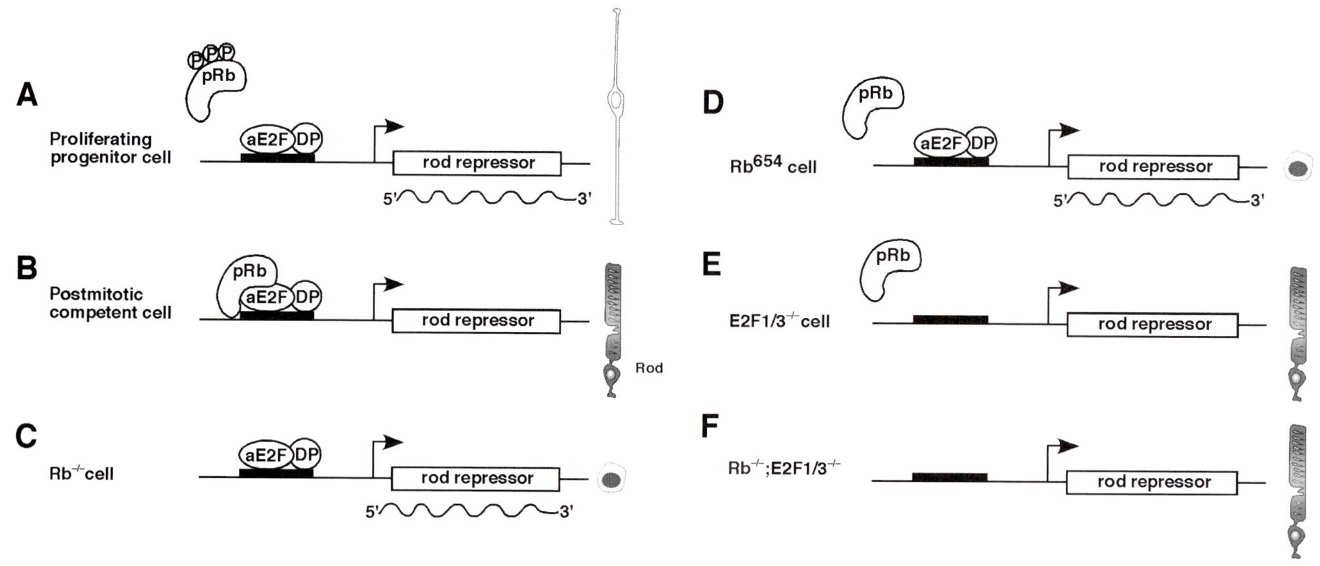

Figure 25.3 The regulation of rod development by Rb/E2F interactions. One hypothesis for the regulation of rod development by Rb is that there is a putative rod repressor gene that is an E2F-regulated gene. *A*, In proliferating RPCs, the rod repressor is expressed to prevent premature differentiation. This is achieved by phosphorylation of Rb by cyclin D/CDK4/6 and cyclin E/CDK2, which releases it from binding to activator E2Fs such as E2F1 and E2F3. *B*, In newly postmitotic cells that are competent to become rods, the putative rod repressor is silenced because Rb is no longer phosphorylated by cyclin/CDK and it can bind and repress the activity of the activator E2Fs. This allows these cells to become rods in response to intrinsic and extrinsic cues but is not sufficient for the rod fate. *C*, In Rb-deficient cells the rod repressor is constitutively expressed in newly postmitotic cells, thereby preventing the rod fate. These cells do not adopt another fate and remain partially quiescent in the ONL. *D*, In the Rb^{654} mutant, Rb cannot bind to the activator E2Fs (E2F1 and E2F3), and this leads to the same phenotype as the Rb null, suggesting that these E2Fs are those responsible for regulating the putative rod repressor. *E*, In the absence of E2F1/3, there would be no rod repressor expressed, and rod development would proceed normally. *F*, Similarly, simultaneous deletion of Rb and E2F1/3 would result in rescue of the rod phenotype using the same rationale. Examples of such hypothetical rod repressors are *Pax6* and *Chx10*. Both of these genes are expressed in RPCs, both are induced in the absence of Rb, and both can inhibit the rod fate.

A third possible mechanism for the role of Rb in regulating rod development is through chromatin organization. It is well established that Rb can recruit histone-modifying enzymes such as histone deacetylases to DNA (Zhang et al., 2000). Among the unique hallmarks of differentiated rod photoreceptors are their condensed chromatin structure and small nuclei. It is not known why rods condense their chromatin in this manner, but one possibility is that rod photoreceptors silence much of their genome through condensation, in order to efficiently express high levels of genes required for phototransduction. Owing to the rapid turnover of rod outer segments, these cells are unique in their metabolic requirements, and an efficiently organized genome may help to ensure that gene transcription is sufficient to maintain proper outer segment homeostasis. It is also possible that rod photoreceptors must condense their chromatin for more efficient packing in the ONL. In either case, it is reasonable to propose that Rb may play a role in this process because Rb-deficient cells in the ONL have an open chromatin conformation (Donovan et al., 2006). Current efforts are focused on determining whether Rb is required for chromatin condensation, and this in turn is required for normal rod differentiation, or whether Rb is required for normal rod differentiation, and this in turn leads to condensation of rod chromatin.

Defects in synaptogenesis in Rb-deficient retinas

Synaptogenesis in the inner plexiform layer (IPL) and outer plexiform layer (OPL) proceeds somewhat independently (McArdle et al., 1977; Hinds and Hinds, 1979; Redburn and Madtes, 1986; Sharma et al., 2003). In the IPL of the mouse retina, ganglion cells and their accompanying interneurons, the amacrine cells, elaborate their processes and form conventional presynaptic and postsynaptic connections before birth. In the OPL, horizontal cells first appear 7–10 days before birth. During the first week after birth, cone axons and then rod axons make synaptic contacts with horizontal cells. Rod synaptic terminals, called spherules, have distinctive features, including a single mitochondrion, and usually a single active zone marked by a synaptic ribbon. In contrast, cone synaptic terminals, called pedicles, are much larger and have multiple mitochondria and multiple active zones, each having a synaptic ribbon. Synaptogenesis of bipolar cells serves to link the two plexiform layers; thus, once the bipolar dendrites join horizontal cell presynaptic and postsynaptic contacts with spherules and pedicles in the OPL and the bipolar axons form ribbon-containing synapses with ganglion cells and amacrine cells in the IPL, the basic wiring of the primary visual pathway in the retina is established for later activity-dependent pruning and other synaptic modifications.

In *Chx10-Cre;Rb*$^{Lox/-}$ retinas, rods failed to differentiate in the patches of retinas lacking Rb. Immunostaining, real-time RT-PCR, and morphological analyses have shown that the cells that would normally differentiate into rod photoreceptors remained as immature cells for the first few weeks after birth (Donovan and Dyer, 2004; Zhang et al., 2004a; Donovan et al., 2006). On TEM those cells exhibited nuclear morphology consistent with immature cells, that is, their chromatin failed to condense, which is a characteristic of rod differentiation (Johnson et al., 2006). Therefore, the *Chx10-Cre;Rb*$^{Lox/-}$ retina represented an ideal model in which to study horizontal cell and bipolar cell synaptogenesis in the absence of mature rods and their inputs.

Immunostaining analysis indicated that calbindin^{+}, neurofilament^{+}, and syntaxin^{+} horizontal cell processes extended as far as the outer limiting membrane (OLM) in P12 *Chx10-Cre;Rb*$^{Lox/-}$ retinas and persisted to adult stages (Donovan and Dyer, 2004; Johnson et al., 2006). The total number of horizontal cells in *Chx10-Cre;Rb*$^{Lox/-}$ retinas was no different from that in control (*Chx10-Cre;Rb*$^{Lox/-}$) retinas, nor was the horizontal cell density, as measured by flat-mount immunostaining and nearest-neighbor analysis, different (Johnson et al., 2006). TEM analysis of the *Chx10-Cre;Rb*$^{Lox/-}$ retinas showed that horizontal cells extend processes apically (beginning at P7) rather than laterally, as seen in control *Chx10-Cre;Rb*$^{Lox/+}$ retinas (Johnson et al., 2006). Frequently, ectopic horizontal cell processes reached the OLM and formed ectopic synapses with rod spherules (Johnson et al., 2006). Using antibodies that label bipolar cells (anti-PKCα, -mGluR6, and -Goα), there was no evidence of ectopic bipolar cell dendrites associated with the ectopic rod–horizontal cell synapses (Johnson et al., 2006). This was confirmed by EM analysis (Johnson et al., 2006). The unique feature of the horizontal cell–rod photoreceptor synaptic dyads in *Chx10-Cre;Rb*$^{Lox/-}$ retinas is that they are ectopically formed deep in the ONL, and in some cases reach the OLM (figure 25.4).

Retinal degeneration or other cellular stressors can lead to reorganization of synaptic connections in the retina (Jones et al., 2003; Marc and Jones, 2003; Marc et al., 2003). One unanswered question is whether *Rb* deficiency causes reorganization of previously normal horizontal cell projections or whether normal projections were never formed. Horizontal cells are born early along the apical surface of the retina and then migrate inward to establish the location of the developing OPL. Previous immunostaining analysis showed that normal horizontal cells extend apical processes during migration and then reorganize their processes into the lateral configuration in the postnatal retina. P4 is a critical stage of development when this reorganization begins. P4 horizontal cells in *Chx10-Cre;Rb*$^{Lox/-}$ and control retinas migrated to the same positions and displayed similar morphology. Even in *Rb*-deficient areas, little difference was observed in horizontal cell bodies in Rb-deficient and control retinas. However,

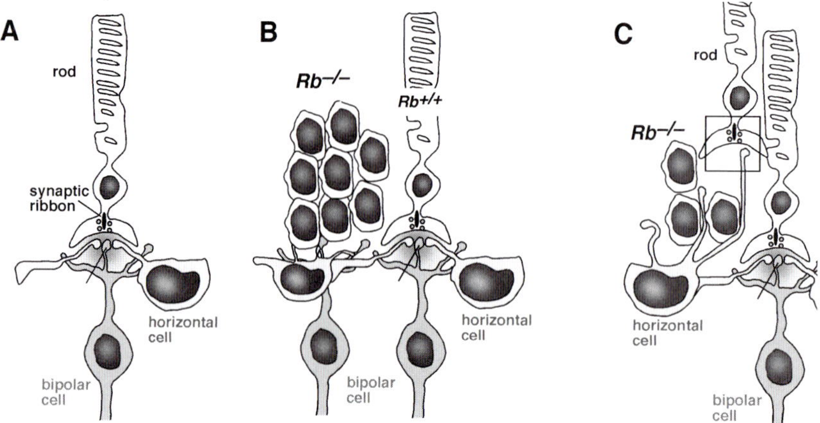

FIGURE 25.4 Ectopic horizontal cell–rod synapses in the absence of Rb. *A*, Horizontal cells are among the first cell types produced in the developing retina. However, two of their synaptic partners, rods and bipolar cells, are among the last cells produced during development. *B*, In the absence of Rb in the *Chx10-Cre;Rb*$^{Lox/Lox}$ retinas, there are mosaic patches in the ONL lacking rod photoreceptors. This is a unique phenotype because these cells do not adopt another cell fate and remain relatively quiescent. This is an ideal model in which to explore the process of synaptogenesis between rods, bipolar cells, and horizontal cells in the absence of direct synaptic contacts apical to the developing INL cells. *C*, In the absence of rod inputs, horizontal cells extend their processes deep into the ONL and form ectopic synapses with normal rods in neighboring mosaic patches of retina. There are no bipolar dendrites in these ectopic synapses.

disruption of developing horizontal processes in the OPL of *Rb*-deficient retinas was evident at P7, when photoreceptor terminals are just beginning to appear. Apically projecting horizontal cell neurites persisted in *Chx10-Cre;Rb*$^{Lox/-}$ retinas, but in control littermates, horizontal processes reorganized into their lateral orientation. Although these studies are useful for identifying changes in synaptogenesis during retinal development, they provide only snapshots of individual stages. Ideally, one should follow maturation and synapse formation of individual horizontal cells throughout retinogenesis to determine whether the apical horizontal cell processes reflect a defect in the normal developmental process or active reorganization of normal lateral horizontal cell process in response to the failure of rods to form in the *Chx10-Cre;Rb*$^{Lox/Lox}$ retinas.

Another important consideration is the role of Rb in horizontal cell development. It is possible that Rb is required for proper horizontal cell differentiation and that the defect in horizontal cell synaptogenesis is due to the absence of Rb in horizontal cells rather than the absence of their rod photoreceptor synaptic partner. As discussed in this chapter, elucidating the cell-autonomous and non-cell-autonomous roles of Rb in retinal development can best be studied using genetic mosaic analysis. The *Chx10-Cre;Rb*$^{Lox/Lox}$*;Z/AP* mouse is ideally suited for this type of analysis. Alkaline phosphatase (AP) is expressed in every cell lacking Rb. By comparing the contribution of AP+ and AP– horizontal cell processes to ectopic synapses using TEM of lead citrate–stained sections of *Chx10-Cre;Rb*$^{Lox/Lox}$*;Z/AP* retinas, we can determine whether Rb is required cell autonomously in developing horizontal cells for proper differentiation and synaptogenesis.

Summary

Until relatively recently, it was assumed that cell cycle genes regulated proliferation during development and that the multiple family members for each gene simply reflected functional redundancy for this essential regulatory network. However, the studies discussed in this chapter emphasize that cell cycle proteins have roles that extend far beyond that of proliferation control, and that individual family members can have both overlapping and unique functions. The Rb family is an excellent example of these principles. Both Rb and p107 regulate RPC proliferation, and they appear to be somewhat interchangeable in this process. Beyond cell cycle regulation, Rb also plays a role in regulating rod photoreceptor development, and p107 cannot substitute for this unique role of Rb in rod photoreceptors. In the absence of Rb, rods fail to form and remain as immature cells in the ONL. The mosaic nature of *Rb* inactivation using *Chx10-Cre;Rb*$^{Lox/Lox}$ mice led to important advances in our understanding of synaptogenesis between rods, horizontal cells, and bipolar cells. Moreover, genetic studies of single and compound knockout mice for the Rb family shed light on the complex redundant and compensatory mechanisms that prevent deregulated proliferation of RPCs during development. These data were used to generate the first knockout mouse models of retinoblastoma and to test new treatments in preclinical models, and they have had direct effects on clinical trials for this debilitating childhood cancer. Both developmental biology and cancer biology benefit when these two traditionally separate fields are brought together in the study of retinal development and of diseases of the retina.

REFERENCES

Akey, D. T., Zhu, X., Dyer, M., Li, A., Sorensen, A., Blackshaw, Fukuda-Kamitani, T., Daiger, S. P., Craft, C. M., et al. (2002). The inherited blindness associated protein AIPL1 interacts with the cell cycle regulator protein NUB1. *Hum. Mol. Genet.* 11(22):2723–2733.

Aslanian, A., Iaquinta, P. J., Verona, R., and Lees, J. A. (2004). Repression of the Arf tumor suppressor by E2F3 is required for normal cell cycle kinetics. *Genes Dev.* 18(12):1413–1422.

Burmeister, M., Novak, J., Liang, M. Y., Basu, S., Ploder, L., Hawes, N. L., Vidgen, D., Hoover, F., Goldman, D., et al. (1996). Ocular retardation mouse caused by Chx10 homeobox null allele: Impaired retinal progenitor proliferation and bipolar cell differentiation. *Nat. Genet.* 112(4):376–384.

Cepko, C. L., Austin, C. P., Yang, X., Alexiades, M., and Ezzeddine, D. (1996). Cell fate determination in the vertebrate retina. *Proc. Natl. Acad. Sci. U.S.A.* 93(2):589–595.

Chen, D., Livne-Bar, I., Vanderluit, J. L., Slack, R. S., Agochiya, M., and Bremner, R. (2004). Cell-specific effects of RB or RB/p107 loss on retinal development implicate an intrinsically death-resistant cell-of-origin in retinoblastoma. *Cancer Cell* 5(6):539–551.

Chen, S., and Dyer, M. (2008). [Identification of Rb target genes in the retina.] Unpublished results.

Clarke, A. R., Maandag, E. R., van Roon, M., van der Lugt, N. M., van der Valk, M., Hooper, M. L., Berns, A., and te Riele, H. (1992). Requirement for a functional Rb-1 gene in murine development. *Nature* 359(6393):328–330.

Coles, B. L., Angenieux, B., Inoue, T., Del Rio-Tsonis, K., Spence, J. R., McInnes, R. R., Arsenijevic, Y., and van der Kooy, D. (2004). Facile isolation and the characterization of human retinal stem cells. *Proc. Natl. Acad. Sci. U.S.A.* 101(44):15772–15777.

Dakubo, G. D., Wang, Y. P., Mazerolle, C., Campsall, K., McMahon, A. P., and Wallace, V. A. (2003). Retinal ganglion cell-derived sonic hedgehog signaling is required for optic disc and stalk neuroepithelial cell development. *Development* 130(13):2967–2980.

Donovan, S. L., and Dyer, M. A. (2004). Developmental defects in Rb-deficient retinae. *Vision Res.* 44(28):3323–3333.

Donovan, S. L., and Dyer, M. A. (2005). Regulation of proliferation during central nervous system development. *Semin. Cell Dev. Biol.* 16(3):407–421.

Donovan, S. L., Schweers, B., Martins, R., Johnson, D., and Dyer, M. A. (2006). Compensation by tumor suppressor genes during retinal development in mice and humans. *BMC Biol.* 4:14.

Dyer, M. A. (2003). Regulation of proliferation, cell fate specification and differentiation by the homeodomain proteins Prox1, Six3, and Chx10 in the developing retina. *Cell Cycle* 2(4): 350–357.

Dyer, M. A. (2004). Mouse models of childhood cancer of the nervous system. *J. Clin. Pathol.* 57(6):561–576.

Dyer, M. A., and Bremner, R. (2005). The search for the retinoblastoma cell of origin. *Nat. Rev. Cancer* 5(2):91–101.

Dyer, M. A., and Cepko, C. L. (2000a). Control of Müller glial cell proliferation and activation following retinal injury. *Nat. Neurosci.* 3(9):873–880.

Dyer, M. A., and Cepko, C. L. (2000b). p57(Kip2) regulates progenitor cell proliferation and amacrine interneuron development in the mouse retina. *Development* 127(16):3593–3605.

Dyer, M. A., and Cepko, C. L. (2001a). p27Kip1 and p57Kip2 regulate proliferation in distinct retinal progenitor cell populations. *J. Neurosci.* 21:4259–4271.

Dyer, M. A., and Cepko, C. L. (2001b). The p57(Kip2) cyclin kinase inhibitor is expressed by a restricted set of amacrine cells in the rodent retina. *J. Comp. Neurol.* 429(4):601–614.

Dyer, M. A., and Cepko, C. L. (2001c). Regulating proliferation during retinal development. *Nat. Rev. Neurosci.* 2(5):333–342.

Dyer, M. A., and Harbour, J. W. (2006). Cellular events in tumorigenesis. In A. D. Singh et al. (Eds.), *Clinical ocular oncology*. London: Elsevier.

Dyer, M. A., Livesey, F. J., Cepko, C. L., and Oliver, G. (2003). Prox1 function controls progenitor cell proliferation and horizontal cell genesis in the mammalian retina. *Nat. Genet.* 34(1):53–58.

Dyer, M. A., Rodriguez-Galindo, C., and Wilson, M. W. (2005). Use of preclinical models to improve treatment of retinoblastoma. *PLoS Med.* 2(10):e332.

Friend, S. H., Bernards, R., Rogelj, S., Weinberg, R. A., Rapaport, J. M., Albert, D. M., and Dryja, T. P. (1986). A human DNA segment with properties of the gene that predisposes to retinoblastoma and osteosarcoma. *Nature* 323(6089):643–646.

Furukawa, T., Morrow, E. M., and Cepko, C. L. (1997). Crx, a novel otx-like homeobox gene, shows photoreceptor-specific expression and regulates photoreceptor differentiation. *Cell* 91(4):531–541.

Gustincich, S., Feigenspan, A., Wu, D. K., Koopman, K. L., and Raviola, E. (1997). Control of dopamine release in the retina: A transgenic approach to neural networks. *Neuron* 18(5):723–736.

Haider, N. B., Naggert, J. K., and Nishina, P. M. (2001). Excess cone cell proliferation due to lack of a functional NR2E3 causes retinal dysplasia and degeneration in rd7/rd7 mice. *Hum. Mol. Genet.* 10(16):1619–1626.

Hinds, J. W., and Hinds, P. L. (1979). Differentiation of photoreceptors and horizontal cells in the embryonic mouse retina: An electron microscopic, serial section analysis. *J. Comp. Neurol.* 187(3):495–511.

Howes, K. A., Ransom, N., Papermaster, D. S., Lasudry, J. G., Albert, D. M., and Windle, J. J. (1994). Apoptosis or retinoblastoma: Alternative fates of photoreceptors expressing the HPV-16 E7 gene in the presence or absence of p53. *Genes Dev.* 8(11):1300–1310.

Jacks, T., Fazeli, A., Schmitt, E. M., Bronson, R. T., Goodell, M. A., and Weinberg, R. A. (1992). Effects of an Rb mutation in the mouse. *Nature* 359(6393):295–300.

Jeon, C. J., Strettoi, E., and Masland, R. H. (1998). The major cell populations of the mouse retina. *J. Neurosci.* 18(21): 8936–8946.

Johnson, D. A., Donovan, S. L., and Dyer, M. A. (2006). Mosaic deletion of Rb arrests rod differentiation and stimulates ectopic synaptogenesis in the mouse retina. *J. Comp. Neurol.* 498(1): 112–128.

JONES, B. W., WATT, C. B., FREDERICK, J. M., BAEHR, W., CHEN, C. K., LEVINE, E. M., MILAM, A. H., LAVAIL, M. M., and MARC, R. E. (2003). Retinal remodeling triggered by photoreceptor degenerations. *J. Comp. Neurol.* 464(1):1–16.

KNUDSON, A. (1971). Mutation and cancer: Statistical study of retinoblastoma. *Proc. Natl. Acad. Sci.* 68:820–823.

LAURIE, N. A., DONOVAN, S. L., SHIH, C. S., ZHANG, J., MILLS, N., FULLER, C., TEUNISSE, A., LAM, S., RAMOS, Y., et al. (2006). Inactivation of the p53 pathway in retinoblastoma. *Nature* 444 (7115):61–66.

LAURIE, N. A., GRAY, J. K., ZHANG, J., LEGGAS, M., RELLING, M., EGORIN, M., STEWART, C., and DYER, M. A. (2005). Topotecan combination chemotherapy in two new rodent models of retinoblastoma. *Clin. Cancer Res.* 11(20):7569–7578.

LEES, E., FAHA, B., DULIC, V., REED, S. I., and HARLOW, E. (1992). Cyclin E/cdk2 and cyclin A/cdk2 kinases associate with p107 and E2F in a temporally distinct manner. *Genes Dev.* 6(10): 1874–1885.

LOBE, C. G., KOOP, K. E., KREPPNER, W., LOMELI, H., GERTSENSTEIN, M., and NAGY, A. (1999). Z/AP, a double reporter for Cre-mediated recombination. *Dev. Biol.* 208(2):281–292.

MA, C., PAPERMASTER, D., and CEPKO, C. L. (1998). A unique pattern of photoreceptor degeneration in cyclin D1 mutant mice. *Proc. Natl. Acad. Sci. U.S.A.* 95(17):9938–9943.

MACLAREN, R. E., PEARSON, R. A., MACNEIL, A., DOUGLAS, R. H., SALT, T. E., AKIMOTO, M., SWAROOP, A., SOWDEN, J. C., and ALI, R. R. (2006). Retinal repair by transplantation of photoreceptor precursors. *Nature* 444(7116):203–207.

MACPHERSON, D., and DYER, M. A. (2007). Retinoblastoma: From the two-hit hypothesis to targeted chemotherapy. *Cancer Res.* 67(16):7547–7550.

MACPHERSON, D., SAGE, J., KIM, T., HO, D., MCLAUGHLIN, M. E., and JACKS, T. (2004). Cell type-specific effects of Rb deletion in the murine retina. *Genes Dev.* 18(14):1681–1694.

MARC, R. E., and JONES, B. W. (2003). Retinal remodeling in inherited photoreceptor degenerations. *Mol. Neurobiol.* 28(2): 139–147.

MARC, R. E., JONES, B. W., WATT, C. B., and STRETTOI, E. (2003). Neural remodeling in retinal degeneration. *Prog. Retin. Eye Res.* 22(5):607–655.

MARINO, S., VOOIJS, M., VAN DER GULDEN, H., JONKERS, J., and BERNS, A. (2000). Induction of medulloblastomas in p53-null mutant mice by somatic inactivation of Rb in the external granular layer cells of the cerebellum. *Genes Dev.* 14(8):994–1004.

MARTINS, R. A., LINDEN, R., and DYER, M. A. (2006). Glutamate regulates retinal progenitors cells proliferation during development. *Eur. J. Neurosci.* 24(4):969–980.

MCARDLE, C. B., DOWLING, J. E., and MASLAND, R. H. (1977). Development of outer segments and synapses in the rabbit retina. *J. Comp. Neurol.* 175(3):253–274.

MEARS, A. J., KONDO, M., SWAIN, P. K., TAKADA, Y., BUSH, R. A., SAUNDERS, T. L., SIEVING, P. A., and SWAROOP, A. (2001). Nrl is required for rod photoreceptor development. *Nat. Genet.* 29(4): 447–452.

REDBURN, D. A., and MADTES, P. (1986). Postnatal development of 3H-GABA-accumulating cells in rabbit retina. *J. Comp. Neurol.* 243(1):41–57.

ROBANUS-MAANDAG, E., DEKKER, M., VAN DER VALK, M., CARROZZA, M. L., JEANNY, J. C., DANNENBERG, J. H., BERNS, A., and TE RIELE, H. (1998). p107 is a suppressor of retinoblastoma development in pRb-deficient mice. *Genes Dev.* 12(11):1599–1609.

ROWAN, S., and CEPKO, C. L. (2004). Genetic analysis of the homeodomain transcription factor Chx10 in the retina using a novel multifunctional BAC transgenic mouse reporter. *Dev Biol.* 271(2):388–402.

SCHWEERS, B. A., and DYER, M. A. (2005). Perspective: New genetic tools for studying retinal development and disease. *Vis. Neurosci.* 22(5):553–560.

SHARMA, R. K., O'LEARY, T. E., FIELDS, C. M., and JOHNSON, D. A. (2003). Development of the outer retina in the mouse. *Brain Res. Dev. Brain Res.* 145(1):93–105.

SKAPEK, S. X., LIN, S. C., JABLONSKI, M. M., MCKELLER, R. N., TAN, M., HU, N., and LEE, E. Y. (2001). Persistent expression of cyclin D1 disrupts normal photoreceptor differentiation and retina development. *Oncogene* 20(46):6742–6751.

SUN, H., CHANG, Y., SCHWEERS, B., DYER, M. A., ZHANG, X., HAYWARD, S. W., and GOODRICH, D. W. (2006). An E2F binding-deficient Rb1 protein partially rescues developmental defects associated with Rb1 nullizygosity. *Mol. Cell Biol.* 26(4):1527–1537.

TROPEPE, V., COLES, B. L., CHIASSON, B. J., HORSFORD, D. J., ELIA, A. J., MCINNES, R. R., and VAN DER KOOY, D. (2000). Retinal stem cells in the adult mammalian eye. *Science* 287(5460): 2032–2036.

VOOIJS, M., TE RIELE, H., VAN DER VALK, M., and BERNS, A. (2002). Tumor formation in mice with somatic inactivation of the retinoblastoma gene in interphotoreceptor retinol binding protein-expressing cells. *Oncogene* 21(30):4635–4645.

ZHANG, H. S., GAVIN, M., DAHIYA, A., POSTIGO, A. A., MA, D., LUO, R. X., HARBOUR, J. W., and DEAN, D. C. (2000). Exit from G1 and S phase of the cell cycle is regulated by repressor complexes containing HDAC-Rb-hSWI/SNF and Rb-hSWI/SNF. *Cell* 101(1):79–89.

ZHANG, J., GRAY, J., WU, L., LEONE, G., ROWAN, S., CEPKO, C. L., ZHU, X., CRAFT, C. M., and DYER, M. A. (2004a). Rb regulates proliferation and rod photoreceptor development in the mouse retina. *Nat. Genet.* 36(4):351–360.

ZHANG, J., SCHWEERS, B., and DYER, M. A. (2004b). The first knockout mouse model of retinoblastoma. *Cell Cycle* 3(7):952–959.

ZHANG, H., XIONG, Y., and BEACH, D. (1993). Proliferating cell nuclear antigen and p21 are components of multiple cell cycle kinase complexes. *Mol. Biol. Cell* 4(9):897–906.

ZHU, C. C., et al. (2002). Six-3 mediated auto repression and eye development requires interaction with members of the Grouch-related family of co-repressors. *Development* 129(12): 2835–2849.

26 Gene Regulatory Networks and Retinal Ganglion Cell Development

XIUQIAN MU AND WILLIAM H. KLEIN

The mammalian retina is an exquisitely patterned neural tissue that arises from an amorphous sheet of dividing neuroblasts during fetal and neonatal life (figure 26.1*A*). By determining the mechanisms that underlie the formation of the retina, we can improve our understanding of CNS development as well as establish more robust methods for the repair and regeneration of damaged retinas (for a recent example, see MacLaren et al., 2006). Impressive advances have been made over the past decade that elucidate many of the crucial features controlling retinal development.

In the broadest sense, two developmental processes work in parallel to construct the retina, cellular lamination and cell type differentiation (figures 26.1*B* and *C*). Contrary to expectation, these processes may be genetically separable (Fu et al., 2006). In this chapter we concentrate primarily on the mechanisms that control the differentiation of retinal cell types, with particular emphasis on retinal ganglion cells (RGCs). In all vertebrates, differentiation of the six retinal neurons (rod, cone, horizontal, bipolar, amacrine, and ganglion) and one glial cell type (Müller) proceeds in a sequential manner, with RGCs the first cells to differentiate and Müller glia the last (for a recent review, see Cayouette et al., 2006). The retinal cell types form as subpopulations of retinal progenitor cells (RPCs) progress through a classical developmental sequence of cell competence, specification/commitment, and differentiation.

The differentiation of each retinal cell type is a highly complex process requiring both extrinsic and intrinsic factors. Recent investigations have emphasized the importance of distinct subpopulations of RPCs, each programmed to generate a limited number of cell types (Mu et al., 2005b; Yan et al., 2005; Cayouette et al., 2006). These subpopulations can easily be observed in the differential expression of a host of transcription factors, which act in combination to control specific retinal cell fates (Furukawa et al., 1997; Brown et al., 1998; Mears et al., 2001; Hatakeyama and Kageyama, 2004; Mu and Klein, 2004; Ohtoshi et al., 2004; Li et al., 2004; Mu et al., 2005a; Feng et al., 2006; Fujitani et al., 2006). Our intention here is to review recent information on the intrinsic genetic program that regulates RGC formation. Studies on RGC development in the mouse and other vertebrates are beginning to reveal the detailed behavior of RPCs during the early stages of retinogenesis. Consequently, we can now follow RGC progression from naive, uncommitted neuroblasts to their ultimate fate as fully differentiated neurons capable of receiving, processing, and transmitting the electrical signals required in the brain for visual perception.

A gene regulatory network for retinal ganglion cell development

To better conceptualize the regulatory events we wish to describe, we rely on a gene regulatory network model for RGC development that we have previously proposed (Mu et al., 2005a) and continue to develop (figure 26.2). It is becoming increasingly apparent that studying the functions of groups of interacting molecules offers novel, more global ways of understanding developmental processes than does studying linear pathways or single elements (see *Nature* 435:1, 2005). Establishing comprehensive networks of interacting molecules can explain emerging behaviors in ways that cannot be done by studies of linear pathways or single elements within a network. Our model is based on analogous gene regulatory networks constructed by Davidson and co-workers for sea urchin development (Davidson et al., 2002, 2003; Amore et al., 2003). In all these models, *cis*-regulatory elements associated with each gene in the network are identified and connected to their corresponding transcription factors, which in turn serve to regulate gene expression through *cis*-regulatory elements on genes encoding other transcription factors. In our RGC gene regulatory network, most *cis*-regulatory elements are predicted to exist based largely on circumstantial evidence, and their existence still requires direct confirmation. Nonetheless, as can be seen in figure 26.2, the RGC gene regulatory network features a downward cascade of transcription factors occupying at least four different tiers. This

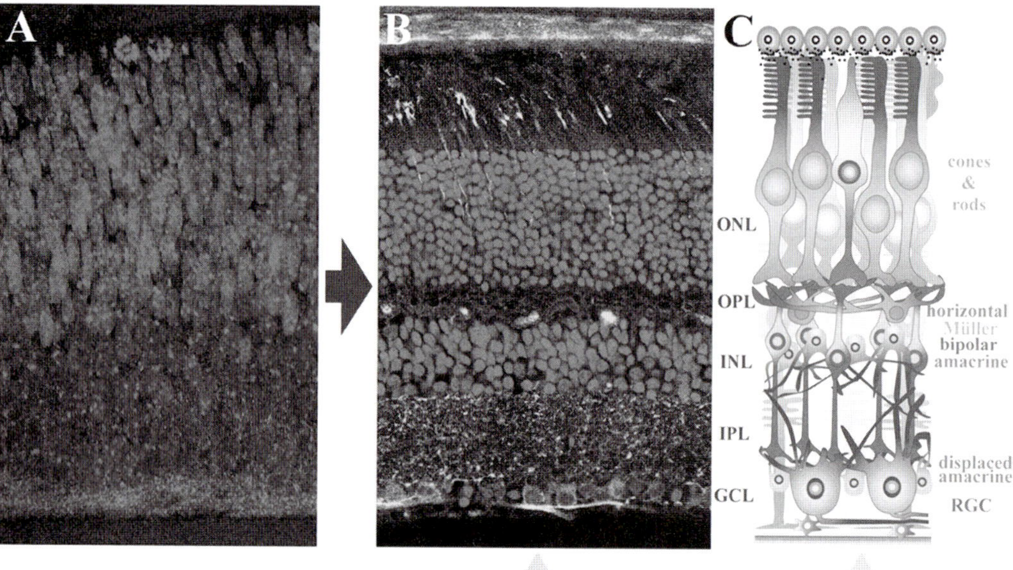

FIGURE 26.1 Developing and mature mouse retinas. *A*, An embryonic retina at E12.5. *B*, A postnatal retina at P16. Nuclei are labeled in red with propidium iodide and represent the positions of the cell soma. Neurite processes are labeled in green and blue with antineurofilament antibody and anticholine acetyltransferase antibody, respectively, and represent axons and dendrites. *C*, Schematic representation of the mature retina. RGCs and displaced amacrine cells are found within the ganglion cell layer (GCL). Intermediate neurons (horizontal, bipolar, and amacrine) are found within the inner nuclear layer (INL), and rod and cone photoreceptor cells are found within the outer nuclear layer (ONL). IPL and OPL are inner plexiform and outer plexiform layers where axons and dendrites synapse. RGC, retinal ganglion cell. See color plate 14.

transcription factor cascade leads ultimately to the expression of downstream genes whose products are required to form a mature, functional RGC. The network is constructed on the basis of results obtained from gene expression profiling, spatiotemporal expression patterns, chromatin immunoprecipitation analyses, and retinal phenotypes associated with various mouse knockout lines (Mu et al., 2005a, 2008).

Early regulatory events in retinogenesis

The retina originates in embryogenesis from the optic vesicle, which forms at the anteriormost portion of the neural tube. For normal eye development to occur, extensive interactions are required between the overlying surface ectoderm (the presumptive lens) and the evaginating optic vesicle. Following the allocation of the optic vesicle into the future retinal pigmented epithelium and the prospective neural retina, a number of important transcription factors are expressed in the neural retina that are required for establishing a field of actively dividing, multipotent RPCs. These so-called panneural retinal determination factors include Rx/Rax, which is essential for the formation of RPCs (Zhang et al., 2000; Bailey et al., 2004), Prox1, Six3, and Chx10, which have roles in regulating RPC proliferation and cell fate specification (Burmeister et al., 1996; Dyer, 2003), and Sox2, a dose-dependent regulator of RPC competence required for Notch1 signaling (Taranova et al., 2006). Retinas from mice harboring either germ line or retina-specific null mutations in the genes encoding any of the previously mentioned transcription factors have severe defects that affect the entire RPC population. This indicates that these factors are positioned upstream of the RGC gene regulatory network and represent genes at the top of the regulatory hierarchy for retinogenesis (see figure 26.2). Despite the strict requirement for these and several other transcription factors in controlling various aspects of RPC proliferation and competence, their precise functions and relationships to each other remain unclear. Nevertheless, it is becoming apparent that a complex retinal determination gene network involving extensive feedback and autoregulatory circuitry underlies the expression of these regulatory genes in the early developing retina and sits above the RGC gene regulatory network (Marquardt, 2003; Silver and Rebay, 2005).

A key retinal determination factor expressed in the early developing retina is Pax6, a pair-rule homeobox-containing transcription factor that is essential for the formation of all retinal cell types with the exception of amacrine cells (Marquardt et al., 2001; Marquardt, 2003). RPCs expressing

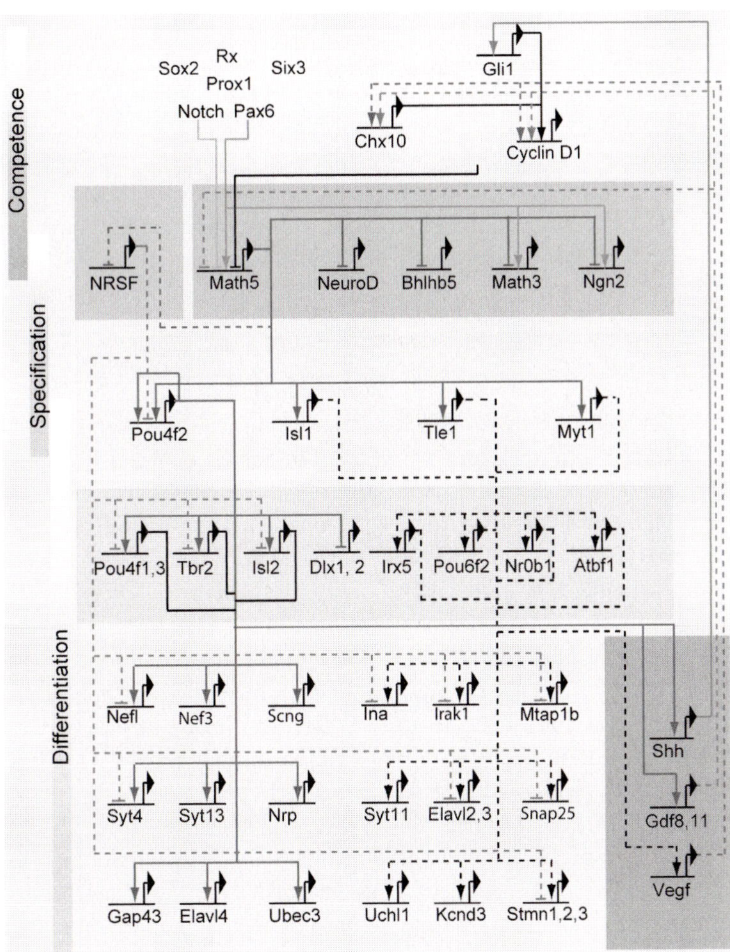

FIGURE 26.2 A gene regulatory network model for RGC development. Genes are depicted such that the right side of the *bent arrow* for each gene indicates the gene product and the left side indicates the transcriptional control region. *Solid lines* connecting genes indicate established upstream-downstream relationships, and *dashed lines* suggest inferred relationships. *Downward-pointing arrows* indicate gene activation, and *downward perpendicular lines* indicate gene repression. In most cases the connections have not been shown to be direct. Genes boxed in yellow represent regulators of general retinal competence and RPC proliferation; genes boxed in orange are proneural bHLH genes associated with establishing competence in RPCs for specific retinal cell fates. The light brown-purple box represents the general repression of RGC genes hypothesized to be mediated by the neural differentiation transcriptional repressor NSRF/REST (Mu et al., 2005b); the blue and purple-blue boxes represent genes encoding RGC-specific upstream (blue) and downstream (purple-blue) transcription factors. Genes boxed in green are those that encode proteins associated with RGC maturation and function. Genes boxed in purple encode secreted signaling molecules. In some cases only representative examples are shown for each box. A more detailed description can be found in Mu et al., 2005b. See color plate 15.

Pax6 represent the first step in the progression toward RGC commitment, although it is clear that Pax6 has broader roles in retinogenesis (Marquardt and Gruss, 2002). Evidence gathered from several vertebrate species indicates that the Notch-Delta signaling pathway, mediated by the basic helix-loop-helix (bHLH) transcription factors Hes1 and Hes5, is essential for maintaining *Pax6*-expressing cells in a proliferative state and inhibiting the differentiation of retinal cell types (Perron and Harris, 2000; Jadhav et al., 2006a). Recent studies suggest that Notch1 not only maintains the progenitor cell state by lateral inhibition, as was previously thought, but is also required to inhibit photoreceptor cell fate; in retinas where Notch1 is removed early in retinogenesis, cone photoreceptor cells differentiate at the expense of other retinal cell types (Jadhav et al., 2006b; Yaron et al., 2006). This provocative result suggests that suppression of cone photoreceptor cell fate by Notch1 allows for the specification of the other retinal cell types (Yaron et al., 2006). Whatever the precise mechanism of Notch1 signaling, it seems clear that an early step in retinogenesis is the loss of Notch1 activity in a subpopulation of RPCs destined to become RGCs (Nelson et al., 2006). The basis on which this subpopulation of RPCs is selectively released from the Notch signal is unclear, but in the absence of Notch1 or Hes1, the intrinsic genetic program required for RGC development is initiated (Jadhav et al., 2006a; Nelson et al., 2006). RPCs in this subpopulation thus acquire the competence for committing to an RGC fate and are the first RPCs in the retina to undergo this transition. As retinogenesis proceeds, Notch1 activity is overridden in other RPC subpopulations, thereby leading to the differentiation of the later retinal cell types (Perron and Harris, 2000; Jadhav et al., 2006a).

Math5 and retinal ganglion cell formation

Math5 and Retinal Ganglion Cell Competence RPCs become competent to form RGCs by activating the expression of the gene encoding the proneural bHLH transcription factor Math5, a mouse orthologue of *Drosophila* Atonal (Brown et al., 1998; Vetter and Brown, 2001; Le et al., 2006). *Math5* expression is first detected at embryonic day 11 (E11) in RPCs distributed throughout the neuroblast layer. Gene knockouts have demonstrated that in the absence of Math5, RGCs do not develop (Brown et al., 2001; Kay et al., 2001; Wang et al., 2001). *Pax6-Math5*-expressing RPCs are believed to define a competence field that permits the subsequent steps of RGC formation to proceed (Wang et al., 2001; Yang et al., 2003). Although expression of *Math5* is necessary, it is not sufficient for RGCs to form. *Math5* is expressed in a larger number of RPCs than would be expected if its sole function were dedicated to RGC development (Wang et al., 2001). Moreover, lineage-tracing experiments indicate that *Math5*-expressing cells can give rise to other retinal cell types besides RGCs (Yang et al., 2003).

Results obtained from mice, *Xenopus*, chicks, and zebrafish have demonstrated the importance of Math5 (Ath5 in *Xenopus*, chick, and zebrafish) in vertebrate retinogenesis (reviewed in Vetter and Brown, 2001). Recent reports have identified a number of downstream genes whose expression is dependent on the presence of Math5 or Ath5 orthologues, including some genes that may be direct targets (Yang et al., 2003; Logan et al., 2005; Mu et al., 2005a). Identifying genes regulated by Math5 has provided valuable information for constructing the RGC gene regulatory network with Math5 positioned as the central node (see figure 26.2). Although understanding the role of Math5 in the developing retina clearly requires further study, a picture is now emerging on how this proneural bHLH transcription factor acts to establish neuronal cell competence.

Math5 and Cell Cycle Progression Math5 has at least three critical functions in RPCs of the developing retina. It promotes cell cycle progression, suppresses non-RGC fates, and activates RGC fate. Math5 and Ath5 orthologues are thought to promote cell cycle progression by causing RPCs to exit the cell cycle and advance to G_0 (Kay et al., 2001; Yang et al., 2003; Matter-Sadzinski et al., 2005; Le et al., 2006). Time-lapse analysis in zebrafish retinas demonstrates a striking correlation in the expression of zebrafish *Ath5*, cell cycle exit, and RGC differentiation (Poggi et al., 2005). In this study, RPCs expressing green fluorescent protein (GFP) under the control of the *Ath5* gene promoter were monitored by three-dimensional time-lapse analysis. *Ath5*-expressing cells divide just once along the circumferential axis to produce two postmitotic daughters, one of which becomes an RGC. However, in *Ath5* mutant retinas, which lack RGCs, *Ath5*-expressing RPCs divide along the central-peripheral axis and produce two RGCs. These results suggest that extrinsic signals act on *Ath5*-expressing RPCs to influence the orientation of cell division and alter normal cell fate (Poggi et al., 2005). Brown and co-workers have suggested a possible mechanism for cell cycle exit (Le et al., 2006). These investigators have shown that Math5 is required for the expression of the cell cycle inhibitor p27/Kip1; RPCs lacking Math5 have diminished and shifted levels of p27/Kip1 and are unable to appropriately exit the cell cycle (Le et al., 2006). Currently, it is not known whether Math5 regulates *p27/Kip1* directly or indirectly. It is also not clear whether Math5 is solely responsible for the cell cycle exit of Math5-expressing cells.

Math5 and Suppression of Non–Retinal Ganglion Cell Fates Math5 also plays a critical role in suppressing the development of other retinal cell types by inhibiting the expression of the genes encoding NeuroD1, Math3, Neurogenin2 (Ngn2), and Bhlhb5, all of which are bHLH transcription factors that play important roles in the formation of rod and cone photoreceptor cells, amacrine cells, and bipolar cells (Hatakeyama and Kageyama, 2004; Mu et al., 2005b; Feng et al., 2006; Le et al., 2006). *NeuroD1* and *Ngn2* are expressed in mitotically active RPCs, and *Ngn2* expression may initially overlap with that of *Math5*. Notably, in chick retinal development, Ngn2 and Ath5 compete to regulate the *Ath5* promoter (Matter-Sadzinski et al., 2001, 2005). In chicks, Ngn2 is thought to be the initial activator of *Ath5* expression following the downregulation of *Hes1* (Matter-Sadzinski et al., 2005). Chick Ath5 autoregulates its own expression after initial activation by Ngn2 (Matter-Sadzinski et al., 2005), but this autoregulatory mechanism does not appear to operate for Math5 in the mouse retina (Hutcheson et al., 2005). The chick results suggest that once *Ath5* is expressed, it represses *Ngn2* expression. Because Ngn2 has the ability to activate *Ath5*, additional control mechanisms must be in place to ensure Ngn2 does not activate *Ath5* inappropriately. It is apparent that during retinogenesis, RPC subpopulations distributed throughout the neuroblast layer are delicately balanced in ways that can be profoundly affected by altering the levels and combinations of bHLH and other transcription factors (Hatakeyama and

Kageyama, 2004; Mu et al., 2005a, 2005b). Thus, *Hes1*-expressing cells remain as multipotent, actively dividing RPCs, *Math5*-expressing cells exit the cell cycle and advance to an RGC competent state, and *Neurod*-, *Math3*-, *Ngn2*-, and *Bhlhb5*-expressing cells assume competence for other retinal cell fates.

Math5 and the Activation of Retinal Ganglion Cell Fate Based on the retinal phenotypes of *Math5* knockout mice, the most conspicuous role for Math5 is the activation of the genetic program responsible for RGC differentiation. The earliest manifestation of Math5's action is the activation of four genes, each of which encodes a transcription factor that is first expressed as RGCs begin to differentiate. The four factors are POU domain factor Pou4f2 (also called Brn3b), LIM homeodomain factor Isl1, transcriptional repressor Groucho family member Tle1, and zinc finger protein Myt1 (see figure 26.2; Mu et al., 2005a). The expression of these factors is dependent on the presence of Math5, as revealed by gene expression profiling experiments that compared *Math5* mutant and wild-type retinas (Mu et al., 2005a). Pou4f2 is the only transcription factor of the four thus far shown to be essential for RGC development. Retinas from *Pou4f2* knockout mice have defects in RGC differentiation but not in the initial specification of RGCs (Gan et al., 1996, 1999; Erkman et al., 2000; Wang et al., 2000). This phenotype is consistent with the placement of *Pou4f2* genetically downstream of *Math5* (see figure 26.2).

Pou4f2, Isl1, Tle1, and Myt1, and possibly other early-expressed transcription factors (Yang et al., 2003; Logan et al., 2005) control the expression of downstream genes that encode additional transcription factors expressed at later times in RGC development (see figure 26.2). Transcription factors whose expression depends on Pou4f2 have been identified by gene expression profiling that compared wild-type retinas with *Pou4f2* mutant retinas (Mu et al., 2004). These Pou4f2-dependent transcription factors and the additional transcription factors whose expression is independent of Pou4f2 represent the next tier in the RGC gene regulatory network. Math5 therefore exerts its function in RGC development largely by initiating a transcription factor cascade, mediated in part by Pou4f2, which ultimately leads to the activation of genes required for the formation of the mature RGC. Because not all *Math5*-expressing cells become committed to an RGC fate, additional factors must participate so that the RGC transcriptional cascade is activated in only a subset of *Math5*-expressing cells.

Regulation of Math5 *expression*

Activation of *Math5* in Retinal Progenitor Cells A critical but unresolved question in retinal development is how different RPC subpopulations come to express distinct combinations of transcription factors. This complex process is made even more complicated by the fact that different RPC subpopulations intermingle and are distributed relatively uniformly throughout the neuroblast layer, appearing and disappearing as retinogenesis proceeds. Extrinsic factors are likely to have roles in establishing the developmental potential of RPCs, but only a few of these factors have been characterized (e.g., Harpavat and Cepko, 2003). It now seems likely that the extrinsic environment may not be the major driver for specifying RPC fates and that RPCs may be developmentally constrained by intrinsic programs set up at very early times in retinogenesis (Livesey and Cepko, 2001; Mu et al., 2005b; Cayouette et al., 2006). Because Math5 is essential for RGC formation and RGCs are the first retinal cell type to differentiate, understanding the intrinsic mechanisms that control the expression of *Math5* is particularly important for developing a meaningful model of retinogenesis.

Math5 is activated in a subpopulation of RPCs as *Hes1* and *Hes5* expression is downregulated. Retinal-specific expression of reporter transgenes using 5′-regulatory DNA from *Math5* or from *Ath5* orthologues from mouse, *Xenopus*, zebrafish, and chicken has been reported (Matter-Sadzinski et al., 2001, 2005; Hutcheson et al., 2005; Poggi et al., 2005). Some of these reports implicate bHLH factor-binding sites (E-boxes) as *cis*-regulatory elements involved in controlling *Ath5* expression. Matter-Sadzinski et al. (2001, 2005) have suggested that Ngn2 binds to an E-box within the chick *Ath5* promoter to activate *Ath5* expression. However, in the mouse, Ngn2's involvement in *Math5* expression has not been demonstrated. In addition, while Ath5 may autoregulate its expression in chicks (Matter-Sadzinski et al., 2001, 2005), *Math5* expression does not appear to be autoregulatory in the mouse retina (Hutcheson et al., 2005). These results suggest that there are significant differences in the mechanisms that control *Math5* and *Ath5* expression among vertebrate species.

Besides E-boxes, additional *cis*-regulatory elements are likely to be required to activate *Math5*/*Ath5* expression, but at present, these elements remain poorly defined. Pax6 must play some role in regulating *Math5* expression in the retina because in the absence of Pax6, *Math5* is not expressed (Marquardt et al., 2001). It is not clear, however, whether Pax6 is a direct activator of *Math5*. Conserved Pax6-binding sites have been found in the 5′-regulatory DNA of *Math5* but it is not clear whether these sites are functional Pax6 regulatory elements (Nadean Brown, pers. comm.).

Regulating the Duration of *Math5* Expression In addition to the mechanisms that control the activation of *Math5* expression, additional mechanisms must operate

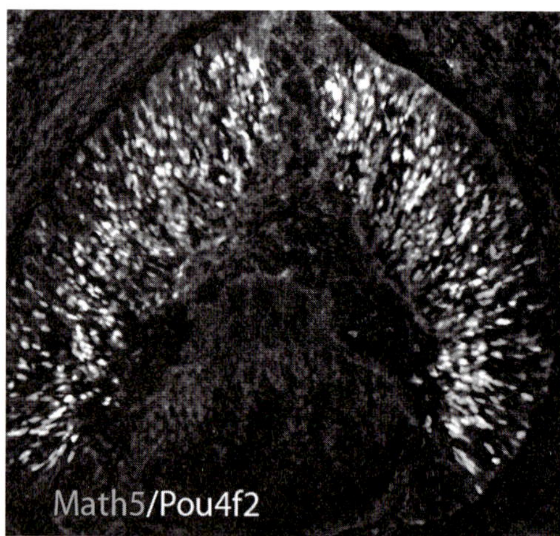

FIGURE 26.3 Segregated expression of Math5 and Pou4f2 in retinogenesis. The image represents an E14.5 retina from a knock-in mouse in which a gene encoding an HA-epitope-tagged Math5 replaces the endogenous *Math5* allele. Math5-HA expression is detected by immunostaining with an anti-HA antibody (red). Pou4f2 expression is detected by immunostaining with an anti-Pou4f2 antibody (green). Yellow staining shows the overlap in expression of Math5 and Pou4f2. See color plate 16.

to maintain *Math5*'s expression over a relatively narrow temporal and spatial window. This is because *Math5* is transiently expressed during retinal development, with a peak between E12.5 and E15.5 (Brown et al., 1998; Kim et al., 2005; Poggi et al., 2005). A subset of *Math5*-expressing RPCs commit to an RGC fate by activating *Pou4f2* and other early expressing transcription factor genes (Mu et al., 2005a). This commitment step correlates with a substantial downregulation in *Math5* expression spatially (Brown et al., 1998; Poggi et al., 2005). Direct visualization of *Pou4f2* activation and *Math5* downregulation is depicted in figure 26.3, which shows an E14.5 retina doubly immunostained for Pou4f2 and HA-tagged Math5. In the neuroblast layer, many *Math5*-expressing cells are detected (figure 26.3). *Math5-Pou4f2*-expressing cells are also seen in the neuroblast layer, although the double-labeled cells tend to be concentrated to a zone more basally located than cells expressing just *Math5* (see figure 26.3). In the emerging ganglion cell layer, *Pou4f2*-expressing cells are readily seen, but in this region, very few *Math5*-expressing cells or *Math5-Pou4f2*-expressing cells are detected. This result supports a model in which Math5 activates the expression of *Pou4f2* in a subset of RPCs in the neuroblast layer. Shortly after *Pou4f2* is activated, *Math5* expression is extinguished as newly differentiating RGCs begin their migration to the ganglion cell layer.

The tightly regulated expression of *Math5* may serve as an important mechanism to coordinate RGC development with other retinal cell types. Recent results suggest that regulating the duration of *Math5* expression is crucial in determining whether an RPC will commit to an RGC fate or some other fate (Kim et al., 2005), and this seems to be mediated by the TGF-β superfamily member GDF11. GDF11 controls the number of RGCs, as well as amacrine and photoreceptor cells that form during retinal development (Kim et al., 2005). GDF11 does not affect the proliferation of RPCs, as it does in other neuronal progenitor cells, but instead it controls the duration of *Math5* expression; retinas lacking GDF11 have prolonged *Math5* expression and produce an excess of RGCs at the expense of other retinal cell types (Kim et al., 2005). GDF11 is expressed in both RPCs and RGCs and appears to work by a feedback mechanism in which the fates of the multipotent RPCs expressing *Math5* can be altered by modulating the duration of *Math5* expression (Kim et al., 2005).

REPRESSING *MATH5* EXPRESSION IN OTHER RETINAL PROGENITOR CELLS Subpopulations of actively dividing, multipotent neuroblasts arise soon after the neural retina first emerges as a distinct neuroepithelial sheet. As discussed earlier, one of these subpopulations contains multipotent RPCs that activate the expression of *Math5* and form a field of RPCs competent to become RGCs. However, other RPC subpopulations programmed to specify other retinal cell fates also arise at this time. These other subpopulations will never express *Math5*. A significant issue that still must be addressed centers on the mechanisms by which individual intrinsic programs are set up in distinct RPC subpopulations.

Recent progress has been made in addressing this issue by the identification of two transcription factors, Foxn4, a winged helix forkhead factor, and Ptf1a, a bHLH factor, which are both required to determine horizontal and amacrine cell fates during mouse retinogenesis (Li et al., 2004; Fujitani et al., 2006). *Foxn4* knockout mice have revealed that Foxn4 controls the formation of amacrine and horizontal cells by activating the expression of *Math3*, *NeuroD1*, and *Prox1*, and that Foxn4 cooperates with Pax6 to perform its functions (Li et al., 2004). Loss of Foxn4 appears to result in an overproduction of rod photoreceptor cells (Li et al., 2004). *Ptf1a* knockout mice have revealed that Ptf1a marks postmitotic RPCs with competence to produce horizontal and amacrine cells exclusively (Fujitani et al., 2006). In this study, *Ptf1a* was identified as a primary downstream target for Foxn4. Notably, the loss of Ptf1a results in an upregulation of *Pou4f2* and an increase in the number of RGCs (Fujitani et al., 2006). Together, the results of Li et al. (2004) and Fujitani et al. (2006) suggest a model for horizontal and amacrine cell formation in which RPCs expressing *Pax6* and *Foxn4* activate the expression of *Ptf1a*. RPCs in this subpopulation can take on one of two pathways; in one,

Prox1 is activated downstream of *Ptf1a* and horizontal cells are specified, and in the other, *Math3* and *NeuroD1* are activated in conjunction with *Ptf1a*, and amacrine cells are specified (Li et al., 2004; Fujitani et al., 2006).

Math5 is not expressed in the *Foxn4-Ptf1a* RPC lineage, and *Foxn4* and *Ptf1a* are not expressed in *Math5*-expressing RPCs. This suggests that negative cross-regulation among these transcription factors is operating to keep *Math5* repressed in *Foxn4-Ptf1a*-expressing RPCs and *Foxn4* and *Ptf1a* repressed in *Math5*-expressing RPCs. Intriguingly, loss of Ptf1a results in upregulation of *Pou4f2* (Fujitani et al., 2006), implying that *Math5* is also upregulated in *Ptf1a* mutant retinas. Indeed, Ptf1a may directly repress *Math5* expression or regulate other transcriptional activity that leads to *Math5* repression. However, the fact that *Foxn4*-null retinas do not upregulate *Pou4f2* is perplexing, since Foxn4 activates the expression of *Ptf1a* (Li et al., 2004; Fujitani et al., 2006). *Ptf1a* null retinas, however, continue to express *Foxn4*, which may indicate that *Ptf1a* null RPCs reflect an altered competence state that differs from that of *Foxn4* null RPCs.

The identification of distinct RPC subpopulations for RGC and horizontal and amacrine cell competence highlights the importance of intrinsic programs that control the fates of RPCs early in retinogenesis. It is remarkable that in the developing retina, these distinct subpopulations are spatially interspersed and temporally overlapped. What remains a mystery is the mechanism that allows one RPC to assume an RGC-competent state while a nearby RPC takes on a horizontal or amacrine cell–competent state. It may be that the intrinsic programs for these RPC subpopulations are set up much earlier than is currently thought, perhaps even before the onset of retinogenesis.

Regulation of retinal ganglion cell differentiation downstream of Math5

Transition from Retinal Ganglion Cell Competence to Retinal Ganglion Cell Commitment The biological significance of *Math5* downregulation in newly differentiating RGCs is not known. However, this downregulation is concurrent with the loss of multipotency and irreversible commitment to RGC differentiation. The regulatory mechanisms underlying RGC commitment are likely to be associated with what has been termed a lockdown state by Davidson and co-workers for irreversible differentiation in embryo development (Davidson et al., 2002, 2003; Levine and Davidson, 2005). Three steps are required for achieving a lockdown state in RGCs. First, Math5 must activate the genes encoding the early-expressing transcription factors Pou4f2, Isl1, Tle1, and Myt1. Second, one or more of these factors must act either directly or indirectly to repress *Math5*'s expression, thereby establishing a negative feedback loop. Third, the early expressing factors must maintain their expression in the absence of Math5 by auto- and cross-regulation, thereby establishing a positive feedback loop.

At present, it is not known whether Math5 is a direct activator of any of the early-expressing transcription factors. In *Xenopus*, a *Pou4f2* orthologue is thought to be a direct target of *Xenopus* Ath5 (Hutcheson and Vetter, 2001), but no evidence has emerged to indicate that *Pou4f2* is a target of Math5 in the mouse retina. Unfortunately, very little is known about the mechanisms that turn off *Math5* in RGCs or that maintain the expression of *Pou4f2*, *Isl1*, *Tle1*, and *Myt1* following downregulation of *Math5* expression. It is possible that Math5 activates the expression of a transcription factor that is positioned genetically upstream of *Pou4f2* and the other early-expressing transcription factors, but to date, no compelling evidence exists for this putative factor. Clearly, much additional work is required before we fully understand the regulatory events that advance a competent RPC to a committed RGC.

Genes Regulated by Pou4f2 The best-studied transcription factor associated with the differentiation of RGCs is Pou4f2, which is essential for RGC differentiation, axon outgrowth and pathfinding, and RGC survival (Erkman et al., 1996, 2000; Gan et al., 1996, 1999; Wang et al., 2000, 2002). Although Pou4f2 clearly plays a crucial role in RGC differentiation, RGCs still form in its absence, but they are abnormal and most undergo apoptosis by E18.5. In addition, the expression of many RGC genes is not affected by the absence of Pou4f2 (Mu et al., 2004). These results indicate that parallel regulatory pathways independent of Pou4f2 contribute to RGC differentiation. These other pathways are likely to involve Isl1, Tle1, and Myt1, each representing a different branch of the RGC gene regulatory network that is controlled ultimately by Math5 (see figure 26.2).

Pou4f2 functions as a transcriptional activator (Trieu et al., 1999; Martin et al., 2005), and gene expression profiling with *Pou4f2* null retinas has identified 87 genes whose expression is significantly altered in the absence of Pou4f2 (Mu et al., 2004). The encoded products of the Pou4f2-dependent genes fall largely into four major functional groups: neural integrity and function, secreted signaling molecules, transcription factors, and cell cycle regulators. As expected, Pou4f2 is required for the expression of many genes in RGCs, but unexpectedly, Pou4f2 is also required for genes that are expressed in proliferating RPCs where Pou4f2 is never expressed. The dependence of a number of RPC genes on Pou4f2 suggests that Pou4f2 has non-cell-autonomous functions. These functions are crucial for maintaining the correct number of RPCs by controlling their rate of proliferation (Mu et al., 2004; Mu et al., 2005b).

Constructing a comprehensive RGC gene regulatory network requires distinguishing genes whose expression depends directly on Pou4f2 from those whose dependence is indirect. Three likely target genes for Pou4f2 have been identified to date. One is *Pou4f1*, which is closely related to Pou4f2 and is expressed in RGCs one day later than *Pou4f2*. Turner and co-workers have reported the presence of a regulatory region upstream of *Pou4f1* containing Pou4f-binding sites that can be activated by either Pou4f1 or Pou4f2 (Trieu et al., 1999). It is possible that Pou4f2 initially activates *Pou4f1*, and its expression is then maintained by both Pou4f1 and Pou4f2.

Our laboratory has recent results using electrophoretic mobility shift assays, transient transactivation of reporter genes in tissue culture cells, and chromatin immunoprecipitation analysis with embryonic retinas suggesting that Pou4f2 binds to and activates transcription from Pou4f-binding sites within regulatory regions associated with the genes encoding Tbr2/Eomes, a T-box transcription factor, and sonic hedgehog (Shh), a secreted signaling molecule (Mu et al., 2004; Mao et al., 2008). Recently, techniques have become available to perform genome-wide chromatin immunoprecipitation analysis for global mapping of transcription factor binding sites and target gene networks (Ji et al., 2006; Zeller et al., 2006). These techniques are ideally suited for genome-wide identification of Math5- and Pou4f2-binding sites, as well as binding sites for other transcription factors in the RGC gene regulatory network.

Regulation of Retinal Ganglion Cell Axon Outgrowth and Pathfinding Retinas from *Pou4f2* null mice contain residual RGCs that survive into adulthood and extend neurites (Gan et al., 1996, 1999; Wang et al., 2000). However, these neurites do not grow normally and have defects in finding their appropriate targets in the brain (Erkman et al., 2000; Wang et al., 2000, 2001). Several genes whose products are involved in axon outgrowth and pathfinding are strongly downregulated in the absence of Pou4f2. These include axon guidance factors Gap43 and neuropilin1, and several components of the axon cytoskeleton, including persyn/gamma-synuculein, neurofilament light chain, neurofilament middle chain, and tau (Mu et al., 2004). These results suggest that Pou4f2 directs a hierarchical program linking signaling events to cytoskeletal changes required for axon outgrowth and pathfinding (Erkman et al., 2000). Recent results from our laboratory indicate that *Tbr2/Eomes*, which appears to be a direct target of Pou4f2, functions in this hierarchical program. RGCs and optic nerves from *Tbr2/Eomes* knockout mice have defects similar to those of *Pou4f2* knockout mice, although somewhat milder (Mao et al., 2008). This suggests that Pou4f2 works partly through Trb2/Eomes to regulate axon outgrowth and pathfinding.

Other aspects of RGC axon outgrowth, pathfinding and retinotectal topographic mapping may depend on regulatory processes not controlled by Pou4f2. Both canonical and noncanonical Wnt signaling have been shown to be involved in the growth and retinotectal projections of RGC axons (Ouchi et al., 2005; Rodriguez et al., 2005; Liu et al., 2006; Schmitt et al., 2006). In these examples, Wnt signaling components are expressed in RGCs, and therefore their expression must be regulated by RGC transcription factors.

Control of Retinal Progenitor Cell Proliferation by Retinal Ganglion Cell–Secreted Signaling Molecules
In the past few years, studies from a number of laboratories have revealed a previously unsuspected function for RGCs in regulating the proliferation rate of RPCs. These studies have shown that in addition to their well-known physiological functions in receiving, processing, and transmitting visual information to the brain, RGCs are also a source of several secreted signaling molecules that modify the extrinsic environment of the developing retina. One of the most important signaling molecules in early retinogenesis is Shh. Wallace and co-workers have demonstrated that RGC-derived Shh controls RPC proliferation and the timing of RGC development in the developing mouse retina (Dakubo and Wallace, 2004; Wang et al., 2005). Shh signaling upregulates the gene encoding CyclinD1, which is known to play an important role in RPC proliferation (Sicinski et al., 1995); in retinas where the *Shh* gene is conditionally knocked out, *CyclinD1* is strongly downregulated (Wang et al., 2005). In zebrafish retinas, Shh produced by newly differentiating RGCs is thought to be required for the central-peripheral propagation wave along which RGCs and other retinal cell types differentiate (Neumann and Nüesslein-Volhard, 2000), but this has not been supported by other studies (Kay et al., 2005; Masai et al., 2005). However, in contrast to the role played by Shh in stimulating RPC proliferation in the mouse retina, Shh appears to negatively regulate the cell cycle and to promote cell cycle exit in the zebrafish retina (Masai et al., 2005; Neumann, 2005). Although the reasons for the discrepancy between zebrafish and mouse are not clear, a more recent report with *Xenopus* retinas indicates that Shh may modulate the cycling rate of RPCs, thereby promoting cell cycle exit (Locker et al., 2006).

Gene expression profiling with *Pou4f2* null and *Math5* null retinas has identified three secreted signaling molecules whose genes are expressed exclusively in RGCs during retinogenesis (Mu et al., 2004; Mu et al., 2005b). *Shh* and *Gdf8/Myostatin*, a close relative of *Gdf11*, were strongly downregulated in *Pou4f2* null and *Math5* null retinas, whereas *Vegf* was downregulated only in *Math5* null retinas. Notably, the absence of Pou4f2 does not alter *Vegf* expression, indicating that *Vegf* is regulated by a non-Pou4f2 branch of the RGC gene regulatory network (see figure 26.2). As discussed earlier in the chapter, it is likely that *Shh* is a direct target gene of Pou4f2 (Mu et al., 2004; Fu et al., 2008). RGC-derived Shh is thought to function by binding to the Patched receptor on the surface of RPCs and initiating a signal transduction pathway mediated through the Gli family of transcription factors. *Gli1* and *Gli3* are expressed in RPCs (Dakubo and Wallace, 2004; Mu et al., 2004), and *Gli1* expression is under the control of the Shh signaling pathway, which reinforces the Shh signal by positive feedback. *Gli1* expression in RPCs is dramatically downregulated in the absence of Shh or Pou4f2 (Dakubo and Wallace, 2004; Mu et al., 2004; Wang et al., 2005). This suggests a model in which Pou4f2 activates the expression of *Shh* in RGCs thereby leading to the secretion of Shh into the extracellular environment. Secreted Shh then binds to Patched on the surface of RPCs, and *Gli1* expression is induced.

In the chick retina, Vegf appears to stimulate RPCs by activating the MEK-ERK pathway as well as by elevating *Hes1* expression (Hashimoto et al., 2006). Vegf ligand secreted by RGCs works through the Flk1 receptor located on the surface of RPCs (Hashimoto et al., 2006). The results with Shh and Vegf suggest that RGCs act in the ganglion cell layer as a developmental signaling center to influence RPC proliferation rates. Other secreted signaling molecules, such as GDF8/myostatin and GDF11, may also contribute to signaling events that are initiated from newly differentiated RGCs.

In a recent investigation, our laboratory asked whether the ablation of RGCs from the developing retina would alter the extracellular environment. We were particularly interested in determining whether the loss of RGCs affected the ability of other retinal cell types to assume their fates. Models have been proposed in which RGCs and other retinal cell types provide feedback signals to the RPCs to alter the extrinsic environment and allow RPCs to advance to new competence states (reviewed in Cayouette et al., 2006). We ablated RGCs genetically by inserting a conditionally expressed gene encoding diphtheria toxin A (DTA) polypeptide into the *Pou4f2* locus and activating the *Dta* gene early in retinogenesis using a *Six3-Cre* recombinase mouse line (Furuta et al., 2000; Mu et al., 2005b). RGC-ablated retinas produced all of the retinal cell types (with the exception of RGCs) in the correct locations and relative proportions. However, the retina was 30%–50% thinner as a result of attenuation in the rate of RPC proliferation (Mu et al., 2005b). Genes encoding cell cycle regulators CyclinD1 and Chx10 are downregulated in RGC-ablated retinas, while *Math5* expression is significantly upregulated. Apparently, the continuous loss of RGCs alters the intrinsic program of RPCs such that they abnormally exit the cell cycle and express *Math5* in a futile attempt to generate more RGCs. The results are consistent with previous findings that secreted signaling molecules produced in RGCs regulate the rate of RPC proliferation and control RGC number and timing of differentiation. The results of Mu et al. (2005b) demonstrate that RGCs are not required for RPC competence change and suggest that intrinsic rather than extrinsic factors play the major role in specifying retinal cell types. However, RGCs do affect RPC proliferation, and this provides a positive feedback mechanism to ensure there is a sufficient supply of RPCs throughout retinogenesis (Mu et al., 2005b).

Future prospects

Developmental Regulation of Retinal Ganglion Cell Subtypes Throughout this review, we have considered RGCs as a uniform cell type, which is an oversimplification. Numerous RGC subtypes have been identified by their morphological and physiological properties in the retinas of several vertebrate species. For instance, RGC axons have different retinotectal projections along the nasal-temporal and dorsal-ventral axes, indicating a functional specialization associated with axial patterning (McLaughlin et al., 2003). Unfortunately, the number of RGC subtypes that are present in the mouse retina is ill-defined, and a lack of agreed-upon criteria for identifying RGC subtypes makes it difficult to address the mechanisms by which they develop. In a recent study, Coombs et al. (2006) used 14 morphological measures to classify mouse RGCs parametrically into different clusters. Their analysis revealed 14 clusters with distinct morphological features. The ability to apply straightforward, reproducible criteria to identifying RGC subtypes should yield a valuable baseline for future studies on RGC development (Coombs et al., 2006).

Because of a lack of functional and molecular definition for most RGC subtypes, virtually nothing is known about the mechanisms that control their formation, although a few studies have described the development of morphological diversity during postnatal stages of retinogenesis (e.g., Diao et al., 2004; Mumm et al., 2006). One extensively investigated RGC subtype was initially identified by its expression of a gene encoding a novel photoreceptor, melanopsin, which was shown to be involved in nonvision light responses (Hattar et al., 2003). *Melanopsin*-expressing RGCs make up about 1% of mouse RGCs and function in circadian photoentrainment and pupil constriction (Hattar et al., 2003). How *Melanopsin*-expressing cells arise is not yet understood, but in *Math5* null retinas, photic entrainment is lost and circadian rhythms are altered, suggesting that Math5 regulates the development of these cells (Wee et al., 2003).

In Vitro Generation of Retinal Ganglion Cells from Embryonic Stem Cells An ultimate objective in research on retinal development is to establish practical methods for repairing and regenerating damaged retinas. A striking example of the progress being made in this area is the recent work of MacLaren et al. (2006), who transplanted photoreceptor precursor cells from late ontogenetic stages into genetically damaged adult mouse retinas and achieved a remarkable degree of repair, as evidenced by the differentiation of the precursors into rod photoreceptor cells, the formation of synaptic connections, and improved visual function. This study emphasized the importance of selecting the appropriate progenitor cells for transplantation. One way to enhance the suitability of RPCs for transplantation is to manipulate them genetically so that they express combinations of transcription factors that confer the desired characteristics. Introducing different combinations of transcription factors associated with different retinal cell fates into naive progenitor cells might be a useful approach to generate precursor cells for transplantation. In a study using *Xenopus*, coexpression of various combinations of transcription factors transfected into developing retinas resulted in retinas in which cell fates were significantly altered according the predicted combinatorial coding (Wang and Harris, 2005). Given our current knowledge of the RGC gene regulatory network, it should now be possible to genetically alter uncommitted progenitor cells using key transcription factors such as Pax6, Math5, Pou4f2, and others to coax progenitors into assuming RGC fates with high efficiency.

A promising method for generating retinal cell types in vitro is through selective differentiation of embryonic stem (ES) cells. This has been achieved by supplying ES cells with the appropriate growth factor medium. The generation of retinal precursors and differentiated retinal neurons has been reported using mouse ES cells (Zhao et al., 2002; Ikeda et al., 2005), and efficient generation of retinal precursors that differentiated primarily into RGCs and amacrine cells was recently reported using human ES cells (Lamba et al., 2006). Procedures for introducing genes into ES cells are well established, thus providing a means to generate ES cells that express transcription factors positioned at key nodes in the RGC network. Within the foreseeable future, it should be possible to efficiently generate large fields of RGCs by differentiating ES cells in vitro with various genetic manipulations.

ACKNOWLEDGMENTS Work was supported by grants nos. EY11930 and EY10608 from the National Eye Institute, and by grants from the Ziegler Foundation and the Robert A. Welch Foundation, G-0010. The generation of genetically engineered mice, maintenance of mice, and DNA sequencing were supported in part by a National Cancer Institute Cancer Center support grant no. CA16672. We are grateful to Nadean Brown of the Children's Hospital Research Foundation, the University of Cincinnati, and Xueyao Fu and Jang-Hyeon Cho of the M. D. Anderson Cancer Center for allowing us to cite their unpublished results.

REFERENCES

AMORE, G., YAVROUIAN, R. G., PETERSON, K. J., RANSICK, A., MCCLAY, D. R., and DAVIDSON, E. H. (2003). Spdeadringer, a sea urchin embryo gene required separately in skeletogenic and oral ectoderm gene regulatory networks. *Dev. Biol.* 261:55–81.

BAILEY, T. J., EL-HODIRI, H., ZHANG, L., SHAH, R., MATHERS, P. H., and JAMRICH, M. (2004). Regulation of vertebrate eye development by Rx genes. *Int. J. Dev. Biol.* 48:761–770.

BROWN, N. L., KANCKAR, S., VETTER, M. L., TUCKER, P. K., GEMZA, D. L., and GLASER, T. (1998). Math5 encodes a murine basic helix-loop-helix transcription factor expressed during early stages of retinal neurogenesis. *Development* 125:4821–4833.

BROWN, N. L., PATEL, S., BRZEZINSKI, J., and GLASER, T. (2001). Math5 is required for retinal ganglion cell and optic nerve formation. *Development* 128:2497–2508.

BURMEISTER, M., NOVAK, J., LIANG, M. Y., BASU, S., PLODER, L., HAWES, N. L., VIDGEN, D., HOOVER, F., GOLDMAN, D., et al. (1996). Ocular retardation mouse caused by Chx10 homeobox null allele: Impaired retinal progenitor proliferation and bipolar differentiation. *Nat. Genet.* 12:376–384.

CAYOUETTE, M., POGGI, L., and HARRIS, W. A. (2006). Lineage in the vertebrate retina. *Trends Neurosci.* 29:563–570.

COOMBS, J., VAN DER LIST, D., WANG, G. Y., and CHALUPA, L. M. (2006). Morphological properties of mouse retinal ganglion cells. *Neuroscience* 140:123–136.

DAKUBO, G. D., and WALLACE, V. A. (2004). Hedgehogs and retinal ganglion cells: Organizers of the mammalian retina. *Neuroreport* 15:479–482.

DAVIDSON, E. H., MCCLAY, D. R., and HOOD, L. (2003). Regulatory gene networks and the properties of the developmental process. *Proc. Natl. Acad. Sci. U.S.A.* 100:1475–1480.

DAVIDSON, E. H., RAST, J. P., OLIVERI, P., RANSICK, A., CALESTANI, C., YUH, C. H., MINOKAWA, T., AMORE, G., HINMAN, V., et al. (2002). A genomic regulatory network for development. *Science* 295:1669–1678.

DIAO, L., DENG, Q., and HE, S. (2004). Development of the mouse retina: Emerging morphological diversity of the ganglion cells. *J. Neurobiol.* 61:236–249.

DYER, M. A. (2003). Regulation of proliferation, cell fate specification and differentiation by the homeodomain proteins Prox1, Six3, and Chx10 in the developing retina. *Cell Cycle* 2: 350–357.

ERKMAN, L., MCEVILLY, R. J., LUO, L., RYAN, A. K., HOOSHMAND, F., O'CONNELL, S. M., KEITHLEY, E. M., RAPAPORT, D. H., RYAN, A. F., et al. (1996). Role of transcription factors Brn-3.1 and Brn-3.2 in auditory and visual system development. *Nature* 381:603–606.

ERKMAN, L., YATES, P. A., MCLAUGHLIN, T., MCEVILLY, R. J., WHISENHUNT, T., O'CONNELL, S. M., KRONES, A. I., KIRBY, M. A., RAPAPORT, D. H., et al. (2000). A POU domain transcription factor-dependent program regulates axon pathfinding in the vertebrate visual system. *Neuron* 28:779–792.

FENG, L., XIE, X., JOSHI, P. S., YANG, Z., SHIBASAKI, K., CHOW, R. L., and GAN, L. (2006). Requirement for Bhlhb5 in the specification of amacrine and cone bipolar subtypes in mouse retina. *Development* 133:4815–4825.

FU, X., KIYAMA, T., MU, X., and KLEIN, W. (2008). [Shh is a target gene for Pontf2 in developing retinal ganglion cells.] Unpublished results.

FU X., SUN, H., KLEIN, W. H., and MU, X. (2006). Beta-catenin is essential for lamination but not neurogenesis in mouse retinal development. *Dev. Biol.* 299:424–437.

Fujitani, Y., Fujitani, S., Luo, H., Qiu, F., Burlison, J., Long, Q., Kawaguchi, Y., Edlund, H., Macdonald, R. J., et al. (2006). Ptf1a determines horizontal and amacrine cell fates during mouse retinal development. *Development* 133:4439–4450.

Furukawa, T., Morrow, E. M., and Cepko, C. L. (1997). Crx, a novel otx-like homeobox gene, shows photoreceptor-specific expression and regulates photoreceptor differentiation. *Cell* 91: 531–541.

Furuta, Y., Lagutin, O., Hogan, B. L., and Oliver, G. C. (2000). Retina- and ventral forebrain-specific Cre recombinase activity in transgenic mice. *Genesis* 26:130–132.

Gan, L., Wang, S. W., Huang, Z., and Klein, W. H. (1999). POU domain factor Brn-3b is essential for retinal ganglion cell differentiation and survival but not for initial cell fate specification. *Dev. Biol.* 210:469–480.

Gan, L., Xiang, M., Zhou, L., Wagner, D. S., Klein, W. H., and Nathans, J. (1996). POU domain factor Brn-3b is required for the development of a large set of retinal ganglion cells. *Proc. Natl. Acad. Sci. U.S.A.* 93:3920–3925.

Harpavat, S., and Cepko, C. L. (2003). Thyroid hormone and retinal development: An emerging field. *Thyroid* 13:1013–1019.

Hashimoto, T., Zhang, X. M., Chen, B. Y., and Yang, X. J. (2006). VEGF activates divergent intracellular signaling components to regulate retinal progenitor cell proliferation and neuronal differentiation. *Development* 133:2201–2210.

Hatakeyama, J., and Kageyama, R. (2004). Retinal cell fate determination and bHLH factors. *Semin. Cell Dev. Biol.* 15:83–89.

Hattar, S., Liao, H. W., Takao, M., Berson, D. M., and Yau, K. W. (2003). Melanopsin-containing retinal ganglion cells: Architecture, projections, and intrinsic photosensitivity. *Science* 295:1065–1070.

Hutcheson, D. A., Hanson, M. I., Moore, K. B., Brown, N. L., and Vetter, M. L. (2005). bHLH-dependent and -independent modes of *Ath5* gene regulation during retinal development. *Development* 132:829–839.

Hutcheson, D. A., and Vetter, M. L. (2001). The bHLH factors Xath5 and XNeuroD can upregulate the expression of XBrn3d, a POU-homeodomain transcription factor. *Dev. Biol.* 232:327–338.

Ikeda, H., Osakada, F., Watanabe, K., Mizuseki, K., Haraguchi, T., Miyoshi, H., Kamiva, D., Honda, Y., et al. (2005). Generation of RX+/Pax6+ neural retinal precursors from embryonic stem cells. *Proc. Natl. Acad. Sci. U.S.A.* 102:11331–11336.

Jadhav, A. P., Cho, S. H., and Cepko, C. L. (2006a). Notch activity permits retinal cells to progress through multiple progenitor states and acquire a stem cell property. *Proc. Natl. Acad. Sci. U.S.A.* 103:18998–19003.

Jadhav, A. P., Mason, H. A., and Cepko, C. L. (2006b). Notch1 inhibits photoreceptor production in the developing mammalian retina. *Development* 133:913–923.

Ji H., Vokes, S. A., and Wong, W. H. (2006). A. comparative analysis of genome-wide chromatin immunoprecipitation data for mammalian transcription factors. *Nucleic Acids Res.* 34:e146.

Kay, J. N., Finger-Baier, K. C., Roeser, T., Staub, W., and Baier, H. (2001). Retinal ganglion cell genesis requires lakritz, a zebrafish atonal homolog. *Neuron* 30:725–736.

Kay, J. N., Link, B. A., and Baier, H. (2005). Staggered cell-intrinsic timing of ath5 expression underlies the wave of ganglion cell neurogenesis in the zebrafish retina. *Development* 132: 2573–2585.

Kim, J., Wu, H. H., Lander, A. D., Lyons, K. M., Matzuk, M. M., and Calof, A. L. (2005). GDF11 controls the timing of progenitor cell competence in developing retina. *Science* 308: 1927–1930.

Lamba, D. A., Karl, M. O., Ware, C. B., and Reh, T. A. (2006). Efficient generation of retinal progenitor cells from human embryonic stem cells. *Proc. Natl. Acad. Sci. U.S.A.* 103:12769–12774.

Le, T. T., Wroblewski, E., Patel, S., Riesenberg, A. N., and Brown, N. L. (2006). Math5 is required for both early retinal neuron differentiation and cell cycle progression. *Dev. Biol.* 295:764–778.

Levine, M., and Davidson, E. H. (2006). Gene regulatory networks for development. *Proc. Natl. Acad. Sci. U.S.A.* 102:4936–4942.

Li S., Mo Z., Yang, X., Price, S. M., Shen, M. M., and Xiang, M. (2004). Foxn4 controls the genesis of amacrine and horizontal cells by retinal progenitors. *Neuron* 43:795–760.

Liu, H., Thurig, S., Mohamed, O., Dufort, D., and Wallace, V. A. (2006). Mapping canonical Wnt signaling in the developing and adult retina. *Invest. Ophthalmol. Vis. Sci.* 47:5088–5097.

Livesey, F. J., and Cepko, C. L. (2001). Vertebrate neural cell-fate determination: Lessons from the retina. *Nat. Rev. Neurosci.* 2:109–118.

Locker, M., Agathocleous, M., Amato, M. A., Parain, K., Harris, W. A., and Perron, M. (2006). Hedgehog signaling and the retina: Insights into the mechanisms controlling the proliferative properties of neural precursors. *Genes Dev.* 20:3036–3048.

Logan, M. A., Steele, M. R., Van Raay, T. J., and Vetter, M. L. (2005). Identification of shared transcriptional targets for the proneural factors Xath5 and XNeuroD. *Dev. Biol.* 285: 570–583.

MacLaren, R. E., Pearson, R. A., MacNeil, A., Douglas, R. H., Salt, T. E., Akimoto, M., Swaroop, A., Sowden, J. C., and Ali, R. R. (2006). Retinal repair by transplantation of photoreceptor precursors. *Nature* 444:203–207.

Mao, C. A., Kiyama, T., Pan, P., Furuta, Y., Hadjantonakis, A. K., and Klein, W. H. (2008). Eomesodermin, a target gene of Pou4f2, is required for retinal ganglion cell and optic nerve development in the mouse. *Development* 135:271–280.

Marquardt, T. (2003). Transcriptional control of neuronal diversification in the retina. *Prog. Retin. Eye. Res.* 22:567–577.

Marquardt, T., Ashery-Padan, R., Andrejewski, N., Scardigli, R., Guillemot, F., and Gruss, P. (2001). *Pax6* is required for the multipotent state of retinal progenitor cells. *Cell* 105:43–55.

Marquardt, M., and Gruss, P. (2002). Generating neuronal diversity in the retina: One for nearly all. *Trends Neurosci* 25:32–38.

Martin, S. E., Mu, X., and Klein, W. H. (2005). Identification of an N-terminal transcriptional activation domain within Brn3b/POU4f2. *Differentiation* 73:18–27.

Masai, I., Yamaguchi, M., Tonou-Fujimori, N., Komori, A., and Okamoto, H. (2005). The hedgehog-PKA pathway regulates two distinct steps of the differentiation of retinal ganglion cells: The cell-cycle-exit of retinoblasts and their neuronal maturation. *Development* 132:1539–1553.

Matter-Sadzinski, L., Matter, J. M., Ong, M. T., Hernandez, J., and Ballivet, M. (2001). Specification of neurotransmitter receptor identity in developing retina: The chick ATH5 promoter integrates the positive and negative effects of several bHLH proteins. *Development* 128:217–231.

Matter-Sadzinski, L., Puzianowska-Kuznicka, M., Hernandez, J., Ballivet, M., and Matter, J. M. (2005). A. bHLH transcriptional network regulating the specification of retinal ganglion cells. *Development* 132:1907–1921.

McLaughlin, T., Hindges, R., and O'Leary, D. D. (2003). Regulation of axial patterning of the retina and topographic mapping to the brain. *Curr. Opin. Neurobiol.* 13:57–69.

Mears, A. J., Kundo, M., Swain, P. K., Takada, Y., Bush, R. A., Saunders, T. L., Sieving, P. A., and Swaroop, A. (2001). Nrl is required for rod photoreceptor development. *Nat. Genet.* 29: 447–453.

Mu, X., Beremand, P. D., Zhao, S., Pershad, R., Sun, H., Scarpa, A., Liang, S., Thomas, T. L., and Klein, W. H. (2004). Discrete gene sets depend on POU domain transcription factor Brn3b/Brn-3.2/POU4f2 for their expression in the mouse embryonic retina. *Development* 131:1197–1210.

Mu, X., Fu, X., Beremand, P. D., Thomas, T. L., and Klein, W. H. (2008). Gene regulation logic in retinal ganglion cell development: Isl1 defines a critical branch distinct from but overlapping with Pou4f2. Submitted for publication.

Mu, X., Fu, X., Sun, H., Beremand, P. D., Thomas, T. L., and Klein, W. H. (2005a). A. gene network downstream of transcription factor Math5 regulates retinal progenitor cell competence and ganglion cell fate. *Dev. Biol.* 280:467–481.

Mu, X., Fu, X., Sun, H., Liang, S., Maeda, H., Frishman, L. J., and Klein, W. H. (2005b). Ganglion cells are required for normal progenitor-cell proliferation but not cell-fate determination or patterning in the developing mouse retina. *Curr. Biol.* 15: 525–530.

Mu, X., and Klein, W. H. (2004). A. gene regulatory hierarchy for retinal ganglion cell specification and differentiation. *Semin. Cell Dev. Biol.* 15:115–123.

Mumm, J. S., Williams, P. R., Godinho, L., Koerber, A., Pittman, A. J., Roeser, T., Chien, C. H., Baier, H., and Wong, R. O. (2006). In vivo imaging reveals dendritic targeting of laminated afferents by zebrafish retinal ganglion cells. *Neuron* 52:609–621.

Nelson, B. R., Gumusen, B., Hartman, B. H., and Reh, T. A. (2006). Notch activity is downregulated just prior to retinal ganglion cell differentiation. *Dev. Neurosci.* 28:128–141.

Neumann, C. J. (2005). Hedgehogs as negative regulators of the cell cycle. *Cell Cycle* 4:1139–1140.

Neumann, C. J., and Nüsslein-Volhard, C. (2000). Patterning of the zebrafish retina by a wave of sonic hedgehog activity. *Science* 289:2137–2139.

Ohtoshi, A., Wang, S. W., Maeda, H., Saszik, S. M., Frishman, L. J., Klein, W. H., and Behringer, R. R. (2004). Regulation of retinal cone bipolar cell differentiation and photopic vision by the CVC homeobox gene *Vsx1*. *Curr. Biol.* 14:530–536.

Ouchi, Y., Tabata, Y., Arai, K., and Watanabe, S. (2005). Negative regulation of retinal-neurite extension by beta-catenin signaling pathway. *J. Cell Sci.* 118:4473–4483.

Perron, M., and Harris, W. A. (2000). Determination of vertebrate retinal progenitor cell fate by the Notch pathway and basic helix-loop-helix transcription factors. *Cell Mol. Life Sci.* 57:215–223.

Poggi, L., Vitorino, M., Masai, I., and Harris, W. A. (2005). Influences on neural lineage and mode of division in the zebrafish retina in vivo. *J. Cell Biol.* 171:991–999.

Rodriguez, J., Esteve, P., Weini, C., Ruiz, J. M., Fermin, Y., Trousse, F., Dwivedy, A., Holt, C., and Bovolenta, P. (2005). SFRP1 regulates the growth of retinal ganglion cell axons through the Fz2 receptor. *Nat. Neurosci.* 8:1281–1282.

Schmitt, A. M., Shi, J., Wolf, A. M., Lu, C. C., King, L. A., and Zou, Y. (2006). Wnt-Ryk signaling mediates medial-lateral retinotectal topographic mapping. *Nature* 439:31–37.

Sicinski, P., Donaher, J. L., Parker, S. B., Li, T., Fazeli, A., Gardner, H., Haslam, S. Z., Bronson, R. T., Elledge, S. J., et al. (1995). Cyclin D1 provides a link between development and oncogenesis in the retina and breast. *Cell* 82:621–630.

Silver, S. J., and Rebay, I. (2005). Signaling circuitries in development: Insights from the retinal determination gene network. *Development* 132:3–13.

Taranova, O. V., Magness, S. T., Fagan, B. M., Wu, Y., Surzenko, N., Hutton, S. R., and Pevny, L. H. (2006). SOX2 is a dose-dependent regulator of retinal progenitor competence. *Genes Dev.* 20:1187–1202.

Trieu, M., Rhee, J. M., Fedtsova, N., and Turner, E. E. (1999). Autoregulatory sequences are revealed by complex stability screening of the mouse Brn-3.0 locus. *J. Neurosci.* 19:6549–6558.

Vetter, M. L., and Brown, N. L. (2001). The role of basic helix-loop-helix genes in vertebrate retinogenesis. *Semin. Cell Dev. Biol.* 12:491–498.

Wang, J. C., and Harris, W. A. (2005). The role of combinatorial coding by homeodomain and bHLH transcription factors in retinal cell fate specification. *Dev. Biol.* 285:101–115.

Wang, S. W., Gan, L., Martin, S. E., and Klein, W. H. (2000). Abnormal polarization and axon outgrowth in retinal ganglion cells lacking the POU-domain transcription factor Brn-3b. *Mol. Cell. Neurosci.* 16:141–156.

Wang, S. W., Kim, B. S., Ding, K., Wang, H., Sun, D., Johnson, R. L., Klein, W. H., and Gan, L. (2001). Requirement for math5 in the development of retinal ganglion cells. *Genes Dev.* 15:24–29.

Wang, S. W., Mu, X., Bowers, W. J., Kim, D. S., Plas, D. J., Crair, M. C., Federoff, H. J., Gan, L., and Klein, W. H. (2003). Brn3b/Brn3c double knockout mice reveal an unsuspected role for Brn3c in retinal ganglion cell axon outgrowth. *Development* 129:467–477.

Wang, Y., Dakubo, G. D., Thurig, S., Mazerolle, C. J., and Wallace, V. A. (2005). Retinal ganglion cell–derived sonic hedgehog locally controls proliferation and timing of RGC development in the embryonic mouse retina. *Development* 132: 5103–5113.

Wee, R., Castrucci, A. M., Provencio, I., Gan, L., and Van Gelder, R. N. (2003). Loss of photic entrainment and altered free-running circadian rhythms on math5$^{-/-}$ mice. *J. Neurosci.* 22:10427–10433.

Yan, R. T., Ma, W., Liang, L., and Wang, S. Z. (2005). bHLH genes and retinal cell fate specification. *Mol. Neurobiol.* 32: 157–171.

Yang, Z., Ding, K., Pan, L., Deng, M., and Gan, L. (2003). Math5 determines the competence state of retinal ganglion cell progenitors. *Dev. Biol.* 264:240–254.

Yaron, O., Farhy, C., Marquardt, T., Applebury, M., and Ashery-Padan, R. (2006). Notch1 functions to suppress cone-photoreceptor fate specification in the developing mouse retina. *Development* 133:1367–1378.

Zeller, K. I., Zhao, X., Lee, C. W., Chiu, K. P., Yao, F., Yustein, J. T., Ooi, H. S., Orlov, Y. L., Shahab, A., et al. (2006). Global mapping of c-Myc binding sites and target gene networks in human B. cells. *Proc. Natl. Acad. Sci. U.S.A.* 103:17834–17839.

Zhang, L., Mathers, P. H., and Jamrich, M. (2000). Function of Rx, but not Pax6, is essential for the formation of retinal progenitor cells in mice. *Genesis* 28:135–142.

Zhao, X., Liu, J., and Ahmad, I. (2002). Differentiation of embryonic stem cells into retinal neurons. *Biochem. Biophys. Res. Commun.* 297:177–184.

27 Cell Death in the Mouse Retina

LUCIA GALLI-RESTA AND MARIA CRISTINA CENNI

Cell loss is commonly observed in the development of vertebrate neural structures. In many regions of the developing nervous system, neurons and their connections are produced in excess of their adult number and then partly eliminated (reviewed in Oppenheim, 1981; Buss and Oppenheim, 2004). In the developing retina, cell death was initially analyzed in vertebrates other than the mouse because their retinal structures were more accessible to manipulation, but in recent years the use of transgenic technologies has made the mouse the elective model in which to test the role of individual molecular components in the death process. In this chapter we refer to both mouse and nonmouse studies to provide an overall view on cell death in the retina. The first part of the chapter describes the time course and locations of cell death in the developing mouse retina; the second part is a brief summary of key experiments investigating the contribution of cell death to circuit maturation. The third part summarizes the role of neurotrophic factors in controlling cell death in retinal development, and the last part looks at current knowledge on the genes and molecules involved in retinal cell death.

Major phases of cell death in the developing mouse retina

Dying cells can be recognized on the basis of morphological or biochemical criteria, the latter being a very powerful tool to identify specific death pathways, the former being most handy for preliminary or quantitative analyses. On light microscopy, neurons that die during normal development exhibit condensation and breakdown of chromatin into fragments, or apoptotic bodies (Wyllie et al., 1980). Cells displaying this morphology (figure 27.1*A*) are called pyknotic. Pyknotic cells have been observed throughout the course of development of the mouse retina (Silver and Hughes, 1973; Young, 1984; Laemle et al., 1999; Pequignot et al., 2003), with three major temporal peaks in terms of density of dying cells. An early phase of cell death affects the retina and the surrounding eye tissues between embryonic day 9 (E9) and E11, around the time of optic vesicle formation and retinal induction. A second peak of cell death is observed between E15.5 and E17.5, when neurogenesis is already under way. Finally, dying neurons are observed in different retinal locations during the first 2 weeks of life, when retinal neurons are differentiating and synaptic connections are being formed.

In the early phase of death, pyknotic cells in the retina are observed mostly in the central region and are likely to be proliferating cells, as almost no neuronal cell has been generated at this age. At this stage, cell death is also observed in the lens and in the non-neuronal epithelium behind the retina. It has been suggested that this early death might contribute to shape the eye, analogous to the role played by death during other morphogenetic events in the organism. In line with this view, both bone morphogenetic proteins (BMPs) and transforming growth factor-β (TGF-β), which have already been involved in morphogenetic events outside the nervous system, appear to regulate retinal cell death at this stage. In the chick, BMP signaling appears to regulate both cell death and cell proliferation around the time of optic vesicle formation (Trousse et al., 2001). In addition, mice deficient in the *Msx2* gene, which is thought to regulate BMP signaling, have increased early death and develop microphthalmia as a consequence of the reduced pool of progenitors in the eye tissues (Wu et al., 2003). Finally, knockout mice for both TGF-β_2 and TGF-β_3 display a significant reduction in early cell death (Dunker and Krieglstein, 2002).

When the second peak of death occurs in the retina, dying cells appear to consist of both early-born retinal ganglion cells (RGCs) and neuroblasts. Pharmacological manipulations in the chick have shown that RGC death in this phase is triggered by nerve growth factor (NGF) binding to its low-affinity receptor, p75 (Frade et al., 1996). In the mouse, many cells express p75 in and along the developing optic nerve at this stage, and death at this time is reduced in embryos carrying deletions in the NGF or the p75 gene (Frade and Barde, 1999). Furthermore, knockout mice for NRIF, a zinc finger protein that interacts with p75 signaling, have reduced cell death in the retina, as do NGF or p75 null mice (Casademunt et al., 1999). NGF/p75-mediated cell death has been found in several instances of neuronal development and in neurodegeneration (Dechant and Barde, 2002). In the developing nervous tissue, death triggered by NGF concentrates in regions that are subsequently crossed by growing nerve fibers (the central region of the ganglion cell layer [GCL] and the future optic nerve head in the retina), leading to the suggestion that this death might clear the way for newly forming axonal pathways (Frade et al., 1996; Frade and Barde, 1999). As for death in the neuroblast layer at this stage, its significance and amount are still largely unclear (reviewed in de la Rosa and de Pablo, 2000).

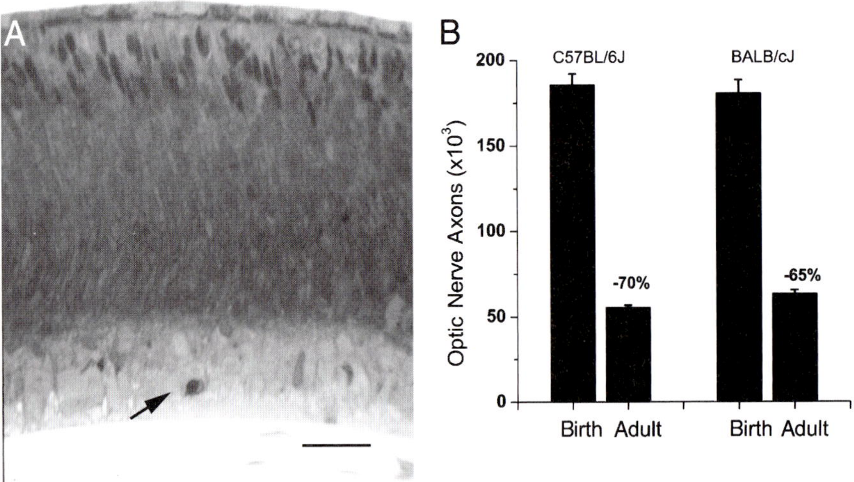

FIGURE 27.1 *A*, Cross section of a P1 retina. *Arrow* points to a dying cell. *B*, Decrease in the number of axons in the optic nerve between birth and adulthood in two common strains of laboratory mice. (Adapted from Strom and Williams, 1998.)

During the first 2 weeks of life in the mouse retina, dying cells are observed at different retinal locations (Young, 1984; Pequignot et al., 2003): at postnatal day 2 (P2), most dying cells are in the GCL; at P9, dying cells are observed mostly in the inner nuclear layer (INL); finally, at P15, dying cells are both in the GCL and in the outer nuclear layer (ONL). The observation of degenerating cells in various retinal layers during retinal differentiation is common to mammals and suggests that most cell populations in the retina undergo phases of cell loss while differentiating. However, verifying this supposition is proving difficult: degenerating cells can be identified on the basis of morphological or biochemical criteria, which commonly include nuclear alterations (see figure 27.1*A*), but these features last for only a brief time (ca. 1 hour in the retina; Cellerino et al., 2000), and furthermore, by the time nuclear morphology is altered, cells have usually lost the differentiation markers necessary to identify their original cell type. To bypass this problem, the total number of cells in some populations has been evaluated at different developmental ages and the amount of cell loss obtained as the difference between the peak and the final number. This may underestimate death contribution in cases where new cell addition and cell loss partially overlap in time, as observed at least in some retinal populations (Galli-Resta and Ensini, 1996; Seecharan et al., 2003; Resta et al., 2005), but it provides at least conservative estimates.

In the study of retinal cell death, much attention has been focused on RGCs. This privileged status is at least partly the result of more reliable cell counts for RGCs than for other developing neuronal populations (since RGCs project outside the retina, they can be retrogradely labeled, and often retain these labels when dying; in addition, RGC counts can be validated by axonal counts in the optic nerve). As well, the accessibility of the retina to external manipulation has made RGCs a popular model not only for naturally occurring death in development, but also for neuronal death after axotomy or in different pathological conditions. On the basis of both RGC counts after injection of retrograde tracers in the RGC targets and axonal counts in the optic nerve, a significant decrement in the number of RGCs has been reported in developing mammalian retinas, ranging between 50% and 75% (figure 27.1*B*, reviewed in Dreher and Robinson, 1988). As we have already mentioned, this decrease in total cell number may underestimate the number of dying cells if death occurs while new cells are being added to the population. Attempts to clarify this matter have led to conflicting estimates of the number of dying RGCs (e.g., 50% for the earliest-born mouse RGCs: Farah and Easter, 2005; 69% for all mouse RGCs: Strom and Williams, 1998; up to 90% for rat GCL neurons: Galli-Resta and Ensini, 1996).

Contribution of cell death to the shaping of retinofugal and retinal circuits

The simultaneous occurrence of cell death and the formation of synaptic connections in the retina and elsewhere has led to the hypothesis that death might contribute to circuit refinements. In particular, death has been hypothesized as an elective process to (1) match the size of interconnected neuronal populations, (2) refine connections and remove projecting errors, and (3) control cell density. Here we consider studies addressing these questions in the development of retinal projections to the brain and in the maturation of intraretinal circuits.

Numerous investigations outside the visual system suggest that death contributes to matching the sizes of interconnected neuronal populations. In the visual system, there is strong experimental evidence that target cells are necessary for the survival of presynaptic cells during development, but these interactions do not lead to a precise quantitative matching between afferent and target cell populations at maturity. In adult monkeys, interindividual variations in the number of RGCs do not correlate with changes in the number of cells in the retinorecipient nuclei (Spear et al., 1996; Suner and Rakic, 1996). Similarly, analysis across adult specimens from 56 mouse strains showed no detectable correlation between the number of neurons in the populations of lateral geniculate neurons and RGCs (Seecharan et al., 2003). In contrast, RGC number correlates significantly with lateral geniculate glial cell number, but how cell death might contribute to this correlation remains to be explored.

The refinement of projection errors during development is a second process to which retinal cell death is hypothesized to contribute. In mammals, initial projections of RGCs to the lateral geniculate nucleus and the superior colliculus display some degree of imprecision. In particular, more cells project ipsilaterally or form topographically incorrect connections than in the adult (reviewed in Cowan et al., 1984). Blocking RGCs' electrical activity during this period reduces the loss of wrongly projecting cells in various species (figure 27.2), indicating a role for cell death in this process (O'Leary et al., 1986b; Pequignot and Clarke, 1992). However, the amount and time course of RGC loss are not affected (O'Leary et al., 1986a), or only marginally so (Scheetz et al., 1995), suggesting that normally, retinal impulse activity makes erroneously projecting RGCs more likely to die, but does not otherwise affect the death process.

It has also been suggested that cell death might contribute to shaping the intraretinal circuitry. RGC removal following optic nerve transection at birth in rats did not significantly affect the density of pyknotic profiles in the remaining retinal layers (Beazley et al., 1987), but when specific amacrine cell populations were analyzed in the adult ferret retina after neonatal optic nerve section, these appeared to be differentially affected, some being increased and others decreased in the absence of RGCs. Thus, cell-cell interactions controlling survival in retinal development appear highly specific for the various cell types, and death might indeed contribute to the fine regulation of cell number in the different populations (Williams et al., 2001).

A particular role of cell death during retinal maturation may indeed be in the control of cell density within individual neuronal populations. In the retina, most neuronal types are organized in orderly arrays known as mosaics, and this organization is thought to ensure even detection and processing of the images impinging on the retina (reviewed in Cook and Chalupa, 2000; Galli-Resta, 2002). Schematically, mosaics can be viewed as cell arrays where density is finely regulated on a local scale, so that each neuron ends up being regularly spaced from its like neighbors. Theoretical studies indicate that death cannot by itself generate regular arrays (Eglen and Willshaw, 2002), but several investigations have shown that cell death contributes to the fine control of local cell density within specific retinal populations. First, it has been demonstrated that refinement of the ON alpha RGCs mosaic in cats coincides with the removal of 20% of these cells, and that blocking electrical activity contrasts the selectivity of cell elimination and leads to less orderly mosaics (Jeyarasasingam et al., 1998). Second, in transgenic mice in which retinal cell death is partially suppressed by *Bcl-2* overexpression, the population of dopaminergic amacrine cells undergoes an almost 10-fold increase in cell density and a decrement in the regularity of cell spacing (Raven et al., 2003). Finally, when extracellular ATP signaling is prevented in the rat retina, death among the cholinergic amacrine cells is reduced, causing an increase in their density (figure 27.2*B*, Resta et al., 2005). In summary, mosaic formation appears to involve two types of processes: lateral cell movements, and

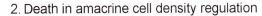

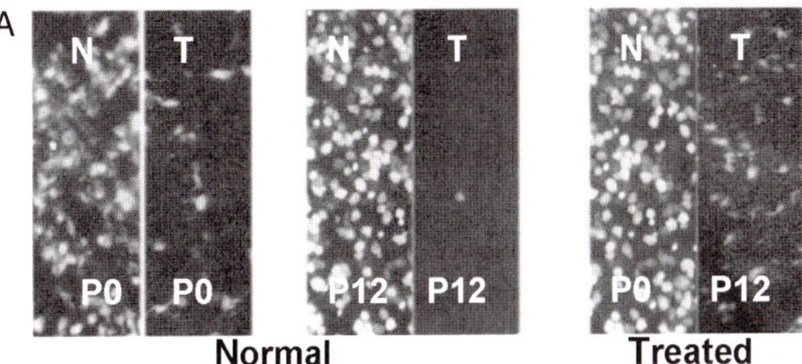

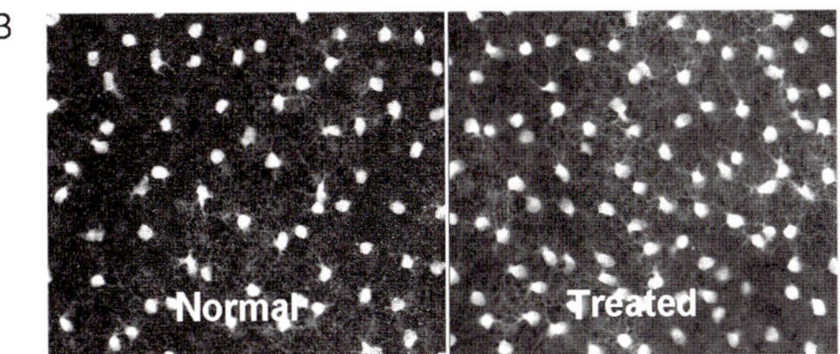

Figure 27.2 *A*, Cell death involvement in the refinement of topographic projections. On P0, both nasal (N) and temporal (T) RGCs project to the posterior contralateral colliculus in rats (*left*). The T contingent is about 14% of the N. The T contingent is almost completely eliminated by P12, after the period of cell death (*center*). However, if RGC impulse activity is blocked, the T contingent is maintained at the P0 value (*right*). (Adapted from O'Leary et al., 1986b.) *B*, Among the cholinergic amacrine cells, death induced by endogenous extracellular ATP contributes to reducing local cell density during development. *Left*, Normal cholinergic cell density. *Right*, Cholinergic cell density 24 hours after extracellular ATP degradation. (From Resta et al., 2005.)

possibly a spatial control on the location of cell genesis aimed at positioning the cell appropriately, while at the same time death eliminates cells, thus keeping local density under control.

The neurotrophic hypothesis

The study of cell death in the different neural regions of the developing organism, and in particular the finding that the survival of postmitotic neurons depends on intercellular interactions, classically exemplified by the need for a target tissue, and the identification of intrinsic trophic factors promoting neuronal survival (initiated with the discovery of NGF), has led to a general hypothesis about cell death regulation. This classic hypothesis in developmental neurobiology, often referred to as the neurotrophic hypothesis, states that during development and differentiation, neuronal survival is contingent on the supply of trophic factors provided by the environment, with a prominent role played by post- and presynaptic tissues (reviewed in Oppenheim, 1991; Bennet et al., 2002; Davies, 2003).

In the retina, current evidence suggests that different neurotrophic factors may be accessible to particular neuronal populations in specific spatiotemporal sequences, so that several neurotrophic interactions may be required for normal development of each neuronal type (Korsching, 1993). Further, as we have already seen, there is also evidence of a death-promoting effect by a classic neurotrophin (endogenous NGF) during embryonic retinal development.

Neurotrophins and their receptors are expressed in the developing retina during the second and the late phases of naturally occurring cell death (reviewed in Frade et al., 1999). Most experimental manipulations concerning the trophic action of neurotrophins on cell death in the retina have been done in the chick. Exogenously applied brain-derived neurotrophic factor (BDNF) reduces RGC death and increases the number of axons in the optic nerve (Frade et al., 1997). Functionally blocking antibodies against neurotrophin-3 (NT-3) prevents the death of a subset of amacrine and ganglion cells in cell culture from E9–E11 dissociated chick retinas (de la Rosa et al., 1994). In vivo, when endogenous NT-3 is neutralized, the retina is reduced in size and abnormal in its organization, showing a narrowing of the inner plexiform layer, most likely as a result of the reduced neuronal number in the adjacent layers (Bovolenta et al., 1996). In the rat, injecting BDNF or NT-4/NT-5 either into the superior colliculus or into the eye limits the death of neonatal RGCs (Cui and Harvey, 1994, 1995; Ma et al., 1998). Similarly, BDNF application has been shown to prevent rat RGC death in culture (reviewed in Frade et al., 1999). Other studies in culture, however, suggest that promoting RGC survival requires simultaneous stimulation by multiple trophic factors (Meyer-Franke et al., 1995). In line with this hypothesis, null mutations for BDNF or NT-4, individually or together, and for their functional receptor TrkB do not display gross defects in the neural retina, suggesting a compensation by other trophic factors (reviewed in Snider, 1994). Finally, recent studies indicate that manipulating the levels of BDNF or its receptor TrkB can modulate the time course of death among RGCs (Pollock et al., 2003), but not their final number (Cellerino et al., 1997; Rohrer et al., 2001).

An additional factor linked to death modulations in the developing retina is insulin-like growth factor (IGF), which, together with IGF-I receptors, is expressed during retinal development (de Pablo and de la Rosa, 1995). Moreover, mRNA and protein expression of the IGF system exhibit temporal and spatial correlation with patterns of cell death during retinal development (Kleffens et al., 1999), and recent evidence suggests that IGF-I modulates RGC death in vivo (Gutierrez-Ospina et al., 2002). Interestingly, a recent study shows that environmental enrichment can modulate the temporal pattern of cell death in the GCL, most likely through modulation of endogenous IGF-I levels (Sale et al., 2007). In addition, it is well established that insulin receptor substrate 2 (Irs2) appears essential for photoreceptor survival in the mouse retina: compared to control littermates, Irs2 knockout mice lose 10% of their photoreceptors 1 week after birth and up to 50% by 2 weeks of age as a result of increased apoptosis (Yi et al., 2005).

Both BMP and TGF-β appear to affect death not only in the earliest phase, but also during postnatal development. Mice deficient in the BMP receptor BMPrIb display higher than normal cell death rates in the INL on P7 (Liu et al., 2003). The addition of neutralizing anti-TGF-β antibodies reduced RGC death in cultured mouse retinas, corresponding to the second and the late death phases (Beier et al., 2006). Finally, several other factors, including interleukin-2 and -4 and TNF-α, have been shown to have neuroprotective effects in the developing retina, but their role in normal cell death, if any, is unclear (reviewed in Linden and Reese, 2006).

In summary, retinal cell survival cannot be linked to individual trophic factors. Individual factors appear to be more pleiotropic and promiscuous than once envisioned, and many interactions occur between members of different families of growth factors. It seems likely that a complex "growth factor homeostasis" occurs in the retina, with a network of factors regulating the survival and maintenance of retinal cells.

Molecules involved in signaling, regulating, and executing programmed cell death

The term *programmed cell death* was initially used to refer to death occurring normally during development, because of its predictable time course and amount. This term has now acquired a more specific meaning, because the unveiling of molecular mechanisms underlying developmental death has made it clear that naturally occurring cell death in development depends on specific gene programs activated by the cells. Almost two decades of study in model organisms, neuronal cultures, and transgenic mice have revealed a central core of conserved molecules that activate, control, and execute the cell death program in many instances (Putcha and Johnson, 2004). In this "central dogma" of apoptosis (as death by activation of a genetic program is often but not always referred to), "thanatins" (Egl-1 in *C. elegans*, BH3-only proteins of the Bcl-2 family in vertebrates) are induced in cells destined to die. They interact with a "death inhibitor" (CED-9 in *C. elegans*, Bcl-2, Bcl-xL in vertebrates), thereby displacing an "adapter" (CED-4 in *C. elegans*, Apaf-1 in vertebrates), which can then promote activation of the "executioner" (CED-3 in *C. elegans*, caspases in vertebrates), which cleaves selected substrates and leads to cell death. This pathway appears remarkably conserved in evolution, but with several fundamental differences: (1) in vertebrates, caspase activation usually requires cytochrome-*c* release from mitochondria; (2) in multiple neuronal populations, cytochrome-*c* release requires expression of at least one multidomain proapoptotic Bcl-2 protein (e.g., Bax); and (3) finally, at least in some neuronal populations, caspase activation requires not only Bax-dependent cytochrome-*c* release but also inactivation of an inhibitor of apoptosis. It is important to point out that, as research proceeds, in addition to this highly conserved death program, alternative death pathways are also becoming known that appear to depend on activation of mechanisms other than the classic caspase-dependent Bcl-2 family–controlled death program.

Evidence for the occurrence of the core apoptotic pathway in retinal cell death during development is still fragmentary, but a number of steps in the core pathways have correlates in the retina.

First, it has been established that naturally occurring cell death in the retina requires gene expression and protein synthesis, since intraocular injections of inhibitors of either transcription or synthesis block RGC death in the neonatal rat retina (Rabacchi et al., 1994).

Second, there is strong evidence for the involvement of both pro- and antiapoptotic proteins of the Bcl-2 family in cell death in the developing retina, although not all these studies support the classic view of the core apoptotic process. Transgenic mice carrying a deletion of the pro-apoptotic *Bax* gene show an almost doubled number of RGCs in adulthood (Mosinger Ogilvie et al., 1998). This correlates with a significant decrease in the percentage of apoptotic cells in the GCL at P2 (Pequignot et al., 2003). However, the overexpression of *Bax* driven by the neuron-specific enolase (NSE) promoter did not affect the numbers of RGCs (Bernard et al., 1998), possibly for the late pattern of *Bax* expression it induced. Bax knockout mice also display lower rates of apoptosis in the INL between P8 and P11, and in the ONL on P15. Furthermore, either *Bax* or *Bak* deletion is sufficient for ectopic photoreceptor PCD during normal development (Hahn et al., 2003). Thus, the Bax-mediated pathway appears to play an important role in retinal cell death during development.

The picture concerning the antiapoptotic Bcl-2 members is more controversial. Gene deletion of the antiapoptotic Bcl-x in the mouse causes massive cell loss in the nervous system, but the retinal phenotype has not been reported. This knockout is lethal to the embryo. On the contrary, one transgenic line lacking the antiapoptotic *Bcl-2* gene showed a 30% loss of RGCs, which, however, occurred after the physiological period of naturally occurring cell death (Cellerino et al., 1999). Naturally occurring RGC death is reduced in transgenic mice overexpressing *Bcl-2* under the control of the NSE promoter (figure 27.3*A*–*C*; Bonfanti

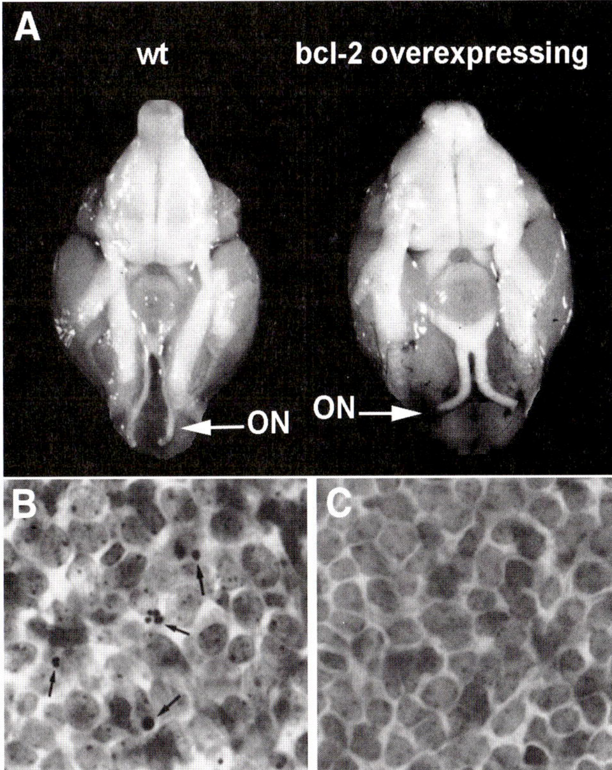

FIGURE 27.3 *A*, Ventral view of the brain of a wild-type (*left*) and *Bcl-2*-overexpressing (*right*) adult mouse. The latter brain is larger than the wild-type mouse brain, and the optic nerve (ON) is clearly larger than normal, as it contains 60% more RGC axons than normal. This increase in RGC number is due to reduced death among these cells during postnatal development. *B*, A field in the wild-type P0 retina showing pyknotic cells (*arrows*). *C*, Almost no dying cell is observed at this stage in the *Bcl-2*-overexpressing retina. (*B* and *C* from Bonfanti et al., 1996.)

et al., 1996). These transgenic mice also display increased numbers of bipolar and some type of amacrine cells, suggesting that Bcl-2 may prevent death in these populations also (Strettoi and Volpini, 2002). However, because different antiapoptotic members of the Bcl-2 family may compensate for one another, interpretation of the alterations observed in knockout mice is complex. In summary, current evidence indicates that antiapoptotic Bcl-2 family members can interfere with programmed cell death in retinal development, but their intrinsic role in this process remains to be elucidated.

As to the BH3-only protein, no evidence of a causal involvement of BH3-only protein in retinal cell death is yet available, but rat RGCs express the BH3-only protein BIM during the period of postnatal programmed cell death, and the relative levels of BIM mRNA in RGCs have a time course correlated with that of RGC death after axotomy (Napankangas et al., 2003).

Finally, many studies indicate the involvement of individual caspases in retinal cell death. Caspases are proteases with selective cleavage sites that execute the death program. In the most characterized death core program, mature caspase-9 recruits and activates downstream caspases, such as caspase-3, resulting in controlled demise of the cell. Caspase-3 activation and the presence of DNA strand breaks due to a caspase-dependent endonuclease are the basis of two popular methods for death detection (activated caspase-3 immunoreactivity and TUNEL, respectively), which, however, do not detect all types of cell death. Mouse embryos deficient in either caspase-3 or caspase-9 display retinal hyperplasia, disorganized cell deployment, and delayed optic fissure closure. These knockout strains have a high level of perinatal death (Kuida et al., 1996). In the few animals that are born, abnormal death kinetics after birth were limited to the inner nuclear layer (Zeiss et al., 2004). In the chick retina, acute treatment with caspase-3 inhibitors reduced to 50% cell death among RGCs in the phase of optic nerve formation (Mayordomo et al., 2003).

In summary, caspase-mediated apoptosis regulated by the Bcl-2 family has been securely established as one way of cell death in the retina, but the causal link between the different molecular players is still less clear than in other model systems. Furthermore, this death paradigm might not be the only one in the developing retina, and the different phases of cell death may not share the same death pathway. In general, as indicated by studies in isolated retinas, there is evidence for multiple posttranslational pathways of death in the developing retina (Guimaraes et al., 2003).

An important aspect of cell death is the complex realm of activators, modulators, and inhibitors of the death program. This field has attracted increasing interest in recent years, but a general picture is still lacking. Much of what is known comes from well-established models of cell death in culture. Very schematically, an emerging picture has been identified that involves (1) extracellular signals that trigger death (NGF/p75 and in the Fas signaling system) and (2) intracellular signaling pathways that regulate activation of the death program. The latter include transcription factors and kinases. In neuronal culture model systems, some of these intracellular effectors appear implicated in the way neurotrophin promotes cell survival, but whether this occurs during retinal development is unknown. As we have seen, NGF/p75 signaling promotes cell death during embryonic retinal development, whereas Fas signaling, another established extracellular death trigger, appears to have little effect on retinal cell death, as *Fas* knockout mice exhibit a delayed period of cell death in retinal development but eventually have normal retinas and appear to lose the same number of retinal cells as do normal mice (Pequignot et al., 2003).

Mutations or deletions of several transcription factors have been shown to induce cell death among developing photoreceptors and RGCs. Of these, Ap3b1, encoding a subunit of the AP-3 adaptor complex, corresponds to the pearl mutation that is associated with an accelerated time course of cell death and CRB1, mutations of which are related to a thickening of the human retina that is probably dependent on alteration of natural cell death (see Linden and Reese, 2006).

Finally, several kinases have been involved in modulating neuronal death (reviewed in Putcha and Johnson, 2004). In the retina, constitutive expression of an activated form of the regulatory subunit of the phosphoinositide 3-kinase causes retinal dysplasia and an increased number of photoreceptors, attributed to reduced death of these neurons during development (Pimentel et al., 2002).

Much effort is being devoted to understanding whether developmental death programs are reactivated during neurodegeneration in retinal pathologies, as well as to elucidate the differences between developmental and pathological death. Reviewing research on pathological cell death in the retina is beyond the scope of the present chapter, but a few aspects deserve consideration. It has been suggested that antiapoptotic "brakes" are set into action to warrant survival of normally maturing neurons. In the retina, downregulation of key pro-apoptotic factors, including pro-apoptotic Bcl-2 family members, Apaf-1, and caspase-3, correlates with maturation, while the expression of XIAP, a potent caspase inhibitor, increases in the adult retina (O'Driscoll et al., 2006), suggesting that adult neurons might survive by switching off elements of the developmental death program. In line with this view, following axotomy, RGCs activate caspase-3 and caspase-9 (Kermer et al., 2000). Experiments testing whether caspase inhibitors prevent RGC death following axotomy, however, have had conflicting results (Kermer et al., 2000; Weishaupt et al., 2003; Spalding et al., 2005;

McKernan et al., 2006). There are also indications that the death of adult retinal cells in neuronal pathologies and related models might involve different mechanisms than those involved in developmental death. For example, *Bax* or *Fas* deletion has no effects on photoreceptor survival in a mouse model of retinitis pigmentosa (Mosinger Ogilvie et al., 1998), whereas during development, *Bax* deletion decreases and *Fas* deletion delays developmental death (Pequignot et al., 2003). Similarly, overexpression of Bcl-2 or Bcl-xL transgenes does not rescue photoreceptor cells in models of retinitis pigmentosa (Joseph and Li, 1996).

Concluding remarks

Despite considerable progress, we are still far from a clear picture of the network of interactions that control retinal development. Cell death is obviously an important component of retinal development, but many aspects of its role and regulation are still obscure. For example, we have little idea of the role of extracellular matrix or of mechanical interactions in regulating cell survival and death in the retina, and we do not know the relevance of pools of dying cells to the evolutionary potential of the system.

Cell death is observed throughout eye and retinal development, with a first peak at the time of optic vesicle formation and two later phases of death, while retinal neurons are generated and when they later differentiate. Much effort has been devoted to understanding the role of cell death in specific processes such as connection refinement and the matching of interconnected cell populations. Most of these studies have shown a modest contribution of cell death, suggesting that death is involved in these processes but is not designed to subserve them. Rather, death appears as one of the fates open to differentiating retinal cells, a fate that is realized with the activation of genetic death programs.

Much current evidence favors the view that cell survival during retinal development is due to trophic intercellular interactions, without which death occurs. This view suggests that death might be a default fate for differentiating neurons.

REFERENCES

Beazley, L. D., Perry, V. H., Baker, B., and Darby, J. E. (1987). An investigation into the role of ganglion cells in the regulation of division and death of other retinal cells. *Brain Res.* 430:169–184.

Beier, M., Franke, A., Paunel-Gorgulu, A. N., Scheerer, N., and Dunker, N. (2006). Transforming growth factor beta mediates apoptosis in the ganglion cell layer during all programmed cell death periods of the developing murine retina. *Neurosci. Res.* 56:193–203.

Bennet, M. R., Gibson, W. G., and Lemon, G. (2002). Neuronal cell death, nerve growth factor and neurotrophic models: 50 years on. *Auton. Neurosci.* 95:1–23.

Bernard, R., Dieni, S., Rees, S., and Bernard, O. (1998). Physiological and induced neuronal death are not affected in NSE-Bax transgenic mice. *J. Neurosci. Res.* 52:247–259.

Bonfanti, L., Strettoi, E., Chierzi, S., Cenni, M., Liu, X., Martinou, J.-C., Maffei, L., and Rabacchi, S. (1996). Protection of retinal ganglion cells from natural and axotomy-induced cell death in neonatal transgenic mice overexpressing Bcl-2. *J. Neurosci.* 16:4186–4194.

Bovolenta, P., Frade, J. M., Marti, E., Rodriguez-Pena, M. A., Barde, Y. A., and Rodriguez-Tebar, A. (1996). Neurotrophin-3 antibodies disrupt the normal development of the chick retina. *J. Neurosci.* 16:4402–4410.

Buss, R. R., and Oppenheim, R. W. (2004). Role of programmed cell death in normal neuronal development and function. *Anat. Sci. Int.* 79:191–197.

Casademunt, E., Carter, B. D., Benzel, I., Frade, J. M., Dechant, G., and Barde, Y. A. (1999). The zinc finger protein NRIF interacts with the neurotrophin receptor p75(NTR) and participates in programmed cell death. *Embo. J.* 18:6050–6061.

Cecconi, F., Alvarez-Bolado, G., Meyer, B. I., Roth, K. A., and Gruss, P. (1998). Apaf1 (CED-4 homolog) regulates programmed cell death in mammalian development. *Cell* 94:727–737.

Cellerino, A., Carroll, P., Thoenen, H., and Barde, Y. A. (1997). Reduced size of retinal ganglion cell axons and hypomyelination in mice lacking brain-derived neurotrophic factor. *Mol. Cell Neurosci.* 9:397–408.

Cellerino, A., Galli-Resta, L., and Colombaioni, L. (2000). The dynamics of neuronal death: A time-lapse study in the retina. *J. Neurosci.* 20:RC92.

Cellerino, A., Michaelidis, T., Barski, J. J., Bahr, M., Thoenen, H., and Meyer, M. (1999). Retinal ganglion cell loss after the period of naturally occurring cell death in *Bcl-2*$^{-/-}$ mice. *Neuroreport* 10:1091–1095.

Cook, J. E., and Chalupa, L. M. (2000). Retinal mosaics: New insights into an old concept. *Trends Neurosci.* 23:26–34.

Cowan, W. M., Fawcett, J. W., O'Leary, D. D., and Stanfield, B. B. (1984). Regressive events in neurogenesis. *Science* 225: 1258–1265.

Cui, Q., and Harvey, A. R. (1994). NT-4/5 reduces naturally occurring retinal ganglion cell death in neonatal rats. *Neuroreport* 5:1882–1884.

Cui, Q., and Harvey, A. R. (1995). At least two mechanisms are involved in the death of retinal ganglion cells following target ablation in neonatal rats. *J. Neurosci.* 15:8143–8155.

Davies, A. M. (2003). Regulation of neuronal survival and death by extracellular signals during development. *Embo. J.* 22:2537–2545.

Dechant, G., and Barde, Y. A. (2002). The neurotrophin receptor p75(NTR): Novel functions and implications for diseases of the nervous system. *Nat. Neurosci.* 5:1131–1136.

de la Rosa, E. J., Arribas, A., Frade, J. M., and Rodriguez-Tebar, A. (1994). Role of neurotrophins in the control of neural development: Neurotrophin-3 promotes both neuron differentiation and survival of cultured chick retinal cells. *Neuroscience* 58:347–352.

de la Rosa, E. J., and de Pablo, F. (2000). Cell death in early neural development: Beyond the neurotrophic theory. *Trends Neurosci.* 23:454–458.

de Pablo, F., and de la Rosa, E. J. (1995). The developing CNS: A scenario for the action of proinsulin, insulin and insulin-like growth factors. *Trends Neurosci.* 18:143–150.

Dreher, B., and Robinson, S. R. (1988). Development of the retinofugal pathway in birds and mammals: Evidence for a common "timetable." *Brain Behav. Evol.* 31:369–390.

Dunker, N., and Krieglstein, K. (2002). Tgfbeta2$^{-/-}$ Tgfbeta3$^{-/-}$ double knockout mice display severe midline fusion defects and early embryonic lethality. *Anat. Embryol. (Berl.)* 206:73–83.

Eglen, S. J., and Willshaw, D. J. (2002). Influence of cell fate mechanisms upon retinal mosaic formation: A modelling study. *Development* 129:5399–5408.

Farah, M. H., and Easter, S. S., Jr. (2005). Cell birth and death in the mouse retinal ganglion cell layer. *J. Comp. Neurol.* 489: 120–134.

Frade, J. M., and Barde, Y. A. (1999). Genetic evidence for cell death mediated by nerve growth factor and the neurotrophin receptor p75 in the developing mouse retina and spinal cord. *Development* 126:683–690.

Frade, J. M., Bovolenta, P., Martinez-Morales, J. R., Arribas, A., Barbas, J. A., and Rodriguez-Tebar, A. (1997). Control of early cell death by BDNF in the chick retina. *Development* 124: 3313–3320.

Frade, J. M., Bovolenta, P., and Rodriguez-Tebar, A. (1999). Neurotrophins and other growth factors in the generation of retinal neurons. *Microsc. Res. Tech.* 45:243–251.

Frade, J. M., Rodriguez-Tebar, A., and Barde, Y. A. (1996). Induction of cell death by endogenous nerve growth factor through its p75 receptor. *Nature* 383:166–168.

Galli-Resta, L. (2002). Putting neurons in the right places: Local interactions in the genesis of retinal architecture. *Trends Neurosci.* 25:638–643.

Galli-Resta, L., and Ensini, M. (1996). An intrinsic limit between genesis and death of individual neurons in the developing retinal ganglion cell layer. *J. Neurosci.* 16:2318–2324.

Guimaraes, C. A., Benchimol, M., Amarante-Mendes, G. P., and Linden, R. (2003). Alternative programs of cell death in developing retinal tissue. *J. Biol. Chem.* 278:41938–41946.

Gutierrez-Ospina, G., Gutierrez de la Barrera, A., Larriva, J., and Giordano, M. (2002). Insulin-like growth factor I partly prevents axon elimination in the neonate rat optic nerve. *Neurosci. Lett.* 325:207–210.

Hahn, P., Lindsten, T., Ying, G. S., Bennett, J., Milam, A. H., Thompson, C. B., and Dunaief, J. L. (2003). Proapoptotic Bcl-2 family members, Bax and Bak, are essential for developmental photoreceptor apoptosis. *Invest. Ophthalmol. Vis. Sci.* 44:3598–3605.

Jeyarasasingam, G., Snider, C. J., Ratto, G. M., and Chalupa, L. M. (1998). Activity regulated cell death contributes to the formation of ON and OFF α ganglion cell mosaics. *J. Comp. Neurol.* 394:335–343.

Joseph, R. M., and Li, T. (1996). Overexpression of Bcl-2 or Bcl-xl transgenes and photoreceptor degeneration. *Invest. Ophthalmol. Vis. Sci.* 37:2434–2446.

Kermer, P., Ankerhold, R., Klocker, N., Krajewski, S., Reed, J. C., and Bahr, M. (2000). Caspase-9: Involvement in secondary death of axotomized rat retinal ganglion cells in vivo. *Brain Res. Mol. Brain Res.* 85:144–150.

Kleffens, M., Groffen, C., Neck, J. W., Vermeij-Keers, C., and Drop, S. L. (1999). mRNA and protein localization of the IGF system during mouse embryonic development in areas with apoptosis. *Growth Horm. IGF Res.* 9:195–204.

Korsching, S. (1993). The neurotrophic factor concept: A reexamination. *J. Neurosci.* 13:2739–2748.

Kuida, K., Zheng, T. S., Na, S., Kuan, C., Yang, D., Karasuyama, H., Rakic, P., and Flavell, R. A. (1996). Decreased apoptosis in the brain and premature lethality in CPP32-deficient mice. *Nature* 384:368–372.

Laemle, L. K., Puszkarczuk, M., and Feinberg, R. N. (1999). Apoptosis in early ocular morphogenesis in the mouse. *Brain Res. Dev. Brain Res.* 112:129–133.

Linden, R., and Reese, B. E. (2006). Programmed cell death in the developing vertebrate retina. In E. Sernagor, S. J. Eglen, W. Harris, and R. O. Wong (Eds.), *Retinal development.* Cambridge: Cambridge University Press.

Liu, J., Wilson, S., and Reh, T. (2003). BMP receptor 1b is required for axon guidance and cell survival in the developing retina. *Dev. Biol.* 256:34–48.

Ma, Y. T., Hsieh, T., Forbes, M. E., Johnson, J. E., and Frost, D. O. (1998). BDNF injected into the superior colliculus reduces developmental retinal ganglion cell death. *J. Neurosci.* 18: 2097–2107.

Mayordomo, R., Valenciano, A. I., de la Rosa, E. J., and Hallbook, F. (2003). Generation of retinal ganglion cells is modulated by caspase-dependent programmed cell death. *Eur. J. Neurosci.* 18:1744–1750.

McKernan, D. P., Caplis, C., Donovan, M., O'Brien, C. J., and Cotter, T. G. (2006). Age-dependent susceptibility of the retinal ganglion cell layer to cell death. *Invest. Ophthalmol. Vis. Sci.* 47: 807–814.

Meyer-Franke, A., Kaplan, M. R., Pfrieger, F. W., and Barres, B. A. (1995). Characterization of the signaling interactions that promote the survival and growth of developing retinal ganglion cells in culture. *Neuron* 15:805–819.

Mosinger Ogilvie, J., Deckwerth, T. L., Knudson, C. M., and Korsmeyer, S. J. (1998). Suppression of developmental retinal cell death but not of photoreceptor degeneration in Bax-deficient mice. *Invest. Ophthalmol. Vis. Sci.* 39:1713–1720.

Napankangas, U., Lindqvist, N., Lindholm, D., and Hallbook, F. (2003). Rat retinal ganglion cells upregulate the pro-apoptotic BH3-only protein Bim after optic nerve transection. *Brain Res. Mol. Brain Res.* 120:30–37.

O'Driscoll, C., Donovan, M., and Cotter, T. G. (2006). Analysis of apoptotic and survival mediators in the early post-natal and mature retina. *Exp. Eye Res.* 83:1482–1492.

O'Leary, D. D., Crespo, D., Fawcett, J. W., and Cowan, W. M. (1986a). The effect of intraocular tetrodotoxin on the postnatal reduction in the numbers of optic nerve axons in the rat. *Brain Res.* 395:96–103.

O'Leary, D. D. M., Fawcett, J. W., and Cowan, W. M. (1986b). Topographical targetting errors in the retinocollicular projection and their elimination by selective ganglion cell death. *J. Neurosci.* 6:3692–3705.

Oppenheim, R. W. (1981). Neuronal cell death and some regressive phenomena during neurogenesis: A selective historical review and progress report. In W. M. Cowan (Ed.), *Studies in developmental neurobiology: Essays in honour of Viktor Hamburger* (pp. 74–133). New York: Oxford University Press.

Oppenheim, R. W. (1991). Cell death during development of the nervous system. *Annu. Rev. Neurosci.* 14:453–501.

Pequignot, M. O., Provost, A. C., Salle, S., Taupin, P., Sainton, K. M., Marchant, D., Martinou, J. C., Ameisen, J. C., Jais, J. P., et al. (2003). Major role of Bax in apoptosis during retinal development and in establishment of a functional postnatal retina. *Dev. Dyn.* 228:231–238.

Pequignot, Y., and Clarke, P. G. (1992). Maintenance of targeting errors by isthmo-optic axons following the intraocular injection of tetrodotoxin in chick embryos. *J. Comp. Neurol.* 321:351–356.

Pimentel, B., Rodriguez-Borlado, L., Hernandez, C., and Carrera, A. C. (2002). A role for phosphoinositide 3-kinase in the control of cell division and survival during retinal development. *Dev. Biol.* 247:295–306.

Pollock, G. S., Robichon, R., Boyd, K. A., Kerkel, K. A., Kramer, M., Lyles, J., Ambalavanar, R., Khan, A., Kaplan, D. R., et al. (2003). TrkB receptor signaling regulates developmental death dynamics, but not final number, of retinal ganglion cells. *J. Neurosci.* 23:10137–10145.

Putcha, G. V., and Johnson, E. M., Jr. (2004). Men are but worms: Neuronal cell death in *C. elegans* and vertebrates. *Cell Death Differ.* 11:38–48.

Rabacchi, S. A., Bonfanti, L., Liu, X. H., and Maffei, L. (1994). Apoptotic cell death induced by optic nerve lesion in the neonatal rat. *J. Neurosci.* 14:5292–5301.

Raven, M. A., Eglen, S. J., Ohab, J. J., and Reese, B. E. (2003). Determinants of the exclusion zone in dopaminergic amacrine cell mosaics. *J. Comp. Neurol.* 461:123–136.

Resta, V., Novelli, E., Di Virgilio, F., and Galli-Resta, L. (2005). Neuronal death induced by endogenous extracellular ATP in retinal cholinergic neuron density control. *Development* 132:2873–2882.

Rohrer, B., LaVail, M. M., Jones, K. R., and Reichardt, L. F. (2001). Neurotrophin receptor TrkB activation is not required for the postnatal survival of retinal ganglion cells in vivo. *Exp. Neurol.* 172:81–91.

Sale, A., Cenni, M. C., Putignano, E., Ciucci, F., Chierzi, S., and Maffei, L. (2007). Maternal enrichment during pregnancy accelerates retinal development of the fetus. *PLoS ONE* 2: e1160.

Scheetz, A. J., Williams, R. W., and Dubin, M. W. (1995). Severity of ganglion cell death during early postnatal development is modulated by both neuronal activity and binocular competition. *Vis. Neurosci.* 12:605–610.

Seecharan, D. J., Kulkarni, A. L., Lu, L., Rosen, G. D., and Williams, R. W. (2003). Genetic control of interconnected neuronal populations in the mouse primary visual system. *J. Neurosci.* 23:11178–11188.

Silver, J., and Hughes, A. F. (1973). The role of cell death during morphogenesis of the mammalian eye. *J. Morphol.* 140:159–170.

Snider, W. D. (1994). Functions of the neurotrophins during nervous system development: What the knockouts are teaching us. *Cell* 77:627–638.

Spalding, K. L., Dharmarajan, A. M., and Harvey, A. R. (2005). Caspase-independent retinal ganglion cell death after target ablation in the neonatal rat. *Eur. J. Neurosci.* 21:33–45.

Spear, P. D., Kim, C. B., Ahmad, A., and Tom, B. W. (1996). Relationship between numbers of retinal ganglion cells and lateral geniculate neurons in the rhesus monkey. *Vis. Neurosci.* 13:199–203.

Strettoi, E., and Volpini, M. (2002). Retinal organization in the *Bcl-2*-overexpressing transgenic mouse. *J. Comp. Neurol.* 446: 1–10.

Strom, R. C., and Williams, R. W. (1998). Cell production and cell death in the generation of variation in neuron number. *J. Neurosci.* 18:9948–9953.

Suner, I., and Rakic, P. (1996). Numerical relationship between neurons in the lateral geniculate nucleus and primary visual cortex in macaque monkeys. *Vis. Neurosci.* 13:585–590.

Trousse, F., Esteve, P., and Bovolenta, P. (2001). Bmp4 mediates apoptotic cell death in the developing chick eye. *J. Neurosci.* 21:1292–1301.

Weishaupt, J. H., Diem, R., Kermer, P., Krajewski, S., Reed, J. C., and Bahr, M. (2003). Contribution of caspase-8 to apoptosis of axotomized rat retinal ganglion cells in vivo. *Neurobiol. Dis.* 13:124–135.

Williams, R. R., Cusato, K., Raven, M. A., and Reese, B. E. (2001). Organization of the inner retina following early elimination of the retinal ganglion cell population: Effects on cell numbers and stratification patterns. *Vis. Neurosci.* 18:233–244.

Wong, R. O., and Godinho, L. (2003). Development of the vertebrate retina. In L. M. Chalupa and J. S. Werner (Eds.), *The visual neurosciences*. Cambridge, MA: MIT Press.

Wu, L. Y., Li, M., Hinton, D. R., Guo, L., Jiang, S., Wang, J. T., Zeng, A., Xie, J. B., Snead, M., et al. (2003). Microphthalmia resulting from MSX2-induced apoptosis in the optic vesicle. *Invest. Ophthalmol. Vis. Sci.* 44:2404–2412.

Wyllie, A. H., et al. (1980). Cell death: The significance of apoptosis. *Int. Rev. Cytol.* 68:251–306.

Yi, X., Schubert, M., Peachey, N. S., Suzuma, K., Burks, D. J., Kushner, J. A., Suzuma, I., Cahill, C., Flint, C. L., et al. (2005). Insulin receptor substrate 2 is essential for maturation and survival of photoreceptor cells. *J. Neurosci.* 25:1240–1248.

Yoshida, H., Kong, Y. Y., Yoshida, R., Elia, A. J., Hakem, A., Hakem, R., Penninger, J. M., and Mak, T. W. (1998). Apaf1 is required for mitochondrial pathways of apoptosis and brain development. *Cell* 94:739–750.

Young, R. W. (1984). Cell death during differentiation of the retina in the mouse. *J. Comp. Neurol.* 229:362–373.

Zeiss, C. J., Neal, J., and Johnson, E. A. (2004). Caspase-3 in postnatal retinal development and degeneration. *Invest. Ophthalmol. Vis. Sci.* 45:964–970.

28 The Function of the Retina prior to Vision: The Phenomenon of Retinal Waves and Retinotopic Refinement

MARLA B. FELLER AND AARON G. BLANKENSHIP

Prior to vision, the developing vertebrate retina spontaneously generates a firing pattern termed retinal waves. During a retinal wave, retinal ganglion cells (RGCs) spontaneously fire correlated bursts of action potentials that propagate across the retina. Retinal waves have been characterized in a wide variety of vertebrate species (for reviews, see Wong, 1999; Firth et al., 2005). In mice, retinal waves have been detected as early as embryonic day 16 (E16) and persist until the time of eye opening at postnatal day 14 (P14).

Retinal waves coincide with a period of visual system development when there is a dramatic level of refinement of the retina's projections to its primary targets in the brain, the superior colliculus (SC) and the lateral geniculate nucleus of the thalamus. In vivo blockade or significant alteration of retinal waves prevents normal refinement of these circuits, indicating that retinal waves are required for normal development of the visual system (reviewed in Torborg and Feller, 2005). However, the mechanisms by which retinal waves drive developmental processes are not fully understood.

In this chapter, we describe (1) the synaptic circuits that mediate retinal waves, (2) the spatial and temporal correlations of retinal waves, and (3) the role of retinal waves in establishing circuits throughout the developing visual system.

Techniques used to measure retinal waves

Several physiological methods have been used to record retinal waves. Spontaneous activity in the developing retina was first detected in vitro in rabbits using extracellular recordings from single RGCs (Masland, 1977). Ten years later, spontaneous correlated bursts of action potentials were detected in vivo in fetal rat pups (Galli and Maffei, 1988). The evidence that these spontaneous bursts of action potentials propagated in the form of waves was provided by a series of experiments using a multielectrode array (MEA), which allowed simultaneous recording from tens of RGCs in ferret retina (Meister et al., 1991; Wong et al., 1993). MEA recordings have been used extensively to characterize spontaneous firing patterns in mice (for recent examples, see Demas et al., 2003; Cang et al., 2005; Torborg et al., 2005).

A large body of work on retinal waves has been conducted using calcium imaging (Wong et al., 1995; Feller et al., 1996), which can monitor activity over larger regions of the retina (up to $2\,mm^2$) than is possible with MEA (less than $0.2\,mm^2$) (Wong, 1998). In calcium imaging, intracellular concentrations of calcium are measured using fluorescent indicators (Wong, 1998). Calcium imaging indirectly measures cell depolarization by monitoring the influx of calcium triggered through voltage-gated calcium channels. Simultaneous electrophysiological recordings from individual RGCs and calcium imaging show that the bursts of action potentials and calcium transients occur simultaneously (Penn et al., 1998; Zhou, 1998; Singer et al., 2001).

Finally, single-cell physiology experiments, such as whole-cell voltage-clamp and current-clamp recordings, have been used to determine the synaptic inputs and membrane potential changes of individual neurons involved in retinal waves (Feller et al., 1996; Zhou, 1998; Butts et al., 1999; Singer et al., 2001).

Cellular mechanisms underlying retinal waves change with retinal development

Retinal waves are detected in mouse retina from a few days before birth until approximately 2 weeks after birth. During this time, the retina itself undergoes a dramatic amount of development (Morgan and Wong, 2006). At E16, the mouse retina consists of a ganglion cell layer that is two to three cell bodies thick and contains both RGCs and cholinergic and GABAergic amacrine cells. Around birth, the first chemical synapses are detectable by electron microscopy (Olney, 1968). These synapses have the morphological characteristics of classic chemical synapses, such as those between amacrine cells and RGCs. At P10, ribbon synapses are first detected in electron micrographs of the inner plexiform layer (IPL), representing the first functional synapses between bipolar cells and RGCs (Fisher, 1979).

The mechanisms underlying retinal waves go through three functional stages as the retina develops (figure 28.1). The stages are defined by the combination of receptor antagonists that block waves (reviewed in Firth et al., 2005; Torborg and Feller, 2005). Stage I retinal waves consist of simultaneous increases in $[Ca^{2+}]_i$ in small clusters of cells that are blocked by gap junction antagonists, and activity that propagates over substantially larger regions that is blocked by nicotinic acetylcholine receptor (nAChR) antagonists. At birth (P0), when chemical synapses are present in the IPL, stage I waves end and stage II waves begin. Stage II waves are blocked by nAChR antagonists and by gap junction antagonists. Stage II waves end and stage III waves begin at P10, when bipolar cells are forming glutamatergic synapses with RGCs. Stage III waves are blocked by ionotropic glutamate receptor antagonists and gap junction antagonists, but not by nAChR antagonists.

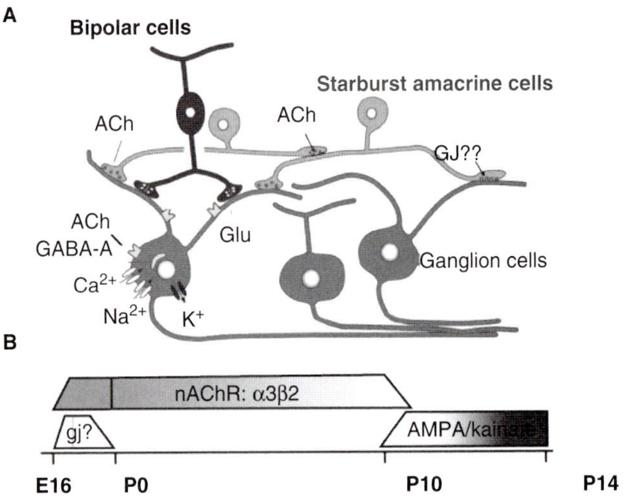

FIGURE 28.1 Three functional stages of retinal wave–generating circuits. *A*, Schematic of circuits that mediate retinal waves. (Modified from Catsicas and Mobbs, 1995.) *B*, Summary of development of the synaptic circuitry that mediates waves in mice. Each color corresponds to a different wave-generating circuit. Yellow corresponds to non-nAChR circuitry, which mediates the nonpropagating events in embryonic mice. There is pharmacological evidence that stage I waves in other species are mediated by gap junctions, but this has not been directly demonstrated in mouse retina. In addition, it is not known which gap junction–coupled networks mediate stage I waves. Red corresponds to stage II circuits, which require activation of nAChRs. Stage II waves are initiated and propagate through a network of starburst amacrine cells. Blue corresponds to stage III circuits, which require activation of ionotropic glutamate receptors. The source of stage III wave initiation and the location of the horizontal coupling that drives coordinated release of glutamate during this stage are not yet known. See color plate 17. (Modified from Bansal et al., 2000.)

The circuitry that underlies stage II retinal waves has been extensively studied and therefore is the best understood. Here we focus primarily on the properties of stage II waves, both their spatial and temporal characteristics and the cellular mechanisms underlying them.

Spatiotemporal properties of stage II retinal waves

A complete description of retinal waves must link the known circuitry that mediates the waves with their global spatial and temporal properties. The spatiotemporal properties of retinal waves have been divided into three parts—wave initiation, propagation, and termination (figure 28.2*A*). Calcium imaging and MEA recording have both been used to describe these properties of stage II retinal waves in mice. Extensive studies have also been conducted in ferrets (Feller et al., 1997; Butts et al., 1999), rabbits (Zhou and Zhao, 2000; Zhou, 2001a), and turtles (Sernagor et al., 2000, 2003) but are not presented here.

How do retinal waves start? Stage II retinal waves begin in random locations in the retina, with all locations having equal probability for wave initiation. Hence, there is no particular region of the retina that functions as a pacemaker for retinal waves. We proposed a computational model that assumes a randomly distributed population of cells with a finite probability of spontaneously depolarizing in which the cells are connected to each other by recurrent excitation (Feller et al., 1997; Butts et al., 1999). When the activity level surpasses a threshold level of depolarization, a retinal wave occurs. After this event, all cells participating in the wave enter a refractory period during which they cannot initiate or participate in subsequent waves. Hence, wave initiation results from a combination of spontaneous depolarization in individual cells and network interactions. Recent evidence supporting this model is presented later in the chapter.

What determines the speed of retinal wave propagation? Stage II retinal waves propagate at a speed of 150 μm/s in mice. This speed is two to three times faster than speeds predicted for the extracellular diffusion of excitatory substances, such as those observed in spreading depression (Martins-Ferreira et al., 1974, 2000; Somjen, 2001), but an order of magnitude slower than epileptic waves that are induced in cortical circuits by blocking all inhibitory synaptic transmission (see, e.g., Prince and Connors, 1986). From these measurements, it has been hypothesized that retinal wave speed is determined by fast chemical synapses, with one step of propagation "slowed" by some diffusive component, such as activation of a G protein–coupled receptor or diffuse release of neurotransmitter.

Stage II retinal waves propagate over a finite region of the retina, stopping at well-defined but shifting boundaries. We

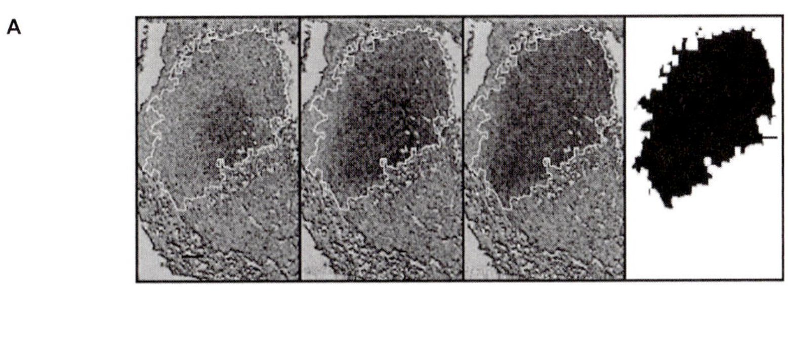

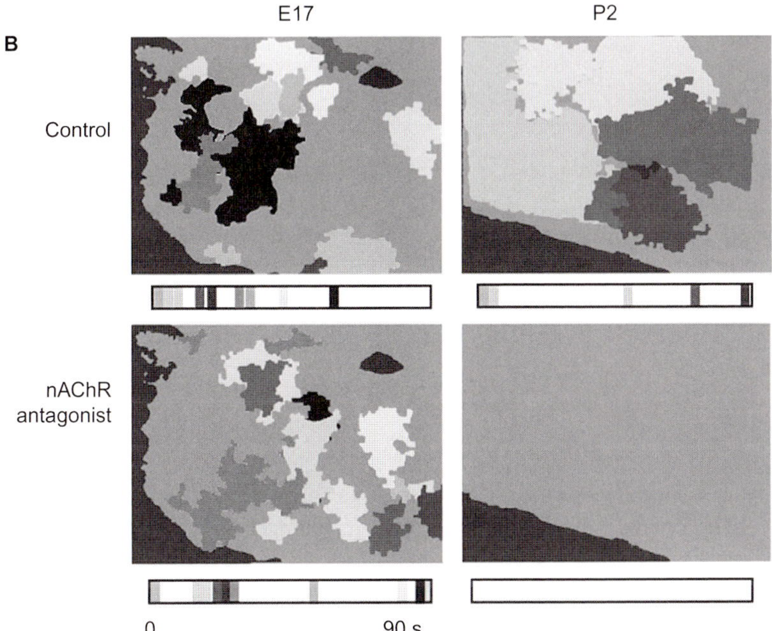

FIGURE 28.2 Calcium imaging reveals spatial and temporal properties of stage I and stage II waves. *A*, Time evolution of a single stage II retinal wave visualized with fluorescence imaging of the calcium indicator fura-2. Decreases in fura-2 fluorescence associated with the increased calcium evoked by waves are shown at successive 0.5 s intervals. The final frame represents the total area of tissue covered by a single wave. *B*, Retinal waves of embryonic day 17 (E17) and postnatal day 2 (P2) retinas. Each frame summarizes 90 s of activity in control ACSF (*top row*) and in 100 μM *d*-tubocurarine, a general nAChR antagonist (*bottom row*). Gray background represents the total retinal surface labeled with fura-2AM. Each color corresponds to individual domains, with a color-coded time bar below each frame to indicate the time of occurrence of each wave. Scale bar = 100 μm. See color plate 18. (Modified from Bansal et al., 2000.)

have shown that these wave boundaries are determined by a "refractory period," defined as a finite period of time lasting 30–40 s after activation of an area of the retina, during which it cannot participate in subsequent waves (Feller et al., 1997). In addition to controlling the distance over which waves propagate, the refractory period acts to define the frequency with which a local region of the retina participates in waves (Feller et al., 1997; Butts et al., 1999).

Mechanisms of stage II retinal waves

A breakthrough in understanding wave-generating mechanisms was the discovery that stage II retinal waves are mediated by a cholinergic circuit. Studies in turtle (Sernagor and Grzywacz, 1999) and in ferret (Feller et al., 1996) showed that curare, a general nAChR antagonist, blocks stage II retinal waves (figure 28.2*B*).

The retina contains many different nAChR subunits. Nicotinic AChRs found in the CNS are either homomultimers consisting entirely of α7 subunits ~~or heteromultimers~~ containing a combination of α and β subunits (Sargent, 1993; McGehee and Role, 1995; Role and Berg, 1996). In heterologous expression systems, α3 subunits form functional nAChRs only in the presence of either the β2 or the β4 subunit (Role and Berg, 1996; Gotti et al., 2005). Which nAChR subunits mediate retinal waves? Antagonists selective for nAChRs containing particular subunits or subunit combinations exist, but these drugs become nonselective at high concentrations.

To identify the functional receptors that mediate retinal waves, a screen of different knockout mice lacking specific nAChR subunits was performed (Bansal et al., 2000). Mice lacking β4-containing nAChRs have normal retinal waves, whereas mice lacking α3-containing nAChRs have altered retinal waves. Mice lacking β2-containing nAChRs do not have stage II retinal waves. Hence, although many classes of nAChRs exist in the retina (Moretti et al., 2004), only β2-containing nAChRs are critical for mediating retinal waves.

Whole-cell voltage-clamp recordings from RGCs show that RGCs receive cholinergic and GABAergic inputs during retinal waves (Feller et al., 1996; Zheng et al., 2004). During development, activation of $GABA_A$ receptors is excitatory (Zhang et al., 2006) and therefore provides some of the depolarization associated with waves (Stellwagen et al., 1999; Wong et al., 2000). However, blockade of $GABA_A$ receptors does not alter the frequency of retinal waves and therefore is not thought to play a critical role in the generation of stage II retinal waves (Stellwagen et al., 1999).

The only source of ACh in the retina is a class of interneurons called starburst amacrine cells (SACs) (Vaney, 1990; Zhou, 2001b), though there is some evidence of transient high expression of ACh in horizontal cells during development (Zhou, 2001b). The properties of SACs and the SAC network are sufficient to explain most characteristics of stage II retinal waves. Direct recordings from SACs indicate they receive synaptic input during waves (Butts et al., 1999; Zheng et al., 2004). In addition, SACs form nAChR-mediated synapses with each other and with RGCs (Zhou, 1998; Zheng et al., 2004, 2006). Paired recordings from SACs show that neighboring SACs monosynaptically release both ACh and GABA onto one another and that each SAC receives input from around 20 other SACs (Zheng et al., 2004, 2006). Current-clamp recordings from SACs show that when all synaptic transmission is blocked, SACs undergo spontaneous depolarizations, followed by long, Ca^{2+}-dependent after-hyperpolarizations (AHPs) (Zheng et al., 2006). The model for how these properties of SACs combine to create stage II retinal waves is as follows (Zheng et al., 2006): (1) Individual SACs spontaneously depolarize and release small amounts of ACh onto other SACs. (2) When a critical mass of neighboring SACs spontaneously depolarize concurrently, they release enough ACh onto other neighboring SACs, causing them to depolarize, and the newly recruited SACs in turn excite other SACs, causing a wave to propagate across the retina. (3) The large calcium influx caused by the depolarization during the wave elicits a large AHP that decays over 30 s. This AHP is the basis of the 30 s refractory period. (4) SACs also synapse onto RGCs, so that when waves of depolarization pass through the SAC network, RGCs receive cholinergic input from the SACs and GABAergic input from SACs or other amacrine cells. ACh and GABA both excite RGCs, causing the RGCs to fire the bursts of action potentials that characterize retinal waves.

Interestingly, in contrast to RGCs, which express nAChRs in the adult retina, expression of nAChRs in SACs decreases with postnatal development (Zheng et al., 2004). Hence, downregulation of nAChRs on SACs may be responsible for the end of stage II retinal waves.

The hypothesis that stage II waves are initiated and propagate through a network of spontaneously active SACs is quite compelling, but there is much left to be explained. First, it is important to note that these experiments have all been done in rabbit retina and have not yet been reproduced in the mouse, though the circuitry is likely to be similar. Second, the channel that underlies the spontaneous depolarization of SACs, and what causes it to be activated, are not yet known. Third, the AHP is mediated by a potassium conductance that is calcium dependent and strongly modulated by cAMP levels; its identity is also unknown. Fourth, it is not known whether these conductances are unique to SACs. In a study of dissociated rat retinal neurons, both cholinergic and noncholinergic amacrine cells exhibited spontaneous, cell-autonomous depolarizations (Firth and Feller, 2006), though these findings have not been reproduced in the intact retina. By verifying this model of stage II retinal wave initiation and propagation in the mouse, targeted gene knockouts will allow the testing of specific hypotheses.

Gap junctions and stage II retinal waves

The role of gap junctions in stage II retinal waves is unclear. Gap junctions coordinate neuronal firing in many brain areas, including the adult retina (Connors and Long, 2004; Sohl et al., 2005), and extensive gap junction coupling exists in the neonatal retina (Penn et al., 1994; Catsicas et al., 1998). Gap junction antagonists have been used extensively to study the role of coupling in retinal waves, but the results of these pharmacological studies are inconsistent: in some studies gap junction antagonists block retinal waves (Hansen et al., 2005), in others they do not (Stacy et al., 2005). Part of the difficulty may arise from the fact that gap junction antagonists have nonspecific effects such as blockade of voltage-gated calcium channels (Vessey et al., 2004). Another limitation to using general pharmacological agents to block gap junctions is that since most cells in the retina are gap junction coupled (Sohl et al., 2005), general gap junction antagonists do not identify specific coupled networks that may mediate retinal waves.

Recent evidence that gap junction coupling can mediate retinal wave propagation under certain conditions came from a study using a transgenic mouse in which SACs located in a large segment of the retina did not produce acetylcholine (ACh) (Stacy et al., 2005). At P3, ACh-knockout regions of the retina did not exhibit retinal waves. However, by P5, waves were recorded in ACh-knockout regions, and these waves were blocked by gap junction receptor antagonists, while retinal waves in wild-type littermates were not. Hence, expression of gap junctions can compensate for an absence of normal synaptic connections.

One way to circumvent the limitations of gap junction antagonists is to study retinal waves in transgenic mice with genes for specific connexins knocked out and reporter genes knocked in. Connexins are the proteins that make up gap junctions. Three connexins have been identified in neurons in the adult retina: Cx36, Cx45, and Cx57 (Sohl et al., 2005). Using a mouse in which the Cx36 gene is replaced by a β-galactosidase reporter (Deans et al., 2001, 2002), we have demonstrated that Cx36 is expressed during retinal development in RGCs, glycinergic AII amacrine cells, and cone bipolar cells (Hansen et al., 2005). Cx36−/− mice have mostly normal stage II retinal waves, though 15% of Cx36−/− RGCs tonically fire action potentials in the normally quiet periods between waves (Hansen et al., 2005; Torborg et al., 2005). Studies of retinal waves in other connexin knockout mice have not yet been completed. Perturbation of gap junctions has more dramatic effects during stage I and stage III retinal waves, as described in the next section.

Properties of stage I and stage III retinal waves

Stage I retinal waves, lasting from E16 to P0 in mice, are characterized by small clusters of synchronous increases in intracellular calcium that are insensitive to nAChR and $GABA_A$ receptor antagonists, as well as larger, nAChR-mediated waves (Bansal et al., 2000) (see figure 28.2*B*). Waves seen in E17 retinas do not always respect refractory boundaries defined by previous waves but do propagate with a similar speed to that of stage II retinal waves. This early activity is blocked by gap junction receptor antagonists (Zhou and Zhao, 2000; Stacy et al., 2005). Hence, the retina follows a similar developmental pattern observed in both the developing spinal cord and cortex in which early network connectivity is mediated by gap junctions, and this electrical coupling is reduced as chemical synapses mature (Roerig and Feller, 2000). Interestingly, mice lacking the nAChR α3 subunit are able to generate retinal waves through an extension of the stage I wave-generating mechanism (Bansal et al., 2000), perhaps similarly to the mice lacking ACh in a segment of the retina (Stacy et al., 2005). Hence, the mechanisms mediating stage I waves can be extended in the absence of normal spontaneously active retinal circuits.

The circuitry underlying stage III waves has not been identified, but it is probable that the SAC network is not the source of correlated activity. Stage III waves are not blocked by nAChR antagonists (Bansal et al., 2000). During stage III waves, SACs no longer undergo spontaneous depolarizations (Zheng et al., 2006). Furthermore, SACs do not express nAChRs, and the GABA they release onto one another is inhibitory (Zheng et al., 2004). These changes in the properties of SACs eliminate all recurrent excitation in the SAC network.

Blockade of $GABA_{A/C}$ and glycine receptors leads to an increase in stage III wave frequency (Zhou, 2001a; Syed et al., 2004), indicating that endogenous GABA release regulates wave initiation but is not critical for the generation of retinal waves. These changes correspond to the same point in development when activation of $GABA_A$ receptors becomes inhibitory (Fischer et al., 1998; Zhang et al., 2006).

The role of gap junctions in stage III retinal waves is not fully elucidated. In Cx36−/− mice, RGCs have a significant increase in asynchronous firing of action potentials in the normally silent periods between retinal waves (Torborg et al., 2005). These extra action potentials are blocked by glutamate receptor antagonists (Hansen et al., 2005), indicating that Cx36-coupled networks normally suppress interwave release of glutamate. Cx36 is highly expressed in glycinergic AII amacrine cells, which make gap junction connections with other AII amacrine cells and cone bipolar cells. In addition, AII amacrine cells have a glycinergic input onto OFF cone bipolar cells (Pourcho and Goebel, 1985; Strettoi et al., 1992; Deans et al., 2002). Since both glycine and glutamate modulate the spontaneous firing of RGCs, one hypothesis is that Cx36 is critical for coordinating the release of these two transmitters.

Where are stage III waves initiated, and how do they propagate? Stage III glutamate receptor–mediated waves propagate at approximately twice the velocity and depolarize individual ganglion cells at approximately twice the frequency as stage II waves (Bansal et al., 2000; Muir-Robinson et al., 2002), consistent with stage III waves being mediated by mechanisms distinct from those mediating stage II waves. Stage III waves are blocked by ionotropic glutamate receptor antagonists (Bansal et al., 2000). Synapses containing ionotropic glutamate receptors are found between photoreceptors and OFF bipolar cells, between bipolar cells and amacrine cells, and between bipolar cells and RGCs. Additionally, a class of amacrine cells expressing vesicular glutamate transporter III at terminals presynaptic to RGCs and other amacrine cells has recently been identified (Haverkamp and Wässle, 2004; Johnson et al., 2004). Which of these components of the various glutamatergic circuits mediates stage III waves remains to be determined.

Retinal waves and the development of visual circuits

Retinal waves exist during a period of development when several different visual circuits are being established (for reviews, see Wong, 1999; Torborg and Feller, 2005). RGCs project to two primary targets in the brain, the SC and the dorsal lateral geniculate nucleus of the thalamus (dLGN). In these targets, RGCs respectively establish an arrangement of connections in target fields, termed a retinotopic map, that reflects the spatial arrangement of the RGCs in the retina, and eye-specific maps with inputs from the two retinas layering in neighboring but nonoverlapping regions. The precise retinotopic and eye-specific targeting of RGC axons observed in the adult mouse emerges prior to visual experience from initially diffuse and overlapping projections. In addition, during the first postnatal week, neurons in the dLGN are forming connections within the visual cortex, where they are also organized in precise retinotopic maps (Cang et al., 2005). In mice, there are no ocular dominance columns, although there is a distinct region of visual cortex where neurons receive inputs strongly driven by one eye or the other.

There is a clear role for both neural activity and molecular factors, such as the ephrins and their corresponding Eph receptors, in the establishment of these maps, though the relative importance of the two throughout the process of axon targeting and refinement is the subject of ongoing research (reviewed in O'Leary and McLaughlin, 2005). Controversy remains as to whether neural activity is instructive or permissive during these developmental events. If retinal waves play an instructive role in retinotopic map refinement, then retinotopic information must be contained within the spontaneous firing pattern (Crair et al., 2001; Eglen et al., 2003), and this information must be used to guide axonal refinement. Retinotopic information is in fact contained in the correlation structure of retinal waves: their propagating nature ensures that cells that are closer together are more temporally correlated in their firing than cells that are farther apart (Meister et al., 1991; Wong, 1993; Eglen et al., 2003). Alternatively, if retinal waves play a permissive role in retinotopic refinement, then the spontaneous firing pattern creates an environment in which molecular cues that contain retinotopic information, such as ephrins/Eph, can function. For example, in developing spinal cord, the periodicity of rhythmic activity affects the expression of axon guidance proteins (Hanson and Landmesser, 2004, 2006). Retinal waves periodically activate the cAMP/PKA pathway (Dunn et al., 2006), which may be critical for modulating protein function in individual RGCs.

Mice lacking β2-nAChRs have become a model system for establishing an instructive role for retinal waves in visual system development. β2-nAChR−/− mice do not have stage II retinal waves (Bansal et al., 2000). MEA recordings reveal that individual β2 RGCs fire bursts of action potentials, but these bursts are not correlated with the firing of neighboring cells (McLaughlin et al., 2003) (figure 28.3*A*). Indeed, the average firing rate of individual RGCs is the same in wild-type and β2 mice, but both the temporal structure within bursts and the nearest-neighbor correlations are significantly reduced. β2 mice have poorly refined retinotopic maps in their retinocollicular (Grubb et al., 2003; McLaughlin et al., 2003; Chandrasekaran et al., 2005; Pfeiffenberger et al., 2006) (figure 28.3*B*) and thalamocortical projections (Cang et al., 2005), as well as altered eye-specific layers in the dLGN (Rossi et al., 2001; Muir-Robinson et al., 2002; Pfeiffenberger et al., 2005), indicating that the correlated firing patterns induced by retinal waves is indeed important for the establishment of visual maps.

One caveat to the findings that visual maps are altered in β2 mice is that β2 mice are global knockouts, meaning β2 is lacking in the target tissue as well as in the retina (Moretti et al., 2004; Gotti et al., 2005). However, the observed phenotypes are likely to be due to the effects of β2 on retinal waves, since (1) they can be reproduced by intraocular injections of nAChR antagonists (Cang et al., 2005; Chandrasekaran et al., 2005; Pfeiffenberger et al., 2005) and (2) the defects are constrained to the time that retinal waves are altered. If the altered visual maps observed in β2 mice were due to, say, a defect in β2-mediated plasticity, this deficit should persist throughout the life of the mouse. However, β2 mice have mostly normal stage III retinal waves, and visual responses are quite robust. These later patterns of activity drive refinement in both the SC and dLGN (Muir-Robinson et al., 2002; Grubb et al., 2003; Chandrasekaran et al., 2005).

Not all manipulations that alter spontaneous retinal firing patterns alter visual map formation. For example, Cx36−/− mice, which have extra action potentials between retinal waves, have normal eye-specific layers (Torborg et al., 2005). In addition, pharmacological manipulations in ferrets that alter different features of the spontaneous firing patterns do not prevent normal eye-specific segregation (Stellwagen and Shatz, 2002; Huberman et al., 2003). Hence, the nature of the instructive signals provided by retinal waves is still controversial. An understanding of the cellular basis of the different features of spontaneous activity patterns, and therefore the ability to precisely manipulate activity patterns, will be critical for resolving this issue. Future studies in which targeted manipulations alter specific features of spontaneous activity patterns should help determine what features of retinal waves drive the normal development of visual circuits.

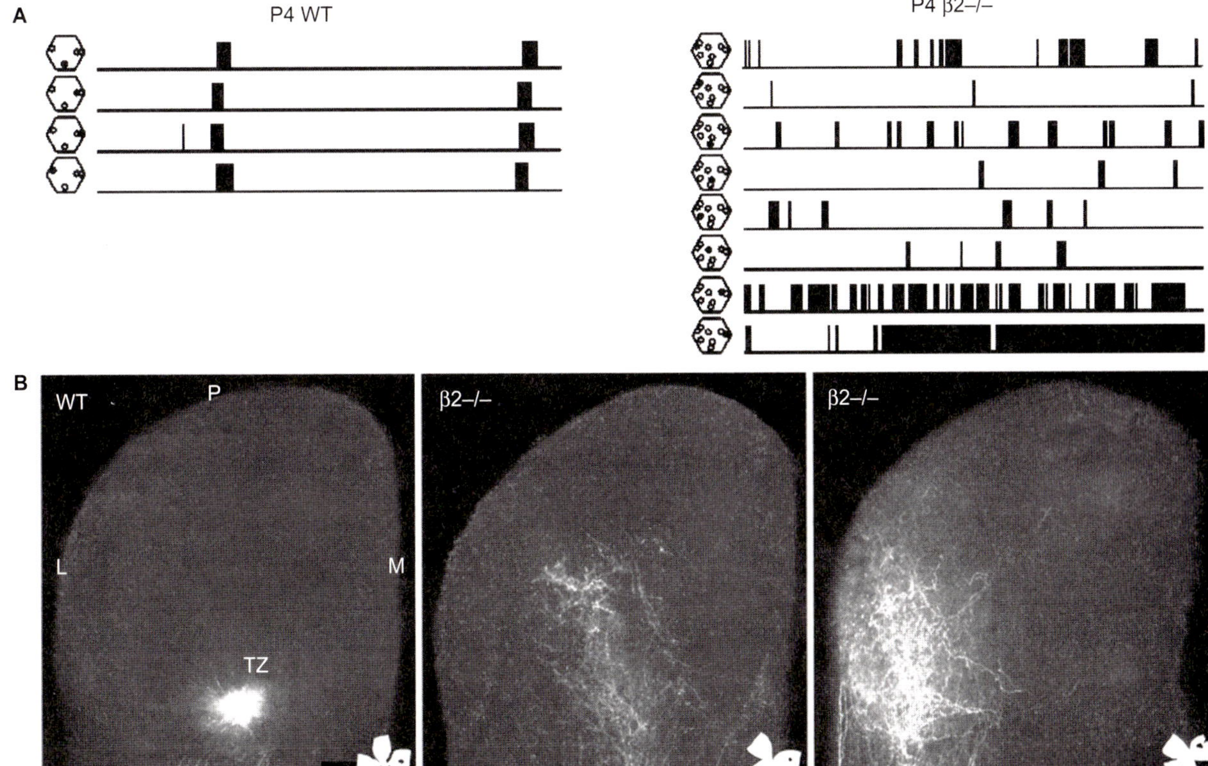

FIGURE 28.3 Knockout mice lacking the β2 subunit of nAChR have disrupted retinal firing patterns and altered retinotopic projections. *A*, β2–/– retinas have altered firing patterns during the first postnatal week. Spike trains were recorded with a multielectrode array (MEA) from four representative cells in a P4 wild-type retina and eight representative cells in a P4 β2–/– retina. Hexagons to the left of each spike train show the position of the electrode on which that unit was recorded (*black circle*) relative to the other represented units (*gray circles*). The maximum extent of the array is 480 μm. *B*, β2–/– mice have defective topographic remodeling of the retinocollicular projection. Fluorescence images of DiI-labeled RGC axons in SC of P8 wild-type (*left*) and β2–/– (*center* and *right*) mice. *Left*, Focal injection of DiI into the temporal retina of a P7 wild-type mouse reveals a single, densely labeled TZ in anterior SC at P8 characteristic of refined topographic organization of the mature retinocollicular projection. *Center* and *right*, Focal DiI injections, similar in size to that in *A*, into temporal retina of P7 β2–/– mice at P8 reveal TZs characterized by large domains of loosely organized arborizations. Temporal is to the right and dorsal is to the top for each retinal tracing. L, lateral; M, medial; P, posterior; Tz, termination zone. Scale bar = 250 μm. (Modified from McLaughlin et al., 2003.)

REFERENCES

BANSAL, A., SINGER, J. H., HWANG, B., and FELLER, M. B. (2000). Mice lacking specific nAChR subunits exhibit dramatically altered spontaneous activity patterns and reveal a limited role for retinal waves in forming ON/OFF circuits in the inner retina. *J. Neurosci.* 20:7672–7681.

BUTTS, D. A., FELLER, M. B., SHATZ, C. J., and ROKHSAR, D. S. (1999). Retinal waves are governed by collective network properties. *J. Neurosci.* 19:3580–3593.

CANG, J., RENTERIA, R. C., KANEKO, M., LIU, X., COPENHAGEN, D. R., and STRYKER, M. P. (2005). Development of precise maps in visual cortex requires patterned spontaneous activity in the retina. *Neuron* 48:797–809.

CATSICAS, M., BONNESS, V., BECKER, D., and MOBBS, P. (1998). Spontaneous Ca^{2+} transients and their transmission in the developing chick retina. *Curr. Biol.* 8:283–286.

CATSICAS, M., and MOBBS, P. (1995). Retinal development: Waves are swell. *Curr. Biol.* 5:977–979.

CHANDRASEKARAN, A. R., PLAS, D. T., GONZALEZ, E., and CRAIR, M. C. (2005). Evidence for an instructive role of retinal activity in retinotopic map refinement in the superior colliculus of the mouse. *J. Neurosci.* 25:6929–6938.

CONNORS, B. W., and LONG, M. A. (2004). Electrical synapses in the mammalian brain. *Annu. Rev. Neurosci.* 27:393–418.

CRAIR, M. C., HORTON, J. C., ANTONINI, A., and STRYKER, M. P. (2001). Emergence of ocular dominance columns in cat visual cortex by 2 weeks of age. *J. Comp. Neurol.* 430:235–249.

DEANS, M. R., GIBSON, J. R., SELLITTO, C., CONNORS, B. W., and PAUL, D. L. (2001). Synchronous activity of inhibitory networks in neocortex requires electrical synapses containing connexin36. *Neuron* 31:477–485.

DEANS, M. R., VÖLGYI, B., GOODENOUGH, D. A., BLOOMFIELD, S. A., and PAUL, D. L. (2002). Connexin36 is essential for transmission of rod-mediated visual signals in the mammalian retina. *Neuron* 36:703–712.

DEMAS, J., EGLEN, S. J., and WONG, R. O. (2003). Developmental loss of synchronous spontaneous activity in the mouse retina is independent of visual experience. *J. Neurosci.* 23:2851–2860.

Dunn, T. A., Wang, C. T., Colicos, M. A., Zaccolo, M., DiPilato, L. M., Zhang, J., Tsien, R. Y., and Feller, M. B. (2006). Imaging of cAMP levels and protein kinase a activity reveals that retinal waves drive oscillations in second-messenger cascades. *J. Neurosci.* 26:12807–12815.

Eglen, S. J., Demas, J., and Wong, R. O. (2003). Mapping by waves: Patterned spontaneous activity regulates retinotopic map refinement. *Neuron* 40:1053–1055.

Feller, M. B., Butts, D. A., Aaron, H. L., Rokhsar, D. S., and Shatz, C. J. (1997). Dynamic processes shape spatiotemporal properties of retinal waves. *Neuron* 19:293–306.

Feller, M. B., Wellis, D. P., Stellwagen, D., Werblin, F. S., Shatz, C. J. (1996). Requirement for cholinergic synaptic transmission in the propagation of spontaneous retinal waves. *Science* 272:1182–1187.

Firth, S. I., and Feller, M. B. (2006). Dissociated GABAergic retinal interneurons exhibit spontaneous increases in intracellular calcium. *Vis. Neurosci.* 23:807–814.

Firth, S. I., Wang, C. T., and Feller, M. B. (2005). Retinal waves: Mechanisms and function in visual system development. *Cell Calcium* 37:425–432.

Fischer, K. F., Lukasiewicz, P. D., and Wong, R. O. (1998). Age-dependent and cell class–specific modulation of retinal ganglion cell bursting activity by GABA. *J. Neurosci.* 18:3767–3778.

Fisher, L. J. (1979). Development of synaptic arrays in the inner plexiform layer of neonatal mouse retina. *J. Comp. Neurol.* 187:359–372.

Galli, L., and Maffei, L. (1988). Spontaneous impulse activity of rat retinal ganglion cells in prenatal life. *Science* 242:90–91.

Gotti, C., Moretti, M., Zanardi, A., Gaimarri, A., Champtiaux, N., Changeux, J. P., Whiteaker, P., Marks, M., Clementi, F., et al. (2005). Heterogeneity and selective targeting of nAChR subtypes expressed on retinal afferents of the superior colliculus and lateral geniculate nucleus: Identification of a new native nAChR subtype α3 β2 (α5 or β3) enriched in retinocollicular afferents. *Mol. Pharmacol.* 68(4):1162–1171.

Grubb, M. S., Rossi, F. M., Changeux, J. P., and Thompson, I. D. (2003). Abnormal functional organization in the dorsal lateral geniculate nucleus of mice lacking the beta 2 subunit of the nicotinic acetylcholine receptor. *Neuron* 40:1161–1172.

Hansen, K. A., Torborg, C. L., Elstrott, J., and Feller, M. B. (2005). Expression and function of the neuronal gap junction protein connexin 36 in developing mammalian retina. *J. Comp. Neurol.* 493:309–320.

Hanson, M. G., and Landmesser, L. T. (2004). Normal patterns of spontaneous activity are required for correct motor axon guidance and the expression of specific guidance molecules. *Neuron* 43:687–701.

Hanson, M. G., and Landmesser, L. T. (2006). Increasing the frequency of spontaneous rhythmic activity disrupts pool-specific axon fasciculation and pathfinding of embryonic spinal motoneurons. *J. Neurosci.* 26:12769–12780.

Haverkamp, S., and Wässle, H. (2004). Characterization of an amacrine cell type of the mammalian retina immunoreactive for vesicular glutamate transporter 3. *J. Comp. Neurol.* 468:251–263.

Huberman, A. D., Wang, G. Y., Liets, L. C., Collins, O. A., Chapman, B., and Chalupa, L. M. (2003). Eye-specific retinogeniculate segregation independent of normal neuronal activity. *Science* 300:994–998.

Johnson, J., Sherry, D. M., Liu, X., Fremeau, R. T., Jr., Seal, R. P., Edwards, R. H., and Copenhagen, D. R. (2004). Vesicular glutamate transporter 3 expression identifies glutamatergic amacrine cells in the rodent retina. *J. Comp. Neurol.* 477:386–398.

Martins-Ferreira, H., De Oliveira Castro, G., Struchiner, C. J., and Rodrigues, P. S. (1974). Circling spreading depression in isolated chick retina. *J. Neurophysiol.* 37:773–784.

Martins-Ferreira, H., Nedergaard, M., and Nicholson, C. (2000). Perspectives on spreading depression. *Brain Res. Brain Res. Rev.* 32:215–234.

Masland, R. H. (1977). Maturation of function in the developing rabbit retina. *J. Comp. Neurol.* 175:275–286.

McGehee, D. S., and Role, L. W. (1995). Physiological diversity of nicotinic acetylcholine receptors expressed by vertebrate neurons. *Annu. Rev. Physiol.* 57:521–546.

McLaughlin, T., Torborg, C. L., Feller, M. B., and O'Leary, D. D. (2003). Retinotopic map refinement requires spontaneous retinal waves during a brief critical period of development. *Neuron* 40:1147–1160.

Meister, M., Wong, R. O., Baylor, D. A., and Shatz, C. J. (1991). Synchronous bursts of action potentials in ganglion cells of the developing mammalian retina. *Science* 252:939–943.

Moretti, M., Vailati, S., Zoli, M., Lippi, G., Riganti, L., Longhi, R., Viegi, A., Clementi, F., and Gotti, C. (2004). Nicotinic acetylcholine receptor subtypes expression during rat retina development and their regulation by visual experience. *Mol. Pharmacol.* 66:85–96.

Morgan, J., and Wong, R. O. L. (2006). Development of cell types and synaptic connections in the retina. In H. Kolb, E. Fernandez, and R. Nelson (Eds.), *Webvision: The organization of the retina and the visual system* (http://webvision.med.utah.edu/index.html).

Muir-Robinson, G., Hwang, B. J., and Feller, M. B. (2002). Retinogeniculate axons undergo eye-specific segregation in the absence of eye-specific layers. *J. Neurosci.* 22:5259–5264.

O'Leary, D. D., and McLaughlin, T. (2005). Mechanisms of retinotopic map development: Ephs, ephrins, and spontaneous correlated retinal activity. *Prog. Brain Res.* 147:43–65.

Olney, J. W. (1968). An electron microscopic study of synapse formation, receptor outer segment development, and other aspects of developing mouse retina. *Invest. Ophthalmol.* 7:250–268.

Penn, A. A., Riquelme, P. A., Feller, M. B., and Shatz, C. J. (1998). Competition in retinogeniculate patterning driven by spontaneous activity. *Science* 279:2108–2112.

Penn, A. A., Wong, R. O., and Shatz, C. J. (1994). Neuronal coupling in the developing mammalian retina. *J. Neurosci.* 14:3805–3815.

Pfeiffenberger, C., Cutforth, T., Woods, G., Yamada, J., Renteria, R. C., Copenhagen, D. R., Flanagan, J. G., and Feldheim, D. A. (2005). Ephrin-As and neural activity are required for eye-specific patterning during retinogeniculate mapping. *Nat. Neurosci.* 8:1022–1027.

Pfeiffenberger, C., Yamada, J., and Feldheim, D. A. (2006). Ephrin-As and patterned retinal activity act together in the development of topographic maps in the primary visual system. *J. Neurosci.* 26:12873–12884.

Pourcho, R. G., and Goebel, D. J. (1985). A combined Golgi and autoradiographic study of (3H)glycine-accumulating amacrine cells in the cat retina. *J. Comp. Neurol.* 233:473–480.

Prince, D. A., and Connors, B. W. (1986). Mechanisms of interictal epileptogenesis. *Adv. Neurol.* 44:275–299.

Roerig, B., and Feller, M. B. (2000). Neurotransmitters and gap junctions in developing neural circuits. *Brain Res. Brain Res. Rev.* 32:86–114.

Role, L. W., and Berg, D. K. (1996). Nicotinic receptors in the development and modulation of CNS synapses. *Neuron* 16: 1077–1085.

Rossi, F. M., Pizzorusso, T., Porciatti, V., Marubio, L. M., Maffei, L., and Changeux, J. P. (2001). Requirement of the nicotinic acetylcholine receptor beta 2 subunit for the anatomical and functional development of the visual system. *Proc. Natl. Acad. Sci. U.S.A.* 98:6453–6458.

Sargent, P. B. (1993). The diversity of neuronal nicotinic acetylcholine receptors. *Annu. Rev. Neurosci.* 16:403–443.

Sernagor, E., Eglen, S. J., and O'Donovan, M. J. (2000). Differential effects of acetylcholine and glutamate blockade on the spatiotemporal dynamics of retinal waves. *J. Neurosci.* 20: RC56(1–6).

Sernagor, E., and Grzywacz, N. M. (1999). Spontaneous activity in developing turtle retinal ganglion cells: Pharmacological studies. *J. Neurosci.* 19:3874–3887.

Sernagor, E., Young, C., and Eglen, S. J. (2003). Developmental modulation of retinal wave dynamics: Shedding light on the GABA saga. *J. Neurosci.* 23:7621–7629.

Singer, J. H., Mirotznik, R. R., and Feller, M. B. (2001). Potentiation of L-type calcium channels reveals nonsynaptic mechanisms that correlate spontaneous activity in the developing mammalian retina. *J. Neurosci.* 21:8514–8522.

Sohl, G., Maxeiner, S., and Willecke, K. (2005). Expression and functions of neuronal gap junctions. *Nat. Rev. Neurosci.* 6:191–200.

Somjen, G. G. (2001). Mechanisms of spreading depression and hypoxic spreading depression-like depolarization. *Physiol. Rev.* 81:1065–1096.

Stacy, R. C., Demas, J., Burgess, R. W., Sanes, J. R., and Wong, R. O. (2005). Disruption and recovery of patterned retinal activity in the absence of acetylcholine. *J. Neurosci.* 25:9347–9357.

Stellwagen, D., and Shatz, C. J. (2002). An instructive role for retinal waves in the development of retinogeniculate connectivity. *Neuron* 33:357–367.

Stellwagen, D., Shatz, C. J., and Feller, M. B. (1999). Dynamics of retinal waves are controlled by cyclic AMP. *Neuron* 24:673–685.

Strettoi, E., Raviola, E., and Dacheux, R. F. (1992). Synaptic connections of the narrow-field, bistratified rod amacrine cell (AII) in the rabbit retina. *J. Comp. Neurol.* 325:152–168.

Syed, M. M., Lee, S., Zheng, J., and Zhou, Z. J. (2004). Stage-dependent dynamics and modulation of spontaneous waves in the developing rabbit retina. *J. Physiol.* 560:533–549.

Torborg, C. L., and Feller, M. B. (2005). Spontaneous patterned retinal activity and the refinement of retinal projections. *Prog. Neurobiol.* 76:213–235. Epub 2005.

Torborg, C. L., Hansen, K. A., and Feller, M. B. (2005). High frequency, synchronized bursting drives eye-specific segregation of retinogeniculate projections. *Nat. Neurosci.* 8:72–78.

Vaney, D. I. (1990). Chapter 2. The mosaic of amacrine cells in the mammalian retina. *Prog. Retin. Res.* 9:49.

Vessey, J. P., Lalonde, M. R., Mizan, H. A., Welch, N. C., Kelly, M. E., and Barnes, S. (2004). Carbenoxolone inhibition of voltage-gated Ca channels and synaptic transmission in the retina. *J. Neurophysiol.* 92:1252–1256.

Wong, R. O. (1993). The role of spatio-temporal firing patterns in neuronal development of sensory systems. *Curr. Opin. Neurobiol.* 3:595–601.

Wong, R. O. (1998). Calcium imaging and multielectrode recordings of global patterns of activity in the developing nervous system. *Histochem. J.* 30:217–229.

Wong, R. O. (1999). Role of retinal waves in visual system development. *Ann. Rev. Neurosci.* 22:29–47.

Wong, R. O., Chernjavsky, A., Smith, S. J., and Shatz, C. J. (1995). Early functional neural networks in the developing retina. *Nature* 374:716–718.

Wong, R. O., Meister, M., and Shatz, C. J. (1993). Transient period of correlated bursting activity during development of the mammalian retina. *Neuron* 11:923–938.

Wong, W. T., Myhr, K. L., Miller, E. D., and Wong, R. O. (2000). Developmental changes in the neurotransmitter regulation of correlated spontaneous retinal activity. *J. Neurosci.* 20:351–360.

Zhang, L. L., Pathak, H. R., Coulter, D. A., Freed, M. A., and Vardi, N. (2006). Shift of intracellular chloride concentration in ganglion and amacrine cells of developing mouse retina. *J. Neurophysiol.* 95:2404–2416.

Zheng, J. J., Lee, S., and Zhou, Z. J. (2004). A developmental switch in the excitability and function of the starburst network in the mammalian retina. *Neuron* 44:851–864.

Zheng, J., Lee, S., and Zhou, Z. J. (2006). A transient network of intrinsically bursting starburst cells underlies the generation of retinal waves. *Nat. Neurosci.* 9:363–371.

Zhou, Z. J. (1998). Direct participation of starburst amacrine cells in spontaneous rhythmic activities in the developing mammalian retina. *J. Neurosci.* 18:4155–4165.

Zhou, Z. J. (2001a). A critical role of the strychnine-sensitive glycinergic system in spontaneous retinal waves of the developing rabbit. *J. Neurosci.* 21:5158–5168.

Zhou, Z. J. (2001b). The function of the cholinergic system in the developing mammalian retina. *Prog. Brain Res.* 131:599–613.

Zhou, Z. J., and Zhao, D. (2000). Coordinated transitions in neurotransmitter systems for the initiation and propagation of spontaneous retinal waves. *J. Neurosci.* 20:6570–6577.

29 ON and OFF Pathways in the Mouse Retina and the Role of Stimulation

NING TIAN

Parallel processing of neuronal signals is a fundamental feature of most if not all sensory systems in vertebrates. In the visual system, the most extensively studied example is the parallel processing of increments and decrements in luminance of visual stimulation by two separate synaptic pathways, the ON and OFF pathways. The separation of these two synaptic pathways starts at the first synapse between photoreceptors and bipolar cells in the outer retina. They remain separated to a large extent in the inner retina, the lateral geniculate nucleus (LGN), and the visual cortex. The separation of ON and OFF signals forms the basis of virtually all visual signal processing in higher centers of visual system.

Although much has been learned about the structures and function of the synaptic pathways in mature retinas, considerably less is known about how retinal synaptic pathways are formed during development and what regulatory mechanisms may guide maturation of the retinal synaptic pathways. It was earlier assumed that retinal synaptic circuitry matures early in development. It is indeed the case that many aspects of synaptic signaling in the retina reach maturity before the retina begins receiving visual stimulation. For example, by the time of eye opening in rodents, rabbits, cats, and ferrets, most of the morphological features of the retina and the expression of synthesizing enzymes, transporters, and receptors for neurotransmitters of retinal neurons resemble those in adult animals (Fisher 1979b; Greiner and Weidman, 1981; Redburn and Madtes, 1987; Sassoe-Pognetto and Wässle, 1997; Pow and Barnett, 2000; Johnson et al., 2003). However, recent studies have demonstrated that connectivity between neurons, synaptic structures and functions, and the neuronal processing of mammalian retina can be modified and refined before and after eye opening during postnatal development.

In this chapter I discuss the development of ON and OFF pathways in the retina and the possible roles of visual stimulation in the maturation of these synaptic pathways. I first highlight the basic cellular/synaptic structure and the developmental processes of ON and OFF pathways, focusing on the developmental segregation of retinal ganglion cell (RGC) dendrites into ON and OFF pathways. I then review the modifications of maturation of ON and OFF pathways induced by alteration of synaptic activity during postnatal development of the mouse retina. Finally, I discuss the possible mechanisms regulating the developmental segregation of ON and OFF pathways in mouse retina. Although some of the evidence discussed in this chapter is from other mammalian species, the major conclusions derived from those data appear to apply well to mouse retina. This is reflected in an excellent review that addressed the similar developmental processes of ON and OFF synaptic pathways primarily based on the observations from cats and ferrets (Chalupa and Günhan, 2004).

Cellular and synaptic structure of retinal ON and OFF pathways

The detailed organization of the mouse retinal synaptic pathways is described in other chapters; here I highlight only the cellular and synaptic structure of the ON and OFF pathways. The separation of ON and OFF pathways originates at the first synapse between photoreceptors (rods and cones) and bipolar cells in the outer retina (figure 29.1). In all vertebrate retinas, light stimulation hyperpolarizes the membrane potentials of photoreceptors and decreases the synaptic release of glutamate from these cells. Glutamate released from photoreceptors activates an ionotropic glutamate receptor on cone OFF bipolar cells and depolarizes their membrane potentials. On cone ON bipolar cells and on all rod bipolar cells, glutamate activates a metabotropic glutamate receptor and hyperpolarizes the membrane potentials of these cells (see chapters 12 and 14, this volume, for details). This sign-reversing and nonreversing action of glutamate on the ON and OFF bipolar cells separates the increment and decrement luminance signals into ON and OFF pathways.

Different from ON and OFF bipolar cells, which have different types of glutamate receptors at their postsynaptic

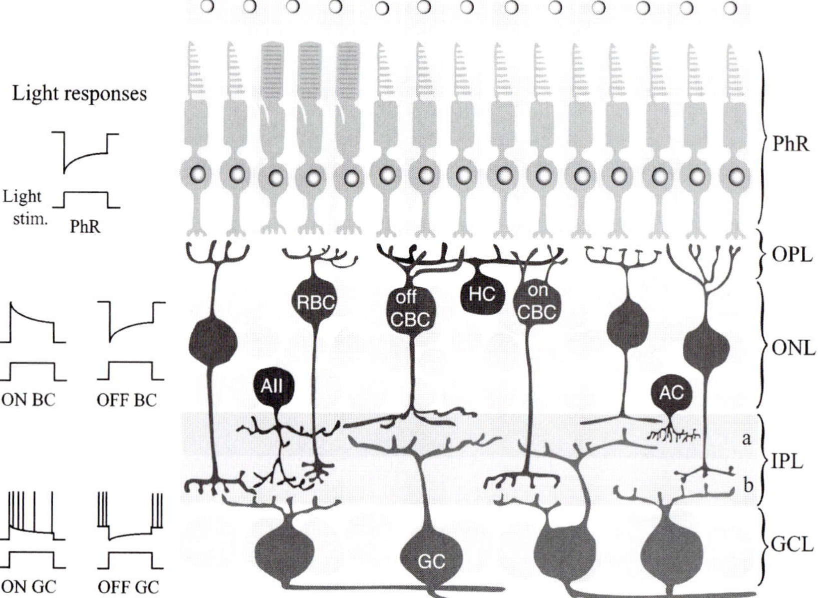

FIGURE 29.1 Schematic drawing of the principal anatomical components, synaptic connections, and representative light responses of ON and OFF pathways of mammalian retina. Photoreceptors (rods and cones) synapse with bipolar and horizontal cells in the OPL. ON and OFF signals are generated in the OPL by the activation of metabotropic and ionotropic glutamate receptors on ON and OFF bipolar cells, respectively. For the cone bipolar cells, whereas all ON bipolar cells synapse with RGCs in sublamina b, all OFF bipolar cells make synapses with RGCs in sublamina a of IPL. A subpopulation of RGCs receives synaptic inputs from both ON and OFF bipolar cells. Bipolar cells that receive rod inputs synapse with AII amacrine cells, which in turn make electrical synapses with cone OFF bipolar cells and chemical synapses with cone ON bipolar cells. Light responses in outer retinal neurons, such as photoreceptors and bipolar and horizontal cells, are graded potentials. In the inner retina, transient signals and spikes originate on RGCs and amacrine cells. AC, amacrine cell; AII, AII amacrine cell; GC, ganglion cell; HC, horizontal cell; Off CBC, cone OFF bipolar cell; On CBC, cone ON bipolar cell; PhR, photoreceptor; RBC, rod bipolar cell. (Adapted from Xu and Tian, 2004.)

sites to transmit visual signals, all RGCs use ionotropic glutamate receptors at their synapses as their primary synaptic receptors to conduct glutamatergic synaptic inputs from bipolar cells. The separation of ON and OFF pathways at the level of synaptic inputs to RGCs relies on the RGC dendritic distribution and selective synaptic connections with ON and OFF bipolar cells in distinct sublaminae of the inner plexus layer (IPL). There are more than a dozen morphologically distinctive subtypes of RGCs in adult mouse retina (Rockhill et al., 2002; Sun et al., 2002; Diao et al., 2004; Kong et al., 2005; Coombs et al., 2006). Despite the enormous diversity in structural and functional properties among different subtypes of RGCs, all ON RGCs ramify their dendrites only in sublamina b (ON layer) of the IPL and synapse with cone ON bipolar cells. In contrast, all OFF RGCs ramify their dendrites only in sublamina a (OFF layer) of the IPL and synapse with cone OFF bipolar cells (Famiglietti and Kolb, 1976; Nelson et al., 1978). Thus, the ON and OFF pathways are maintained functionally and structurally separated. A subset of RGCs, the ON-OFF RGCs, ramify their dendrites in both sublaminae, synapse with both ON and OFF bipolar cells, and signal both the onset and termination of light (Amthor et al., 1984).

The rod bipolar cells, on the other hand, do not directly synapse with RGCs. Instead, they synapse with a specific group of amacrine cells, the AII amacrine cells, and depolarize these cells when light is on. The latter then depolarize cone ON bipolar cells through gap junction connections and hyperpolarize cone OFF bipolar cells and OFF RGCs by releasing the inhibitory neurotransmitter glycine onto these cells (Bloomfield and Dacheux, 2001). Therefore, the separation of rod-driven ON and OFF signals starts at the synaptic connections between AII amacrine cells and cone bipolar cells.

Development of retinal synaptic circuitry and the segregation of ON and OFF pathways

The development of mammalian retinal synaptic circuitry is commonly described as a two-step process. The first step includes the commitment of major cell types and the establishment of an initial synaptic circuitry. The second step includes remodeling of the fine structure of cell-cell connections to form specific synaptic pathways. In rodents, most of the cellular and molecular machinery required for synaptic transmission between retinal neurons develops during the period shortly before and after birth (figure 29.2*A*). RGCs are the first neurons to differentiate, followed by cones, amacrine, and horizontal cells before birth, and then rods, bipolar cells, and Müller cells after birth (Marquardt and Gruss, 2002; Xu and Tian, 2004). Synaptogenesis follows a somewhat similar order as neurogenesis (Maslim and Stone, 1986; Nishimura and Rakic, 1987). Morphologically identified conventional synapses between amacrine and RGCs in the IPL appear during the first postnatal week. Then cones and rods establish synaptic connectivity with horizontal cells in the outer plexus layer (OPL). The last element to establish synaptic connectivity during development is the bipolar cells, which provide postsynaptic dendrites to photoreceptors and horizontal cells in the OPL and presynaptic axons to amacrine cells and RGCs in the IPL. In mouse retina, bipolar cells start to form synapses in the OPL and IPL early in the second postnatal week (Fisher, 1979b). At this time a synaptic link is completed that is needed to elicit light responses in RGCs (Maslim and Stone, 1986; Nishimura and Rakic, 1987). Consistent with the time course of synaptogesis characterized by morphology, functional synaptic transmission carried by vesicular γ-aminobutyric acid (GABA) and glycine release from amacrine cells was found preceding vesicular glutamate transmission from bipolar cells in developing mouse retina, and the spontaneous glutamatergic synaptic inputs from bipolar cells in mouse RGCs were recorded as early as P7 (Johnson et al., 2003).

Synaptogenesis continues for several weeks after establishment of the initial synaptic connections from photoreceptor to RGCs (figure 29.2*B*). In mouse, the density of conventional synapses in the IPL increases rapidly from 85 synapses/1,000 μm^3 at the ages of P3–P10 to 223 synapses/1,000 μm^3 around the time of eye opening (P11–P15), which is very close to the adult level. The density of ribbon synapses between bipolar cells and RGCs in the IPL, on the other hand, is low around the time of eye opening (45 synapses/1,000 μm^3) and increases about 2.5-fold 3 weeks after eye opening to reach the adult level (Fisher, 1979b). Consistently, functional features of synaptic maturation, measured as the frequency of vesicle-mediated spontaneous synaptic transmitter release, increase continuously with synaptogenesis (see figure 29.2*B*). The rates of AMPA receptor–mediated spontaneous excitatory postsynaptic currents and GABA/glycine receptor–mediated spontaneous inhibitory postsynaptic currents remain constant for a few days after eye opening and then surge fourfold around 2 weeks after eye opening, reaching a plateau by P60 (Tian and Copenhagen, 2001).

In addition to the developmental increase in the number of synapses and the frequency of spontaneous synaptic transmitter release, the initially established retinal synaptic circuitry is profoundly refined morphologically and functionally during postnatal development to form specific synaptic pathways, such as ON and OFF pathways. Early in postnatal development, the dendrites of RGCs ramify diffusely throughout the IPL in mammalian retinas (Maslim and Stone, 1988; Bodnarenko and Chalupa, 1993; Bodnarenko et al., 1995, 1999; Bansal et al., 2000; Wang et al., 2001;

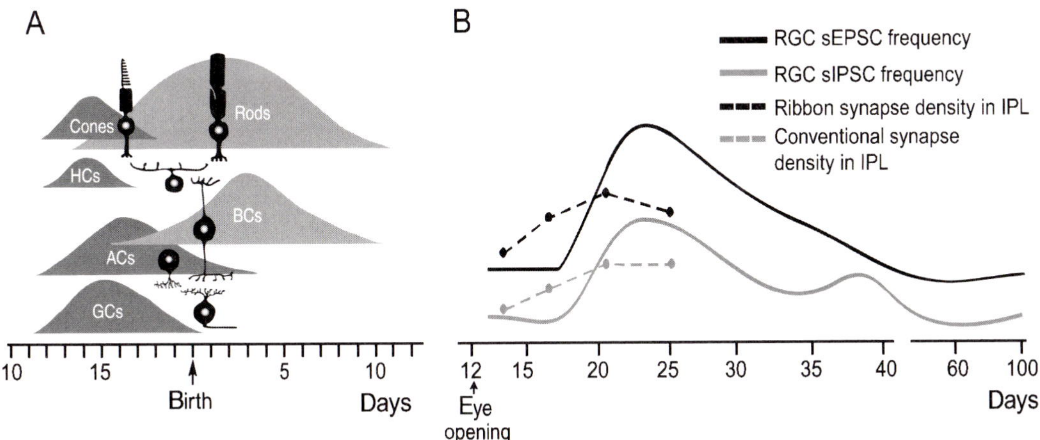

FIGURE 29.2 Neurogenesis and synaptogenesis in developing retina. *A*, Neurogenesis in rodent retina begins before birth and is largely completed shortly after birth. There are roughly two waves in retinal neurogenesis. The differentiation of RGCs, horizontal cells, amacrine cells, and cones starts early during prenatal development and is mostly completed before birth. The differentiation of rods and bipolar cells, however, starts shortly before birth and continues for 1–2 weeks after birth. (Modified from Young, 1985.) *B*, Synaptogenesis of mouse retina starts before eye opening and continues for several weeks after eye opening. The density of both ribbon and conventional synapse in IPL reaches a peak at age P21. (Modified from Fisher, 1979a.) The frequency of RGC spontaneous synaptic inputs increases with age and peaks around 2 weeks after eye opening. (Modified from Tian and Copenhagen, 2001.) The curves show the relative cell populations, synaptic densities, and frequencies of spontaneous synaptic inputs as functions of time. Numbers indicate prenatal and postnatal days of murine development. sEPSC, spontaneous excitatory postsynaptic current; sIPSC, spontaneous inhibitory postsynaptic current.

Diao et al., 2004), where they could synapse with both ON and OFF bipolar cells. With subsequent maturation, RGC dendrites are seen to be much more narrowly stratified, with most or all of the arbors restricted to sublamina a or b. This laminar refinement predicts there is an age-dependent decrease in the number of RGCs receiving synaptic inputs from both ON and OFF bipolar cells. Indeed, analysis of RGC dendritic arborization in mouse retina shows that whereas 53% of RGCs in P10-aged animals ramify in both sublaminae a and b of IPL, only 29% of mouse RGCs in P30-aged animals ramify in both sublaminae a and b (Tian and Copenhagen, 2003).

The developmental stratification of RGC dendritic arbors is reflected physiologically as an age-dependent decrease in the number of RGCs that respond with spikes at the onset and termination of a light. This maturational decline in the percentages of ON-OFF responding RGCs has been observed electrophysiologically in mouse, cat, and ferret retinas (Bisti et al., 1998; Wang et al., 2001; Tian and Copenhagen, 2003). These results serve to illuminate the observation that, because the ON and OFF sublaminae of the IPL are so well regulated, the retina is one of the best places in the nervous system to directly link structural characteristics with functional responsiveness at the cellular level.

As a technical note, it should be mentioned that the morphological characterization of RGC dendritic patterns has been facilitated significantly by the availability of mouse lines in which GFP or YFP is driven by the Thy1 promoter (Feng et al., 2000). In line H of the Thy1-YFP-expressing mice, several dozen YFP-labeled RGCs are randomly distributed throughout the retina (figure 29.3*A*) with minimal overlap of their dendritic fields (figure 29.3*B*). Confocal microscopy of these individual cells in whole mounted retinas provides a precise measurement of the fine structure of the arborization patterns of RGC dendrites and the distribution in the IPL (figure 29.3*C–F*).

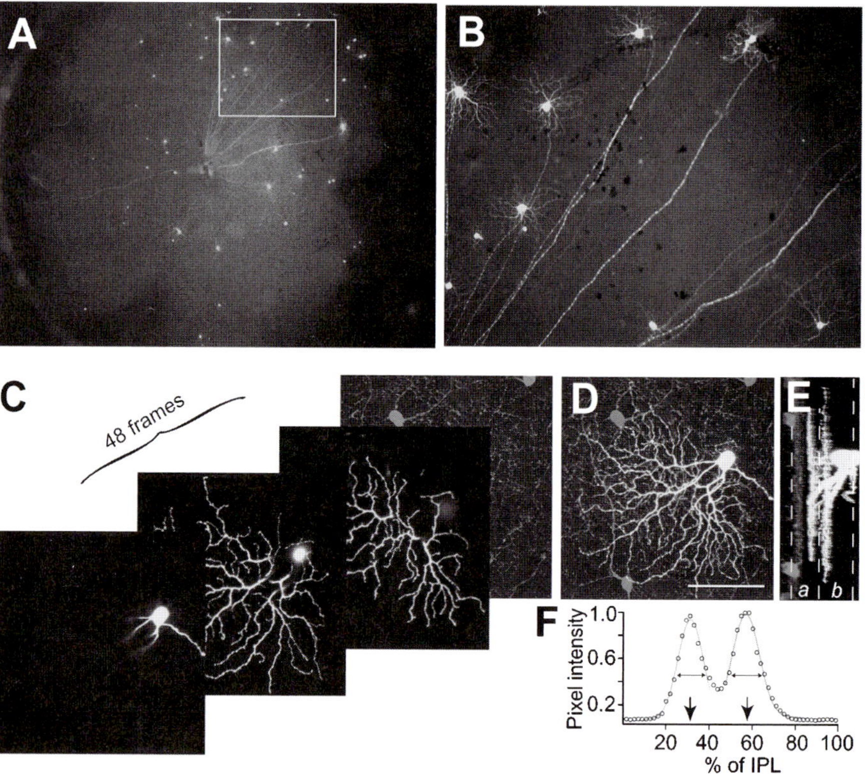

Figure 29.3 Dendritic ramification patterns of YFP expressing RGCs in the IPL can be determined using confocal microscopy from Thy1-YFP transgenic mouse retina. *A*, View from vitreal side of a flat-mounted retina harvested from a Thy1-YFP-expressing mouse. *B*, Enlarged view of the area inside the *box* in *A*. Axons from individual RGCs cross the retina from each soma to the optic nerve head. *C*, Four frames taken from a representative stack of confocal images of a bistratified RGC showing the soma and axon, the dendrites ramified in sublamina b (blue), the dendrites ramified in sublamina a (green) of the RGC, and immunolabeling of dopaminergic amacrine cells (red). *D*, A stacked image of the same cell as shown in panel *C*. *E*, The 90° rotation view of the cell in *D*. Three *dashed lines* indicate the inner border of the IPL, the boundary of sublaminae a and b, and the outer border of the IPL. *F*, Normalized pixel intensity of the dendrites of each frame (*open circles*) plotted as a function of IPL depth of the cell in panel *C*. The data were fitted with two Gaussian distributions (green and blue lines). *Double-arrow lines* indicate widths. *Single arrows* indicate the locations of the two peaks of dendritic density. See color plate 19.

How is the RGC dendritic stratification regulated in developing retina? It is postulated that RGCs achieve their mature stratified patterns by removing "misplaced" dendrites from diffuse ramification patterns. This pruning of RGC dendrites is one of the best examples of the maturational reorganization of neuronal processes (Wong and Ghosh, 2002) and has been found in cat (Dann et al., 1988; Maslim and Stone, 1988; Bodnarenko and Chalupa, 1993; Bodnarenko et al., 1995), ferret (Bodnarenko et al., 1999), rabbit (Wong, 1990), rat (Yamasaki and Ramoa, 1993), and mouse (Bansal et al., 2000; Diao et al., 2004). Although the exact underlying synaptic and molecular mechanisms regulating the RGC dendritic stratification are not clear, accumulating evidence suggests that this developmental refinement crucially depends on synaptic activities, including both spontaneous and visually evoked activities, before and after eye opening.

Synaptic activity and the developmental segregation of ON and OFF pathways

Both the spontaneous activity present early in postnatal development and visually evoked activity occurring later in postnatal development have been reported to influence the developmental refinement of RGC dendrites. In early developing retina, before an animal can respond to visual stimulation, RGCs fire periodic bursts of action potentials that are highly correlated and propagate across the RGC layer in a wavelike fashion (Wong, 1999). These spontaneous burst activities—namely, retina waves—are mediated by mainly excitatory neurotransmission, with a developmental shift from cholinergic to glutamatergic in mammalian retina (Wong, 1999; Wong et al., 2000). The retina wave had been implicated to direct the RGC axonal projections to their thalamus targets in LGN (see chapter 28, this volume, for details). Recent studies suggest that these spontaneous activities might also regulate RGC dendritic maturation, dendritic filopodial movement, and the maintenance or elimination of existing processes (Wong and Wong, 2000; Wong and Ghosh, 2002). Genetic deletion of the β subunit of nicotinic acetylcholine receptors diminished the retina wave mediated by acetylcholine receptors and slowed the stratification and segregation of RGC dendrites in the IPL during early (before P8) postnatal development. The retinas of the mutant mice had significantly narrower IPL, and RGC dendrites were not stratified or only weakly stratified into two distinct sublaminae. Between P8 and eye opening (P14), when retinal waves are mediated by ionotropic glutamate receptor–mediated transmission, the IPL of the mutant mice approximately doubled in size and RGC dendrites segregated into four or five distinguishable strata like those of wild-type animals, suggesting that both early cholinergic and later glutamatergic synaptic transmission contribute to the developmental refinement of RGC dendrites (Bansal et al., 2000).

The critical roles of glutamatergic synaptic inputs from bipolar cells to the developmental stratification and segregation of RGC dendrites into ON and OFF pathways were also demonstrated in another set of experiments. During the time period of normal dendritic stratification of RGCs, intraocular injection of APB, an agonist for class III metabotropic glutamate receptors exclusively expressed on the rod bipolar and cone ON bipolar cells, hyperpolarized these bipolar cells and blocked the glutamate release from these neurons, resulting in an arrest of the developmental stratification and segregation of RGC dendrites into ON or OFF layer of the IPL. About 40% of the RGCs in APB-treated adult retina have their dendrites multistratified in both sublaminae a and b of IPL, a significantly higher percentage than that seen in untreated age-matched controls (Bodnarenko and Chalupa, 1993; Bodnarenko et al., 1995, 1999), and this effect is irreversible with prolonged APB treatment (Deplano et al., 2004). In contrast, APB treatment did not alter the RGC density or somata and dendritic field size, demonstrating that excitatory synaptic inputs from bipolar cells have a highly selective impact on RGC dendritic stratification.

The role of visually evoked activity in the developmental segregation of RGC dendrites into ON and OFF pathways is shown by the finding that light deprivation retards the maturational conversion of RGCs ramified in both sublaminae a and b of the IPL into cells ramified only in sublamina a or b of the IPL. Tian and Copenhagen (2003) compared the lamination patterns of RGCs in cyclic light–reared mice to those in dark-reared mice. At P30, 53% of the RGCs ramified in both sublaminae a and b of the IPL in the dark-reared mice versus 29% in cyclic light–reared mice. This difference was highly significant. However, this percentage was very close to the P10-aged mice raised in cyclic light (53%). These anatomical findings predicted that many more RGCs in P30 dark-reared mice should be ON-OFF-responsive RGCs in comparison with age-matched controls. Multielectrode array recordings of light responses from RGCs verified this prediction. In the P27–P30-aged mice raised in constant darkness, the percentage of ON-OFF-responsive RGCs was more than fourfold higher than in age-matched controls raised in cyclic light but comparable to the percentage of ON-OFF-responsive RGCs in P10–P12-aged mice. These results demonstrated that light stimulation is critical for the developmental segregation of RGC dendrites into ON and OFF pathways.

Visual stimulation also influences other morphological and functional attributes of RGCs. In dark-reared mice, the density of conventional synapses in IPL is greater than in mice reared under cyclic light conditions (Fisher, 1979a). Light deprivation also blocked the age-dependent increase in spontaneous synaptic inputs to RGCs after eye opening in mouse retina (Tian and Copenhagen, 2001) and an age-dependent remodeling of dendritic complexity of a class of RGCs in hamster retina (Wingate and Thompson, 1994). In dark-reared turtle retina, receptive field areas of RGCs expanded to more than twice the size of those observed in animals reared under normal conditions, suggesting that visual experience plays a role in controlling the outgrowth of turtle RGC dendrites (Sernagor and Grzywacz, 1996). In developing rat retina, the expression of brain-derived neurotrophic factor, a factor that controls RGC dendrites arborization, is also modulated by visual experience (Seki, 2003).

Possible mechanisms of activity-dependent developmental segregation of ON and OFF pathways in the retina

It is unclear how synaptic activity regulates the developmental segregation of RGC dendrites into ON and OFF pathways. Chalupa and colleagues (1998) proposed two possible general synaptic mechanisms. In the first model, they assumed that RGCs synapse functionally with only ON or OFF bipolar cells in early postnatal development, although their dendrites ramify in both the inner and outer IPL (see figure 29.5*A*). The asymmetrical synaptic inputs from ON or OFF bipolar cells could "instruct" those RGCs to sever uninnervated dendrites during later postnatal development. If this were the case, one would expect to find RGCs stratified in both the inner and outer IPL but responding only to the onset or offset of light stimulation in the early postnatal developing retina. Recent results obtained with simultaneous patch-clamp and morphological recordings of ferret RGCs revealed that all RGCs with dendrites ramifying in both the inner and outer IPL responded to both the onset and offset of light in both young and adult animals, indicating that RGCs with dendrites ramifying in both inner and outer IPL are innervated by both ON and OFF bipolar cells (Wang et al., 2001). Consistent with these results, intraocular injection of APB or light deprivation increased both the ON-OFF-responsive and multistratified RGCs in cat (Bodnarenko and Chalupa, 1993; Bodnarenko et al., 1995; Bisti et al., 1998) and mouse (Tian and Copenhagen, 2003) retina, respectively. Thus, it appears unlikely that an asymmetry of ON and OFF synaptic inputs is responsible for the elimination of exuberant processes in immature RGCs.

In the second model, it was assumed that synaptic transmission from bipolar cells triggers an intrinsic program in RGCs ramifying in both inner and outer IPL that leads to the retraction of one or another set of their dendritic processes (see figure 29.5*B*). This model relies on cell-specific intrinsic genetic programs that activate differential pruning of an individual cell's dendrites in either sublamina a or b. No molecular or genetic mechanisms that would mediate this selective pruning have been identified.

These two models are proposed based on the common assumption that RGCs achieve their mature stratified patterns from early diffuse ramification patterns by selective pruning of "misplaced" dendrites. Although it is well documented that the dendrites of RGCs are diffusely ramified in the IPL in early development and then gradually stratified into narrow strata during postnatal development in many species of mammals, including mice, two recent studies showed that the dendrites of most RGCs in mouse retina are narrowly stratified in the IPL, similar to that of adult animals before eye opening (Bansal et al., 2000; Diao et al., 2004), suggesting that dendritic pruning is largely completed at the time of eye opening. Insofar as the percentage of RGCs responding to both the onset and offset of light declined from 40%–76% at the time of eye opening to around 20% in adult ferrets and mice (Wang et al., 2001; Tian and Copenhagen, 2003) and the population of RGCs with dendrites ramifying in both sublaminae a and b of the IPL decreased from 53% at eye opening to 29% 2–3 weeks after eye opening (Tian and Copenhagen, 2003), these results strongly suggest that the developmental segregation of RGC dendrites into ON and OFF pathways after eye opening is unlikely to be achieved by simply removing some "misplaced" dendrites from already narrowly stratified dendritic plexus.

How could a narrowly stratified RGC dendritic plexus reorganize synaptic connections with ON and OFF bipolar cells in different strata of the IPL in developing retina? A recent study of developing zebrafish retina using in vivo time-lapse imaging demonstrated that the lamina-restricted dendritic plexus of RGCs could "migrate" from the inner border of the IPL to the outer border of the IPL in 2–3 days without diffusely elaborating their dendrites throughout the IPL (Mumm et al., 2006). This redistribution of stratified dendritic plexus involves simultaneous adding dendrites in one stratum and eliminating dendrites in another stratum of the IPL during the course of development. Unfortunately, the same technique has not been successfully applied to the study of developing mammalian retina, and therefore it has not been directly demonstrated whether mammalian RGCs could take the same developmental strategy as zebrafish RGCs to redistribute their dendrites in the IPL (Chalupa, 2006).

Recently, we quantitatively analyzed the dendritic stratification and ramification patterns of RGCs of developing mouse retinas fixed at different developmental time points (Xu and Tian, 2007). Our results showed that the majority of mouse RGCs have narrowly stratified dendrites at the time of eye opening and a large portion of them have their dendrites located near the center of the IPL (figure 29.4*B*). Therefore, these RGCs could synapse with both ON and OFF bipolar cells and respond to both onset and offset of

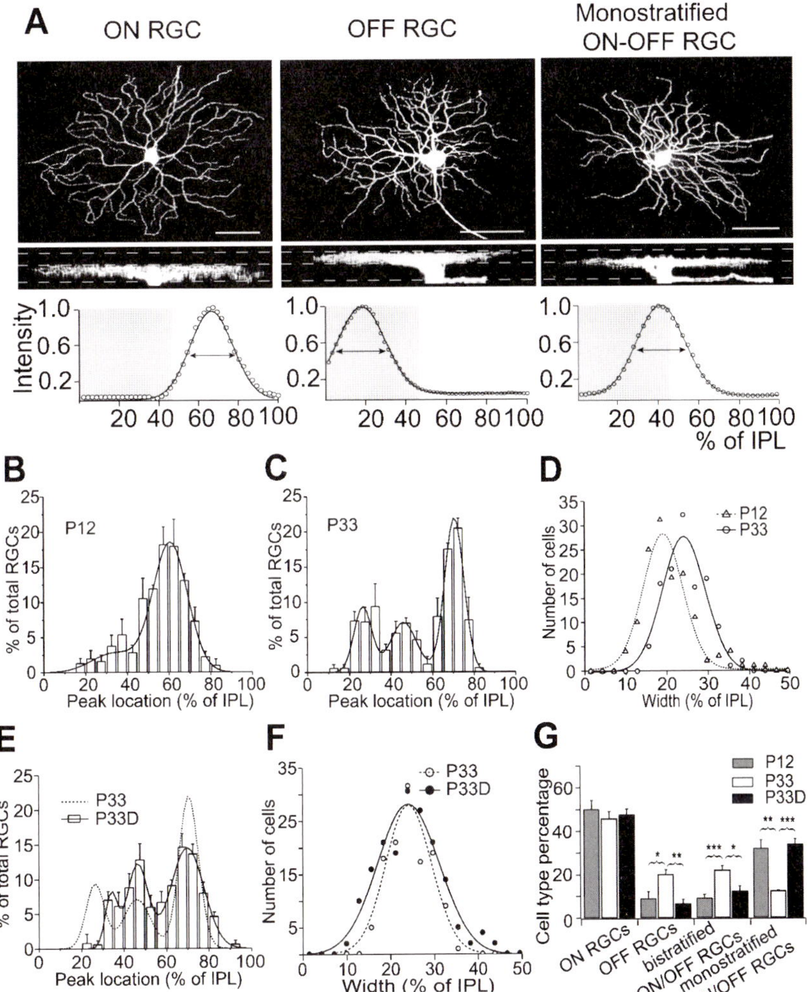

Figure 29.4 The developmental redistribution of RGC dendrites that altered the relative populations of RGCs receiving synaptic inputs from ON and OFF BC RGCs were classified into ON, OFF, monostratified ON-OFF, and bistratified ON-OFF RGCs based on their dendritic distribution patterns in the IPL. *A*, *Upper panels*, Stacked images of an ON RGC (*left*), an OFF RGC (*center*), and a monostratified ON-OFF RGC (*right*). *Middle panels*, 90° rotation views of the same three cells. *Lower panels*, Normalized dendritic distribution of each cell (*open circles*) and the Gaussian fitting of the data (*line*). *Shaded area* indicates the sublamina a. Scale bars = 100 µm. *B*, Average histogram of the peak dendritic location of all monostratified RGCs of P12-aged mice. The histogram fitted well with a double Gauss distribution, with a major peak located at 60% of IPL thickness and a minor peak located at 35% of IPL thickness, respectively ($\chi^2 = 0.536$, $r^2 = 0.984$). *C*, Average histogram of peak dendritic location of all monostratified RGCs of P33-aged mice. The histogram fitted well with a triple Gaussian distribution, with three peaks located at 25%, 50%, and 70% of IPL thickness, respectively ($\chi^2 = 0.686$, $r^2 = 0.989$). *D*, Distributions of the dendritic widths of monostratified RGCs from P12- and P33-aged mice and Gaussian fittings of the data. *E*, Average histogram of the peak dendritic distribution of monostratified RGCs of dark-reared mice and age-matched controls. The histogram of dark-reared mice fitted well with a triple Gaussian distribution ($\chi^2 = 0.603$, $r^2 = 0.982$). *F*, Distribution of dendritic widths of all three groups of monostratified RGCs of dark-reared and control mice and Gaussian fittings of the data. *G*, Average percentages of ON, OFF, bistratified ON-OFF, and monostratified ON-OFF RGCs of P12- and P33-aged mice raised in cyclic light (P33) and constant darkness (P33D). (Modified from Xu and Tian, 2007.)

light stimulation. After eye opening, the RGCs with dendrites located at the center of the IPL redistributed their dendrites close to the inner or outer border of the IPL (figure 29.4*C*) and therefore become ON or OFF cells, without a further reduction in the width of their dendritic stratification (figure 29.4*D* and *G*). Similar to the effects induced by long-term treatment of cats' eyes with intraocular injection of APB (Deplano et al., 2004), light deprivation preferentially retarded the dendritic redistribution of mouse RGCs from the center of the IPL to the OFF layer of the IPL (figure 29.4*E*) without changing the width of dendritic distribution (figure 29.4*F*), which resulted in more RGCs having dendrites located near the center of the IPL and receiving synaptic inputs from both ON and OFF bipolar cells (figure

29.4*G*). These results suggest that the dendritic refinement of mouse RGCs after eye opening requires both targeted dendritic growth and selective dendritic elimination, similar to what was reported in zebrafish by Mumm et al. (2006), and probably driven by visually evoked synaptic activity. It is also worth noting that the number of RGCs ramified in both sublaminae a and b of the IPL with a single layer of dendritic plexus (figure 29.4*A*, *right*) decreased with age, while the number of RGCs ramified in both sublaminae a and b of the IPL with clear bistratified dendritic patterns (see figure 29.3*E*) increased with age (see figure 29.4*G*), suggesting that monostratified and bistratified ON-OFF RGCs are likely to be in different developmental status.

When all of these findings are considered together, it appears that the maturation of mouse RGC dendrites and the developmental segregation of ON and OFF pathways in the retina undergo a multistage process during postnatal development. In early postnatal development, RGCs restrict their dendrites from a diffusely ramified pattern into narrowly stratified patterns, primarily through dendritic pruning before eye opening (figure 29.5*C*, step 1). At this stage, some of the RGCs ramify their dendrites only in sublamina a or b of the IPL, but a large number of RGCs still synapse with both ON and OFF bipolar cells in both sublaminae a and b. This initial dendritic pruning is at least in part regulated by spontaneous retinal activity. Later during postnatal development, narrowly stratified RGCs further refine their dendritic distribution in the IPL and synaptic connections with ON and OFF bipolar cells (figure 29.5*C*, step 2). This later refinement further segregates the RGC dendrites into ON and OFF pathways after eye opening and is regulated by visually evoked synaptic inputs from bipolar cells.

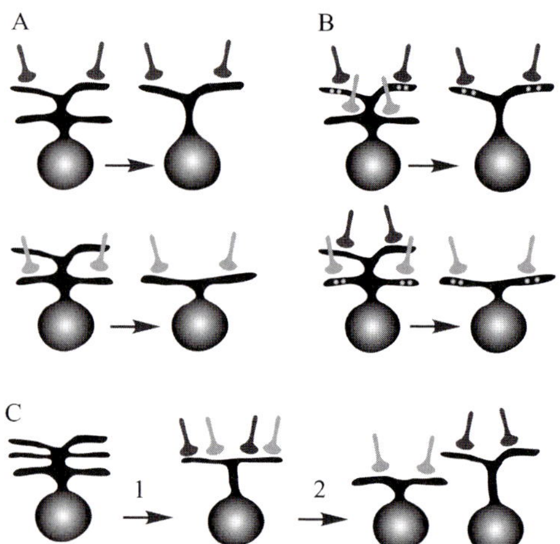

FIGURE 29.5 Schematic diagram illustrating possible mechanisms underlying RGC dendritic stratification and segregation. *A*, Asymmetrical afferent innervation model. RGCs have their dendrites initially bistratified in both ON and OFF sublaminae of IPL and have asymmetrical synaptic inputs. During development, dendrites that receive afferent inputs are maintained, whereas those that do not receive afferent input are eliminated. *B*, Intrinsic program model. Signal inputs from both ON and OFF bipolar cells trigger an intrinsic program in the bistratified RGCs, leading to elimination of the dendrites in either ON or OFF sublamina. *C*, Multistage model. The dendrites of mouse RGCs initially ramify diffusely throughout the IPL and then gradually are restricted to a narrowly stratified pattern before eye opening. After eye opening, RGCs further redistribute their dendrites into the ON or OFF layer of the IPL, probably guided by visually evoked synaptic activity.

REFERENCES

AMTHOR, F. R., OYSTER, C. W., and TAKAHASHI, E. S. (1984). Morphology of ON-OFF direction-selective ganglion cells in the rabbit retina. *Brain Res.* 298:187–190.

BANSAL, A., SINGER, J. H., HWANG, B. J., XU, W., BEAUDET, A., and FELLER, M. B. (2000). Mice lacking specific nicotinic acetylcholine receptor subunits exhibit dramatically altered spontaneous activity patterns and reveal a limited role for retinal waves in forming ON and OFF circuits in the inner retina. *J. Neurosci.* 20:7672–7681.

BISTI, S., GARGINI, C., and CHALUPA, L. M. (1998). Blockade of glutamate-mediated activity in the developing retina perturbs functional segregation of ON and OFF pathways. *J. Neurosci.* 18:5019–5025.

BLOOMFIELD, S. A., and DACHEUX, R. F. (2001). Rod vision: Pathways and processing in the mammalian retina. *Prog. Retin. Eye Res.* 20:351–384.

BODNARENKO, S. R., and CHALUPA, L. M. (1993). Stratification of ON and OFF ganglion cell dendrites depends on glutamate-mediated afferent activity in the developing retina. *Nature* 364: 144–146.

BODNARENKO, S. R., JEYARASASINGAM, G., and CHALUPA, L. M. (1995). Development and regulation of dendritic stratification in retinal ganglion cells by glutamate-mediated afferent activity. *J. Neurosci.* 15:7037–7045.

BODNARENKO, S. R., YEUNG, G., THOMAS, L., and MCCARTHY, M. (1999). The development of retinal ganglion cell dendritic stratification in ferrets. *Neuroreport* 10:2955–2959.

CHALUPA, L. M. (2006). Developing dendrites demonstrate unexpected specificity. *Neuron* 52:567–568.

CHALUPA, L. M., and GÜNHAN, E. (2004). Development of ON and OFF retinal pathways and retinogeniculate projections. *Prog. Retin. Eye Res.* 23:31–51.

CHALUPA, L. M., JEYARASASINGAM, G., SNIDER, C. J., and BODNARENKO, S. R. (1998). Development of ON and OFF retinal ganglion cell mosaics. In L. M. Chalupa and B. L. Finlay, (Eds.), *Development and organization of the retina: From molecules to function* (pp. 77–89). New York: Plenum Press.

COOMBS, J., VAN DER LIST, D., WANG, G. Y., and CHALUPA, L. M. (2006). Morphological properties of mouse retinal ganglion cells. *Neuroscience* 140:123–136.

DANN, J. F., BUHL, E. H., and PEICHL, L. (1988). Postnatal dendritic maturation of alpha and beta ganglion cells in cat retina. *J. Neurosci.* 8:1485–1499.

DEPLANO, S., GARGINI, C., MACCARONE, R., CHALUPA, L. M., and BISTI, S. (2004). Long-term treatment of the developing retina with the metabotropic glutamate agonist APB induces long-term changes in the stratification of retinal ganglion cell dendrites. *Dev. Neurosci.* 26:396–405.

Diao, L., Sun, W., Deng, Q., and He, S. (2004). Development of the mouse retina: Emerging morphological diversity of the ganglion cells. *J. Neurobiol.* 61:236–249.

Famiglietti, E. W., and Kolb, H. (1976). Structure basis for ON- and OFF-center responses in retinal ganglion cells. *Science* 194:193–195.

Feng, G., Mellor, R. H., Bernstein, M., Keller-Peck, C., Nguyen, Q. T., Wallace, M., Nerbonne, J. M., Lichtman, J. W., and Sanes, J. R. (2000). Imaging neuronal subsets in transgenic mice expressing multiple spectral variants of GFP. *Neuron* 28:41–51.

Fisher, L. J. (1979a). Development of retinal synaptic arrays in the inner plexiform layer of dark-reared mice. *J. Embryol. Exp. Morphol.* 54:219–227.

Fisher, L. J. (1979b). Development of synaptic arrays in the inner plexiform layer of neonatal mouse retina. *J. Comp. Neurol.* 187: 359–372.

Greiner, J. V., and Weidman, T. A. (1981). Histogenesis of the ferret retina. *Exp. Eye Res.* 33:315–332.

Johnson, J., Tian, N., Caywood, M. S., Reimer, R. J., Edwards, R. H., and Copenhagen, D. R. (2003). Vesicular neurotransmitter transporter expression in developing postnatal rodent retina: GABA and glycine precede glutamate. *J. Neurosci.* 23:518–529.

Kong, J. H., Fish, D. R., Rockhill, R. L., and Masland, R. H. (2005). Diversity of ganglion cells in the mouse retina: Unsupervised morphological classification and its limits. *J. Comp. Neurol.* 489:293–310.

Marquardt, T., and Gruss, P. (2002). Generating neuronal diversity in the retina: One for nearly all. *Trends Neurosci.* 25:32–38.

Maslim, J., and Stone, J. (1986). Synaptogenesis in the retina of the cat. *Brain Res.* 373:35–48.

Maslim, J., and Stone, J. (1988). Time course of stratification of the dendritic fields of ganglion cells in the retina of the cat. *Dev. Brain Res.* 44:87–93.

Mumm, J. S., Willams, P. R., Godinho, L., Kroeber, A., Pittman, A. J., Roeser, T., Chien, C. B., Bailer, H., and Wong, R. O. L. (2006). In vivo imaging reveals dendritic targeting of laminated afferents by zebrafish retinal ganglion cells. *Neuron* 52:609–621.

Nelson, R., Famiglietti, E. V. J., and Kolb, H. (1978). Intracellular staining reveals different levels of stratification for on- and off-center ganglion cells in cat retina. *J. Neurophysiol.* 41:472–483.

Nishimura, Y., and Rakic, P. (1987). Synaptogenesis in the primate retina proceeds from the ganglion cells towards the photoreceptors. *Neurosci. Res. Suppl.* 6:S253–S68.

Pow, D. V., and Barnett, N. L. (2000). Developmental expression of amino acid transporter 5: A photoreceptor and bipolar cell glutamate transporter in rat retina. *Neurosci. Lett.* 280:21–24.

Redburn, D. A., and Madtes, P. (1987). GABA: Its roles and development in retina. *Prog. Retin. Eye Res.* 6:69–84.

Rockhill, R. L., Daly, F. J., MacNeil, M. A., Brown, S. P., and Masland, R. H. (2002). The diversity of ganglion cells in a mammalian retina. *J. Neurosci.* 22:3831–3843.

Sassoe-Pognetto, M., and Wässle, H. (1997). Synaptogenesis in the rat retina: Subcellular localization of glycine receptors, GABA(A) receptors, and the anchoring protein gephyrin. *J. Comp. Neurol.* 381:158–174.

Seki, M., Nawa, H., Fukuchi, T., Abe, H., and Takei, N. (2003). BDNF is upregulated by postnatal development and visual experience: Quantitative and immunohistochemical analyses of BDNF in the rat retina. *Invest. Ophthalmol. Vis. Sci.* 44: 3211–3218.

Sernagor, E., and Grzywacz, N. M. (1996). Influence of spontaneous activity and visual experience on developing retinal receptive fields. *Curr. Biol.* 6:1503–1508.

Sun, W., Li, N., and He, S. (2002). Large-scale morphological survey of mouse retinal ganglion cells. *J. Comp. Neurol.* 451: 115–126.

Tian, N., and Copenhagen, D. R. (2001). Visual deprivation alters development of synaptic function in inner retina after eye opening. *Neuron* 32:439–443.

Tian, N., and Copenhagen, D. R. (2003). Visual stimulation is required for refinement of ON and OFF pathways in postnatal retina. *Neuron* 39:85–96.

Wang, G. Y., Liets, L. C., and Chalupa, L. M. (2001). Unique functional properties of ON and OFF pathways in the developing mammalian retina. *J. Neurosci.* 21:4310–4317.

Wingate, R. J. T., and Thompson, I. D. (1994). Targeting and activity-related dendritic modification in mammalian retinal ganglion cells. *J. Neurosci.* 14:6621–6637.

Wong, R. O. L. (1990). Differential growth and remodelling of ganglion cell dendrites in the postnatal rabbit retina. *J. Comp. Neurol.* 294:109–132.

Wong, R. O. L. (1999). Retinal waves and visual system development. *Annu. Rev. Neurosci.* 22:29–47.

Wong, R. O. L., and Ghosh, A. (2002). Activity-dependent regulation of dendritic growth and patterning. *Nat. Rev. Neurosci.* 3: 303–312.

Wong, W. T., Myhr, K. L., Miller, E. D., and Wong, R. O. L. (2000). Developmental changes in the neurotransmitter regulation of correlated spontaneous retinal activity. *J. Neurosci.* 20:351–360.

Wong, W. T., and Wong, R. O. L. (2000). Rapid dendritic movements during synapse formation and rearrangement. *Curr. Opin. Neurobiol.* 10:118–124.

Xu, H. P., and Tian, N. (2004). Pathway-specific maturation, visual deprivation, and development of retinal pathway. *Neuroscientist* 10:337–346.

Xu, H. P., and Tian, N. (2007). Retinal ganglion cell dendrites undergo a visual activity-dependent redistribution after eye-opening. *J. Comp. Neurol.* 503:244–259.

Yamasaki, E. N., and Ramoa, A. S. (1993). Dendritic remodelling of retinal ganglion cells during development of the rat. *J. Comp. Neurol.* 329:277–289.

Young, R. W. (1985). Cell differentiation in the retina of the mouse. *Anat. Rec.* 212:199–205.

30 Retinoic Acid Function in Central Visual Pathways

URSULA C. DRÄGER, TUANLIAN LUO, AND ELISABETH WAGNER

From the time the mouse grew into an acceptable species for brain research, it incorporated an ambitious purpose that distinguished it from other low-cost neurobiological model systems. Its small size, rapid breeding cycle, genetic accessibility, and structurally representative mammalian brain designated it as model species for breaking down the confines of brain research, with the ultimate goal of facilitating access to the genetic basis of functions and diseases of the human brain (Sidman et al., 1965). As neurobiological experimentation in its early days was insulated from cell biological and molecular biological research by a total gap in language, methods, and concepts, the mouse was instrumental in dissolving the boundaries with both these fields successively. Cell-biological neuroscience flourished in mice long before such techniques were adapted to other species, and the genetic insight from simpler molecular model species, such as *Drosophila*, expanded into vertebrate neuroscience by way of screens in the mouse for important invertebrate genes. The advance of transgenic techniques, including gene replacements and conditional null mutants, then made the mouse the foremost model in which to study gene function.

This unique standing of the mouse has only recently been challenged by the analysis of naturally occurring neurological mutations in humans: both in sheer number of living specimens and in sophistication of brain functions, laboratory mice cannot compete with humans. Nevertheless, with respect to higher visual functions, the mouse continues to be an indispensable animal model, even in the pursuit of a genetic understanding of higher cognitive functions that are considered characteristically human. A surprising result from the sequencing of entire genomes over recent years is the remarkable similarity in protein-coding genes between phenotypically different species such as mice and men. It is now apparent that the differences must be somehow inherent in the regulation of gene expression. Here we want to show that the compact mouse brain uniquely facilitates the discovery of large-scale organizational principles for the regulation of gene expression. In the current postgenomic era, however, the mouse cannot be appraised in isolation. Rather, neurobiological discoveries made in the mouse must be integrated with relevant facts collected in other species.

The first recordings from single neurons in visual centers of the mouse established that its brain is not only anatomically but also functionally very similar to that of other mammals, including primates (Dräger, 1975; Dräger and Hubel, 1975). The frontier in exploration of higher visual functions progressed over the following years from recordings in anesthetized animals to studies of awake, behaving monkeys and then to integrating these findings with insights from psychophysical observations in humans. Although it would be futile for mouse vision research to attempt to replicate studies in primates, the anatomical investigations described in chapter 20 of this volume establish that the mouse cortex contains the anatomical requisites for higher visual processing originally defined in primates. In this chapter we show that the regulation of gene expression in higher visual pathways is part of a novel transcriptional parcellation of the cerebral cortex that undoubtedly exists in humans as well. Because our argument for the validity of the mouse in cognitive research is based on studies of the retinoid system, about which very little is known with respect to the brain, a brief introduction to the topic is provided.

It is well known that vitamin A is exceptionally important for vision, but available evidence points exclusively to the eye: vitamin A deficiency causes inborn eye malformations in developing embryos and night blindness in visual function. Whether vitamin A also plays a role in the development and function of the central visual pathways is not known. Because efforts to understand vitamin A actions in the brain tend to become hampered by several unexplained difficulties, a general review of retinoids in the brain is in order, with an emphasis on the functional dorsal telencephalon. We then describe how we use our own data to extract information from the large Web-based data banks that have aggregated information on the mouse and human genomes (Magdaleno et al., 2006; Lein et al., 2007). Finally, we explain how this combined information points to an integral role for vitamin A in selected higher visual and cognitive functions.

The retinoid system

The biological effects of vitamin A are mediated through its two active derivatives, retinaldehyde and retinoic acid (RA): retinaldehyde forms the visual chromophore bound to opsin, which makes vision possible, and RA regulates gene transcription. Although the high rhodopsin content of photoreceptors makes the functional retina the organ of highest vitamin A content in the adult, the developing eye is the RA-richest site in the embryo, as it contains very high levels of the retinaldehyde dehydrogenases (RALDHs), which oxidize retinaldehyde to RA (Dräger et al., 2001; Luo et al., 2006). Also expressed in the eye are the CYP26 enzymes, which catabolize RA and limit its spread. RA acts by binding to nuclear receptors that are members of the large family of ligand-regulated transcription factors (Mark and Chambon, 2003). Binding of RAs to their receptors that reside at RA response elements (RAREs) in gene promoters causes conformational changes, which allows recruitment of co-activators to the transcriptional machinery. Dissociation of RA from the receptors causes recruitment of transcriptional corepressors. The RA receptors include eight major RAR-α, -β, and -γ isoforms and six major RXR-α, -β, and -γ isoforms, and RA-sensitive gene expression is regulated by RAR/RXR heterodimers (Mark and Chambon, 2003). In addition, the RXRs form heterodimers with a wide range of other nuclear receptors, including the thyroid hormone and vitamin D receptors. Owing to the large number of isoforms and the enormous number of different heterodimeric combinations, RA-binding receptors constitute by far the most elaborate subgroup of the nuclear receptor transcription factors.

Both vitamin A deficiency and excess can result in severe malformations that are created in growing embryos at specific sites and critical developmental stages, indicating that normal RA actions are distinctly localized. The determinants for this localization are apparent from observations of null mutant mice generated for practically every retinoid gene (Mark and Chambon, 2003): most of the retinoid mutants do not have dramatic phenotypes except for null mutants for the metabolic enzymes, which tend to have severe deformities at the sites that are also vulnerable to nutritional vitamin A deficiency. This suggests that the most important criteria for the localization of RA signaling are locally regulated RA levels, which are synthesized by locally expressed RALDHs and catabolized by CYP26s. A major role for the RALDHs in localizing RA actions is consistent with their widely dispersed and sparse expression: the enzymes are restricted to a few sites in the body, with much of the intervening tissue being free of RA-synthesizing enzymes, which is especially true for the brain. Other retinoid factors, in particular the many RARs that convey the immense transcriptional complexity, are expressed profusely in overlapping ways and serve partially redundant functions, so that their role in simple localization is relatively minor.

Actions of retinoic acid in the brain

From in vitro studies on human stem cells, it is estimated that RAs can influence the mRNA levels of about 15% of all protein-coding genes by twofold or more (Cawley et al., 2004). Since the actual RA actions in vivo are determined by their cellular and developmental context, however, one cannot predict which of the many possibilities of RA-regulated gene expression will occur at a particular site. What constitutes this context needs to be characterized in vivo for each condition, as has been done in detail for the RA-rich retina. RA actions in the brain are mostly studied in very early embryos, and only limited information is available for the postnatal, functioning brain. The brain ranks among the regions of lowest RA production in the body; its overall RA synthesis is more than 100-fold lower than in the embryonic retina. Most components of the retinoid system are expressed in the postnatal brain, and in many cases their expression patterns differ from those in the embryo, which points to unique RA contributions to brain function (Lane and Bailey, 2005). Compelling evidence exists for critical RA involvement in important neurobiological activities, including learning, memory, and sleep (Chiang et al., 1998; Misner et al., 2001; Maret et al., 2005). Although these functions are major fields of investigation in neuroscience, the RA evidence is rarely considered, because it is not clear how it is integrated with the neurobiological mechanisms of these activities.

We first summarize the results of several studies on the brain and emphasize some unique, puzzling features that hint at unknown mechanisms through which RA signaling is reinforced in the brain and integrated with neurobiological events. We then describe patterns of elevated RA levels that emerge during postnatal development in the cortex and delineate the dorsal visual stream and the pathway for visual attention (Wang and Burkhalter, 2004; Wagner et al., 2006). Using these RA patterns, we searched gene expression data banks, which have recently become available as a public resource for the mouse, to identify genes that are potentially regulated by RA in the context of the brain. Because the genomes of mice and humans are very similar and the basic brain organization is conserved, mouse data can provide clues to human diseases. Among the genes whose expression is differentially regulated along the RA band are many implicated in cognitive diseases and abnormalities of dorsal stream function. We suggest that the uneven distribution of RA is part of normal postnatal pattern formation in the cerebral cortex; elevated RA levels designate which cortical territories remain relatively more plastic, by boosting gene expression in response to rapid neuronal and physiological changes, which impinge via signaling cascades onto a common combinatorial transcriptional network (Rosenfeld et al., 2006).

Retinoic acid reporter mice

Colocalization of RA signaling with sites of RALDH expression is strikingly obvious in studies of RA reporter mice that are transgenic for the RA-sensitive promoter of the RAR-β gene driving β-galactosidase (lacZ) (Rossant et al., 1991; Smith et al., 2001; Luo et al., 2004). In early embryos, when RA is exclusively synthesized by RALDH2 expressed in the trunk and the eye anlage, the RALDH sites are matched by high lacZ expression in the reporter embryo (figure 30.1*A*). This differential RA distribution can be independently verified by explant assays with RARE-lacZ reporter cells, which are F9 embryonic stem cells transfected with a RARβ-lacZ construct similar to that used for the transgenic RA reporter mice (Wagner et al., 1992) (see the three culture wells between the embryos in figure 30.1*A*). High lacZ induction in RA reporter mice serves as a general, reliable indicator for RALDH expression throughout most of the body in early embryos except for the brain. Although the RA content of the brain is very low, several different RA reporter strains all show consistently very high RA signaling at specific brain sites (Misner et al., 2001; Luo et al., 2004). This strong RA signaling in the reporter brains is not, however, matched by locally elevated RA levels measured using several different methods, including RA reporter cell responses to supernatants of cultured brain explants (figure 30.1*B*), and no RALDHs are expressed in these regions.

These discrepancies indicate that the early embryonic brain responds to RA that diffuses from elsewhere, most likely from RALDHs expressed in the optic vesicle and stalk, and by convection via the cerebrospinal fluid in the ventricular lumen, which is wide open at this early stage (Luo et al., 2004). Consistent with such a route, lacZ at this stage is highest in the ventricular layer. Surprisingly, however, not all the brain ventricular zones are labeled, but in the telencephalon RA signaling is restricted to the dorsal part, and in the di- and mesencephalon it exhibits distinct, changing patterns, some of which suggest a role in visual development. For example, the tectal target regions for the RALDH-rich

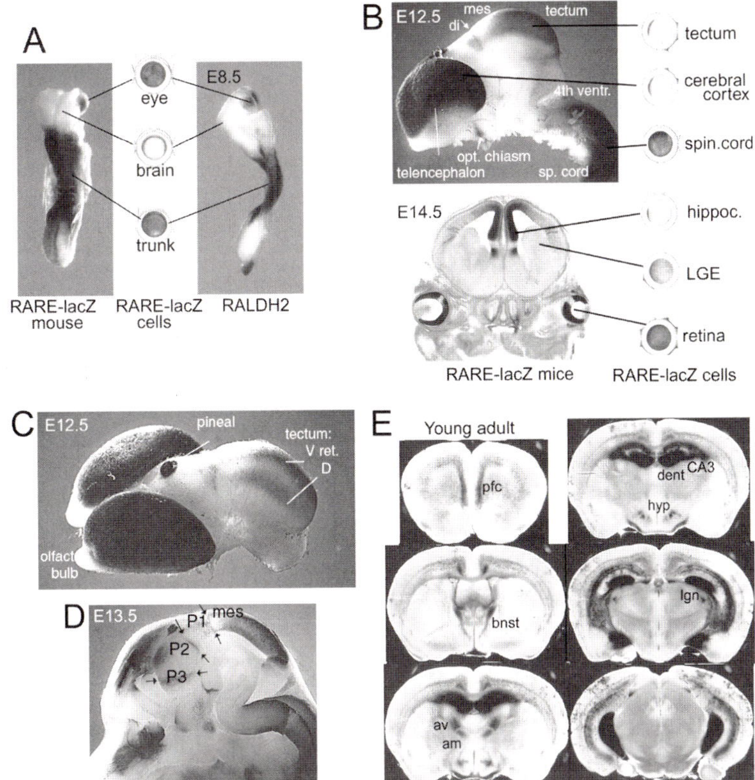

FIGURE 30.1 *A* and *B*, RA signaling in RA reporter mice (RARE-lacZ mice) (Rossant et al., 1991) is compared with RALDH2 expression by in situ hybridization (1A) and with RA measurement by RA reporter cells (RARE-lacZ cells) (Wagner et al., 1992). *C*, Ventricular layer lacZ expression in target areas of axons from dorsal (D) and ventral (V) retina is visible through the thin tectal roof of this E12.5 whole-brain preparation. *D*, E13.5 head hemisected along the midsagittal plane to show the lacZ-marked borders between the diencephalic prosomers (P1–P3) and the mesencephalon (mes) in the ventricular layer (Luo et al., 2004). *E*, Coronal slices through adult RA reporter brain to illustrate RA signaling in the optic axons, the hippocampus, and the anterior thalamus. For other details, see Luo et al., 2004.

axon bundles from the dorsal and ventral retina compartments are delineated by lacZ before the axons arrive (figure 30.1*C*). In the diencephalon, lacZ outlines the segmental (prosomeric) boundaries (figure 30.1*D*), which represent borders along which the growth trajectories of the dorsal and ventral optic axon bundles are differentially deviated during the primary innervation of optic targets. This phenomenon points to a role for RA-regulated factors in the proportioning of the dorsal and ventral retina compartments to the di- and mesencephalic visual projection maps (Luo et al., 2004). LacZ expression in reporter mice marks sites implicated in RA actions also in the postnatal brain, most prominently the hippocampus (figure 30.1*E*). In the thalamus, lacZ marks the anteroventral and anteromedial nuclei, which project to the medial RALDH3-expressing cortex (van Groen et al., 1999). Measurements with several different techniques show that hippocampal RA levels are only slightly higher than the low background in the brain, and no RALDHs are expressed in the lacZ-positive anterior thalamic nuclei (Luo et al., 2004). The observations in RA reporter mice thus indicate that RA signaling is selectively amplified in the brain at sites where independent evidence also points to preferential RA actions.

Role of retinoic acid in dorsal telencephalon function

Part of the evidence for a role for RA in neurobiological activities comes from functional studies on RAR knockout mice. RAR-β null mutants lack long-term potentiation (LTP) in recordings from hippocampal slices; behaviorally, their long-term memory is severely impaired, and they have abnormal sleep and sleep EEG (Chiang et al., 1998; Maret et al., 2005). Curiously, however, RAR-β is expressed only in low amounts in the hippocampus, cerebral cortex, or thalamus, where these functions are generated (Lane and Bailey, 2005). RA is required for the formation of new neurons in the postnatal dentate gyrus, a process involved in normal learning and memory (Jacobs et al., 2006). Nutritional vitamin A deficiency impairs memory and hippocampal LTP in mice, and these defects can be cured by vitamin A supplementation (Misner et al., 2001). The cortex of deprived rats accumulates β-amyloid deposits and other signs that parallel those in Alzheimer's disease (Corcoran et al., 2004), and normal memory loss in aging rats due to naturally occurring reductions in retinoid function with age can be alleviated with vitamin A supplements (Etchamendy et al., 2001). Unfortunately, these observations do not suggest a simple way to enhance memory, because dentate neurogenesis is also decreased in response to RA excess: chronic exposure of mice to elevated RA levels reduces the formation of new neurons here, and the mice exhibit impaired memory and depression-like behaviors (Crandall et al., 2004; O'Reilly et al., 2006). Similarly, some humans treated with Accutane (13-*cis* RA) for acne develop symptoms of clinical depression.

Impaired dentate neurogenesis cannot account for the loss of hippocampal LTP, and cortical memory does not depend on the formation of new neurons. Changes of gene expression in learning and memory require that information about rapid physiological events be converted faithfully into specific transcriptional processes. However, RA levels do not show any rapid physiological fluctuations, nor do any other retinoid components undergo changes on a neurophysiological time scale. Without doubt, the strictly defined retinoid system does not possess the dynamic properties required for learning and memory. Instead, most information about dynamic events in the nervous system is conveyed via signaling cascades to the cAMP response element–binding (CREB) protein and its family members of transcription factors, which function as key mediators of stimulus-induced nuclear responses (Lonze and Ginty, 2002; Carlezon et al., 2005). Several arguments point to CREB and the transcriptional coregulator level, at which RA actions in the brain are integrated with neurobiological functions and amplified. On the one hand, RA was shown to activate CREB directly by causing its phosphorylation at Ser-133 via nongenomic mechanisms (Canon et al., 2004). On the other hand, the discrepancies in the RA reporter responses point to CREB. The promoter of the RAR-β gene, which drives lacZ expression in the transgenic mice, contains a functional CREB-binding site (Kruyt et al., 1992). A synergistic enhancement of RA responses by CREB has been suggested for bronchial epithelial cells (Aggarwal et al., 2006). In a similar manner, the spatially selective amplification of RA signaling in the reporter brains might be mediated via physiologically activated CREB at the same sites. CREB-stimulated RAR-β enhancement could also explain the observations that RAR-β null mutants show profound functional defects at sites in the brain, where normal RAR-β expression is very low (Chiang et al., 1998; Maret et al., 2005).

Both pCREB and RA-dependent gene expression depend on the transcriptional co-activator CREB-binding protein (CBP), which contains a domain for CREB interaction and a separate nuclear receptor–interacting domain. CBP, which has histone acetyl transferase (HAT) activity that facilitates access to the DNA, is one of many transcriptional coregulators with different enzymatic activities that are recruited by a wide range of DNA-binding transcription factors in a combinatorial transcriptional code. The signaling cascades that convey information about dynamic events to CREB are now recognized to target in addition other transcriptional components and to influence a network of sequentially exchanged coregulator complexes that execute diverse enzymatic modifications of the transcriptional apparatus, which are required for context-specific gene expression (Johannessen et al., 2004; Rochette-Egly, 2005; Lonard and O'Malley, 2006; Rosenfeld et al., 2006).

RALDH2

Both the hippocampus and cerebral cortex of the adult brain are derived from the dorsal telencephalic wall of the embryo. To address the question of which genes are responsive to RA in the context of the functional brain, we compared the topography of gene expression with the RA distribution inferred from RALDH expression sites, focusing on the postnatal cerebral cortex because of its distinct RALDH patterns. A large fraction of the total RA content of the brain is supplied by passive exchange with the low levels in the circulation, which perfuses the brain evenly (Kurlandsky et al., 1995). Two RALDHs expressed in the cerebral cortex, RALDH2 and RALDH3, can be assumed to impart spatial RA patterns on top of the diffuse RA distribution provided by the circulation (Wagner et al., 2002). The RALDH2 enzyme is expressed in the meninges covering the cortical surface, from where it is likely to generate an outside-in RA decline in the cortex but no marked RA-level differences in the tangential dimension, as its expression is relatively uniform. RALDH2 is activated rather late during embryonic development; its levels increase to a maximum for about a week perinatally and then decrease. Low RALDH2 levels persist in the meninges throughout life. The changing RALDH2 expression over the life cycle is illustrated by Northern blots of isolated telencephala (Smith et al., 2001) (figure 30.2, *left*); histologically in coronal sections through an adult brain, the RALDH2-labeled meninges are best visible in the meningeal channels of the stratum lacunare in the hippocampus (Wagner et al., 2002) (figure 30.2, *right*).

RALDH3

RALDH3 begins to be expressed by selected neurons a day before birth, when a faint trace becomes detectable at the most medial edge of the cingulate cortex (figure 30.3, *arrows*). In newborns at postnatal day 0.5 (P0.5), the expression has intensified and expanded, and a day later it covers the entire rostrocaudal extent of the medial limbic cortex. By P3 the RALDH3 territory has expanded laterally beyond the limbic cortex into a narrow band of adjoining neocortex. Over the following days, RALDH3 expression decreases selectively in the caudal and intermediate limbic cortex and eventually disappears completely from there. Strong expression persists, however, in the rostral part of the medial limbic lobe and in a chain of neocortical regions that border the entire medial limbic cortex. Throughout the rest of postnatal life, the RALDH3 topography remains constant, but enzyme levels decrease slowly. The part of the limbic lobe from which RALDH3 disappears is the retrosplenial cortex, including all its anatomical subdivisions. The lasting RALDH3 expression in the caudal third of the neocortex is localized in the medial extrastriate region (see the color code in color plate 20). In the intermediate third, RALDH3 marks parietal association areas and motor cortex, and in the rostral third the enzyme is expressed in the limbic cingulate and prefrontal cortex and the adjoining secondary motor cortex (Wagner et al., 2002, 2006). The medial extrastriate cortex contains the dorsal visual stream (Wang and Burkhalter, 2004), which is best characterized in primates as the pathway for spatial vision and motion perception as distinct from the ventral visual stream for color and form perception (Merigan and Maunsell, 1993; Goodale and Westwood, 2004), and the entire medial RALDH3 band in the mouse corresponds to the cortical network for visual attention and spatial imagery in humans (Dolan, 2002; Knauff et al., 2002).

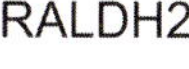

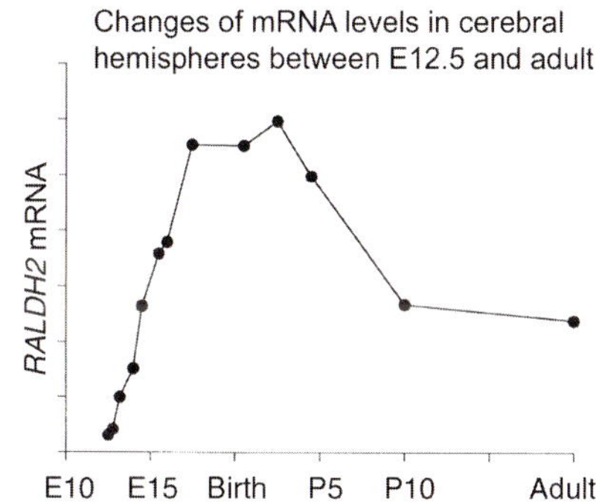

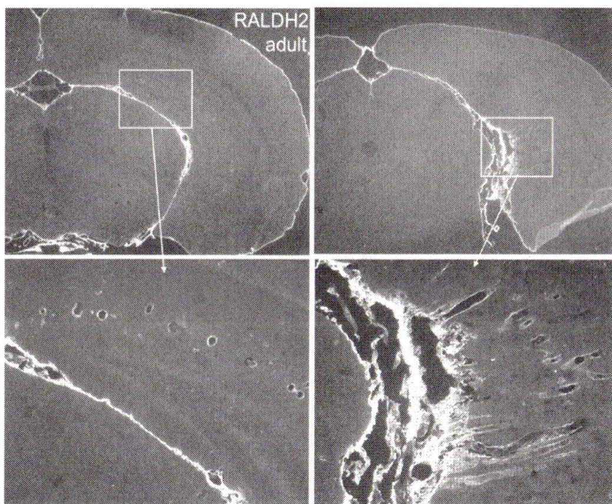

FIGURE 30.2 Changes in total RALDH2 mRNA in cerebral hemispheres (Smith et al., 2001). Here the enzyme is expressed in the meninges at all ages, as shown in the antiserum-labeled coronal sections from an adult brain (Wagner et al., 2002).

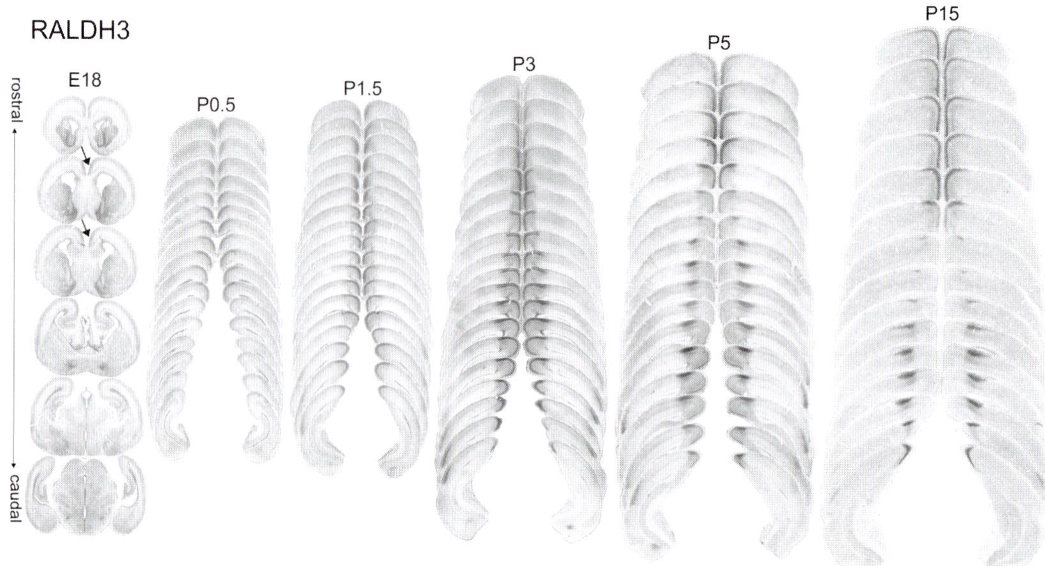

FIGURE 30.3 Stacks of coronal brain sections at six ages labeled with a RALDH3 antiserum (Wagner et al., 2006).

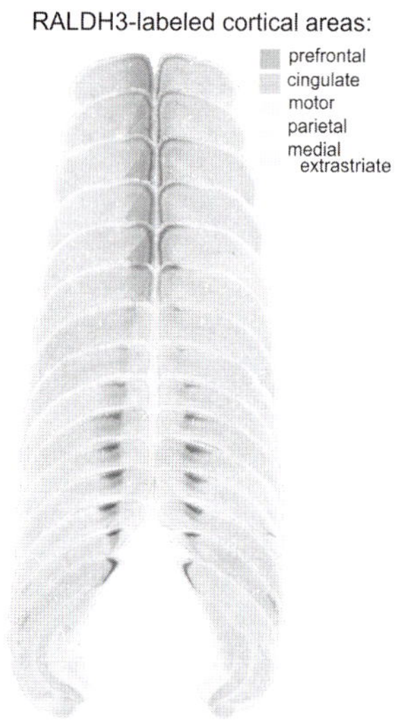

FIGURE 30.4 The anatomical locations of the medial RALDH3 band are indicated for P15 in the form of a color code (visible in color plate 20), in which *prefrontal* includes the prelimbic and medial orbital cortices; *cingulate* includes areas 1 and 2 of the cingulate cortex; *motor* designates mostly the secondary motor cortex, in addition to a small caudal part of the primary motor cortex; *parietal* includes the medial and lateral parietal association cortices; and *medial extrastriate* extends from a location where the rostral extrastriate region abuts the parietal association cortex all the way caudally, an elongated region also called area 18b or V2M (Wagner et al., 2006). See color plate 20.

RALDH3 colocalizes with markers for neuronal plasticity

When the shifted stable RALDH3 band is compared with a range of cytoarchitectonic characteristics at different postnatal ages, some of the markers show strikingly differential expression at corresponding tangential locations along the entire rostrocaudal extent (figure 30.5). Some late-maturing features, including expression of parvalbumin and the SMI32 neurofilament epitope, are delayed, and some immature characteristics are preferentially maintained, as illustrated for the polysialated form of the neural cell adhesion molecule PSA-NCAM (Wagner et al., 2006). This indicates that RALDH3 colocalizes with a band of cortex that has cytoarchitectonic attributes of a relatively less mature and more plastic neuronal circuitry and that extends along the whole rostrocaudal dimension of the cerebral cortex.

Relationship between RALDH3 and neurotrophin-3

The RALDH3 band represents a tangential pattern that emerges very late, only after the first postnatal week in mice. Because the tangential organization of the cortex is determined irreversibly already during embryonic development but the results of the early determination events become visible only postnatally (Grove and Fukuchi-Shimogori, 2003), we wondered which factors act upstream of RALDH3 and bring about its postnatal pattern (Wagner et al., 2006). One of these appears to be neurotrophin-3 (NT-3), whose normal expression is compared to RALDH3 in figure 30.6. Strong NT-3 along the medial embryonic cortex precedes RALDH3; during P1–P2 the territories of the two markers overlap briefly, but over the next few days they change into tangentially complementary domains. Along the rostromedial limbic cortex, where RALDH3 remains strong, NT-3 expression fades, and caudomedially, where RALDH3 shifts from medial limbic regions into adjoining neocortex, strong

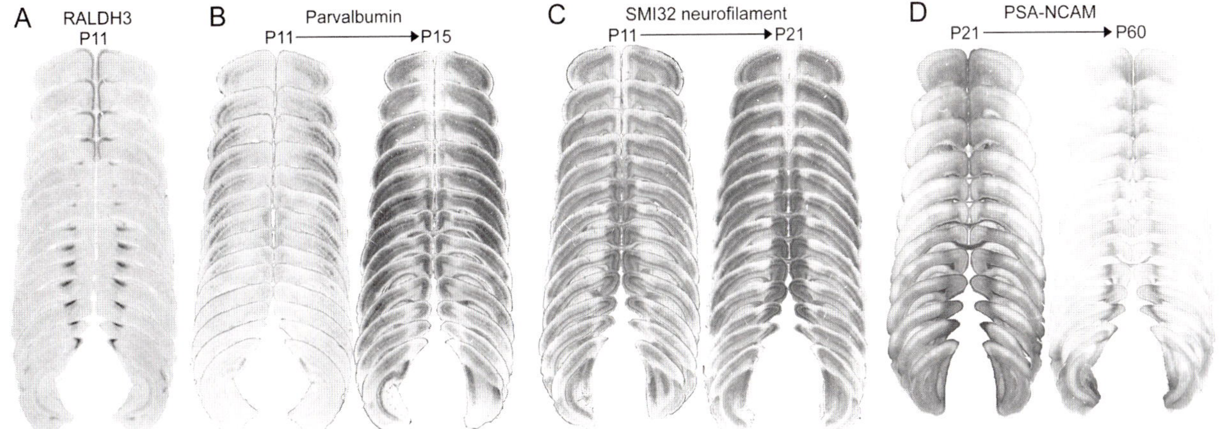

FIGURE 30.5 *A–D*, Stacks of coronal cortex sections illustrating the delay in maturation of parvalbumin and neurofilaments along the RALDH3 band, as well as the persistence of the immature form of the neural cell adhesion molecule PSA-NCAM (Wagner et al., 2006).

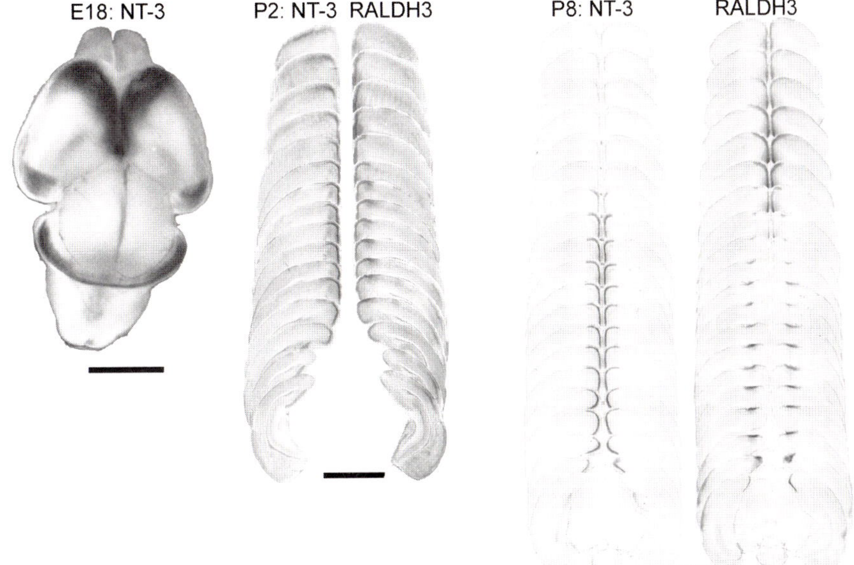

FIGURE 30.6 Comparisons of NT-3 and RALDH3 maturation in the medial cortex (Wagner et al., 2006). NT-3 expression precedes RALDH3; after a transient overlap, the two markers occupy complementary territories. Scale bars = 2 mm.

NT-3 expression persists in all retrosplenial areas. Like RALDH3, the NT-3 pattern seems to remain constant throughout life, but its levels diminish. Because of this intriguing relationship between the two markers, we tested RALDH3 expression in conditional NT-3 knockout mice (Wagner et al., 2006): in the absence of NT-3, RALDH3 is present but fails to undergo its normal lateral shift, instead maintaining its normally transient early postnatal expression pattern. The cytoarchitectonic markers with differential expression along the RALDH3 band in normal cortex shift to match the abnormal RALDH3 in the NT-3 null mutants (not shown here).

RALDH3 and NT-3 define distinct maturation patterns in the postnatal cortex

Figure 30.7 (*left*) summarizes the topographical changes in RALDH3 expression and its relationship to NT-3, as projected onto the postnatal cortex surface. At P2 the two markers transiently occupy the same territory along the medial edge of the cortex, but subsequently their expressions change gradually into two topographically complementary patterns. In coronal brain sections the stable, shifted patterns can be adequately diagnosed from three samples: sections at the level of the cingulate cortex, the parietal association

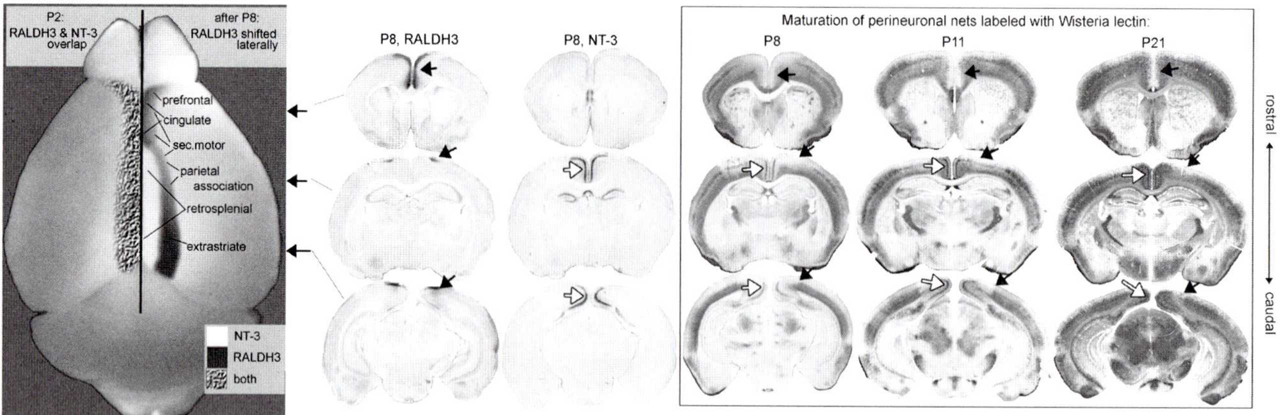

FIGURE 30.7 *Left*, Schematic surface view of the transient cortical territories occupied by RALDH3 and NT-3 early postnatally and of the shifted stable expression patterns. *Right*, Neighboring coronal sections through a P8 normal mouse brain labeled for RALDH3, NT-3, and perineuronal nets, illustrated for three anteroposterior levels at the cingulate, parietal cortex, and dorsal visual stream, as indicated by the *horizontal arrows*. Sections at the corresponding levels are also shown for perineuronal nets at P11 and P21. Note that perineuronal-net maturation is delayed at RALDH3 (*black arrows*) and accelerated at NT-3 (*white arrows*).

cortex, and the medial peristriate cortex, which contains the dorsal visual stream (figure 30.7, *right*). A comparison of the patterns with several cytoarchitectonic characteristics shows that both RALDH3 and NT-3 colocalize with developmental expression differentials, which are often opposite in direction. This point is illustrated for the maturation of perineuronal nets detected with Wisteria lectin; the appearance of these extracellular structures is known to gradually limit the plasticity of cortical neurons by cementing synapses in place and restricting the perineuronal diffusion space (Koppe et al., 1997). At the sites of RALDH3 expression, which are indicated by the *black arrows* in figure 30.7, maturation of perineuronal nets is suppressed, and at the NT-3 sites (*white arrows*), their maturation is relatively advanced.

These colocalizations do not allow the conclusion that either RALDH3 or NT-3 induces these patterns; rather, the two factors delineate in the postnatal cortex distinct topographical territories with separate maturation properties that may be opposite in direction. Since the patterns are reflected in several very ordinary and commonly studied cytoarchitectonic characteristics, we expected that they would have been identified and named in classic neuroanatomy. However, while all the details that we observe are in agreement with known features of particular cortical regions, the entire RALDH3-colocalized band has not been recognized previously or given a comprehensive name, and we adhere here to our preliminary nomenclature.

BGEM data bank searches

To explore at what time in development a shifted pattern can first be detected for any gene, we turned to the Brain Gene Expression Map (BGEM) database (www.stjudebgem.org/web/mainPage/mainPage.php). This site contains in situ hybridization images for four ages: E10, E17, P7, and P42. We searched through all the 2,200 genes that were included soon after the Web site was published (Magdaleno et al., 2006). Although this search was necessarily cursory, no shifted patterns were detectable for any gene among the embryonic data. Among the P7 data, most of the genes with differential expression in the medial cortex still resemble the early transient patterns shown for P2 in figure 30.7, but for several genes, some shifted characteristics are apparent. Among the P42 data, however, multiple genes display strikingly shifted, RALDH3-colocalized expression patterns. From the BGEM searches we concluded that the patterns we observe are clearly the main patterns for all genes with differential expression along the medial cortex, and that a shifted, RALDH3-colocalized pattern emerges only relatively late during postnatal cortex maturation.

Allen Brain Atlas searches

Because the BGEM data bank is limited with respect to adult ages, we searched the Web site of the Allen Brain Atlas (www.brainatlas.org/aba/), which lists expression data for 21,000 mouse genes (Lein et al., 2007). This Web site contains an enormous amount of data collected by nonradioactive in situ hybridizations of fully adult (P56) brains and photographed at low and higher magnifications. Because we are trying to characterize patterning across the entire postnatal cortex, we chose low-resolution dark-field pictures, which are sufficient for detection of transcortical patterns. For figure 30.8 the same three levels as in figure 30.7

were selected out of the serial sections available in the Allen database, while the full evaluation was based on inspection of all sections. The Allen data show that the transient midline patterns present at P2 have practically disappeared by P56 and are replaced by the two stable patterns represented by RALDH3 and NT-3. Within both territories a gene can be differentially up- or downregulated, and if differential expression is visible for both regions, it is most often in the opposite direction. A few genes, however, are regulated in the same directions in the two territories.

So far, we have found 370 genes whose mRNA levels are upregulated (304 genes) or downregulated (66 genes) along the entire RALDH3 band. Figure 30.8 shows a few examples of genes from the Allen Brain Atlas Web site that are differentially up- or downregulated along RALDH3, in addition to three genes whose expression is upregulated within the NT-3 territory. For multiple technical reasons, the search results up to now represent only a fraction of all the genes that must be differentially regulated along the cortical midline, and chance was involved in the detection of patterned expression. First, the patterns can only be satisfactorily distinguished in coronal sections, but the Allen team screened all genes initially in parasagittal sections; only when potentially interesting patterns became detectable were the genes also processed for visualization in the coronal plane. Second, for many genes, expression is difficult to evaluate even in coronal sections owing to underexposure of the preparations with respect to the cortex. Third, all the Allen data are on P56, whereas we found that some differences are more pronounced earlier during cortex maturation.

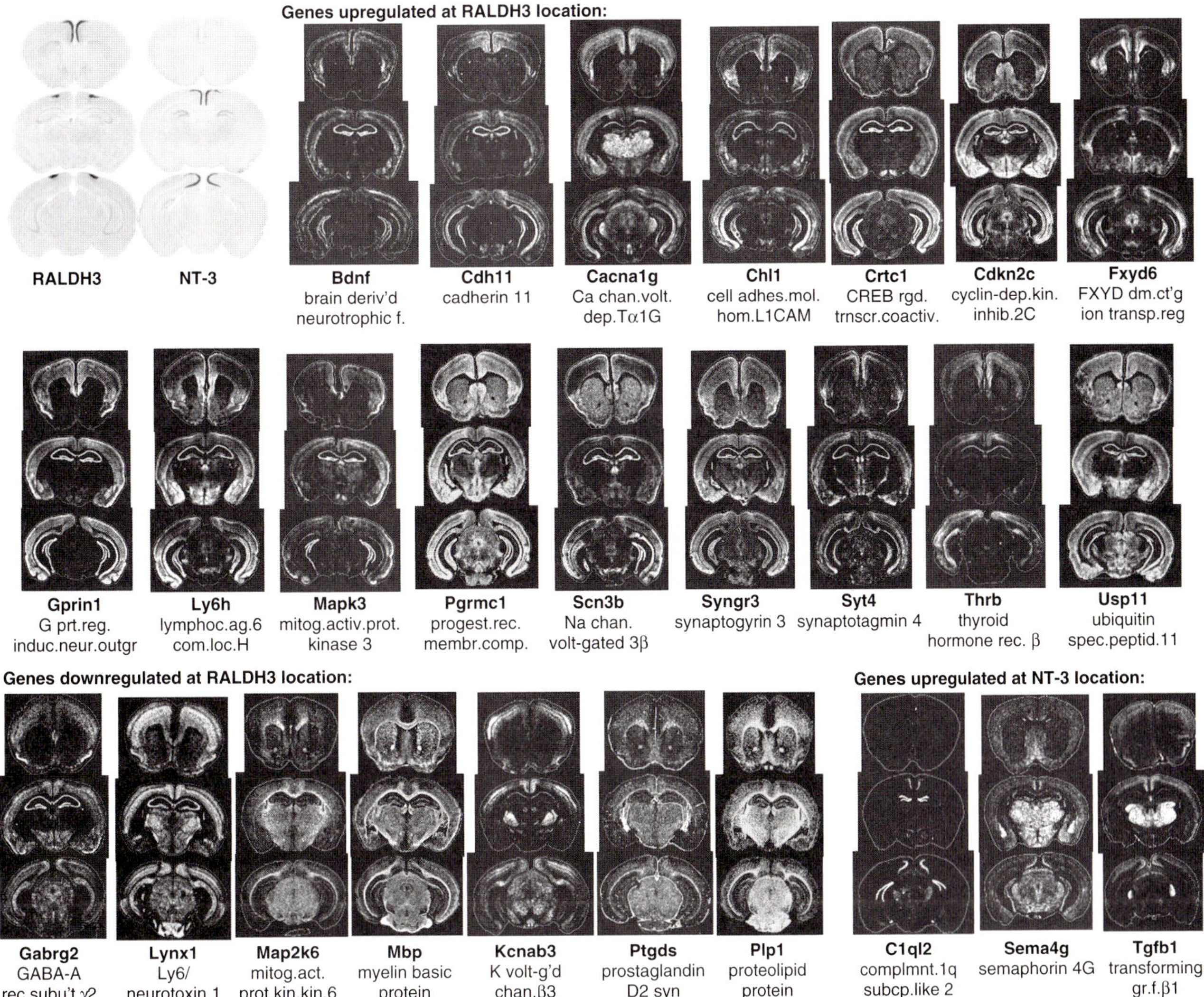

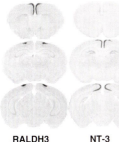

FIGURE 30.8 Coronal sections through an adult mouse brain labeled for RALDH3 and NT-3 by immunohistochemistry are compared with dark-field views from the Allen Web site of representative coronal sections, labeled by in situ hybridizations for different genes. The medial RALDH3 and NT-3 expression patterns are enhanced to accentuate the topographical parallels between these low-magnification images.

Evaluations of the data bank searches

To detect a trend in the assortment of identified genes, we performed ontology searches with the Pathway Express program for the RALDH3 colocalized genes (Draghici et al., 2003). The most common pathways are neuroactive ligand-receptor interactions and the MAPK and CamK signaling pathways. This result differs from corresponding ontology searches performed by Balmer and Blomhoff (2002) for all the genes they found to be regulated by RA in the most recent literature survey: they obtained a flat ontology distribution, indicative of RA roles in many different cellular functions throughout the body. If one assumes that RA causes the differential expression of the genes along the RALDH3 band, the differences between the ontology searches point to unique properties of RA signaling in the brain. Our assumption that RA itself represents a significant factor is supported by the similarity in regulation that apparently occurs in response to RA diffusing from either RALDH3 or RALDH2, as is obvious in the thumbnail views in figure 30.8 and in other images from the data banks: in most cases, the expression of the genes that are upregulated along the RALDH3 band is also strong in upper cortical regions close to the RALDH2 expression in the meninges. Among the patterns of downregulated genes, both the RALDH3 band and the uppermost cortical layers appear relatively empty.

The ontology search results relate to the notion, explained earlier, that we think the unusually strong RA signaling in the brain is due to a convergence with CREB-activated gene expression and a mutual amplification. Canon et al. (2004) describe that RA can rapidly activate CREB via ERK (MAPK) phosphorylation in a nongenomic pathway; interestingly, they report that RA-mediated CREB activation lasts much longer than neurotrophin-mediated activation. In preliminary comparisons of the group of shifted genes with CREB-regulated genes (Lonze and Ginty, 2002; Cawley et al., 2004; Carlezon et al., 2005), we find a significant overlap. As the activation of CREB-dependent gene expression requires Ser-133 phosphorylation of CREB, we performed preliminary Western blots with a pCREB antibody, which showed that pCREB levels are elevated along both the RALDH3 and the NT-3 bands compared with other cortical regions (Luo et al., 2008).

One of the known factors contributing to CREB's enormous range of highly specific gene expression is that it causes transcription of other transcription factors, with which it collaborates in combinatorial transcriptional codes (Lonze and Ginty, 2002; Cawley et al., 2004). Among the best characterized examples are the immediate early genes, including *c-fos*, whose mRNA levels rise within minutes of CREB activation but always return to baseline within a brief time even if CREB phosphorylation persists. Canon et al. (2004) report that *c-fos* is also rapidly upregulated following RA applications to neuronal cultures and that this occurs via nongenomic mechanisms, because the *c-fos* promoter does not contain an RA response element. *c-Fos* is known to form heterodimers with members of the jun family of transcription factors and to bind to AP1 sites contained in the promoters of many genes. Searches through the Allen database show that both *c-fos* and *junB* are upregulated along the RALDH3 band (not shown here). This chronic elevation of immediate early genes, which cannot be explained by CREB activation alone, is one of the arguments in support of the notion that RA and CREB act in concert along the shifted location.

A related intriguing property of the preliminary shifted gene list is that it contains a high fraction of factors directly or indirectly involved in transcription, which has also been recognized as a common characteristic of genes implicated in cognitive diseases (Hong et al., 2005). Examples are several other transcription factors, as well as coregulators with enzymatic activities implicated in epigenetic mechanisms, including acetylation, methylation, phosphorylation, ADP-ribosylation, ubiquitination, and ATP-dependent chromatin remodeling. A differential expression of components in the transcriptional apparatus is bound to influence gene transcription, a process known to be exquisitely sensitive to protein levels and gene dosage, as is apparent in the rapid proteasome-mediated turnover of all transcriptional components and in the severe consequences of CBP coactivator reduction in Rubinstein-Taybi syndrome (Hong et al., 2005; Rochette-Egly, 2005; Lonard and O'Malley, 2006; Rosenfeld et al., 2006). The RALDH3 colocalized genes contain many that are compromised in different cognitive diseases, including genes implicated in mental retardation syndromes, Alzheimer's disease, candidate genes for autism, schizophrenia, and other psychiatric disorders. An interesting example is the *Chd7* gene, a chromodomain helicase recently identified as being mutated in CHARGE syndrome (Vissers et al., 2004), a form of mental retardation in which one-third of the cases also show autism. The CHARGE syndrome consists of a nonrandom association of ocular coloboma (C), heart anomaly (H), choanal atresia (A), retarded growth or development (R), genital hypoplasia (G), and ear anomalies or hearing impairment (E). This combination of malformations is practically identical to retinoid embryopathy (Wilson et al., 1953; Shenefelt, 1972); in fact, choanal atresia is the reason that simple RALDH3 null mutant mice die shortly after birth (Dupe et al., 2003). Localization of the *Chd7* gene has been described by in situ hybridization both for human and mouse embryos (Bosman et al., 2005): its levels are highest at sites with RALDH expression or lacZ labeling in the RA-reporter mice. The Allen data show that *Chd7* is upregulated in the adult cortex along the RALDH3 band, as is also the case for the *Mecp2* gene mutated in Rett syndrome, another form of syndromic autism.

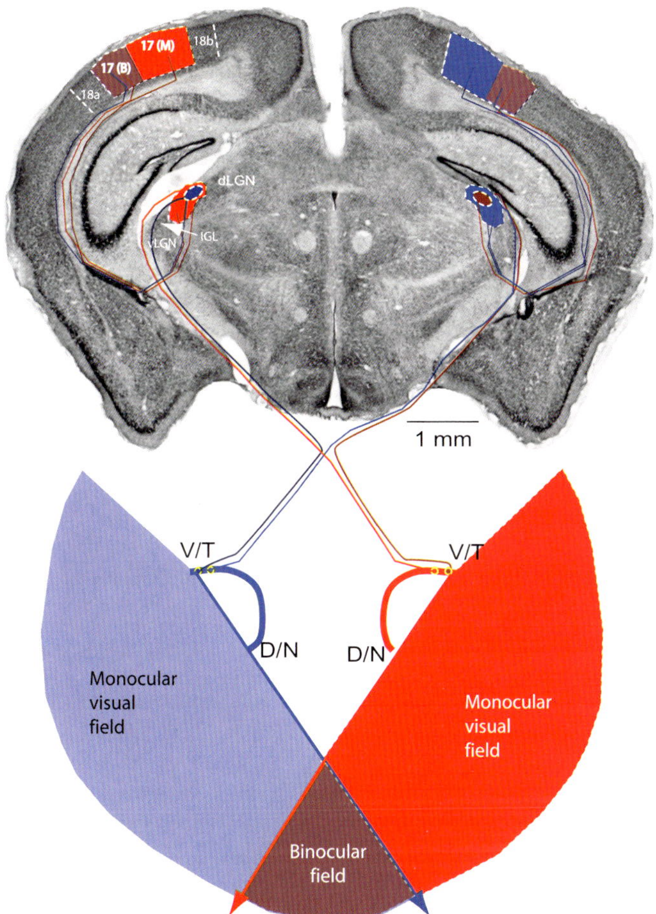

PLATE 1 Schematic diagram showing the organization of the ipsilateral and contralateral visual pathways in mice. Blue and red indicate fibers and regions representing the left and right eyes, respectively. Purple indicates binocular regions. Ipsilateral projections arising from the ventrotemporal retina terminate in dorsomedial dLGN. Contralateral retinal projections fill the rest of the dLGN. The locations of other retinorecipient nuclei in the dorsal thalamus, the intergeniculate leaflet (IGL), and ventral LGN (vLGN) are also shown. The dLGN projects topographically to primary visual cortex (area 17). The medial two-thirds of area 17 receives monocular input from the contralateral eye (17M). The lateral one-third receives binocular inputs (17B). Adjacent to area 17 laterally is area 18a; area 18b is medial. (See figure 3.3.)

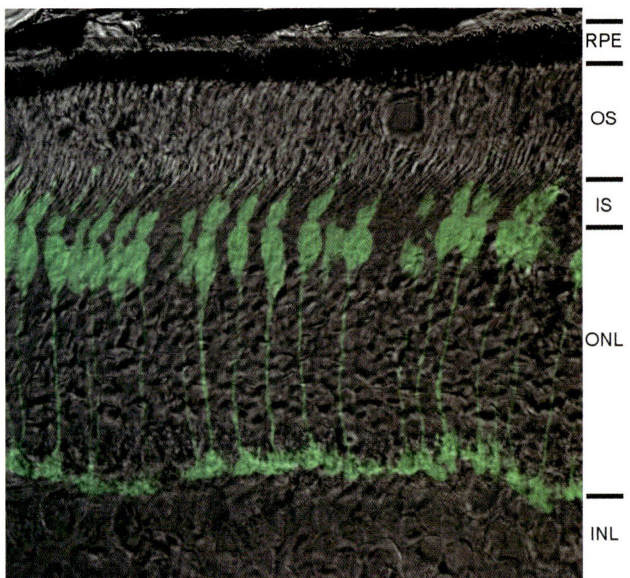

PLATE 2 Disposition and numerosity of mouse cones. The image superimposes confocal DIC and fluorescence image of a frozen section of the photoreceptor and RPE cell layer of a mouse retina. The mouse from whose eye the section was made expressed EGFP under the human M/L cone promoter (Fei and Hughes, 2001). (See figure 10.1.)

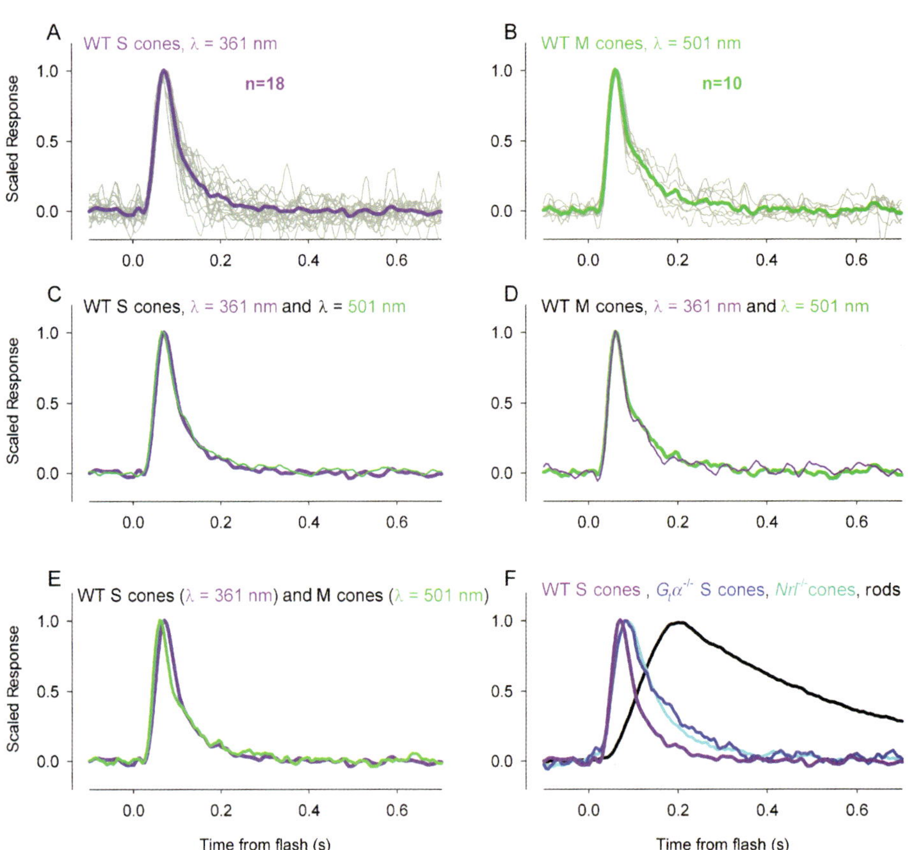

PLATE 3 Dim-flash responses of single mouse cones. Average dim-flash response data of S-dominant (*A* and *C*) and M-dominant (*B* and *D*) cones, stimulated with either UV (361 nm) or midwave (501 nm) flashes, are shown. In each case, analysis of the action spectrum reveals that the UV flash activates only the S-opsin in the cone, while the midwave flash activates M-opsin (the two being coexpressed). *F*, The averaged responses in *A* and *B* are compared with those of the cones of $G_t\alpha^{-/-}$ and $Nrl^{-/-}$ mice and with responses from wild-type mouse rods recorded under the same conditions (Nikonov et al., 2006). The midwave background light required to suppress rod responses in the wild-type mouse is not needed in experiments with $G_t\alpha^{-/-}$ and $Nrl^{-/-}$ cones and is at least partially responsible for the faster response kinetics of the wild-type cones. (See figure 10.5.)

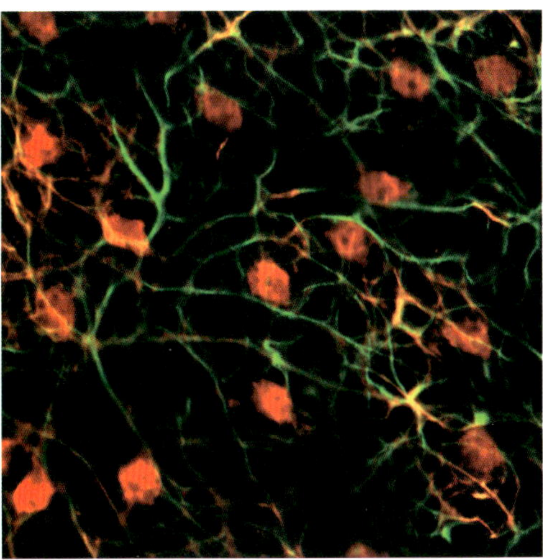

PLATE 4 Confocal image of a whole mount mouse retina in which horizontal cells are revealed with antibodies against calbindin D (red signal), while their axonal complexes are labeled with antineurofilament antibodies (green staining). (See figure 12.5.)

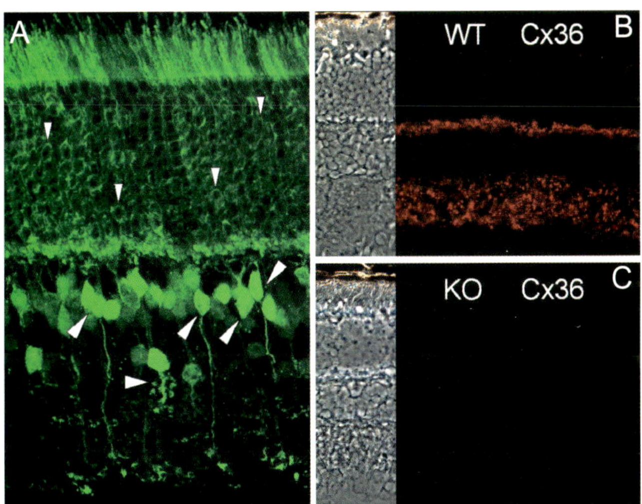

PLATE 5 *A*, β-Gal reporter in transgenic mouse retina indicates that Cx36 is expressed by photoreceptors in the ONL and by bipolar cells and amacrine cells in the INL. *Small arrowheads* indicate photoreceptor somata; *large arrowheads* indicate somata of an AII amacrine cell and bipolar cells. *B*, Transverse view of immunolabeling of the wild-type mouse retina for Cx36. Labeling is confined to the plexiform layers, consistent with the known locations of gap junctions between retinal neurons. *C*, Immunolabeling for Cx36 is absent in the Cx36 KO mouse retina. (See figure 13.1.) (*A*, Adopted from Deans et al., 2002, with permission. *B* and *C*, Adopted from Deans et al., 2001, with permission.)

A

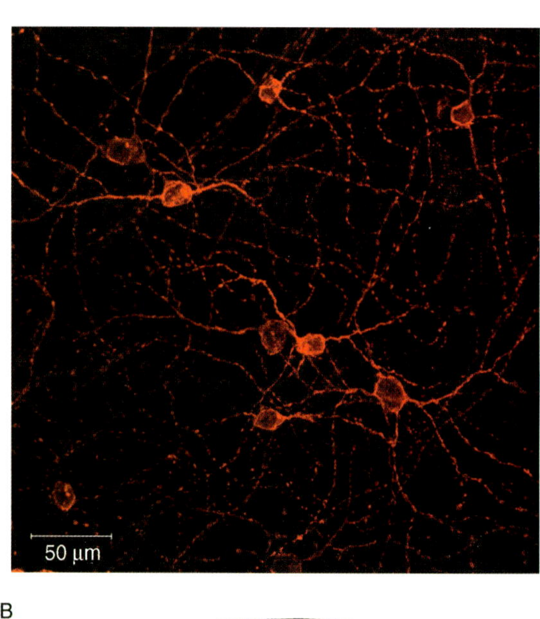

B

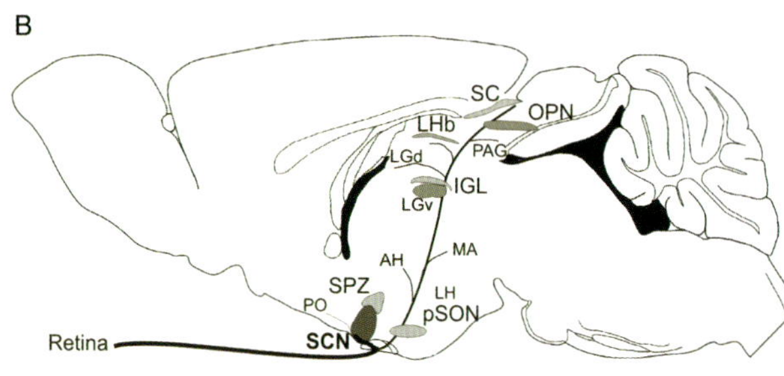

Plate 6 Morphology and projections of mRGCs in mouse. *A*, Retina flat mount stained with a polyclonal antimouse melanopsin antibody showing specific staining of dendrites, somata, and axons of a small subset of retinal ganglion cells. *B*, Schematic drawing showing direct axonal projections of mRGCs to several brain regions. (Results from Hattar et al., 2006, are redrawn here.) Brain regions receiving significant projections are represented in large, bold letters. AH, anterior hypothalamic nucleus; IGL, intergeniculate leaflet; LGd, lateral geniculate nucleus, dorsal division; LGv, lateral geniculate nucleus, ventral division; LH, lateral hypothalamus; LHb, lateral habenula; MA, median amygdaloid nucleus; OPN, olivary pretectal nucleus; PAG, periaqueductal gray; PO, preoptic; pSON, perisupraoptic nucleus; SC, superior colliculus; SCN, suprachiasmatic nucleus; SPZ, subparaventricular zone. (See figure 17.2.)

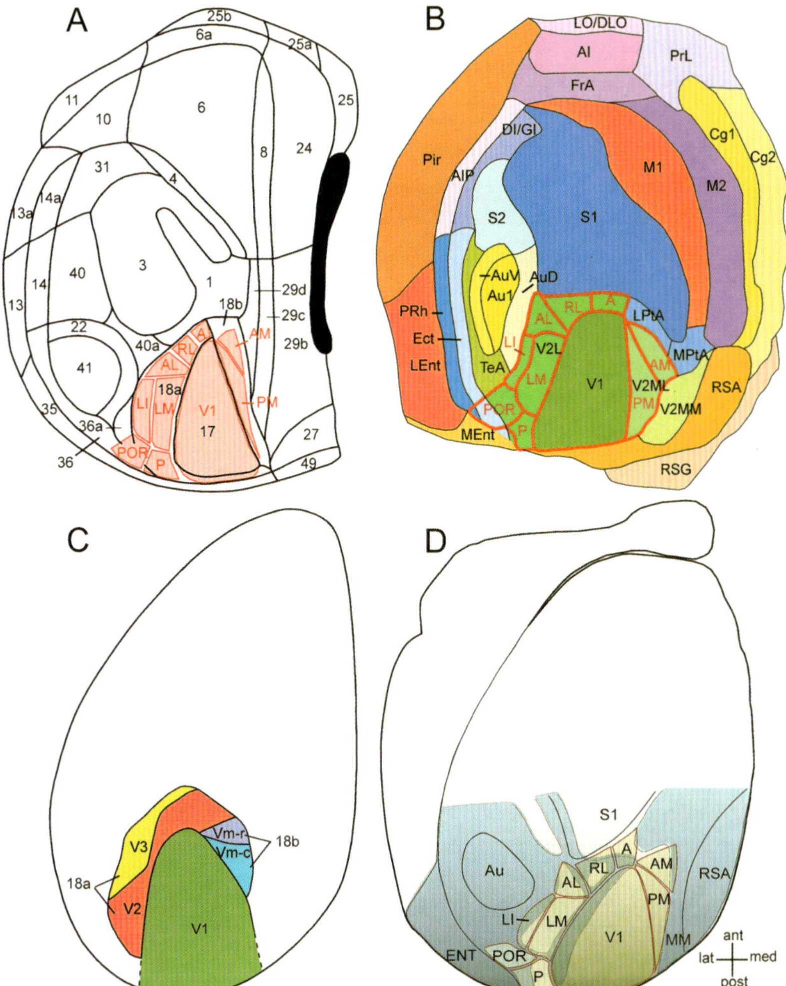

PLATE 7 Different maps of mouse visual cortex. *A*, Flat map of cytoarchitectonic areas (*black outlines*) in the left hemisphere of mouse cerebral cortex published by Caviness and Frost (1980). *Red shaded regions* represent schematic outlines of visuotopically organized areas, identified by Wang and Burkhalter (2006). Note that areas 18a and 18b contain multiple visuotopic areas. *B*, Flat map of cytoarchitectonic areas of the left mouse cerebral cortex constructed by David C. Van Essen by unfolding coronal sections taken from the atlas of Paxinos and Franklin (2001). *Red outlines* represent schematic borders of visuotopically defined areas identified by Wang and Burkhalter (2007). Note that areas V2L and V2ML contain multiple visuotopically organized areas. *C*, Visuotopic organization of the left mouse visual cortex derived by mapping of receptive fields, published by Wagor et al. (1980). In this map, cytoarchitectonic area 18a contains areas V2 and V3 and cytoarchitectonic area 18b contains the rostral and caudal medial visual areas, Vm-r and Vm-c. *D*, Area map of left mouse visual cortex derived by topographic mapping of V1 connections and receptive field mapping (Wang and Burkhalter, 2007). *Blue shading* represents the distribution of callosal connections in superficial layers. (See figure 20.1.)

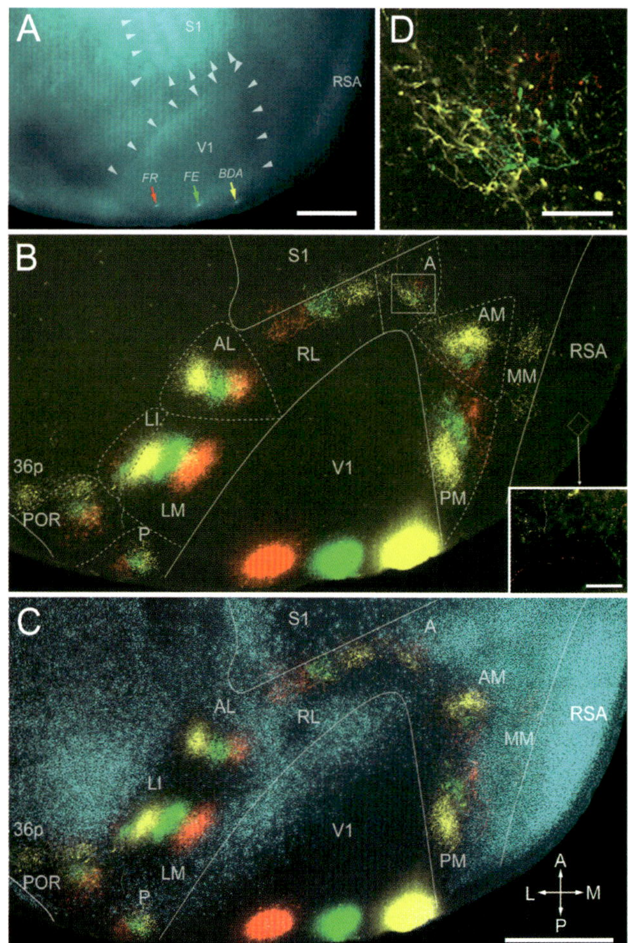

Plate 8 Topographic maps of V1 connections in mouse visual cortex. Representation of azimuth in extrastriate visual cortex is shown in horizontal sections of left occipital cortex. The maps were generated by making three simultaneous injections of fluororuby (FR, red), fluoroemerald (FE, green), and biotinylated dextran amine (BDA, yellow) into V1, followed by triple-anterograde tracing of intracortical connections. *A*, Darkfield image showing heavy myelination in primary visual cortex (V1) and the barrel field of primary somatosensory cortex (S1). *Arrowheads* indicate myeloarchitectonic borders. *Arrows* indicate injection sites in V1. *B*, Fluorescently labeled axonal connections after injections of FR, FE, and BDA at different nasotemporal locations (azimuth) of the upper visual field representation in V1. *Dashed lines* indicate areal borders, which were determined by mapping inputs from the perimeter of V1. *Solid lines* indicate myeloarchitectonic borders. *C*, Overlay of BDA-labeled axonal projections shown in *B* and bisbenzimide-labeled callosally projecting neurons (blue). *D*, Higher magnification image of axonal labeling shown in area A (inset in *B*). A, anterior; L, lateral; M, medial; P, posterior. Scale bar = 1 mm (*A–C*), 0.1 mm (*B, inset*), and 0.3 mm (*D*). (See figure 20.2.)

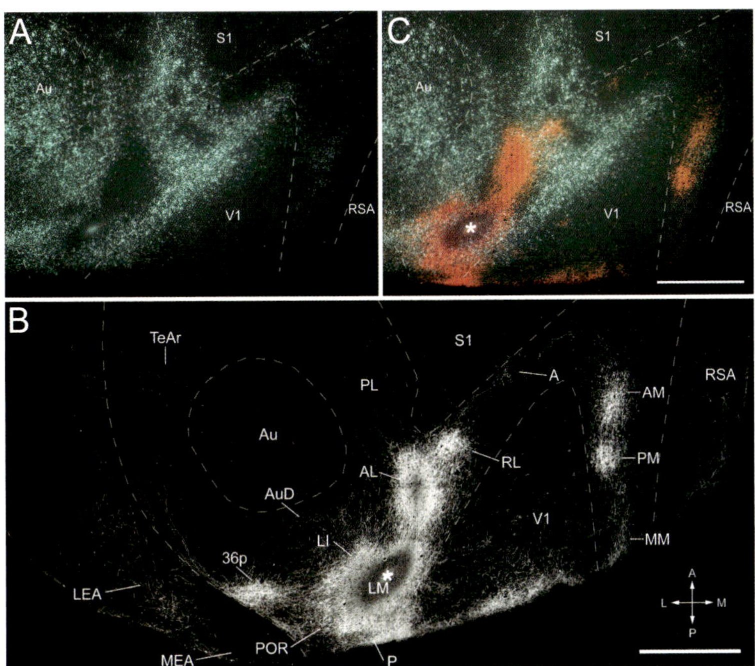

Plate 9 Intracortical connections of the extrastriate lateromedial area (LM) in mouse visual cortex, shown in tangential sections through the flattened posterior cerebral cortex. *A*, Fluorescence image showing the distribution of retrogradely labeled callosal connections. *Dashed lines* represent the myeloarchitectonic borders of V1, S1, and RSA. *B*, Darkfield image of biotinylated dextran amine (BDA)–labeled axonal connections of area LM. *Asterisk* indicates the injection site. Note the strong connections to areas POR and 36p. *C*, Superimposition of BDA-labeled LM connections (gold) with callosal connections (blue somata). A, anterior; L, lateral; M, medial; P, posterior. Scale bar = 1 mm in all images. (See figure 20.3.)

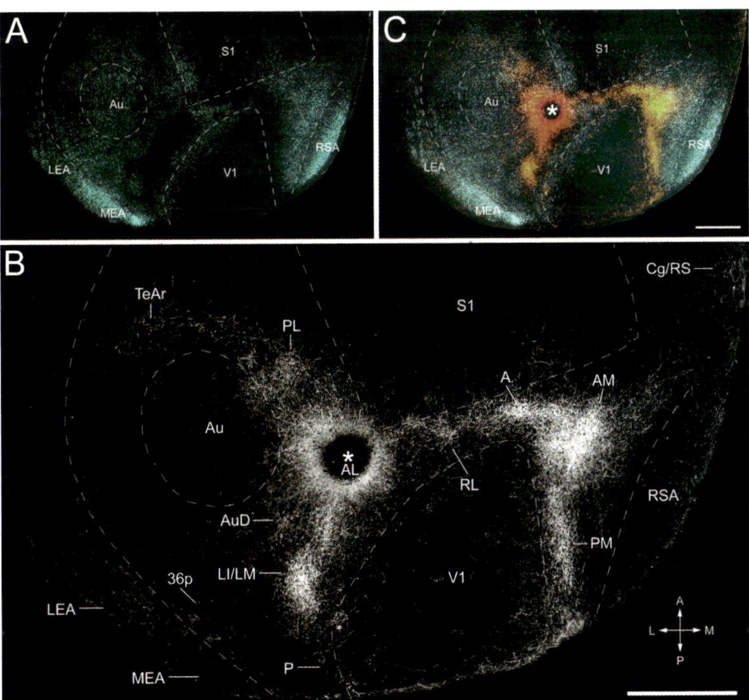

Plate 10 Intracortical connections of the extrastriate lateromedial area (AL) in mouse visual cortex, shown in tangential sections through the flattened posterior cerebral cortex. *A*, Fluorescence image showing the distribution of retrogradely labeled callosal connections. *Dashed lines* represent the myeloarchitectonic borders of V1, S1, and RSA. *B*, Darkfield image of biotinylated dextran amine (BDA)–labeled axonal connections of area AL. *Asterisk* indicates injection site. Note the strong connections to areas PL, A, and Cg/RS. *C*, Superimposition of BDA-labeled LM connections (gold) with callosal connections (blue somata). A, anterior; L, lateral; M, medial; P, posterior. Scale bar = 1 mm in all images. (See figure 20.4.)

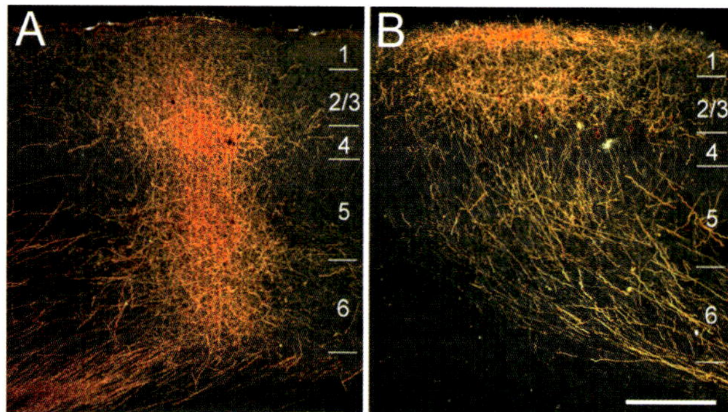

Plate 11 Laminar organization of inter-areal feedforward and feedback connections in mouse visual cortex labeled by anterograde tracing with BDA. *A*, Coronal section showing feedforward axons that originate from the lower area V1 and terminate in the higher extrastriate area LM. The projection column includes layers 2/3 to 6, and inputs to layer 1 are sparse. *B*, Coronal section showing feedback axons that originate from area LM and terminate in V1. The projections to layer 1, 2/3, and 5 are dense, whereas inputs to layer 4 are sparse. Scale bar = 0.2 mm. (See figure 20.5.)

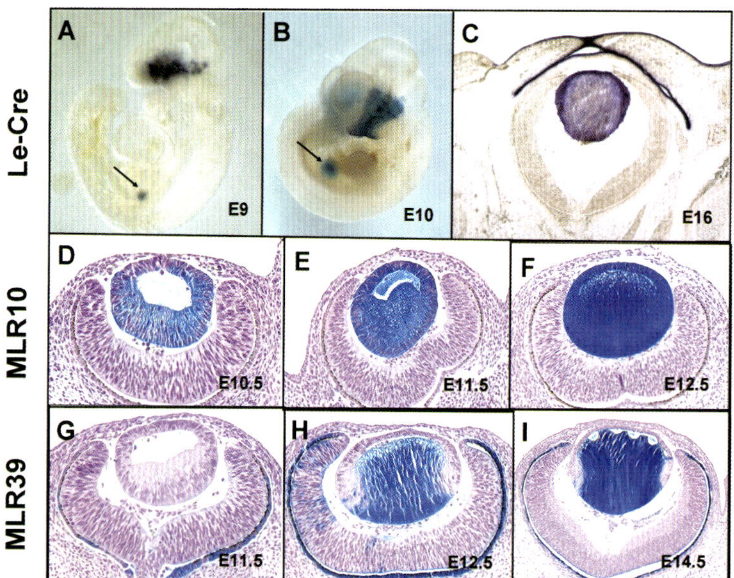

Plate 12 Cre expression patterns in three different transgenic strains: Le-Cre (*A–C*), MLR10 (*D–F*), and MLR39 (*G–I*). Cre expression in whole-mount (*A* and *B*) or tissue sections (*C–I*) is indicated by blue (*B* and *D–I*) or purple (*A* and *C*) staining following histochemical detection of a Cre-activated reporter allele. *Arrows* in *A* and *B* indicate Cre expression in the developing pancreas of Le-Cre mice. Developmental time points are indicated. (See figure 22.2.) (Adapted from Ashery-Padan et al., 2000, and Zhao et al., 2004.)

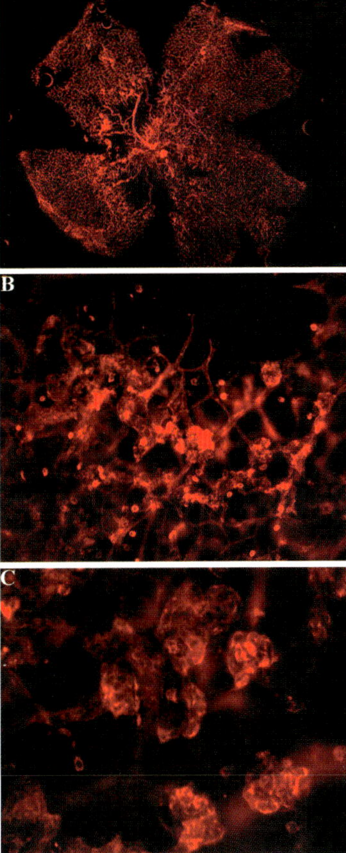

Plate 13 Visualization of vessels in P17 retinal flat-mount preparations stained with GS-lectin from a mouse model of OIR. *A*, Low-power (magnification ×25) image of the retina shows areas of central vaso-obliteration, as well as neovascular tufts. *B*, Higher magnification (×200) shows neovascular tuft formation at the transition zone between vascular and central avascular retina. *C*, At even greater magnification (×400), multiple neovascular tufts are evident. (See figure 23.4.)

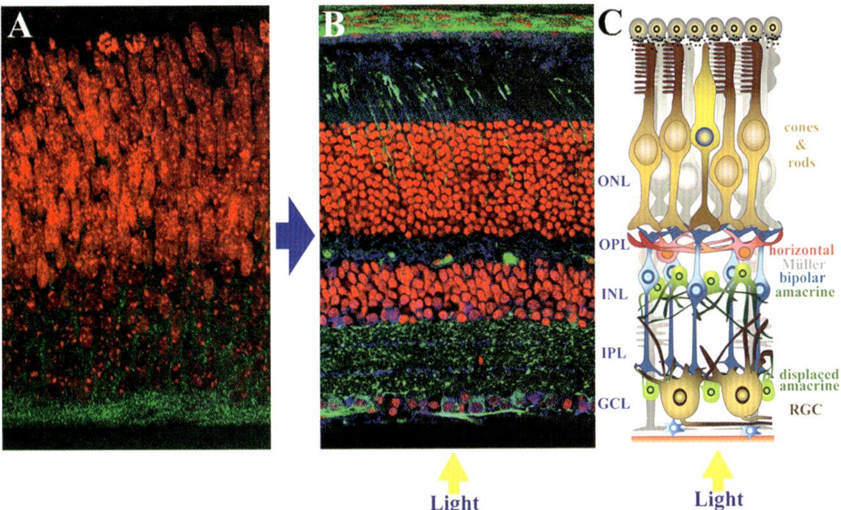

Plate 14 Developing and mature mouse retinas. *A*, An embryonic retina at E12.5. *B*, A postnatal retina at P16. Nuclei are labeled in red with propidium iodide and represent the positions of the cell soma. Neurite processes are labeled in green and blue with antineurofilament antibody and anticholine acetyltransferase antibody, respectively, and represent axons and dendrites. *C*, Schematic representation of the mature retina. RGCs and displaced amacrine cells are found within the ganglion cell layer (GCL). Intermediate neurons (horizontal, bipolar, and amacrine) are found within the inner nuclear layer (INL), and rod and cone photoreceptor cells are found within the outer nuclear layer (ONL). IPL and OPL are inner plexiform and outer plexiform layers where axons and dendrites synapse. RGC, retinal ganglion cell. (See figure 26.1.)

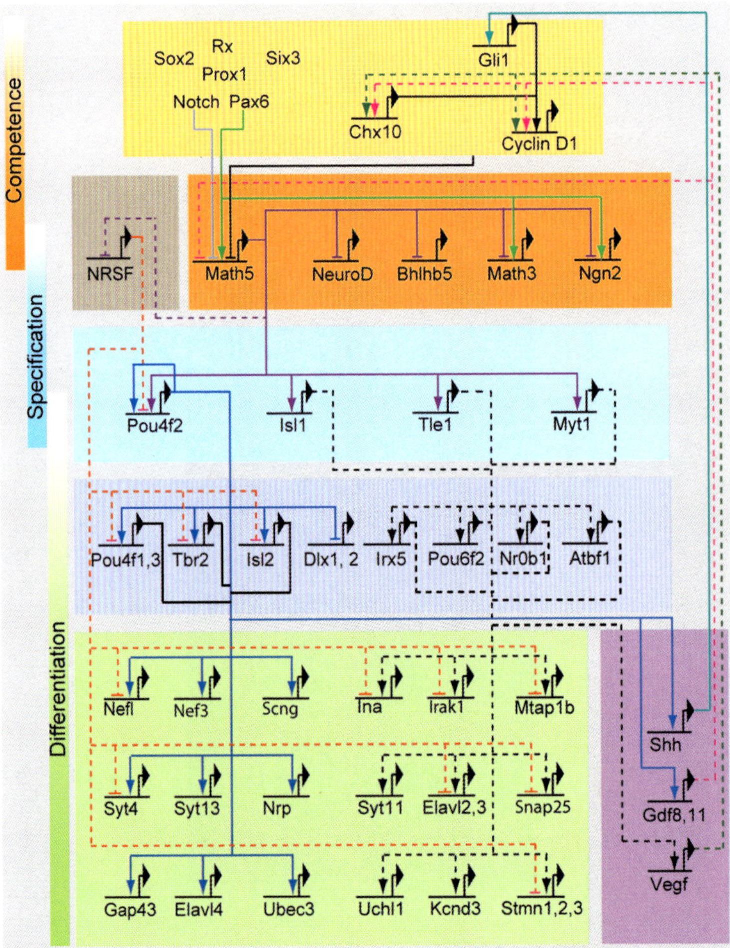

Plate 15 A gene regulatory network model for RGC development. Genes are depicted such that the right side of the *bent arrow* for each gene indicates the gene product and the left side indicates the transcriptional control region. *Solid lines* connecting genes indicate established upstream-downstream relationships, and *dashed lines* suggest inferred relationships. *Downward-pointing arrows* indicate gene activation, and *downward perpendicular lines* indicate gene repression. In most cases the connections have not been shown to be direct. Genes boxed in yellow represent regulators of general retinal competence and RPC proliferation; genes boxed in orange are proneural bHLH genes associated with establishing competence in RPCs for specific retinal cell fates. The light brown-purple box represents the general repression of RGC genes hypothesized to be mediated by the neural differentiation transcriptional repressor NSRF/REST (Mu et al., 2005b); the blue and purple-blue boxes represent genes encoding RGC-specific upstream (blue) and downstream (purple-blue) transcription factors. Genes boxed in green are those that encode proteins associated with RGC maturation and function. Genes boxed in purple encode secreted signaling molecules. In some cases only representative examples are shown for each box. A more detailed description can be found in Mu et al., 2005b. (See figure 26.2.)

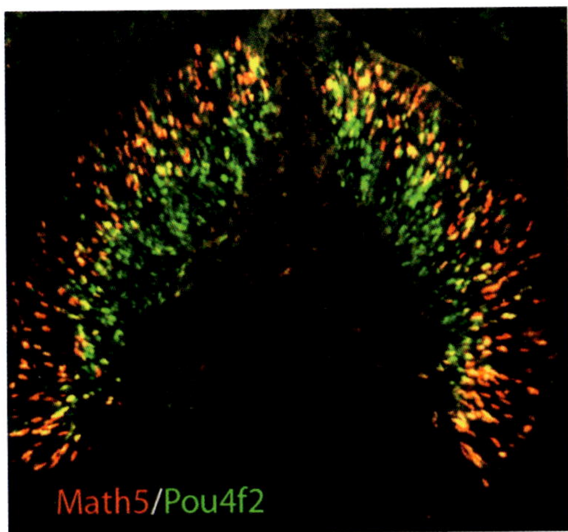

Plate 16 Segregated expression of Math5 and Pou4f2 in retinogenesis. The image represents an E14.5 retina from a knock-in mouse in which a gene encoding an HA-epitope-tagged Math5 replaces the endogenous *Math5* allele. Math5-HA expression is detected by immunostaining with an anti-HA antibody (red). Pou4f2 expression is detected by immunostaining with an anti-Pou4f2 antibody (green). Yellow staining shows the overlap in expression of Math5 and Pou4f2. (See figure 26.3.)

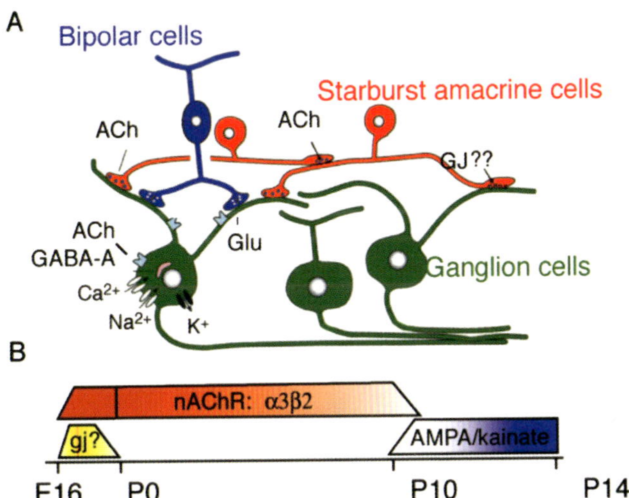

Plate 17 Three functional stages of retinal wave–generating circuits. *A*, Schematic of circuits that mediate retinal waves. (Modified from Catsicas and Mobbs, 1995.) *B*, Summary of development of the synaptic circuitry that mediates waves in mice. Each color corresponds to a different wave-generating circuit. Yellow corresponds to non-nAChR circuitry, which mediates the nonpropagating events in embryonic mice. There is pharmacological evidence that stage I waves in other species are mediated by gap junctions, but this has not been directly demonstrated in mouse retina. In addition, it is not known which gap junction–coupled networks mediate stage I waves. Red corresponds to stage II circuits, which require activation of nAChRs. Stage II waves are initiated and propagate through a network of starburst amacrine cells. Blue corresponds to stage III circuits, which require activation of ionotropic glutamate receptors. The source of stage III wave initiation and the location of the horizontal coupling that drives coordinated release of glutamate during this stage are not yet known. (See figure 28.1.) (Modified from Bansal et al., 2000.)

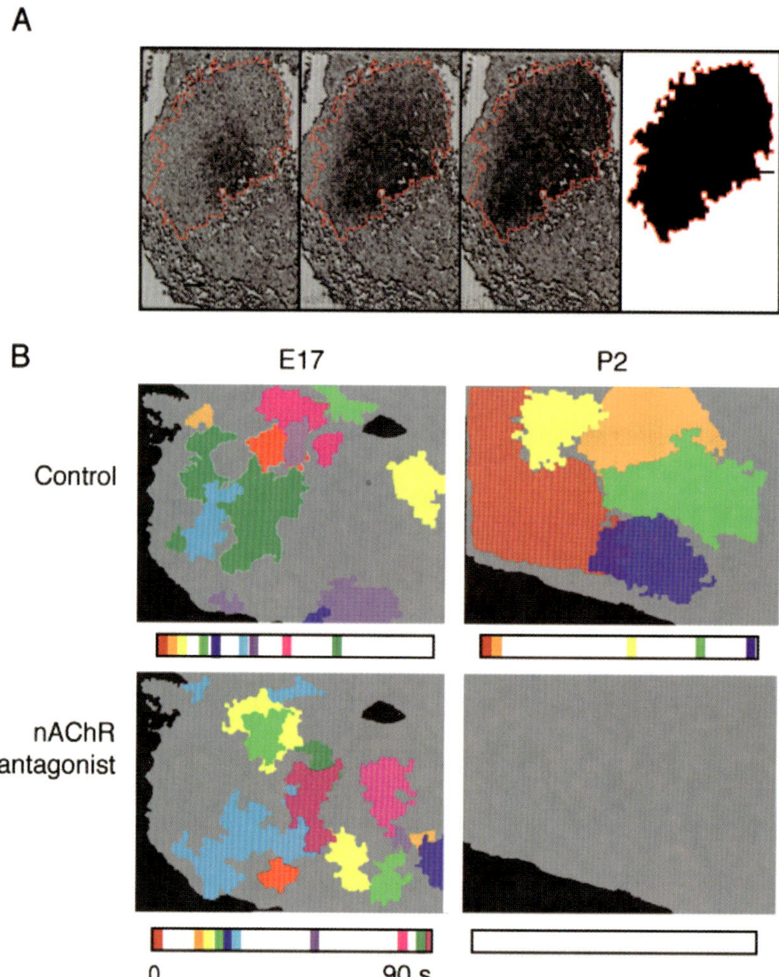

PLATE 18 Calcium imaging reveals spatial and temporal properties of stage I and stage II waves. *A*, Time evolution of a single stage II retinal wave visualized with fluorescence imaging of the calcium indicator fura-2. Decreases in fura-2 fluorescence associated with the increased calcium evoked by waves are shown at successive 0.5 s intervals. The final frame represents the total area of tissue covered by a single wave. *B*, Retinal waves of embryonic day 17 (E17) and postnatal day 2 (P2) retinas. Each frame summarizes 90 s of activity in control ACSF (*top row*) and in 100 μM *d*-tubocurarine, a general nAChR antagonist (*bottom row*). Gray background represents the total retinal surface labeled with fura-2AM. Each color corresponds to individual domains, with a color-coded time bar below each frame to indicate the time of occurrence of each wave. Scale bar = 100 μm. (See figure 28.2.) (Modified from Bansal et al., 2000.)

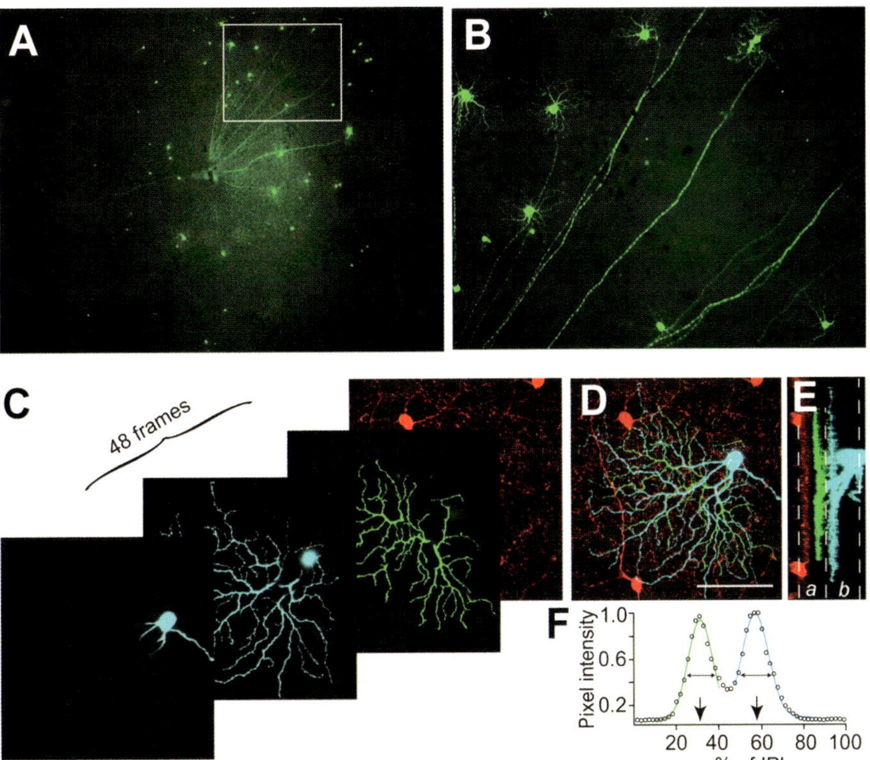

PLATE 19 Dendritic ramification patterns of YFP expressing RGCs in the IPL can be determined using confocal microscopy from Thy1-YFP transgenic mouse retina. *A*, View from vitreal side of a flat-mounted retina harvested from a Thy1-YFP-expressing mouse. *B*, Enlarged view of the area inside the *box* in *A*. Axons from individual RGCs cross the retina from each soma to the optic nerve head. *C*, Four frames taken from a representative stack of confocal images of a bistratified RGC showing the soma and axon, the dendrites ramified in sublamina b (blue), the dendrites ramified in sublamina a (green) of the RGC, and immunolabeling of dopaminergic amacrine cells (red). *D*, A stacked image of the same cell as shown in panel *C*. *E*, The 90° rotation view of the cell in *D*. Three *dashed lines* indicate the inner border of the IPL, the boundary of sublaminae a and b, and the outer border of the IPL. *F*, Normalized pixel intensity of the dendrites of each frame (*open circles*) plotted as a function of IPL depth of the cell in panel *C*. The data were fitted with two Gaussian distributions (green and blue lines). *Double-arrow lines* indicate widths. *Single arrows* indicate the locations of the two peaks of dendritic density. (See figure 29.3.)

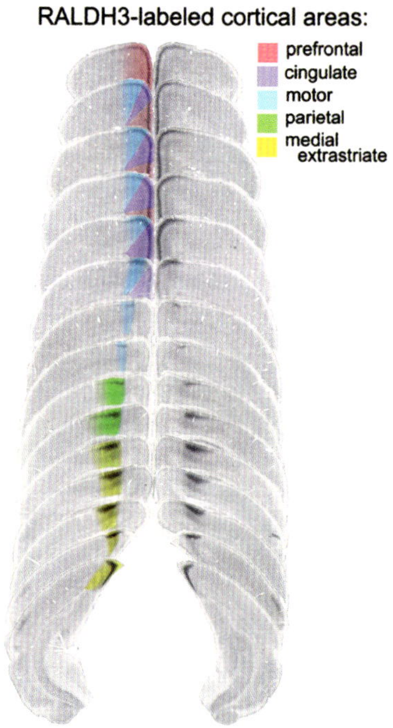

RALDH3-labeled cortical areas:

prefrontal
cingulate
motor
parietal
medial extrastriate

Plate 20 The anatomical locations of the medial RALDH3 band are indicated for P15 in the form of a color code, in which *prefrontal* includes the prelimbic and medial orbital cortices; *cingulate* includes areas 1 and 2 of the cingulate cortex; *motor* designates mostly the secondary motor cortex, in addition to a small caudal part of the primary motor cortex; *parietal* includes the medial and lateral parietal association cortices; and *medial extrastriate* extends from a location where the rostral extrastriate region abuts the parietal association cortex all the way caudally, an elongated region also called area 18b or V2M (Wagner et al., 2006). (See figure 30.4.)

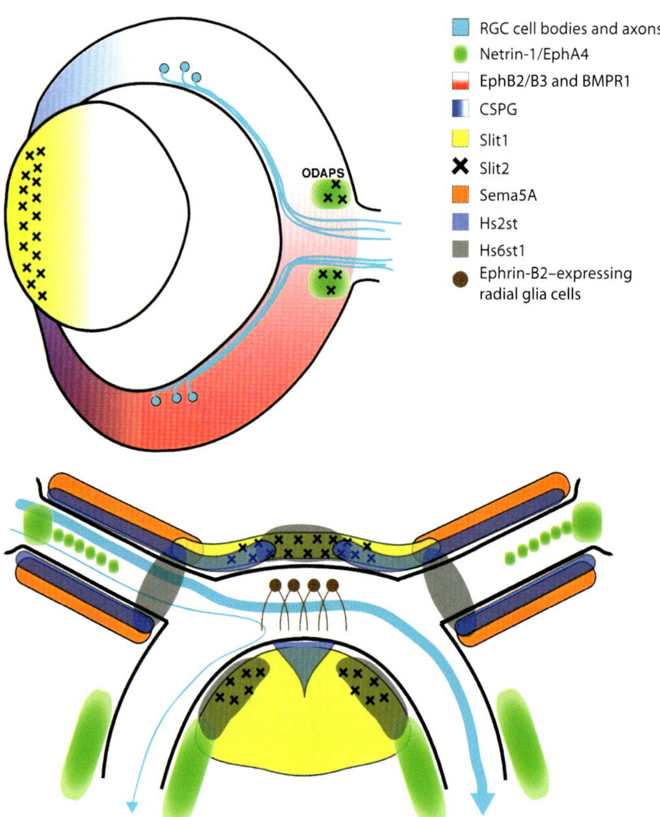

Plate 21 Cues that guide RGC axons through the visual pathway. *Top*, RGC axons (blue) express many receptors for a number of cues in the retina that guide them toward the optic disc and out of the retina. *Bottom*, A variety of cues surrounding the optic nerve, chiasm, and tract help to funnel RGC axons properly through the ventral diencephalon toward their final targets, the LGN and SC. ODAPs, optic disc astrocyte precursor cells. (See figure 32.2.)

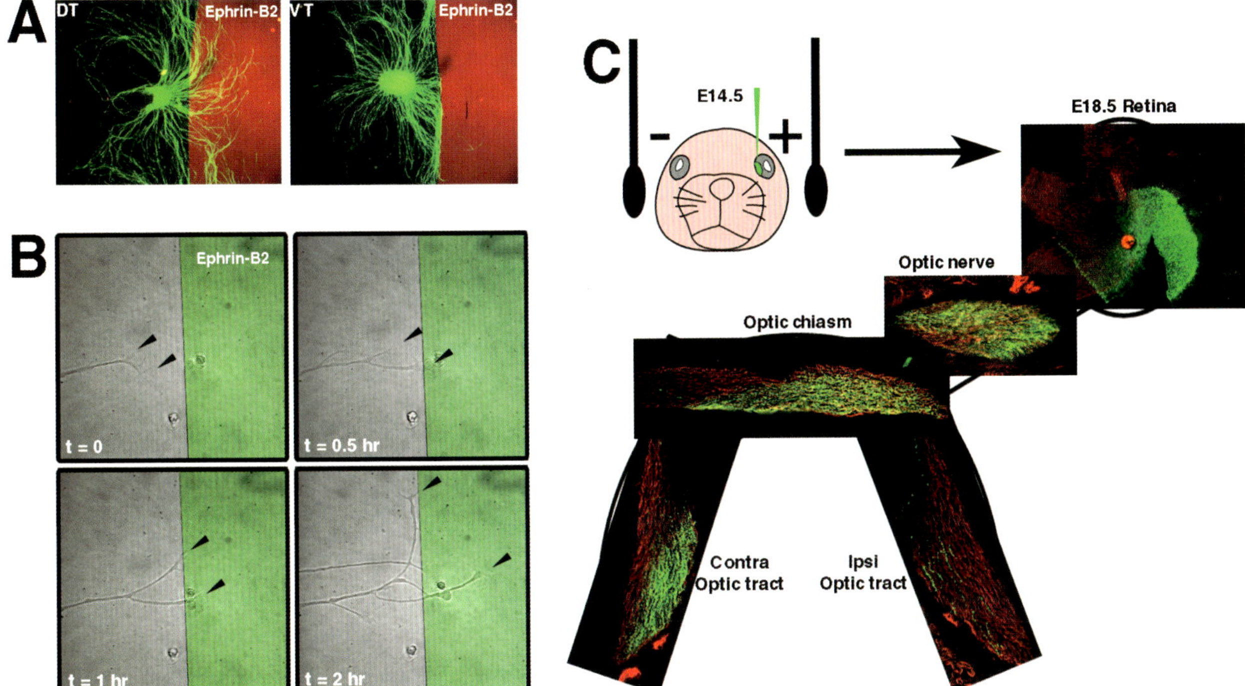

Plate 22 Important techniques for studying RGC projections in the developing mouse visual system. *A*, DT and VT retinal explants plated near a border of 0.5 μg/mL ephrin-B2 (red). Axons from DT explants project into the ephrin-B2 region, while VT axons are clearly inhibited. *B*, Time-lapse imaging can be used to study RGC growth cone behavior in real time as they encounter a border, in this case ephrin-B2. *Arrowheads* highlight two growth cones, one of which projects into the ephrin-B2 region and the other of which is repelled and travels parallel to the ephrin-B2 border. *C*, Diagram depicting in utero retinal electroporation. Briefly, DNA is injected into embryonic retina. Current is passed through electroporation paddles, and embryos are allowed to survive for several days. Embryos are perfused, the retina is collected, and heads are cryosectioned. In this case, GFP-positive cells can be seen in the retina, and many GFP-positive RGC projections are visible through the optic nerve, chiasm, and tract. Red denotes neurofilament. (See figure 32.5.) (All images courtesy of T. Petros and C. Mason.)

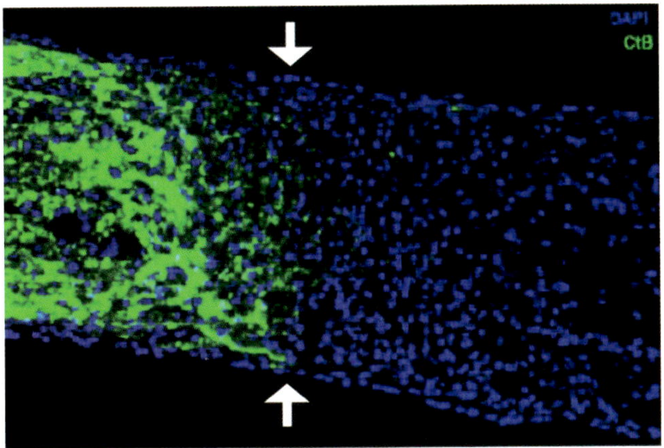

Plate 23 After an optic nerve crush injury, RGC axons were labeled with an intravitreal injection of fluorophore-conjugated cholera toxin B. The bright axons (green) failed to regrow across the lesion site (*arrows*) after 8 days in vivo. Optic nerve nuclei are counterstained with a nuclear dye, DAPI. (See figure 33.6.) (Y. Duan and J. L. Goldberg. [2008]. Unpublished data.)

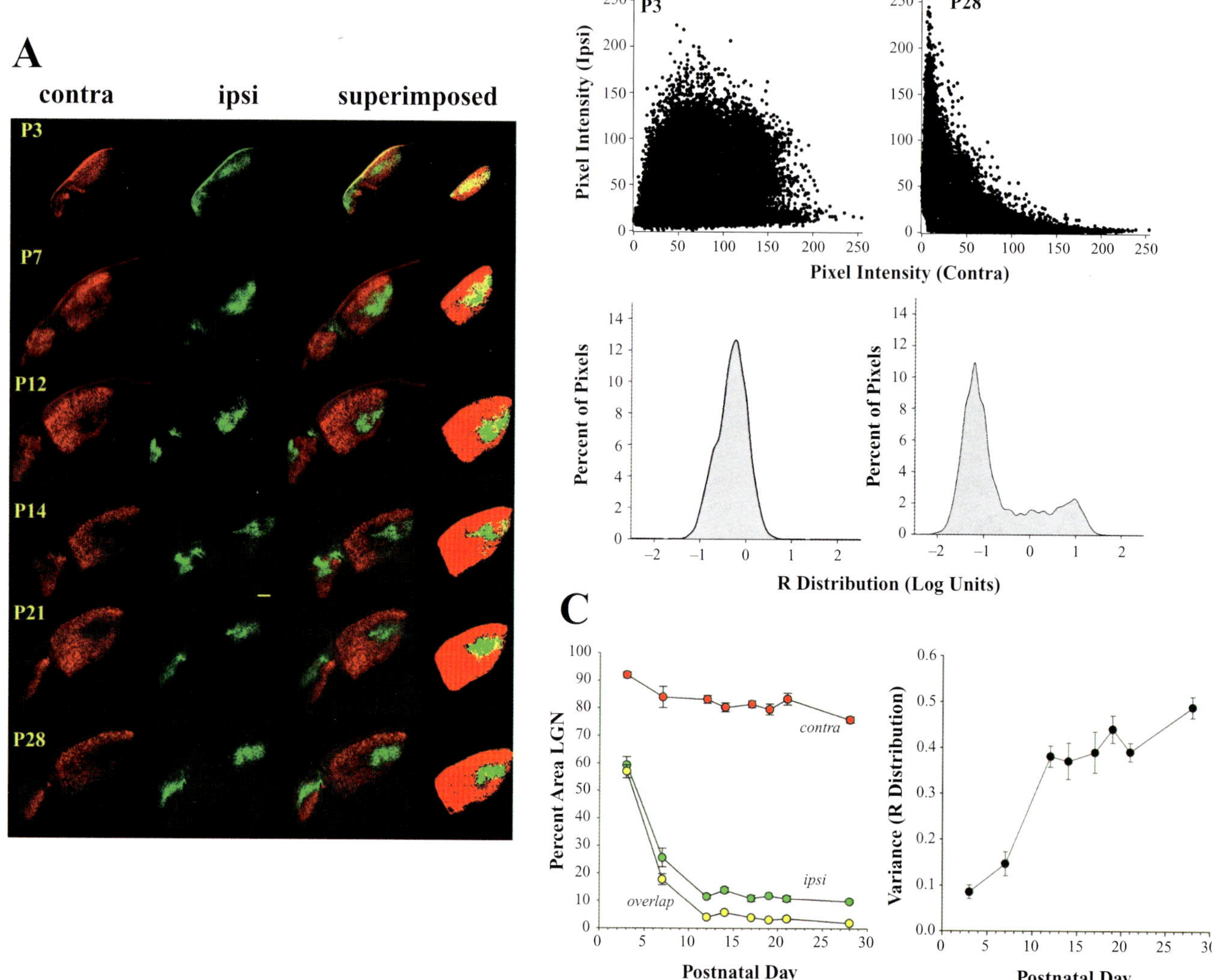

PLATE 24 Retinogeniculate axon segregation in the developing mouse. *A*, Anterograde transport of CTβ conjugated to Alexa Fluor 594 (red) labels contralateral eye projections, and anterograde transport of CTβ conjugated to Alexa Fluor 488 (green) labels ipsilateral eye projections. Panels from left to right depict red and green fluorescence labeling of the same section of LGN. Adjacent to these are the superimposed fluorescent pattern and corresponding pseudo-colored image, where pixel intensity is assigned a single value above a defined threshold. Pixels that contain both red and green fluorescence are considered areas of overlap and are represented in yellow. Scale bar = 100 μm. *B*, Pixel intensity analysis reveals degree of eye-specific segregation in the developing LGN. *Top*, Scatterplots of pixel intensity for a single section through LGN at P3 and P28. Each point represents a pixel in which the fluorescence intensity of the ipsilateral projection is plotted against the intensity of the contralateral projection. At P3, when projections overlap, pixel intensities show a positive correlation. At P28, projections are segregated and pixel intensities show a negative correlation. *Bottom*, Corresponding *R* distributions of pixel intensity. For each pixel the logarithm of the intensity ratio ($R = \log_{10} F_I/F_C$) is plotted as a frequency histogram (bin size = 0.1 log units). A narrow *R* distribution (P3) shows an unsegregated pattern; a wide one (P28) shows a segregated pattern. *C*, Summary plots showing the spatial extent of retinal projections (*left*) and the variance of *R* distributions (*right*) at different ages. *Left*, Percent area in LGN occupied by contralateral, ipsilateral, and overlapping terminal fields at different ages. Each point represents the mean and SEM for a group of same-aged animals. Note that ipsilateral projections and the degree of overlap recede between P3 and P12. *Right*, Mean and SEM variance values obtained from *R* distributions. Changes in spatial extent are accompanied by a parallel increase in variance and reflect a progressive increase in the degree of eye-specific segregation between P3 and P12. (See figure 34.2.) (Adapted from Jaubert-Miazza et al., 2005.)

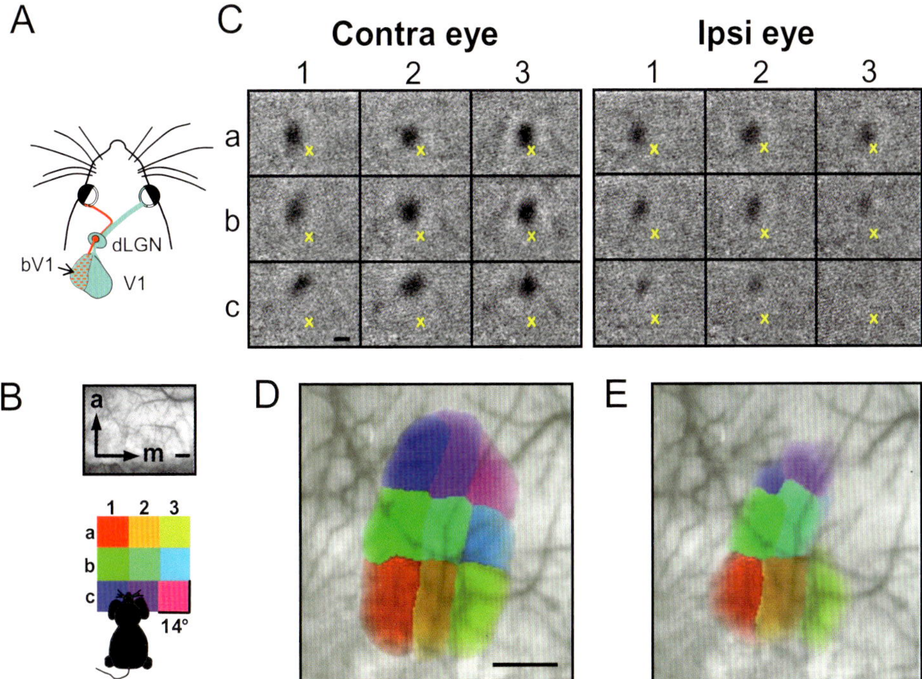

Plate 25 Retinotopic mapping of mouse binocular visual cortex using optical imaging of intrinsic signals. *A*, Schematic illustration of primary visual pathway in the mouse, depicting the location of the dorsal lateral geniculate nucleus (dLGN) and the primary visual cortex (V1), with the binocular zone (bV1) located laterally. *B*, *Top*, Cortical blood vessel pattern as imaged through the skull. *Bottom*, Arrangement of grating stimuli used to map the central visual field. Color denotes stimulus position. *C*, Individual activity maps displaying responses to the 3 × 3 stimulus grid depicted in *B* are presented separately to the two eyes. The coordinates of the yellow cross are fixed in each map. *D* and *E*, Color-coded maps of the combined responses to contralateral (*D*) and ipsilateral (*E*) eye stimulation superimposed on the cortical blood vessel pattern, revealing the extent of the binocular zone. Color indicates stimulus position eliciting the strongest response at each pixel. Scale bars = 0.5 mm. (See figure 36.1.)

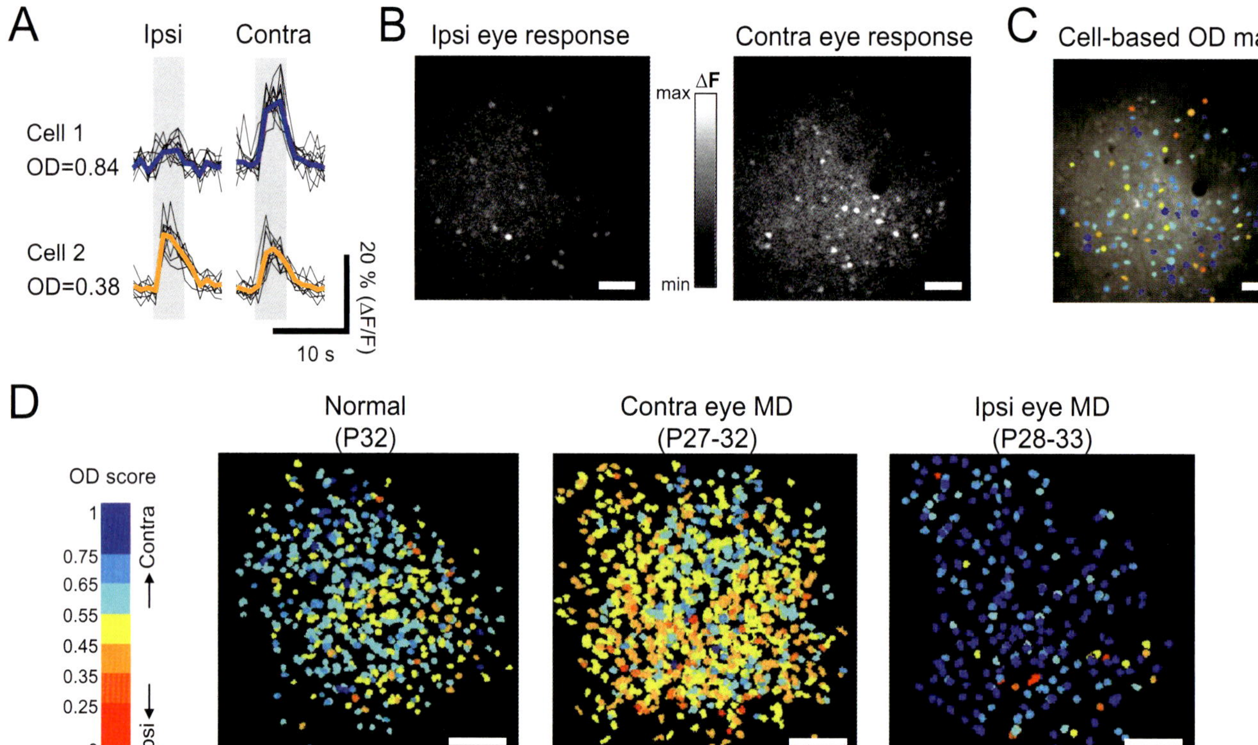

Plate 26 Mapping OD in mouse binocular visual cortex by two-photon calcium imaging. *A*, Examples of visually evoked calcium transients (fluorescent change, ΔF/F) recorded from two different neurons in the binocular visual cortex loaded with the calcium indicator dye OGB-1AM. *Thin traces* show individual responses to stimulation of each eye; *thick traces* are average responses to eight stimulus presentations. Stimulation periods are indicated by gray bars. *B*, Response maps (ΔF) for the contralateral (*left panel*) and ipsilateral (*right panel*) eye 230 μm below the pial surface in a normal mouse. *C*, A cell-based OD map computed from the single-eye response maps in *B*. Individual neurons are color coded by the OD score, as indicated by the labels in *D*. OD score of 1 or 0 denotes exclusive response to contralateral or ipsilateral eye stimulation, respectively, and a value of 0.5 indicates an equal response to both eyes. *D*, Overlay of cell-based OD maps at different depths for a normal mouse (*left*, four depths, 190–290 μm), after a 5-day contralateral MD (*center*, six depths, 195–410 μm), and after a 5-day ipsilateral MD (*right*, two depths, 200 and 225 μm). Note weak clustering of cells with similar OD values in the normal mouse. Scale bars = 50 μm. (See figure 36.3.)

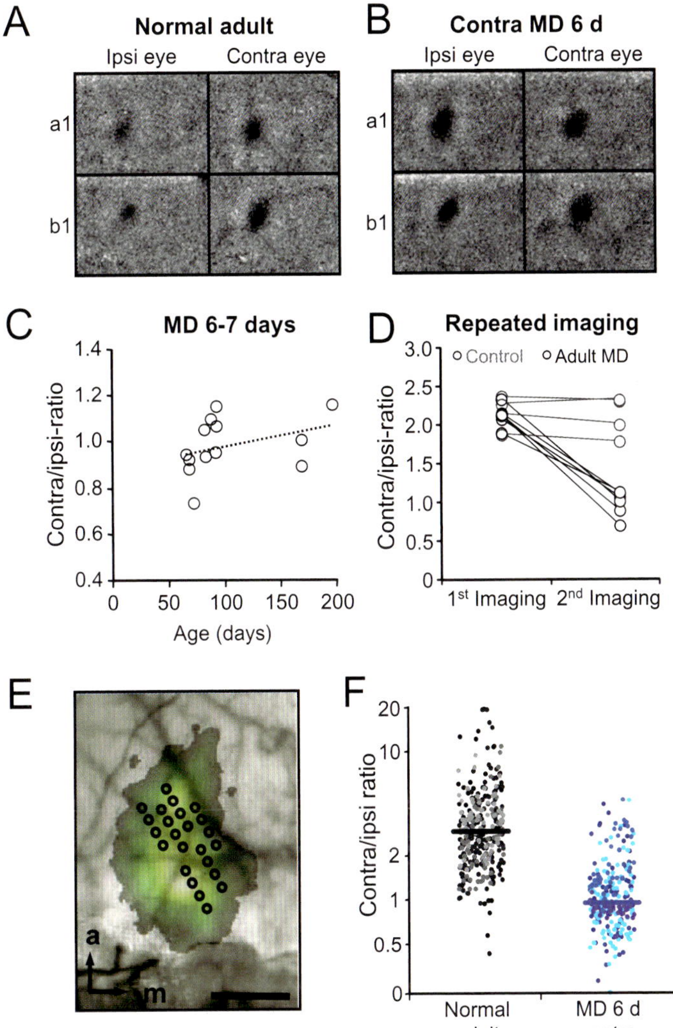

Plate 27 OD plasticity in adult visual cortex assessed with intrinsic signal imaging and multielectrode recordings. *A* and *B*, Ipsilateral and contralateral eye responses in the same mouse before (*A*, P80, contralateral/ipsilateral ratio = 2.21) and after 6 days of MD (*B*, P92, contralateral/ipsilateral ratio = 1.09). Stimulus arrangement as in figure 36.2*A*. *C*, Ratio of contralateral to ipsilateral eye response strength after 6–7 days of MD in normal adult mice plotted against age shows no significant correlation. $R^2 = 0.12$, $P = 0.24$. *D*, Contralateral/ipsilateral ratio values from repeated experiments in adult control animals (gray, interimaging period 1–3 weeks) and in deprived adult animals before and after 6 days of MD in the contralateral eye (black). *E*, Functional map of the binocular region (green corresponds to the ipsilateral eye representation), used for targeting electrode penetrations (*circles*). Scale bar = 0.5 mm. *F*, Distribution of contralateral/ipsilateral ratio values from all recording sites in adult control (2.99 ± 0.28, mean ± SEM, 324 recording sites, 4 mice) and deprived (1.05 ± 0.12, 260 recording sites, 5 mice) animals, showing strong OD shifts in response to MD. Each color represents a different animal. *Horizontal lines* indicate mean group values. (See figure 36.4.)

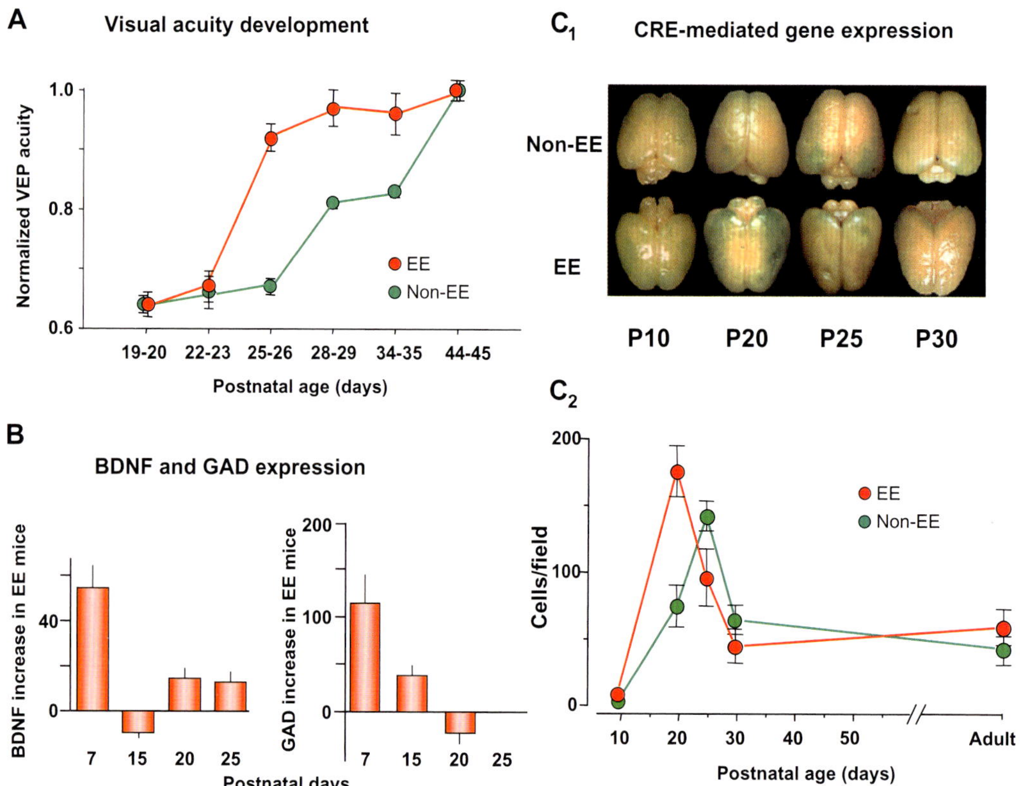

Plate 28 Acceleration of visual system development by environmental enrichment. *A*, EE accelerates the maturation of visual acuity. Visual acuity of non-EE (green) and EE (red) rats has been assessed by means of visual evoked potentials (VEPs) recorded from the binocular portion of the visual cortex at different ages during postnatal development. VEP acuity is normalized to the acuity value at P44–P45 and is plotted as a function of age for each experimental group to show the leftward shift of the curve for EE animals. *B*, Higher levels of BDNF and GAD65/67 expression in EE pups. ELISA and Western blot analysis have been used to measure, respectively, BDNF and GAD65/67 protein levels in the visual cortex of EE and non-EE animals at different postnatal ages. Data are plotted as percentage of variation between the two groups, with positive values indicating higher levels in EE mice. *C*, Accelerated CRE-mediated gene expression development in the visual cortex of EE mice. C_1, Examples of brains at different ages (P10–P30) from CRE-lacZ transgenic mice reared in non-EE or EE conditions. X-gal histochemistry has been used to reveal the occurrence of CRE-mediated gene expression (blue precipitate). C_2, Quantification of the density of X-gal-positive cells for non-EE (green) and EE (red) mice at the indicated ages. Fields were chosen to sample layers II–VI of the binocular visual cortex. CRE-mediated gene expression is developmentally regulated in both groups, but its peak is accelerated in EE mice. (See figure 37.1.) (*A*, Modified from Landi et al., 2007b. *B* and *C*, Modified from Cancedda et al., 2004.)

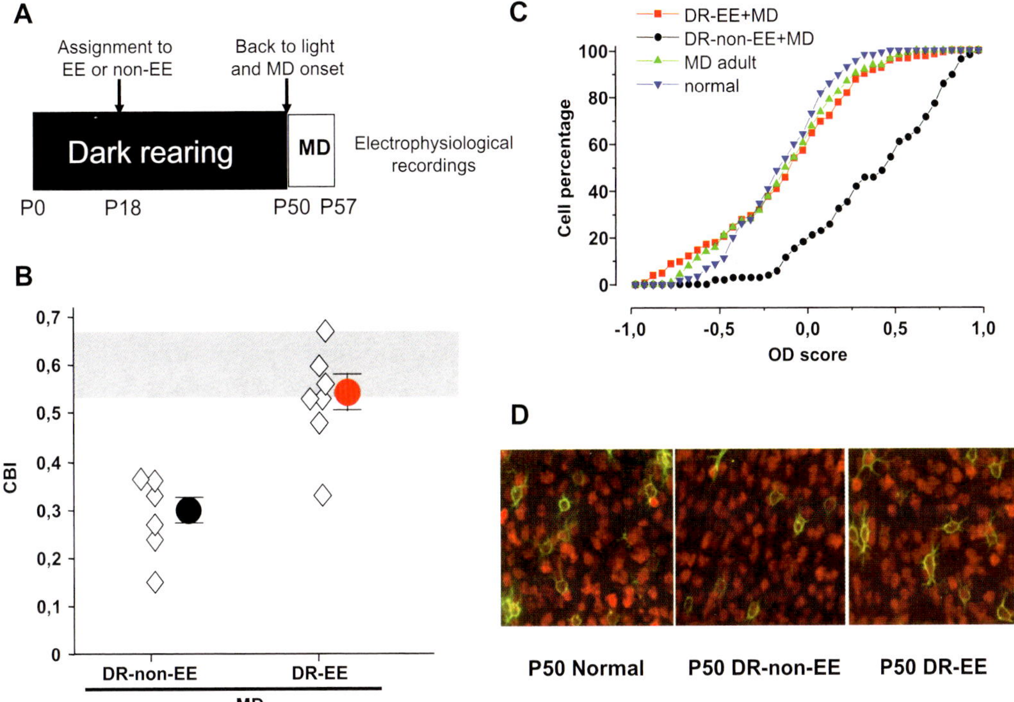

PLATE 29 Environmental enrichment promotes consolidation of visual cortical connections in dark-reared rats. *A*, Schematic diagram of the dark-rearing (DR) protocol combined with EE. Newborn rats were reared in complete darkness from P0 until P50. Together with DR, they were maintained, starting from P18, in either non-EE or EE conditions. Rats were then subjected to 1 week of MD, in normal light conditions. *B* and *C*, Normal closure of the critical period for MD in EE rats. *B*, Summary of MD effects in all DR animals. The OD distribution of each animal has been summarized with the contralateral bias index (CBI = {[N(1) – N(7)] + 1/2[N(2/3) – N(5/6)] + N(Tot)}/2N(Tot), where N(tot) is the total number of recorded cells and N(i) is the number of cells in class (i) (*open diamonds* denote individual data; *circles* denote mean of the group ± SE). CBI scores in DR-non-EE + MD rats differ from those in DR-EE + MD rats, which do not differ from those in normal adults (*shaded rectangle*). *C*, Cumulative fractions for OD scores. For each cell, an OD score was computed as {[Peak(ipsi) – baseline(ipsi)] – [Peak(contra) – baseline(contra)]}/{[Peak(ipsi) – baseline(ipsi)] + [Peak(contra) – baseline(contra)]} (Rittenhouse et al., 1999). This score is –1 for class 1 cells, +1 for class 7 cells, and around 0 for class 4 cells. Only the curve for DR + non-EE MD animals significantly differs from that in normal rats. *D*, Examples of staining for Wisteria floribunda agglutinin (which labels perineural nets, green) and NeuN (neuronal marker, red) in Oc1B of a normal rat, a DR-non-EE rat, and a DR-EE rat at P50. The decrease caused by DR in the number of perineural net–surrounded neurons is reduced in EE-DR animals. Calibration bar = 100 μm. (See figure 37.2.) (Modified from Bartoletti et al., 2004.)

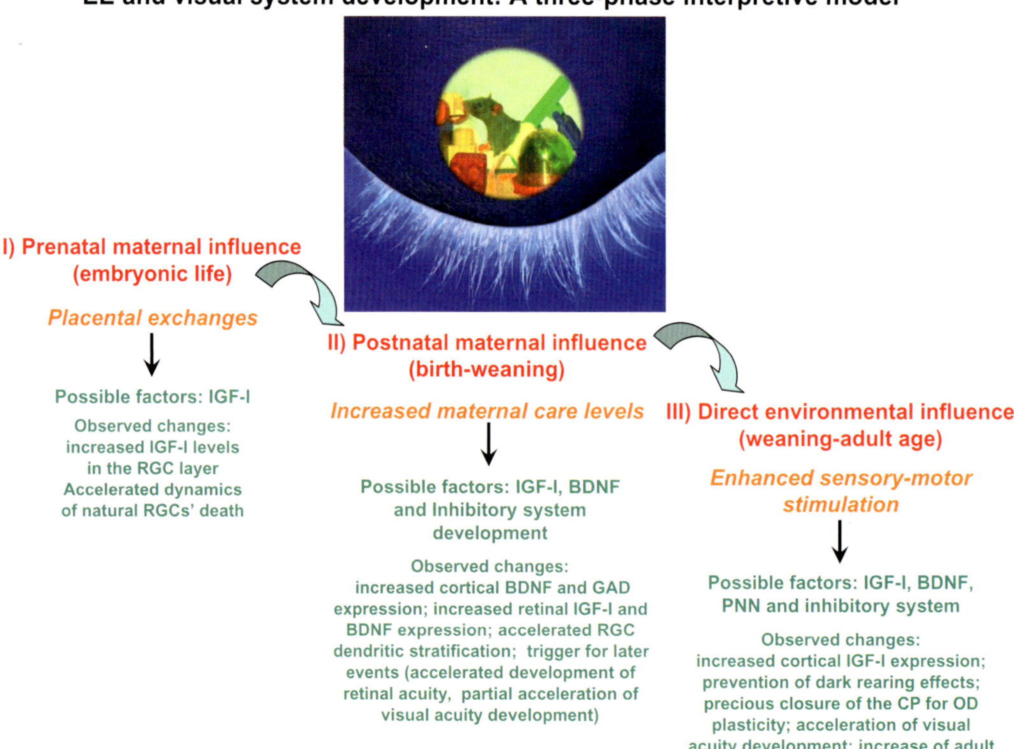
EE and visual system development: A three-phase interpretive model
I) Prenatal maternal influence (embryonic life)
Placental exchanges
Possible factors: IGF-I
Observed changes: increased IGF-I levels in the RGC layer Accelerated dynamics of natural RGCs' death
II) Postnatal maternal influence (birth-weaning)
Increased maternal care levels
Possible factors: IGF-I, BDNF and Inhibitory system development
Observed changes: increased cortical BDNF and GAD expression; increased retinal IGF-I and BDNF expression; accelerated RGC dendritic stratification; trigger for later events (accelerated development of retinal acuity, partial acceleration of visual acuity development)
III) Direct environmental influence (weaning-adult age)
Enhanced sensory-motor stimulation
Possible factors: IGF-I, BDNF, PNN and inhibitory system
Observed changes: increased cortical IGF-I expression; prevention of dark rearing effects; precious closure of the CP for OD plasticity; acceleration of visual acuity development; increase of adult visual cortical plasticity

Plate 30 Model of environmental enrichment effects on visual system development and plasticity. Shown is an interpretive framework for understanding the data on EE influence on the developing visual system. The effects elicited by EE on visual system development and plasticity are due not only to changes in the levels of sensory visual stimulation but also to very early factors activated even in the absence of vision. The available data support a model in which three distinct temporal phases during pup development are differently controlled by the richness of the environment: a prenatal phase in which the mother mediates the influence of the environment through placental exchanges with the fetus, an early postnatal phase in which higher levels of maternal care in EE stimulate the expression of experience-dependent factors in the visual system, and a third (and final) phase in which the autonomous interaction of the developing pup with the enriched environment further promotes the maturation of visual functions (see the text for details). (See figure 37.5.)

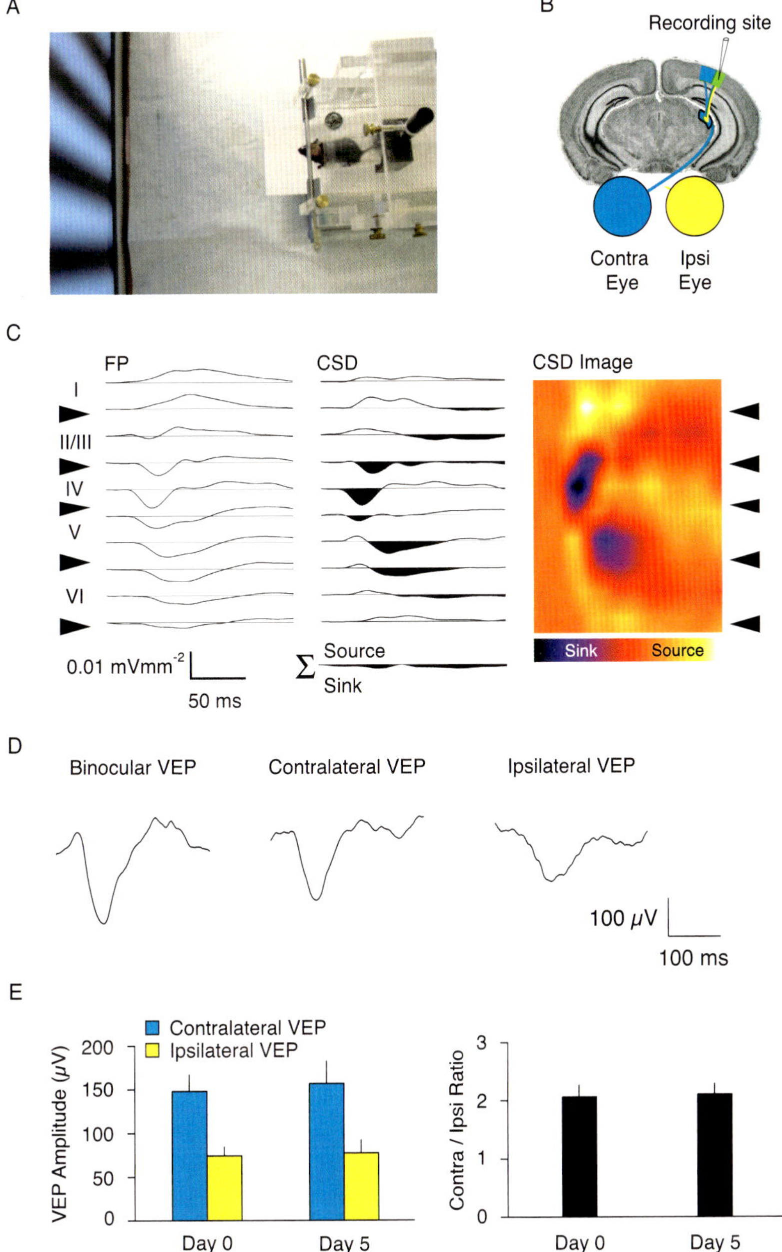

Plate 31 The extended duration VEP recording technique is a reliable method to assess OD plasticity in mice. *A*, Representation of VEP recording setup. A mouse previously implanted with recording electrodes in Oc1 is placed in a restraint apparatus in front of a computer monitor displaying visual stimuli. Mice are fully awake and alert during all recording sessions. *B*, Schematic diagram of the mouse visual system. Input from the stronger contralateral eye arrives via the LGN to the monocular and binocular zones of V1, whereas input from the weaker ipsilateral eye projects only to the small binocular zone. *C*, Current source density profile of VEPs for an adult mouse. Binocular VEP depth profile is shown in the *left panel*, with the corresponding cortical layers designated by *arrowheads*. *Middle panel* shows the CSD profile. Current sinks are negative-going and shaded black. The color image plot in the *right panel* is an interpolation of CSD traces. The earliest latency current sink is observed in layer 4, followed by longer latency sinks in layers 2/3 and 5. Cold and warm colors represent current sinks and sources, respectively. *D*, Typical VEP responses obtained during the three viewing conditions used in all experiments. Each trace is an average of 100 presentations of a reversing (1 Hz) sinusoidal grating. *E*, VEPs recorded from awake mice are stable over several days. Displayed in the *left panel* are the average VEP amplitude (n = 6 mice) in response to contralateral eye (*blue bars*) and ipsilateral eye (*yellow bars*) stimulation at baseline (day 0) and after 5 days of normal visual experience. *Right panel* shows the stability of contralateral/ipsilateral ratios over days. (See figure 38.1.)

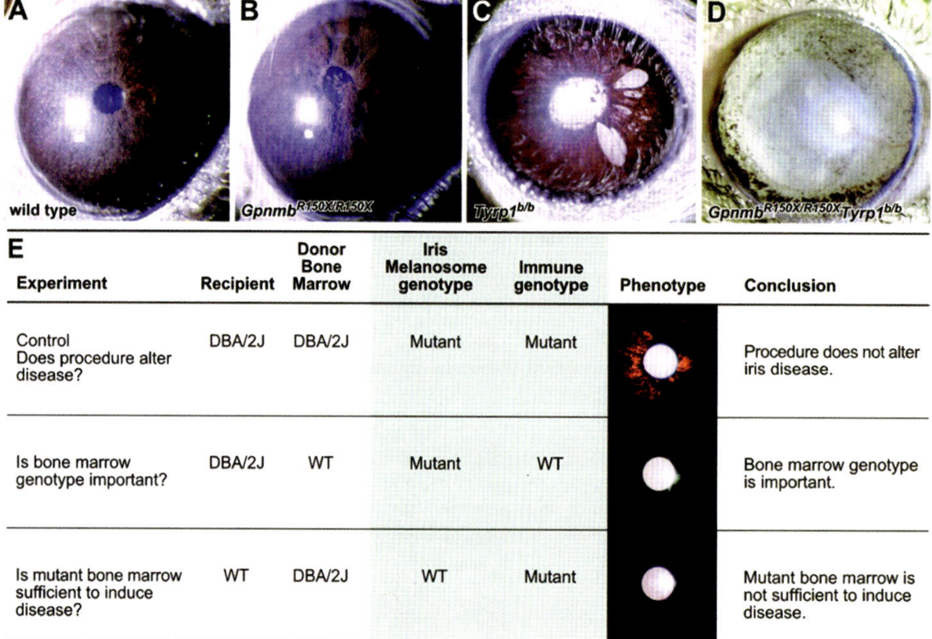

Experiment	Recipient	Donor Bone Marrow	Iris Melanosome genotype	Immune genotype	Phenotype	Conclusion
Control Does procedure alter disease?	DBA/2J	DBA/2J	Mutant	Mutant		Procedure does not alter iris disease.
Is bone marrow genotype important?	DBA/2J	WT	Mutant	WT		Bone marrow genotype is important.
Is mutant bone marrow sufficient to induce disease?	WT	DBA/2J	WT	Mutant		Mutant bone marrow is not sufficient to induce disease.

PLATE 32 Melanosomes contribute to DBA/2J pigment dispersion. *A–D*, Mutations in genes encoding the melanosomal proteins TYRP1 and GPNMB cause iris disease. DBA/2J mice that are homozygous mutant for both genes have the most severe disease (*D*). All images are from 24-month-old mice. *E*, Evidence of an immune contribution to DBA/2J pigment dispersion. Bone marrow genotype has an important effect on the phenotype. (See figure 39.1.) (Modified from John, 2005. *A–D*, Reproduced from Mo et al., 2003 [*Journal of Experimental Medicine*, 2003, 197:1335–1344. Copyright 2003, Rockefeller University Press]. *E*, Reproduced from John, 2005 [*Investigative Ophthalmology and Visual Science*, 2005, 46:2650–2661. Copyright 2005, Association for Research in Vision and Ophthalmology].)

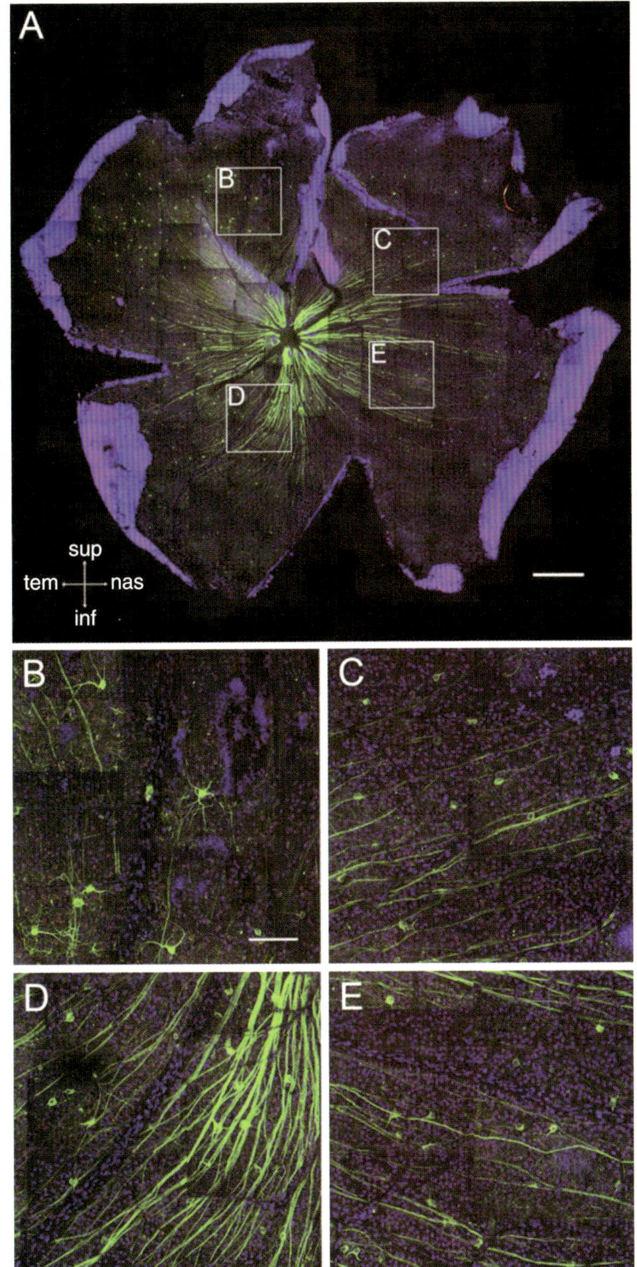

PLATE 33 Whole-mounted glaucomatous retina showing fan-shaped patterns of RGC loss and survival. *A*, High-resolution survey of a whole-mounted retina from a moderately affected eye stained for axons (green, Smi32) and amacrine cells (red, ChAT) and nuclei counterstained with TOPRO (blue). The axon bundles entering the optic nerve head are markedly reduced and show sectors of relatively high axon densities alternating with sectors with almost no persisting axons. Scale bar = 500 µm. *B–E*, High-power views of the boxed areas outlined in *A*. Scale bar = 100 µm. (See figure 39.3.) (Reproduced from Jacobs et al., 2005 [*Journal of Cell Biology*, 2005, 171:313–325. Copyright © 2005, Rockefeller University Press].)

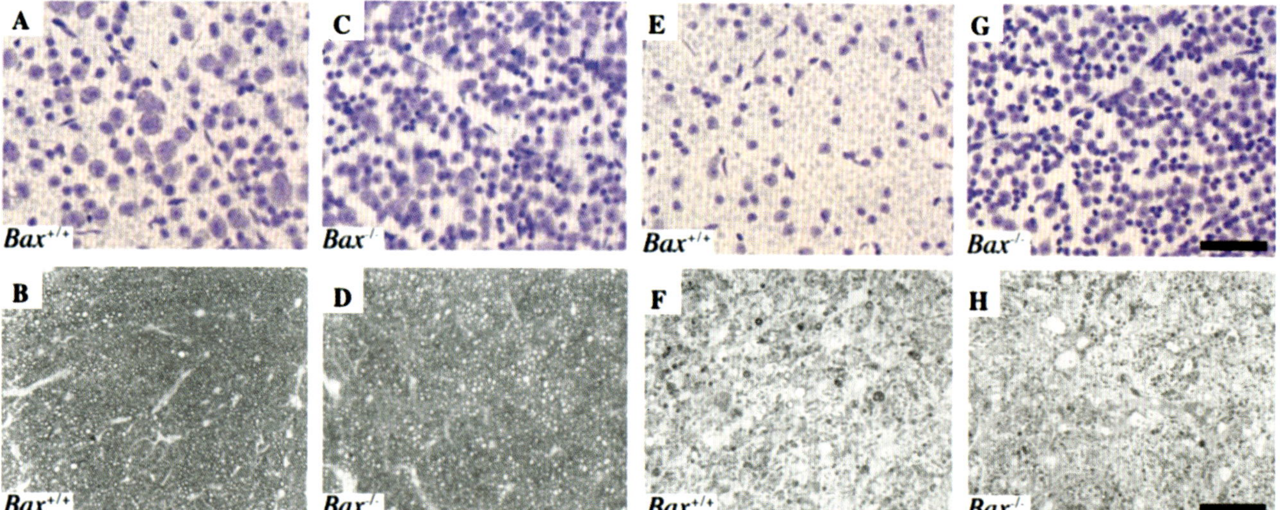

PLATE 34 *Bax* deficiency prevents glaucomatous RGC death but is not required for optic nerve degeneration. RGC layers (*A*, *C*, *E*, and *G*) and optic nerves (*B*, *D*, *F*, and *H*) were analyzed in *Bax*-sufficient and *Bax*-deficient DBA/2J mice (genotype indicated). Mice were analyzed at preglaucomatous (*A–D*) and severe glaucomatous (*E–H*) stages. *Bax*-deficient DBA/2J mice had severe optic nerve damage but no RGC death. (See figure 39.4.) (Modified from Libby et al., 2005c.)

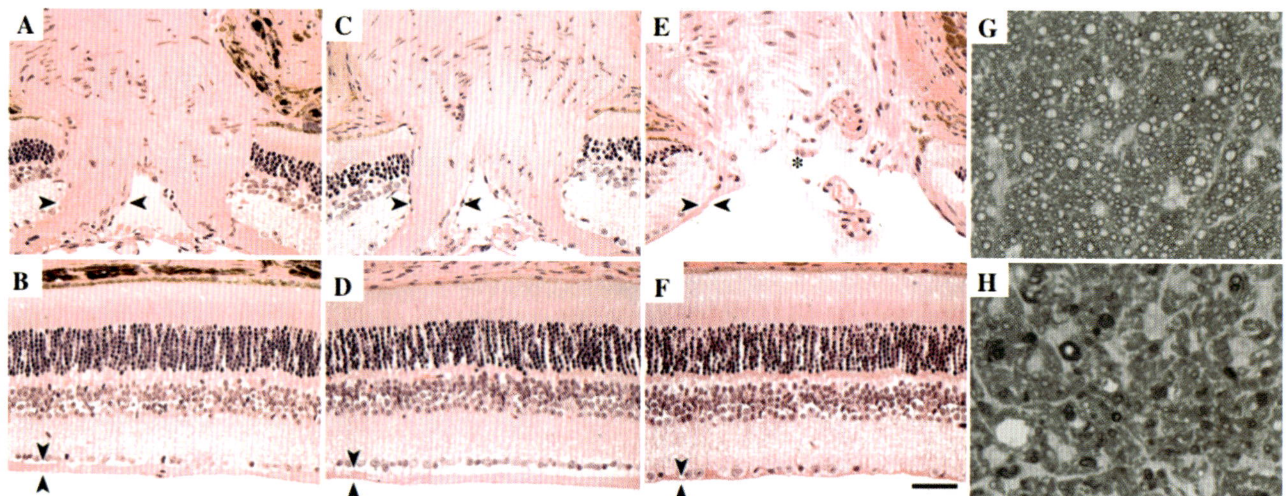

PLATE 35 Radiation treatment prevents glaucomatous optic nerve excavation. *A–F*, Hematoxylin-eosin-stained sections of untreated and treated DBA/2J mouse eyes (*A* and *B*). Optic nerve head (ONH) (*A*) and retina (*B*) from nonglaucomatous DBA/2J mice showing large numbers of axons as evidenced by a thick nerve fiber layer (NFL) (*arrowheads*). ONH (*C*) and retina (*D*) of a treated DBA/2J mouse (14 months old) is indistinguishable from nonglaucomatous controls. *E* and *F*, In contrast, untreated DBA/2J mice show severe excavation of ONH (*) and no NFL. Cross sections of the optic nerve from treated (*G*) and untreated (*H*) DBA/2J mice stained with PPD, a stain that labels myelin sheath and sick or dying axons. The severe axon loss and scarring in the untreated eye are absent in the treated eye. The vast majority (>96%) of eyes from radiation-treated DBA/2J mice were completely rescued from glaucoma. (See figure 39.5.) (Modified from Anderson et al., 2005. Reproduced from *Proceedings of the National Academy of Sciences of the USA*, 2005, 102:4566–4571. Copyright © 2005 National Academy of Sciences.)

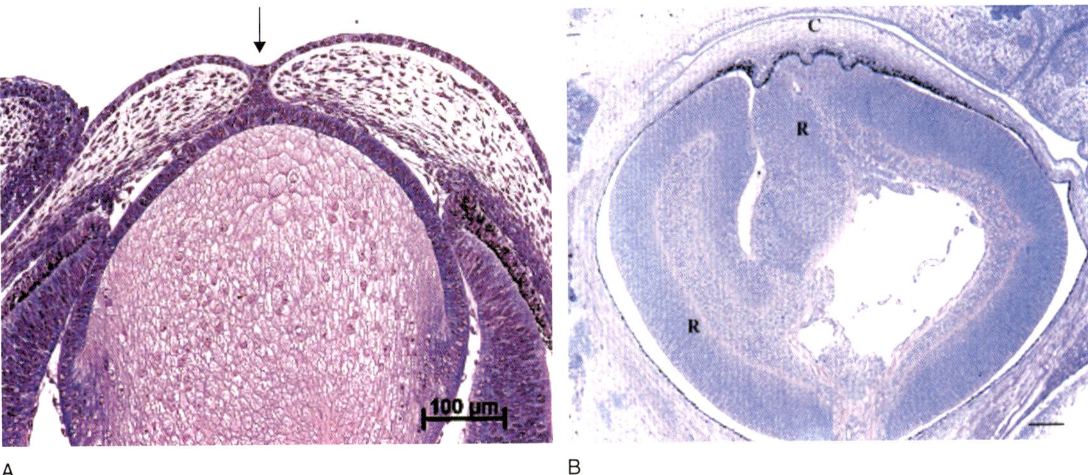

Plate 36 Mutations in transcription factors and their effect on lens development. *A*, Histological section through a developing eye of a Pax6 mutant (*Pax6*^{Aey11}; E17.5) clearly demonstrates the persisting lens stalk (*arrow*), the connection between the lens and the cornea. *B*, Histological section of the developing eye of the *aphakia* mouse (deletions in the *Pitx3* promoter) shows absence of the lens at E18.5; the eyeball is filled with retinal derivatives. C, cornea; R, retina. (See figure 40.1.) (*A*, From Graw et al., 2005. *B*, From Semina et al., 2000.)

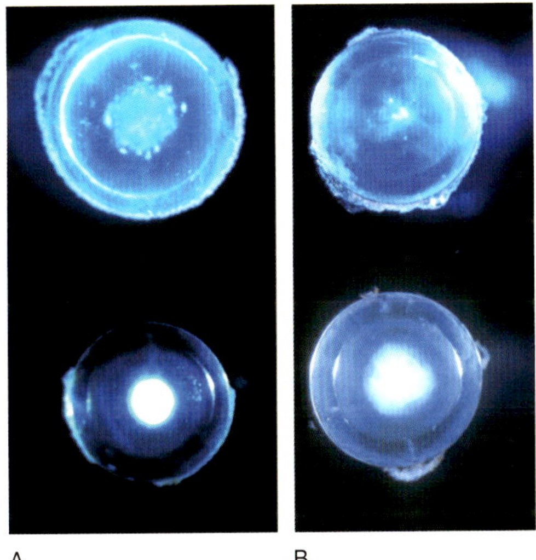

Plate 37 Mutations in *Gja8* and *Cryaa*. Gross appearance of lenses of the *Gja8*^{Aey5} mutant mouse (*A*) compared with lenses from a *Cryaa*^{Aey7} mutant mouse (*B*). The upper row indicates the phenotype for the heterozygotes and the lower row that for the homozygous mutants. In both cases, a gene dose effect can be observed. (See figure 40.2.)

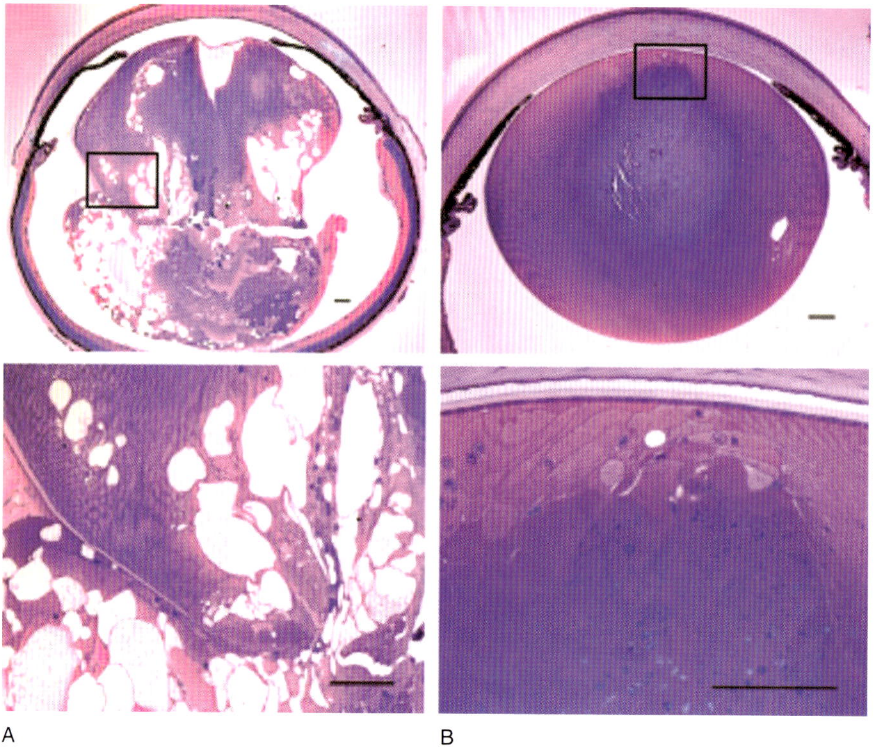

PLATE 38 Mutations in *Cryg*. Histological sections of cataractous lenses from two different mutant lines are shown. The mutations have been induced by ENU in the *Cryga* gene (*A*) or in the *Crygd* gene (*B*). Inset in the overview marks the magnification, which is given below. The differences in severity are apparent. Bars = 100 μm. (See figure 40.3.) (From Graw et al., 2004.)

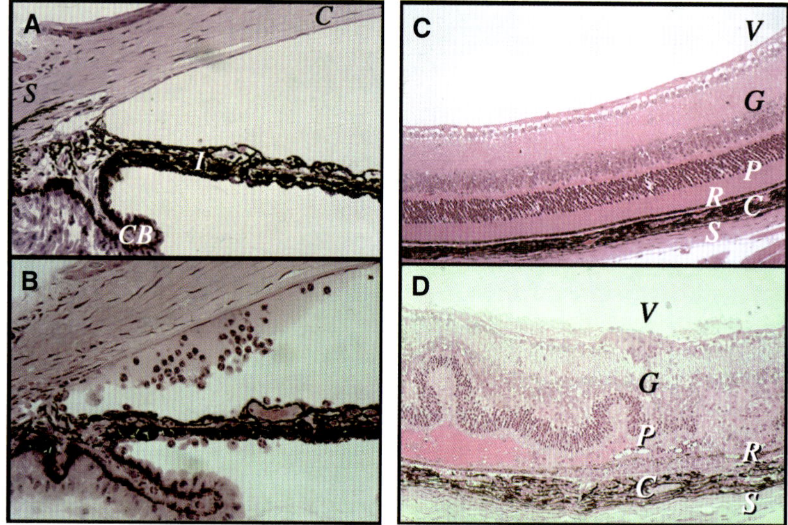

PLATE 39 Typical histology of EIU and EAU in the mouse. Healthy compared to diseased eye tissue in EIU (*A* and *B*) and in EAU (*C* and *D*). *A*, Healthy anterior chamber. Shown is the angle where the iris and ciliary body connect to the sclera. C, cornea; CB, ciliary body; I, iris; S, sclera. *B*, EIU in a C3H mouse induced by subcutaneous injection of LPS. Note infiltration of inflammatory cells in the angle and around the iris and ciliary processes. Original magnification ×1200. *C*, Healthy mouse retina. C, choroid; G, ganglion cell layer; P, photoreceptor cell layer; R, retinal pigment epithelium; S, sclera; V, vitreous. *D*, EAU in the B10.RIII mouse induced by immunization with IRBP. Note structural disorganization and loss of nuclei in the ganglion and photoreceptor cell layers, retinal folds, subretinal exudate, vasculitis, damage to the retinal pigment epithelium, and choroid inflammation. Original magnification ×1000. (See figure 42.2.) (Photomicrographs courtesy of Dr. Chi-Chao Chan, NEI, NIH.)

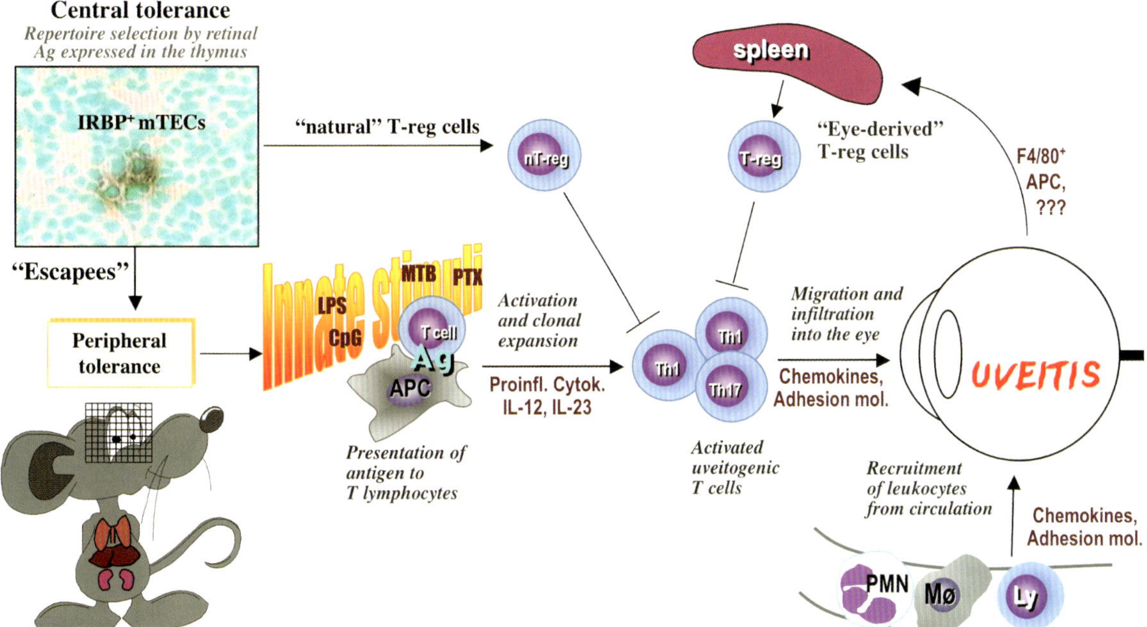

Plate 40 Critical checkpoints in EAU pathogenesis. Schematic representation of critical events and checkpoints in the pathogenesis of EAU as revealed by studies in mouse models. (See figure 42.3.) (This figure was previously published in Caspi, 2006. Copyright does not apply.)

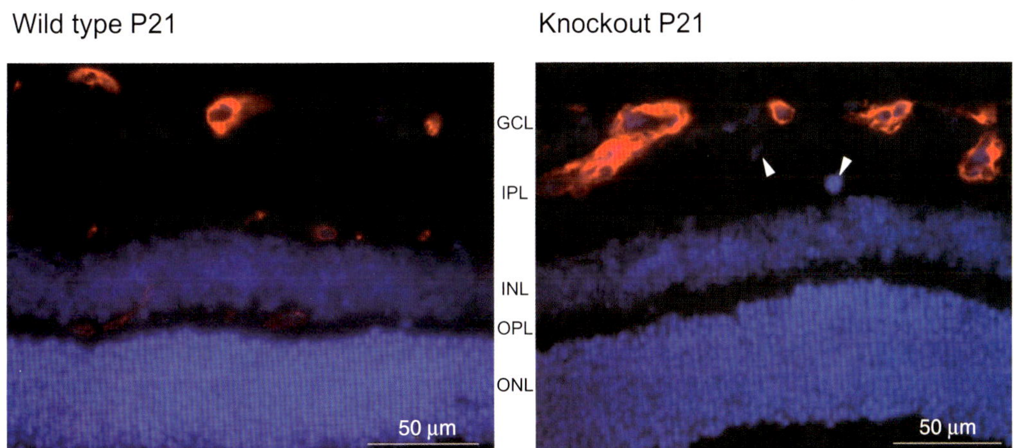

Plate 41 Sections of the central retina from wild-type and knockout mice at P21 after staining with a collagen IV antibody (red), which detects the extracellular matrix of endothelial cells, and diamidinophenylindol/DAPI (blue), which labels cell nuclei. Blood vessels (red) in wild-type mice are present in three layers, indicating completed development of the superficial (ganglion cell layer [GCL]), deep (outer plexiform layer [OPL]), and intermediate (border between the inner plexiform layer [IPL] and inner nuclear layer [INL]) vessel networks. In contrast, age-matched knockout mice show only enlarged superficial vessels, while the deeper and intermediate networks failed to develop. In addition, the presence of nuclei in the IPL (*white arrowheads*) may reflect the characteristic disorganization in the GCL. (See figure 43.2.) (Images acquired and provided courtesy of Nikolaus Schäfer, Division of Medical Molecular Genetics, Institute of Medical Genetics, University of Zurich, Switzerland.)

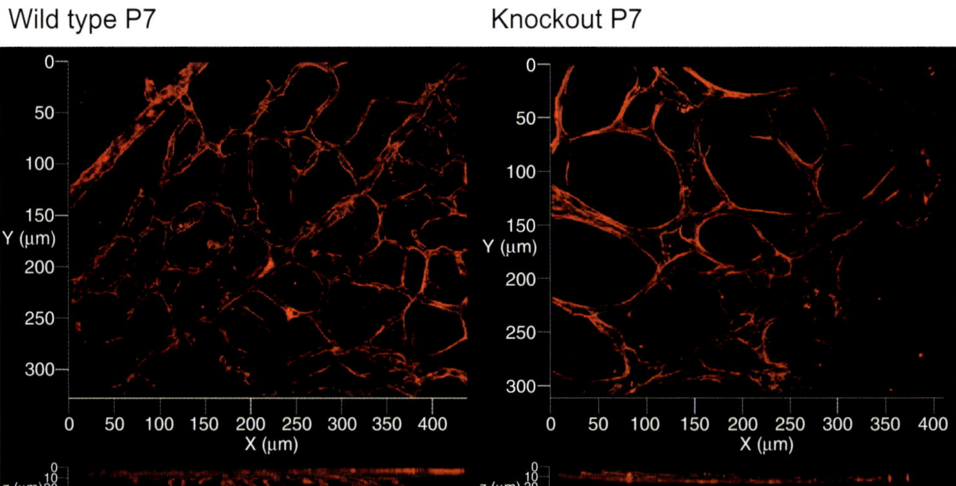

PLATE 42 Three-dimensional microscopy of retinal flat mounts stained with anticollagen IV from wild-type and knockout mice at P7. *Top panels* show an area of approximately 300 × 400 µm from wild-type and knockout mice. Vessels in the knockout are dilated, and the capillary network is less dense than in the wild-type control. *Bottom panels* (*z*-axis) show how blood vessels enter the deeper retinal layers in wild-type mice by angiogenic sprouting. In contrast, this process is abolished in knockout mice, and the vessels do not invade the deeper retinal layers. (See figure 43.3.) (Images acquired using the Zeiss ApoTome technology and provided courtesy of Nikolaus Schäfer, Division of Medical Molecular Genetics, Institute of Medical Genetics, University of Zurich, Switzerland.)

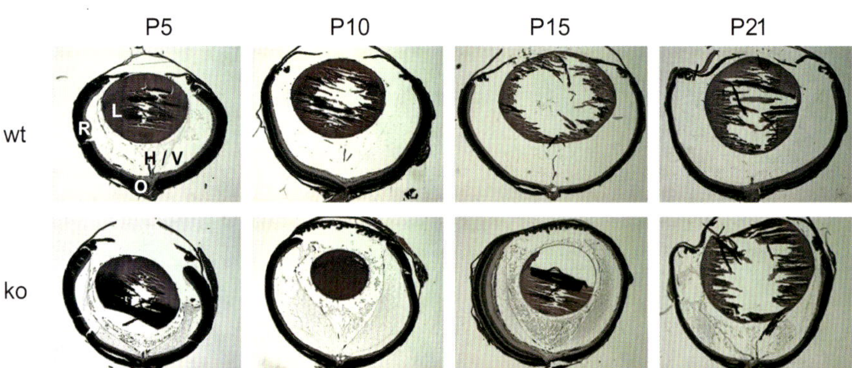

PLATE 43 Hematoxylin-eosin-stained sections of whole eyes from wild-type (wt) and norrin knockout (ko) mice at P5, P10, P15, and P21. The hyaloid vessel system (H) in the vitreous body (V) is clearly present in wild-type mice at P5 and P10, and remnants are evident at P15. In knockout mice, the hyaloid vasculature persists through P21 and beyond, and regression of this vascular network is profoundly delayed. L, lens; O, optic nerve; R, retina. (See figure 43.4.) (Images acquired and provided courtesy of Dr. Ulrich Luhmann, Division of Medical Molecular Genetics, Institute of Medical Genetics, University of Zurich, Switzerland.)

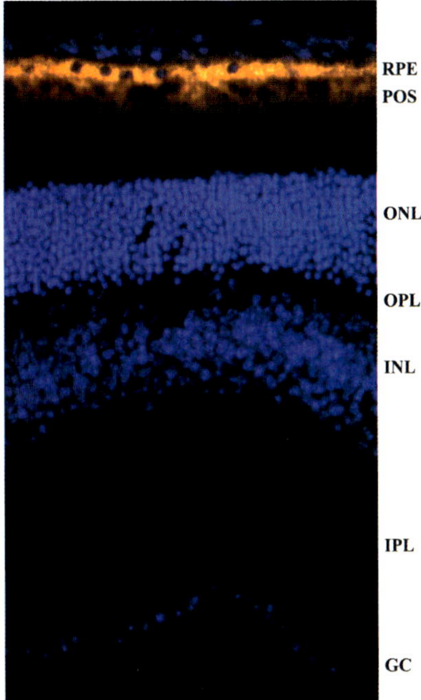

Plate 44 Autofluorescence of RPE lipofusin in *Abca4/Abcr*$^{-/-}$ mouse retina. Cross section of mouse retina viewed by epifluorescence microscopy (excitation 425 ± 45 nm, emission 510 nm long pass). Nuclei are stained with DAPI. The yellow-gold autofluorescence in RPE cells is associated with lipofuscin in RPE cells. The less pronounced autofluorescence in photoreceptor outer segments (POS) is attributable to lipofuscin precursors that form in this location. The albino mouse was 8 months old and homozygous for leucine at amino acid 450 of Rpe65. GC, ganglion cell layer; INL, inner nuclear layer; IPL, inner plexiform layer; ONL, outer nuclear layer; OPL, outer plexiform layer; RPE, retinal pigment epithelium. (See figure 44.3.)

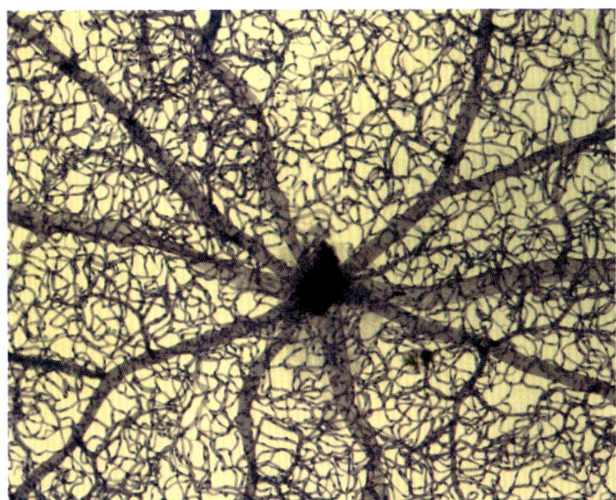

Plate 45 The retinal vasculature of the mouse, following isolation by proteolytic digestion of the formalin-fixed retina. (See figure 45.1.)

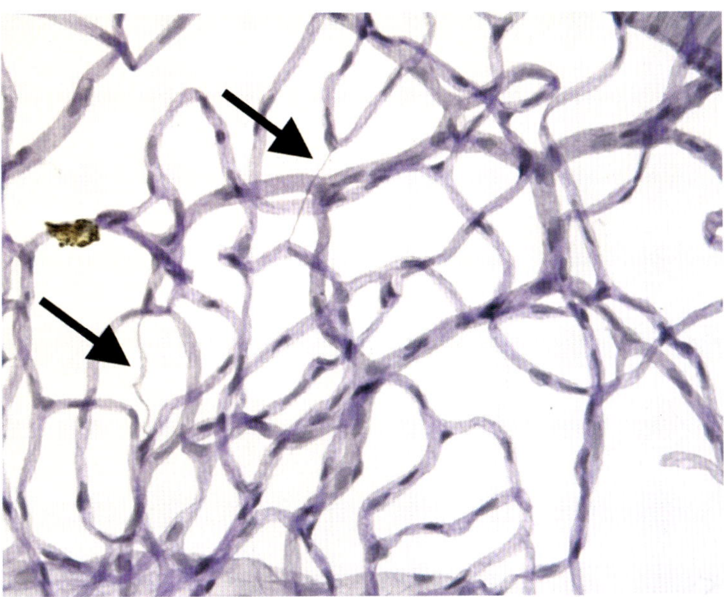

Plate 46 Degenerate (acellular) capillaries (*arrows*) in the diabetic mouse retina. The degenerate vessels lack vascular cell nuclei and have an irregular or shrunken diameter compared to surrounding healthy capillaries. (See figure 45.2.)

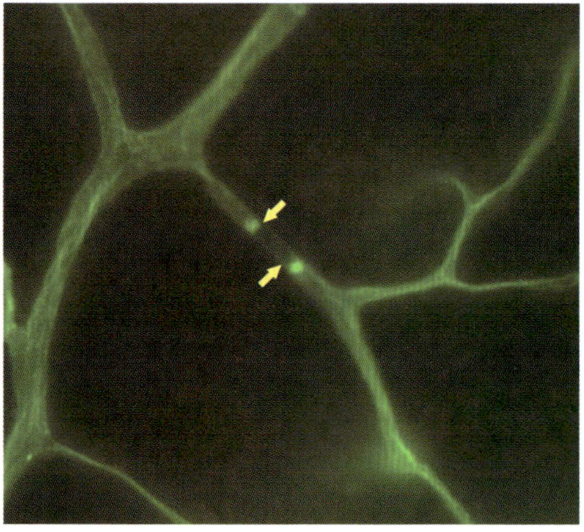

PLATE 47 Leukocyte adherence, or leukostasis (*arrows*), in the retinal microvasculature of the diabetic mouse. (See figure 45.4.)

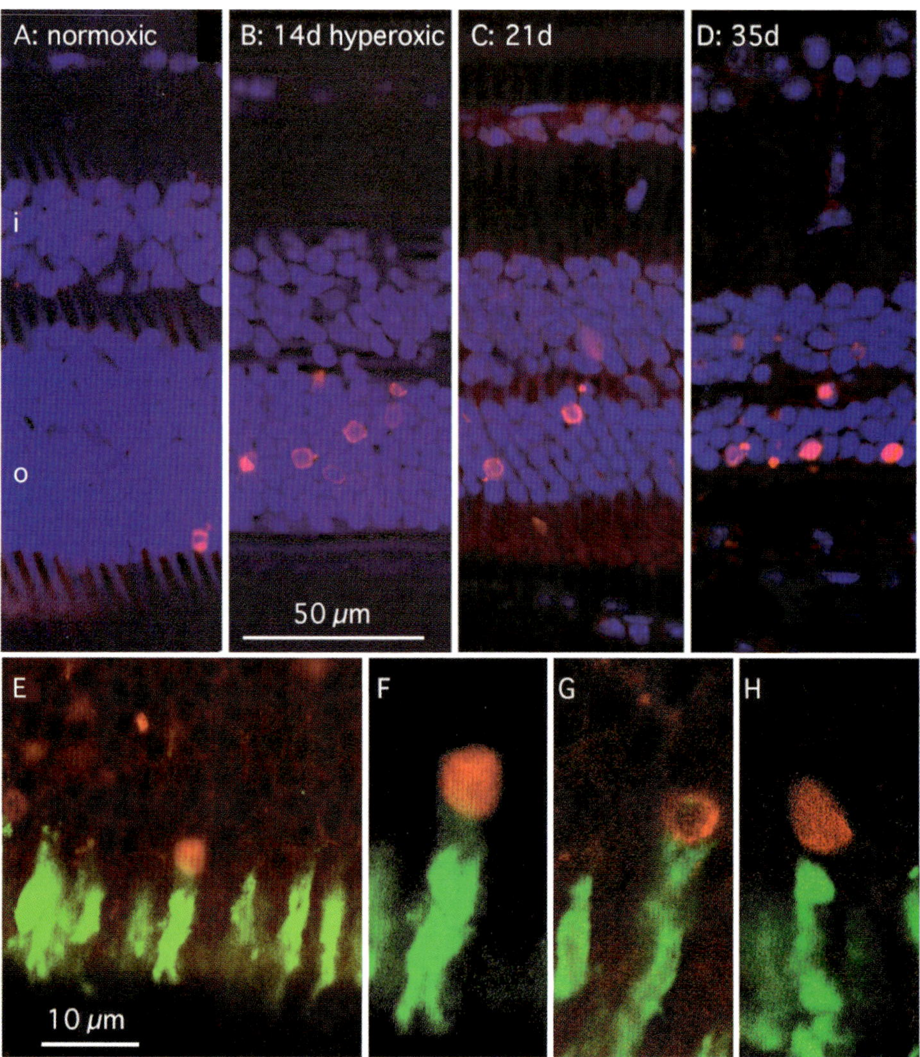

PLATE 48 Oxygen is selectively toxic to photoreceptors. *A–D*, Sections across the retina of C57BL/6 mice exposed to high oxygen levels in inhaled air. Before exposure, dying (red, TUNEL-labeled) cells were rare. Exposure to hyperoxia for 14–35 days (*B–D*) increased the frequency of dying cells, selectively in the ONL (o). By 35 days, the ONL had thinned and TUNEL+ debris appeared in the inner nuclear layer (i), probably ingested by Müller cells. The blue dye is a DNA label (bisbenzamide). *E* and *F*, When the sheaths of cones were labeled with PNA lectin, the nuclei of some were TUNEL labeled (red), indicating that cones as well as rods were oxygen sensitive. (See figure 46.3.) (From Geller et al., 2006.)

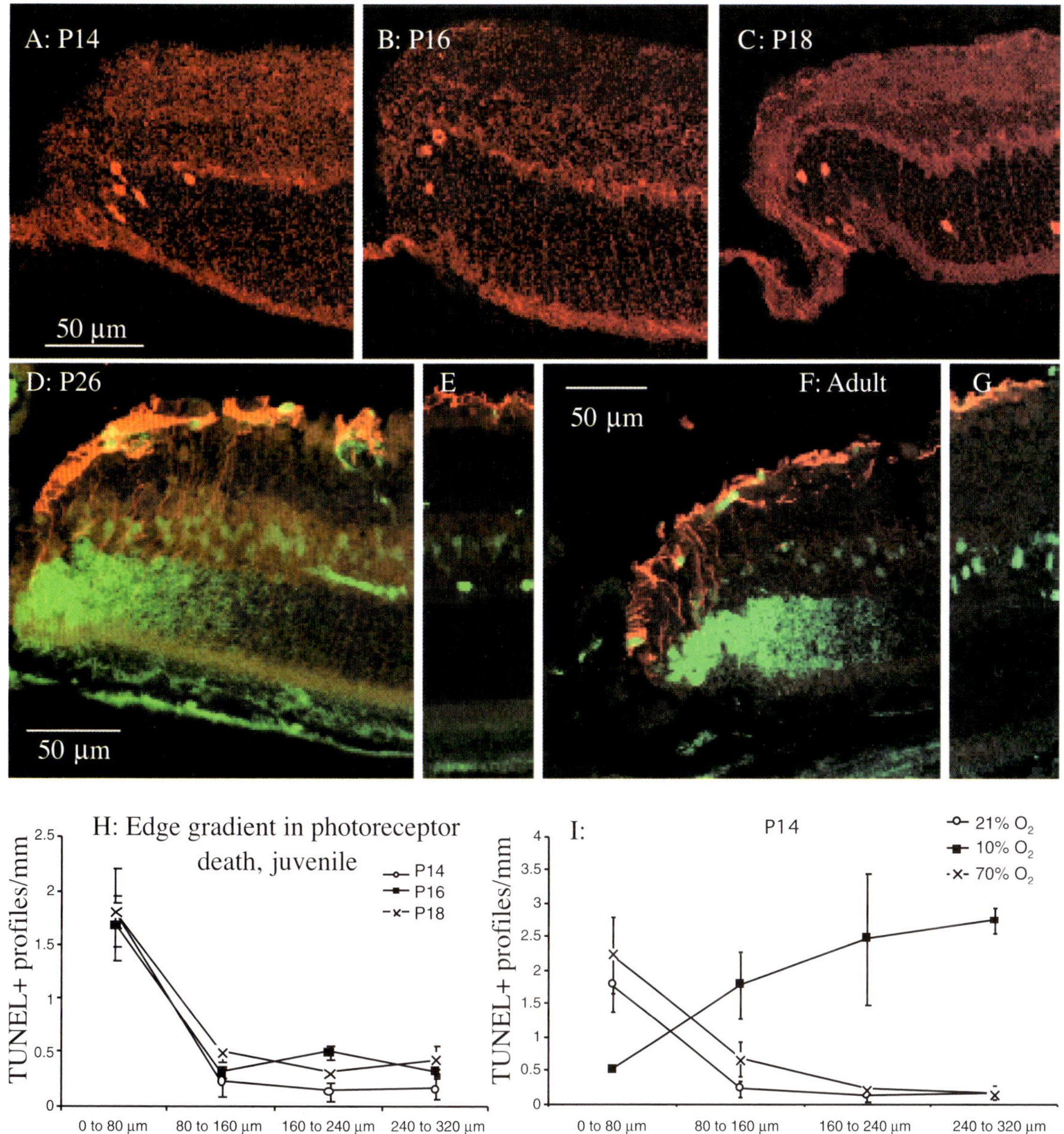

PLATE 49 Photoreceptors at the most peripheral margin of the retina are subject to stress from early postnatal life. *A–C*, The edge of the retina of C57BL/6 mouse retina, with dying cells (bright red, TUNEL labeled) clustering at the edge of P14, P16, and P18. All are in the ONL. *D* and *E*, This cluster of dying cells colocalizes with the upregulation of two stress-induced proteins. GFAP is normally expressed (red) only at the inner surface of the retina, by astrocytes (*E* and *G*). At the edge, GFAP is upregulated also in Müller cells. FGF-2 is strongly upregulated (green) in photoreceptors, in a gradient that is maximal at the end. *H*, Quantification of the frequency of dying cells in the peripheral-most 100 μm of retina. *I*, Oxygen influences this distribution of dying cells at the edge of the early postnatal retina. Hypoxia increases photoreceptor death throughout most of the retina; at the edge, however, hyperoxia reduces death, suggesting that the edge-related death is driven by oxygen stress (see the text). Hyperoxia causes a small increase in the frequency of dying cells at the edge of the retina. (See figure 46.4.) (From Mervin and Stone, 2002a, 2002b.)

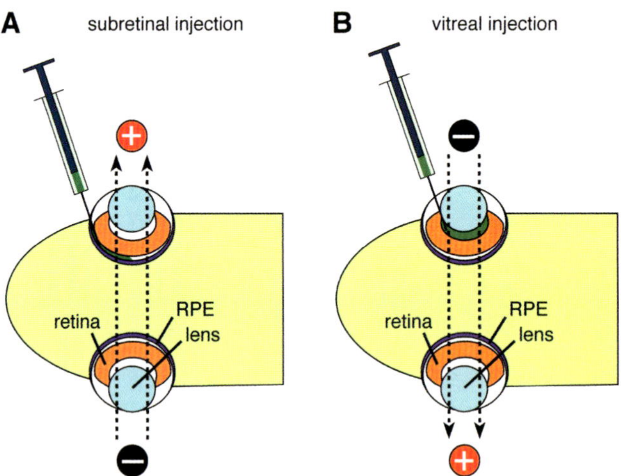

Plate 50 Strategy for in vivo electroporation *A*, Electroporation to the scleral (RPE) side of the retina. *B*, Electroporation to the vitreal side of the retina. (See figure 51.1.)

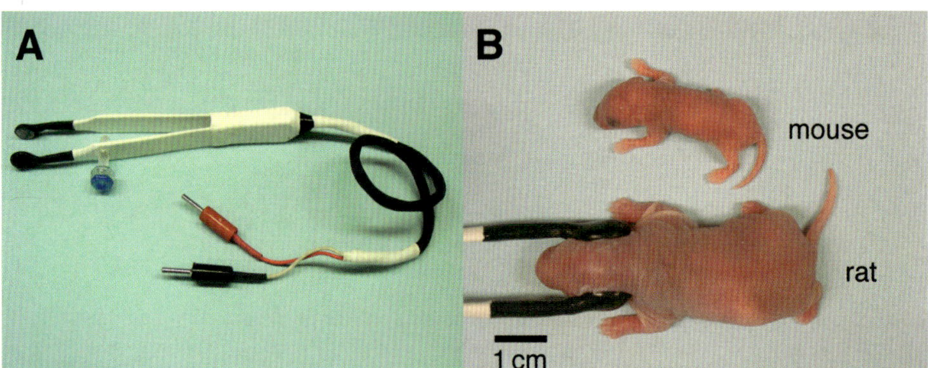

Plate 51 Electrodes and procedure for in vivo electroporation. Tweezer-type electrodes (*A*) are placed to hold the head of newborn (P0) rat or mouse (*B*). (See figure 51.2.)

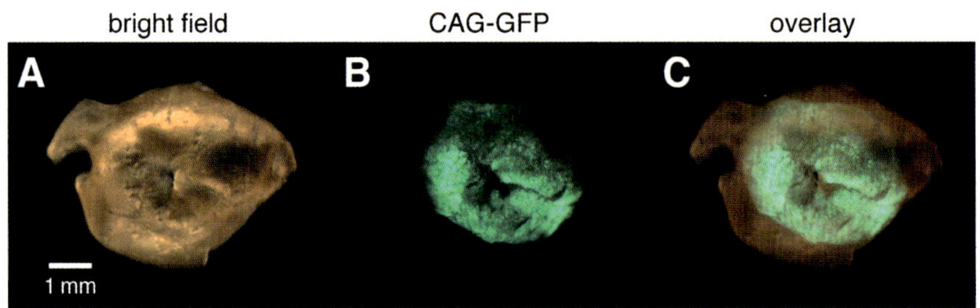

Plate 52 Whole-mount preparation of rat retina in vivo electroporated at P0 with CAG-GFP (Matsuda and Cepko, 2004), a GFP expression vector driven by the CAG (chicken β-actin promoter with cytomegalovirus enhancer) promoter and harvested at P21. Images are from the scleral side. Bright-field (*A*), GFP (*B*), and merged (*C*) images are shown. (See figure 51.3.)

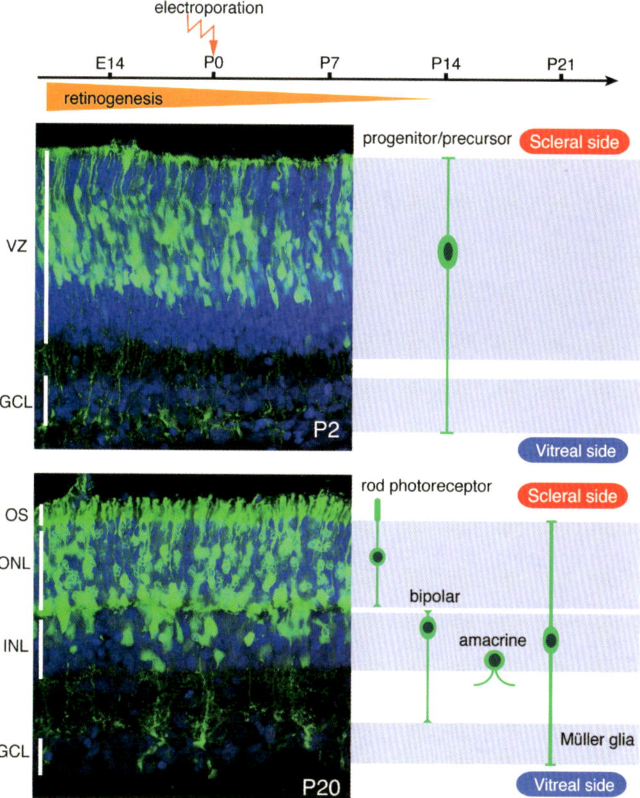

PLATE 53 In vivo electroporated retina (P0 electroporation, section). Rat retinas were in vivo electroporated with CAG-GFP at P0 and harvested at P2 (*top panel*) or P20 (*bottom panel*). At P2, most of the GFP-positive cells have the morphology of progenitor/precursor cells, suggesting that DNAs are preferentially transfected to progenitor/precursor cells. Retinogenesis is completed within the first 2 weeks after birth. At P20, GFP is observed in four differentiated cell types: rod photoreceptors, bipolar cells, amacrine cells, and Müller glia. Early-born cell types (cone, horizontal, and ganglion cells) are not labeled by P0 electroporation. GCL, ganglion cell layer; INL, inner nuclear layer; ONL, outer nuclear layer; OS, outer segment; VZ, ventricular zone. (See figure 51.4.)

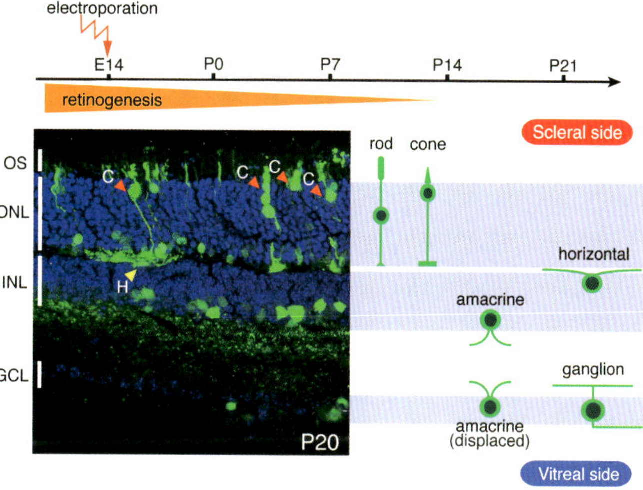

PLATE 54 In vivo electroporated retina (E14 electroporation, section). Mouse embryonic retinas were electroporated with UB-GFP (Matsuda and Cepko, 2004), a GFP expression vector driven by the human ubiquitin promoter, at E14 in utero, and harvested at P20. Early-born cell types (cone, amacrine, horizontal, and ganglion cells) are clearly labeled with GFP, while late-born cell types (bipolar and Müller glial cells), which are generated from E14 RPCs after several rounds of cell division, are poorly labeled. This is probably due to dilution of introduced plasmids. *Red arrowheads* indicate the labeled cone photoreceptors. *Yellow arrowhead* indicates the labeled horizontal cell. GCL, ganglion cell layer; INL, inner nuclear layer; ONL, outer nuclear layer; OS, outer segment. (See figure 51.6.)

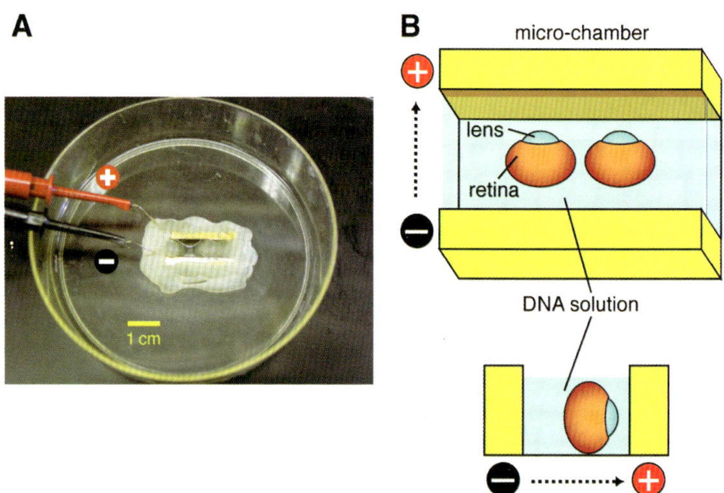

PLATE 55 *A*, Microchamber for in vitro electroporation. *B*, Orientation of the retina in the chamber. Maximum transduction efficiency can be obtained when the scleral side is facing the minus electrode. (See figure 51.7.)

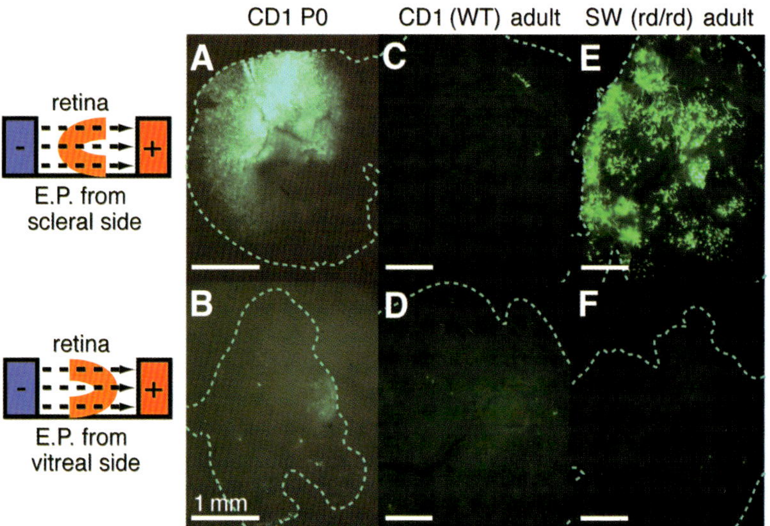

PLATE 56 In vitro electroporated retinal explant (whole mount). Mouse retinas of P0 CD1 (*A* and *B*), adult CD1 (*C* and *D*), or adult Swiss Webster mice with a retinal degeneration mutation (*E* and *F*) were in vitro electroporated with CAG-GFP from the scleral side (*A*, *C*, and *E*) or from the vitreal side (*B*, *D*, and *F*) and cultured for 5 days. Images *A*, *C*, and *E* are from the scleral side and images *B*, *D*, and *F* are from the vitreal side. Note that only the scleral side of developing retina or of degenerated retina is highly transfectable. In *E*, most of the GFP-positive cells are Müller glial cells. (See figure 51.8.)

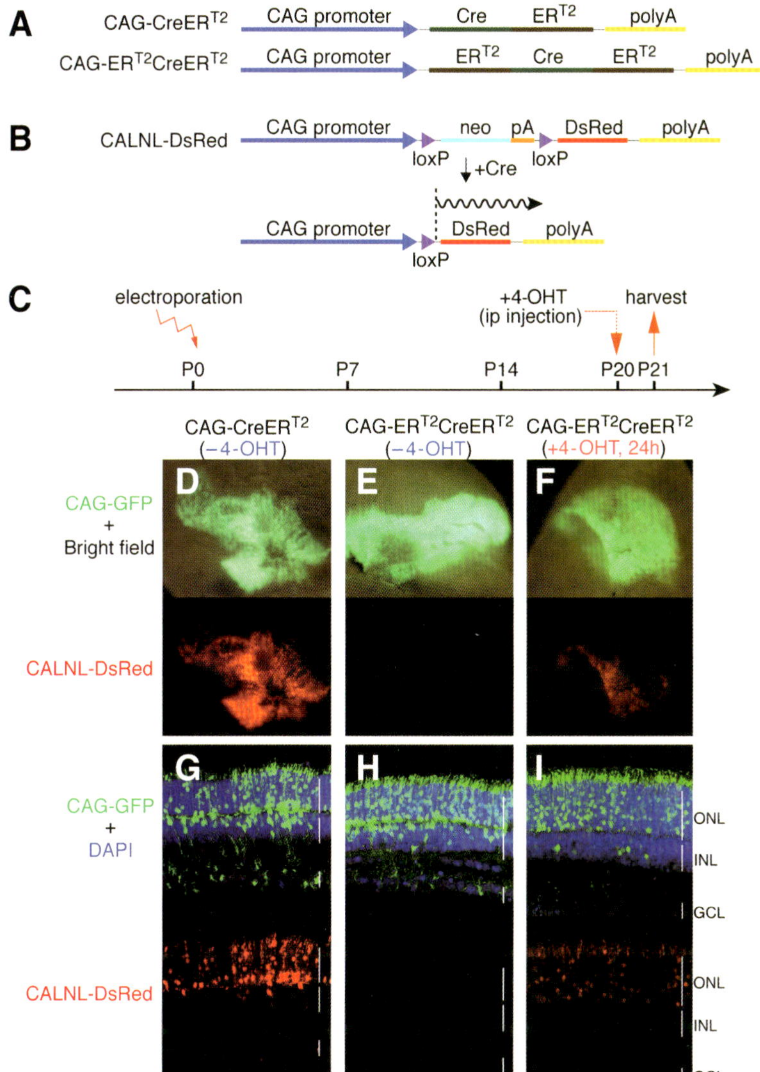

PLATE 57 Temporal regulation of gene expression in the retina using inducible Cre recombinases. *A*, CAG-CreER^{T2}: Fusion protein (CreER^{T2}) between Cre recombinase and the mutated ligand-binding domain (ER^{T2}) of the human estrogen receptor is expressed under the control of the CAG promoter. CAG-ER^{T2}CreER^{T2}: Fusion protein (ER^{T2}CreER^{T2}) composed of Cre and two ER^{T2} domains is expressed under the control of the CAG promoter. CreER^{T2} and ER^{T2}CreER^{T2} are conditionally activated in response to 4-OHT. *B*, CALNL-DsRed: Cre/loxP-dependent inducible expression vector. DsRed is expressed only in the presence of Cre. *C*, A scheme of the experiment. *D–I*, P0 rat retinas were coelectroporated with three plasmids: CAG-GFP (transfection control), CALNL-DsRed (recombination indicator), and CAG-CreER^{T2} (*D*) or CAG-ER^{T2}CreER^{T2} (*E* and *F*). The retinas were stimulated without 4-OHT (*D* and *E*) or with 4-OHT (*F*) by IP injection at P20 and then harvested at P21. Whole-mount preparations of the harvested retinas are shown. *G–I*, Sections of the retinas shown in *D–F*. Cell nuclei were stained with DAPI. When CreER^{T2} was used, significant background recombination was observed even in the absence of 4-OHT. On the other hand, ER^{T2}CreER^{T2} had no detectable basal activity in the absence of 4-OHT. GCL, ganglion cell layer; INL, inner nuclear layer; ONL, outer nuclear layer. (See figure 51.9.)

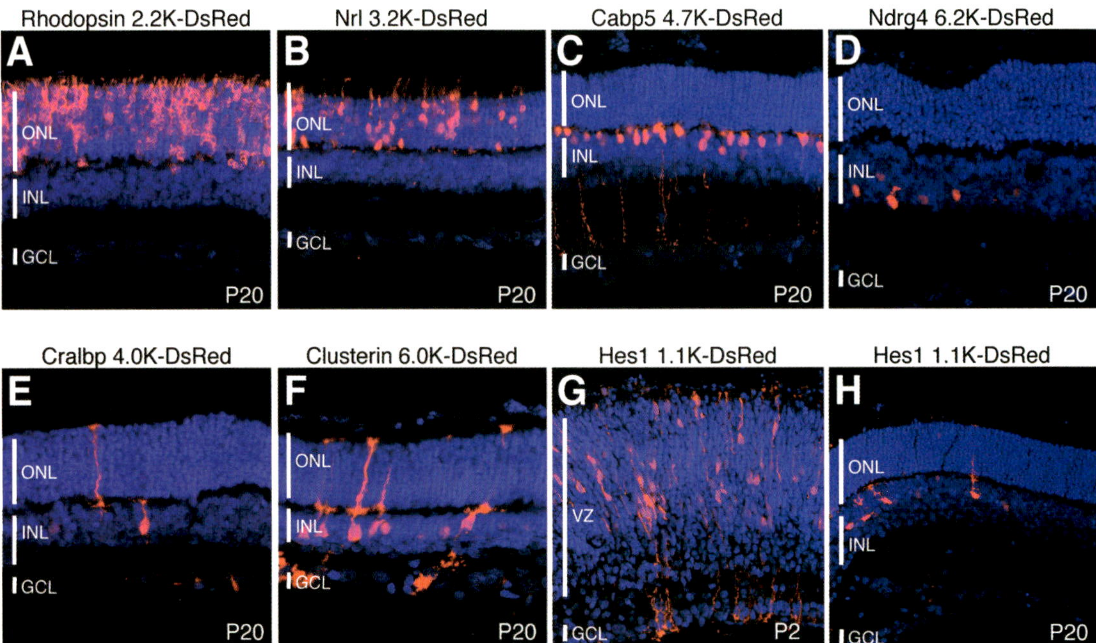

Plate 58 Spatial regulation of gene expression in the retina using cell type–specific promoters. Retinal cell type–specific promoters were fused to DsRed cDNA and electroporated into P0 rat retinas. The retinas were harvested at P20 (*A–F* and *H*) or P2 (*G*), sectioned, and stained with DAPI. Promoters of rhodopsin (*A*), Nrl (*B*), Cabp5 (*C*), Ndrg4 (*D*), Cralbp (*E*), clusterin (*F*), and Hes1 (*G* and *H*) were used to express DsRed. GCL, ganglion cell layer; INL, inner nuclear layer; ONL, outer nuclear layer. (See figure 51.10.)

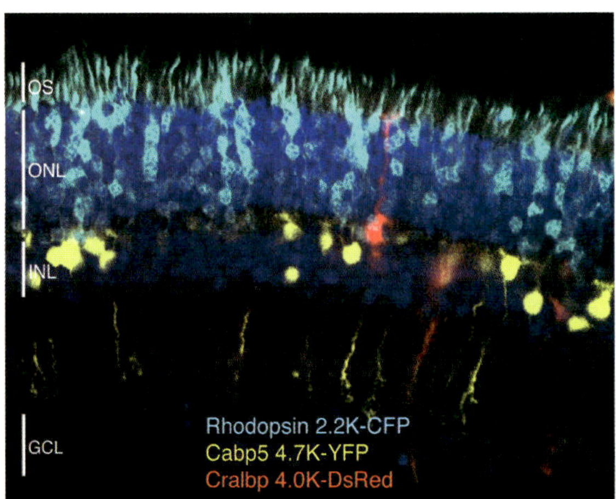

Plate 59 Multicolor labeling of the retina using cell type–specific promoters. P0 rat retina was electroporated with three reporter constructs: rhodopsin promoter 2.2K-CFP (specific for rods), Cabp5 promoter 4.7K-YFP (specific for a subset of bipolar cells), and Cralbp promoter 4.0K-DsRed (specific for Müller glia). The retina was harvested at P20, sectioned, and stained with DAPI. GCL, ganglion cell layer; INL, inner nuclear layer; ONL, outer nuclear layer; OS, outer segment. (See figure 51.11.)

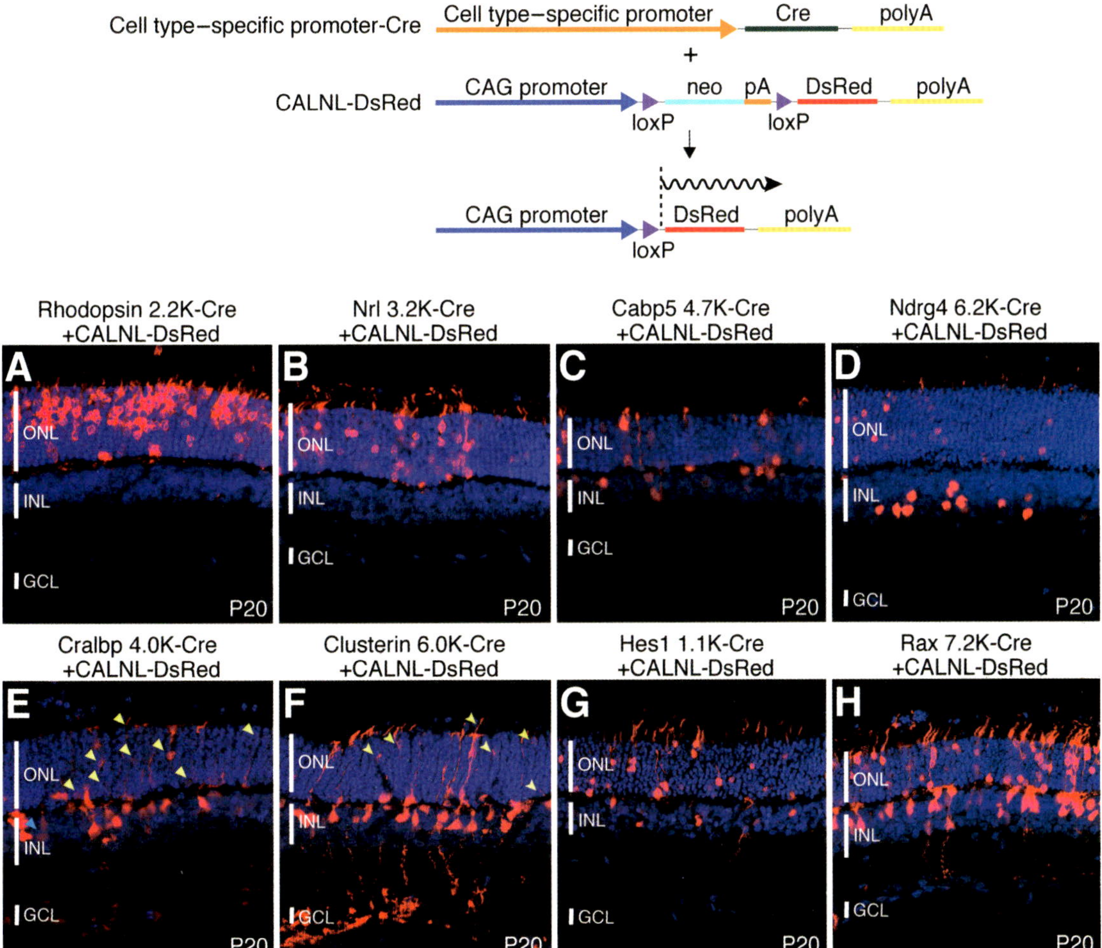

Plate 60 Lineage tracing experiments in the retina using the Cre/loxP system and cell type–specific promoters. P0 rat retinas were coelectroporated with retinal cell type–specific promoter Cre and CALNL-DsRed (recombination indicator). DsRed expression, induced by Cre/loxP-mediated recombination, was driven by the ubiquitous CAG promoter. The retinas were harvested at P20, sectioned, and stained with DAPI. Promoters of rhodopsin (*A*), Nrl (*B*), Cabp5 (*C*), Ndrg4 (*D*), Cralbp (*E*), clusterin (*F*), Hes1 (*G*), and Rax (*H*) were used to express Cre. *Yellow arrowheads* indicate the labeled rods. *Blue arrowhead* indicates the labeled bipolar cell. GCL, ganglion cell layer; INL, inner nuclear layer; ONL, outer nuclear layer. (See figure 51.12.)

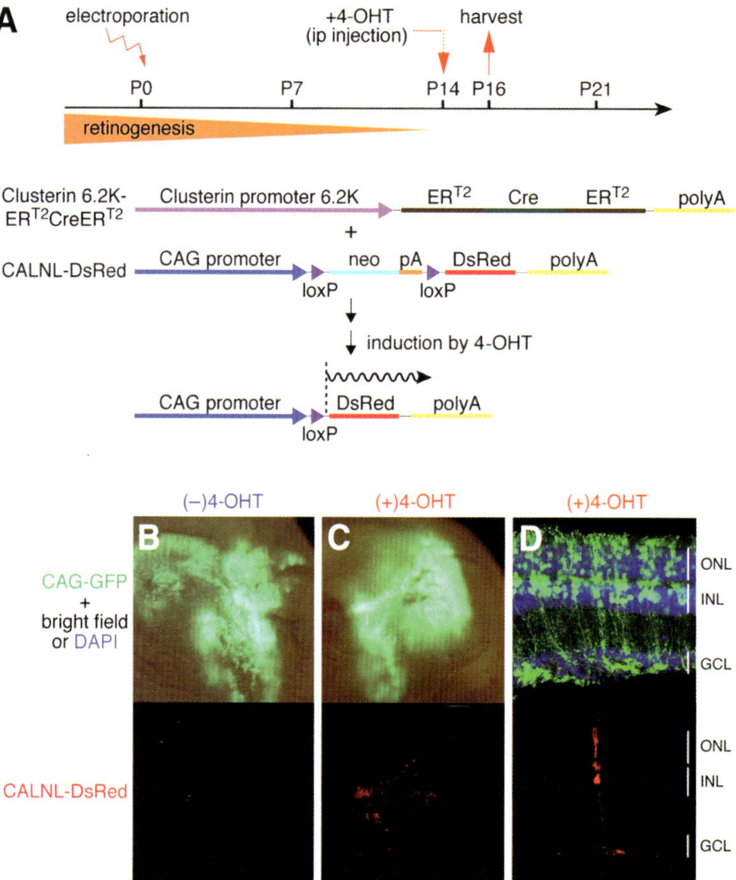

Plate 61 Inducible expression in the differentiated Müller glia (*A*). Clusterin promoter was fused to $ER^{T2}CreER^{T2}$ cDNA and co-electroporated into P0 rat retinas with CALNL-DsRed (recombination indicator) and CAG-GFP (transfection control). Retinas were stimulated with or without 4-OHT at P14 by IP injection, then harvested at P16. *B*, Whole-mount preparation of the transfected retina harvested at P16 without 4-OHT stimulation. No DsRed expression was detected. *C*, Whole-mount preparation of the transfected retina stimulated with 4-OHT at P14 and harvested at P16. *D*, The retina shown in *C* was sectioned and stained with DAPI. Only Müller glial cells are labeled with DsRed. (See figure 51.13.)

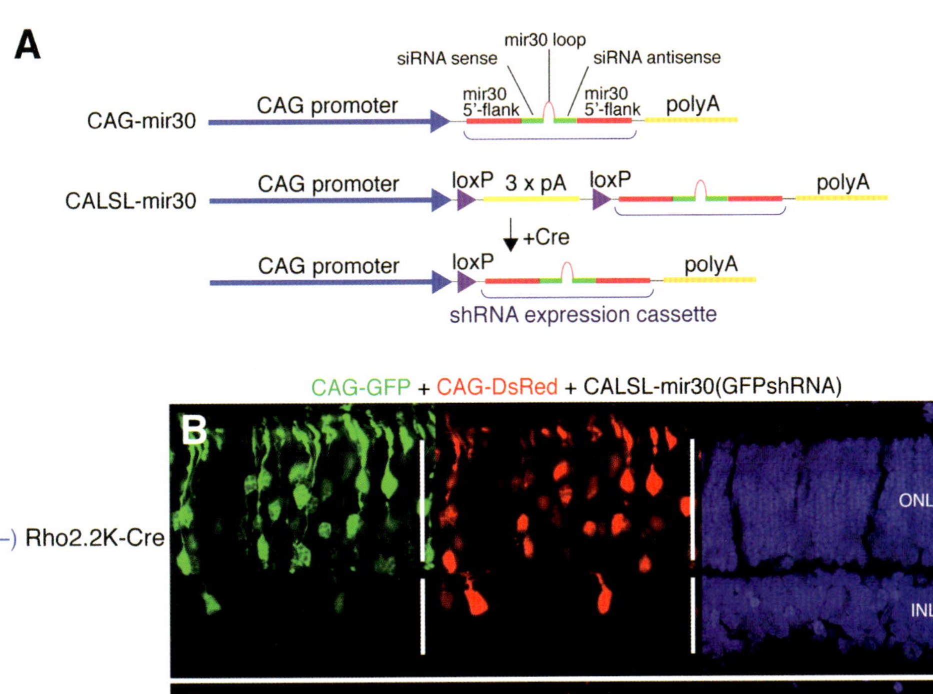

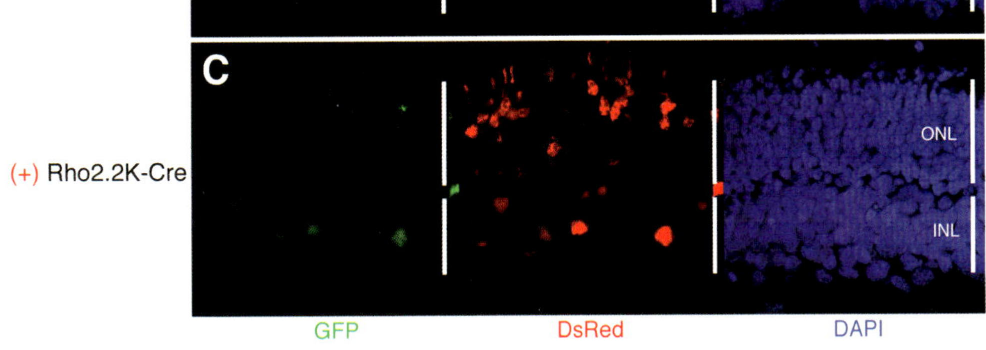

Plate 62 Inducible RNAi in the retina. *A*, CAG-mir30: The mir30 expression cassette is expressed under the control of the CAG promoter. The mir30 expression cassette has the hairpin stem composed of siRNA sense and antisense strands (22nt each), a loop derived from human mir30 (19nt), and 125nt mir30 flanking sequences on both sides of the hairpin. The mir30 primary transcript is processed to generate the mature shRNA. CALSL-mir30: Cre-dependent inducible shRNA expression vector carrying a floxed transcriptional stop cassette (3xpolyA signal sequences). Only in the presence of Cre, the mir30 expression cassette is expressed under the control of the CAG promoter. *B* and *C*, Conditional GFP knockdown in the retina. CAG-GFP and CAG-DsRed and CALSL-mir30(GFPshRNA) expressing an shRNA against GFP were coelectroporated without (*B*) or with (*C*) the rhodopsin promoter Cre into P0 rat retinas. The retinas were harvested at P20, sectioned, and stained with DAPI. Rod-specific GFP knockdown was observed in the presence of the rhodopsin promoter Cre. (See figure 51.14.)

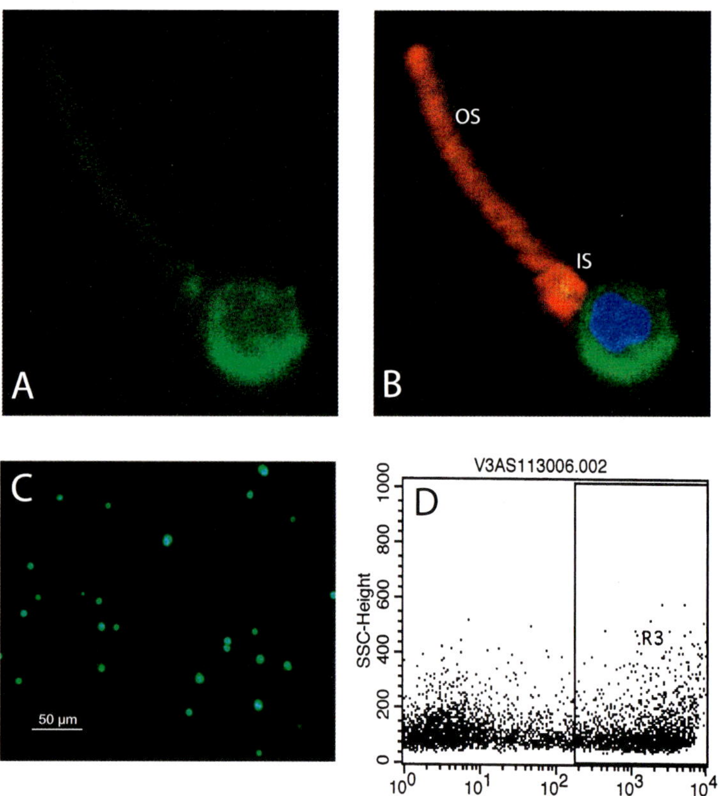

Plate 63 *A*, A single rod photoreceptor isolated from adult *wt-Gfp* mice shows the expression of GFP. *B*, The same cell shows staining for rhodpsin (red) in the outer segment (OS) and inner segment (IS) regions and bis-benzimide staining (blue) for the nucleus. *C*, Samples of dissociated cells are viewed under the microscope before (shown) and after flow sorting. *D*, Flow cytometry allows the GFP-positive population of cells to be gated (R3) and sorted separately. (See figure 55.1.)

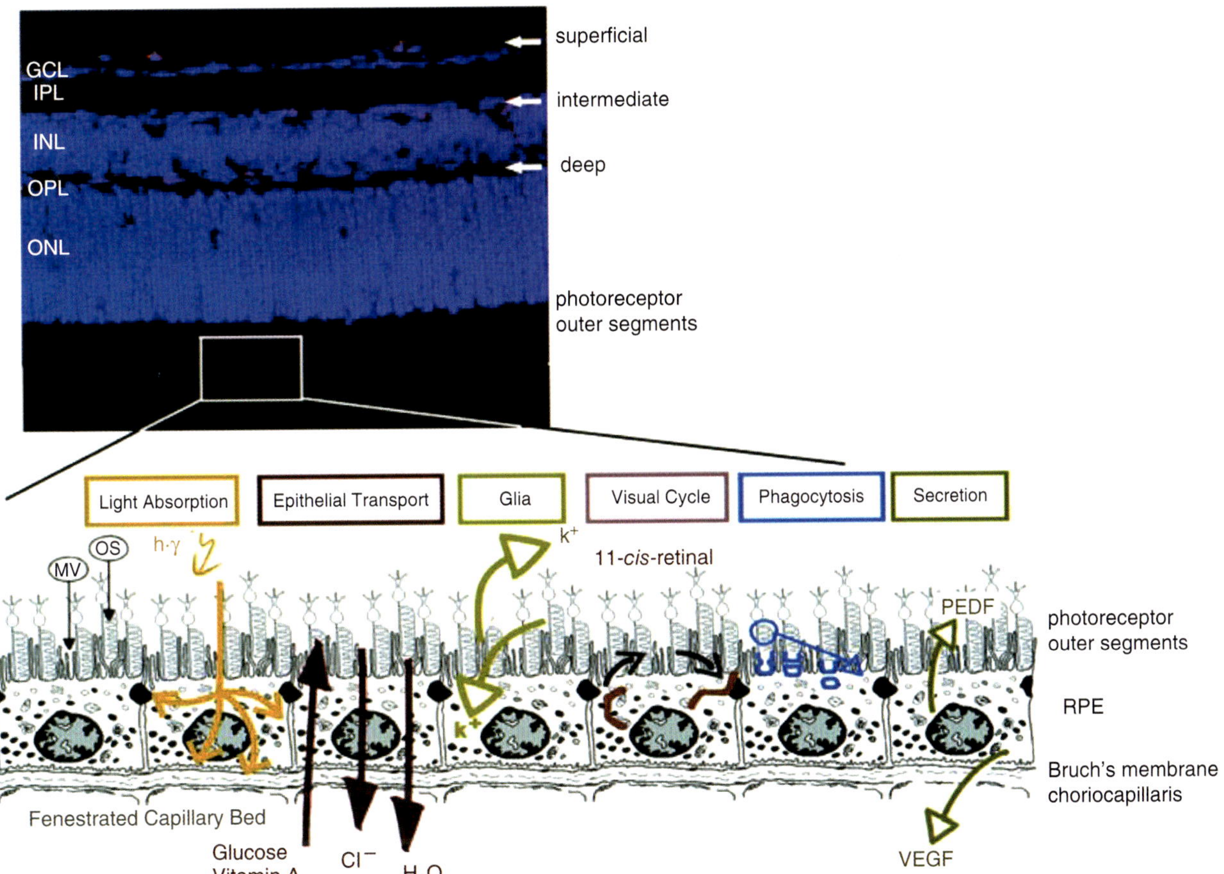

Plate 64 *Top*, The retina is a complex, striated tissue with highly organized neuronal layers. The inner retinal vasculature forms three distinct plexuses: The superficial plexus forms within the ganglion cell layer (GCL), the intermediate plexus forms at the inner edge of the inner nuclear layer (INL), and the deep plexus forms at the outer edge of the INL. *Bottom*, Posterior to the retina are the RPE, Bruch's membrane, and the choriocapillaris. The RPE performs many functions that are critical to retinal function. (See figure 56.1.) (*Top*, From Dorrell and Friedlander, 2006. *Bottom*, From Strauss, 2005.)

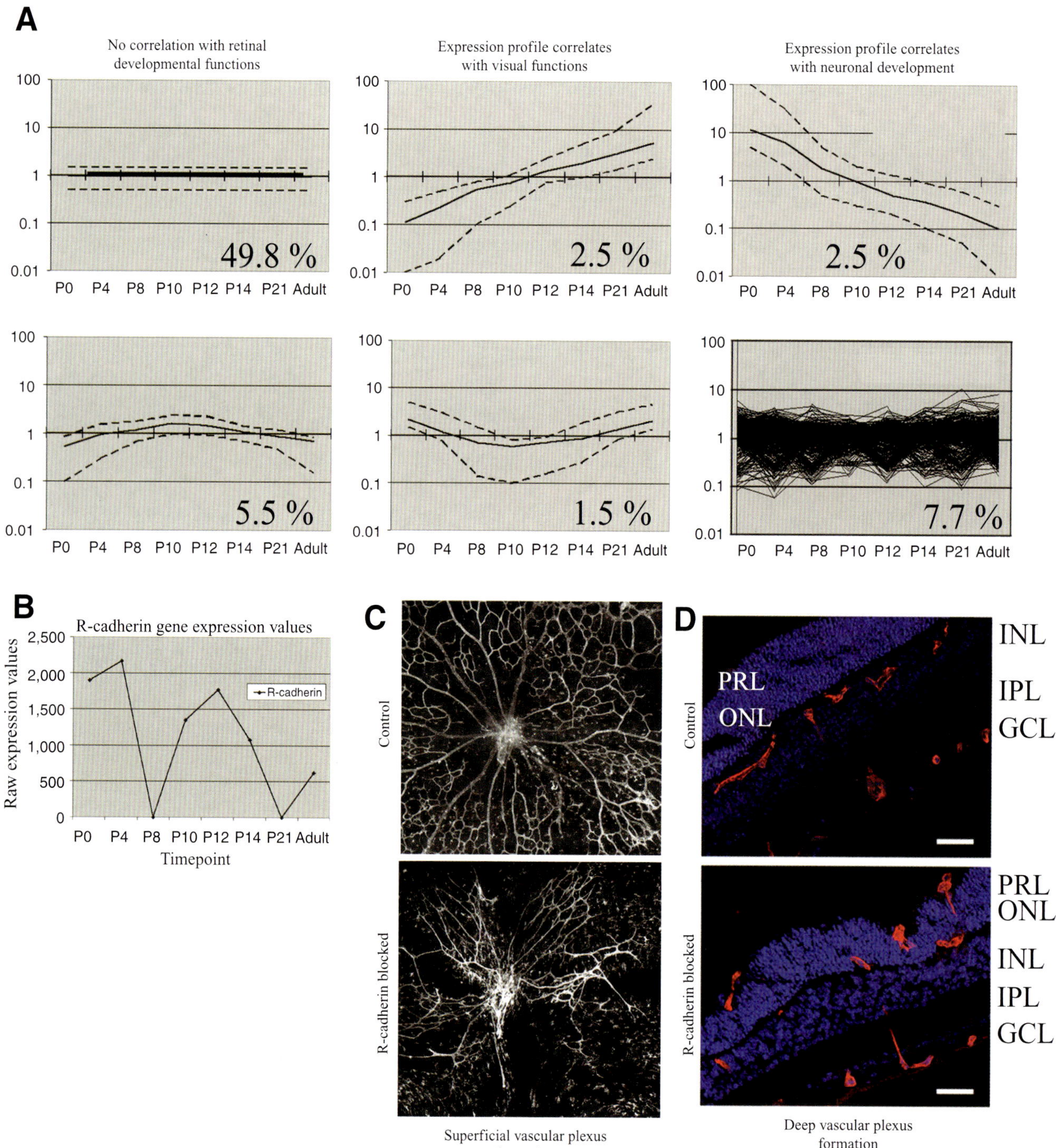

PLATE 65 *A*, Gene expression profile clustering of mRNA from whole mouse retinas at different postnatal developmental stages. Based on expression profile, gene function could be classified as having probable involvement in the onset of vision (mouse retinal development nears completion and vision begins around P14), neuronal development and differentiation (nears completion around P14), or potential involvement in postnatal retinal vascular development (a process that undergoes multiple changes during these times, and thus gene expression would vary throughout). *B*, The expression profile of R-cadherin was determined to have a potential relationship to retinal vascular development. When R-cadherin function was blocked, the retinal vasculature failed to form normally in the superficial plexus (*C*), and guidance to the normal deep vascular plexuses was disrupted (*D*). Vessels migrated through the photoreceptor layer and into the subretinal space. (See figure 56.2.) (Adapted from Dorrell et al., 2002, 2004.)

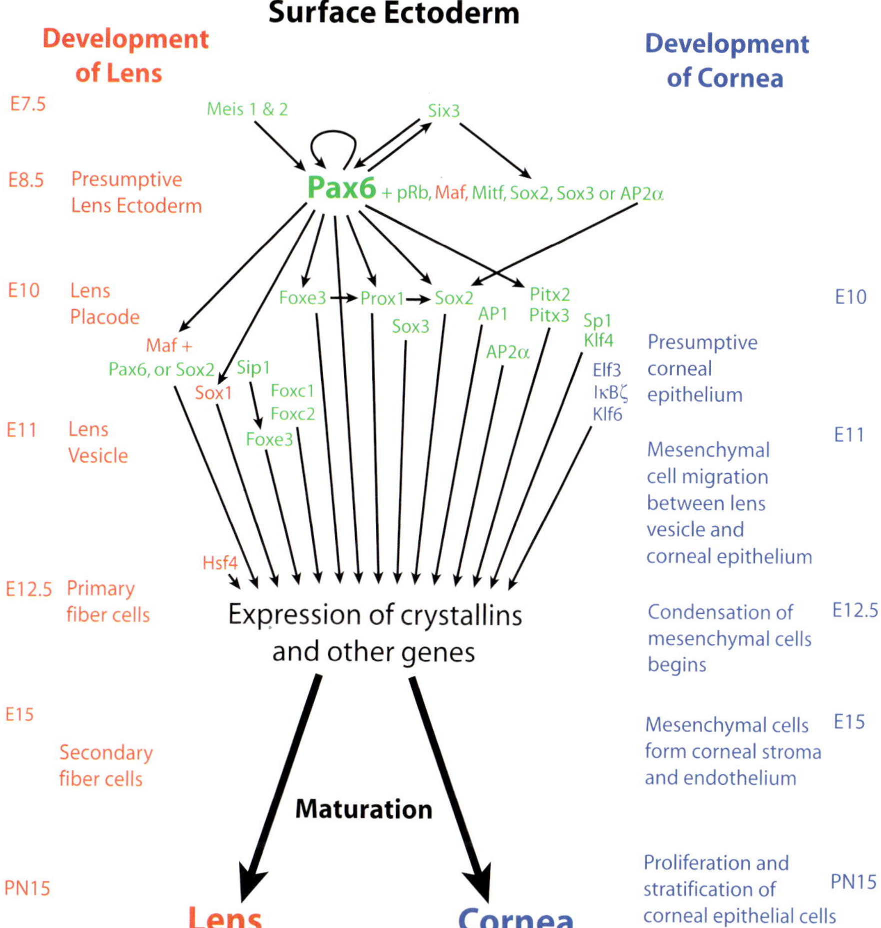

Plate 66 Transcription factors regulating the development of mouse lens and cornea. The network of transcription factors regulating the development of lens (red), or cornea (blue), or both (green) is shown, along with the embryonic age and the developmental stages of lens and cornea. Many of these transcription factors remain active in the mature lens and cornea. (See figure 57.2.)

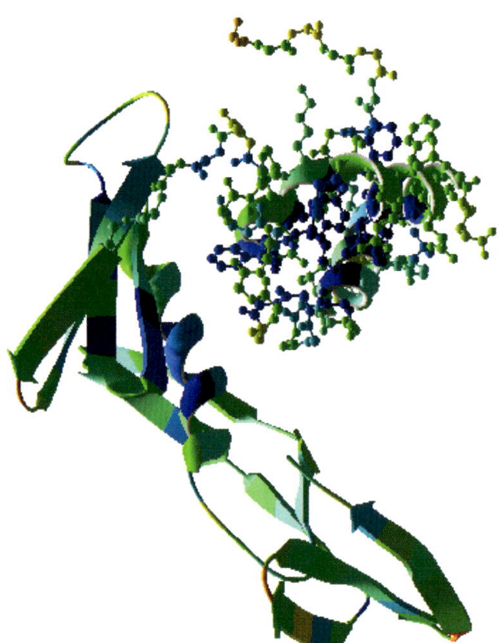

PLATE 67 Model of αA-crystallin secondary and tertiary structure, colored according to the hydrophobicity of its amino acid residues. The most hydrophobic residues are colored dark blue; the least hydrophobic residues are colored red. The Rosetta algorithm on the HMMSTR server (www.bioinfo.rpi.edu/~bystrc/hmmstr/server.php) (Bystroff and Shao, 2002) available on the ExPASY (http://au.expasy.org/) home page was used for molecular modeling. Full-length αA-crystallin secondary structure was calculated at 29.5% α helix and 32% β sheet content. The N-terminal globular domain is organized into three helices, displayed as ribbons with hydrophobic side chains buried. Structure-function regions identified earlier (Smith et al., 1996; Pasta et al., 2003) make up the first two of these N-terminal α helices. The highly conserved residues 102–117 of the "α crystallin domain" (Caspers et al., 1995), containing the substantial first part of a DNA-binding motif (Singh et al., 1998), as well as an arginine residue 116 shown to be critical for molecular integrity (Bera et al., 2002), are predicted to have α-helical conformation and are displayed as ribbons. This is consistent with an older 3D model (Farnsworth et al., 1998) and makes the α-helical prediction that is somewhat higher than previous calculations (Farnsworth et al., 1997; Horwitz et al., 1998; Bova et al., 2000) seem plausible. However, it is inconsistent with site-directed spin label studies that demonstrate β sheet conformation for residues 109–120 (Berengian et al., 1997). The model confirms the β sheet secondary structure of residues 67–101, determined to be an alcohol dehydrogenase (ADH) and 1,1′-bi (4-anilino) naphtalene-5,5′-disulfonic acid (bis-ANS) binding site and to exhibit extensive chaperone activity (Farnsworth and Singh, 2004). (See figure 58.1.)

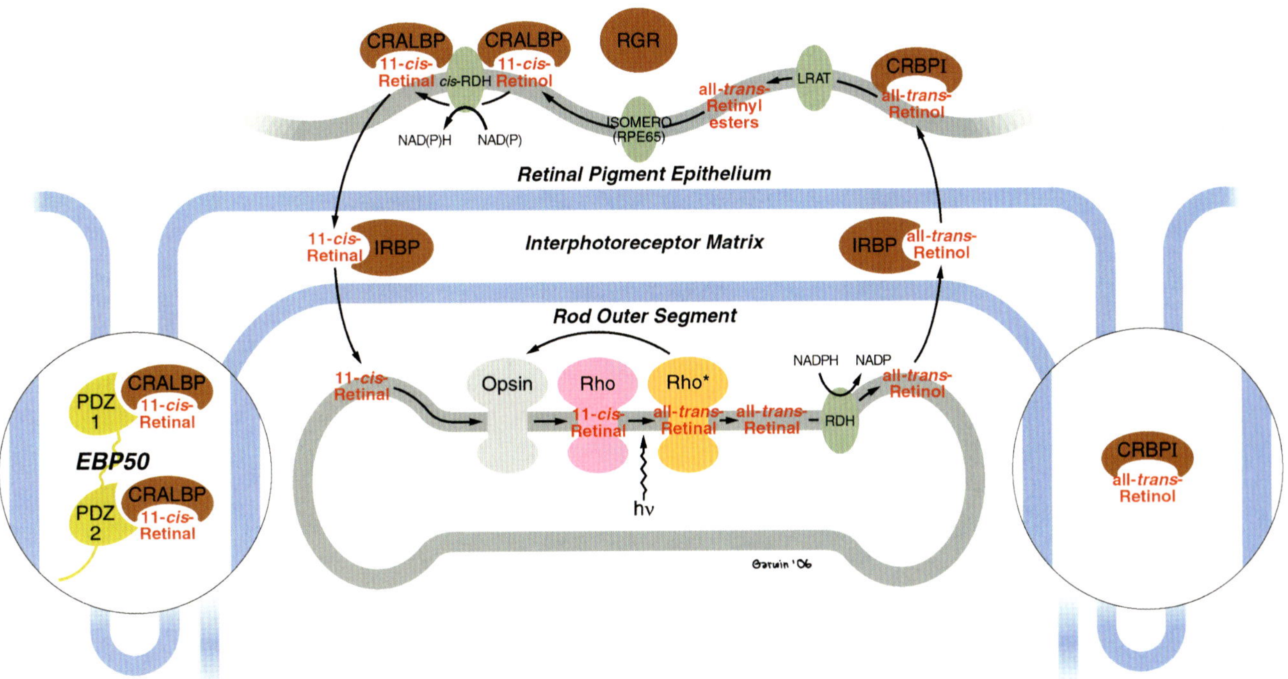

Plate 68 Hypothetical schematic of the rod photoreceptor visual cycle. Transcellular diffusion and intracellular enzymatic processing of visual cycle retinoids are shown. A retinal pigmented epithelial (RPE) cell is depicted with apical process extending toward a rod outer segment, with one disc membrane. Reactions and processes are as discussed in the text. *Circular insets* depict putative roles of components in RPE apical processes. *cis*-RDH, 11-*cis*-retinal dehydrogenase; CRALBP, cellular retinaldehyde-binding protein; CRBPI, cellular retinol-binding protein type I; EBP50, ERM-binding phosphoprotein of 50 kd, also known as NHERF-1 (sodium hydrogen exchanger regulatory factor type 1); IRBP, interphotoreceptor retinoid-binding protein; ISOMERO, isomerohydrolase, recently identified as RPE65; LRAT, lecithin : retinol acyltransferase; PDZ, a scaffold domain protein; RGR, retinal G protein–coupled receptor; RDH, all-*trans*-retinol dehydrogenase; Rho, rhodopsin; Rho*, activated rhodopsin (metarhodopsin II); RPE65, retinal pigmented epithelial protein of 65 kd. (See figure 59.1.)

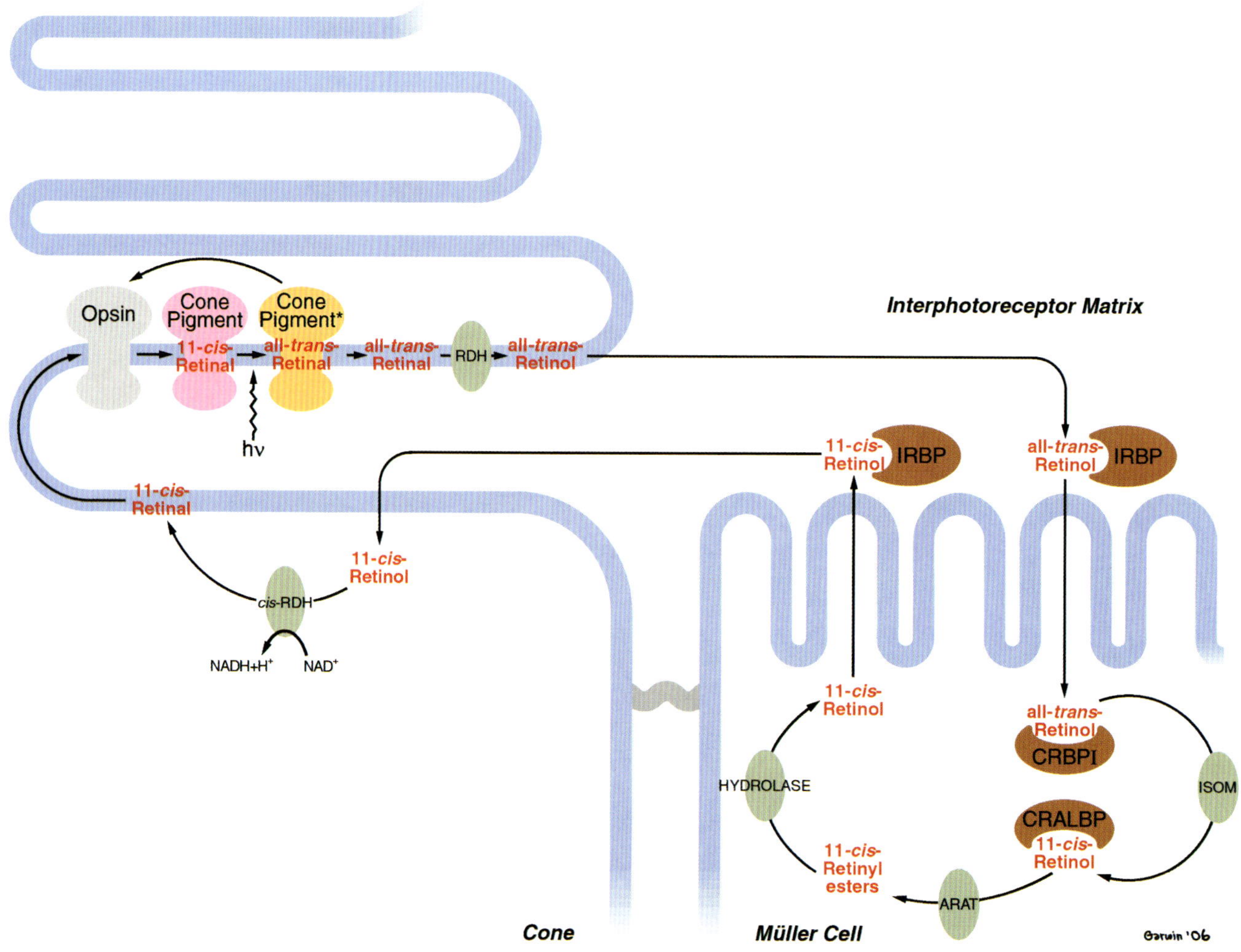

PLATE 69 Hypothetical schematic of the cone photoreceptor visual cycle. Transcellular diffusion and intracellular enzymatic processing of cone visual cycle retinoids are shown. Structure at *left* depicts a portion of the inner and outer segments of a cone photoreceptor cell. Structure at *right* depicts the apical end of a Müller cell. The cells are joined by structures of the external limiting membrane (*short wavy line*). ARAT, acylCoA:retinol acyltransferase; HYDROLASE, 11-*cis*-retinyl ester hydrolase; ISOM, isomerase. See also the abbreviation key for figure 59.1. (See Figure 59.2.) (After Mata et al., 2002.)

The dorsal visual stream

The visual system of mice is organized according to the same basic plan found in all mammals and best characterized in primates. A main difference between mice and primates is the amount of space the brain devotes to the projections from different parts of the retina. Whereas in primates the central visual representations of the fovea are disproportionately magnified, mice do not have a fovea but a broad horizontal region of the retina that is relatively enlarged in central visual maps. Although this streak-like specialization is not apparent in simple histological preparations of the retina, it is strikingly obvious as differential RA distribution in retinas of RA reporter mice (Dräger et al., 2001; Luo et al., 2006). Like primates, mice have retinal ganglion cells of different sizes and functional properties that convey different aspects of visual information in the parallel magno- and parvocellular pathways to the cortex (Merigan and Maunsell, 1993). In higher peristriate areas the two visual pathways feed into physically divergent systems (Wang and Burkhalter, 2004). The dorsal stream that receives the magnocellular input acts in spatial and motion perception; it contains the information about "where" a stimulus is located. The ventral stream, by contrast, functions as cognitive pathway that carries the information about "what" a stimulus is (Merigan and Maunsell, 1993; Goodale and Westwood, 2004; Wang and Burkhalter, 2004). The dorsal visual stream integrates with other sensory input in parietal regions, and the combined information is propagated rostrally into areas in which attentional and executive processes are generated (Coogan and Burkhalter, 1993; Dolan, 2002; Wang and Burkhalter, 2004).

As described earlier, the caudal part of the RALDH3 band contains the dorsal visual stream (Wang and Burkhalter, 2004), which is likely relevant for its higher neuronal plasticity and late maturation in humans (Braddick et al., 2003; Goodale and Westwood, 2004). These characteristics were demonstrated in psychophysical studies of specific visual skills in children: dorsal stream function, including perception of motion and vernier acuity, develops later and remains plastic for a much longer time than color and form vision, which are processed in the ventral stream (Skoczenski and Norcia, 2002; Mitchell and Neville, 2004). Moreover, dorsal stream function is known to be selectively affected in several human cognitive syndromes (Braddick et al., 2003). Visual impairments restricted to the dorsal stream in the presence of normal ventral stream function accompany Williams syndrome (Braddick et al., 2003; Meyer-Lindenberg et al., 2006), dyslexia (Buchholz and McKone, 2004), autism (Pellicano et al., 2005), and schizophrenia (Schechter et al., 2003; Keri et al., 2004), and they are also a prominent defect in low-birth-weight children (Downie et al., 2003). Premature birth is a classic condition of vitamin A deficiency, because the retinol storage capacity of the human liver develops late: it is always insufficient in premature babies and slowly reaches its capacity only later in childhood (Shenai, 1999).

The etiology of some of the syndromes with dorsal stream abnormalities involves both genetic and environmental contributions, including schizophrenia (Schechter et al., 2003; Keri et al., 2004) and autism (Pellicano et al., 2005); others are mainly due to mutations, including Williams syndrome, which is caused by a hemizygous microdeletion of about 28 genes (Meyer-Lindenberg et al., 2006). Because the size and location of the deletion can vary between individuals affected with Williams syndrome, the critical genes for the cognitive symptoms have been identified; using fMRI, Meyer-Lindenberg et al. (2006) mapped the locations of functional abnormalities to the dorsal visual stream of the human brain (figure 30.9, *left*). Comparisons of the human data with the

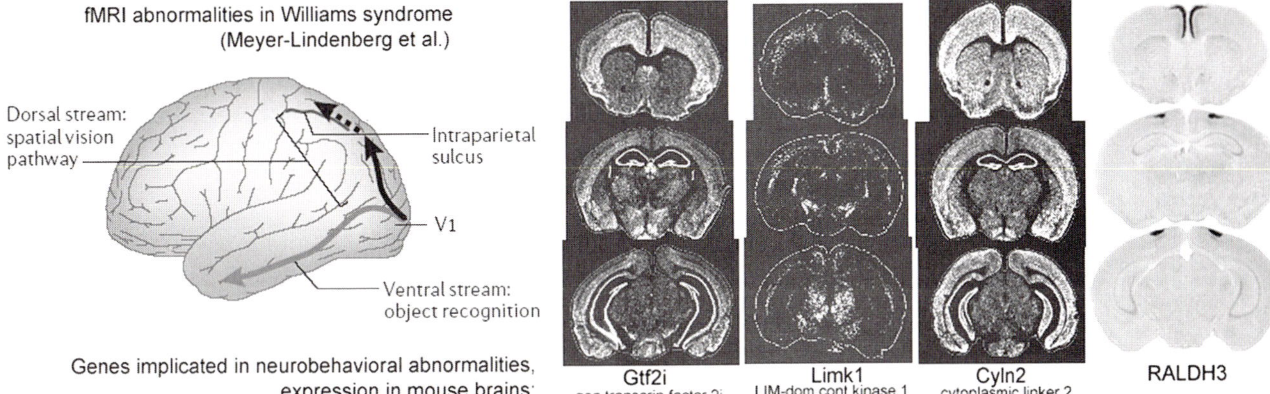

FIGURE 30.9 *Left*, Illustration from a review by Meyer-Lindenberg et al., (2006) on Williams syndrome. *Interrupted arrow* indicates the localization of functional abnormalities. *Right*, Allen data bank expressions of the three genes in the mouse cortex that have been linked to the cognitive defects in humans, and comparison with RALDH3.

localizations in the Allen atlas show that the expression of all three cognition-linked genes is differentially regulated along the RALDH3 band (figure 30.9, *right*): the general transcription factor *Gtf2i* and the cytoplasmic linker *Cyln2* are slightly higher, and the LIM domain containing kinase *Limk1* is slightly lower in this territory. Although all three genes are expressed throughout the cortex, as are most of the genes implicated in cognitive functions, we suggest that their differential expression along the RALDH3 band ought to differentially accentuate this anatomical location with respect to functional abnormalities that are caused by the halved gene dosage in Williams syndrome.

Conclusion

From our own histological examinations and the gene expression data searches we conclude that the postnatally emerging RALDH3 band along the medial cortex demarcates a pivotal postnatal patterning event for functional characteristics that has not previously been recognized as a coherent arrangement. The entire complement of genes with differential regulation along the shifted, RALDH3-colocalized location can be assumed to contain some that are directly influenced by RA, some that might act upstream of RALDH3 expression, and others that might be mainly responsive to any one of the shifted genes. Available information does not allow placing a gene in any of these three categories, and recent advances in the molecular biology of transcriptional specificity indicate that these categories are not clear-cut alternatives (Rochette-Egly, 2005; Lonard and O'Malley, 2006; Rosenfeld et al., 2006). This point has been most thoroughly investigated for the transcription factor CREB, which represents the site of convergence for about 300 physiological and pathological stimuli (Lonze and Ginty, 2002; Cawley et al., 2004; Johannessen et al., 2004). Each one of these stimuli results in the same CREB phosphorylation at Ser-133, which then initiates nuclear responses that are, however, different and appropriate for every stimulus. This amazing specificity of gene expression is now believed to be largely generated at the level of gene transcription, on which intracellular signaling cascades converge together with other determinants, including the ligand availability for nuclear receptors, to influence dynamically changing coregulator interactions with the basic transcriptional apparatus (Kadonaga, 2004; Rosenfeld et al., 2006). From the observations that RA responses are preferentially amplified in the brain, we suspect that the combinatorial mechanisms for specific gene expression must be unusually complex in the brain.

ACKNOWLEDGMENTS Experimental work was supported by grants EY01938 and EY13272 from the National Eye Institute. For the gene expression data in the mouse brain, we are greatly indebted to the team of the Allen Brain Atlas (www.brain-map.org) and the BGEM team (www.stjudebgem.org/web/mainPage/mainPage.php). We thank Yasuo Sakai for the NT-3 reporter brains (figure 30.6) and James Crandall and Peter McCaffery for reading the manuscript.

REFERENCES

Aggarwal, S., Kim, S. W., Cheon, K., Tabassam, F. H., Yoon, J. H., and Koo, J. S. (2006). Nonclassical action of retinoic acid on the activation of the cAMP response element-binding protein in normal human bronchial epithelial cells, *Mol. Biol. Cell.* 17:566–575.

Balmer, J. E., and Blomhoff, R. (2002). Gene expression regulation by retinoic acid. *J. Lipid Res.* 43:1773–1808.

Bosman, E. A., Penn, A. C., Ambrose, J. C., Kettleborough, R., Stemple, D. L., and Steel, K. P. (2005). Multiple mutations in mouse Chd7 provide models for CHARGE syndrome. *Hum. Mol. Genet.* 14:3463–3476.

Braddick, O., Atkinson, J., and Wattam-Bell, J. (2003). Normal and anomalous development of visual motion processing: Motion coherence and 'dorsal-stream vulnerability.' *Neuropsychologia* 41: 1769–1784.

Buchholz, J., and McKone, E. (2004). Adults with dyslexia show deficits on spatial frequency doubling and visual attention tasks. *Dyslexia* 10:24–43.

Canon, E., Cosgaya, J. M., Scsucova, S., and Aranda, A. (2004). Rapid effects of retinoic acid on CREB and ERK phosphorylation in neuronal cells. *Mol. Cell. Biol.* 15:5583–5592.

Carlezon, W. A., Duman, R. S., and Nestler, E. J. (2005). The many faces of CREB. *Trends Neurosci.* 28:436–445.

Cawley, S., Bekiranov, S., Ng, H. H., Kapranov, P. E., Sekinger, A., Kampa, D., Piccolboni, A., Sementchenko, V., Cheng, J., et al. (2004). Unbiased mapping of transcription factor binding sites along human chromosomes 21 and 22 points to widespread regulation of noncoding RNAs. *Cell* 116:499–509.

Chiang, M. Y., Misner, D., Kempermann, G., Schikorski, T., Giguere, V., Sucov, H. M., Gage, F. H., Stevens, C. F., and Evans, R. M. (1998). An essential role for retinoid receptors RARβ and RXRγ in long-term potentiation and depression. *Neuron* 21:1353–1561.

Coogan, T. A., and Burkhalter, A. (1993). Hierarchical organization of areas in rat visual cortex. *J Neurosci.* 13:3749–3772.

Corcoran, J. P., So, P. L., and Maden, M. (2004). Disruption of the retinoid signalling pathway causes a deposition of amyloid beta in the adult rat brain. *Eur. J. Neurosci.* 20:896–902.

Crandall, J., Sakai, Y., Zhang, J., Koul, O., Mineur, Y., Crusio, W. E., and McCaffery, P. (2004). 13-*cis*-retinoic acid suppresses hippocampal cell division and hippocampal-dependent learning in mice. *Proc. Natl. Acad. Sci. U.S.A.* 101:5111–5116.

Dolan, R. J. (2002). Emotion, cognition, and behavior. *Science* 298:1191–1194.

Downie, A. L., Jakobson, L. S., Frisk, V., and Ushycky, I. (2003). Periventricular brain injury, visual motion processing, and reading and spelling abilities in children who were extremely low birthweight. *J. Int. Neuropsychol. Soc.* 9:440–449.

Dräger, U. C. (1975). Receptive fields of single cells and topography in mouse visual cortex. *J. Comp. Neurol.* 160:269–290.

Dräger, U. C., and Hubel, D. H. (1975). Responses to visual stimulation and relationship between visual, auditory, and somatosensory inputs in mouse superior colliculus. *J. Neurophysiol.* 38:690–713.

Dräger, U. C., Li, H., Wagner, E., and McCaffery, P. (2001). Retinoic acid synthesis and breakdown in the developing mouse retina. *Progr. Brain Res.* 131:579–588.

Draghici, S., Khatri, P., Bhavsar, P., Shah, A., Krawetz, S. A., and Tainsky, M. A. (2003). Onto-Tools, the toolkit of the modern biologist: Onto-Express, Onto-Compare, Onto-Design and Onto-Translate. *Nucleic Acids Res.* 31:3775–3781.

Dupe, V., Matt, N., Garnier, J. M., Chambon, P. Mark, M., and Ghyselinck, N. B., (2003). A newborn lethal defect due to inactivation of retinaldehyde dehydrogenase type 3 is prevented by maternal retinoic acid treatment. *Proc. Natl. Acad. Sci. U.S.A.* 100:410–421.

Etchamendy, N., Enderlin, V., Marighetto, A., Vouimba, R. M., Pallet, V., Jaffard, R., and Higueret, P. (2001). Alleviation of a selective age-related relational memory deficit in mice by pharmacologically induced normalization of brain retinoid signaling. *J. Neurosci.* 21:6423–6429.

Goodale, M. A., and Westwood, D. A. (2004). An evolving view of duplex vision: Separate but interacting cortical pathways for perception and action. *Curr. Opin. Neurobiol.* 14:203–211.

Grove, E. A., and Fukuchi-Shimogori, T. (2003). Generating the cerebral cortical area map. *Annu. Rev. Neurosci.* 26:355–380.

Hong, E. J., West, A. E., and Greenberg, M. E. (2005). Transcriptional control of cognitive development. *Curr. Opin. Neurobiol.* 15:21–28.

Jacobs, S., Lie, D. C., DeCicco, K. L., Shi, Y., DeLuca, L. M., Gage, F. H., and Evans, R. M. (2006). Retinoic acid is required early during adult neurogenesis in the dentate gyrus. *Proc. Natl. Acad. Sci. U.S.A.* 103:3902–3907.

Johannessen, M., Delghandi, M. P., and Moens, U. (2004). What turns CREB on? *Cell Signal* 16:1211–1127.

Kadonaga, J. T. (2004). Regulation of RNA polymerase II transcription by sequence-specific DNA binding factors. *Cell* 116: 247–257.

Keri, S., Kelemen, O., Benedek, G., and Janka, Z. (2004). Vernier threshold in patients with schizophrenia and in their unaffected siblings. *Neuropsychology* 18:537–542.

Knauff, M., Mulack, T., Kassubek, J., Salih, H. R., and Greenlee, M. W. (2002). Spatial imagery in deductive reasoning: A functional MRI study. *Brain Res. Cogn. Brain Res.* 13: 203–212.

Koppe, G., Bruckner, G., Brauer, K., Hartig, W., and Bigl, V. (1997). Developmental patterns of proteoglycan-containing extracellular matrix in perineuronal nets and neuropil of the postnatal rat brain. *Cell Tissue Res.* 288:33–41.

Kruyt, F. A., Folkers, G., van den Brink C. E., and van der Saag, P. T. (1992). A cyclic AMP response element is involved in retinoic acid-dependent RAR beta 2 promoter activation. *Nucleic Acids Res.* 20:6393–6399.

Kurlandsky, S. B., Gamble, M. V., Ramakrishnan, R., and Blaner, W. S. (1995). Plasma delivery of retinoic acid to tissues in the rat. *J. Biol. Chem.* 270:17850–17857.

Lane, M. A., and Bailey, S. J. (2005). Role of retinoid signalling in the adult brain. *Prog. Neurobiol.* 75:275–293.

Lein, E. S., Hawrylycz, M. J., Ao, N., Ayres, M., Bensinger, A., Bernard, A., Boe, A. F., Boguski, M. S., Brockway, K. S, et al. (2007). Genome-wide atlas of gene expression in the adult mouse brain. *Nature* 445:168–176.

Lonard, D. M., and O'Malley, B. W. (2006). The expanding cosmos of nuclear receptor coactivators. *Cell* 125:411–414.

Lonze, B. E., and Ginty, D. D. (2002). Function and regulation of CREB family transcription factors in the nervous system. *Neuron* 35:605–623.

Luo, T., Sakai, Y. Wagner, E., and Dräger, U. C. (2006). Retinoids, eye development and maturation of visual function. *J. Neurobiol.* 66:677–686.

Luo, T., Wagner, E., and Dräger, U. C. (2008). Unpublished results.

Luo, T., Wagner, E., Grün, F., and Dräger, U. C. (2004). Retinoic acid signaling in the brain marks formation of optic projections, maturation of the dorsal telencephalon, and function of limbic sites. *J. Comp. Neurol.* 470:297–316.

Magdaleno, S., Jensen, P., Brumwell, C. L., Seal, A., Lehman, K., Asbury, A., Cheung, T., Cornelius, T., Batten, D. M, et al. (2006). BGEM: An in situ hybridization database of gene expression in the embryonic and adult mouse nervous system. *PLoS Biol.* 4:e86.

Maret, S., Franken, P., Dauvilliers, Y., Ghyselinck, N. B., Chambon P., and Tafti, M. (2005). Retinoic acid signaling affects cortical synchrony during sleep. *Science* 310:111–113.

Mark, M., and Chambon, P. (2003). Functions of RARs and RXRs in vivo: Genetic dissection of the retinoid signaling pathway. *Pure Appl. Chem.* 75:1709–1732.

Merigan, W. H., and Maunsell, J. H. (1993). How parallel are the primate visual pathways? *Annu. Rev. Neurosci.* 16:369–402.

Meyer-Lindenberg, A., Mervis, C. B., and Faith Berman, K. (2006). Neural mechanisms in Williams syndrome: A unique window to genetic influences on cognition and behaviour. *Nat. Rev. Neurosci.* 7:380–893.

Misner, D. L., Jacobs, S., Shimizu, Y., de Urquiza, A. M., Solomin, L., Perlmann, T., De Luca, L. M., Stevens, C. F., and Evans, R. M. (2001). Vitamin A deprivation results in reversible loss of hippocampal long-term synaptic plasticity. *Proc. Natl. Acad. Sci. U.S.A.* 98:11714–11719.

Mitchell, T. V., and Neville, H. J. (2004). Asynchronies in the development of electrophysiological responses to motion and color. *J. Cogn. Neurosci.* 16:1363–1674.

O'Reilly, K. C., Shumake, J., Gonzalez-Lima, F., Lane, M. A., and Bailey, S. J. (2006). Chronic administration of 13-*cis*-retinoic acid increases depression-related behavior in mice. *Neuropsychopharmacology* 31:1919–1927.

Pellicano, E., Gibson, L., Maybery, M., Durkin, K., and Badcock, D. R. (2005). Abnormal global processing along the dorsal visual pathway in autism: A possible mechanism for weak visuospatial coherence? *Neuropsychologia* 43:1044–1053.

Rochette-Egly, C. (2005). Dynamic combinatorial networks in nuclear receptor-mediated transcription. *J. Biol. Chem.* 280: 32565–32568.

Rosenfeld, M. G., Lunyak, V., and Glass, C. K. (2006). Sensors and signals: A coactivator/corepressor/epigenetic code for integrating signal-dependent programs of transcriptional response. *Genes Dev.* 20:1405–1428.

Rossant, J., Zirngibl, R., Cado, D., Shago M., and Giguère, V. (1991). Expression of a retinoic acid response element-hsplacZ transgene defines specific domains of transcriptional activity during mouse embryogenesis. *Genes Dev.* 5:1333–1344.

Schechter, I., Butler, P. D., Silipo, G., Zemon, V., and Javitt, D. C. (2003). Magnocellular and parvocellular contributions to backward masking dysfunction in schizophrenia. *Schizophr. Res.* 64:91–101.

Shenai, J. P. (1999). Vitamin A supplementation in very low birth weight neonates: Rationale and evidence. *Pediatrics* 104:1369–1374.

Shenefelt, R. E. (1972). Morphogenesis of malformations in hamsters caused by retinoic acid. *Teratology* 5:403–418.

Sidman, R. L., Green, M. C., and Appel, S. H. (1965). *Catalog of the Neurological Mutants of the Mouse.* Cambridge, MA: Harvard University Press.

Skoczenski, A. M., and Norcia, A. M., (2002). Late maturation of visual hyperacuity. *Psychol. Sci.* 13:537–541.

Smith, D., Wagner, E., Koul, O., McCaffery, P., and Dräger, U. C. (2001). Retinoic acid synthesis for the developing telencephalon. *Cereb. Cortex* 11:894–905.

van Groen, T., Kadish, I., and Wyss, J. M. (1999). Efferent connections of the anteromedial nucleus of the thalamus of the rat. *Brain Res. Brain Res. Rev.* 30:1–26.

Vissers, L. E., van Ravenswaaij, C. M., Admiraal, R., Hurst, J. A., de Vries, B. B., Janssen, I. M., van der Vliet, W. A., Huys, E. H., de Jong, P. J., et al. (2004). Mutations in a new member of the chromodomain gene family cause CHARGE syndrome. *Nat. Genet.* 36:955–957.

Wagner, E., Luo, T., and Dräger, U. C. (2002). Retinoic acid synthesis in the postnatal mouse brain marks distinct developmental stages and functional systems. *Cereb. Cortex* 12:1244–1253.

Wagner, E., Luo, T., Sakai, Y., Parada L. F., and Dräger, U. C. (2006). Retinoic acid delineates the topography of neuronal plasticity in postnatal cerebral cortex. *Eur. J. Neurosci.* 24:329–340.

Wagner, M., Han, B., and Jessell, T. M. (1992). Regional differences in retinoid release from embryonic neural tissue detected by an in vitro reporter assay. *Development* 116:55–66.

Wang, Q., and Burkhalter, A. (2004). Dorsal and ventral streams for processing of visual information in mouse cerebral cortex. *Soc. Neurosci. Abstr.* 300.5.

Wilson, J. G., Roth, C. B., and Warkany, J. (1953). An analysis of the syndrome of malformations induced by maternal vitamin A deficiency: Effects of restoration of vitamin A at various times during gestation. *Am. J. Anat.* 92:189–217.

V DEVELOPMENT AND PLASTICITY OF RETINAL PROJECTIONS AND VISUOTOPIC MAPS

31 Intraretinal Axon Guidance

LYNDA ERSKINE AND HANNAH THOMPSON

Visual information is relayed from the eye to the central nervous system (CNS) via the axons of retinal ganglion cells (RGCs). These connections are established early in development by the guidance of RGC axons along a highly stereotypical pathway to reach and innervate visual targets. The first pathfinding task faced by RGC axons is to navigate from their site of origin to their exit point from the eye, the optic fissure/disc (figure 31.1). In mice, this occurs from approximately embryonic day (E) 11 to E18 in a center-to-peripheral wave that reflects the differentiation of the developing retina (Dräger, 1985). The first RGCs to be generated are located within dorsocentral retina, a short distance from the developing optic disc. However, axons from later-generated RGCs are located more peripherally and must travel a significant distance to exit the eye. Nevertheless, the growth of all RGC axons is directed toward the optic disc from the outset, forming a highly ordered, radial array that converges on the optic disc (see figure 31.1).

As they extend toward the optic disc, RGC axons are restricted to the optic fiber layer (OFL) at the inner (vitreal) surface of the retina (see figure 31.1). Here they grow along the pial endfeet of surrounding neuroepithelial cells and, in the case of later-formed RGCs, a scaffold of previously formed axons (Silver and Sidman, 1980; Silver and Sapiro, 1981). The mechanisms that restrict RGC axons to the OFL and control disc-directed growth are beginning to be unraveled. Studies in mice, particularly of naturally occurring and targeted mutations, have been instrumental in revealing the cellular and molecular basis of intraretinal pathfinding. A surprising finding in these studies has been the degree of complexity and regional variability in the mechanisms used to direct RGC axons out of the eye.

This chapter focuses on our current understanding of the mechanisms directing intraretinal guidance in mice. The growth of RGC axons within the retina involves a number of distinct processes: restriction to the OFL, control of the initial polarity of axon outgrowth within the OFL, directed growth toward the optic disc, and targeting to the optic disc/exit from the eye. Each of these processes is considered in turn. Dorsal-ventral differences in the mechanisms regulating intraretinal guidance are also discussed.

Growth cones and guidance cues

Developing axons are tipped by growth cones, highly dynamic structures that play an active role in directing outgrowth. Growth cones are both motor and sensory in nature, providing the machinery for outgrowth and searching the environment for signals that convey guidance information. These guidance signals can be either attractive or repulsive and act either at short or long range to influence the direction of axon outgrowth. Considerable progress has been made in elucidating the molecular basis of axon guidance, including the identification of several conserved families of guidance cues and their cognate receptors (reviewed by Dickson, 2002). Interactions between many of the molecules, acting simultaneously or sequentially, underlie correct axon pathfinding within the retina.

Restriction of retinal ganglion cell axons to the optic fiber layer

RGC axons are restricted to the OFL by a combination of the growth-promoting properties of the neuroepithelial endfeet localized to this region (Stier and Schlosshauer, 1998) and inhibitory properties of the outer retinal layers. In vitro, removal of the pial endfeet of the neuroepithelial cells but not preexisting RGC axons blocks growth of new axons into the OFL, demonstrating that it is the growth-promoting properties of the endfeet rather than fasciculation with previously generated axons that supports the extension of RGC axons within the OFL (Stier and Schlosshauer, 1995). This growth-promoting property of the neuroepithelial endfeet is mediated in part by the cell adhesion molecule NCAM. In rat retinas, NCAM is expressed strongly by the endfeet and is required, at least by a subset of RGC axons, to drive their forward extension (Brittis and Silver, 1995; Brittis et al., 1995). Avoidance of the outer retina also plays an important role in restricting RGC axons to the OFL. This is not due to the lack of growth-promoting molecules within the outer retina but is a result of an active avoidance of this region driven by the presence of inhibitory guidance cues (Stier and Schlosshauer, 1995). One family of guidance cues involved in mediating this process are the Slits (Thompson et al., 2006b).

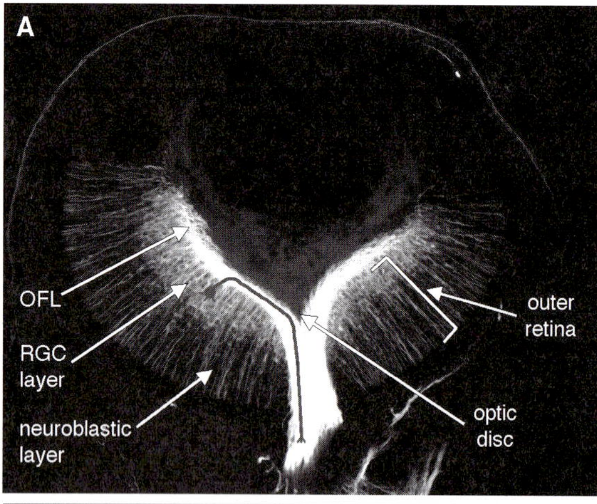

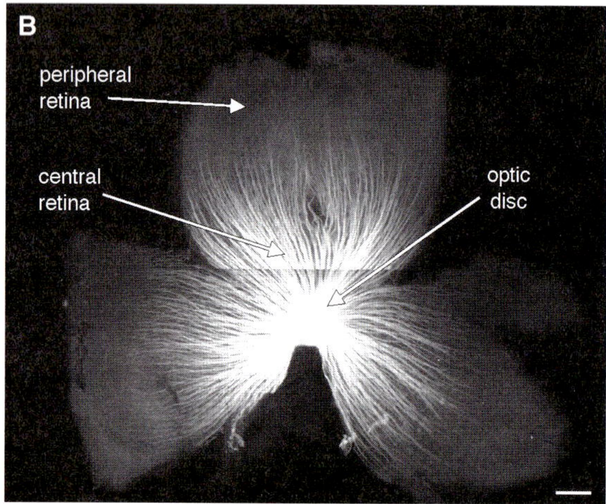

FIGURE 31.1 Organization of RGC axons within the developing mouse retina. *A*, Cross section of an E13.5 mouse retina stained with TUJ1 to label the RGCs and their axons. At this age, the retina is composed of three layers: the OFL at the inner surface of the retina, the RGC layer, and an outer neuroblastic region containing dividing cells. RGC axons extend exclusively within the OFL, where they grow directly toward the optic disc. *B*, Flat-mount of E18.5 mouse retina in which the RGC axons have been back-labeled from the optic chiasm with DiI. From the outset, the growth of retinal axons is oriented directly toward the optic disc, forming a highly organized radial array over the retinal surface. Scale bar = 50 μm (*A*), 500 μm (*B*).

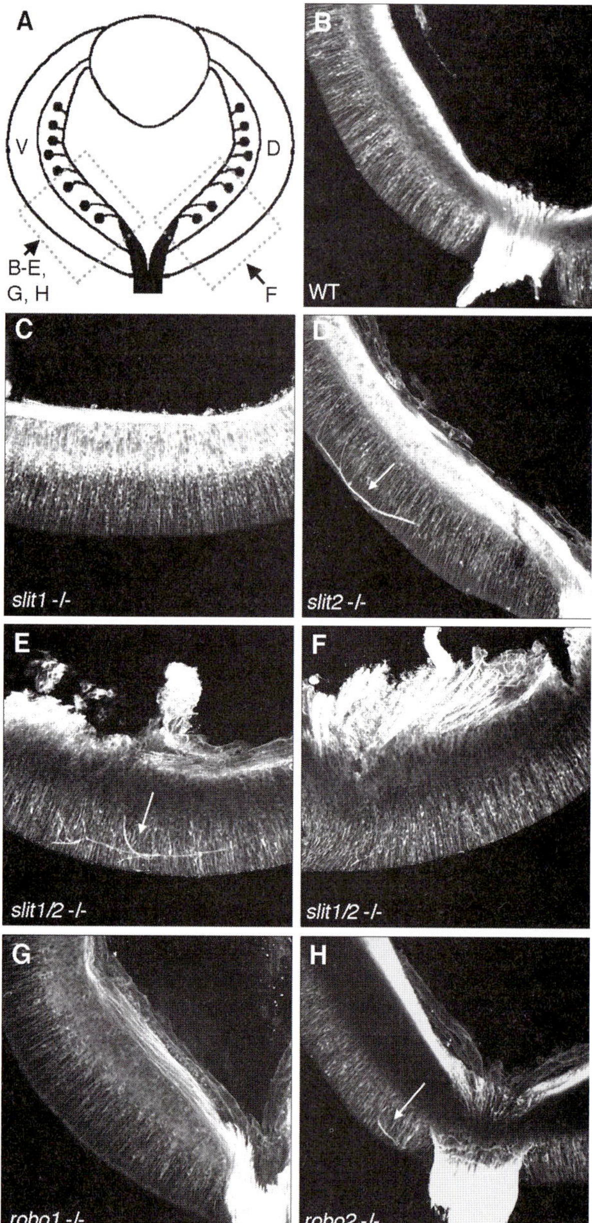

FIGURE 31.2 Robo-Slit signaling helps restrict RGC axons to the OFL. *A*, Diagram showing the areas imaged. D, dorsal; V, ventral. *B–H*, Coronal sections of E16.5 mouse retinas stained with TUJ1. In mice lacking *slit2* (alone or in combination with *slit1*) or *robo2*, subsets of RGC axons (*arrows*) extend aberrantly through the outer layers of ventral retina. Scale bar = 100 μm.

Slits are secreted guidance molecules that, acting through their roundabout (Robo) receptors, play a key role in directing axon guidance and cell migration (reviewed by Nguyen-Ba-Charvet and Chédotal, 2002). There are three Slits in vertebrates (Slit1–3) and four Robos (Robo1–4), subsets of which are expressed in the developing mouse visual system. One member of the Robo family, Robo2, is expressed by RGCs from the time their axons first start to extend within the retina. *robo1* also is expressed in the retina but from slightly later in development (E14.5) and is restricted to a scattered subpopulation of cells. Slits also are expressed in the retina in a pattern consistent with a role in directing intraretinal pathfinding. Throughout the period when RGC axons are navigating in the eye, both *slit1* and *slit2* are expressed strongly in the inner region of the retina (Erskine et al., 2000).

In mice lacking *slit2*, and to a much greater extent in mice lacking both *slit1* and *slit2*, a subset of RGC axons extends aberrantly away from the OFL through the outer layers of the retina (Thompson et al., 2006b; figure 31.2*A–F*). Surprisingly, although located in the outer retina, these ectopic axons still extend in a relatively directed fashion toward the optic disc and exit the eye, demonstrating that the guidance cues that determine disc-directed growth are not localized exclusively to the OFL (Goldberg, 1977). Similar defects are found in mice lacking *robo2*, whereas in *robo1*-deficient mice intraretinal axon pathfinding occurs normally (Thompson et al., 2008; figure 31.2*G* and *H*).

Axons of RGCs arise from the basal processes of recently differentiated cells that still retain their neuroepithelial-like morphology and extend directly into the OFL (Hinds and Hinds, 1974). In the absence of Slit-Robo signaling, the aberrant axons in the outer retina originate from cells located in the RGC layer, indicating that the polarity of the retina is not perturbed as occurs in rat retinas following overexpression or removal of chondroitin sulfates (Brittis et al., 1992; Brittis and Silver, 1994). The overall organization of the retina is also normal (Thompson et al., 2006b). However, whether the position on the cell body on which the axon arises is altered has not been established. Nevertheless, this demonstrates that an important function of Slit-Robo signaling is to help restrict RGC axons to the OFL.

Although it cannot be excluded formally that Slits act to promote growth within the OFL (Jin et al., 2003), all the evidence supports an inhibitory role for these molecules in the mouse retina. In vitro, both Slit1 and Slit2 are potent inhibitors of RGC axon outgrowth, and their expression in the RGC and presumptive inner nuclear layers places them in an ideal location to act as a barrier to RGC axon extension as occurs in other regions of the developing optic pathway (Erskine et al., 2000; Plump et al., 2002; Thompson et al., 2006a). Furthermore, Slits are expressed by RGCs rather than by neuroepithelial cells (Thompson et al., 2006b), suggesting they are unlikely to be involved in promoting growth in the OFL (Stier and Schlosshauer, 1998).

Slits clearly are not the only factors that restrict RGC axons to the OFL since in the absence of Slit-Robo signaling, only a small subset of axons project aberrantly through the outer retina (see figure 31.2). As they extend through the outer retina, the aberrant axons form tightly grouped bundles, a behavior characteristic of axons growing though an inhibitory environment. This suggests that other inhibitory signals are present in the outer retina and act in parallel to Robos/Slits to define the OFL. The identity of these signals is not known and is the focus of ongoing work.

Control of the initial polarity of retinal ganglion cell axon outgrowth within the optic fiber layer

Following their differentiation, RGCs transiently extend small processes in random directions until one process, which invariably originates on the side of the cell closest to the optic disc, develops into the mature axon (Brittis and Silver, 1995). This initial polarity of axon outgrowth could, in theory, be controlled either by inhibitory factors in the peripheral retina preventing extension or by growth-promoting factors on the optic disc side of the cell "pulling" axons in this direction. Several lines of evidence support a model whereby initial axon polarity is controlled by a "push" away from the peripheral retina.

Prior to axon outgrowth, the entire retinal neuroepithelium is inhibitory to RGC axon extension (Halfter, 1996). As development proceeds, this inhibitory activity recedes peripherally and, in rats, this correlates with a wave of chondroitin sulfate proteoglycan (CSPG) expression (Brittis et al., 1992). The CSPGs are a heterogeneous family of molecules composed of a protein core to which carbohydrate moieties (chondroitin sulfate chains) are attached. CSPGs are components of the extracellular matrix and can act either directly to influence axon outgrowth or indirectly, by modulating the function of other guidance cues (Kantor et al., 2004). In vitro, CSPGs inhibit RGC axon extension, and removal of endogenous chondroitin sulfates with chondroitinase ABC lyase from developing rat retinas results in ectopic differentiation of RGCs and impairment of the initial direction of axon outgrowth (Brittis et al., 1992). Many RGCs differentiate prematurely in the retinal periphery and are located ectopically, at the outer (ventricular) surface of the retina. RGC axon extension is also perturbed, with looping axons found in the retinal periphery and extending in random directions along the ventricular surface (Brittis et al., 1992). This suggests that CSPGs play two important roles in the retina: (1) control of the timing and location of RGC differentiation, and (2) by inhibiting axon extension into the retinal periphery, helping direct the initial polarity of RGC axon outgrowth.

Slit signaling also plays a key role in controlling the initial direction of RGC axon outgrowth. In mice lacking either *slit2* or *robo2*, the organization of the OFL layer is perturbed, with many axons initially extending into the peripheral retina (Thompson et al., 2006b; Erskine et al., 2008; figure 31.3). At all developmental stages, these defects occur specifically in the most peripheral part of the retina where recently differentiated RGCs are located. However, only the initial direction of growth is affected, and the axons ultimately loop around and extend toward the optic disc and out of the eye (Thompson et al., 2006b). This demonstrates that Slit signaling plays an important role in determining the initial polarity of RGC axon outgrowth but that other factors are the key determinants of overall disc-directed growth.

At least at the mRNA level, *slit2* is uniformly expressed throughout the central-peripheral axis of the developing mouse retina (Erskine et al., 2000). How, then, might Slit signaling act to control axon polarity? One possibility is that an extraretinal source of Slit is the major player in this process. In vitro assays have demonstrated that the lens is a potent inhibitor of RGC axon extension, and an important component of this inhibitory activity is Slit2 (Ohta et al., 1999; Thompson et al., 2006b). As a result of its location in the eye, factors secreted by the lens accumulate at higher concentrations in the retinal periphery, making this tissue an ideal source of signaling molecules involved in controlling RGC axon polarity (figure 31.3*H*). Thus, similar to the roof-plate in the developing spinal cord (Augsberger et al., 1999), the lens may function as the principal regulator of the initial direction of RGC axon outgrowth. An additional possibility is that Slit signaling in the retina is regulated differentially by the restricted expression of other molecules. Heparan sulfate proteoglycans are required for Slit localization and function (Hu, 2001; Inatani et al., 2003). RGCs also express CXCR4, the receptor for stromal cell–derived factor-1 (SDF-1), an inhibitor of Slit signaling (Chalasani et al., 2003a, 2003b). However, whether these molecules are expressed in graded fashion across the retina is not known.

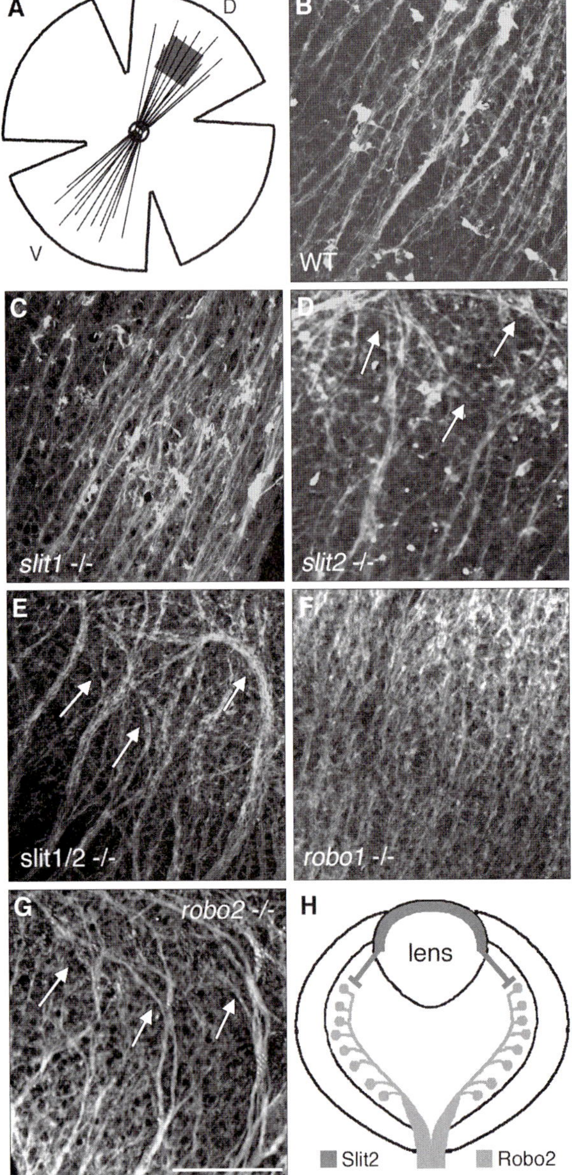

FIGURE 31.3 Robo-Slit signaling controls the initial polarity of RGC axon outgrowth. *A*, Diagram of a flat-mounted retina showing the region imaged (*gray box*). D, dorsal; V, ventral. *B–G*, Flat-mounted E16.5 mouse retinas stained with TUJ1. In mice lacking *slit2* or *robo2*, the organization of the dorsal but not ventral OFL is perturbed, with axons from recently differentiated RGCs projecting aberrantly into the retinal periphery. *Arrows* indicate examples of disorganized bundles of RGC axons. Bar = 100 µm. *H*, The lens secretes Slit2, raising the possibility it is this extraretinal source of Slit that, by blocking growth of Robo2-positive RGC axons into the retinal periphery, controls the initial direction of RGC axon outgrowth.

Directed growth of retinal ganglion cell axons toward the optic disc

The growth of RGC axons toward the optic disc is highly directed and organized, resulting in groups of tightly bundled, centrally oriented axons forming a radial array over the surface of the retina (see figure 31.1*B*). Ultrastructural studies of the mouse retina at early stages of development revealed a series of interconnected tunnels, formed by the endfeet of neuroepithelial cells, that are oriented toward the optic fissure and predict the path taken by pioneer RGC axons (Silver and Sidman, 1980). It has been proposed that these tunnels provide directional information to the RGC axons and channel them into the optic nerve. However, because the tunnels are localized to the central retina, as development proceeds, such channels are unlikely to be the major determinant of disc-directed growth (Brittis and Silver, 1995). Grafting experiments in chick also demonstrated that the optic disc does not have significant chemotropic activity, suggesting that short- rather than long-range cues direct intraretinal pathfinding (Halfter, 1996). With a few exceptions, the identity of these signals remains largely unknown.

The cell adhesion molecule BEN (also called DM-GRASP/SC1/neurolin) mediates both homophilic and heterophilic interactions and has been implicated in directing outgrowth and guidance of a number of different axonal subtypes. In the mouse retina, BEN is expressed by RGCs shortly after they begin to extend axons and is present on RGC axons in the OFL. Much lower levels of BEN expression are found on the distal segments of axons in the optic nerve, suggesting a potential role for this molecule in directing growth toward the optic disc (Weiner et al., 2004). However, mice lacking BEN show only subtle defects in intraretinal pathfinding (figure 31.4*C*). In BEN-deficient mice, the tight bundling together of RGC axons is impaired, resulting in significantly broader fascicles. Only rarely do pathfinding errors occur, with a very small number of axons

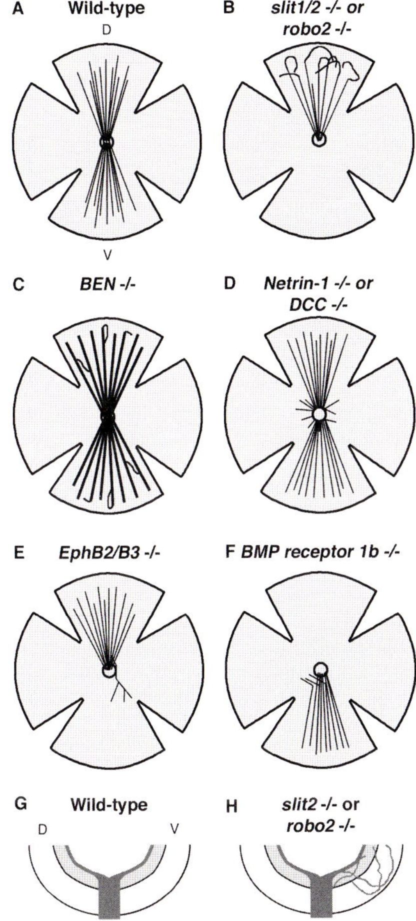

FIGURE 31.4 Diagrams illustrating the intraretinal pathfinding defects that occur in mice lacking specific signaling molecules or their receptors. Some molecules (e.g., BEN, netrin-1) are required for the guidance of RGC axons originating throughout the retina (*C* and *D*). Other factors function in a regionally restricted manner (*B* and *E–H*).

looping back to extend in the wrong direction (Weiner et al., 2004). Similar but more severe guidance errors are seen in the goldfish retina following inhibition of neurolin/BEN function (Ott et al., 1998).

One explanation for the relatively subtle defects observed following loss of BEN is compensation by other cell adhesion molecules. In rat retinas, the cell adhesion molecule L1 is expressed exclusively on developing neurons and is highly enriched in regions where actively extending RGC axons make contact with previously formed, more centrally located axons (Brittis and Silver, 1995). Blocking L1 function in cultured rat retinas results in loss of disc-directed growth, with many axons turning 90° and running parallel to the retinal circumference. Thus, L1-mediated contact with previously formed axons is an important factor controlling the overall direction of RGC axon outgrowth (Brittis et al., 1995).

Several other environmental factors also have been implicated in helping direct RGC axons toward the optic disc. In chick retinas a wave of sonic hedgehog (Shh) expression dissipates across the retina, the front of which lies central relative to newly differentiated RGCs (Kolpak et al., 2005). In addition to its well-characterized role in patterning, Shh can act directly on RGC axons to influence their rate and direction of outgrowth (Trousse et al., 2001). In vivo, blocking or overexpressing Shh has a striking effect on intraretinal pathfinding. The OFL becomes extremely disorganized and populated with axons that extend in random directions rather than directly toward the optic disc (Kolpak et al., 2005). Differentiation and patterning of the retina are normal following modulation of Shh signaling, suggesting these are primary guidance defects. Furthermore, since both gain and loss of Shh function induced essentially identical phenotypes (Kolpak et al., 2005), the precise level of Shh protein in the retina appears to be the critical factor underlying the directionality of RGC axon extension.

In vitro, Shh can function as a positive or negative regulator of RGC axon outgrowth, depending on its concentration (Kolpak et al., 2005). It has not been possible to determine the relative concentration of Shh in the developing retina. However, based on its expression profile and the level of Shh mRNA in the retina relative to that in other tissues, it appears likely that it acts as a positive factor in vivo. This suggests a model whereby a local gradient of Shh in the retina acts to promote growth in a central direction and, in combination with L1-mediated axon fasciculation and the growth-promoting properties of the neuroepithelial endfeet, controls the directed extension of RGC axons toward the optic disc.

The positive gradient of Shh in the chick retina is balanced as well by a negative gradient of guidance cues under the control of the zinc finger transcription factor Zic3 (Zhang et al., 2004). In the retina, Zic3 is expressed in a high peripheral-low central gradient, and in vitro it induces the expression of factors inhibitory to RGC axon outgrowth. Overexpression of Zic3 in the developing chick retina has no effect on general patterning but blocks RGC axon extension toward the optic disc (Zhang et al., 2004). The guidance cues regulated by Zic3 are enigmatic and are not factors known to regulate intraretinal pathfinding as netrins, Slits, or CSPGs do, indicating that many factors essential for intraretinal pathfinding remain to be determined. Whether Shh and Zic3 serve similar functions in the mouse retina also needs to be established.

Factors that act cell autonomously within RGCs to regulate intraretinal pathfinding have also been identified. The POU domain transcription factor Brn-3.2 (other names: Brn-3b, Pou4f2) is expressed by RGCs, and in mice lacking Brn-3.2, the fasciculation and guidance of RGC axons within the retina are impaired. The extent of RGC axon fasciculation is decreased substantially, and many axons adopt abnormal trajectories and fail to reach the optic disc (Erkman et al., 2000). This results in optic nerve hypoplasia and, ultimately, RGC death. Several downstream targets of Brn-3.2 have been identified, including ab-LIM, an actin-binding protein (Erkman et al., 2000). Blocking ab-LIM function in developing chick retinas results in axon guidance errors similar to those in Brn-3.2-deficient mice (Erkman et al., 2000), suggesting that ab-LIM is a component of the guidance program activated by Brn-3.2. Other genes linked to axon guidance are likely to be activated by Brn-3.2. Further work is required to determine the precise molecular cascade linking this transcription factor to changes in axon outgrowth.

Targeting of retinal ganglion cell axons to the optic disc, and exit from the eye

Once they reach the central retina, the next challenge faced by RGC axons is to locate and enter the optic disc. Oriented channels formed by neuroepithelial endfeet have been suggested to play a key role in directing this process (Silver and Sidman, 1980). Several guidance cues critical for targeting and entry into the optic disc also have been identified.

A major regulator of axon exit from the eye is netrin-1. Netrins are a family of secreted, laminin-related molecules that, acting via their DCC (deleted in colorectal carcinoma) and UNC5 receptors, function as bifunctional guidance cues that attract some axons while repelling others. Netrins can act either at short or long range, the extent of diffusion being regulated by interaction with the extracellular matrix (reviewed by Barallobre et al., 2005). In the developing mouse retina, netrin-1 is expressed specifically by the glial cells lining the optic fissure/disc, whereas DCC is present on RGC axons (Deiner et al., 1997). In netrin-1- or DCC-deficient mice, large numbers of RGC axons fail to exit the eye, resulting in optic nerve hypoplasia (Deiner et al., 1997; figure 31.4*D*). The axons grow normally toward the region of the optic disc but then, rather than exiting the eye, splay out and extend aberrantly into other regions of the retina. In the region of the disc, some axons also extend away from the OFL, through the thickness of the retina and along the ventricular surface. In vitro, netrin-1 acts as a positive regulator of RGC axon outgrowth (Wang et al., 1996; Deiner et al., 1997). Together with the tight localization of netrin-1 protein to the glial cells surrounding the optic disc and the phenotype of the netrin-1- and DCC-deficient mice, this suggests that netrin-1 acts locally to attract RGC axons to the optic disc and out of the eye (Deiner et al., 1997).

Since netrin-1 is a potent attractant for RGC axons, why do RGC axons not normally get stuck at the optic disc instead of entering the optic nerve? One explanation for this has come from studies in *Xenopus*. At the optic nerve head of the developing *Xenopus* retina, laminin-1, a component of the extracellular matrix, is confined to the retinal surface. In vitro, laminin-1 can convert netrin-1-mediated attraction to repulsion and, by adding exogenous laminin peptides in vivo, impairs RGC axon guidance into the optic nerve (Höpker et al., 1999). Thus, local modulation of netrin-1 function by other factors in the environment, such as laminin-1, may play a critical role in helping drive RGC axons out of the eye.

Several other factors also have been implicated in helping to guide RGC axons into the optic disc. Ephrins are a large family of receptor tyrosine kinases involved in regulating a number of different developmental processes, including the establishment of the topographic map formed by RGC axons in their targets (reviewed by Kullander and Klein, 2002). There are 13 ephrins in mammals, divided into A and B classes, based on their binding specificity for GPI-linked (ephrin-A) or transmembrane (ephrin-B) ligands. In addition to the classic kinase-dependent "forward" signaling mediated by ephrin receptors, these molecules also function in a kinase-independent fashion and act as ligands for ephrin-expressing cells (reviewed by Kullander and Klein, 2002). "Reverse" signaling from specific EphBs (EphB2 and EphB3) acting as guidance cues plays a role in the local targeting of RGC axons to the optic disc.

During early stages of development (E12.5–E14.5), when RGC axons are pathfinding to the optic disc, EphB2 and EphB3 are expressed uniformly along the dorsoventral axis of the mouse retina. EphB3 is restricted to the RGC layer, whereas EphB2 also is expressed in the outer retina (Birgbauer et al., 2000; Williams et al., 2003). Their binding partners, ephrin-Bs, also are expressed in the developing retina. In mice lacking EphB3 but not EphB2 alone, a small number of RGC axons make guidance errors in the region of the optic disc (figure 31.4*E*). As they approach the central retina, a small subset of RGC axons deviate away from their normal trajectory and bypass the optic disc, resulting in axons extending for variable distances into the opposite side of the retina (Birgbauer et al., 2000). These defects are similar to but occur much less frequently than those seen in the netrin-1- and DCC-deficient mice (Deiner et al., 1997). In double mutants lacking both EphB2 and EphB3, the incidence and the severity of guidance defects are increased substantially compared with what is seen in single mutants. Mice lacking EphB3 and the intracellular kinase domain of EphB2 show a similar level of targeting errors to EphB3 as single mutants do, suggesting that the extracellular domain of EphB2 is sufficient to mediate targeting to the optic disc and, in this instance, is functioning as a guidance cue rather than as a receptor (Birgbauer et al., 2000). In support of this conjecture, in vitro, the extracellular domains of EphBs function as inhibitory guidance factors for RGC axons (Birgbauer et al., 2001).

Bone morphogenic protein (BMP) receptor 1b also plays an important role in controlling the targeting of RGC axons to the optic disc. BMPs are members of the TGF-β family of signaling molecules known to play important roles during development, including eye formation. BMPs signal by binding to a complex formed from type I and type II receptors. On binding, the type II receptor activates the type I receptor, resulting in the phosphorylation of specific Smads that translocate into the nucleus and activate target genes. There are two type I receptors for BMPs, BMP receptor 1A (ALK3) and BMP receptor 1B (ALK6; Kawabata et al., 1998). In the developing mouse retina, both BMP receptor 1A and receptor 1B are strongly expressed in the outer neuroblastic layer, with much lower expression in the RGC layer. BMP receptor 1A is uniformly distributed, whereas BMP receptor 1B is expressed exclusively in the ventral retina (Liu et al., 2003). In mice lacking BMP receptor 1B, a subset of RGC axons originating in ventral retina make targeting errors in the region of the optic disc (Liu et al., 2003). These errors are similar in frequency and severity to those seen in EphB2/B3 knockout mice (Deiner et al., 1997; Birgbauer et al., 2000) and result in a small subset of axons failing to enter the optic disc and extending aberrantly into the opposite side of the retina (figure 31.4*F*). Since BMP receptor 1B is most strongly expressed in undifferentiated cells, it is unlikely this reflects a direct role for BMPs in directing RGC axon pathfinding (Augsberger et al., 1999). Additionally, although in the absence of BMP receptor 1B the overall patterning of the dorsoventral axis of the retina is normal, the expression of specific signaling molecules known to regulate intraretinal pathfinding (Brn-3.2, netrin-1; Erkman et al., 2000; Deiner et al., 1997) is decreased significantly. This suggests that a key function of BMP signaling in the retina is to control the expression of guidance cues such as netrin-1, critical for axon exit from the eye.

A number of other genes and signaling molecules also act indirectly to control the growth of RGC axons out of the eye. The *kidney and retinal defects* (*krd*) mouse has a deletion in chromosome 19 that includes the Pax2 locus. Pax2 is expressed normally by the glial cells of the optic disc and stalk, and in heterozygous *krd* mice many RGC axons fail to exit the optic disc (Otteson et al., 1998). Similar guidance defects are found in a subpopulation of anophthalmic mice (ZRDCT-AN) that develop microphthalmia (Silver et al., 1984), heterozygous *belly spot and tail* (*Bst*) mice (Rice et al., 1997), and conditional Shh mutants lacking Shh in RGCs (Dakubo et al., 2003). In all of these mice, the underlying defect is a failure in development or closure of the optic fissure, highlighting the importance of this structure for the normal guidance of RGC axons out of the eye.

Dorsal-ventral differences in the mechanisms that regulate intraretinal axon pathfinding

There is a considerable degree of diversity in the mechanisms regulating intraretinal pathfinding in the ventral and dorsal halves of the retina (see figure 31.4). In some instances this can be explained by selective expression of specific guidance cues in defined regions of the retina, in other cases the underlying cause is not so obvious.

BMP receptor 1B is expressed exclusively in the ventral part of the retina and, not unexpectedly, in mice lacking this molecule, guidance errors occur specifically in RGC axons originating in ventral retina (Liu et al., 2003). Similar guidance errors occur in EphB2/B3-deficient mice but are found more frequently from axons from dorsal retina (Birgbauer et al., 2000). This again can be explained by differential expression. From E15.5 on, EphB2 is expressed in a high ventral-low dorsal gradient (Birgbauer et al., 2000). Dorsal RGC axons growing toward the optic disc therefore encounter an increasing gradient of inhibitory EphB proteins that helps to prevent their extension away from the optic disc and into the ventral half of the retina. Thus, within dorsal and ventral retina, distinct families of signaling molecules are expressed differentially and function in parallel to help guide RGC axons out of the eye.

Other guidance cues act in a region-specific manner that cannot easily be explained on the basis of expression alone. Slit proteins are expressed throughout the dorsoventral axis of the developing mouse retina, and in vitro, both dorsal and ventral RGC axons respond similarly to Slits (Erskine et al., 2000; Thompson et al., 2006b). Despite this, Slits regulate distinct aspects of intraretinal pathfinding in dorsal and ventral retina (see figure 31.4). In ventral retina, Slit signaling helps restrict RGC axons to the OFL, whereas in dorsal retina it controls the initial polarity of RGC axon outgrowth. Region-specific differences, independent of differential expression, also are seen in the goldfish retinas following block of neurolin/BEN or the L1-like antigen, E587, function. Both molecules are expressed uniformly throughout the retina; however, following loss of function, RGC axon guidance defects occur exclusively in dorsal retina (Ott et al., 1998). The simplest explanation for the regional specificity of these guidance cues is that it reflects the action of other signaling molecules that act differentially within dorsal or ventral retina to compensate for their loss. These studies highlight the complexities of the mechanisms regulating intraretinal pathfinding and demonstrate that cooperative or redundant interactions between multiple coexpressed guidance cues are critical for the normal guidance of RGC axons toward the optic disc and out of the eye.

Why is there such disparity in the mechanisms regulating intraretinal pathfinding in dorsal and ventral retina? It is likely this reflects the different developmental histories of

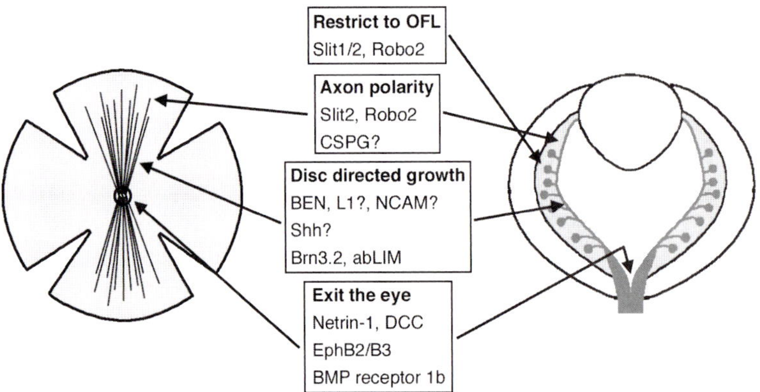

FIGURE 31.5 Summary of the signaling molecules known to be required for intraretinal axon guidance and their site of action. The ? symbol indicates molecules for which a role has been demonstrated in other species (chick, rat) but has not been established formally in the mouse. See the text for details.

these regions and later the role of specific signaling molecules in wiring the mature visual system. Differences across the dorsoventral axis of the retina are established early in development by the restricted expression of transcription factors and signaling molecules with distinct downstream targets. For example, the homeodomain transcription factor Vax2 is expressed exclusively within ventral retina, whereas Tbx5 is localized to dorsal retina (Barbieri et al., 1999; Sowden et al., 2001). Retinoid-metabolizing enzymes also are expressed differentially along the dorsoventral axis (Wagner et al., 2000). The developmental program underlying the patterning of the dorsal and ventral retina is therefore distinct from early stages, resulting in numerous differences between these regions. There are differences in the timing of RGC differentiation and in the rate of expansion of the dorsal and ventral OFL (Halfter et al., 1985). Many guidance cues are differentially expressed along the dorsoventral axis, most likely reflecting their later role in the establishment of functional topographic maps in visual targets.

There also are important functional differences. As a result of the position of the eyes in the head, the dorsal and ventral regions of the mature mouse retina respond to different parts of the visual world, and this is reflected in the distribution of the various classes of cone photoreceptors, a feature of retinal organization that is more striking in the mouse than in any other species (Szel et al., 1996). Thus, given the myriad differences between dorsal and ventral retina, it is perhaps not surprising that the repertoire of signaling molecules regulating intraretinal pathfinding in these disparate regions is distinct. Dorsal and ventral RGC axons also follow different trajectories as they navigate the optic chiasm and tract (Chan and Guillery, 1994), suggesting that the use of distinct guidance mechanisms to direct the outgrowth of dorsal and ventral RGC axons is a conserved feature of the entire optic pathway.

Conclusion

The cellular and molecular mechanisms that guide RGC axons in the retina, the first critical step in the formation of functional visual connections, are beginning to come into focus (figure 31.5). Because of its genetic tractability, the mouse as a study model has been instrumental in this process and has provided key insights into the genes and signaling molecules underlying intraretinal pathfinding. However, we have only begun to scratch the surface, and much work remains to be done to learn the full repertoire of signals critical for intraretinal axon pathfinding, as well as the upstream factors controlling their temporal and spatial expression. Another key challenge is to investigate the multiple redundant or cooperative interactions that occur between coexpressed signaling molecules and their relative importance in different regions of the retina. With the cloning of the genomes of many species, including the mouse, advances in understanding the molecular mechanisms regulating axon guidance are occurring rapidly. The ability to generate mouse strains lacking specific genes, combined with several large-scale mouse mutagenesis programs, means that mice will continue to play a pivotal role in this process. Much remains to be learned about the complex signaling mechanisms underlying this important early event in the establishment of functional neuronal connections in the developing visual system.

REFERENCES

AUGSBERGER, A., SCHUCHARDT, A., HOSKINS, S., DODD, J., and BUTLER, S. (1999). BMPs as mediators of roof plate repulsion of commissural neurons. *Neuron* 24:127–141.

BARALLOBRE, M. J., PASCUAL, M., DEL RIO, J. A., and SORIANO, E. (2005). The netrin family of guidance factors: Emphasis on Netrin-1 signalling. *Brain Res. Brain Res. Rev.* 49:22–47.

Barbieri, A. M., Lupo, G., Bulfone, A., Andreazzoli, M., Mariani, M., Fougerousse, F., Consalez, G. G., Borsani, G., Beckmann, J. S., et al. (1999). A homeobox gene, *vax2*, controls the patterning of the eye dorsoventral axis. *Proc. Natl. Acad. Sci. U.S.A.* 96:10729–10734.

Birgbauer, E., Cowan, C. A., Sretavan, D. W., and Henkemeyer, M. (2000). Kinase independent function of EphB receptors in retinal axon pathfinding to the optic disc from dorsal but not ventral retina. *Development* 127:1231–1241.

Birgbauer, E., Oster, S. F., Severin, C. G., and Sretavan, D. W. (2001). Retinal axon growth cones respond to EphB extracellular domain as inhibitory guidance cues. *Development* 128:3041–3048.

Brittis, P. A., Canning, D. R., and Silver, J. (1992). Chondroitin sulfate as a regulator of neuronal patterning in the retina. *Science* 255, 733–736.

Brittis, P. A., Lemmon, V., Rutishauser, U., and Silver, J. (1995). Unique changes of ganglion cell growth cone behaviour following cell adhesion molecule perturbations: A time-lapse study of the living retina. *Mol. Cell. Neurosci.* 6:333–339.

Brittis, P. A., and Silver, J. (1994). Exogenous glycosaminoglycans induce complete inversion of retinal ganglion cell bodies and their axons within the retinal neuroepithelium. *Proc. Natl. Acad. Sci. U.S.A.* 91:7539–7542.

Brittis, P. A., and Silver, J. (1995). Multiple factors govern intraretinal axon guidance: A time-lapse study. *Mol. Cell. Neurosci.* 6:413–432.

Chalasani, S. H., Baribaud, F., Coughlan, C. M., Sunshine, M. J., Lee, V. M., Doms, R. W., Littman, D. R., and Raper, J. A. (2003a). The chemokine stromal cell-derived factor-1 promotes the survival of embryonic retinal ganglion cells. *J. Neurosci.* 23:4601–4612.

Chalasani, S. H., Sabelko, K. A., Sunshine, M. J., Littman, D. R., and Raper, J. A. (2003b). A chemokine, SDF-1, reduces the effectiveness of multiple axonal repellents and is required for normal axon pathfinding. *J. Neurosci.* 23:1360–1371.

Chan, S. O., and Guillery, R. W. (1994). Changes in fiber order in the optic nerve and tract of rat embryos. *J. Comp. Neurol.* 344:20–32.

Dakubo, G. D., Wang, Y. P., Mazerolle, C., Campbell, K., McMahon, A. P., and Wallace, V. A. (2003). Retinal ganglion cell-derived sonic hedgehog signaling is required for optic disc and stalk neuroepithelial cell development. *Development* 130: 2967–2980.

Deiner, M. S., Kennedy, T. E., Fazeli, A., Serafini, T., Tessier-Lavigne, M., and Sretavan, D. W. (1997). Netrin-1 and DCC mediate axon guidance locally at the optic disc: Loss of function leads to optic nerve hypoplasia. *Neuron* 19:575–589.

Dickson, B. J. (2002). Molecular mechanisms of axon guidance. *Science* 298:1959–1964.

Dräger, U. C. (1985). Birth dates of retinal ganglion cells giving rise to the crossed and uncrossed optic projections in the mouse. *Proc. R. Soc. Lond. B. Biol. Sci.* 224:57–77.

Erkman, L., Yates, P. A., McLaughlin, T., McEvilly, R. J., Whisenhunt, T., O'Connell, S. M., Krones, A. I., Kirby, M. A., Rapaport, D. H., et al. (2000). A POU domain transcription factor-dependent program regulates axon pathfinding in the vertebrate visual system. *Neuron* 28:779–792.

Erskine, L., Williams, S. E., Brose, K., Kidd, T., Rachel, R. A., Goodman, C. S., Tessier-Lavigne, M., and Mason, C. A. (2000). Retinal ganglion cell axon guidance in the mouse optic chiasm: Expression and function of Robos and Slits. *J. Neurosci.* 20:4975–4982.

Goldberg, S. (1977). Unidirectional, bidirectional and random growth of embryonic optic axons. *Exp. Eye Res.* 25:399–404.

Halfter, W. (1996). Intraretinal grafting reveals growth requirements and guidance cues for optic axons in the developing avian retina. *Dev. Biol.* 177:160–177.

Halfter, W., Deiss, S., and Schwarz, U. (1985). The formation of the axonal pattern in the embryonic avian retina. *J. Comp. Neurol.* 232:466–480.

Hinds, J. W., and Hinds, P. L. (1974). Early ganglion cell differentiation in the mouse retina: An electron microscopic analysis utilizing serial sections. *Dev. Biol.* 37:381–416.

Höpker, V. H., Shewan, D., Tessier-Lavigne, M., Poo, M. M., and Holt, C. (1999). Growth cone attraction to netrin-1 is converted to repulsion by laminin-1. *Nature* 401:69–73.

Hu, H. (2001). Cell-surface heparan sulfate is involved in the repulsive guidance activities of Slit2 protein. *Nat. Neurosci.* 4: 695–701.

Inatani, M., Irie, F., Plump, A. S., Tessier-Levigne, M., and Yamaguchi, Y. (2003). Mammalian brain morphogenesis and midline axon guidance require heparan sulfate. *Science* 302: 1044–1046.

Jin, Z., Zhang, J., Klar, A., Chédotal, A., Rao, Y., Cepko, C. L., and Bao, Z. Z. (2003). Irx4-mediated regulation of Slit1 expression contributes to the definition of early axonal paths inside the retina. *Development* 130:1037–1048.

Kantor, D. B., Chivatakarn, O., Peer, K. L., Oster, S. F., Inatani, M., Hansen, M. J., Flanagan, J. G., Yamaguchi, Y., Sretavan, D. W., et al. (2004). Semaphroin 5A is a bifunctional axon guidance cue regulated by heparan and chondroitin sulfate proteoglycans. *Neuron* 44:961–975.

Kawabata, M., Imamura, T., and Miyazono, K. (1998). Signal transduction by bone morphogenetic proteins. *Cytokine Growth Factor Rev.* 9:49–61.

Kolpak, A., Zhang, J., and Bao, Z. Z. (2005). Sonic hedgehog has a dual effect on the growth of retinal ganglion axons depending on its concentration. *J. Neurosci.* 25:3432–3441.

Kullander, K., and Klein, R. (2002). Mechanisms and function of Eph and ephrin signalling. *Nat. Rev. Mol. Cell Biol.* 3:475–486.

Liu, J., Wilson, S., and Reh, T. (2003). BMP receptor 1b is required for axon guidance and cell survival in the developing retina. *Dev. Biol.* 256:34–47.

Nguyen-Ba-Charvet, K. T., and Chédotal, A. (2002). Role of Slit proteins in the vertebrate brain. *J. Physiol. Paris* 96:91–98.

Ohta, K., Tannahill, D., Yoshida, K., Johnson, A. R., Cook, G. M. W., and Keynes, R. J. (1999). Embryonic lens repels retinal ganglion cell axons. *Dev. Biol.* 211:124–132.

Ott, H., Bastmeyer, M., and Stuermer, C. A. O. (1998). Neurolin, the goldfish homolog of DM-GRASP, is involved in retinal axon pathfinding to the optic disk. *J. Neurosci.* 18:3363–3372.

Otteson, D. C., Sheldon, E., Jones, J. M., Kameoka, J., and Hitchcock, P. F. (1998). Pax2 expression and retinal morphogenesis in the normal and *Krd* mouse. *Dev. Biol.* 193:209–224.

Plump, A. S., Erskine, L., Sabatier, C., Brose, K., Epstein, C. J., Goodman, C. S., Mason, C. A., and Tessier-Lavigne, M. (2002). Slit1 and Slit2 cooperate to prevent premature midline crossing of retinal axons in the mouse visual system. *Neuron* 33:219–232.

Rice, D. S., Tang, Q., Williams, R. W., Harris, B. S., Davisson, M. T., and Goldowitz, D. (1997). Decreased retinal ganglion cell number and misdirected axon growth associated with fissure defects in *Bst/+* mutant mice. *Invest. Ophthalmol. Vis. Sci.* 38:2112–2124.

Silver, J., Puck, S. M., and Albert, D. M. (1984). Development and aging of the eye in mice with inherited optic nerve aplasia: Histopathological studies. *Exp. Eye Res.* 38:257–266.

Silver, J., and Sapiro, J. (1981). Axonal guidance during development of the optic nerve: The role of pigmented epithelia and other extrinsic factors. *J. Comp. Neurol.* 202:521–538.

Silver, J., and Sidman, R. L. (1980). A mechanism for the guidance and topographic patterning of retinal ganglion cell axons. *J. Comp. Neurol.* 189:101–111.

Sowden, J. C., Holt, J. K., Meins, M., Smith, H. K., and Bhattacharya, S. S. (2001). Expression of *Drosophila* omb-related T-box genes in the developing human and mouse neural retina. *Invest. Ophthalmol. Vis. Sci.* 42:3095–3102.

Stier, H., and Schlosshauer, B. (1995). Axonal guidance in the chicken retina. *Development* 121:1443–1454.

Stier, H., and Schlosshauer, B. (1998). Different cell surface areas of polarized radial glia having opposite effects on axonal outgrowth. *Eur. J. Neurosci.* 10:1000–1010.

Szel, A., Rohlich, P., Caffe, A. R., and van Veen, T. (1996). Distribution of cone photoreceptors in the mammalian retina. *Microsc. Res. Tech.* 35:445–462.

Thompson, H., Andrews, B., Parnavelas, J., and Erskine, L. (2008). [Robo2 but not Robol is required for intraretinal axon pathfinding.] Unpublished results.

Thompson, H., Barker, D., Camand, O., and Erskine, L. (2006a). Slits contribute to the guidance of retinal ganglion cell axons in the mammalian optic tract. *Dev. Biol.* 296:476–484.

Thompson, H., Camand, O., Barker, D., and Erskine, L. (2006b). Slit proteins regulate distinct aspects of retinal ganglion cell axon guidance within dorsal and ventral retina. *J. Neurosci.* 26: 8082–8091.

Trousse, F., Marti, E., Gross, P., Torres, M., and Bivalent, P. (2001). Control of retinal ganglion cell axon growth: A new role for Sonic hedgehog. *Development* 128:3927–3936.

Wagner, E., McCaughey, P., and Dräger, U. C. (2000). Retinoic acid in the formation of the dorsoventral retina and its central projections. *Dev. Biol.* 222:460–470.

Wang, L. C., Rachel, R. A., Marcus, R. C., and Mason, C. A. (1996). Chemo suppression of retinal axon growth by the mouse optic chiasm. *Neuron* 17:849–862.

Weiner, J. A., Koop, S. J., Nicolas, S., Faribault, S., Pfaff, S. L., Pursue, O., and Sans, J. R. (2004). Axon fasciculation defects and retinal dysphasia in mice lacking the immunoglobulin super family adhesion molecule BEN/ALCAM/SC1. *Mol. Cell. Neurosci.* 27:59–69.

Williams, S. E., Mann, F., Erskine, L., Sakurai, T., Wei, S., Rossi, D. J., Gale, N. W., Holt, C. E., Mason, C. A., et al. (2003). Ephrin-B2 and EphB1 mediate retinal axon divergence at the optic chiasm. *Neuron* 39:919–935.

Zhang, J., Jin, Z., and Bao, Z. Z. (2004). Disruption of gradient expression of Zic3 resulted in abnormal intraretinal axon projection. *Development* 131:1553–1562.

32 Early Development of the Optic Stalk, Chiasm, and Astrocytes

TIMOTHY J. PETROS AND CAROL A. MASON

Visual information is conveyed from the retina to higher brain regions by retinal ganglion cells (RGCs), the only output from the retina. RGCs project toward the ventral diencephalon, where fibers from both retinas converge to form the X-shaped optic chiasm. RGC divergence at the chiasm establishes a binocular projection, which is essential for information from one point of visual space to be observed by both retinas yet converge at the same loci in higher visual areas. Throughout the animal kingdom, the extent of RGC divergence closely correlates with the degree of binocular vision. Uncrossed RGC axons always arise from the temporal portion of the retina, whereas crossed RGC axons always arise from nasal retina. In humans, a highly binocular species, about 40% of all RGC axons project ipsilaterally, whereas this percentage drops to around 15% in ferrets. In most birds and fishes, uncrossed projections are absent because the lateral location of their eyes does not allow for any overlap in visual space.

Mice are a poor binocular species, with a very small population of uncrossed RGC fibers (ca. 3%–5%, depending on the strain of mice). These uncrossed axons arise from the peripheral ventrotemporal (VT) crescent. Despite the small number of uncrossed axons, the murine retina is an excellent model for developmental studies (Guillery et al., 1995). Over the past three decades, research on the mouse, in conjunction with work on fish, frog, and chick models, has uncovered molecules that pattern the retina and guide RGC axons through the visual pathway to their final destination. Moreover, in vitro and in vivo assays utilizing the murine visual system have been successfully combined with genetic approaches to study the molecular mechanisms guiding retinal divergence at the optic chiasm.

In this chapter, we examine the development of RGC projections from the retina through the optic tract. First, we review the development of ipsilaterally and contralaterally projecting RGCs during the early, middle, and late period of growth. Next we emphasize the cells, guidance cues, and regulatory genes that direct RGC projections throughout the visual pathway. We then discuss differences between mechanisms guiding uncrossed versus crossed projections by focusing on recent studies that have uncovered molecular mechanisms important for axon divergence at the chiasm. Throughout, we highlight perturbations of molecular expression in the retina that alter the proportion of crossed to uncrossed fibers. These perturbations are of special interest in albino mutants, a unique case in which both the proportion of ipsilateral projections and the line of decussation (the border in the temporal retina demarcating the ipsilaterally projecting RGCs) are altered. The work reviewed in this chapter highlights the mouse visual system as an excellent model for understanding the development of retinal projections.

Development of retinal ganglion cell projections: Early, middle, and late stages

In the murine retina, RGCs differentiate shortly after optic fissure closure, around embryonic day 11 (E11), and continue to differentiate until about P0. RGC differentiation occurs in a central to peripheral gradient, such that the youngest RGCs are added in the peripheral retina. RGC projections can be divided into three phases, with each phase displaying different trajectories at the optic chiasm.

Early Phase The earliest-born RGCs are located in the dorsocentral (DC) retina and are referred to as "pioneer axons" because they are thought to help establish the projection pathways of later-born RGC axons. The DC fibers enter the ventral diencephalon at E12–E13, where they give rise to both crossed and uncrossed projections (Colello and Guillery, 1990; Marcus et al., 1995). The crossing fibers project through the radial glia palisade and follow the contour of a population of early-born chiasm neurons, which forms an inverted V-shaped array at the posterior boundary of the future X-shaped optic chiasm (figure 32.1*A*). During this early phase, uncrossed axons do not approach the midline glial palisade and instead project directly into the ipsilateral optic tract upon entering the ventral diencephalon. The pioneering ipsilateral projections from DC retina are transient, but whether the cells die or migrate to the VT retina, the site of mature ipsilateral projections, remains unknown.

Middle Phase RGC projections continue to enter the ventral diencephalon from E14.5 to E16.5, the peak phase

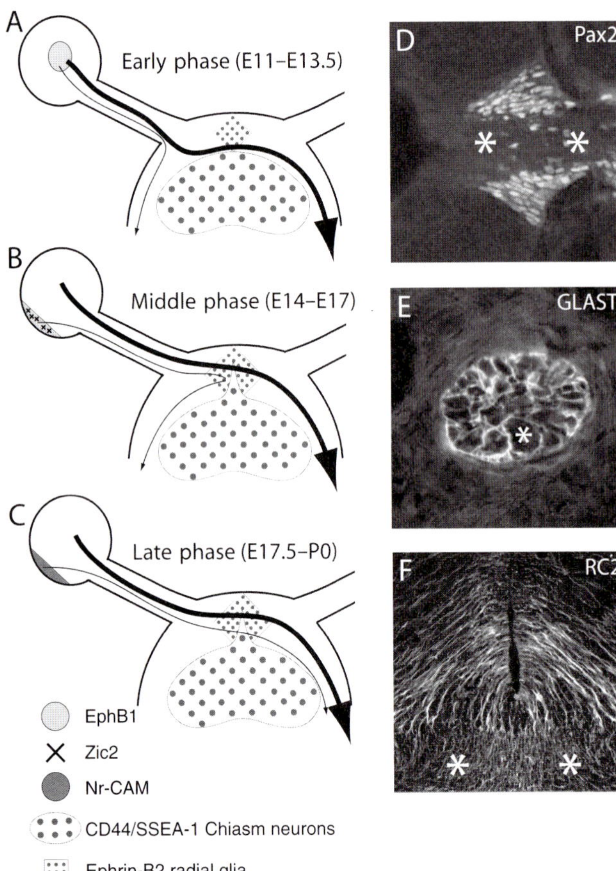

FIGURE 32.1 The three phases of RGC projections, and cell populations encountered by RGC axons. *A*, During the early phase of RGC axonogenesis, crossed projections (EphB1$^-$) and transient uncrossed projections (EphB1$^+$) arise from the dorsocentral retina. The uncrossed fibers do not interact with the midline radial glia, instead projecting directly into the ipsilateral optic tract, while the crossed projections follow the border of the early-born chiasm neurons. *B*, EphB1 and Zic2 are upregulated in the VT crescent during the middle phase, giving rise to the uncrossed RGC projections found in the adult. *C*, At later ages, RGC projections from VT retina cross the chiasm, concurrent with Nr-CAM upregulation in the VT crescent. *D*, Coronal section through optic disc immunostained for Pax2 highlights the optic disc astrocyte precursor (ODAPs) population surrounding RGC axons exiting the retina (Courtesy of T. Petros and C. Mason.) *E*, Interfascicular glia are clearly visible surrounding axon bundles in this transverse section through the optic nerve, as visualized with GLAST immunostaining (Courtesy of T. Petros.) *F*, RC2$^+$ processes of midline radial glia extend from the base of the third ventricle to the pial surface of the ventral diencephalon, directly through the pathway of RGC projections (Courtesy of S. Williams.) *White asterisks* indicate location of RGC axons.

of RGC outgrowth. RGC axons arising from non-VT retina project through the optic chiasm into the contralateral optic tract. Unlike in the early phase, uncrossed RGC fibers arise from the peripheral VT crescent and enter the glial palisade near the midline (figure 32.1*B*). Time-lapse imaging of DiI-filled RGCs demonstrates that growth cones from VT retina pause, often for hours, and undergo dynamic extension and retraction before making a U-turn back into the ipsilateral optic tract. Although growth cones from non-VT RGCs also pause before crossing, they do not display such extensive exploratory behavior (Godement et al., 1994; Mason and Wang, 1997).

LATE PHASE Crossed RGC projections arise from the expanding peripheral retina until birth (E19), and their projections follow earlier-born RGC axons into the contralateral optic tract. During this late phase (E17–P0) of RGC development, the vast majority of newly born VT RGCs project contralaterally rather than ipsilaterally (Dräger, 1985) (figure 32.1*C*). This temporal change in projection pattern mimics the late development of the cat retina (Reese et al., 1991), in which early-born temporal RGCs project ipsilaterally and later-born temporal axons project contralaterally, implying a conserved evolutionary mechanism.

Glia in the retinal ganglion cell axon projection pathway

OPTIC DISC ASTROCYTE PRECURSOR CELLS The majority of RGC projections exit the retina before a glial network develops. However, optic disc astrocyte precursor cells (ODAPs) are a specialized population of Pax2$^+$ astrocyte precursor cells (APCs) that encircle RGC axons as they exit the retina (figure 32.1*D*). ODAPs give rise to astrocytes that migrate into the retina at later ages and populate the RGC fiber layer (Watanabe and Raff, 1988; Dakubo et al., 2003; Petros et al., 2006). Mice lacking ODAPs display hypoplasia and severe RGC projection errors in the retina (Dakubo et al., 2003), demonstrating the importance of these cells in guiding RGCs out of the retina.

ASTROCYTE PROGENITORS/ASTROCYTES IN OPTIC NERVE Upon entering the optic nerve, RGC axons fasciculate and form bundles as they project toward the ventral diencephalon. These bundles are ensheathed by interfascicular glia (Colello and Guillery, 1992), which are most likely APCs that give rise to the astrocytes that populate the mature optic nerve (figure 32.1*E*). The molecular mechanisms by which these interfascicular glia organize and guide RGC axons toward the optic chiasm are unknown. Around E18, specialized astrocytes at the optic nerve head form a tight meshwork that appears to act as a barrier to oligodendrocytes migrating toward the retina (similar to the lamina cribrosa in other species). Although these specialized glia become reactive in retinal diseases such as glaucoma (reviewed in Hernandez, 2000), their role in the development of RGC projections has not been addressed.

MIDLINE RADIAL GLIA The organization of RGC axon bundles ensheathed by interfascicular glia changes at the optic nerve–chiasm junction, at which point interfascicular glia are no longer observed. Instead, radial glia cell bodies line the base of the third ventricle and extend dense processes from the ventricular zone to the pial surface of the ventral diencephalon on either side of the midline (reviewed in Mason and Sretavan, 1997; figure 32.1*F*). These radial glia cells express proteins common to immature radial glia such as RC2 (specific to mouse radial glia), brain lipid-binding protein (BLBP), and the glutamate transporter GLAST (Williams et al., 2003). DiI labeling reveals that newly arrived RGC growth cones dive toward the pial surface and extend along the endfeet of the radial glia (Colello and Coleman, 1997; Chung et al., 2008). As RGC axons enter this palisade of glial processes, they segregate into crossed and uncrossed components (Marcus et al., 1995). Crossing axons traverse the midline midway along the radial glial processes, whereas uncrossed axons make their turn above the pial endfeet (Chung et al., 2008). Axon outgrowth from VT but not DT explants is substantially decreased when grown on dissociated chiasm midline cells (Wang et al., 1995), making these radial glia cells of primary interest for studying molecular mechanisms of axon divergence.

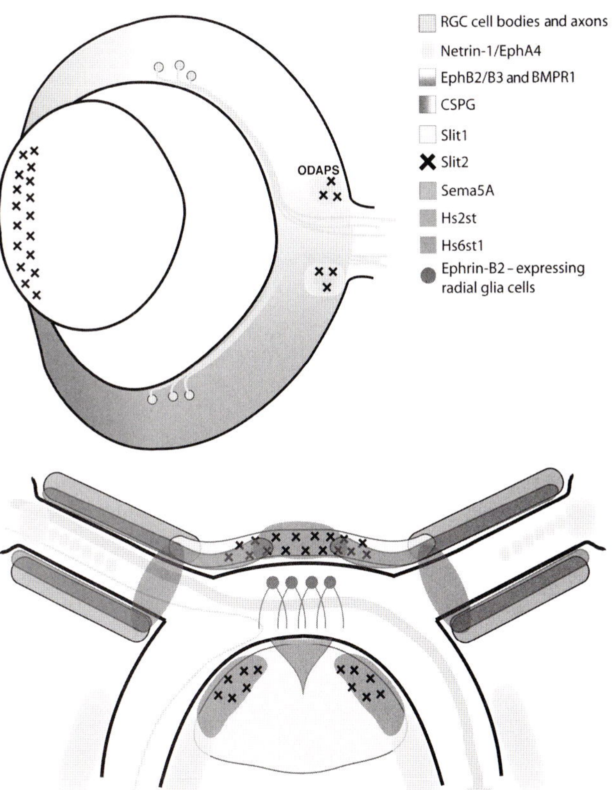

Figure 32.2 Cues that guide RGC axons through the visual pathway. *Top*, RGC axons (blue) express many receptors for a number of cues in the retina that guide them toward the optic disc and out of the retina. *Bottom*, A variety of cues surrounding the optic nerve, chiasm, and tract help to funnel RGC axons properly through the ventral diencephalon toward their final targets, the LGN and SC. ODAPs, optic disc astrocyte precursor cells. See color plate 21.

Guidance cues and their role in retinal ganglion cell axon navigation through the visual pathway

In the past decade, the identification of guidance factors in numerous species and systems has led to characterization of their role in the mouse retinal axon pathway (reviewed in Williams et al., 2004; figure 32.2). In this section, the discussion is limited to cues that are important for general RGC growth through the chiasm but that do not influence divergence at the chiasm. As detailed in the next several sections, studies of these guidance factors have relied on analysis of mutant mice, leading to several characteristic phenotypes such as axon stalling, projection errors, and axon defasciculation (figure 32.3).

Exiting the Retina In the retina, RGC growth cones must correctly integrate many guidance cues to properly orient toward the optic disc, where they turn 90° and enter the optic nerve. Chondroitin sulfate proteoglycans expressed in a high peripheral-low central gradient are required for orienting RGC axons toward the optic disc and away from the peripheral retina (Brittis et al., 1992). Both the BMP-1B receptor and EphB2/B3 receptors are expressed in a high ventral-low dorsal gradient. It is interesting that RGC axons from ventral retina make projection errors at the optic disc in *Bmpr1b*$^{-/-}$ mice (Liu et al., 2003), whereas *EphB2/B3*$^{-/-}$ display guidance errors from dorsal retina (Birgbauer et al., 2000). Two members of the immunoglobulin gene family, L1 and NCAM, are highly expressed on RGC axons, and perturbation of these molecules causes RGC growth cones to misproject or stall in the retina (Brittis et al., 1995). ODAPs express several molecules that potentially interact with RGC axons at the optic disc, such as netrin-1 (Deiner et al., 1997), EphA4 (Petros et al., 2006), and Slit2 (Erskine et al., 2000). Whereas netrin-1 is clearly required for RGC axons to properly exit the retina (Deiner et al., 1997), the role of EphA4, Slit2, and other unidentified guidance cues in ODAPs remains unknown. Recently it has been demonstrated that the repulsive action of *Slit1/2* expressed by the lens is important for several aspects of intraretinal RGC projections via interaction with roundabout (Robo) receptors on RGC axons (Thompson et al., 2006b).

Projecting through the Optic Nerve Once the RGC axons exit the retina, less is known about cues that guide projections through the optic nerve. Sema5A is expressed by neuroepithelial cells surrounding the optic nerve, and blocking Sema5A signaling leads to RGC axons straying out of the optic nerve (Oster et al., 2003; figure 32.3*B*). RGC axons project through the interfascicular glia/APCs that express several guidance cues, such as EphA4 (Petros et al., 2006) and netrin-1 (Deiner et al., 1997), but it is unclear how these cues support RGC axon extension through the optic nerve.

Shaping the Chiasm RGC axons are guided toward the optic chiasm by cues expressed by the ventral diencephalic cells. Netrin-1, expressed by cells caudal to the chiasm, is required for RGC axons to enter the optic chiasm at the proper angle (Deiner and Sretavan, 1999; figure 32.3*C*). *Slit1* is expressed by cells anterior to the chiasm, channeling RGC axons toward the chiasm midline (Plump et al., 2002). *Slit2* is strongly expressed directly dorsal and anterior to the proximal optic chiasm and is inhibitory to RGC axons (Erskine et al., 2000). Although *Slit1* and *Slit2* single-knockout mice display relatively normal phenotypes, *Slit1/2* double mutants display an ectopic chiasm just anterior to the normal chiasm (through the normally *Slit2*$^+$ region) and a subset of RGC axons misproject just lateral to the optic nerve–chiasm junction (through the normally *Slit1*$^+$ regions) (Plump et al., 2002; figure 32.3*D*). Thus, *Slit1/2* act as repulsive cues funneling Robo$^+$ RGC axons toward the chiasm midline and optic tracts. Of note, RGC axons in mice lacking Mena, an actin regulatory protein expressed in RGC growth cones,

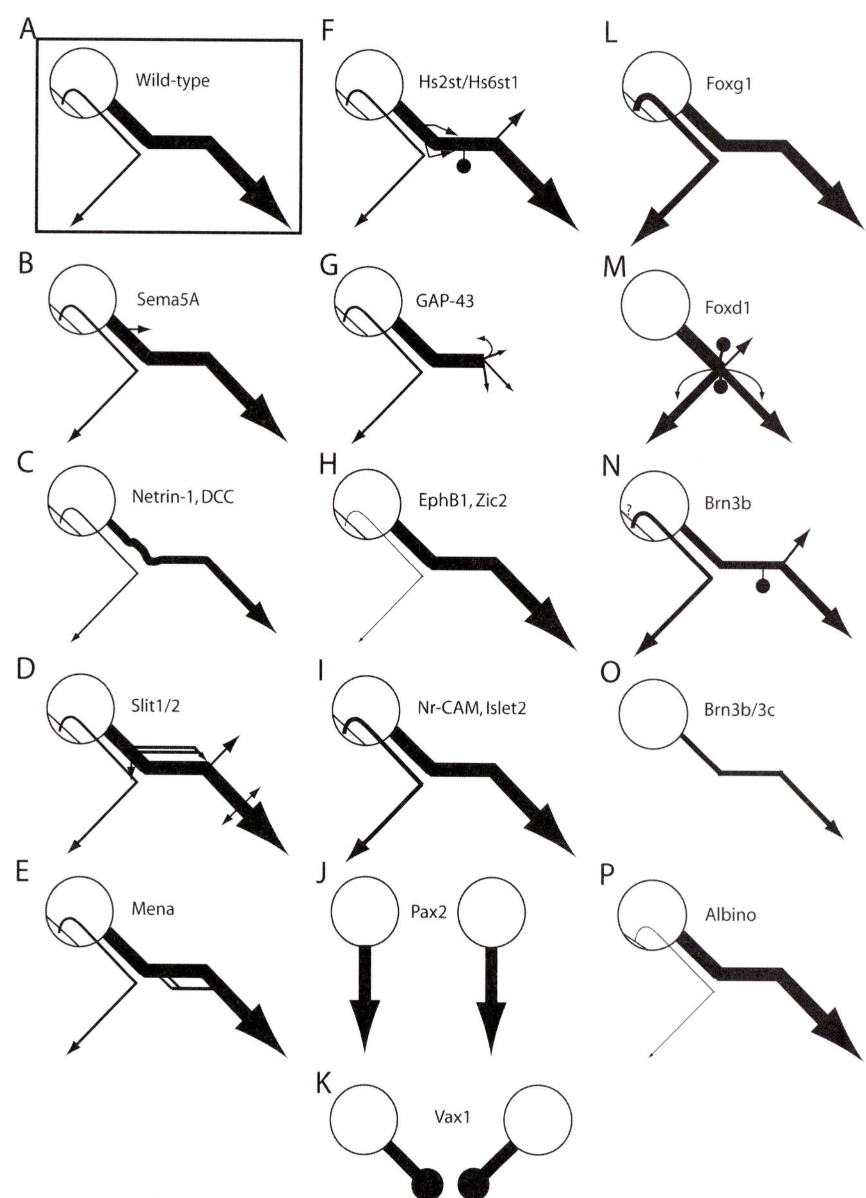

Figure 32.3 Defects in RGC projections observed in mutant mice. *A*, The normal projection pattern observed in WT mice. *B–P*, RGC misprojections observed in mutant mice. (See the text for details.)

defasciculate at the chiasm and form an ectopic posterior chiasm, similar to the ectopic anterior chiasm observed in *Slit1/2*$^{-/-}$ mice (Menzies et al., 2004; figure 32.3*E*); however, the role of Mena in this signaling pathway is not understood.

An enzyme involved in the addition of sulfates to heparan sulfate (HS) sugars (Hs2st) is expressed just posterior to the optic chiasm midline, and RGC projections in *Hs2st*$^{-/-}$ mice wander posterior to the chiasm midline (Pratt et al., 2006; figure 32.3*F*). *Hs6st1* is expressed directly anterior and posterior to the optic chiasm, mimicking *Slit1/2* expression patterns (Pratt et al., 2006), and *Hs6st1*$^{-/-}$ RGCs are less sensitive to Slit2 repulsion.

Optic Tract GAP-43 is an integral membrane bound protein that is highly expressed by developing neurons during axon growth. In *GAP-43*$^{-/-}$ mice, RGC axons appear to reach the chiasm normally, but they stall at the chiasm, and their projections into the optic tract are grossly perturbed (Strittmatter et al., 1995; figure 32.3*G*). Subsequent studies found that GAP-43 is required in RGC axons for mediating interactions with unknown guidance cues at the chiasm–optic tract junction, as *GAP-43*$^{-/-}$ axons display decreased outgrowth on lateral diencephalon cell membranes (Zhang et al., 2000). Whereas *GAP-43* is required at the chiasm–optic tract junction, *Slit1* and *Slit2* appear to be required in more dorsal segments of the optic tract (see figure 32.3*D*). In *Slit1*$^{-/-}$ and *Slit1/2*$^{-/-}$ mice, aberrant branches of RGC axons project into the telencephalon at several points along the optic tract (Thompson et al., 2006a).

These findings highlight the fact that RGC growth cones must integrate a wide variety of attractive and repulsive cues to properly navigate from the retina through the chiasm and into the optic tracts (summarized in figure 32.2). This analysis does not include the primary termination sites of RGC projections, the lateral geniculate nucleus (LGN) and superior colliculus (SC), where many guidance cues play an important role in establishing retinotopic organization and eye-specific projections (reviewed in this volume; see chapters 28, 31, and 34.)

Axon-axon interactions, which likely play a major role in guiding axons through the visual pathway, should be mentioned even though the molecular bases of these interactions are not understood. Fasciculation and bundling are important for neighbor-neighbor interactions, while defasciculation may play a role in reorganizing axons, as occurs before and after traversing the midline (Chan and Chung, 1999). Axon-axon interactions are quite challenging to analyze both in vitro and in vivo, largely because the molecules most often implicated in axon-axon signaling are cell adhesion molecules (CAMs), a large family whose members can function through homophilic and heterophilic interactions. Since many cells express several members of this family, the function of one member may be compensated for by other members, thus masking a functional role for certain CAMs in RGC guidance. For example, CAM family members L1, neurofascin, contactin, TAG-1 and NB-2 are all expressed in similar (though not identical) patterns in RGCs during development (Williams et al., 2006). Characterizing the molecular components involved in RGC axon-axon interactions for extension through the visual pathway and possibly for regulating divergence at the chiasm remains a major issue for understanding the development of RGC projections.

Molecules important for axon divergence at the chiasm: The uncrossed projection

Over the past several years, substantial progress has been made toward understanding the development of the uncrossed pathway. Initial identification of molecular cues that guide RGC axon divergence at the optic chiasm came from *Xenopus*. Ephrin-B expression was detected at the *Xenopus* optic chiasm when ipsilateral projections develop during metamorphosis, but it is absent at earlier stages when all RGCs project contralaterally. Ectopic expression of ephrinBs at the midline leads to a precocious ipsilateral projection (Nakagawa et al., 2000). These findings in *Xenopus* were extended to the developing visual projections in mice.

Ephrin-B1/ephrin-B2 A screen of Eph receptors and ephrins in the retina and ventral diencephalon identified two candidates for guiding ipsilateral projections (figure 32.4*A*). Ephrin-B2 expression in the chiasm region is first observed at E13 in radial glia cells at the chiasm midline, and expression remains high until E16, after which it is downregulated (Williams et al., 2003; figure 32.4*A*). This temporal expression pattern correlates precisely with the generation of mature ipsilateral projections (E13.5–E16.5). Perturbation of ephrin-B2 leads to a decrease in the number of ipsilateral projections, further supporting a role for ephrin-B2 as an important midline repulsive cue for uncrossed RGC axons (Williams et al., 2003).

In the retina, EphB1 is the only Eph receptor specifically expressed in VT crescent RGCs from E13.5 to E16 (Williams et al., 2003; figure 32.4*A*). From E12.5 to E14, EphB1 is also expressed in the DC retina, the source of the transient early-born uncrossed RGC projections. However, DC projections do not approach ephrin-B2-expressing radial glia cells at the chiasm midline, and thus the function of EphB1 in these early-born RGCs remains unknown. *EphB1*$^{-/-}$ mice display a significant reduction in ipsilateral RGC projections (see figures 32.3*H* and 32.4*A*), and perturbations of EphB1 in vitro causes chiasm cells to be less repulsive to VT axons (Williams et al., 2003). Although *EphB2* and *EphB3* are

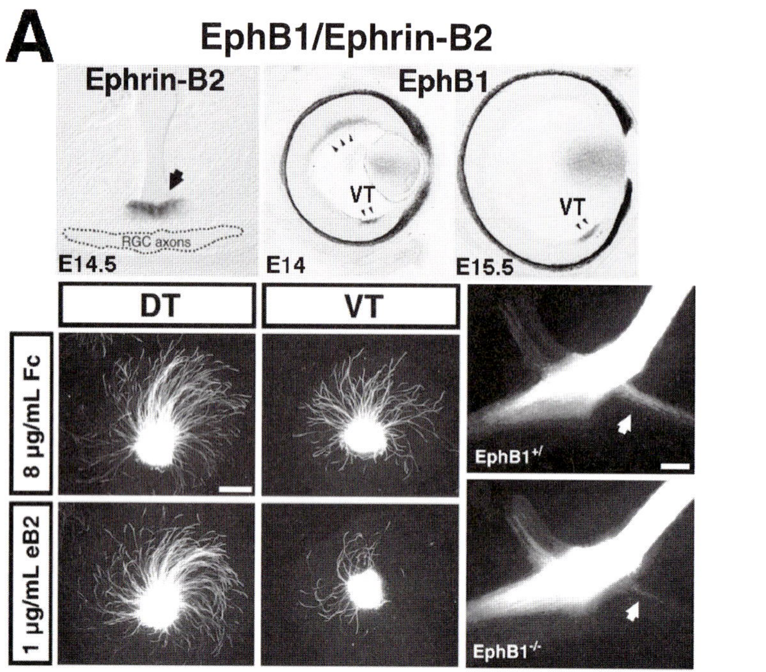

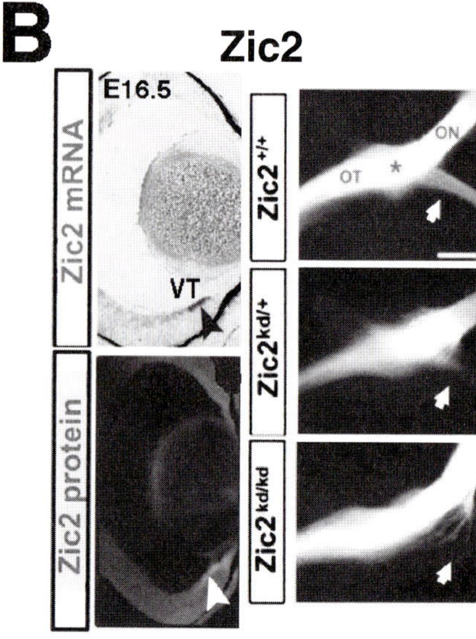

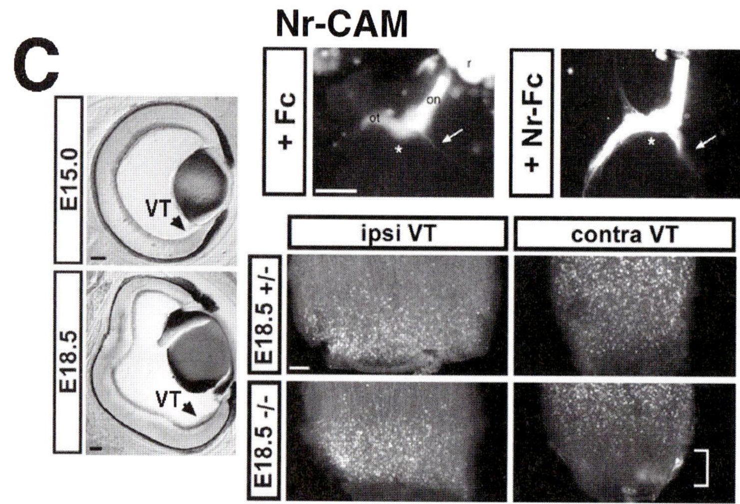

FIGURE 32.4 Cues that guide RGC projections from the VT crescent. *A*, *Top*, In situ hybridizations highlighting *ephrin-B2* expression at the chiasm and *EphB1* in DC and VT retina at E14, but restricted to VT retina by E15.5. *Bottom left and center*, Retinal explant cultures from VT retina display decreased axon outgrowth when grown on ephrin-B2 substrates compared to DT explants, an effect not observed with high concentrations of Fc. *Bottom right*, Whole-retina DiI fills reveal a significant decrease in uncrossed projections in *EphB1*$^{-/-}$ mice compared to wild-type or *EphB1*$^{+/-}$ mice. (Reprinted from Williams et al. [2003]. Ephrin-B2 and EphB1 mediate retinal axon divergence at the optic chiasm. *Neuron* 39:919–935, copyright 2003, with permission from Elsevier.) *B*, *Left*, Sections through E16.5 retina reveal Zic2 mRNA and protein specifically expressed in VT retina. *Right*, Whole-retina DiI fills demonstrate a significant decrease in uncrossed projections in *Zic2*$^{kd/+}$ mice that is further enhanced in *Zic2*$^{kd/kd}$ mice (Reprinted from Herrera et al. [2003]. Zic2 patterns binocular vision by specifying the uncrossed retinal projection. *Cell* 114: 545–557, copyright 2003, with permission from Elsevier.) *C*, *Left*, *Nr-CAM* is weakly expressed in VT during the peak-phase of RGC projections, but *Nr-CAM* is strongly upregulated in VT during the late phase. *Top right*, When semi-intact preps are cultured in the presence of function-blocking Nr-CAM-Fc, a large increase in ipsilateral projections is observed (as revealed by whole-retina DiI fills). *Bottom right*, Rhodamine-dextran retrograde backfills reveal a decrease in contralaterally projecting RGCs from VT at E18.5 and a corresponding increase in ipsilateral projections, which is not observed at earlier ages. (Reprinted from Williams et al. [2006]. A role for Nr-CAM in the patterning of binocular visual pathways. *Neuron* 50:535–547, copyright 2006, with permission from Elsevier.)

expressed in a high ventral-low dorsal gradient, *EphB2/EphB3*$^{-/-}$ mice have normal ipsilateral projections. These findings demonstrate that EphB1 is critical for the formation of the uncrossed projection. A small population of uncrossed fibers remains in *EphB1* mutants, indicating that other factors may also influence ipsilateral projections.

Zic2 The zinc finger transcription factor Zic2 was found to be necessary for directing ipsilateral projections at the chiasm (figure 32.4*B*). Like EphB1, Zic2 is expressed in VT retina primarily during the formation of uncrossed projections, from E13.5 to E16 (Herrera et al., 2003). *Zic2* knockdown mice display significantly reduced ipsilateral projections (see figure 32.3*H*), while Zic2 overexpression is sufficient to render contralaterally projecting RGCs to be inhibited by chiasm cells (Herrera et al., 2003). Zic2 and EphB1 appear to colocalize in VT RGCs (Pak et al., 2004), and Zic2 overexpression upregulates EphB1 mRNA in RGCs (Lee et al., 2008). Thus, Zic2 appears to regulate EphB1 expression in VT retina, which in turn interacts with ephrin-B2 at the chiasm midline, resulting in repulsion and ipsilateral projections. Surprisingly, Zic2 is not expressed by the EphB1^{+} early-born DC RGCs that project ipsilaterally, highlighting a significant difference between the pioneering, transient DC RGCs growing during the early period and VT RGCs that form the permanent ipsilateral projection (figure 32.1*A–C*).

Molecules important for axon divergence at the chiasm: The crossed projection

The characterization of EphB1/ephrin-B2 as the principal repulsive receptor-ligand pair for uncrossed axons has elucidated the molecular mechanisms guiding crossed projections. Recent work examining late-born crossed VT RGCs has provided some insight into the molecular mechanisms of crossed projections, but identification of cues associated with crossing fibers from non-VT retina has proved more elusive.

Nr-CAM Late-born RGCs from VT project contralaterally. Concurrent with the development of these late-born crossed projections, EphB1 and ephrin-B2, which are required for the uncrossed projection, are downregulated in VT and chiasm, respectively, by E17 (Williams et al., 2003). During the middle phase of RGC projections, Nr-CAM is highly expressed throughout the RGC layer except for the VT crescent, where its levels are reduced (Williams et al., 2006). By E17, Nr-CAM expression is upregulated in VT retina, coincident with the production of late-born contralateral VT projections (figure 32.4*C*). *Nr-CAM*$^{-/-}$ mice display an increase in the number of late-born ipsilateral projections arising from VT and a corresponding decrease in contralateral projections (Williams et al., 2006; see figures 32.3*I* and 32.4*C*). However, contralateral projections from non-VT retina appear normal in *Nr-CAM*$^{-/-}$ mice, indicating that Nr-CAM is required for mediating the crossing of late-born VT RGCs but not non-VT crossed RGC axons, even though both populations express significant levels of Nr-CAM. It is worth noting that CAM family members neurofascin and TAG-1 are also upregulated in VT retina at E17.5, both of which may interact with Nr-CAM to guide late-born uncrossed projections (Williams et al., 2006).

Islet2 The LIM-homeodomain transcription factor Isl2 is expressed in RGCs in a high dorsal-low ventral gradient during the peak phase of RGC differentiation (Pak et al., 2004). Similar to Nr-CAM, Isl2 expression in the VT crescent is weak at E15.5 but greatly increases during the late phase of RGC projections at E17.5. In a lacZ reporter mouse, all Isl2-positive RGCs project contralaterally (Pak et al., 2004). *Isl2*$^{-/-}$ mice display a significant increase in ipsilateral projections specifically from VT retina (see figure 32.3*I*), while no ectopic ipsilateral projections are seen arising from other parts of the retina, mimicking the phenotype of *Nr-CAM*$^{-/-}$ mice (Williams et al., 2006). Whether Isl2 regulates Nr-CAM expression remains to be analyzed.

Default Mechanism versus Crossing-Promoting Molecules in Non-VT Retina Late-born crossed RGC projections from VT retina are molecularly distinct from crossed RGCs outside the VT crescent. Both *Nr-CAM* and *Isl2* are expressed throughout the RGC layer during the peak phase of RGC growth and become upregulated in VT retina during the late phase, but *Nr-CAM* and *Isl2* mutants display RGC projection defects only from this late-born VT population. To date, there are few clues as to the molecular mechanisms that guide contralateral projections from non-VT retina.

Is crossing by non-VT retina a "default mechanism"—that is, do RGC axons that lack receptors to repulsive cues freely traverse the chiasm midline and enter the contralateral optic tract? Or are there as yet unidentified cues expressed at the chiasm that direct RGC axons to cross the midline? If so, would perturbation of these cues result in ectopic ipsilateral projections from non-VT retina? The failure to identify guidance cues that promote crossed projections in the mouse optic chiasm supports the idea that midline crossing occurs by default. However, the observations that RGC growth cones from non-VT retina pause and expand at the chiasm midline before crossing (Godement et al., 1994) and that RGC axons from all retinal regions are inhibited by chiasm cells in vitro (Wang et al., 1995) imply that the crossing mechanism is more complex. The CAMs L1, Nr-CAM, TAG-1, and neurofascin show strong expression in non-VT retina during the middle period of RGC growth, suggesting that these L1 family members may have redundant or co-active roles in midline crossing. Additionally, CAMs are known to directly interact with other guidance families in CNS and PNS pathways (Bechara et al, 2000), thus complicating the issue even further.

Other guidance factors have been characterized in zebrafish, in which all RGCs normally cross the midline and project to the contralateral tectum. *Sema3d* is expressed anterior and posterior to the chiasm (Halloran et al., 1999), similar to *Slit1/2* in mice. Both overexpression and knockdown of *Sema3d* produce ectopic ipsilateral RGC projections, causing RGC growth cones to pause and display exploratory behavior at the chiasm midline, a behavior not observed in wild-type embryos (Sakai and Halloran, 2006). In the zebrafish mutant *belladonna (lhx2)*, the optic chiasm does not form and all RGC axons project to the ipsilateral tectum, making the transcription factor Lhx2 a possible upstream regulator of Sema3d (Karlstrom et al., 1996; Seth et al., 2006). Thus, at least in zebrafish, crossing does not occur simply from a lack of receptors for repulsive cues, but instead there are specific cues and regulatory genes that direct RGC axons across the midline into the contralateral optic tract.

The Belgian sheepdog has a recessive mutation that, similar to belladonna, results in an achiasmatic RGC projection (Williams et al., 1994). Furthermore, there are several reports of achiasmatic humans (Victor et al., 2000), providing evidence that crossing the chiasm may not be a default mechanism in primates. Are there similar mutations in mice that might shed light on molecular mechanisms that guide crossed RGC axons? The transcription factor Pax2 is expressed at the optic disc and throughout the optic stalk during development (Nornes et al., 1990). Among other defects, *Pax2*$^{-/-}$ mice are achiasmatic, with *all* RGCs projecting into the ipsilateral optic tract (Torres et al., 1996; see figure 32.3*J*). This finding sheds light on potential signaling components for midline crossing at the chiasm, but identifying molecular mechanisms that direct contralateral projections remains one of the most important and least understood questions regarding the developing retinal projections.

Regulatory genes in the retina and chiasm important for chiasm patterning

Recent studies have uncovered a number of regulatory genes important for patterning the retina, several of which also play an important role in mediating RGC axon divergence at the chiasm. Many of these genes are also expressed in the ventral diencephalon, and knockout models of these genes can display moderate to severe defects in the optic chiasm environment. Although it can be difficult to determine the cause of RGC misprojections (i.e., defects in RGCs, the chiasm, or both), these studies provide insight into the development of RGC projections and the chiasm. They can also be useful in establishing a catalogue of phenotypes for ongoing genetic screens, which are becoming more common in the mouse nervous system.

Vax1/2 Two members of the ventral anterior homeobox family, *Vax1* and *Vax2*, are expressed in the ventral retina during development. *Vax1* expression is confined to cells in the optic disc and optic stalk during RGC differentiation (Mui et al., 2005), similar to the transcription factor Pax2 (Nornes et al., 1990) and EphA4 (Petros et al., 2006). RGC axons of *Vax1*$^{-/-}$ mice stall at the optic nerve–chiasm junction and fail to enter the ventral diencephalon (Bertuzzi et al., 1999; see figure 32.3*K*). *Vax2* is expressed in a high ventral-low nasal gradient in the mouse retina, similar to EphB2 (Birgbauer et al., 2000), and *Vax2*$^{-/-}$ mice display defects in retinal patterning and targeting in the SC (Barbieri et al., 2002; Mui et al., 2002). However, the first group reported that ipsilateral RGC projections are eliminated in *Vax2*$^{-/-}$ mice (Barbieri et al., 2002), while the line of *Vax2*$^{-/-}$ mice used by the second group had no defects in ipsilateral projections at the chiasm (Mui et al., 2002). These differences in RGC divergence at the chiasm could result from the strain variations (mixed 129/C57Bl6 vs. C57Bl6, respectively) or from differences in *Vax2* gene-targeting deletions.

Foxg1/Foxd1 The winged helix transcription factors Foxg1 and Foxd1 (also known as BF-1 and BF-2) have complementary expression patterns in the retina, with Foxd1 being restricted to the VT quadrant and Foxg1 expressed primarily in the nasal retina (Herrera et al., 2004; Pratt et al., 2004). *Foxg1*$^{-/-}$ mice display a large increase in ipsilateral projections, although the expression of EphB1 and the source of these ectopic ipsilateral projections remain unknown (Pratt et al., 2004; see figure 32.3*L*). Surprisingly, *Foxd1*$^{-/-}$ mice also have an abnormally large ipsilateral projection even though EphB1 and Zic2 expression in VT retina are absent in these mice (Herrera et al., 2004; see figure 32.3*M*). Unlike WT retina, ipsilateral projections in *Foxd1*$^{-/-}$ mice originate from the entire retina. These findings are complicated by the fact that Foxd1 is also expressed in the ventral diencephalon, and the optic chiasm region is grossly perturbed in *Foxd1*$^{-/-}$ mice (Herrera et al., 2004).

Brn-3b/3c The POU domain transcription factor Brn-3b is essential for the proper differentiation and survival of RGCs. *Brn-3b*$^{-/-}$ mice have substantially fewer RGCs than wild-type mice, and the surviving RGCs display guidance errors at many regions of the visual pathway (Erkman et al., 2000; see figure 32.3*N*). Of note, *Brn-3b*$^{-/-}$ mice display a significant increase in ipsilateral projections (Erkman et al., 2000; Wang et al., 2002), although it is not known from which retinal region these ectopic ipsilateral projections arise. Surprisingly, the misrouted ipsilateral axons were not observed in *Brn-3b*$^{-/-}$/*3c*$^{-/-}$ mice (Wang et al., 2002), while many of the other defects observed in *Brn-3b*$^{-/-}$ mice remain (see figure 32.3*O*). This finding implicates Brn-3c in promoting ipsilateral RGC projections, even through only 50% of RGCs express Brn-3c and *Brn-3c*$^{-/-}$ mice are not reported to have any retinal or RGC projection defects.

One confounding factor with the interpretation of such phenotypes is that a given gene may be expressed in both the retina and the optic chiasm (i.e., *Foxd1*). The presence of a gene in both RGCs and chiasm cells consequently makes it difficult to determine whether the RGC projection errors arise from perturbations in RGC axons, chiasm cells, or both. One way to address this issue is by performing in vitro mix-and-match cultures, whereby wild-type retinal explants are cultured with mutant chiasm cells, and vice versa (Herrera et al., 2004; Williams et al., 2006). Thus, chiasm phenotypes must be analyzed with regard to retinal perturbations and the topographic source of RGCs, as well as perturbations of chiasm cells and the ventral diencephalon.

The albino

Albinism, also known as congenital hypopigmentary disease, is caused by a defect in the synthesis or packaging of melanin. The lack of pigment in the retinal pigment epithelium (RPE) leads to a variety of defects in the retina and visual projections, one of which is a decrease in the number of uncrossed RGCs (for a review, see Jeffrey and Erskine, 2005). Several studies utilizing various techniques have identified that the percentage of uncrossed RGC projections correlates with the degree of RPE pigmentation (LaVail et al., 1978; Rachel et al., 2002), with albino mice having about 40%–50% fewer ipsilateral projections (Rice et al., 1995). Of note, albino mice show a reduction in the number of Zic2-expressing cells, in agreement with a diminished ipsilateral projection.

Albino organisms provide a unique model because they are the only known mouse mutation in which there is both a decrease in the proportion of uncrossed axons and a shift in the line of decussation that divides uncrossed and crossed regions of retina (see figure 32.3*P*). All of the RGC projection errors at the chiasm described earlier result in an increase or decrease in the number of ipsilaterally projecting RGCs, but in none of these cases is there a shift in the dividing line between uncrossed and crossed RGCs. The uncrossed RGCs in the albino arise from the most peripheral VT retina, resulting in a temporal shift in the line of decussation. In contrast, embryonic monocular enucleations result in a decrease in uncrossed projections from the intact eye that is similar to the levels seen in albinism, but enucleations do not alter the line of decussation (Chan and Guillery, 1993). In albino humans, the line of decussation shifts between 6° and 14° into the temporal retina (Hoffmann et al., 2003).

The precise location of the line of decussation is essential for establishing the proper organization of visual space, and its location in different species correlates well with the degree of binocular vision. However, genes that define the line of decussation are not known. Moreover, it remains unclear how perturbations in melanin biosynthesis affect retinal gene expression and RGC divergence at the midline.

One interesting theory for establishing the line of decussation is that a signal expressed by nonretinal tissue at the temporal pole of the retina could control gene expression important for uncrossed projections. As binocular vision evolved and eyes rotated from the side to the front of the head, this signal could have altered the patterning of the retina to increase the number of uncrossed fibers and shift the line of decussation nasally (Lambot et al., 2005). To investigate this theory, it would be of interest to examine the expression of transcription factors and diffusible cues in tissue adjacent to VT or temporal retina in various species, especially albinos, that display different degrees of binocularity.

New approaches for studying mouse visual system development

As evidenced earlier, although mice are a poor binocular species with a very small percentage of uncrossed axons, they are a useful organism for studying the development of RGC projections. The ability to manipulate mouse genetics is a powerful tool that can be combined with in vitro assays for studying molecular mechanisms guiding RGC axon growth and guidance. Different regions of the retina can be cultured either adjacent to a zone (border assay) or on alternating stripes (stripe assay) of a substrate, or in the presence of chiasm cells (Williams et al., 2003; Petros et al., 2006; figure 32.5*A*). Time-lapse imaging provides a means for observing RGC growth cones in real time as they interact with cues in vitro that they may contact in their projection pathway in vivo (figure 32.5*B*).

It has been technically challenging to express genes of interest into RGCs in vivo. Recently, in utero electroporation has been successfully adapted for gene delivery into the embryonic retina (Garcia-Frigola et al., 2007; figure 32.5*C*). Expression remains high for weeks, and GFP is clearly visible throughout RGC axons. The ability to ectopically express genes in RGCs and follow their trajectory provides a powerful technique for studying murine RGC projections.

Conclusion

Over the past two decades, progress has been made toward understanding visual system development, with a focus on optic chiasm patterning. The murine system provides an

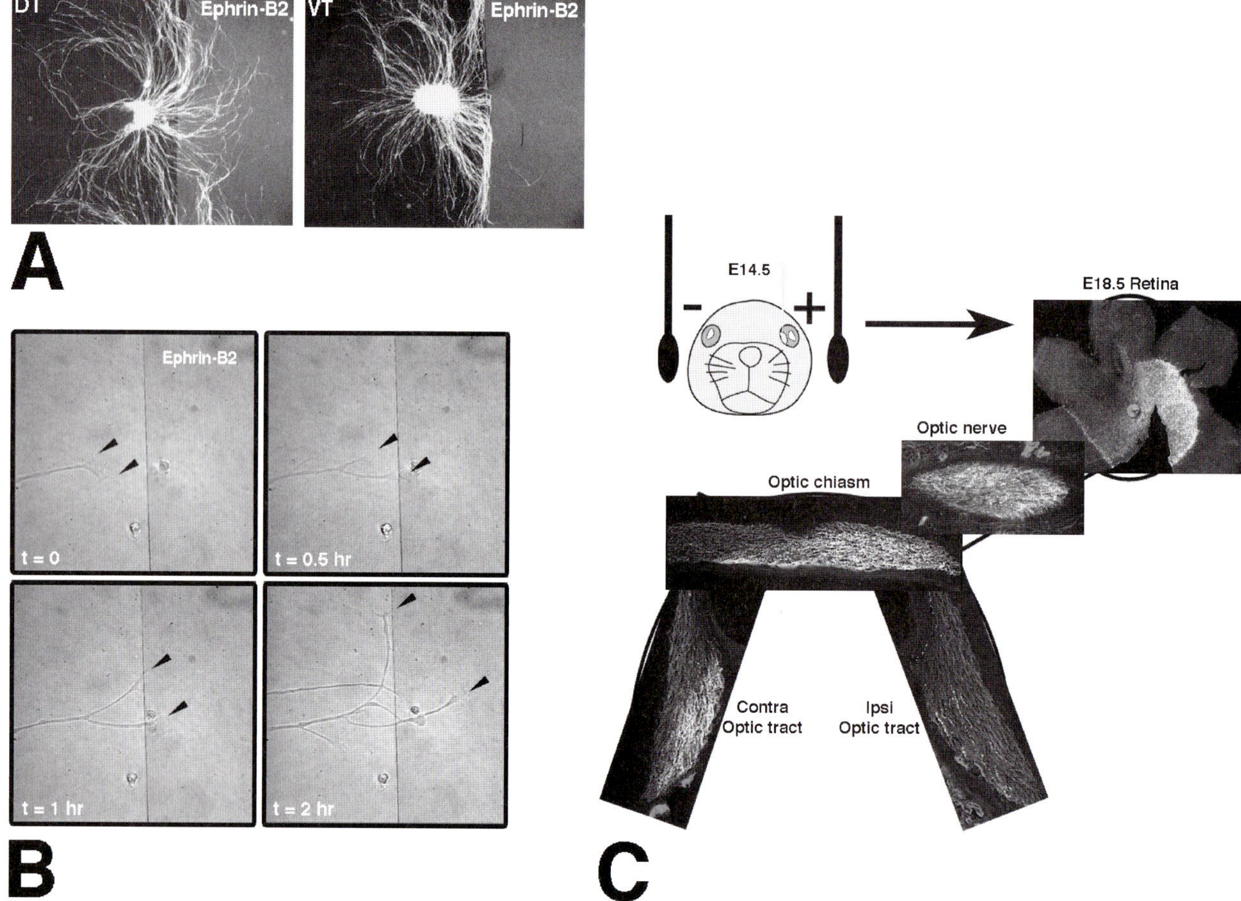

FIGURE 32.5 Important techniques for studying RGC projections in the developing mouse visual system. *A*, DT and VT retinal explants plated near a border of 0.5 μg/mL ephrin-B2 (red). Axons from DT explants project into the ephrin-B2 region, while VT axons are clearly inhibited. *B*, Time-lapse imaging can be used to study RGC growth cone behavior in real time as they encounter a border, in this case ephrin-B2. *Arrowheads* highlight two growth cones, one of which projects into the ephrin-B2 region and the other of which is repelled and travels parallel to the ephrin-B2 border. *C*, Diagram depicting in utero retinal electroporation. Briefly, DNA is injected into embryonic retina. Current is passed through electroporation paddles, and embryos are allowed to survive for several days. Embryos are perfused, the retina is collected, and heads are cryosectioned. In this case, GFP-positive cells can be seen in the retina, and many GFP-positive RGC projections are visible through the optic nerve, chiasm, and tract. Red denotes neurofilament. See color plate 22. (All images courtesy of T. Petros and C. Mason.)

excellent model in which to study retinal specification and axon guidance. Guidance cues and regulatory genes have been uncovered in the retina, optic nerve, chiasm, and tract whose combined interactions help to guide RGC axons from the retina toward their targets. Perturbation of these molecules can result in a wide variety of projection errors at the chiasm, ranging from an increase or decrease in the size of ipsilateral projections to axon defasciculation and ectopic projections.

Significant progress has been made in identifying molecular mechanisms that guide RGC axon divergence at the optic chiasm, an essential step for the development of binocular vision. Zic2 appears to regulate EphB1 in VT retina, which directs ipsilateral projections via interaction with ephrin-B2 at the chiasm midline. At later stages, Islet2 and Nr-CAM are required for crossed projections from VT retina. It will be of interest to test these mice mutants for changes in visual acuity, to link RGC projection errors with functional consequences.

Despite this progress, there are still many questions that remain unanswered. What are the molecular mechanisms that guide crossed projections from non-VT retina—the bulk of the crossed projection? What is the role of the pioneer axons? How do axon-axon interactions help direct RGC projections? And are these findings in mice relevant to the human visual system? Although there is new evidence that ephrin-B2 expression is analogous in humans and mice (Lambot et al., 2005), further studies are needed to answer these questions and identify how many developmental principles in mice can be extended to the human visual pathway.

ACKNOWLEDGMENTS Work was supported by NIH grant nos. EY012736, EY015290, and F31 NS051008. We are grateful to members of the Mason Lab, both past and present, for their comments on this manuscript and for contributions to this body of work.

REFERENCES

Barbieri, A. M., Broccoli, V., Bovolenta, P., Alfano, G., Marchitiello, A., Mocchetti, C., Crippa, L., Bulfone, A., Marigo, V., et al. (2002). Vax2 inactivation in mouse determines alteration of the eye dorsal-ventral axis, misrouting of the optic fibres and eye coloboma. *Development* 129:805–813.

Bechara, A., Falk, J., Moret, F., and Castellani, V. (2007). Modulation of semaphorin signaling by Ig superfamily cell adhesion molecules. *Adv. Exp. Med. Biol.* 600:61–72.

Bertuzzi, S., Hindges, R., Mui, S. H., O'Leary, D. D., and Lemke, G. (1999). The homeodomain protein vax1 is required for axon guidance and major tract formation in the developing forebrain. *Genes Dev.* 13:3092–3105.

Birgbauer, E., Cowan, C. A., Sretavan, D. W., and Henkemeyer, M. (2000). Kinase independent function of EphB receptors in retinal axon pathfinding to the optic disc from dorsal but not ventral retina. *Development* 127:1231–1241.

Brittis, P. A., Canning, D. R., and Silver, J. (1992) Chondroitin sulfate as a regulator of neuronal patterning in the retina. *Science* 255:733–736.

Brittis, P. A., Lemmon, V., Rutishauser, U., and Silver, J. (1995). Unique changes of ganglion cell growth cone behavior following cell adhesion molecule perturbations: A time-lapse study of the living retina. *Mol. Cell. Neurosci.* 6:433–449.

Chan, S. O., and Chung, K. Y. (1999). Changes in axon arrangement in the retinofugal pathway of mouse embryos: Confocal microscopy study using single- and double-dye label. *J. Comp. Neurol.* 406:251–262.

Chan, S. O., and Guillery, R. W. (1993). Developmental changes produced in the retinofugal pathways of rats and ferrets by early monocular enucleations: The effects of age and the differences between normal and albino animals. *J. Neurosci.* 13: 5277–5293.

Chung, K. Y., Blazeski, R., and Mason, C. A. (2008). [Retinal axon growth cone relationships with cells of the optic chiasm.] Unpublished results.

Colello, S. J., and Coleman, L. A. (1997). Changing course of growing axons in the optic chiasm of the mouse. *J. Comp. Neurol.* 379:495–514.

Colello, R. J., and Guillery, R. W. (1990). The early development of retinal ganglion cells with uncrossed axons in the mouse: Retinal position and axonal course. *Development* 108: 515–523.

Colello, R. J., and Guillery, R. W. (1992). Observations on the early development of the optic nerve and tract of the mouse. *J. Comp. Neurol.* 317:357–378.

Dakubo, G. D., Wang, Y. P., Mazerolle, C., Campsall, K., McMahon, A. P., and Wallace, V. A. (2003). Retinal ganglion cell–derived Sonic hedgehog signaling is required for optic disc and stalk neuroepithelial cell development. *Development* 130: 2967–2980.

Deiner, M. S., Kennedy, T. E., Fazeli, A., Serafini, T., Tessier-Lavigne, M., and Sretavan, D. W. (1997). Netrin-1 and DCC mediate axon guidance locally at the optic disc: Loss of function leads to optic nerve hypoplasia. *Neuron* 19:575–589.

Deiner, M. S., and Sretavan, D. W. (1999). Altered midline axon pathways and ectopic neurons in the developing hypothalamus of netrin-1- and DCC-deficient mice. *J. Neurosci.* 19:9900–9912.

Dräger, U. C. (1985). Birth dates of retinal ganglion cells giving rise to the crossed and uncrossed optic projections in the mouse. *Proc. R. Soc. Lond. B Biol. Sci.* 224:57–77.

Erkman, L., Yates, P. A., McLaughlin, T., McEvilly, R. J., Whisenhunt, T., O'Connell, S. M., Krones, A. I., Kirby, M. A., Rapaport, D. H., et al. (2000). A POU domain transcription factor-dependent program regulates axon pathfinding in the vertebrate visual system. *Neuron* 28:779–792.

Erskine, L., Williams, S. E., Brose, K., Kidd, T., Rachel, R. A., Goodman, C. S., Tessier-Lavigne, M., and Mason, C. A. (2000). Retinal ganglion cell axon guidance in the mouse optic chiasm: Expression and function of robos and slits. *J. Neurosci.* 20:4975–4982.

Garcia-Frigola, C., Carreres, M. I., Vegar, C., Herrera, E. (2007). Gene delivery into mouse retinal ganglion cells by in utero electroporation. *BMC Dev. Biol.* 7:103.

Godement, P., Wang, L. C., Mason, C. A. (1994). Retinal axon divergence in the optic chiasm: Dynamics of growth cone behavior at the midline. *J. Neurosci.* 14:7024–7039.

Guillery, R. W., Mason, C. A., and Taylor, J. S. (1995). Developmental determinants at the mammalian optic chiasm. *J. Neurosci.* 15:4727–4737.

Halloran, M. C., Severance, S. M., Yee, C. S., Gemza, D. L., Raper, J. A., and Kuwada, J. Y. (1999). Analysis of a Zebrafish semaphorin reveals potential functions in vivo. *Dev. Dyn.* 214: 13–25.

Hernandez, M. F. (2000). The optic nerve head in glaucoma: Role of astrocytes in tissue remodeling. *Prog. Retin. Eye. Res.* 19:297–321.

Herrera, E., Brown, L., Aruga, J., Rachel, R. A., Dolen, G., Mikoshiba, K., Brown, S., and Mason, C. A. (2003). Zic2 patterns binocular vision by specifying the uncrossed retinal projection. *Cell* 114:545–557.

Herrera, E., Marcus, R., Li, S., Williams, S. E., Erskine, L., Lai, E., and Mason, C. (2004). Foxd1 is required for proper formation of the optic chiasm. *Development* 131:5727–5739.

Hoffmann, M. B., Tolhurst, D. J., Moore, A. T., and Morland, A. B. (2003). Organization of the visual cortex in human albinism. *J. Neurosci.* 23:8921–8930.

Jeffrey, G., and Erskine, L. (2005). Variations in the architecture and development of the vertebrate optic chiasm. *Prog. Retin. Eye. Res.* 24:721–753.

Karlstrom, R. O., Trowe, T., Klostermann, S., Baier, H., Brand, M., Crawford, A. D., Grunewald, B., Haffter, P., Hoffmann, H., et al. (1996). Zebrafish mutations affecting retinotectal axon pathfinding. *Development* 123:427–438.

Lambot, M. A., Depasse, F., Noel, J. C., and Vanderhaeghen, P. (2005). Mapping labels in the human developing visual system and the evolution of binocular vision. *J. Neurosci.* 25: 7232–7237.

LaVail, J. H., Nixon, R. A., and Sidman, R. L. (1978). Genetic control of retinal ganglion cell projections. *J. Comp. Neurol.* 182:399–421.

Lee, R., Garcia-Frigola, C., Carreres, M. I., Vegar, C., Mason, C., and Herrera, E. (2008). Zic2 promotes axonal divergence at the optic chiasm midline by regulation of the EphB1 receptor. Submitted.

Liu, J., Wilson, S., and Reh, T. (2003). BMP receptor 1b is required for axon guidance and cell survival in the developing retina. *Dev. Biol.* 256:34–48.

Marcus, R. C., Blazeski, R., Godement, P., and Mason, C. A. (1995). Retinal axon divergence in the optic chiasm: Uncrossed axons diverge from crossed axons within a midline glial specialization. *J. Neurosci.* 15:3716–3729.

Mason, C. A., and Sretavan, D. W. (1997). Glia, neurons, and axon pathfinding during optic chiasm development. *Curr. Opin. Neurobiol.* 7:647–653.

Mason, C. A., and Wang, L. (1997). Growth cone form is behavior-specific and, consequently, position-specific along the retinal axon pathway. *J. Neurosci.* 17:1086–1100.

Menzies, A. S., Aszodi, A., Williams, S. E., Pfeifer, A., Wehman, A. M., Goh, K. L., Mason, C. A., Fassler, R., and Gertler, F. B. (2004). Mena and vasodilator-stimulated phosphoprotein are required for multiple actin-dependent processes that shape the vertebrate nervous system. *J. Neurosci.* 24:8029–8038.

Mui, S. H., Hindges, R., O'Leary, D. D., Lemke, G., and Bertuzzi, S. (2002). The homeodomain protein Vax2 patterns the dorsoventral and nasotemporal axes of the eye. *Development* 129:797–804.

Mui, S. H., Kim, J. W., Lemke, G., and Bertuzzi, S. (2005). Vax genes ventralize the embryonic eye. *Genes Dev.* 19:1249–1259.

Nakagawa, S., Brennan, C., Johnson, K. G., Shewan, D., Harris, W. A., and Holt, C. E. (2000). Ephrin-B regulates the ipsilateral routing of retinal axons at the optic chiasm. *Neuron* 25: 599–610.

Nornes, H. O., Dressler, G. R., Knapik, E. W., Deutsch, U., and Gruss, P. (1990). Spatially and temporally restricted expression of Pax2 during murine neurogenesis. *Development* 109: 797–809.

Oster, S. F., Bodeker, M. O., He, F., and Sretavan, D. W. (2003). Invariant Sema5A inhibition serves an ensheathing function during optic nerve development. *Development* 130: 775–784.

Pak, W., Hindges, R., Lim, Y. S., Pfaff, S. L., and O'Leary, D. D. (2004). Magnitude of binocular vision controlled by islet-2 repression of a genetic program that specifies laterality of retinal axon pathfinding. *Cell* 119:567–578.

Petros, T. J., Williams, S. E., and Mason, C. A. (2006). Temporal regulation of EphA4 in astroglia during murine retinal and optic nerve development. *Mol. Cell. Neurosci.* 32:49–66.

Plump, A. S., Erskine, L., Sabatier, C., Brose, K., Epstein, C. J., Goodman, C. S., Mason, C. A., and Tessier-Lavigne, M. (2002). Slit1 and Slit2 cooperate to prevent premature midline crossing of retinal axons in the mouse visual system. *Neuron* 33:219–232.

Pratt, T., Conway, C. D., Tian, N. M., Price, D. J., and Mason, J. O. (2006). Heparan sulphation patterns generated by specific heparan sulfotransferase enzymes direct distinct aspects of retinal axon guidance at the optic chiasm. *J. Neurosci.* 26: 6911–6923.

Pratt, T., Tian, N. M., Simpson, T. I., Mason, J. O., and Price, D. J. (2004). The winged helix transcription factor Foxg1 facilitates retinal ganglion cell axon crossing of the ventral midline in the mouse. *Development* 131:3773–3784.

Rachel, R. A., Mason, C. A., and Beermann, F. (2002). Influence of tyrosinase levels on pigment accumulation in the retinal pigment epithelium and on the uncrossed retinal projection. *Pigment Cell Res.* 15:273–281.

Reese, B. E., Guillery, R. W., Marzi, C. A., and Tassinari, G. (1991). Position of axons in the cat's optic tract in relation to their retinal origin and chiasmatic pathway. *J. Comp. Neurol.* 306:539–553.

Rice, D. S., Williams, R. W., and Goldowitz, D. (1995). Genetic control of retinal projections in inbred strains of albino mice. *J. Comp. Neurol.* 354:459–469.

Sakai, J. A., and Halloran, M. C. (2006). Semaphorin 3d guides laterality of retinal ganglion cell projections in zebrafish. *Development* 133:1035–1044.

Seth, A., Culverwell, J., Walkowicz, M., Toro, S., Rick, J. M., Neuhauss, S. C., Varga, Z. M., and Karlstrom, R. O. (2006). Belladonna/(Ihx2) is required for neural patterning and midline axon guidance in the zebrafish forebrain. *Development* 133: 725–735.

Strittmatter, S. M., Fankhauser, C., Huang, P. L., Mashimo, H., and Fishman, M. C. (1995). Neuronal pathfinding is abnormal in mice lacking the neuronal growth cone protein GAP-43. *Cell* 80:445–452.

Thompson, H., Barker, D., Camand, O., and Erskine, L. (2006a). Slits contribute to the guidance of retinal ganglion cell axons in the mammalian optic tract. *Dev. Biol.* 296:476–484.

Thompson, H., Camand, O., Barker, D., and Erskine, L. (2006b). Slit proteins regulate distinct aspects of retinal ganglion cell axon guidance within dorsal and ventral retina. *J. Neurosci.* 26:8082–8091.

Torres, M., Gomez-Pardo, E., and Gruss, P. (1996). Pax2 contributes to inner ear patterning and optic nerve trajectory. *Development* 122:3381–3391.

Victor J. D., Apkarian, P., Hirsch, J., Conte, M. M., Packard, M., Relkin, N. R., Kim, K. H. S., and Shapley, R. (2000). Visual function and brain organization in non-decussating retinal-fugal fiber syndrome. *Cereb. Cortex* 10:2–22.

Wang, L. C., Dani, J., Godement, P., Marcus, R. C., and Mason, C. A. (1995). Crossed and uncrossed retinal axons respond differently to cells of the optic chiasm midline in vitro. *Neuron* 15:1349–1364.

Wang, S. W., Mu, X., Bowers, W. J., Kim, D. S., Plas, D. J., Crair, M. C., Federoff, H. J., Gan, L., and Klein, W. H. (2002). Brn3b/Brn3c double knockout mice reveal an unsuspected role for Brn3c in retinal ganglion cell axon outgrowth. *Development* 129:467–477.

Watanabe, T., and Raff, M. C. (1988). Retinal astrocytes are immigrants from the optic nerve. *Nature* 332:834–837.

Williams, R. W., Hogan, D., and Garraghty, P. E. (1994). Target recognition and visual maps in the thalamus of achiasmatic dogs. *Nature* 367:637–639.

Williams, S. E., Grumet, M., Colman, D. R., Henkemeyer, M., Mason, C. A., and Sakurai, T. (2006). A role for Nr-CAM in the patterning of binocular visual pathways. *Neuron* 50: 535–547.

Williams, S. E., Mann, F., Erskine, L., Sakurai, T., Wei, S., Rossi, D. J., Gale, N. W., Holt, C. E., Mason, C. A., et al. (2003). Ephrin-B2 and EphB1 mediate retinal axon divergence at the optic chiasm. *Neuron* 39:919–935.

Williams, S. E., Mason, C. A., and Herrera, E. (2004). The optic chiasm as a midline choice point. *Curr. Opin. Neurobiol.* 14:51–60.

Zhang, F., Lu, C., Severin, C., and Sretavan, D. W. (2000). GAP-43 mediates retinal axon interaction with lateral diencephalon cells during optic tract formation. *Development* 127:969–980.

33 Axon Growth and Regeneration of Retinal Ganglion Cells

JEFFREY L. GOLDBERG

How do retinal ganglion cell (RGC) axons grow during development, and why do they fail to regrow when injured? RGCs extend long axons carrying all of the visual information through the optic nerve, across the optic chiasm, and into the brain. Our understanding of the essential regulators of this process has advanced considerably in recent years. Investigating the regulation of axon growth is crucial to understanding why axons fail to regenerate in the central nervous system (CNS) after injury or in disease, and rodent model systems have proved invaluable to expanding our understanding of axon growth and regeneration.

What signals induce axon growth?

Do Neurons Need Specific Extrinsic Signals for Axon Growth? Because the same signals that induce axon growth are generally critical for neuronal survival, these two functions have been difficult to disentangle—remove putative axon growth signals in vitro or in vivo, and the neurons die. The development of genetic tools to block apoptosis in neurons made it possible to address this question (Goldberg and Barres, 2000). For example, RGCs can be purified and cultured in the complete absence of glial cells; elevating the expression of the antiapoptotic protein Bcl-2 maintains neuronal survival after all trophic signals are withdrawn (Goldberg et al., 2002a). Despite high levels of survival in the absence of exogenous signals, Bcl-2-overexpressing RGCs fail to elaborate axons or dendrites unless axon growth-inducing signals are present, clearly demonstrating that axon growth is not a default function of a surviving neuron but must be specifically signaled (figure 33.1).

RGCs are similar to other neurons in this requirement for extrinsic signals to signal axon growth. For example, when developing dorsal root ganglion (DRG) sensory neurons from transgenic mice that lack the pro-apoptotic protein Bax are cultured in vitro, withdrawal of neurotrophic factors does not induce apoptosis. These $Bax^{-/-}$ DRG sensory neurons grow rudimentary axons, but neurotrophins greatly increase axon outgrowth in vitro (Lentz et al., 1999). Even embryonic peripheral neurons that survive in culture without added trophic factors fail to extend neurites (Lindsay et al., 1985), and adult DRG neurons that do not appear to depend on neurotrophic factors for survival still respond to such factors by increasing axon outgrowth (Lindsay, 1988). Taken together, these findings indicate that surviving neurons do not constitutively extend axons and that axon growth must be specifically signaled by extracellular signals.

What Are the Extracellular Signals That Induce Axon Growth? A great variety of extracellular signals have been found to induce axon growth. The most potent signals are peptide trophic factors. Many different families have been studied intensively and have widespread roles in regulating the developing and adult nervous system. Different neurons are frequently responsive to different trophic factors, and multiple trophic factors can often combine to induce even greater axon growth.

The best studied peptide trophic factors for RGC axon growth in vitro (and regeneration in vivo) are brain-derived neurotrophic factor (BDNF), ciliary neurotrophic factor (CNTF), insulin-like growth factor (IGF), basic fibroblast growth factor (bFGF), and glial cell line–derived neurotrophic factor (GDNF). Interestingly, each of these belongs to a different family, acts on different receptors, and activates different downstream signaling molecules, but all appear to converge on similar regulators of axon growth (table 33.1).

RGCs extend axons well in response to BDNF and CNTF, but both together induce more axon growth than either does alone (Goldberg et al., 2002a; Jo et al., 1999; Logan et al., 2006; Loh et al., 2001). Interestingly, in studies that dissociate survival from axon growth, the peptides that most strongly promote cell survival are the same ones that most strongly promote axon growth (Mansour-Robaey et al., 1994; Mey and Thanos, 1993). This is even more remarkable in light of data suggesting that the survival and axon growth responses to trophic factors diverge inside the neuron, using different intracellular signaling pathways (Atwal et al., 2000; Goldberg et al., 2002a). Recent evidence has extended the list of trophic signaling molecules beyond these traditional families. For example, a small, macrophage-derived, calcium-binding protein named oncomodulin binds RGCs and strongly promotes RGC axon growth in vitro and in vivo (Yin et al., 2006).

Are extracellular signals other than peptide trophic factors sufficient to induce axon elongation? Extracellular matrix molecules such as laminin and heparin sulfate proteoglycans, and cell adhesion molecules such as L1 and N-cadherin, are expressed in the visual pathway (Lafont et al., 1992; Reichardt and Tomaselli, 1991) and help promote axon growth in vitro and in vivo. Eliminating N-cadherin expression, for example, clearly decreases RGC axon growth in vivo (Riehl et al., 1996). Although these signaling interactions can potentiate axon outgrowth in purified CNS neurons if soluble glial or peptide trophic signals are present, so far they do not appear to be sufficient to induce axon growth on their own (Goldberg et al., 2002a). Rather, they appear to provide a critical substrate along which axons extend, thereby strongly potentiating axon outgrowth. Other adhesion and guidance molecules that normally direct RGC axons as they steer through the visual pathway to their targets in the brain (Oster et al., 2004) may also contribute to the signaling of axon elongation. For example, netrin-1, a well-described axon guidance molecule homologous to laminin that guides early RGC axons to the optic nerve head as they exit the retina (de la Torre et al., 1997), may also stimulate elongation (Serafini et al., 1994), although it may not be as effective in stimulating RGC axon growth on its own (Goldberg et al., 2002a). As axon guidance molecules activate the same growth cone mechanisms discussed earlier, it is not surprising that their effects may overlap with effects on elongation as well. Finally, other extracellular signals as simple as purine nucleotides may be critical to inducing axon growth, although the mechanism of this activity is still mysterious (Benowitz et al., 1998). Therefore, peptide trophic factors appear to most strongly induce axon outgrowth, but adhesion molecules can greatly potentiate this growth, and molecules thought to be primarily involved in growth cone guidance may also have some elongation-promoting activity.

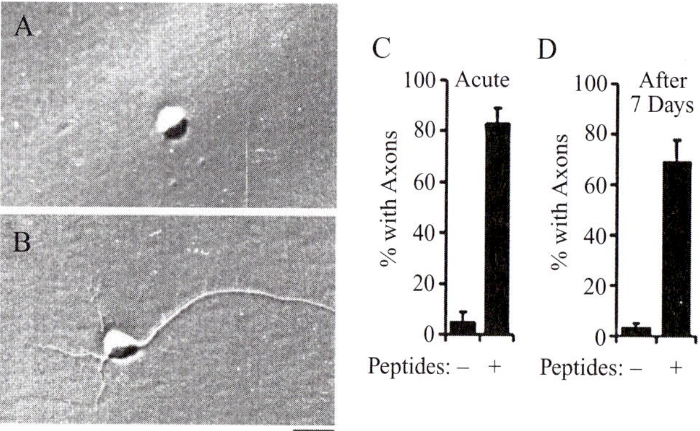

FIGURE 33.1 RGCs require extrinsic signals to extend axons. *A* and *B*, Purified rat RGCs were infected acutely with a virus carrying the antiapoptotic gene *Bcl-2* and cultured in media without (*A*) or with (*B*) peptide trophic factors. Scale bar = 30 μm. *C*, Population data showing the percent of purified RGCs extending axons more than 15 μm from the cell body (mean ± SEM). *D*, Population data as in *C*, for *Bcl-2*-expressing RGCs first cultured 1 week in minimal media lacking peptide trophic factors and then returned to media with or without trophic factors, as marked. (Reprinted from Goldberg, J. L., Espinosa, J. S., Xu, Y., Davidson, N., Kovacs, G. T., Barres, B. A. [2002]. Retinal ganglion cells do not extend axons by default: Promotion by neurotrophic signaling and electrical activity. *Neuron* 33(5):689–702. Copyright 2002, with permission from Elsevier.)

WHERE DO EXTRACELLULAR SIGNALS ACT TO INDUCE AXON ELONGATION? Where do trophic peptides act, at the cell body or on the axons themselves? Local application of neurotrophins to a growth cone is sufficient to enhance the rate of growth cone extension in vitro (Letourneau, 1978) and in vivo (Tucker et al., 2001). The definitive answer, however, has come from experiments using Campenot chambers, a powerful technique in which neurons are cultured with their cell bodies in one compartment while their axons grow under a wall into a separate compartment, with the culture media in each compartment kept separated. Classic experiments using cultures of peripheral neurons in these chambers demonstrated the necessity for trophic peptides to signal at the axons and growth cones themselves for the axons to survive and grow (figure 33.2) (Campenot, 1994). Trophic peptides in the cell body compartment keep the neurons alive, but the axons in the peripheral compartment die back. Amazingly, in these experiments, the

TABLE 33.1

Example peptide trophic factors that stimulate RGC survival and axon growth

Trophic Factor	Family	Approx. Mol. Wt.	Receptor
BDNF	Neurotrophins	27 kd (dimer)	Trk-B
CNTF	Cytokines	22 kd	CNTFR-α/GP130/LIFR-β
IGF-I	IGFs	7.5 kd (free form)	IGF-1R
bFGF	FGFs	24 kd	FGF-Rs
GDNF	Neurturins	22–55 kd	GFR-α/RET
Oncomodulin	EF-hand	11.7 kd	Unknown

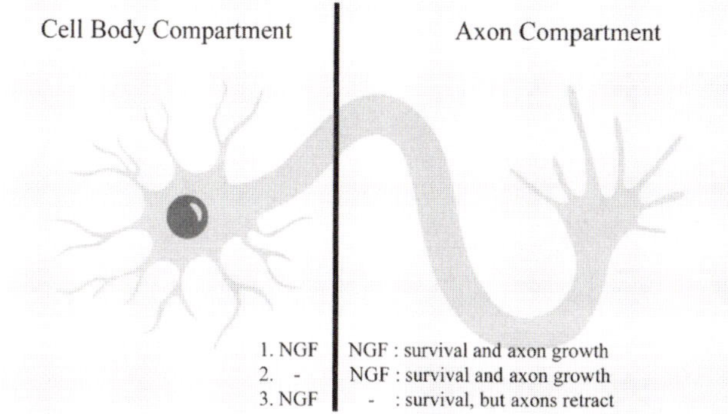

FIGURE 33.2 Campenot chambers have proven invaluable in dissecting the functions important to axons from those important to the cell body. In these experiments, a wall separates the culture dish into two or more compartments, and although the axons can grow under the wall into the distal compartment, the contents of the culture media do not diffuse from one side to the other. In this way, factors can be added exclusively to the axons or cell bodies to the exclusion of the other. For example, in the classic experiments dissociating cellular survival from axon growth, neurotrophins such as NGF added to the axon or cell body compartments supported neuronal survival, but the neurotrophin had to be added specifically to the axon compartment to support the survival and growth of the axons themselves (see the text). (Reprinted from Goldberg, J. L. [2003]. How does an axon grow? *Genes and Development* 17(8):941–958. Copyright 2003, with permission from Cold Spring Harbor Press.)

presence of trophic peptides only in the peripheral (axon) compartment is sufficient to induce survival of the cell body. Therefore, the provision of proper growth signals to the axons is as important as providing survival signals to the cell body and points to the importance of providing developing neurons with axon growth signals all along the growth pathway. For example, RGC axon growth is stimulated by soluble signals from the retina, optic nerve, and superior colliculus (Goldberg et al., 2002b), and these are likely to stimulate passing axons in vivo.

Although trophic factors may act solely at the axon, to induce axon elongation they must also activate processes at the cell body. How do growth signals at the axon get passed along to the distant cell body, where gene transcription and translation are induced to support survival and axon growth? Neurotrophin-mediated activation of tyrosine kinase (Trk) receptors leads to endocytosis of activated, ligand-bound receptors into clathrin-coated vesicles. These signaling endosomes carry with them the machinery of the ras-raf-MAP kinase signaling cascades and can continue to activate these pathways once inside the cell (Howe et al., 2001). Neurotrophin signaling endosomes may then be retrogradely transported along microtubules back to the cell body, where they can activate transcriptional regulators and induce new gene expression (Riccio et al., 1997; Watson et al., 1999). In addition, there may be retrograde signaling of neurotrophin-mediated survival signals without retrograde transport of NGF-containing endosomes (MacInnis and Campenot, 2002), raising an interesting hypothesis that survival signals and axon growth or other signals may be carried along separate but complementary pathways. It is not yet known whether the retrograde transport of signals from the growth cone is necessary for axon growth if similar signals are already acting at the cell body, as is likely to happen in vivo. Retrograde carriage of neurotrophic signals may modify the signal to carry more information, for example by changing signaling components in different cellular compartments, and may provide crucial signals along the way, for example for maintenance of axonal structure along its length, or for suppression or support of axon branching. Experiments tackling the relationship between vesicle localization and signaling effects will help shed light on these important questions.

How Do Extracellular Signals Induce Axon Elongation? We know surprisingly little about the intracellular mechanisms by which neurotrophic signals elicit axon growth. Two relevant questions can be addressed in this domain: what are the intermediate signaling pathways that receptors activate to elicit growth, and what are the specific aspects of axon growth that this signaling pathway regulates? A few models have been particularly fruitful in defining which signaling cascades are important for axon growth. Campenot chamber experiments similar to those described earlier showed that for peripheral neurons, both ras-raf-MAP kinase and PI3-kinase-Akt signaling pathways downstream of neurotrophin receptors contribute to axon outgrowth (Atwal et al., 2000). In recent years, significant progress has been made in identifying how these two signaling pathways are activated by neurotrophin receptors; details of these experiments have been reviewed extensively elsewhere (Kaplan and Miller, 2000). A second type of experiment takes advantage of neurons in which apoptosis is blocked by knocking out Bax or overexpressing Bcl-2. In Bcl-2-overexpressing RGCs, pharmacologic inhibition of either MAP kinase or PI3 kinase partially reduces axon outgrowth, but inhibiting both together is necessary to block axon elongation altogether (Goldberg et al., 2002a). Although the specifics may vary from neuron to neuron, these data hint at a fascinating complexity of the regulation of these different parameters of axon growth that remains to be more fully studied.

How does the activation of these signaling pathways actually regulate axon growth? Regulation of the transcription and translation of genes needed for general cellular growth, axonal cytoskeletal dynamics, supply and insertion of membrane and cytoplasmic building blocks, translation of axonally localized mRNAs, and proteosome activity have all been implicated and have been reviewed in depth elsewhere (Goldberg, 2003). Much of this work has been initiated in models outside the visual system, but early indications are that many of these regulatory pathways are shared by all neurons. Interestingly, in purified RGC cultures, both BDNF and CNTF induce similar rates of axon growth, but the two together induce more than either does alone, raising the hypothesis that different trophic factors may be responsible for different facets of axon growth (Goldberg et al., 2002a).

Control of Neuronal Responsiveness to Trophic Peptides An interesting difference between the ability of trophic peptides to promote axon growth by CNS neurons such as RGCs and by peripheral nervous system (PNS) neurons has been identified. Peptide trophic factors such as neurotrophins are sufficient to induce axon growth by purified PNS neurons in culture. In contrast, to elicit axon growth from CNS neurons in culture, peptide trophic signals alone are insufficient. For instance, RGCs fail to survive in the presence of such trophic signals as BDNF or CNTF unless their cAMP levels are elevated, either pharmacologically or by depolarization (Meyer-Franke et al., 1995). Cyclic AMP elevation and depolarization do not promote axon growth on their own. Similarly, RGCs kept alive with Bcl-2 overexpression extend axons only poorly in response to BDNF, but this axon growth is greatly potentiated by cAMP elevation or by physiological levels of electrical activity, either from endogenous retinal activity or from direct electrical stimulation when cultured on a silicon chip (Goldberg et al., 2002a) (figure 33.3).

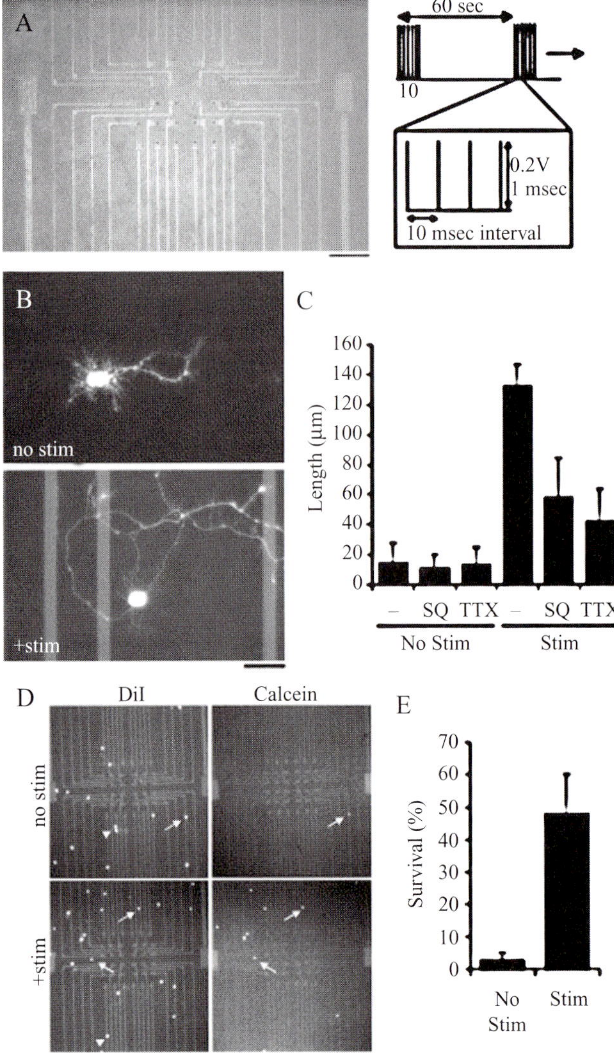

Figure 33.3 Effects of electrical activity on axon growth and survival in response to BDNF. *A*, Photograph of silicon chip growth substrate and diagram of burst-stimulation protocol. *B*, DiI-labeled RGCs cultured on silicon chips extended rudimentary axons in response to BDNF (*top*). Axon growth was enhanced if the neurons were stimulated with electrical activity (*bottom*). *C*, Mean longest axon/RGC ± SEM measured after 16 hours in the presence of BDNF, with stimulation, SQ, or TTX, as marked and as described in the text. *D*, DiI-labeled RGCs (*left panels*) were plated in media containing BDNF and stimulated by electrical activity as marked. RGC survival was assessed 48 hours later by labeling with calcein-AM (*right panels*). DiI-labeled RGCs stained with calcein are alive (*arrows*); those lacking calcein are dead (*arrowheads*). *E*, RGC survival in response to BDNF was enhanced 10-fold by electrical stimulation. Scale bar = 50 μm (*B*) or 200 μm (*D*). (Reprinted from Goldberg, J. L., Espinosa, J. S., Xu, Y., Davidson, N., Kovacs, G. T., Barres, B. A. [2002]. Retinal ganglion cells do not extend axons by default: Promotion by neurotrophic signaling and electrical activity. *Neuron* 33(5):689–702. Copyright 2002, with permission from Elsevier.)

Do neurons have to be electrically active to respond to trophic activities for axon growth? Experiments in vivo suggest that electrical activity is not absolutely required: injecting tetrodotoxin into the eye to block action potentials (Shatz and Stryker, 1988) or studying the munc-18 knockout mouse in which synaptic release of neurotransmitters is essentially eliminated (Verhage et al., 2000) both reveal that RGCs and other CNS neurons successfully elongate their axons to their targets. Recent studies, however, also highlight the possible effects of electrical activity in sculpting axonal morphology. Activity regulates growth cone responsiveness to guidance cues, enhancing netrin responsiveness and inhibiting myelin repulsion (Ming et al., 2001). In addition, activity shapes the specificity of local connectivity of axons, for example in the selection and elimination of cortical innervation targets (Catalano and Shatz, 1998; Kalil et al., 1986; Katz and Shatz, 1996). Data on the effect of activity on axon growth have been more controversial. Neuronal activity may increase the rate of axon arborization in vitro and in vivo by stabilizing growing branches (Cantallops et al., 2000; Cohen-Cory, 1999; Rashid and Cambray-

Deakin, 1992). On the other hand, growth cones may collapse acutely in response to electrical stimulation, but then desensitize and recommence axon growth (Fields et al., 1990). Therefore, after a brief accommodation at the growth cone, the longer-term effects of electrical stimulation appear to promote axon growth.

This trophic dependence contrasts with PNS neurons, which survive and regenerate their axons in response to trophic peptides in the absence of cAMP elevation or electrical activity, raising the hypothesis that the trophic signaling of axon growth may differ between CNS and PNS neurons. Could this difference contribute to their different abilities to regenerate in vivo? Previous studies have suggested that neither trophic factor delivery alone nor electrical stimulation alone induces CNS axonal regeneration. If axon growth normally depends on activity in vivo, and if damaged cells are less active or elevate cAMP less effectively in response to activity, a CNS neuron's ability to regenerate its axon could be impaired. Therefore, it may be crucial to provide trophic peptides as well as signals such as cAMP elevation to ensure an optimal axon growth response. Although cAMP elevation has been implicated in overcoming inhibitory signals at the growth cone (Ming et al., 2001), it is interesting to speculate whether some of the effect of cAMP in promoting regeneration in vivo is actually attributable to improving the neuron's response to trophic or other positive peptide signals (Hu et al., 2006; Qui et al., 2002).

Intrinsic control of axon growth

Intrinsic Growth Ability of Central Nervous System Neurons Is Developmentally Regulated Are the rate and extent of axon growth purely dependent on extracellular signals and substrates, or do they also depend on the intrinsic state of the neuron? This is a critical if largely unanswered question in research on axon growth and regeneration. Embryonic CNS neurons can regenerate their axons quite readily, but they lose their capacity to regenerate with age. For example, in the spinal cord, axons lose the ability to regenerate between P4 and P20 (Kalil and Reh, 1982; Reh and Kalil, 1982; Saunders et al., 1992). This developmental loss of regenerative ability has generally been attributed to the maturation of CNS glial cells, both astrocytes and oligodendrocytes, and to the production of CNS myelin, all of which strongly inhibit regenerating axons after injury. In experiments in which the inhibitory environment is removed or molecularly blocked, however, only a few percent of axons regenerate, and functional recovery typically proceeds remarkably slowly. For example, RGCs take 2 months to regenerate through a peripheral nerve graft (Aguayo et al., 1987; Bray et al., 1987). These experiments indicate that an inhibitory environment is likely only part of the explanation.

Are the neurons themselves partly responsible? Axons from P2 or older hamster retinas have lost the ability to reinnervate even embryonic tectal explants (Chen et al., 1995). Similar explant preparations have shown a developmental loss of regenerative ability in cerebellar Purkinje cells and brainstem neurons (Blackmore and Letourneau, 2006; Dusart et al., 1997). This suggests that changes in a CNS neuron's intrinsic ability to grow could also explain this developmental loss of regenerative ability. The inability of postnatal neurons to reextend their axons might also be explained by the development of glial cells, however, which are largely generated postnatally. Therefore, the ability to separate neurons from CNS glia remains critical to determining whether CNS neurons actually change in their intrinsic axon growth ability during development.

When cultured in strongly trophic environments in the complete absence of CNS glia and at clonal density, embryonic RGCs extend axons up to 10 times faster than postnatal RGCs (figure 33.4) (Goldberg et al., 2002b). The evidence for this decreased growth ability being intrinsically maintained is twofold. First, embryonic RGCs grow at a faster rate than postnatal RGCs in a variety of environments that should facilitate growth, including in media containing neurotrophic factors, in media conditioned by cells from the embryonic visual pathway, and after transplantation into developing pathways in vivo. In all cases, embryonic RGCs extended their axons at rates substantially higher than did the postnatal RGCs, suggesting that any extrinsic growth-promoting environment is dependent on an intrinsically set maximal growth rate. Second, RGCs purified from either embryonic or postnatal ages and cultured away from all of the other cell types with which they normally interact retained their faster or slower growth phenotypes, respectively. Therefore, the difference in the abilities of embryonic and postnatal RGCs to elongate axons is not dependent on continued signaling by neighboring cell types but is intrinsically maintained.

Do these neurons lose their axon growth ability as the result of intrinsic aging? Embryonic RGCs aged up to 10 days in purified cultures, to the age they would decrease their axon growth ability in vivo, continue to elongate their axons rapidly, suggesting that the change in axon growth ability is signaled by an extrinsic cue (Goldberg et al., 2002b). The decrease in axon growth ability occurs sharply at birth during the period of target innervation, but E20 RGCs cocultured with superior collicular slices retain their rapid axon growth ability, suggesting that target contact is not responsible for this change. Indeed, retinal maturation, and specifically a membrane-associated signal from retinal amacrine cells, was shown to be sufficient to induce the developmental decrease in RGC axon growth ability. Thus, a membrane-associated cue from these presynaptic amacrine cells signals embryonic

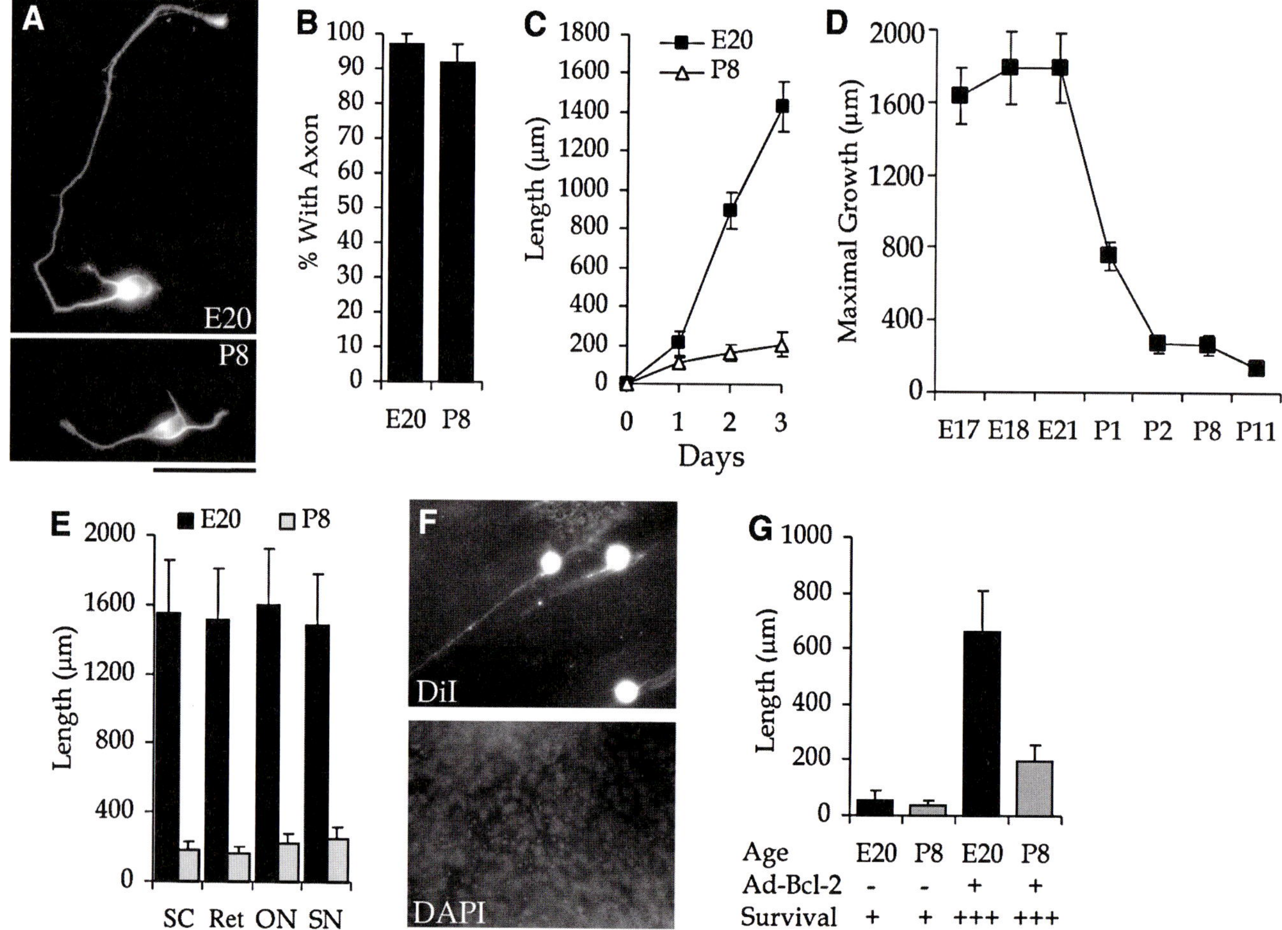

Figure 33.4 Difference in axon growth ability of E20 and P8 RGCs. *A–D*, RGCs purified by immunopanning were cultured at clonal density (<5/mm^2) on poly-D-lysine (PDL) and laminin in growth medium containing BDNF, ciliary neurotrophic factor (CNTF), insulin, and forskolin (GM). *A*, RGC axons immunolabeled for the axonal protein-tubulin III after 18 hours. *B*, Percentage of RGCs at each age elaborating at least one axon more than 20 μm after 3 days. *C*, Average length of each neuron's longest axon at days 1, 2, and 3. E20 and P8 axon lengths did not differ statistically at day 1. P8 axon lengths at days 2 and 3 were longer than on the day before (Dunnett's $P < 0.05$). *D*, Time course of change in intrinsic axon growth ability of RGCs purified simultaneously from rats of different ages and cultured in target-conditioned growth medium. Means ± SEM. *E*, RGC axon length after 3 days at clonal density in minimal medium conditioned by superior collicular (SC), retinal (Ret), optic nerve (ON), or sciatic nerve (SN) cells. Scale bars = 50 μm. (Reprinted from Goldberg, J. L., Klassen, M. P., Hua, Y., Barres, B. A. [2002]. Amacrine-signaled loss of intrinsic axon growth ability by retinal ganglion cells. *Science* 296: 1860–1864. Copyright 2002, with permission from Science Publishing.)

RGCs to decrease their axon growth ability, but once this signal is sent, the loss is permanent: removal of the amacrine cells does not allow the RGCs to speed up again.

Does Dendrite Growth Ability Replace Axon Growth Ability? Why would a presynaptic cell type signal these CNS neurons to decrease their intrinsic axon growth ability? Remarkably, at about the same time that neonatal RGCs lose their ability to rapidly elongate axons, they gain the ability to rapidly generate dendrites (Goldberg et al., 2002b). This increase in dendritic growth ability is not an RGC-autonomous result of intrinsic aging, because RGCs do not increase their dendrite growth ability with time in purified cultures, but rather is signaled by a retinal cue (Goldberg et al., 2002a). Therefore, retinal cues trigger neonatal RGCs to irreversibly switch from an axonal to a dendritic growth mode. Whether the increase in dendritic growth ability and the decrease in axon growth ability are the result of the same signal is not yet known, but an interesting implication of these data is that the control of axon versus dendrite growth may be largely intrinsic, rather than determined by separate extracellular cues (figure 33.5). Axons and dendrites appear to respond to many, or possibly all, of the same growth and guidance signals. It is

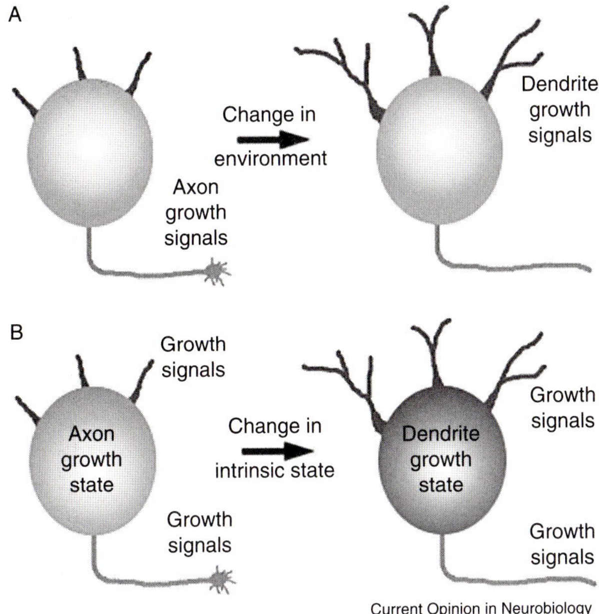

Figure 33.5 Is axon versus dendrite growth a function of environment, a function of the intrinsic growth state of the neuron, or both? *A*, In the extrinsic control hypothesis, axon-specific and dendrite-specific growth signals are presented to the neuron at different developmental windows or locations. *B*, In the intrinsic control hypothesis, growth signals are available in general, and the neuron's intrinsic growth state, either axonal or dendritic, determines which processes are preferentially responsive to extrinsic trophic signals. The change in intrinsic state could come from an intrinsic, preprogrammed clock or aging mechanism or could be elicited by an extrinsic signal; for example, amacrine cells are able to signal RGCs to decrease their intrinsic axon growth ability (Goldberg et al., 2002b). Note, however, that the amacrine signal does not have to be present in an ongoing fashion: Once it signals RGCs to decrease their axon growth ability, they retain this new phenotype intrinsically. (Reprinted from Goldberg, J. L. [2004]. Intrinsic neuronal regulation of axon and dendrite growth. *Current Opinion in Neurobiology* 14(5):551–557. Copyright 2004, with permission from Elsevier.)

unknown whether some of the signals found previously to increase dendrite outgrowth, such as bone morphogenic protein-7 (Higgins et al., 1997), actually modulate the growth mode of the neuron from axonal to dendritic, rather than stimulating dendritic growth cones preferentially. Many of the previous studies that have shown that presynaptic cell types stimulate dendritic growth may reflect a switch in the neurons from axonal to dendritic growth modes, after which the neurons extend dendrites in response to growth signals already present. Thus, the ability of neurotrophic factors to stimulate axon and dendrite growth may strongly depend on whether a neuron is in an axonal or dendritic growth state, and raises the question of the identity of the extracellular signal that induces a dendritic growth mode (Goldberg et al., 2002b).

What Molecular Changes Underlie the Developmental Loss in Rapid Axon Growth Ability? In response to this amacrine cell-associated cue, RGCs could gradually increase the expression of genes that limit axon growth or decrease the expression of genes necessary for faster axonal elongation, or both. For instance, in the developing chick, RGCs lose axon growth responsiveness to laminin either by downregulating specific integrins (laminin receptors) (Cohen et al., 1989; de Curtis and Reichardt, 1993; de Curtis et al., 1991) or by downregulating the activation of such integrins (Ivins et al., 2000), although they continue to respond to laminin-2 (merosin) (Cohen and Johnson, 1991). At least for mammalian RGCs, such changes are not responsible for the observed decrease in growth ability, as postnatal RGCs continue to be responsive to laminin-1, as well as a variety of other substrates, and laminin-2 is no more effective than laminin-1 in promoting postnatal RGC axon growth (Goldberg et al., 2002a). Similarly, a difference in trophic receptor levels or responsiveness to trophic signals could explain these differences. For example, depolarization rapidly elevates Trk-B receptors on the surface of CNS neurons (Du et al., 2000; Meyer-Franke et al., 1998). Exogenously elevating Trk-B levels, however, fails to increase P8 axon growth rates to embryonic levels (Goldberg et al., 2002a). The antiapoptotic protein Bcl-2 was proposed as an intrinsic genetic switch that decreases axon growth rate by RGCs (Chen et al., 1997), but Bcl-2 overexpression by purified RGCs in culture neither promotes axon growth nor enhances axon growth in response to neurotrophic signaling in vitro or in vivo (Goldberg et al., 2002a), a result consistent with other findings (Goldberg and Barres, 2000; Chierzi et al., 1999; Greenlund et al., 1995; Lodovichi et al., 2001; Michaelidis et al., 1996).

What molecular mechanisms could regulate the axonal or dendritic growth mode of a neuron? If properly regulated, almost any molecule in the cell could be crucial to determining axon versus dendrite growth (Goldberg, 2003). It is attractive to first consider transcription factors that could activate the expression of whole programs of axon or dendrite growth and could also maintain an intrinsic phenotype in the absence of ongoing extrinsic signaling. For example, the POU domain transcription factor Brn-3b is essential for RGC development. In *Brn-3b*$^{-/-}$ mice, RGCs fail to extend axons properly, and 80% die before birth; in addition, *Brn-3b*$^{-/-}$ RGCs in culture extend only rudimentary axons and instead elaborate abnormal, dendrite-like processes (Erkman et al., 1996, 2000; Gan et al., 1996, 1999; Wang et al., 2000). RGCs also express the related family members Brn-3a and Brn-3c: about 50% of RGCs express both Brn-3b and Brn-3c. The *Brn-3b*$^{-/-}$ *Brn-3c*$^{-/-}$ double knockout shows an almost total loss of axon outgrowth from explanted retinas, suggesting that both Brn-3b and Brn-3c contribute to controlling RGC axon growth (Wang et al., 2002). In these experiments, the only neurons that were found to elaborate neurites were those that did not express the alkaline phosphatase marker from the mutated Brn-3c locus, which suggests that, in RGCs that do not normally express Brn-3c, alternative transcription factors drive axon outgrowth. Thus, transcription factors involved in cell fate determination, which is often defined by cell morphology, may act directly via the control of axon and dendrite growth ability.

What are the genes downstream of Brn-3b that could effect changes in the intrinsic axon growth state of a neuron? Recently, *Brn-3b*$^{-/-}$ retinas were compared with wild-type retinas in microarray experiments to determine which genes depend on Brn-3b for their expression, and several genes linked to axon guidance were found to be downregulated in *Brn-3b*$^{-/-}$ retinas (Mu et al., 2004). Furthermore, the NGF receptor Trk-A was identified as a transcriptional target of Brn-3a (Ma et al., 2003) providing a direct link from transcription factor expression to trophic responsiveness. These experiments point to the power of using focused microarray experiments in relation to established phenotypic models.

Transcription factors are not the only master regulators in a cell. Levels of specific complements of proteins can be regulated posttranslationally by ubiquitination and degradation. Because there are hundreds of ubiquitin ligases in mammalian genomes, the potential for subcellular regulation of the levels of specific proteins is vast. Recently, exciting data have demonstrated that the ubiquitin ligase anaphase-promoting complex (APC) has a significant role in regulating the axon growth rate of cerebellar granule neurons. APC was originally found to be essential for mitosis in dividing cells, but it is also highly expressed in postmitotic neurons. Blocking APC or its activator Cdh1 with RNAi or dominant negative approaches led to a greater than twofold increase in axon length but not to a change in dendrite length, suggesting that Cdh1-APC complexes normally inhibit axon but not dendrite growth (Konishi et al., 2004). Furthermore, APC normally binds to and leads to the proteasomal degradation of the transcriptional corepressor SnoN, and knocking down SnoN itself led to a decrease in axon growth (Stegmuller et al., 2006). What are the targets of SnoN that regulate axon growth? Whether these specific proteins will be relevant for axon growth or regeneration in RGCs remains to be examined, but the principle of illuminating such regulatory pathways is very exciting.

How does the intrinsic state of neuron allow the same extrinsic cues to induce axon or dendrite growth preferentially (see figure 33.5)? Cytoplasmic kinases or phosphatases may provide an axon- or dendrite-specific interpretation of extrinsic cues. For example, electrical activity seems to be crucial to potentiate both axon and dendrite growth in various neurons in response to trophic signals (Goldberg, 2003). The influx of Ca^{2+} during depolarization activates a family of Ca^{2+}-dependent signaling kinases, calmodulin kinases (CaMKs), which have now been implicated in both axon- and dendrite-specific growth. For axon growth, overexpression of a dominant-negative variant of CaMKI in embryonic hippocampal and postnatal cerebellar granule neurons decreases axon outgrowth, whereas expression of cytosolic dominant-negative CaMKII or nuclear dominant-negative CaMKIV constructs has no effect on axon growth in these cells (Wayman et al., 2004). In other studies, CaMKII-β and nuclear CaMKIV have been found to stimulate dendrite but not axon growth in hippocampal or cortical cultures (Fink et al., 2003; Redmond et al., 2002). Thus, CaMK isoforms can differentially control axon- and dendrite-specific outgrowth in hippocampal neurons. Further experiments should point to mechanisms of either developmental or subcellular regulation, or both, for these kinases.

The levels of second messengers such as cAMP and cGMP, if intrinsically maintained, could affect axon and dendrite growth differentially. As discussed earlier, cAMP is crucial for RGCs to extend axons in response to neurotrophic factors (Goldberg et al., 2002a), and a developmental decrease in cAMP levels has been proposed to underlie the developmental loss of axon regeneration in the presence of inhibitory myelin-associated cues (Cai et al., 2001). In a strongly trophic, noninhibitory environment, however, an increase in cAMP does not revert the slow axon growth of postnatal RGCs to the fast growth of their embryonic state (Goldberg et al., 2002b).

Thus, critical questions remain. What is the molecular basis for the developmental loss of intrinsic axon growth ability in RGCs? And how does such a loss relate to the failure of RGCs to regenerate in vivo?

Axon regeneration in the mature visual system

Axons that get cut either by injury or disease in the PNS reinitiate the whole process of axon growth, elongating back to their peripheral targets and restoring sensorimotor function. Yet when axons in the adult mammalian CNS are severed, they largely fail to regenerate. This appears to occur independent of the mode of axon injury, whether traumatic, ischemic, immunologic, or degenerative: in all cases, RGCs fail to regenerate into the optic nerve. Furthermore, RGCs (and other CNS neurons) typically die after axon injury. After an optic nerve crush injury behind the eye, 95% of postnatal rodent RGCs die within 2–3 days, and a similar number die in the adult rodent within 2 weeks (Berkelaar et al., 1994; Villegas-Perez et al., 1993). Thus, there are multiple issues to address when considering approaches to improve RGC regeneration and survival and axon growth past the injury site first, and later guidance and target innervation.

Although it was once believed that adult CNS neurons intrinsically lacked any ability to regenerate, this view was disproved 25 years ago by elegant experiments demonstrating that at least some RGCs could regenerate their axons through fragments of peripheral nerve grafts (So and Aguayo, 1985). The failure of RGCs and other CNS neurons to regenerate their axons is generally ascribed to an inhibitory glial environment; however, the lack of successful regeneration in experiments designed to overcome inhibitory CNS glial cues also hints at other extrinsic or intrinsic regulation of axon growth.

How Is Retinal Ganglion Cell Regeneration Studied? Although traumatic optic neuropathy is one of the least common human scenarios in which RGC axons are injured, it has been the best studied model in rodents by far. Typically, the optic nerve is surgically cut or crushed within the orbit behind the eye, although experiments crushing the nerve intracranially have also been studied. The regenerative response is assayed by labeling RGC axons and determining whether any extend past the lesion site into the optic nerve (figure 33.6), or into a peripheral nerve graft in experiments styled after Aguayo's early work (So and Aguayo, 1985). Interestingly, although injuring the optic nerve at increasing distances from the eye delays the onset of RGC cell death (Berkelaar et al., 1994), there may be less regenerative response with more distal injury (You et al., 2000).

Other optic neuropathies are also beginning to be modeled in rodents. In optic neuritis, optic nerve oligodendrocytes demyelinate from RGC axons in concert with an autoimmune reaction. This has been modeled in rat and mouse models of experimental autoimmune encephalomyelitis, in which rodents' immune system is stimulated to react against myelin-associated proteins. Immunization against myelin-oligodendrocyte glycoprotein (MOG) induces multiple sclerosis-like demyelination throughout the brain, including in the optic nerve (Storch et al., 1998), but creating transgenic mice with T cells directed against MOG, or passively transferring anti-MOG T cells in rats, creates demyelinating disease largely confined to the optic nerve, mimicking optic neuritis (Bettelli et al., 2003; Shao et al., 2004). In such models, RGC axons are incidentally severed and fail to regenerate, and, as after optic nerve trauma, RGCs die with a 1- to 2-week delay (Guan et al., 2006).

Ischemic optic neuropathy—a stroke of the optic nerve—is exceedingly common in humans, and taking an old technology for creating strokes in the brain and applying it to the optic nerve has allowed the study of ischemic optic neuropathy in rodents. In this photothrombotic model, the photosensitizing dye rose bengal is injected into the tail vein and the surgically exposed optic nerve is illuminated with a 514 nm or 535 nm wavelength laser. Photoactivation of the intravascular rose bengal leads to free radical generation, endothelial damage, and platelet degranulation, creating a focal thrombosis in the optic nerve. This model has been studied recently to examine the RGC and optic nerve response to ischemic axon injury (Bernstein et al., 2003), and future work may be directed at enhancing RGC survival and regeneration in such models.

Finally, the second most common cause of irreversible blindness in the world is glaucomatous optic neuropathy. Glaucoma is a neurodegenerative disease, and lowering intraocular pressure often slows its progression. Glaucomatous optic neuropathy has been extensively studied in rodent models (reviewed in Morrison et al., 2005; Whitmore et al., 2005), although the primary concern in these studies is usually RGC survival, not RGC axon regeneration, and as such is not considered in this chapter.

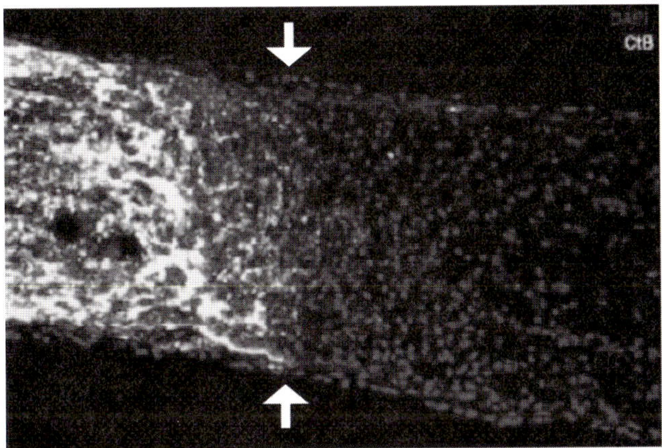

Figure 33.6 After an optic nerve crush injury, RGC axons were labeled with an intravitreal injection of fluorophore-conjugated cholera toxin B. The bright axons failed to regrow across the lesion site (*arrows*) after 8 days in vivo. Optic nerve nuclei are counterstained with a nuclear dye, DAPI. See color plate 23. (Y. Duan and J. L. Goldberg. [2008]. Unpublished data.)

Intrinsic and Extrinsic Regulation of Adult Retinal Ganglion Cell Regeneration Since RGCs do not extend axons in the absence of specific extracellular signals, regenerative failure might be explained in part by a relative inability of mature CNS astrocytes and oligodendrocytes to secrete trophic signals after injury. Indeed, ample evidence exists to support a role for neurotrophins in stimulating axon growth in vivo. The same peptide trophic factors that stimulate RGC axon growth in vitro enhance RGC survival and axon regeneration in vivo (Aguayo et al., 1996; Cui et al., 1999; Yip and So, 2000). Furthermore, as was seen for RGCs in vitro (Goldberg et al., 2002a), elevation of cAMP levels in RGCs enhances their regenerative ability after optic nerve injury in vivo (Cui et al., 2003; Monsul et al., 2004; Watanabe et al., 2003).

Our understanding of the mechanisms of axon growth has led to progress in understanding regenerative failure. For example, understanding that the regulation of both repulsion and collapse of growth cones by inhibitory molecules relies on the same intracellular signaling pathways suggests that manipulating these common regulators can increase regeneration. Thus, blocking the growth cone collapsing activity of the small GTPase rho increases RGC regeneration in the inhibitory environment of the optic nerve in vivo (Lehmann et al., 1999), an effect that may be caused in part by blockade of inhibitory signaling at the growth cone, but also in part by increasing the intrinsic growth ability of the neurons themselves. Such manipulations may be combined with cAMP elevation and trophic factor delivery to enhance regeneration even further (Hu et al., 2006).

Does the loss of intrinsic axon growth ability by RGCs (Goldberg et al., 2002b) contribute to their failure to regenerate after injury in the adult? As mentioned earlier, a loss of intrinsic axon growth ability could explain why in many previous experiments, regeneration proceeded remarkably slowly, even when glial inhibitory cues were removed. For example, most RGCs take 2–3 months to regenerate through peripheral nerve grafts to the superior colliculus (Aguayo et al., 1987; Bray et al., 1987), although the fastest RGCs may extend 1–2 mm/day into peripheral nerve grafts. This is approximately the rate they extend axons in vitro (Goldberg et al., 2002b), and far slower than the 10 days they would take if they elongated their axons at an embryonic growth rate of 10 mm/day. It is not clear whether this developmental switch is reversible either: soluble signals from optic nerve glia or peripheral nerve glia, or from retinal or superior collicular cells, were not able to reverse the loss of rapid axon growth ability in RGCs in vitro, suggesting that the developmental switch may normally be permanent (Goldberg et al., 2002b). There remains the possibility, however, that other signals, or the discovery and manipulation of genes involved in this transition, may revert the postnatal neurons to their embryonic axon growth ability, and that this may be critical to increase regeneration in the CNS. Thus, a combined approach may be required—both the intrinsic neuronal growth state and the extrinsic environment may have to be optimized for successful regeneration after injury.

Conclusion

Our understanding of how RGC axons grow and the regulation of RGC axon regeneration is still in its infancy. Although a great deal of progress has been made recently in understanding the nature of the extracellular signals that induce axon growth, we still know relatively little about the intracellular molecular mechanisms by which these signals are transduced into the neuron and ultimately how they elicit growth. Fortunately, new molecular tools, including genomics, proteomics, and RNAi, should help us elucidate novel components of the axon growth machinery that couple transmembrane signaling receptors at the growth cone to the axonal cytoskeleton. In particular, these methods should soon reveal the underlying transcriptional program elicited by peptide trophic factors that triggers axon growth. Determining the full roster of genes induced during axon growth, which genes are needed for axon elongation both during development and for regeneration, and whether developmental differences in intrinsic axon growth ability between embryonic and postnatal RGCs underly the failure of RGC regeneration should help in developing new approaches to enhancing RGC regeneration in the mouse and, ultimately, in the human visual system.

ACKNOWLEDGMENTS Portions of this chapter are reprinted with permission from earlier publications (Goldberg, 2003, 2004). Figures 33.1 to 33.5 and their accompanying captions are reprinted by permission of the publishers. Figure 33.6 was generated in experiments supported by a grant from the National Eye Institute.

REFERENCES

Aguayo, A. J., Clarke, D. B., Jelsma, T. N., Kittlerova, P., Friedman, H. C., and Bray, G. M. (1996). Effects of neurotrophins on the survival and regrowth of injured retinal neurons. *Ciba Found. Symp.* 196:135–144.

Aguayo, A. J, Vidal-Sanz, M., Villegas-Perez, M. P., and Bray, G. M. (1987). Growth and connectivity of axotomized retinal neurons in adult rats with optic nerves substituted by PNS grafts linking the eye and the midbrain. *Ann. N.Y. Acad. Sci.* 495:1–9.

Atwal, J. K., Massie, B., Miller, F. D., and Kaplan, D. R. (2000). The TrkB-Shc site signals neuronal survival and local axon growth via MEK and P13-kinase. *Neuron* 27:265–277.

Benowitz, L. I., Jing, Y., Tabibiazar, R., Jo, S. A., Petrausch, B., Stuermer, C. A., Rosenberg, P. A., and Irwin, N. (1998). Axon outgrowth is regulated by an intracellular purine-sensitive mechanism in retinal ganglion cells. *J. Biol. Chem.* 273: 29626–29634.

Berkelaar, M., Clarke, D. B., Wang, Y. C., Bray, G. M., and Aguayo, A. J. (1994). Axotomy results in delayed death and apoptosis of retinal ganglion cells in adult rats. *J. Neurosci.* 14:4368–4374.

Bernstein, S. L., Guo, Y., Kelman, S. E., Flower, R. W., and Johnson, M. A. (2003). Functional and cellular responses in a novel rodent model of anterior ischemic optic neuropathy. *Invest. Ophthalmol. Vis. Sci.* 44:4153–4162.

Bettelli, E., Pagany, M., Weiner, H. L., Linington, C., Sobel, R. A., and Kuchroo, V. K. (2003). Myelin oligodendrocyte glycoprotein-specific T cell receptor transgenic mice develop spontaneous autoimmune optic neuritis. *J. Exp. Med.* 197: 1073–1081.

Blackmore, M., and Letourneau, P. C. (2006). Changes within maturing neurons limit axonal regeneration in the developing spinal cord. *J. Neurobiol.* 66:348–360.

Bray, G. M., Villegas-Perez M. P., Vidal-Sanz, M., and Aguayo, A. J. (1987). The use of peripheral nerve grafts to enhance neuronal survival, promote growth and permit terminal reconnections in the central nervous system of adult rats. *J. Exp. Biol.* 132:5–19.

Cai, D., Qiu, J., Cao, Z., McAtee, M., Bregman, B. S., and Filbin, M. T. (2001). Neuronal cyclic AMP controls the developmental loss in ability of axons to regenerate. *J. Neurosci.* 21:4731–4739.

Campenot, R. B. (1994). NGF and the local control of nerve terminal growth. *J. Neurobiol.* 25:599–611.

Cantallops, I., Haas, K., and Cline, H. T. (2000). Postsynaptic CPG15 promotes synaptic maturation and presynaptic axon arbor elaboration in vivo. *Nat. Neurosci.* 3:1004–1011.

Catalano, S. M., and Shatz, C. J. (1998). Activity-dependent cortical target selection by thalamic axons. *Science* 281:559–562.

Chen, D. F., Jhaveri, S., and Schneider, G. E. (1995). Intrinsic changes in developing retinal neurons result in regenerative failure of their axons. *Proc. Natl. Acad. Sci. U.S.A.* 92:7287–7291.

Chen, D. F., Schneider, G. E., Martinou, J. C., and Tonegawa, S. (1997). Bcl-2 promotes regeneration of severed axons in mammalian CNS. *Nature* 385:434–439.

Chierzi, S., Strettoi, E., Cenni, M. C., and Maffei, L. (1999). Optic nerve crush: Axonal responses in wild-type and bcl-2 transgenic mice. *J. Neurosci.* 19:8367–8376.

Cohen, J., and Johnson, A. R. (1991). Differential effects of laminin and merosin on neurite outgrowth by developing retinal ganglion cells. *J. Cell Sci. Suppl.* 15:1–7.

Cohen, J., Nurcombe, V., Jeffrey, P., and Edgar, D. (1989). Developmental loss of functional laminin receptors on retinal ganglion cells is regulated by their target tissue, the optic tectum. *Development* 107:381–387.

Cohen-Cory, S. (1999). BDNF modulates, but does not mediate, activity-dependent branching and remodeling of optic axon arbors in vivo. *J. Neurosci.* 19:9996–10003.

Cui, Q., Lu, Q., So, K. F., and Yip, H. K. (1999). CNTF, not other trophic factors, promotes axonal regeneration of axotomized retinal ganglion cells in adult hamsters. *Invest. Ophthalmol. Vis. Sci.* 40:760–766.

Cui, Q., Yip, H. K., Zhao, R. C., So, K. F., and Harvey, A. R. (2003). Intraocular elevation of cyclic AMP potentiates ciliary neurotrophic factor-induced regeneration of adult rat retinal ganglion cell axons. *Mol. Cell. Neurosci.* 22:49–61.

de Curtis, I., Quaranta, V., Tamura, R. N., and Reichardt, L. F. (1991). Laminin receptors in the retina: Sequence analysis of the chick integrin alpha 6 subunit. Evidence for transcriptional and posttranslational regulation. *J. Cell Biol.* 113:405–416.

de Curtis, I., and Reichardt, L. F. (1993). Function and spatial distribution in developing chick retina of the laminin receptor alpha 6 beta 1 and its isoforms. *Development* 118:377–388.

de la Torre, J. R., Hopker, V. H., Ming, G. L., Poo, M. M., Tessier-Lavigne, M., Hemmati-Brivanlou, A., and Holt, C. E. (1997). Turning of retinal growth cones in a netrin-1 gradient mediated by the netrin receptor DCC. *Neuron* 19:1211–1224.

Du, J., Feng, L., Yang, F., and Lu, B. (2000). Activity- and Ca(2+)-dependent modulation of surface expression of brain-derived neurotrophic factor receptors in hippocampal neurons. *J. Cell Biol.* 150:1423–1434.

Dusart, I., Airaksinen, M. S., and Sotelo, C. (1997). Purkinje cell survival and axonal regeneration are age dependent: An in vitro study. *J. Neurosci.* 17:3710–3726.

Erkman, L., McEvilly, R. J., Luo, L., Ryan, A. K., Hooshmand, F., O'Connell, S. M., Keithley, E. M., Rapaport, D. H., Ryan, A. F., and Rosenfeld, M. G. (1996). Role of transcription factors Brn-3.1 and Brn-3.2 in auditory and visual system development. *Nature* 381:603–606.

Erkman, L., Yates, P. A., McLaughlin, T., McEvilly, R. J., Whisenhunt, T., O'Connell, S. M., Krones, A. I., Kirby, M. A., Rapaport, D. H., et al. (2000). A POU domain transcription factor-dependent program regulates axon pathfinding in the vertebrate visual system. *Neuron* 28:779–792.

Fields, R. D., Neale, E. A., and Nelson, P. G. (1990). Effects of patterned electrical activity on neurite outgrowth from mouse sensory neurons. *J. Neurosci.* 10:2950–2964.

Fink, C. C., Bayer, K. U., Myers, J. W., Ferrell, J. E., Jr., Schulman, H., and Meyer, T. (2003). Selective regulation of neurite extension and synapse formation by the beta but not the alpha isoform of CaMKII. *Neuron* 39:283–297.

Gan, L., Wang, S. W., Huang, Z., and Klein, W. H. (1999). POU domain factor Brn-3b is essential for retinal ganglion cell differentiation and survival but not for initial cell fate specification. *Dev. Biol.* 210:469–480.

Gan, L., Xiang, M., Zhou, L., Wagner, D. S., Klein, W. H., and Nathans, J. (1996). POU domain factor Brn-3b is required for the development of a large set of retinal ganglion cells. *Proc. Natl. Acad. Sci. U.S.A.* 93:3920–3925.

Goldberg, J. L. (2003). How does an axon grow? *Genes Dev.* 17:941–958.

Goldberg, J. L. (2004). Intrinsic neuronal regulation of axon and dendrite growth. *Curr. Opin. Neurobiol.* 14:551–557.

Goldberg, J. L., and Barres, B. A. (2000). The relationship between neuronal survival and regeneration. *Annu. Rev. Neurosci.* 23:579–612.

Goldberg, J. L., Espinosa, J. S., Xu, Y., Davidson, N., Kovacs, G. T., and Barres, B. A. (2002a). Retinal ganglion cells do not extend axons by default: Promotion by neurotrophic signaling and electrical activity. *Neuron* 33:689–702.

Goldberg, J. L., Klassen, M. P., Hua, Y., and Barres, B. A. (2002b). Amacrine-signaled loss of intrinsic axon growth ability by retinal ganglion cells. *Science* 296:1860–1864.

Greenlund, L. J., Korsmeyer, S. J., and Johnson, E. M., Jr. (1995). Role of BCL-2 in the survival and function of developing and mature sympathetic neurons. *Neuron* 15:649–661.

Guan, Y., Shindler, K. S., Tabuena, P., Rostami, A. M. (2006). Retinal ganglion cell damage induced by spontaneous autoimmune optic neuritis in MOG-specific TCR transgenic mice. *J. Neuroimmunol.* 178:40–48.

Higgins, D., Burack, M., Lein, P., and Banker, G. (1997). Mechanisms of neuronal polarity. *Curr. Opin. Neurobiol.* 7:599–604.

Howe, C. L., Valletta, J. S., Rusnak, A. S., and Mobley, W. C. (2001). NGF signaling from clathrin-coated vesicles: Evidence that signaling endosomes serve as a platform for the Ras-MAPK pathway. *Neuron* 32:801–814.

Hu, Y., Cui, Q., and Harvey, A. R. (2006). Interactive effects of C3, cyclic AMP and ciliary neurotrophic factor on adult retinal ganglion cell survival and axonal regeneration. *Mol. Cell. Neurosci.* 34:88–98.

Ivins, J. K., Yurchenco, P. D., Lander, A. D. (2000). Regulation of neurite outgrowth by integrin activation. *J. Neurosci.* 20: 6551–6560.

Jo, S. A., Wang, E., and Benowitz, L. I. (1999). Ciliary neurotrophic factor is and axogenesis factor for retinal ganglion cells. *Neuroscience* 89:579–591.

Kalil, K., and Reh, T. (1982). A light and electron microscopic study of regrowing pyramidal tract fibers. *J. Comp. Neurol.* 211: 265–275.

Kalil, R. E., Dubin, M. W., Scott, G., and Stark, L. A. (1986). Elimination of action potentials blocks the structural development of retinogeniculate synapses. *Nature* 323:156–158.

Kaplan, D. R., and Miller, F. D. (2000). Neurotrophin signal transduction in the nervous system. *Curr. Opin. Neurobiol.* 10:381–391.

Katz, L. C., and Shatz, C. J. (1996). Synaptic activity and the construction of cortical circuits. *Science* 274:1133–1138.

Konishi, Y., Stegmuller, J., Matsuda, T., Bonni, S., and Bonni, A. (2004). Cdh1-APC controls axonal growth and patterning in the mammalian brain. *Science* 303:1026–1030.

Lafont, F., Rouget, M., Triller, A., Prochiantz, A., and Rousselet, A. (1992). In vitro control of neuronal polarity by glycosaminoglycans. *Development* 114:17–29.

Lehmann, M., Fournier, A., Selles-Navarro, I., Dergham, P., Sebok, A., Leclerc, N., Tigyi, G., and McKerracher, L. (1999). Inactivation of Rho signaling pathway promotes CNS axon regeneration. *J. Neurosci.* 19:7537–7547.

Lentz, S. I., Knudson, C. M., Korsmeyer, S. J., Snider, W. D. (1999). Neurotrophins support the development of diverse sensory axon morphologies. *J. Neurosci.* 19:1038–1048.

Letourneau, P. C. (1978). Chemotactic response of nerve fiber elongation to nerve growth factor. *Dev. Biol.* 66:183–196.

Lindsay, R. M. (1988). Nerve growth factors (NGF, BDNF) enhance axonal regeneration but are not required for survival of adult sensory neurons. *J. Neurosci.* 8:2394–2405.

Lindsay, R. M., Thoenen, H., and Barde, Y. A. (1985). Placode and neural crest–derived sensory neurons are responsive at early developmental stages to brain-derived neurotrophic factor. *Dev. Biol.* 112:319–328.

Lodovichi, C., Di Cristo, G., Cenni, M. C., and Maffei, L. (2001). Bcl-2 overexpression per se does not promote regeneration of neonatal crushed optic fibers. *Eur. J. Neurosci.* 13:833–838.

Logan, A., Ahmed, Z., Baird, A., Gonzalez, A. M., and Berry, M. (2006). Neurotrophic factor synergy is required for neuronal survival and disinhibited axon regeneration after CNS injury. *Brain* 129:490–502.

Loh, N. K., Woerly, S., Bunt, S. M., Wilton, S. D., and Harvey, A. R. (2001). The regrowth of axons within tissue defects in the CNS is promoted by implanted hydrogel matrices that contain BDNF and CNTF producing fibroblasts. *Exp. Neurol.* 170: 72–84.

Ma, L., Lei, L., Eng, S. R., Turner, E., and Parada, L. F. (2003). Brn3a regulation of TrkA/NGF receptor expression in developing sensory neurons. *Development* 130:3525–3534.

MacInnis, B. L., and Campenot, R. B. (2002). Retrograde support of neuronal survival without retrograde transport of nerve growth factor. *Science* 295:1536–1539.

Mansour-Robaey, S., Clarke, D. B., Wang, Y. C., Bray, G. M., and Aguayo, A. J. (1994). Effects of ocular injury and administration of brain-derived neurotrophic factor on survival and regrowth of axotomized retinal ganglion cells. *Proc. Natl. Acad. Sci. U.S.A.* 91:1632–1636.

Mey, J., and Thanos, S. (1993). Intravitreal injections of neurotrophic factors support the survival of axotomized retinal ganglion cells in adult rats in vivo. *Brain Res.* 602:304–317.

Meyer-Franke, A., Kaplan, M. R., Pfrieger, F. W., and Barres, B. A. (1995). Characterization of the signaling interactions that promote the survival and growth of developing retinal ganglion cells in culture. *Neuron* 15:805–819.

Meyer-Franke, A., Wilkinson, G. A., Kruttgen, A., Hu, M., Munro, E., Hanson, M. G., Jr., Reichardt, L. F., and Barres, B. A. (1998). Depolarization and cAMP elevation rapidly recruit TrkB to the plasma membrane of CNS neurons. *Neuron* 21: 681–693.

Michaelidis, T. M., Sendtner, M., Cooper, J. D., Airaksinen, M. S., Holtmann, B., Meyer, M., and Thoenen, H. (1996). Inactivation of bcl-2 results in progressive degeneration of motoneurons, sympathetic and sensory neurons during early postnatal development. *Neuron* 17:75–89.

Ming, G., Henley, J., Tessier-Lavigne, M., Song, H., and Poo, M. (2001). Electrical activity modulates growth cone guidance by diffusible factors. *Neuron* 29:441–452.

Monsul, N. T., Geisendorfer, A. R., Han, P. J., Banik, R., Pease, M. E., Skolasky, R. L., Jr., and Hoffman, P. N. (2004). Intraocular injection of dibutyryl cyclic AMP promotes axon regeneration in rat optic nerve. *Exp. Neurol.* 186:124–133.

Morrison, J. C., Johnson, E. C., Cepurna, W., and Jia, L. (2005). Understanding mechanisms of pressure-induced optic nerve damage. *Prog. Retin. Eye Res.* 24:217–240.

Mu, X., Beremand, P. D., Zhao, S., Pershad, R., Sun, H., Scarpa, A., Liang, S., Thomas, T. L., and Klein, W. H. (2004). Discrete gene sets depend on POU domain transcription factor Brn3b/Brn-3.2/POU4f2 for their expression in the mouse embryonic retina. *Development* 131:1197–1210.

Oster, S. F., Deiner, M., Birgbauer, E., and Sretavan, D. W. (2004). Ganglion cell axon pathfinding in the retina and optic nerve. *Semin. Cell. Dev. Biol.* 15:125–136.

Qiu, J., Cai, D., Dai, H., McAtee, M., Hoffman, P. N., Bregman, B. S., and Filbin, M. T. (2002). Spinal axon regeneration induced by elevation of cyclic AMP. *Neuron* 34:895–903.

Rashid, N. A., and Cambray-Deakin, M. A. (1992). *N*-methyl-D-aspartate effects on the growth, morphology and cytoskeleton of individual neurons in vitro. *Brain Res. Dev. Brain Res.* 67:301–308.

Redmond, L., Kashani, A. H., and Ghosh, A. (2002). Calcium regulation of dendritic growth via CaM kinase IV and CREB-mediated transcription. *Neuron* 34:999–1010.

Reh, T., and Kalil, K. (1982). Functional role of regrowing pyramidal tract fibers. *J. Comp. Neurol.* 211:276–283.

Reichardt, L. F., and Tomaselli, K. J. (1991). Extracellular matrix molecules and their receptors: Functions in neural development. *Annu. Rev. Neurosci.* 14:531–570.

Riccio, A., Pierchala, B. A., Ciarallo, C. L., and Ginty, D. D. (1997). An NGF-TrkA-mediated retrograde signal to transcription factor CREB in sympathetic neurons. *Science* 277:1097–1100.

Riehl, R., Johnson, K., Bradley, R., Grunwald, G. B., Cornel, E., Lilienbaum, A., and Holt, C. E. (1996). Cadherin function is required for axon outgrowth in retinal ganglion cells in vivo. *Neuron* 17:837–848.

Saunders, N. R., Balkwill, P., Knott, G., Habgood, M. D., Mollgard, K., Treherne, J. M., and Nicholls, J. G. (1992). Growth of axons through a lesion in the intact CNS of fetal rat maintained in long-term culture. *Proc. R. Soc. Lond. B Biol. Sci.* 250:171–180.

Serafini, T., Kennedy, T. E., Galko, M. J., Mirzayan, C., Jessell, T. M., and Tessier-Lavigne, M. (1994). The netrins define a family of axon outgrowth-promoting proteins homologous to *C. elegans* UNC-6. *Cell* 78:409–424.

Shao, H., Huang, Z., Sun, S. L., Kaplan, H. J., and Sun, D. (2004). Myelin/oligodendrocyte glycoprotein-specific T-cells induce severe optic neuritis in the C57BL/6 mouse. *Invest. Ophthalmol. Vis. Sci.* 45:4060–4065.

Shatz, C. J., and Stryker, M. P. (1988). Prenatal tetrodotoxin infusion blocks segregation of retinogeniculate afferents. *Science* 242:87–89.

So, K. F., and Aguayo, A. J. (1985). Lengthy regrowth of cut axons from ganglion cells after peripheral nerve transplantation into the retina of adult rats. *Brain Res.* 328:349–354.

Stegmuller, J., Konishi, Y., Huynh, M. A., Yuan, Z., Dibacco, S., and Bonni, A. (2006). Cell-intrinsic regulation of axonal morphogenesis by the Cdh1-APC target SnoN. *Neuron* 50:389–400.

Storch, M. K., Stefferl, A., Brehm, U., Weissert, R., Wallstrom, E., Kerschensteiner, M., Olsson, T., Linington, C., and Lassmann, H. (1998). Autoimmunity to myelin oligodendrocyte glycoprotein in rats mimics the spectrum of multiple sclerosis pathology. *Brain Pathol.* 8:681–694.

Tucker, K. L., Meyer, M., and Barde, Y. A. (2001). Neurotrophins are required for nerve growth during development. *Nat. Neurosci.* 4:29–37.

Verhage, M., Maia, A. S., Plomp, J. J., Brussaard, A. B., Heeroma, J. H., Vermeer, H., Toonen, R. F., Hammer, R. E., van den Berg, T. K., et al. (2000). Synaptic assembly of the brain in the absence of neurotransmitter secretion. *Science* 287: 864–869.

Villegas-Perez, M. P., Vidal-Sanz, M., Rasminsky, M., Bray, G. M., and Aguayo, A. J. (1993). Rapid and protracted phases of retinal ganglion cell loss follow axotomy in the optic nerve of adult rats. *J. Neurobiol.* 24:23–36.

Wang, S. W., Gan, L., Martin, S. E., and Klein, W. H. (2000). Abnormal polarization and axon outgrowth in retinal ganglion cells lacking the POU-domain transcription factor Brn-3b. *Mol. Cell. Neurosci.* 16:141–156.

Wang, S. W., Mu, X., Bowers, W. J., Kim, D. S., Plas, D. J., Crair, M. C., Federoff, H. J., Gan, L., and Klein, W. H. (2002). Brn3b/Brn3c double knockout mice reveal an unsuspected role for Brn3c in retinal ganglion cell axon outgrowth. *Development* 129:467–477.

Watanabe, M., Tokita, Y., Kato, M., and Fukuda, Y. (2003). Intravitreal injections of neurotrophic factors and forskolin enhance survival and axonal regeneration of axotomized beta ganglion cells in cat retina. *Neuroscience* 116:733–742.

Watson, F. L., Heerssen, H. M., Moheban, D. B., Lin, M. Z., Sauvageot, C. M., Bhattacharyya, A., Pomeroy, S. L., and Segal, R. A. (1999). Rapid nuclear responses to target-derived neurotrophins require retrograde transport of ligand-receptor complex. *J. Neurosci.* 19:7889–7900.

Wayman, G. A., Kaech, S., Grant, W. F., Davare, M., Impey, S., Tokumitsu, H., Nozaki, N., Banker, G., and Soderling, T. R. (2004). Regulation of axonal extension and growth cone motility by calmodulin-dependent protein kinase I. *J. Neurosci.* 24:3786–3794.

Whitmore. A. V., Libby, R. T., and John, S. W. (2005). Glaucoma: Thinking in new ways. A role for autonomous axonal self-destruction and other compartmentalised processes? *Prog. Retin. Eye Res.* 24:639–662.

Yin, Y., Henzl, M. T., Lorber, B., Nakazawa, T., Thomas, T. T., Jiang, F., Langer, R., and Benowitz, L. I. (2006). Oncomodulin is a macrophage-derived signal for axon regeneration in retinal ganglion cells. *Nat. Neurosci.* 9:843–852.

Yip, H. K., and So, K, F. (2000). Axonal regeneration of retinal ganglion cells: Effect of trophic factors. *Prog. Retin. Eye Res.* 19: 559–575.

You, S. W., So, K. F., and Yip, H. K. (2000). Axonal regeneration of retinal ganglion cells depending on the distance of axotomy in adult hamsters. *Invest. Ophthalmol. Vis. Sci.* 41:3165–3170.

34 Development of the Retinogeniculate Pathway

WILLIAM GUIDO

Much of our present understanding of the mechanisms underlying the development of sensory connections is based on work done in the mammalian retinogeniculate pathway. In recent years, the mouse has come to the forefront as a model system in which to study visual system development, largely because modern molecular biology allows targeted genetic manipulation. The advent of transgenic mouse models has brought forth abundant new information about the molecular mechanisms involved in early pathfinding, visual map formation, and the subsequent activity-dependent refinement of connections. Although other vertebrate systems also allow genetic dissection, the mouse is particularly well suited for such study because its visual system has some of the rudimentary features found in higher mammals, including humans (see chapter 21).

With the emergence of mouse models, basic information about the structural and functional composition of the developing retinogeniculate pathway is needed. This chapter provides a detailed examination of the changes that occur during late prenatal and early postnatal life, when retinal axons innervate the lateral geniculate nucleus (LGN) and establish and then rearrange their connections with relay cells to form adult patterns of connectivity. This review focuses largely on studies done in a common pigmented strain (C57BL/6) and on the neural elements and related events associated specifically with the retinogeniculate pathway. Topics addressed include the pattern of retinal innervation in the LGN, the structural and functional composition of relay cells and interneurons, their associated patterns of connectivity, and the potential mechanisms underlying the remodeling of connections. The LGN also receives rich innervation from a variety of nonretinal sources, including the brainstem, thalamic reticular nucleus, and layer VI of visual cortex. Virtually nothing is known about how such nonretinal circuitry develops or how such input contributes to the maturation of retinogeniculate connections. Therefore, these aspects of LGN circuitry, while important, are not discussed.

The development of eye-specific segregation in the lateral geniculate nucleus

The topographic representation of visual fields in the retina and central visual targets is a hallmark feature of vision. Visuotopic maps are defined by an orderly series of connections that link neighboring retinal ganglion cells (RGCs) with neighboring neurons in their primary targets, such as the dorsal LGN of thalamus. For example, in the mouse, the nasal-temporal visual axis maps in a medial to lateral plane of the LGN, while upper to lower visual fields map in a dorsal to ventral direction (Grubb et al., 2003; Wagner et al., 2000). A defining feature of these maps is the segregation of inputs from the two eyes. In the LGN of carnivores and primates, retinal projections from the two eyes are divided by cytoarchitectonic laminae. LGN cells within each lamina receive monocular input from the contralateral or ipsilateral eye. However, as is the case with many nocturnal rodents, the LGN of the mouse lacks an obvious lamination pattern (figure 34.1*A*; Reese, 1988; Van Hooser and Nelson, 2006). Instead, retinal projections are organized into non-overlapping territories called eye-specific domains that can be visualized only with anterograde labeling of RGCs (figure 34.1*B*; Godement et al., 1984; Jaubert-Miazza et al., 2005).

In the adult mouse, axons from nasal retina and most of temporal retina cross at the optic chiasm and project contralaterally to the lateral and ventral regions of the LGN. Since the mouse has laterally placed eyes and poor binocular vision, in pigmented strains, the majority of retinal fibers (95%) cross at the optic chiasm (Dräger and Olsen, 1980). Crossed projections representing the contralateral eye occupy as much as 85%–90% of the total area in LGN. A much smaller group of RGCs (5%) that arise from the ventrotemporal region, known as the temporal crescent, have axons that do not cross at the optic chiasm but instead project ipsilaterally and terminate in the anteromedial region of the LGN. These uncrossed projections representing the ipsilateral eye form a patchy cylinder that runs through the

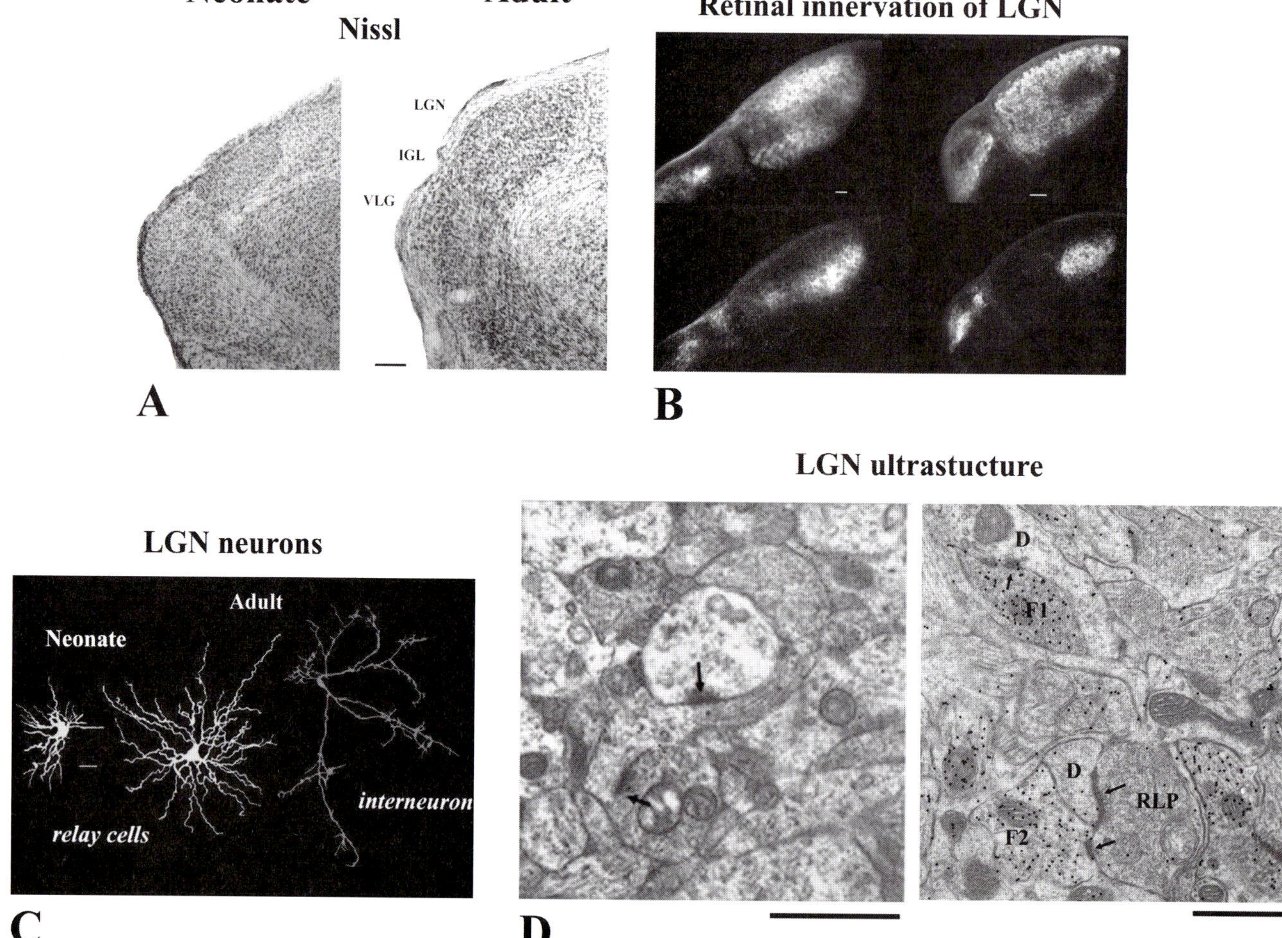

FIGURE 34.1 Anatomical organization of the developing LGN in the C57BL/6 mouse. Neonatal and adult features are shown. *A*, Coronal sections through the LGN with a Nissl stain. At early postnatal ages (P7), the LGN can be distinguished from the intrageniculate leaflet (IGL) and ventral geniculate nuclei (VLG). The cytoarchitecture of the LGN lacks an obvious eye-specific laminar pattern. Scale bar = 100 μm. *B*, Anterograde labeling of retinal projections with fluorescent conjugates of cholera toxin β subunit reveals eye-specific patterning in LGN. Shown are coronal sections through the same section of LGN. The injection of two different fluorescent conjugates reveals both the contralateral eye (crossed, images at *top*) and ipsilateral eye (uncrossed, images at *bottom*) projections. At early ages, projections show substantial overlap. In the adult, uncrossed projections form a nonoverlapping patch that is confined to the anteromedial region of LGN. Scale bars = 100 μm. *C*, Camera lucida reconstructions of biocytin-filled LGN cells. Shown are two filled relay cells (P7 and adult) and one adult interneuron. Relay cells and interneurons are readily distinguished. Developing relay cells have smaller somata and fewer arbors with shorter branches. Scale bar = 20 μm. *D*, EM micrographs showing the synaptic structure in LGN. At P7 (*left*), synapses can be identified (*arrows*), but it is not possible to categorize their composite terminals on the basis of their ultrastructure. At older ages (>P14), the ultrastructure of retinal terminals (RLP), the dendrites (D) of relay cells, and the dendritic terminals (F2) of interneurons are distinct. Note the triadic arrangement of these elements. Axon terminals (F1) of interneurons also make synaptic contact with the dendrites of relay cells. F1 and F2 GABAergic profiles are immunostained with gold particles. Scale bars = 1 μm. (*A*, *B*, and *C*, Adapted from Jaubert-Miazza et al., 2005. *D*, Adapted from Guido et al., 2008.)

rostrocaudal axis of LGN and occupies about 10%–15% of the nucleus. This form of eye-specific patterning is not apparent during the early stages of target innervation and visual map formation but emerges sometime near the end of the first postnatal week (figures 34.1*B* and 34.2*A*; see also figure 34.5; Godement et al., 1984; Jaubert-Miazza et al., 2005). Initially, crossed and uncrossed fibers innervate the LGN at different times, with crossed projections arriving earlier (at E16, about 5 days before birth) than uncrossed ones (P0). At these perinatal ages, crossed retinal projections span almost the entire LGN. Uncrossed projections also begin to fill the LGN in a widespread manner, but by P2 a rudimentary patch of terminal arbors is evident in the anteromedial sector. Between P2 and P5, the inputs from the two eyes still share a substantial amount of terminal space. By P7, retinal projections from the two eyes begin to

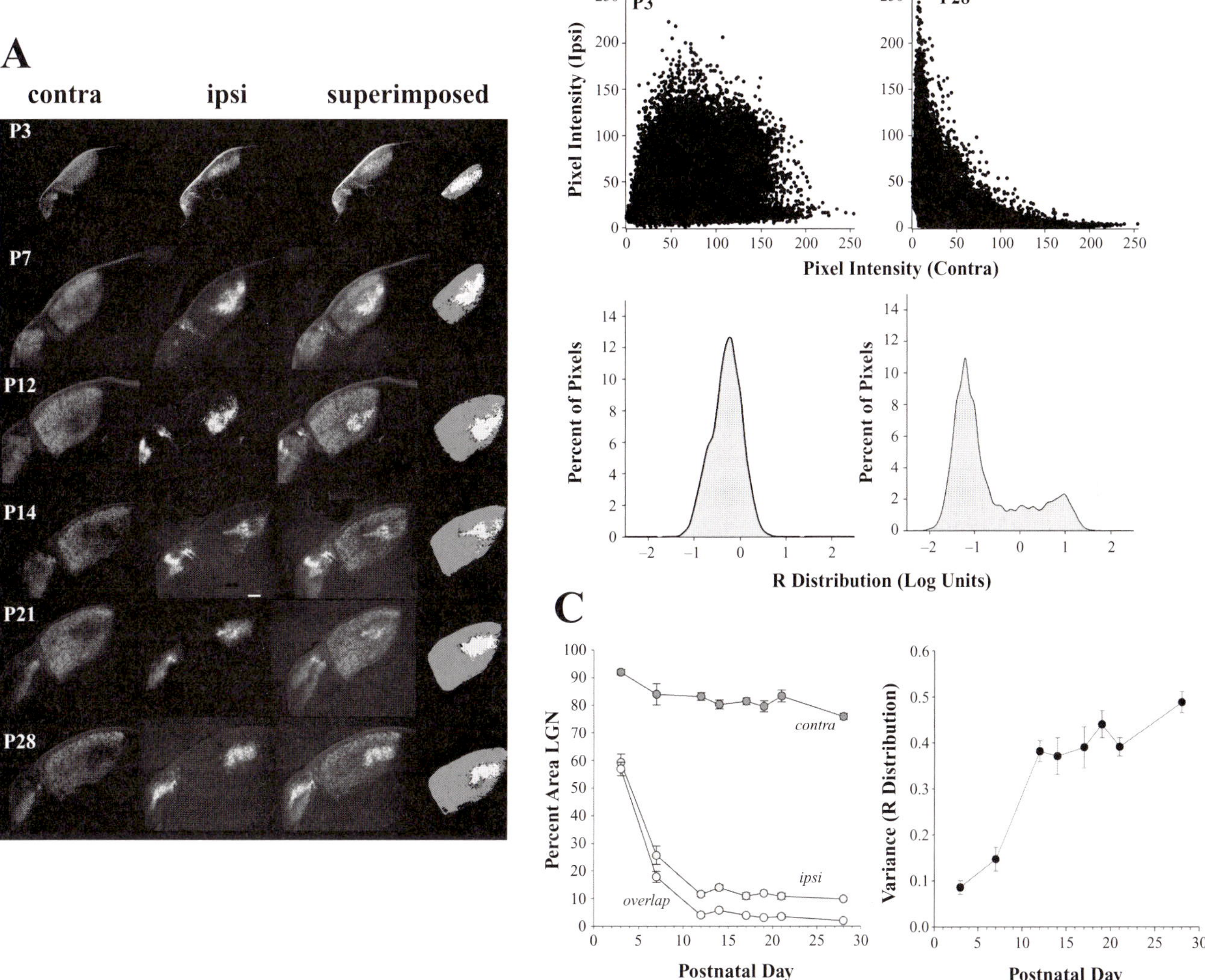

FIGURE 34.2 Retinogeniculate axon segregation in the developing mouse. *A*, Anterograde transport of CTβ conjugated to Alexa Fluor 594 (red) labels contralateral eye projections, and anterograde transport of CTβ conjugated to Alexa Fluor 488 (green) labels ipsilateral eye projections. Panels from left to right depict red and green fluorescence labeling of the same section of LGN. Adjacent to these are the superimposed fluorescent pattern and corresponding pseudo-colored image, where pixel intensity is assigned a single value above a defined threshold. Pixels that contain both red and green fluorescence are considered areas of overlap and are represented in yellow. Scale bar = 100 µm. *B*, Pixel intensity analysis reveals degree of eye-specific segregation in the developing LGN. *Top*, Scatterplots of pixel intensity for a single section through LGN at P3 and P28. Each point represents a pixel in which the fluorescence intensity of the ipsilateral projection is plotted against the intensity of the contralateral projection. At P3, when projections overlap, pixel intensities show a positive correlation. At P28, projections are segregated and pixel intensities show a negative correlation. *Bottom*, Corresponding *R* distributions of pixel intensity. For each pixel the logarithm of the intensity ratio ($R = \log_{10} F_I/F_C$) is plotted as a frequency histogram (bin size = 0.1 log units). A narrow *R* distribution (P3) shows an unsegregated pattern; a wide one (P28) shows a segregated pattern. *C*, Summary plots showing the spatial extent of retinal projections (*left*) and the variance of *R* distributions (*right*) at different ages. *Left*, Percent area in LGN occupied by contralateral, ipsilateral, and overlapping terminal fields at different ages. Each point represents the mean and SEM for a group of same-aged animals. Note that ipsilateral projections and the degree of overlap recede between P3 and P12. *Right*, Mean and SEM variance values obtained from *R* distributions. Changes in spatial extent are accompanied by a parallel increase in variance and reflect a progressive increase in the degree of eye-specific segregation between P3 and P12. See color plate 24. (Adapted from Jaubert-Miazza et al., 2005.)

show clear signs of segregation, and by natural eye opening (P12–P14), they are well segregated and resemble the pattern found in the adult.

In recent years, the cholera toxin β subunit (CTB) has been used extensively as an effective and reliable anterograde tracer (Angelucci et al., 1996; Jaubert-Miazza et al., 2005; Muir-Robinson et al., 2002; Torborg and Feller, 2004; Torborg et al., 2005). When CTB conjugated to different fluorescent dyes is injected into the eyes, retinal projections from both eyes can be visualized simultaneously in a single section of the LGN. This allows the spatial extent for crossed and uncrossed projections to be estimated and the degree of overlap that exists between them to be captured (see figure 34.2). For these types of labeling experiments, estimates of spatial extent are based on the density of pixels that express a given fluorescence intensity above some threshold value (figure 34.2*C*). At P3, uncrossed projections occupy about 60% of the LGN and overlap with crossed ones by as much as 57%. By P7, the uncrossed projections are receding but still occupy about 25% and share 20% of LGN with crossed projections. By P12–P14, the time of natural eye opening, uncrossed projections take on the adult profile, occupying around 12% of LGN and sharing little (<2%), if any, territory with crossed projections.

The difference between unsegregated and segregated retinal projections is better understood by analyzing the fluorescence intensity of individual pixels (figure 34.2*B* and *C*; see chapter 28). These measures have advantages over those that rely on spatial extent because they provide an unbiased or threshold-independent index of segregation (Torborg and Feller, 2004). Scatterplots of pixel intensity underscore a major difference between unsegregated and segregated patterns (see figure 34.2*B*). For these functions, each point represents a pixel in which the fluorescence intensity of the uncrossed projection is plotted against the intensity of the crossed one. When uncrossed and crossed projections overlap, pixel intensities are high for both and show a positive correlation. However, when projections from the two eyes segregate, pixel intensities show an inverse relationship and a negative correlation. Pixel intensity can also be expressed as the logarithm of the ratio fluorescence intensities (e.g., $R = \log_{10} F_I/F_C$) (Torborg and Feller, 2004). These ratio or *R* values can be plotted as a frequency distribution (see figure 34.2*B*). At young postnatal ages, *R* distributions tend to be narrow and unimodal because the majority of pixels have intensity values that are not dominated by one projection or the other. In contrast, at older ages, when eye-specific patterns are well developed, distributions become skewed, wide, and bimodal. The variance of *R* distributions can be used statistically to compare the relative widths of distributions across mice of different ages (see figure 34.2*C*; Jaubert-Miazza et al., 2005) or to assess differences between wild-type mice and transgenic strains (Torborg and Feller, 2004; Torborg et al., 2005; see chapter 28). In the case of retinogeniculate development, a marked increase in variance occurs between P3 and P10–P12. Interestingly, this time course parallels the changes that occur in spatial extent (see figure 34.2*C*). Taken together, they indicate that axon segregation stabilizes just prior to the period of natural eye opening. In the case of transgenic mouse models, application of these techniques has proved to be extremely powerful because it allows one to assess segregation independent of other aspects of visual map formation and refinement (Torborg and Feller, 2004; Torborg et al., 2005; see chapter 28).

The mechanisms underlying eye-specific segregation have been the topic of intense study, and transgenic mouse models have been particularly fruitful in this area (see chapters 28 and 35). Briefly, what has emerged is that molecular cues, in the form of the ephrin family of receptor tyrosine kinases and their cell surface–bound ligands, the ephrin As, play an essential role in the establishment of topographic maps and the location of eye-specific modules (Pfeiffenberger et al., 2005). However, the refinement of eye-specific segregation into nonoverlapping domains is due to the high-frequency burst discharges (Torborg and Feller, 2005; Torborg et al., 2005; see also chapter 28) associated with the wavelike patterns of spontaneous retinal activity that prevail during early postnatal life (Demas et al., 2003). At least two types of spontaneous retinal activity seem involved, an early phase (P0–P8) of cholinergic transmission that contributes to large-scale rearrangements of eye-specific territories and a late phase (P10–P14) involving glutamate signaling that drives local patterns of segregation (Muir-Robinson et al., 2002). Moreover, it appears that late phases of spontaneous retinal activity are important to maintain and stabilize newly established eye-specific patterns (Demas et al., 2006). In *nob* mutant mice, known for a defect at the rod–bipolar cell synapse, retinal axons actually desegregate following the onset of abnormal spontaneous retinal activity close to the time of natural eye opening. Finally, a recent electrophysiological report shows that newly established adultlike connections continue to remain labile well after the period of anatomical segregation. Indeed, they show a remarkable sensitivity to patterned visual activity (Hooks and Chen, 2006; see also chapter 35). Visual deprivation 1 week after natural eye opening leads to synaptic weakening and the recruitment of additional retinal inputs. Whether these fine-scale changes in connectivity can be detected with anatomical labeling techniques remains to be tested.

Structural composition of the developing retinogeniculate pathway

As in most rodent species, the LGN in the mouse is a bean-shaped nucleus that resides in the dorsolateral aspect of the thalamus. In Nissl-stained material, the nucleus is a homogeneous structure with cytoarchitectural boundaries that separate it from the ventral basal complex, medial geniculate nucleus, the intrageniculate leaflet, and the ventral geniculate nuclei (see figure 34.1*A*), although "hidden laminae" do exist in the form of eye-specific patterns of retinal innervation and as a biochemically distinct dorsolateral shell that contains small calbindin-positive cells presumed to receive input from the superior colliculus (Grubb and Thompson, 2004; Reese, 1988).

In the developing LGN, neurons differentiate between E10 and E13 (Angevine, 1970). By E16, the nucleus is visible with a Nissl stain and composed of a narrow strip of cells along the dorsolateral edge of the thalamus (Godement et al., 1984). Between E18 and early postnatal days, the LGN is readily distinguished from other adjacent nuclei (Godement et al., 1984; Jaubert-Miazza et al., 2005) and resembles the adult profile (see figure 34.1*A*).

The cellular composition of mouse LGN is similar to that of higher mammals. There are two basic cell types, thalamocortical relay cells and interneurons. In rodents, the LGN is the only sensory nucleus of thalamus that contains intrinsic interneurons. Both cell types receive retinal input, but only relay cells have axons that exit LGN and project to the visual areas of cortex. Relay cells are excitatory and utilize glutamate as a neurotransmitter, while intrinsic interneurons are inhibitory and use γ-aminobutyric acid (GABA). The morphology of neurons in the rodent LGN has been examined from Golgi-impregnated material (Grossman et al., 1973; Parnavelas et al., 1977; Rafols and Valverde, 1973) and more recently from intracellular fills performed during in vitro recording experiments (Jaubert-Miazza et al., 2005; Ziburkus and Guido, 2006). Overall, these studies show that relay cells have type I or Class A morphology, which consists of a thick unbranched axon, large, spherical somata, and complex multipolar dendritic arbors that are studded with spinelike protrusions (see figure 34.1*C*). Although relay cells display some morphological variation in soma size and dendritic complexity and orientation, it is not clear whether they can be grouped into distinct subclasses, as observed in other species such as the cat (X, Y, and W cells) or primate (M, P, and K cells). Interestingly, most relay cells in the mouse LGN show linear spatial summation in their visual response, a feature that is consistent with X cells (Grubb and Thompson, 2003). Interneurons, with type II or Class B morphology, have a smaller spindle-shaped soma and just a few long sinuous dendrites oriented in a dorsoventral plane that follows the boundaries of the LGN (see figure 34.1*C*). These cells lack a conventional axonal projection, but embedded in their dendritic trees are thin axonlike processes with terminal swellings. Relay cells and interneurons can be distinguished at early postnatal ages by using these morphological criteria or with immunocytochemical markers (Jaubert-Miazza et al., 2005) that stain for the neurofilament protein SMI-32 (relay cells) or the synthesizing enzyme for GABA (interneurons). Compared to their adult counterparts, developing cells have smaller somata and a simpler dendritic architecture comprised of fewer arbors with short branches (see figure 34.1*C*; Jaubert-Miazza et al., 2005; Rafols and Valverde, 1973). A detailed morphometric analysis in the developing mouse is presently lacking. However, in the rat, relay cells undergo two notable "growth spurts" characterized by marked changes in soma size and dendritic complexity (Parnavelas et al., 1977). One occurs at P4–P6, and the other occurs close to the time of eye natural opening (P12–P14). Interneurons seem to develop more slowly and gradually, and do not reach their mature state until P18. What remains to be examined is how the dynamic changes in dendritic complexity are coordinated with the retraction of retinal projections to form adult patterns of connectivity.

In adult mouse, the synaptic arrangements of retinal axons, relay cells, and interneurons have a highly conserved and stereotypic ultrastructure (see figure 34.1*D*; Rafols and Valverde, 1973). At the EM level, retinal (RLP) terminals make synaptic contacts with the proximal portions of relay cell dendrites. Interneurons have a conventional synaptic output via an axon that makes contact (F1 profile) with a dendrite of a relay cell. They also have presynaptic terminals (F2) that arise from their dendrites. The latter form part of a specialized triadic arrangement that involves three synapses: one between a retinal terminal and an F2 terminal, one between the same retinal terminal and the dendrite of a relay cell, and one between the F2 terminal and same dendritic appendage of a relay cell. This triadic arrangement is found within a glomerulus and provides the basis for excitatory responses in relay cells and interneurons, as well as feedforward inhibition between interneurons and relay cells. Although synapses can be readily identified at early ages (P7), it remains difficult to categorize them on the basis of their ultrastructure (see figure 34.1*D*; Slusarczyk et al., 2006). Pale mitochondria characteristic of RLP terminals can be identified, but vesicles are sparsely distributed. Further, it becomes even more difficult to distinguish inhibitory profiles even when GABA-labeled gold particles are used to identify inhibitory elements. By P14, all classes of terminals become recognizable and resemble those found in the adult (see figure 34.1*D*).

Functional composition of the developing retinogeniculate pathway

The morphological changes in cellular composition and synaptic morphology noted in the previous section are accompanied by several functional changes that occur in the membrane properties, the receptor composition of synaptic responses, and patterns of connectivity. The membrane properties of rodent LGN cells have been studied extensively using in vitro intracellular recordings in thalamic slices (Crunelli et al., 1988; Jaubert-Miazza et al., 2005; MacLeod et al., 1997). Adult LGN cells are equipped with several voltage-gated ion conductances. When active, they give rise to complex firing patterns that greatly affect the gain of retinogeniculate signal transmission (figure 34.3*A*). The most notable ones include a mixed cation conductance (I_H) that results in a strong inward rectification during membrane hyperpolarization; a low-threshold, T-type Ca^{2+} conductance that produces a large triangular depolarization (LT Ca^{2+} spike) and burst firing when the membrane is repolarized from a hyperpolarized state; a transient A-type K^+ conductance that leads to an outward rectification during membrane depolarization, thereby introducing a significant delay in spike firing; and a family of other K^+ conductances that become active during repetitive spike firing, producing after-hyperpolarizing (AHPs) responses between spikes and frequency accommodation.

Recordings done at prenatal ages indicate that thalamic cells exhibit inward and outward rectifying responses to current injection as early as E17, but rudimentary action potentials are not evident until P0 (MacLeod et al., 1997). Between P0 and P7, action potentials continue to mature, showing decreases in spike width and increases in amplitude. Sustained levels of depolarization can evoke spike trains that exhibit delays in spike firing and spike frequency accommodation. Membrane depolarization from hyperpolarized states also evokes large low-threshold Ca^{2+} spikes and burst firing. Additionally, high-threshold Ca^{2+}-mediated "spikes" can be elicited at depolarized levels. This response is transient and is observed only at early postnatal ages. By P7–P14, the full complement of active membrane properties is evident, and the voltage responses resemble those seen in the adult (Jaubert-Miazza et al., 2005; MacLeod et al., 1997). Thus, during early postnatal life, relay neurons possess many of the requisite membrane properties needed to receive, respond, and transmit afferent patterns of stimulation. In fact, developing cells are remarkably efficient at doing this. In a novel in vitro preparation in which the eyes, optic pathways, and part of the diencephalon remained intact, it was shown that spontaneous retinal activity generates periodic bursts of action potentials that are temporally coupled to the frequency of the retinal waves (Mooney et al., 1996). Thus, functional if morphologically immature synapses are present even at the earliest stages of postnatal development. However, despite the early presence of synaptic responses, the receptor composition of postsynaptic activity undergoes marked changes during the period of retinogeniculate axon segregation.

In vitro intracellular recordings made in mature LGN cells reveal that retinal stimulation evokes an excitatory postsynaptic potential (EPSP) that is typically followed by inhibitory postsynaptic (IPSP) activity (figure 34.3*B*; Blitz and Regehr, 2005; Jaubert-Miazza et al., 2005; Ziburkus et al., 2003). This EPSP/IPSP sequence reflects the pattern of triadic synaptic arrangements described earlier. Retinal axons make excitatory connections with relay cells. They also have collateral branches that make excitatory connections with interneurons, which in turn form feedforward inhibitory connections with relay cells. IPSP activity serves many functions in LGN, including shaping the center-surround antagonistic receptive field (RF) structure of relay cells, regulating tonic and burst firing patterns, and establishing the overall gain of signal transmission.

As the ultrastructure suggests, these inhibitory aspects of synaptic circuitry are not fully developed at birth. At this time, the majority of synaptic responses are purely excitatory and involve the coactivation of two ionotropic glutamate receptor subtypes, AMPA and NMDA (Chen and Regehr, 2000; Ziburkus et al., 2003). AMPA receptors mediate an early fast-rising, brief depolarization, whereas NMDA receptors contribute to a slower and longer form of excitation. The unique aspect of NMDA activity is its voltage dependency. That is, at resting membrane potentials, NMDA receptors are inactive due to a voltage-dependent blockade of the channel pore by Mg^{2+} ions. However, in the presence of strong postsynaptic depolarization, one that is likely brought about by the activation of AMPA receptors, the Mg^{2+} blockade is relieved and NMDA activation ensues. In many developing sensory structures, the voltage dependency of NMDA receptor activation serves as a "co-incident detector," allowing for an influx of Ca^{2+} ions during periods of strong postsynaptic activation. The activity-dependent influx of Ca^{2+} triggers long-term changes in synaptic strength and a series of signaling cascades that leads to the eventual consolidation of active connections, as well as the elimination of less active ones. At early ages, the excitatory responses of LGN cells are composed largely of NMDA activity (Chen and Regehr, 2000). However, during postnatal development this prevalence gradually wanes, and AMPA responses become more prominent. In fact, by P23 there is a fourfold increase in the AMPA to NMDA ratio, which contributes to the excitatory response. During this transition, NMDA responses also show reduced activation times, possibly reflecting a shift in subunit composition from NR2B to NR2A. During retinogeniculate development, NMDA responses may facilitate synapse strengthening (Chen and Regehr, 2000; Mooney et al., 1993) or contribute to the activation of other nonsynaptic, voltage-dependent events.

Although it has yet to be tested in the mouse LGN, it seems unlikely that NMDA activation leads directly to the activity-dependent refinement of eye-specific connections. Correlated firing between RGCs and LGN relay cells per-

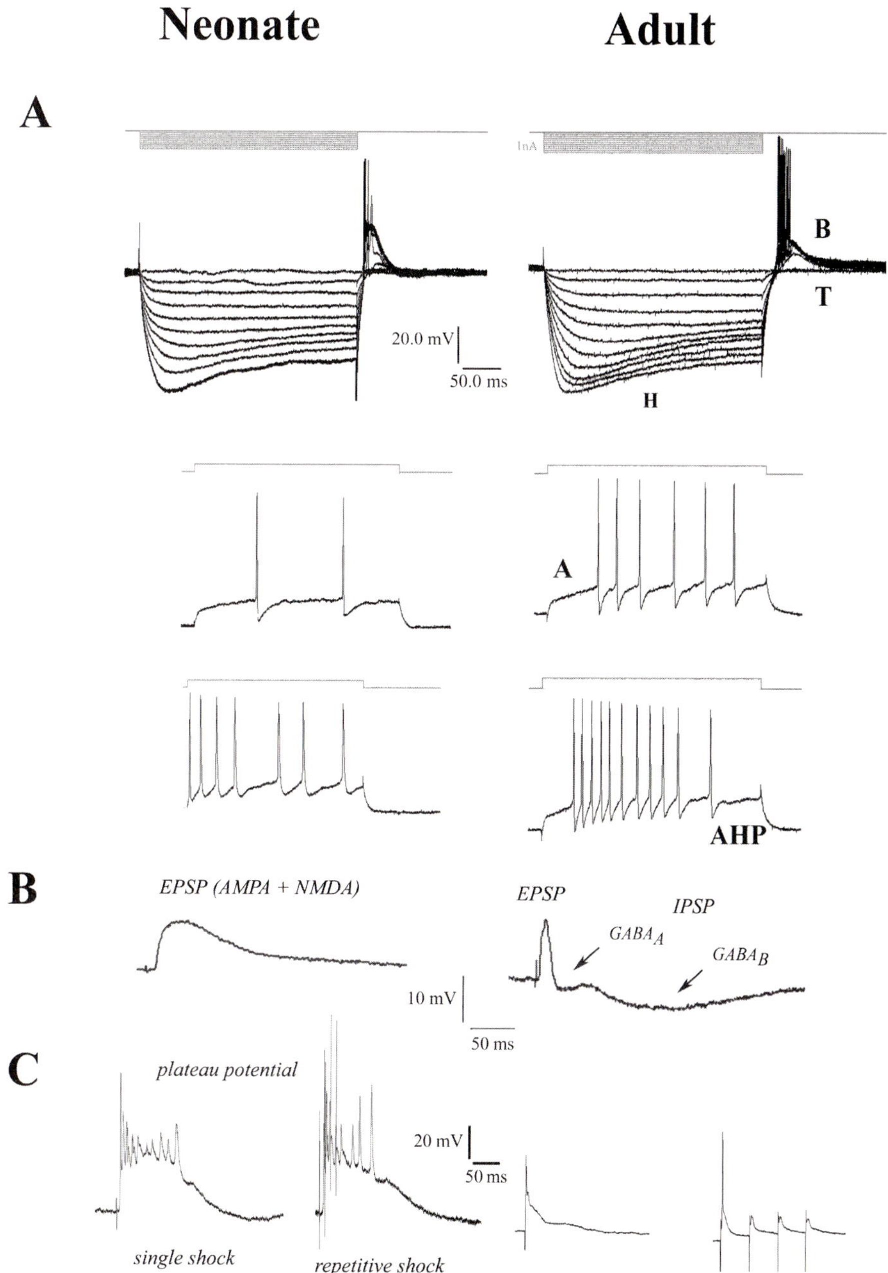

FIGURE 34.3 Electrophysiological and synaptic properties of developing LGN cells. Neonatal responses are shown on the left, and adult responses are shown on the right. *A*, Examples are shown of the voltage responses (*bottom traces*) to current pulse injections (*top traces*). Even at early postnatal ages, the voltage responses of LGN reflect the activation of a number of voltage conductances. Membrane hyperpolarization activates a mixed cation conductance (H) that results in inward rectification. Cessation of the hyperpolarizing pulses leads to the activation of a T-type Ca^{2+} conductance that produces a "rebound" triangular-shaped, low-threshold Ca^{2+} spike (T) and burst firing (B). Membrane depolarization activates a transient A-type K^+ conductance that results in outward rectification and delays spike firing. Large and sustained depolarizing pulses elicit repetitive spiking with frequency accommodation. The repolarization following between each spike activates additional K^+ conductances (AHP). *B*. Examples of postsynaptic activity (EPSP and IPSP) evoked by electrical stimulation of the optic tract. Initially evoked responses are excitatory and take the form of a long-duration EPSP that contains a large NMDA component. At later ages, the EPSP is shorter in duration and typically followed by a pair of IPSPs. The short one occurs just after the EPSP and is mediated by $GABA_A$ receptors. The longer slower one follows the early IPSP and is mediated by $GABA_B$ receptors. *C*, Synaptically evoked plateau potentials in the developing LGN. Shown are responses evoked by single or repetitive stimulation of optic tract. At early ages, suprathreshold stimulation evokes a high-amplitude, long-duration plateau potential. This response is transient and rarely observed after P14. Even strong levels of stimulation fail to evoke such a response. Single and repetitive (25–100 Hz) are shown separately. All responses were recorded between −55 and −67 mV. (Adapted from Jaubert-Miazza et al., 2005.)

sists in the absence of NMDA receptor function (Mooney et al., 1996), and in other mammals, NMDA receptor blockade does not seem to interfere with eye-specific segregation (Smetters et al., 1994), although it may be involved in more subtle forms of anatomical remodeling, such as the refinement of ON and OFF sublaminae (Hahm et al., 1991).

During the time when the receptor composition of excitatory responses is changing, inhibitory responses begin to emerge, but such activity does not fully mature until P10 (Ziburkus et al., 2003). Inhibitory responses in LGN involve two types of GABA receptors (Crunelli et al., 1988; Ziburkus et al., 2003). The first to appear is an early, fast hyperpolarizing response that involves a Cl^- conductance acting through the $GABA_A$ receptor subtype. These early fast $GABA_A$-mediated IPSPs immediately follow EPSP activity and often curtail the late NMDA component of the excitatory response. A second type of IPSP appears near the end of the first week and involves a G protein-activated K^+ conductance acting through a $GABA_B$ receptor subtype. It follows the $GABA_A$ IPSP and is slower and longlasting. Often, the slow decay of the $GABA_B$ response gives rise to a rebound LT spike and bursting.

Thus, the balance of excitatory and inhibitory responses develops at different rates, with excitatory ones maturing faster than inhibitory ones. The functional significance of this sequence is not clear, but the delayed onset of inhibitory activity may promote an increased level of excitatory postsynaptic events implicated in synaptic remodeling (e.g., NMDA and high-threshold voltage-gated Ca^{2+} channel activity) or help to mediate the transmission of strong and sustained levels of depolarization brought about by retinal wave activity (Lo et al., 2002; Mooney et al., 1996).

Finally, of notable significance is the discovery of a transient synaptic event that prevails during early postnatal life. Strong or repetitive retinal stimulation of retinal fibers evokes EPSPs that activate a high-amplitude, longlasting, slow-decaying depolarization (figure 34.3*C*). These "plateau potentials" have a voltage dependency and pharmacology consistent with the activation of high-threshold L-type (longlasting) Ca^{2+} channels (Kammermeier and Jones, 1998; Lo et al., 2002). L-type Ca^{2+} channels are found throughout the nervous system and have been implicated in a variety of cellular events, including the presynaptic release of transmitter substance, activity-dependent gene expression, cell excitability, synaptic plasticity, and cell survival (Lipscombe et al., 2004). In the rodent LGN, L-type channels are located primarily on somata and proximal dendrites (Budde et al., 1998; Jaubert-Miazza et al., 2005). Indeed, these channels reside in the same vicinity as retinal terminals (Rafols and Valverde, 1973; Slusarczyk et al., 2006), thus placing them in an ideal location to amplify retinally evoked events. Plateau potentials in LGN are encountered far more frequently between P0 and P7 (90%), then decline gradually with age so, that by P18–P21 they are rarely observed (Jaubert-Miazza et al., 2005).

At least two factors have been identified that contribute to the developmental regulation of plateau potentials (Ziburkus et al., 2003). First, the high degree of retinal convergence, coupled with heightened NMDA activity, favors the spatial and temporal summation of EPSPs. These synaptic events lead to sustained levels of depolarization and thereby greatly increase the likelihood that high-threshold L-type channels are activated. Interestingly, the episodic barrages of retinal EPSPs associated with the transmission of spontaneous retinal waves (Mooney et al., 1996) are well suited to activate L-type-mediated plateau potentials. Indeed, repetitive stimulation of retinal afferents in a manner that approximates the high-frequency discharge of retinal waves triggers robust plateau-like activity (Lo et al., 2002). Second, the density of L-type Ca^{2+} channels found among LGN cells changes with postnatal age. Using an antibody that recognizes the pore forming α_{1C} subunit of the L-type channel, Jaubert-Miazza et al. (2005) showed that expression peaks between P0 and P7 and then gradually declines, so that by P28 there is a fourfold reduction in the density of labeled cells. Finally, it is worth noting that L-type activity recorded in LGN is identical to the synaptically evoked plateau potentials recorded in developing neurons of the rodent superior colliculus (Lo and Mize, 2000) and brainstem trigeminal complex (Lo and Erzurumlu, 2002). It also bears a similarity to the high-threshold Ca^{2+} activity reported in some brainstem nuclei (Rekling and Feldman, 1997), spinal cord (Kien and Eken, 1998), and invertebrate motor neurons (Dicaprio, 1997). Thus, this event may reflect a highly conserved mechanism by which cells can acquire large amounts of Ca^{2+} in an activity-dependent manner.

Patterns of synaptic connectivity in the developing lateral geniculate nucleus

The age-related changes in postsynaptic receptor and channel function are accompanied by major modifications in the pattern of synaptic connectivity. In vivo recordings in mature mice indicate that relay cells receive monocular input (Grubb and Thompson, 2003). However, at early postnatal ages, when the inputs from the two eyes have overlapping projections, a high incidence of binocular responses is observed (Jaubert-Miazza et al., 2005; Ziburkus and Guido, 2006). In an in vitro explant preparation in which LGN circuitry and large segments of each optic nerve remained intact, separate and distinct EPSPs could be evoked by stimulating either optic nerve (figure 34.4*A*). In addition to binocular responses, another transient feature in synaptic connectivity is the high incidence of synaptic responses, reflecting the convergence of multiple RGC inputs onto a single LGN cell (Chen and Regehr, 2000; Jaubert-Miazza

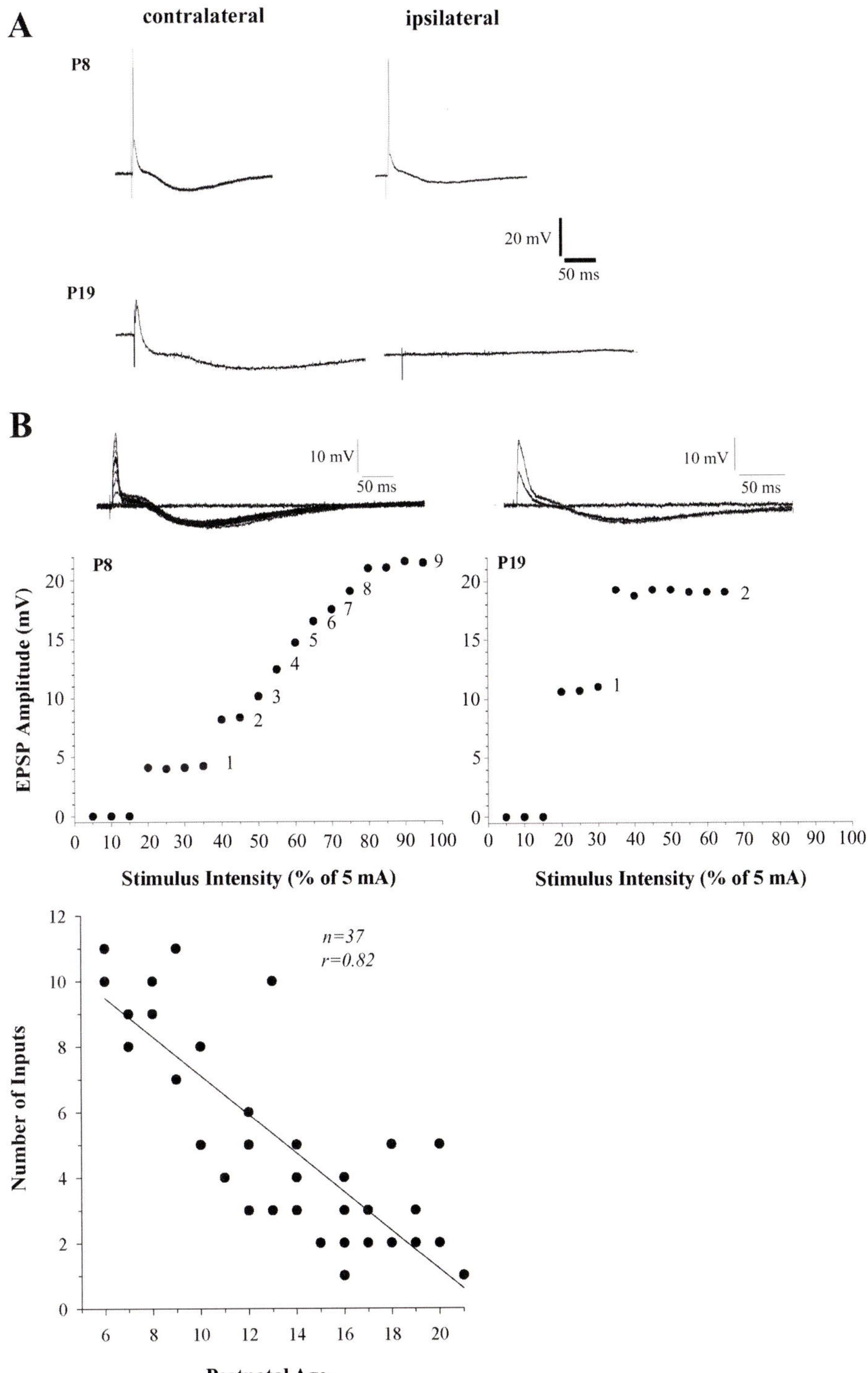

FIGURE 34.4 Synaptic connectivity in the developing LGN. *A*, Examples of EPSPs evoked by the separate stimulation of either the contralateral (*left*) or ipsilateral (*right*) optic nerve. Shown is an example of a binocular response at P8 and a monocular contralateral eye response at P19. Responses at P8 have a spike riding the peak of the EPSP. Binocular responses are frequently encountered before the period of natural eye opening. *B*, Examples of synaptic responses at P8 and P19 evoked by stimulating optic tract (OT) fibers at progressively higher levels of stimulation. Below each response is the corresponding amplitude by stimulus intensity plot. Each step is numbered and corresponds to the recruitment of a separate input. At P8, a progressive increase in stimulus intensity leads to nine incremental gradations in amplitude. At P19, increases in stimulus intensity produce only two steps. The scatterplot below plots estimates of the number of retinal inputs LGN cells receive as a function of age. Each point represents a single cell. There is an age-related decrease in retinal convergence. All responses were recorded between −60 and −67 mV. (Adapted from Jaubert-Miazza et al., 2005.)

et al., 2005; Ziburkus and Guido, 2006; see also chapter 35). Estimates of the number of synaptic inputs a relay cell receives can be obtained by gradually increasing the stimulus intensity applied to retinal fibers and then measuring the amplitude of the evoked response (figure 34.4*B*). In developing LGN cells, progressive increases in stimulus intensity often give rise to multiple stepwise increases in EPSPs (see figure 34.4*B*). These graded changes reflect the successive recruitment of active inputs innervating a single cell. In mature LGN cells tested with an identical protocol, EPSP amplitude shows far fewer steps. In general, these studies reveal a gradual reduction in retinal convergence with age (see figure 34.4*B*). During the first postnatal weeks, cells are reported to receive as many as 12–20 inputs (Chen and Regehr, 2000; Hooks and Chen, 2006; Jaubert-Miazza et al., 2005). Studies in the rat reveal that many developing cells receive up to 4–6 inputs from each eye (Ziburkus and Guido, 2006). Sometime between the second and third postnatal week, monocular responses prevail, and the number of inputs declines to 1–3, thus resembling the adult pattern of connectivity. During this pruning process, there are corresponding changes in synaptic strength. As weak inputs are eliminated, the remaining ones show as much as a 50-fold increase in synaptic strength (Chen and Regehr, 2000). Although not yet demonstrated in the developing mouse, these reported changes in retinal convergence may contribute to the postnatal maturation of RF properties. In the cat and ferret, immature RFs are binocular, quite large, irregularly shaped, and lack distinct ON and OFF subregions (Shatz and Kirkwood, 1984; Tavazoie and Reid, 2000). In contrast, mature RFs are monocular, much smaller, and have well-defined concentric center-surround organization.

The changes in synaptic connectivity described earlier persist after anatomical segregation is complete. Thus, there may be two phases of axonal remodeling: an early coarse phase, best captured by bulk anterograde labeling techniques, that involves eye-specific segregation, and another fine-scale functional form of refinement that involves the physiological strengthening of some synapses and elimination of others.

Potential mechanisms underlying the remodeling of retinogeniculate connections

While retinal waves are thought to play a prominent role in driving the refinement of retinogeniculate connections, the postsynaptic mechanisms responsible for the implementation of these changes remains unresolved. One likely mechanism is based on a Hebbian model of synaptic modification in which temporally correlated activity between pre- and postsynaptic elements leads to a strengthening (i.e., long-term potentiation, LTP) and consolidation of synapses, whereas asynchronous or absent activity results in synapse weakening (i.e., long-term depression, LTD) and synapse elimination. Hebbian-based changes in synaptic strength have been noted in several developing sensory structures, including the mammalian neocortex and the optic tectum of *Xenopus*. In some instances they also seem to contribute to the structural refinement of connections (Malenka and Bear, 2004; Ruthazer and Cline, 2004). Long-term changes in synaptic strength may also be involved in stabilizing retinogeniculate connections. Clearly, retinal waves are sufficient to generate robust postsynaptic activity in LGN (Lo et al., 2002; Mooney et al., 1996), and the "nearest-neighbor, same-eye relations" underlying the spatiotemporal patterning of wave activity seems well suited for promoting Hebbian synaptic plasticity (Torborg and Feller, 2005; see also chapters 28 and 35). Developing LGN cells also exhibit long-term changes in synaptic strength (Mooney et al., 1993) although the exact nature and polarity of these changes await further testing.

Most models of activity-dependent synaptic plasticity rely on coincident detection via NMDA receptor activation. However, a role for NMDA in driving eye-specific refinement seems unlikely. Instead, a more plausible substrate is the L-type Ca^{2+} channel. Patterned retinal activity similar to retinal waves evokes longlasting L-type-mediated plateau potentials in developing LGN cells (Lo et al., 2002). L-type activity can induce long-term changes in synaptic strength in a number of structures, including the hippocampus (Magee and Johnston, 1997), developing superior colliculus (Lo and Mize, 2000), and trigeminal principal nucleus of the brainstem (Guido et al., 2001). Additionally, synaptically evoked Ca^{2+} influx through L-type channels is particularly effective at activating transcription factors that lead to the expression of genes linked to synaptic plasticity (Lonze and Ginty, 2002; West et al., 2002). One in particular involves the cAMP response element (CRE/CREB) transcription pathway (Dolmetsch et al., 2001; Mermelstein et al., 2000). In mouse LGN, CRE-mediated gene expression peaks during early postnatal life (Pham et al., 2001). Moreover, retinofugal projections of mutant mice that show reduced levels of L-type Ca^{2+} channel activity or decreased levels of CRE expression fail to segregate properly (Cork et al., 2001; Green et al., 2004; Pham et al., 2001).

Conclusion

The structural and functional composition of the retinogeniculate pathway undergoes a rapid and dramatic period of remodeling during the first 2 weeks of life (figure 34.5). At or near the time of birth, retinal axons have already innervated the LGN, and within the first few days of postnatal life they establish a coarse topographic map. However, eye-specific domains are not yet present, and retinal projections from the two eyes are diffusely organized, having overlap-

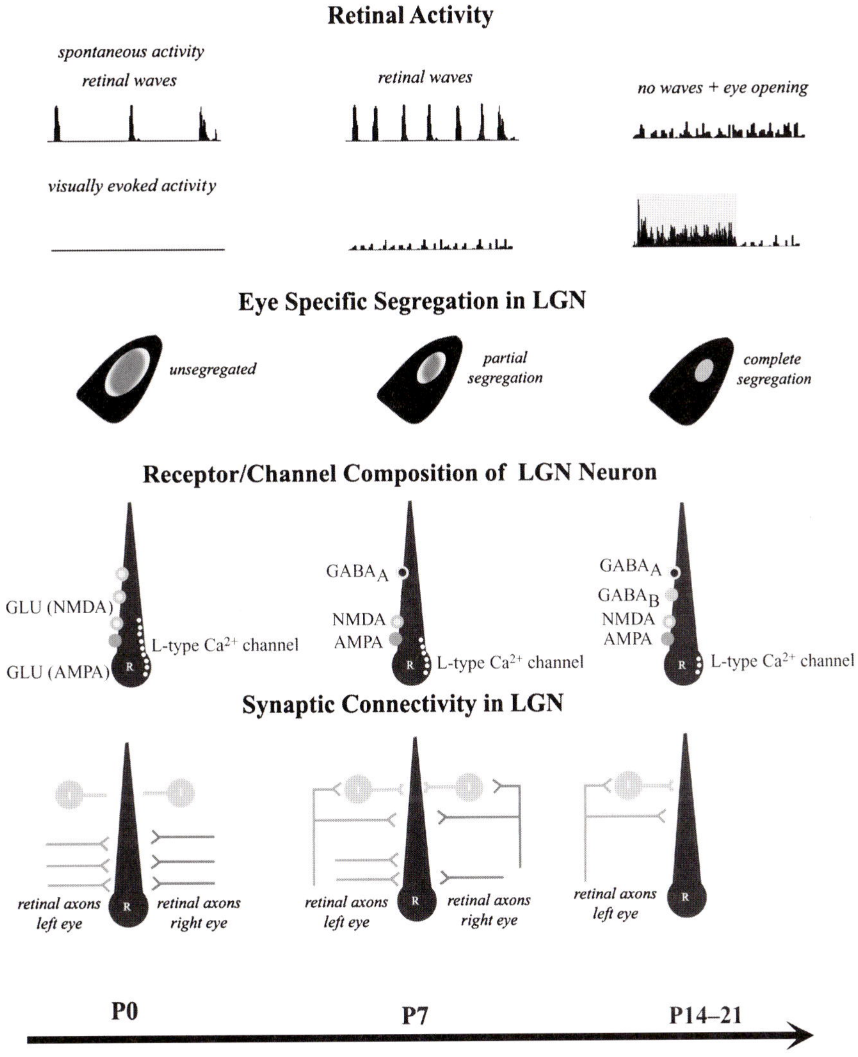

FIGURE 34.5 Summary of major developmental events occurring in the retinogeniculate pathway. *Top to bottom*, Retinal activity, degree of eye-specific segregation in LGN, receptor/channel composition of relay cells, and the pattern of synaptic connectivity are shown at three developmental time periods.

ping terminal fields in LGN. During the first postnatal week, LGN cells are growing in size and complexity and the ultrastructural features of synapses are taking shape. Functional synapses are present, and LGN cells possess the rudimentary membrane properties sufficient to fire bursts of action potentials at frequencies that match the temporal structure of retinal waves. Postsynaptic activity is largely excitatory and comprised of NMDA receptor activation. LGN cells are binocularly responsive, receiving multiple inputs from the two eyes. This high degree of retinal convergence, coupled with an elevated density of L-type Ca^{2+} channels, gives rise to plateau-like depolarizations. The large Ca^{2+} influx associated with L-type channel activation and plateau potentials may contribute to long-term changes in synaptic strength and signaling events involved in the remodeling and stabilization of developing retinogeniculate connections.

After the first postnatal week, retinal inputs from the two eyes show clear signs of segregation, while the membrane properties and spike firing continue to mature. NMDA responses, the density of L-type Ca^{2+} channels, and plateau activity also begin to subside. Inhibitory activity emerges and grows stronger through the formation of a feedforward circuit involving intrinsic interneurons. Finally, before natural eye opening (P12–P14), retinogeniculate axon segregation is complete; there occur a loss of binocular responsiveness, a further reduction in retinal convergence, and a decline in the expression of L-type Ca^{2+} channels, which ultimately contributes to elimination of plateau potential activity. After 2 weeks of age, retinal waves disappear, and visual activity provides the primary drive for newly established connections.

Although a great deal is known on the development of the mouse retinogeniculate pathway, a number of issues remained unresolved. For example, additional morphological information is needed on the growth and maturation of retinogeniculate synapses and the dendrites of relay cells. How are such changes regulated, how are they coordinated with retinal axon segregation, and to what extent do they contribute to the remodeling process? What factors govern whether certain retinal inputs are preserved and strengthened while others are weakened and eventually eliminated? Do such changes rely on retinal activity and a Hebbian form of synaptic plasticity? If so, what neural elements and signaling cascades are involved? These are but a few areas of inquiry, and further investigation is expected to shed light on the mechanisms underlying mammalian sensory development.

ACKNOWLEDGMENTS Work was supported by the National Eye Institute (grant no. EY12716). I thank Fu-Sun Lo, Martha Bickford, Erick Green, Lisa Jaubert-Miazza, Jeremy Mills, and Kim Bui for their contributions, as well as Tania Seabrook for editorial assistance.

REFERENCES

Angelucci, A., Clasca, F., and Sur, M. (1996). Anterograde axonal tracing with the subunit B of cholera toxin: A highly sensitive immunohistochemical protocol for revealing fine axonal morphology in adult and neonatal brains. *J. Neurosci. Methods* 65(1):101–112.

Angevine, J. B., Jr. (1970). Time of neuron origin in the diencephalon of the mouse: An autoradiographic study. *J. Comp. Neurol.* 139(2):129–187.

Blitz, D. M., and Regehr, W. G. (2005). Timing and specificity of feed-forward inhibition within the LGN. *Neuron* 45(6): 917–928.

Budde, T., Munsch, T., and Pape, H. C. (1998). Distribution of L-type calcium channels in rat thalamic neurones. *Eur. J. Neurosci.* 10(2):586–597.

Chen, C., and Regehr, W. G. (2000). Developmental remodeling of the retinogeniculate synapse. *Neuron* 28(3):955–966.

Cork, R. J., Namkung, Y., Shin, H. S., and Mize, R. R. (2001). Development of the visual pathway is disrupted in mice with a targeted disruption of the calcium channel beta(3)-subunit gene. *J. Comp. Neurol.* 440(2):177–191.

Crunelli, V., Haby, M., Jassik-Gerschenfeld, D., Leresche, N., and Pirchio, M. (1988). Cl^- and K^+ dependent inhibitory postsynaptic potentials evoked by interneurones of the rat lateral geniculate nucleus. *J. Physiol.* 399:153–176.

Demas, J., Eglen, S. J., and Wong, R. O. (2003). Developmental loss of synchronous spontaneous activity in the mouse retina is independent of visual experience. *J. Neurosci.* 23(7):2851–2860.

Demas, J., Sagdullaev, B. T., Green, E., Jaubert-Miazza, L., McCall, M. A., Gregg, R. G., Wong, R. O., and Guido, W. (2006). Failure to maintain eye-specific segregation in nob, a mutant with abnormally patterned retinal activity. *Neuron* 50 (2):247–259.

DiCaprio, R. (1997). Plateau potentials in motor neurons in the ventilatory system of the crab. *J. Exp. Biol.* 200(Pt. 12):1725–1736.

Dolmetsch, R. E., Pajvani, U., Fife, K., Spotts, J. M., and Greenberg, M. E. (2001). Signaling to the nucleus by an L-type calcium channel-calmodulin complex through the MAP kinase pathway. *Science* 294(5541):333–339.

Dräger, U. C., and Olsen, J. F. (1980). Origins of crossed and uncrossed retinal projections in pigmented and albino mice. *J. Comp. Neurol.* 191(3):383–412.

Godement, P., Salaun, J., and Imbert, M. (1984). Prenatal and postnatal development of retinogeniculate and retinocollicular projections in the mouse. *J. Comp. Neurol.* 230(4):552–575.

Gomez-Ospina, N., Tsuruta, F., Barreto-Chang, O., Hu, L., and Dolmetsch, R. (2006). The C terminus of the L-type voltage-gated calcium channel Ca(V)1.2 encodes a transcription factor. *Cell* 127(3):591–606.

Green, E., Bui, K., Mills, J., Shin, H., Gregg, R. G., and Guido, W. (2004). Anomalous retinal projections and altered L-type calcium channel expression in the LGN of calcium channel β3 subunit deficient mice. *Soc. Neurosci. Abstr.* 613.12.

Grossman, A., Lieberman, A. R., and Webster, K. E. (1973). A Golgi study of the rat dorsal lateral geniculate nucleus. *J. Comp. Neurol.* 150(4):441–466.

Grubb, M. S., Rossi, F. M. Changeux, J. P., and Thompson, I. D. (2003). Abnormal functional organization in the dorsal lateral geniculate nucleus of mice lacking the beta 2 subunit of the nicotinic acetylcholine receptor. *Neuron* 40(6):1161–1172.

Grubb, M. S., and Thompson, I. D. (2003). Quantitative characterization of visual response properties in the mouse dorsal lateral geniculate nucleus. *J. Neurophysiol.* 90(6):3594–3607.

Grubb, M. S., and Thompson, I. D. (2004). Biochemical and anatomical subdivision of the dorsal lateral geniculate nucleus in normal mice and in mice lacking the beta2 subunit of the nicotinic acetylcholine receptor. *Vision Res.* 44(28):3365–3376.

Guido, W., Lo, F. S., and Erzurumlu, R. S. (2001). Synaptic plasticity in the trigeminal principal nucleus during the period of barrelette formation and consolidation. *Brain Res. Dev. Brain Res.* 132(1):97–102.

Hahm, J. O., Langdon, R. B., and Sur, M. (1991) Disruption of retinogeniculate afferent segregation by antagonists to NMDA receptors. *Nature* 351:568–570.

Hooks, B. M., and Chen, C. (2006). Distinct roles for spontaneous and visual activity in remodeling of the retinogeniculate synapse. *Neuron* 52(2):281–291.

Jaubert-Miazza, L., Green, E., Lo, F. S., Bui, K., Mills, J., and Guido, W. (2005). Structural and functional composition of the developing retinogeniculate pathway in the mouse. *Vis. Neurosci.* 22(5):661–676.

Kammermeier, P. J., and Jones, S. W. (1998). Facilitation of L-type calcium current in thalamic neurons. *J. Neurophysiol.* 79(1):410–417.

Kiehn, O., and Eken, T. (1998). Functional role of plateau potentials in vertebrate motor neurons. *Curr. Opin. Neurobiol.* 8(6):746–752.

Lipscombe, D., Helton, T. D., and Xu, W. (2004). L-type calcium channels: The low down. *J. Neurophysiol.* 92(5):2633–2641.

Lo, F. S., and Erzurumlu, R. S. (2002). L-type calcium channel-mediated plateau potentials in barrelette cells during structural plasticity. *J. Neurophysiol.* 88(2):794–801.

LO, F. S., and MIZE, R. R. (2000). Synaptic regulation of L-type Ca(2+) channel activity and long-term depression during refinement of the retinocollicular pathway in developing rodent superior colliculus. *J. Neurosci.* 20(3):RC58.

LO, F. S., ZIBURKUS, J., and GUIDO, W. (2002). Synaptic mechanisms regulating the activation of a Ca^{2+} mediated plateau potential in developing relay cells of the LGN. *J. Neurophysiol.* 87(3):1175–1185.

LONZE, B. E., and GINTY, D. D. (2002). Function and regulation of CREB family transcription factors in the nervous system. *Neuron* 35(4):605–623.

MACLEOD, N., TURNER, C., and EDGAR, J. (1997). Properties of developing lateral geniculate neurones in the mouse. *Int. J. Dev. Neurosci.* 15(2):205–224.

MAGEE, J. C., and JOHNSTON, D. (1997). A synaptically controlled, associative signal for Hebbian plasticity in hippocampal neurons. *Science* 275(5297):209–213.

MALENKA, R. C., and BEAR, M. F. (2004). LTP and LTD: An embarrassment of riches. *Neuron* 44(1):5–21.

MERMELSTEIN, P. G., BITO, H., DEISSEROTH, K., and TSIEN, R. W. (2000). Critical dependence of cAMP response element-binding protein phosphorylation on L-type calcium channels supports a selective response to EPSPs in preference to action potentials. *J. Neurosci.* 20(1):266–273.

MOONEY, R., MADISON, D. V., and SHATZ, C. J. (1993). Enhancement of transmission at the developing retinogeniculate synapse. *Neuron* 10(5):815–825.

MOONEY, R., PENN, A. A., GALLEGO, R., and SHATZ, C. J. (1996). Thalamic relay of spontaneous retinal activity prior to vision. *Neuron* 17(5):863–874.

MUIR-ROBINSON, G., HWANG, B. J., and FELLER, M. B. (2002). Retinogeniculate axons undergo eye-specific segregation in the absence of eye-specific layers. *J. Neurosci.* 22(13):5259–5264.

PARNAVELAS, J. G., MOUNTY, E. J., BRADFORD, R., and LIEBERMAN, A. R. (1977). The postnatal development of neurons in the dorsal lateral geniculate nucleus of the rat: A Golgi study. *J. Comp. Neurol.* 171(4):481–499.

PFEIFFENBERGER, C., CUTFORTH, T., WOODS, G., YAMADA, J., RENTERIA, R. C., COPENHAGEN, D. R., FLANAGAN, J. G., and FELDHEIM, D. A. (2005). Ephrin-As and neural activity are required for eye-specific patterning during retinogeniculate mapping. *Nat. Neurosci.* 8(8):1022–1027.

PHAM, T. A., RUBENSTEIN, J. L., SILVA, A. J., STORM, D. R., and STRYKER, M. P. (2001). The CRE/CREB pathway is transiently expressed in thalamic circuit development and contributes to refinement of retinogeniculate axons. *Neuron* 31(3):409–420.

RAFOLS, J. A., and VALVERDE, F. (1973). The structure of the dorsal lateral geniculate nucleus in the mouse: A Golgi and electron microscopic study. *J. Comp. Neurol.* 150(3):303–332.

REESE, B. E. (1988). "Hidden lamination" in the dorsal lateral geniculate nucleus: The functional organization of this thalamic region in the rat. *Brain Res.* 472(2):119–137.

REKLING, J. C., and FELDMAN, J. L. (1997). Calcium-dependent plateau potentials in rostral ambiguus neurons in the newborn mouse brain stem in vitro. *J. Neurophysiol.* 78(5):2483–2492.

RUTHAZER, E. S., and CLINE, H. T. (2004). Insights into activity-dependent map formation from the retinotectal system: A middle of the brain perspective. *J. Neurobiol.* 59(1):134–146.

SHATZ, C. J., and KIRKWOOD, P. A. (1984). Prenatal development of functional connections in the cat's retinogeniculate pathway. *J. Neurosci.* 4:1378–1397.

SLUSARCZYK, A. S., KUCUK, C., CHOMSUNG, R., EISENBACK, M. A., GUIDO, W., and BICKFORD, M. E. (2006). Synaptic organization of the adult and neonatal mouse dorsal lateral geniculate nucleus. *Soc. Neurosci. Abstr.* 241.3.

SMETTERS, D. K., HAHM, J., and SUR, M. (1994). An *N*-methyl-D aspartate receptor antagonist does not prevent eye-specific segregation in the ferret retinogeniculate pathway. *Brain Res.* 658:168–178.

TAVAZOIE, S. F., and REID, R. C. (2000). Diverse receptive fields in the lateral geniculate nucleus during thalamocortical development. *Nat. Neurosci.* 3(6):608–616.

TORBORG, C. L., and FELLER, M. B. (2004). Unbiased analysis of bulk axonal segregation patterns. *J. Neurosci. Methods* 135(1–2):17–26.

TORBORG, C. L., and FELLER, M. B. (2005). Spontaneous patterned retinal activity and the refinement of retinal projections. *Prog. Neurobiol.* 76(4):213–235.

TORBORG, C. L., HANSEN, K. A., and FELLER, M. B. (2005). High frequency, synchronized bursting drives eye-specific segregation of retinogeniculate projections. *Nat. Neurosci.* 8(1):72–78.

VAN HOOSER, S. D., and NELSON, S. B. (2006). The squirrel as a rodent model of the human visual system. *Vis. Neurosci.* 23(5):765–778.

WAGNER, E., MCCAFFERY, P., and DRÄGER, U. C. (2000). Retinoic acid in the formation of the dorsoventral retina and its central projections. *Dev. Biol.* 222(2):460–470.

WEBSTER, M. J., and ROWE, M. H. (1984). Morphology of identified relay cells and interneurons in the dorsal lateral geniculate nucleus of the rat. *Exp. Brain Res.* 56(3):468–474.

WEST, A. E., GRIFFITH, E. C., and GREENBERG, M. E. (2002). Regulation of transcription factors by neuronal activity. *Nat. Rev. Neurosci.* 3(12):921–931.

ZIBURKUS, J., and GUIDO, W. (2006). Loss of binocular responses and reduced retinal convergence during the period of retinogeniculate axon segregation. *J. Neurophysiol.* 96(5):2775–2784.

ZIBURKUS, J., LO, F. S., and GUIDO, W. (2003). Nature of inhibitory postsynaptic activity in developing relay cells of the lateral geniculate nucleus. *J. Neurophysiol.* 90(2):1063–1070.

35 Developmental Synaptic Remodeling: Insights from the Mouse Retinogeniculate Synapse

CHINFEI CHEN

What is synaptic remodeling?

Synapses, the connections between neurons of the nervous system, have a remarkable ability to change in strength over a wide range of time scales. This process allows an organism to adapt to its external environment throughout life. During development, the large-scale rearrangement of initially redundant neuronal connections involves a combination of strengthening, weakening, elimination, and reformation of synapses. Such synaptic remodeling—the making and breaking of connections in a neuronal circuit—is crucial for proper development of the nervous system. Developmental synaptic remodeling occurs throughout the animal kingdom, in peripheral and central nervous systems, and the mechanisms underlying this process are of great interest to researchers (Katz and Shatz, 1996; Constantine-Paton and Cline, 1998).

The visual system is a powerful model for studying synaptic remodeling. The visual system is one of the best understood sensory systems and an elegant example of brain adaptation during development (Hübel and Wiesel, 1979; Hübel, 1988). Visual information is initially encoded in the retina, and the output of this processing is specific firing patterns of retinal ganglion cells (RGCs). This information is then transmitted to thalamic relay neurons in the lateral geniculate nucleus (LGN), also known as the visual thalamus, via the retinogeniculate synapse. Relay neurons in turn project to the primary visual cortex and subsequently to neighboring regions of the cortex involved in higher-order processing. At all levels of the visual system, synaptic features can be modified in response to changes in neural activity. In the retina, refinement of RGC dendritic arborization is disrupted on visual deprivation (Tian and Copenhagen, 2003). In the LGN, normal developmental segregation of retinal axons into eye-specific layers is disrupted with blockade of neuronal activity (Sretavan and Shatz, 1986; Shatz and Stryker, 1988). In the visual cortex, changes in sensory experience have profound effects on the structure and function of ocular dominance columns (Wiesel and Hubel, 1963a, 1965; Blakemore et al., 1978). Thus, the visual system is a useful model for studying synaptic remodeling over development and in response to changes in the external environment (Hubel, 1988). This review focuses largely on synaptic remodeling of the mouse LGN, where the ease of monitoring morphological changes in retinal projections and recording functional changes at synaptic connections, combined with the power of mouse genetics, has provided insight into this developmental process.

Synapses of the mouse lateral geniculate nucleus

The mouse, a nocturnal animal, has lower visual acuity than the cat, ferret, or primate. Yet examination of the cellular and synaptic organization of neurons at different levels of the mouse visual system reveals many similarities with other mammals. For example, different regions of the mouse LGN are innervated exclusively by one or the opposite eye, much like the eye-specific layers found in monkey, ferret, and cat LGN (Rakic, 1976; Linden et al., 1981; Shatz, 1983; Godement et al., 1984). Similar to the ferret, mice have their eyes positioned on the side of their head, and thus their visual system is more monocular than binocular. The majority of the mouse LGN receives retinal projections from the opposite (contralateral) eye, with only a small region in the LGN representing ipsilateral projections. This bias toward contralateral projections persists in the visual cortex, which has a relatively small binocular region, a territory where cortical pyramidal cells can be driven by visual stimuli in either eye.

At the cellular level, electron microscopy (EM) studies of the mouse LGN reveal a similar architecture to that of the cat and monkey (Szentagothai, 1963; Colonnier and Guillery, 1964; Peters and Palay, 1966; Rafols and Valverde, 1973; Lieberman, 1974). Two general classes of neurons are seen in the mouse LGN: (1) excitatory thalamic relay neurons that project to the visual cortex and (2) intrinsic interneurons. As in other mammals, thalamic relay neurons outnumber the intrinsic interneurons by approximately four to one (Steriade et al., 1997). While thalamic relay neurons are further classified based on their summation response to visual stimulation into X and Y cells in cat or primates (Cleland et al., 1971; Hoffmann et al., 1972; Shapley et al., 1981), this specialization is still unclear in the mouse. However, the majority of mouse relay neurons recorded in vivo exhibit linear spatial summation responses most similar to the characteristics of X cells (Grubb and Thompson, 2003).

RGC axons synapse on dendritic shafts as well as dendritic spines of thalamic relay neurons in the mouse (Rafols and Valverde, 1973; Lieberman, 1974). They also terminate on presynaptic dendritic structures of intrinsic interneurons that, in turn, form dendrodendritic synapses with thalamic relay neurons. This unusual configuration of synaptic structures, called triads, is thought to play a role in a fast ionotropic negative feedback circuit in cat and monkey (Famiglietti, 1970; Pasik et al., 1973; Hamos et al., 1985; Koch, 1985). An in vitro study from mouse LGN recently demonstrated activation of inhibitory current in relay neurons within 1 ms of glutamatergic retinal axon activation, consistent with a fast inhibitory output of triadic synapses (Blitz and Regehr, 2005).

At the synaptic level, the retinogeniculate synapse is glutamatergic, containing both AMPA and NMDA receptors (Chen and Regehr, 2000). Thus, neurotransmission in the mouse is similar to that in the ferret (Mooney et al., 1993), cat (Kemp and Sillito, 1982), monkey (Molinar-Rode and Pasik, 1992), and rat (Salt, 1986). Elegant EM studies in cats demonstrate that the majority of retinal axons terminate in the proximal third of the dendritic tree, while glutamatergic corticothalamic projections synapse more distally, on the thalamic relay neuron (Hamos et al., 1985; Wilson et al., 1984). Although an analogous study is lacking in the mouse, patch-clamp recordings of excitatory postsynaptic currents (EPSCs) at retinogeniculate synapses demonstrate a very rapid AMPA receptor EPSC decay time course ($\tau = 1$–2 ms), consistent with a proximal location of the synapses (Chen and Regehr, 2000). In contrast, EPSCs from corticothalamic synapses exhibit slower decay kinetics, which most likely reflects their distal position in the relay neuron dendritic tree (Golshani et al., 1998).

Robust synapse remodeling in the mouse lateral geniculate nucleus

Our current understanding of developmental synaptic remodeling in the LGN, shaped from work from many laboratories, is that synapse development and maturation can be separated into at least three distinct phases: (1) coarse mapping and rearrangement of RGC axons in the LGN, (2) fine-scale refinement of neuronal circuitry and functional maturation of synaptic connections, and (3) maintenance of mature synaptic connections (figure 35.1). In the first phase, axons from presynaptic RGCs must map to the postsynaptic relay neurons, distinguishing their proper targets from inappropriate targets. At the retinogeniculate synapse, presynaptic neurons can be labeled in retina, and thus the first phase of remodeling has been elegantly visualized in many species (Rakic, 1976; Linden et al., 1981; Shatz, 1983; Jeffery, 1984; Ziburkus and Guido, 2006), including the mouse (Godement et al., 1984; Muir-Robinson et al., 2002; Jaubert-Miazza et al., 2005). These studies demonstrate that the mapping of retinal axons is initially diffuse, and then, over development, there is a large-scale rearrangement of RGC axon terminals into their eye-specific layers (Sretavan and Shatz, 1984, 1986; see also chapters 28 and 34).

By the time the bulk of eye-specific segregation is complete (P0 in cat, P8–P12 in ferret, mouse, and rat), synaptic contacts have formed and are functional (Shatz and

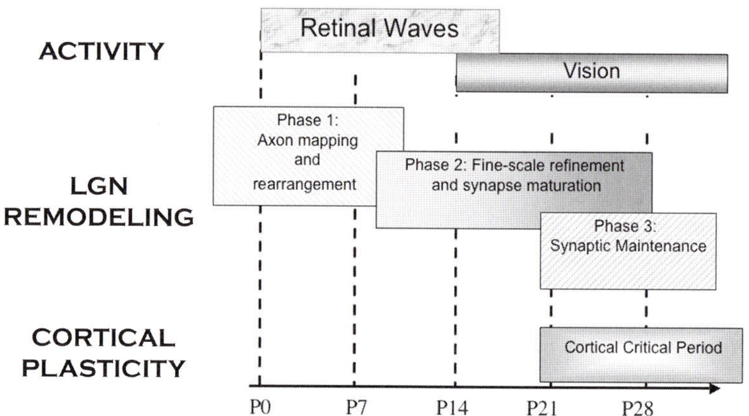

FIGURE 35.1 Timeline of three phases of synapse remodeling in the mouse lateral geniculate nucleus. The initial phase involves retinal axon mapping and coarse rearrangement of axons into eye-specific layers. In the second phase, synaptic connectivity refines, as many synapses are functionally eliminated while others strengthen. During the third phase, synaptic maintenance depends on vision. Time windows for different forms of activity and the cortical critical period are superimposed for comparison.

Kirkwood, 1984; Ramoa and McCormick, 1994; Chen and Regehr, 2000; Jaubert-Miazza et al., 2005; Ziburkus and Guido, 2006). However, a number of features suggest that these synapses are immature at this time (Ramoa and McCormick, 1994; Chen and Regehr, 2000). Synaptic strength is weak, as assessed by the amplitude of the AMPA receptor currents, while the AMPAR/NMDAR current ratio is low. Moreover, the time course of NMDA receptor decay kinetics is slow, consistent with a lack of NR2A receptor, a subunit of NMDAR that is inserted as the synapse matures (Carmignoto and Vicini, 1992; Hestrin, 1992; Monyer et al., 1992, 1994; Vicini et al., 1998). Studies using in vitro preparations of the mouse LGN demonstrate that subsequent synaptic development after axons have segregated into eye-specific layers involves an increase in AMPAR/NMDAR current ratio, an acceleration of NMDAR decay time course, and intense remodeling of the connectivity between RGC and LGN relay neurons (Chen and Regehr, 2000; Jaubert-Miazza et al., 2005).

In a region of the mouse LGN that receives mainly projections from the contralateral retina by P7, 10–15 RGC inputs are estimated to innervate a given LGN neuron between P9 and P11, while the average synaptic strength is weak (Chen and Regehr, 2000). Over the next 2 weeks, spanning the time of eye opening (P12–P14), the number of inputs decreases, or prunes, down to one to three inputs, while the average strength of the remaining inputs increases 20-fold (figure 35.2). Insofar as sharpening of LGN receptive fields (RFs) occurs after eye opening in the cat, ferret, and monkey (Daniels et al., 1978; Blakemore and Vital-Durand, 1986; Tavazoie and Reid, 2000), it is plausible that the large-scale synaptic rearrangement described in mice contributes to this sharpening process. Surprisingly, although the bulk of synaptic remodeling during this second phase of remodeling occurs around eye opening, it does not depend on vision. Instead, spontaneous activity is the driving force of synaptic remodeling during this developmental phase (Hooks and Chen, 2006).

The third phase of remodeling of the retinogeniculate synapse is notable for its dependence on vision (Hooks and Chen, 2006). Dark rearing from birth in mice does not appear to alter the normal developmental remodeling of the retinogeniculate synapse. In contrast, deprivation after a week of vision results in a dramatic change in connectivity. When mice are dark reared from P20 for more than a week (also referred to as late dark rearing), the number of inputs increases from about 3–4 at P20 to about 10 at P27–P32. Concurrently, the strength of the average retinal input decreases by more than half. Thus, visual experience is necessary to maintain LGN circuitry during the third phase of synaptic remodeling. It is currently unclear whether this rearrangement is a reflection of reactivation of previously "eliminated" synapses or the sprouting of de novo synapses.

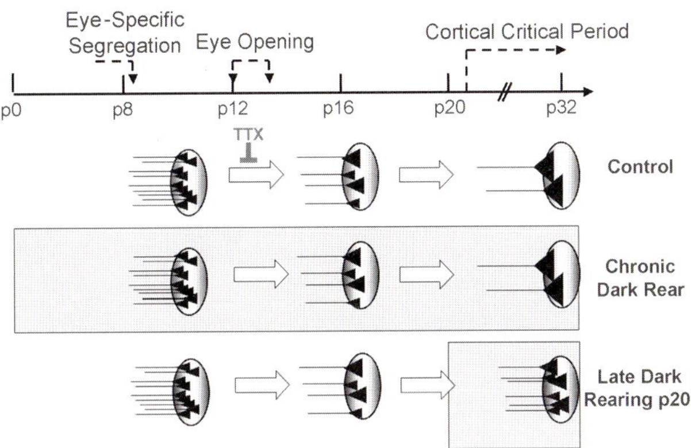

FIGURE 35.2 Role of activity in retinogeniculate development. Shown are changes in the strength and number of RGC axons that innervate an LGN relay neuron over development. Visual deprivation from birth does not appear to disrupt the normal developmental process. However, after exposure to visually evoked activity, the synaptic connections become dependent on vision.

Activity and the three phases of synapse remodeling

Studies in mice thus reveal three phases of plasticity that appear to be regulated by different mechanisms. All are activity dependent, but the relationship between activity and plasticity is different in each case. Both activity and molecular cues play an important role in axon mapping in the first phase of remodeling (Katz and Shatz, 1996). Careful studies involving pharmacological manipulations in the eye and the use of mouse mutants have demonstrated that segregation of these fibers is dependent on retinal waves, synchronous bursts of neuronal activity that march across the retina with a periodicity of 1–2 minutes (Galli and Maffei, 1988; Meister et al., 1991; Wong et al., 1993; Feller et al., 1997; Penn et al., 1998; Muir-Robinson et al., 2000), see also chapters 28 and 34. In addition to retinal waves, axon guidance cues, notably the ephrins, play an important role in axon mapping (Feldheim et al., 1998, 2000; Lyckman et al., 2001; Huberman et al., 2005). Eye-specific layering defects are greater in ephrin-A2, -A3, and -A5 knockout mice that have disruption of retinal waves than in the same mice with normal retinal waves or in mice with abnormal retinal waves (Pfeiffenberger et al., 2005, 2006). Thus, retinal waves and axon guidance cues appear to have distinct roles in dictating the final location of RGC axon terminals.

The second phase of synapse remodeling, between P9 and P20 in mice, is also dependent on spontaneous activity, although the relationship between activity and remodeling is not linear. Inhibiting retinal activity for 12 hours per day over 4 days did not disrupt synaptic remodeling (unpublished observations). Instead, continuous blockade of all activity in the retina over 4 days is necessary for significant retardation of developmental synapse pruning and strengthening (Hooks and Chen, 2006). Thus, the threshold of activity necessary for the second phase of remodeling at the retinogeniculate synapse is very low.

How the first developmental phase of eye-specific segregation relates to the functional synapse plasticity seen during the second phase is unclear. Specific features of retinal waves appear to drive the morphological rearrangement of retinal axon arbors to the proper region of the mouse LGN (Torborg et al., 2005; Demas et al., 2006; but see also Huberman et al., 2003; Grubb and Thompson, 2004; Huberman and Chapman, 2006). However, it is unclear which aspect of these patterns is important for the subsequent functional remodeling of synapses. Indeed, genetically altered mice lacking the nicotinic acetylcholine receptor β_2 subunit (nAChR-β_2; beta 2 mice) exhibit disrupted retinal waves and eye-specific segregation (Muir-Robinson et al., 2002), but only mild abnormalities in LGN RF properties (Grubb et al., 2003; Cang et al., 2005). At the synaptic level, preliminary studies from our laboratory show that developmental input pruning and strengthening of the retinogeniculate synapse are not significantly disrupted at mature ages (>P25) in either beta 2 mice or ephrin-A2/A5 knockout mice (unpublished observations; Hooks et al., 2004). Thus, the second phase of synaptic remodeling is not simply a continuation of the rearrangement of retinal axon fibers seen before P8. The mechanisms underlying the first and second phases of developmental remodeling are likely to be different.

Two aspects of the third phase of plasticity are activity dependent. During this period, maintenance of synaptic connections requires visually evoked activity. Thus, expression of this phase of synaptic remodeling is vision dependent. However, the expression of synaptic plasticity during the third phase is not dependent on cumulative levels of activity. In chronically dark-reared animals, a slowing of NMDA receptor decay time course occurs, but only after P21 in age; deprivation after P21 results in the same effects. Thus, deprivation experiments in mice clearly demonstrate a specific window of development when synaptic function becomes sensitive to visual deprivation.

The dependence on vision occurs only with a history of prior visual experience, suggesting that patterned visually evoked activity, but not spontaneous activity, is necessary for induction of the third phase of synaptic remodeling. It is unclear whether the feature of vision that is important for induction is a specific pattern of activity or whether a threshold level of absolute activity is necessary. The sensory conditions for chronic and late dark-reared animals are identical after P20, yet the response of the retinogeniculate synapse is quite distinct. Thus the difference between the two conditions lies in the period between eye opening and P20. In mice, retinal waves persist for a few days after eye opening, begin to break down by P15, and have completely disappeared by P21 (Demas et al., 2003). Thus there is a short time between eye opening and P21 when both retinal waves and visually evoked activity are seen by LGN relay neurons. Dark rearing during this period does not significantly disrupt retinal wave activity yet may reduce the total level of activity. It is tempting to hypothesize that the induction of vision-dependent synaptic remodeling depends on the total level of activity.

Plasticity in the lateral geniculate nucleus: Comparing the mouse to other species

Data from the mouse suggest there is a great deal of functional plasticity in the LGN, especially during the third phase of remodeling. Is there plasticity in the LGN of other species? Chronic dark-rearing studies in kittens from birth to 4 months of age (a time that corresponds to the end of the cortical critical period in this species) revealed normal RF responses from X cells (Kratz et al., 1979). However, there appeared to be a reduction in the number of physiologically identifiable Y cells in both the monocular and binocular regions of the LGN. These findings were consistent with morphological studies showing an increase in neurons containing laminated bodies, thought to represent X cells, in dark-reared cats (LeVay and Ferster, 1977; Kalil and Worden, 1978). Because neurons of the mouse LGN have not been classified into X and Y cell categories, direct comparisons of the effects of chronic dark rearing in mouse and cat are difficult. If, however, there is a predominance of X cells in mice (Grubb and Thompson, 2003), the lack of dramatic synaptic remodeling at the mouse retinogeniculate synapse in response to chronic dark rearing would be consistent with that previously described in cat. In ferrets, dark rearing at P16 through closed eyelids resulted in convergence of ON- and OFF-center responses. Whether abnormalities in ON/OFF segregation correspond directly to changes in retinogeniculate connectivity or to changes in RGC dendritic arborization (or both) is not clear (Ackerman et al., 2002; Tian and Copenhagen, 2003).

There are remarkably few studies in the LGN examining the physiological consequences to dark rearing during the cortical critical period in cat or monkey that could be compared directly to the third phase of synaptic remodeling in mice. Most studies in these larger mammals have involved monocular or binocular deprivation. The classic work of Wiesel and Hubel demonstrated that only 20% of relay neurons displayed irregular RF properties in the LGN in monocularly deprived kittens during the period when ocular dominance plasticity is robust (Wiesel and Hübel, 1963a, 1963b). However, these studies focused mainly on the midline area of the LGN, representing the region of the visual field that is projected on both left and right retinas (Hübel, 1988). It is unclear whether recordings in the LGN representing the temporal part of the visual field, presumably receiving monocular innervation, would have revealed a different physiology. Interestingly, a study examining monocular deprivation of the rabbit, a species in which more than 90% of the LGN receives monocular innervation, demonstrated a specific developmental time window during which visual deprivation results in disrupted RF properties (Baumbach and Chow, 1978). Moreover, these authors described a later phase of development when vision is needed for maintenance of the RF.

Surprisingly, binocular eyelid suturing in cats elicited different responses than dark rearing or monocular deprivation. For example, monocular deprivation results in a reduction of the size of geniculate neuron somata in the binocular segment of the LGN (Wiesel and Hübel, 1963a), although relay neurons in the monocular segment of the same layer (the region that receives innervation from the deprived eye but not the nondeprived eye) are unaffected (Guillery, 1972). In contrast, binocular suturing results in milder effects on soma size in the binocular region of the LGN, with a greater effect on the monocular segment of the LGN (Wiesel and Hübel, 1965; Guillery, 1972; Hickey et al., 1977). Finally, dark rearing does not significantly affect geniculate soma size. Although it is still unclear why there should be a difference in results of binocular eye suturing and dark rearing, recent data from ferret raise the possibility that light perceived through closed eyelids may represent a differentiating factor (Akerman et al., 2002).

Comparison of remodeling in the lateral geniculate nucleus to other regions of the visual system

The Vision-Sensitive Phase of Lateral Geniculate Nucleus Remodeling and the Cortical Critical Period The vision-dependent period of synaptic remodeling during development of the mouse retinogeniculate synapse corresponds strikingly to the cortical critical period in mouse (Gordon and Stryker, 1996; Hensch, 2004), despite differences in the form of visual deprivation (dark rearing vs. monocular deprivation). Similar to the findings in the LGN, visual deprivation elicits a change in the response of cortical neurons only during a specific developmental window. The analogous change in the binocular region of the visual cortex involves a shift in the responsiveness of cortical neurons to stimulation of one eye or the other, that is, a shift in the ocular dominance (OD) preference of cortical neurons. It is still unclear how the plasticity between the LGN and cortex relate to each other during this developmental period. Both feedback and feedforward processes may influence the response of the LGN and cortex to visual deprivation.

In the mouse visual cortex, changes in OD plasticity depend strongly on the balance of excitatory and inhibitory circuit interactions (Hensch, 2005). The maturation of inhibitory circuits plays an important role in this balance. Manipulations of the level of GABAergic inhibition in the visual cortex can alter the onset of the critical period, consistent with the idea that the induction of OD plasticity is dependent on the maturation of inhibitory synapses (Hensch et al., 1998; Fagiolini and Hensch, 2000). In the future, it will be interesting to determine whether activation of the inhibitory circuitry in the LGN is also important in the induction of the third phase of remodeling in the LGN.

In contrast to the weakening and change in connectivity of retinogeniculate synapses in response to late dark rearing, intracortical glutamatergic synapses onto pyramidal neurons in the monocular region of the visual cortex are unchanged in response to 3 days of deprivation during the cortical critical period (Maffei et al., 2006). Instead, synapses between inhibitory fast-spiking basket cells and star pyramidal neurons strengthen, consistent with a role for LTP of inhibitory circuits in the expression of OD plasticity. However, longer periods of monocular deprivation (40 days) result in the shrinkage of thalamocortical axon arbors serving the deprived eye and further shift OD preference (Antonini et al., 1999). Moreover, some forms of OD plasticity have been shown to be NMDA receptor dependent (Sawtell et al., 2003). This finding, along with studies that demonstrate occlusion of long-term synaptic depression (LTD) in the binocular visual cortex by previous monocular deprivation, suggests that LTD of excitatory synapses may also be involved in synapse remodeling in the cortex (Heynen et al., 2003; Crozier et al., 2007).

The Superior Colliculus Many axons of RGCs bifurcate and innervate both the LGN and superior colliculus (SC; Illing, 1980; Yamadori et al., 1989). Despite their having the same presynaptic neurons, however, there are notable differences in the developmental remodeling of the retinal synapses onto the two subcortical regions. In genetically altered mice with disrupted retinal axon mapping, such as those lacking ephrin-A2/A3/A5, nAChR-β_2, serotonergic receptor 5-HT_{1B}, or the serotonin transporter, mapping defects are greater in the SC than in the LGN (Upton et al., 1999, 2002; Feldheim et al., 2000; Pfeiffenberger et al., 2005, 2006). Consistent with axon mapping defects, RFs in the mice with disrupted retinal waves (beta 2 mice) are more distorted in the SC than in the LGN (Grubb et al., 2003; Chandrasekaran et al., 2005; Mrsic-Flogel et al., 2005).

In vitro studies of rat SC demonstrate that glutamatergic inputs onto superficial collicular neurons also prune at the synaptic level during development (Lu and Constantine-Paton, 2004). In contrast to the LGN, acceleration of this normal process occurs within 24 hours after eye opening. However, in the brain slice preparation of the superficial laminae of the rodent colliculus, it is difficult to selectively stimulate inputs from the cortex, retina, and brainstem.

Thus, the specific class of inputs innervating the collicular neurons that exhibit sensitivity to visual activity during development is still not clear. Moreover, the bulk of pruning still occurs in visually deprived rats, although with a lag when compared with rats reared in a 12-hour light-dark cycle (Lu and Constantine-Paton, 2004). Thus, vision accelerates the time course of the pruning in the colliculus, although the process can occur at a slower rate without sensory experience. These differences between the LGN and the SC during the first and second phases of synapse remodeling suggest that the rules governing developmental synaptic remodeling may also be cell-type specific for RGC targets.

Despite differences in synaptic maturation between different visual system areas, similarities also exist with respect to the role of vision. As for the LGN, the role of sensory experience in the development of the SC varies among species. Chronic visual deprivation does not disrupt the average RF properties of neurons in hamster SC (Rhoades and Chalupa, 1978; Chalupa and Rhoades, 1978) or rabbit (Chow and Spear, 1974). In contrast, binocular eyelid closure in kittens results in significant changes in direction sensitivity in collicular neurons, consistent with a reduction in the Y indirect and direct pathways (Hoffmann and Sherman, 1975). In addition, a recent study examining a number of developmental time points during prolonged chronic dark rearing revealed that collicular RFs gradually become larger (Carrasco et al., 2005). Thus, the role of vision in the maintenance of synapses or synaptic circuits may be a common theme at the retinogeniculate, retinotectal, and cortical synapses of the visual system across species (Crair et al., 1998; Carrasco et al., 2005; Hooks and Chen, 2006).

Genes involved in synapse remodeling

There is a great deal of interest in identifying the genes involved in synaptic remodeling. The power of mouse genetics can be harnessed to this end. Because this field is quite extensive, I cannot do justice to all the candidate genes for developmental synaptic remodeling. Thus, in this chapter, I highlight only some genes that are proposed to play a role in synapse remodeling in the LGN.

Two recent studies using unbiased differential gene expression screens in the visual cortex identified groups of activity-dependent genes that had relatively little overlap (Majdan and Shatz, 2006; Tropea et al., 2006). However, a number of themes emerged from these studies. Both groups found that although there is a set of genes that appear to be regulated by general changes in activity, there are also sets of genes regulated by reducing visually evoked activity in both eyes (dark rearing) that differed from those identified by altering the balance of activity between the two eyes (monocular deprivation or enucleation). Moreover, certain genes are regulated only during a particular developmental window, such as during the cortical critical period, and still others require previous visual experience for normal regulation of gene expression. In the future, it will be interesting to assess whether synaptic remodeling in the different regions of the visual system, in particular the visual cortex and LGN, share common regulatory gene mechanisms.

Other activity-dependent gene expression screens have identified candidates that may contribute to the large-scale synaptic remodeling observed at the retinogeniculate synapse. One gene of interest, cpg15 (candidate plasticity gene 15), was identified from a forward genetic screen in the rat hippocampus after seizure induction (Nedivi et al., 1993). Cpg15 is an activity-dependent gene expressed in the visual system of the cat, rat, mice, and tadpole (Nedivi et al., 1996, 2001; Corriveau et al., 1999) that encodes a secreted protein that binds to the extracellular membrane via glycosylphosphatidylinositol linkage (Naeve et al., 1997). In *Xenopus laevis*, infection of cpg15 in tectal neurons enhances dendritic arbor growth (Nedivi et al., 1998). In the rat, cpg15 is expressed at high levels in the LGN in the first 2 postnatal weeks and then declines with age. At a corresponding developmental period when cgp15 levels are high in cat (prenatally), infusion of the sodium channel inhibitor tetrodotoxin (TTX) into the cerebrospinal fluid or injection of TTX into the eye does not alter cgp15 levels in the contralateral LGN. In contrast, monocular TTX injections at a time corresponding to the onset of the cortical critical period (P18+ in the cat) results in a decrease in LGN cpg15 levels (Corriveau et al., 1999). Expression of cpg15 also occurs in the cortex, lagging developmentally behind that in the LGN. In rat, cpg15 levels are detected at P10 and increase between the second and third postnatal weeks before decreasing in the adult (Nedivi et al., 1996). At the peak of the cortical critical period, cgp15 expression gradually becomes dependent on retinal-driven action potentials. Dark rearing during that time decreases the peak levels of cpg15, but, more interestingly, it prevents the normal developmental decline in cpg15 levels in adulthood. Moreover, previous visual experience during a specific developmental window is important for proper regulation of cpg15 expression (Lee and Nedivi, 2002). Thus, cpg15 exhibits an expression pattern that shares many developmental features of the sensitive/critical period in both LGN and cortex. It will be interesting to examine whether this gene plays a role in glutamatergic synapse remodeling.

Another screen for genes whose expression in the cat LGN changes when spontaneous activity is blocked with intracranial infusion of TTX identified the class I major histocompatibility complex (MHC I) antigen (Corriveau et al., 1998), a protein previously shown to play a role in cell-mediated immune recognition. TTX injected monocularly in the cat reduced the expression of MHC I mRNA. In mice, MHC I is present in the LGN at P6, and the expression decreases by P40. In addition to the visual system,

MHC I is also found in the hippocampus and cortex. Genetically modified mice deficient in either MHC I or a subunit of the MHC receptor (CD3ζ) demonstrate defects in eye-specific layer formation (Huh et al., 2000). Moreover, hippocampal LTP in these mutant mice is enhanced, while LTD is absent. These findings suggest that MHC I plays a role in the developmental remodeling of neuronal axon morphology as well as functional synapses. It will be interesting to determine whether MHC I plays a role in remodeling of the retinogeniculate synapse, and if so, what phase of remodeling it regulates.

Another group of molecules of interest are the neuronal pentraxins, a family of synaptic proteins that have homology to acute phase proteins (pentraxins) of the immune system. Neuronal pentraxins (NP1 and NP2) are present in the mouse LGN at P7, a developmental time when eye-specific layering is nearly complete. The levels of NP1 decrease by P14. In contrast, NP2 is still highly expressed in retinal axons, and NP receptor expression increases during this developmental period. Although NP1/2 knockout mice exhibit abnormal segregation of eye-specific layers, the number of synaptic contacts, assessed in cultures of purified RGCs from these mutant animals, was not different from that seen in cultures from wild-type mice. However, the normal developmental increase in the frequency of mEPSCs did not occur in cultures from the knockout mice, suggesting that although synapses were present, they did not mature normally (Bjartmar et al., 2006).

With growing evidence of different phases of developmental synapse remodeling, it will be important to determine the stage of remodeling each identified candidate gene regulates. For example, neuronal pentraxin affects the early stage of eye-specific layering and possibly synapse maturation (the first and second phase of remodeling). In contrast, mutant mice lacking paired-immunoglobulin-like receptors (PirB mice), a class I MHC receptor, exhibit normal developmental changes of eye-specific inputs in the LGN and cortex (Syken et al., 2006). However, in PirB mice, OD plasticity, as measured indirectly by arc labeling (Tagawa et al., 2005), persists past the normal critical period (Syken et al., 2006). These findings suggest that PirB plays a role in the cortical critical period. It will be interesting to examine whether PirB also plays a role in the third phase of synaptic remodeling at the retinogeniculate synapse.

Conclusion

Our understanding of synaptic remodeling in the CNS continues to grow. Future work will benefit from the power of well-established mouse models of visual development and from mouse genetics. With increasing evidence of distinct phases of synaptic maturation, it is likely that future studies will be able to identify distinct phases of active pruning and maintenance that appear to be governed by different genes and forms of activity.

A number of questions have yet to be answered. One basic question is, what is the purpose of developmental synaptic remodeling? Although some synaptic connections in the CNS exhibit large-scale changes over the course of development, others develop with striking specificity and do not exhibit an early period of refinement (Callaway and Lieber, 1996; Bender et al., 2003; Bureau et al., 2004). One proposed model suggests that transient connections in the LGN are used to establish fine-tuned, oriented RFs in the visual cortex (Tavazoie and Reid, 2000). An alternative model arises from an observation applicable to many areas of the brain, namely, that the ability to adapt to changes is enhanced by previous experience (Knudsen et al., 2000; Hofer et al., 2006b). Perhaps the "memory" of previously pruned synaptic connections provides a scaffold for potential changes in the adult brain (DeBello et al., 2001; Linkenhoker et al., 2005; Hofer et al., 2006a). This may be a principle that is generalizable to the entire CNS.

ACKNOWLEDGMENTS Work was supported by the National Eye Institute (grant no. EY013613) and by the Children's Hospital, Boston, Mental Retardation and Developmental Disabilities Research Center (grant no. PO1 HD18655). I thank B. M. Hooks, Xiaojin Liu, James Choi, Alan Mardinly, Brett Carter, and Whitney Blair for their contributions.

REFERENCES

Akerman, C. J., Smyth, D., and Thompson, I. D. (2002). Visual experience before eye-opening and the development of the retinogeniculate pathway. *Neuron* 36:869–879.

Antonini, A., Fagiolini, M., and Stryker, M. P. (1999). Anatomical correlates of functional plasticity in mouse visual cortex. *J. Neurosci.* 19:4388–4406.

Baumbach, H. D., and Chow, K. L. (1978). Receptive field development in the dorsal lateral geniculate nucleus in rabbits subjected to monocular eyelid suture. *Brain Res.* 159:69–83.

Bender, K. J., Rangel, J., and Feldman, D. E. (2003). Development of columnar topography in the excitatory layer 4 to layer 2/3 projection in rat barrel cortex. *J. Neurosci.* 23:8759–8770.

Bjartmar, L., Huberman, A. D., Ullian, E. M., Renteria, R. C., Liu, X., Xu, W., Prezioso, J., Susman, M. W., Stellwagen, D., et al. (2006). Neuronal pentraxins mediate synaptic refinement in the developing visual system. *J. Neurosci.* 26:6269–6281.

Blakemore, C., Garey, L. J., and Vital-Durand, F. (1978). The physiological effects of monocular deprivation and their reversal in the monkey's visual cortex. *J. Physiol.* 283:223–262.

Blakemore, C., and Vital-Durand, F. (1986). Organization and post-natal development of the monkey's lateral geniculate nucleus. *J. Physiol.* 380:453–491.

Blitz, D. M., and Regehr, W. G. (2005). Timing and specificity of feed-forward inhibition within the LGN. *Neuron* 45:917–928.

Bureau, I., Shepherd, G. M. G., and Svoboda, K. (2004). Precise development of functional and anatomical columns in the neocortex. *Neuron* 42:789–801.

Callaway, E. M., and Lieber, J. L. (1996). Development of axonal arbors of layer 6 pyramidal neurons in ferret primary visual cortex. *J. Comp. Neurol.* 376:295–305.

Cang, J., Kaneko, M., Yamada, J., Woods, G., Stryker, M. P., and Feldheim, D. A. (2005). Ephrin-As guide the formation of functional maps in the visual cortex. *Neuron* 48:577–589.

Carmignoto, G., and Vicini, S. (1992). Activity-dependent decrease in NMDA receptor responses during development of the visual cortex. *Science* 258:1007–1011.

Carrasco, M. M., Razak, K. A., and Pallas, S. L. (2005). Visual experience is necessary for maintenance but not development of receptive fields in superior colliculus. *J. Neurophysiol.* 94:1962–1970.

Chalupa, L. M., and Rhoades, R. W. (1978). Directional selectivity in hamster superior colliculus is modified by strobe-rearing but not by dark-rearing. *Science* 199:998–1001.

Chandrasekaran, A. R., Plas, D. T., Gonzalez, E., and Crair, M. C. (2005). Evidence for an instructive role of retinal activity in retinotopic map refinement in the superior colliculus of the mouse. *J. Neurosci.* 25:6929–6938.

Chen, C., and Regehr, W. G. (2000). Developmental remodeling of the retinogeniculate synapse. *Neuron* 28:955–966.

Chow, K. L., and Spear, P. D. (1974). Morphological and functional effects of visual deprivation on the rabbit visual system. *Exp. Neurol.* 42:429–447.

Cleland, B. G., Dubin, M. W., and Levick, W. R. (1971). Sustained and transient neurones in the cat's retina and lateral geniculate nucleus. *J. Physiol.* 217:473–496.

Colonnier, M., and Guillery, R. W. (1964). Synaptic organization in the lateral geniculate nucleus of the monkey. *Z. Zellforsch. Mikrosk. Anat.* 62:333–355.

Constantine-Paton, M., and Cline, H. T. (1998). LTP and activity-dependent synaptogenesis: The more alike they are, the more different they become. *Curr. Opin. Neurobiol.* 8:139–148.

Corriveau, R. A., Huh, G. S., and Shatz, C. J. (1998). Regulation of class I MHC gene expression in the developing and mature CNS by neural activity. *Neuron* 21:505–520.

Corriveau, R. A., Shatz, C. J., and Nedivi, E. (1999). Dynamic regulation of cpg15 during activity-dependent synaptic development in the mammalian visual system. *J. Neurosci.* 19:7999–8008.

Crair, M. C., Gillespie, D. C., and Stryker, M. P. (1998). The role of visual experience in the development of columns in cat visual cortex. *Science* 279:566–570.

Crozier, R. A., Wang, Y., Liu, C. H., and Bear, M. F. (2007). Deprivation-induced synaptic depression by distinct mechanisms in different layers of mouse visual cortex. *Proc. Natl. Acad. Sci. U.S.A.* 104:1383–1388.

Daniels, J. D., Pettigrew, J. D., and Norman, J. L. (1978). Development of single-neuron responses in kitten's lateral geniculate nucleus. *J. Neurophysiol.* 41:1373–1393.

DeBello, W. M., Feldman, D. E., and Knudsen, E. I. (2001). Adaptive axonal remodeling in the midbrain auditory space map. *J. Neurosci.* 21:3161–3174.

Demas, J., Eglen, S. J., and Wong, R. O. (2003). Developmental loss of synchronous spontaneous activity in the mouse retina is independent of visual experience. *J. Neurosci.* 23:2851–2860.

Demas, J., Sagdullaev, B. T., Green, E., Jaubert-Miazza, L., McCall, M. A., Gregg, R. G., Wong, R. O., and Guido, W. (2006). Failure to maintain eye-specific segregation in nob, a mutant with abnormally patterned retinal activity. *Neuron* 50:247–259.

Fagiolini, M., and Hensch, T. K. (2000). Inhibitory threshold for critical-period activation in primary visual cortex. *Nature* 404:183–186.

Famiglietti, E. V., Jr. (1970). Dendro-dendritic synapses in the lateral geniculate nucleus of the cat. *Brain Res.* 20:181–191.

Feldheim, D. A., Kim, Y. I., Bergemann, A. D., Frisen, J., Barbacid, M., and Flanagan, J. G. (2000). Genetic analysis of ephrin-A2 and ephrin-A5 shows their requirement in multiple aspects of retinocollicular mapping. *Neuron* 25:563–574.

Feldheim, D. A., Vanderhaeghen, P., Hansen, M. J., Frisen, J., Lu, Q., Barbacid, M., and Flanagan, J. G. (1998). Topographic guidance labels in a sensory projection to the forebrain. *Neuron* 21:1303–1313.

Feller, M. B., Butts, D. A., Aaron, H. L., Rokhsar, D. S., and Shatz, C. J. (1997). Dynamic processes shape spatiotemporal properties of retinal waves. *Neuron* 19:293–306.

Galli, L., and Maffei, L. (1988). Spontaneous impulse activity of rat retinal ganglion cells in prenatal life. *Science* 242:90–91.

Godement, P., Salaun, J., and Imbert, M. (1984). Prenatal and postnatal development of retinogeniculate and retinocollicular projections in the mouse. *J. Comp. Neurol.* 230:552–575.

Golshani, P., Warren, R. A., and Jones, E. G. (1998). Progression of change in NMDA, non-NMDA, and metabotropic glutamate receptor function at the developing corticothalamic synapse. *J. Neurophysiol.* 80:143–154.

Gordon, J. A., and Stryker, M. P. (1996). Experience-dependent plasticity of binocular responses in the primary visual cortex of the mouse. *J. Neurosci.* 16:3274–3286.

Grubb, M. S., Rossi, F. M., Changeux, J. P., and Thompson, I. D. (2003). Abnormal functional organization in the dorsal lateral geniculate nucleus of mice lacking the beta 2 subunit of the nicotinic acetylcholine receptor [see comment]. *Neuron* 40:1161–1172.

Grubb, M. S., and Thompson, I. D. (2003). Quantitative characterization of visual response properties in the mouse dorsal lateral geniculate nucleus. *J. Neurophysiol.* 90:3594–3607.

Grubb, M. S., and Thompson, I. D. (2004). The influence of early experience on the development of sensory systems. *Curr. Opin. Neurobiol.* 14:503–512.

Guillery, R. W. (1972). Binocular competition in the control of geniculate cell growth. *J. Comp. Neurol.* 144:117–129.

Hamos, J. E., Van Horn, S. C., Raczkowski, D., Uhlrich, D. J., and Sherman, S. M. (1985). Synaptic connectivity of a local circuit neurone in lateral geniculate nucleus of the cat. *Nature* 317:618–621.

Hensch, T. K. (2004). Critical period regulation. *Annu. Rev. Neurosci.* 27:549–579.

Hensch, T. K. (2005). Critical period plasticity in local cortical circuits. *Nat. Rev. Neurosci.* 6:877–888.

Hensch, T. K., Fagiolini, M., Mataga, N., Stryker, M. P., Baekkeskov, S., and Kash, S. F. (1998). Local GABA circuit control of experience-dependent plasticity in developing visual cortex. *Science* 282:1504–1508.

Hestrin, S. (1992). Developmental regulation of NMDA receptor-mediated synaptic currents at a central synapse. *Nature* 357:686–689.

Heynen, A. J., Yoon, B. J., Liu, C. H., Chung, H. J., Huganir, R. L., and Bear, M. F. (2003). Molecular mechanism for loss of visual cortical responsiveness following brief monocular deprivation. *Nat. Neurosci.* 6:854–862.

Hickey, T. L., Spear, P. D., and Kratz, K. E. (1977). Quantitative studies of cell size in the cat's dorsal lateral geniculate nucleus following visual deprivation. *J. Comp. Neurol.* 172:265–282.

Hofer, S. B., Mrsic-Flogel, T. D., Bonhoeffer, T., and Hubener,

M. (2006a). Lifelong learning: Ocular dominance plasticity in mouse visual cortex. *Curr. Opin. Neurobiol.* 16:451–459.

Hofer, S. B., Mrsic-Flogel, T. D., Bonhoeffer, T., and Hubener, M. (2006b). Prior experience enhances plasticity in adult visual cortex. *Nat. Neurosci.* 9:127–132.

Hoffmann, K. P., and Sherman, S. M. (1975). Effects of early binocular deprivation on visual input to cat superior colliculus. *J. Neurophysiol.* 38:1049–1059.

Hoffmann, K. P., Stone, J., and Sherman, S. M. (1972). Relay of receptive-field properties in dorsal lateral geniculate nucleus of the cat. *J. Neurophysiol.* 35:518–531.

Hooks, B. M., and Chen, C. (2006). Distinct roles for spontaneous and visual activity in remodeling of the retinogeniculate synapse. *Neuron* 52:281–291.

Hooks, B. M., Feldheim, D., Flanagan, J. G., and Chen, C. (2004). Mechanisms of synaptic remodeling. Paper presented at a satellite symposium meeting of ARVO, "Mouse Visual System," Fort Lauderdale.

Hübel, D. H. (1988). *Eye, brain, and vision.* Scientific American Library. Distibuted by W. H. Freeman, New York.

Hübel, D. H., and Wiesel, T. N. (1979). Brain mechanisms of vision. *Sci. Am.* 241:150–162.

Huberman, A. D., and Chapman, B. (2006). Making and breaking eye-specific projections to the lateral geniculate nucleus. In R. Erzurumlu, W. Guido, and Z. Molnar (Eds.), *Development and plasticity in sensory thalamus and cortex* (pp. 247–270). New York: Springer Science + Business Media.

Huberman, A. D., Murray, K. D., Warland, D. K., Feldheim, D. A., and Chapman, B. (2005). Ephrin-As mediate targeting of eye-specific projections to the lateral geniculate nucleus. *Nat. Neurosci.* 8:1013–1021.

Huberman, A. D., Wang, G. Y., Liets, L. C., Collins, O. A., Chapman, B., and Chalupa, L. M. (2003). Eye-specific retinogeniculate segregation independent of normal neuronal activity. *Science* 300:994–998.

Huh, G. S., Boulanger, L. M., Du, H. P., Riquelme, P. A., Brotz, T. M., and Shatz, C. J. (2000). Functional requirement for class I MHC in CNS development and plasticity. *Science* 290:2155–2159.

Illing, R. B. (1980). Axonal bifurcation of cat retinal ganglion cells as demonstrated by retrograde double labelling with fluorescent dyes. *Neurosci. Lett.* 19:125–130.

Jaubert-Miazza, L., Green, E., Lo, F. S., Bui, K., Mills, J., and Guido, W. (2005). Structural and functional composition of the developing retinogeniculate pathway in the mouse. *Vis. Neurosci.* 22:661–676.

Jeffery, G. (1984). Retinal ganglion cell death and terminal field retraction in the developing rodent visual system. *Brain Res.* 315:81–96.

Kalil, R., and Worden, I. (1978). Cytoplasmic laminated bodies in the lateral geniculate nucleus of normal and dark reared cats. *J. Comp. Neurol.* 178:469–485.

Katz, L. C., and Shatz, C. J. (1996). Synaptic activity and the construction of cortical circuits. *Science* 274:1133–1138.

Kemp, J. A., and Sillito, A. M. (1982). The nature of the excitatory transmitter mediating X and Y cell inputs to the cat dorsal lateral geniculate nucleus. *J. Physiol.* 323:377–391.

Knudsen, E. I., Zheng, W., and DeBello, W. M. (2000). Traces of learning in the auditory localization pathway. *Proc. Natl. Acad. Sci. U.S.A.* 97:11815–11820.

Koch, C. (1985). Understanding the intrinsic circuitry of the cat's lateral geniculate nucleus: Electrical properties of the spine-triad arrangement. *Proc. R. Soc. Lond. B. Biol. Sci.* 225:365–390.

Kratz, K. E., Sherman, S. M., and Kalil, R. (1979). Lateral geniculate nucleus in dark-reared cats: Loss of Y cells without changes in cell size. *Science* 203:1353–1355.

Lee, W. C., and Nedivi, E. (2002). Extended plasticity of visual cortex in dark-reared animals may result from prolonged expression of cpg15-like genes. *J. Neurosci.* 22:1807–1815.

LeVay, S., and Ferster, D. (1977). Relay cell classes in the lateral geniculate nucleus of the cat and the effects of visual deprivation. *J. Comp. Neurol.* 172:563–584.

Lieberman, A. R. (1974). Comments on the fine structural organization of the dorsal lateral geniculate nucleus of the mouse. *Anat. Embryol. (Berl.)* 145:261–267.

Linden, D. C., Guillery, R. W., and Cucchiaro, J. (1981). The dorsal lateral geniculate nucleus of the normal ferret and its postnatal development. *J. Comp. Neurol.* 203:189–211.

Linkenhoker, B. A., von der Ohe, C. G., and Knudsen, E. I. (2005). Anatomical traces of juvenile learning in the auditory system of adult barn owls. *Nat. Neurosci.* 8:93–98.

Lu, W., and Constantine-Paton, M. (2004). Eye opening rapidly induces synaptic potentiation and refinement. *Neuron* 43:237–249.

Lyckman, A. W., Jhaveri, S., Feldheim, D. A., Vanderhaeghen, P., Flanagan, J. G., and Sur, M. (2001). Enhanced plasticity of retinothalamic projections in an ephrin-A2/A5 double mutant. *J. Neurosci.* 21:7684–7690.

Maffei, A., Nataraj, K., Nelson, S. B., and Turrigiano, G. G. (2006). Potentiation of cortical inhibition by visual deprivation. *Nature* 443:81–84.

Majdan, M., and Shatz, C. J. (2006). Effects of visual experience on activity-dependent gene regulation in cortex. *Nat. Neurosci.* 9:650–659.

Meister, M., Wong, R. O., Baylor, D. A., and Shatz, C. J. (1991). Synchronous bursts of action potentials in ganglion cells of the developing mammalian retina. *Science* 252:939–943.

Molinar-Rode, R., and Pasik, P. (1992). Amino acids and *N*-acetyl-aspartyl-glutamate as neurotransmitter candidates in the monkey retinogeniculate pathways. *Exp. Brain Res.* 89:40–48.

Monyer, H., Burnashev, N., Laurie, D. J., Sakmann, B., and Seeburg, P. H. (1994). Developmental and regional expression in the rat brain and functional properties of four NMDA receptors. *Neuron* 12:529–540.

Monyer, H., Sprengel, R., Schoepfer, R., Herb, A., Higuchi, M., Lomeli, H., Burnashev, N., Sakmann, B., and Seeburg, P. H. (1992). Heteromeric NMDA receptors: Molecular and functional distinction of subtypes. *Science* 256:1217–1221.

Mooney, R., Madison, D. V., and Shatz, C. J. (1993). Enhancement of transmission at the developing retinogeniculate synapse. *Neuron* 10:815–825.

Mrsic-Flogel, T. D., Hofer, S. B., Creutzfeldt, C., Cloez-Tayarani, I., Changeux, J. P., Bonhoeffer, T., and Hübener, M. (2005). Altered map of visual space in the superior colliculus of mice lacking early retinal waves. *J. Neurosci.* 25:6921–6928.

Muir-Robinson, G., Hwang, B. J., and Feller, M. B. (2002). Retinogeniculate axons undergo eye-specific segregation in the absence of eye-specific layers. *J. Neurosci.* 22:5259–5264.

Naeve, G. S., Ramakrishnan, M., Kramer, R., Hevroni, D., Citri, Y., and Theill, L. E. (1997). Neuritin: A gene induced by neural activity and neurotrophins that promotes neuritogenesis. *Proc. Natl. Acad. Sci. U.S.A.* 94:2648–2653.

Nedivi, E., Fieldust, S., Theill, L. E., and Hevron, D. (1996). A set of genes expressed in response to light in the adult cerebral cortex and regulated during development. *Proc. Natl. Acad. Sci. U.S.A.* 93:2048–2053.

Nedivi, E., Hevroni, D., Naot, D., Israeli, D., and Citri, Y. (1993). Numerous candidate plasticity-related genes revealed by differential cDNA cloning. *Nature* 363:718–722.

Nedivi, E., Javaherian, A., Cantallops, I., and Cline, H. T. (2001). Developmental regulation of CPG15 expression in *Xenopus*. *J. Comp. Neurol.* 435:464–473.

Nedivi, E., Wu, G. Y., and Cline, H. T. (1998). Promotion of dendritic growth by CPG15, an activity-induced signaling molecule. *Science* 281:1863–1866.

Pasik, T., Pasik, P., Hamori, J., and Szentagothai, J. (1973). "Triadic" synapses and other articulations of interneurons in the lateral geniculate nucleus of rhesus monkeys. *Trans. Am. Neurol. Assoc.* 98:293–295.

Penn, A. A., Riquelme, P. A., Feller, M. B., and Shatz, C. J. (1998). Competition in retinogeniculate patterning driven by spontaneous activity. *Science* 279:2108–2112.

Peters, A., and Palay, S. L. (1966). The morphology of laminae A and A1 of the dorsal nucleus of the lateral geniculate body of the cat. *J. Anat.* 100:451–486.

Pfeiffenberger, C., Cutforth, T., Woods, G., Yamada, J., Renteria, R. C., Copenhagen, D. R., Flanagan, J. G., and Feldheim, D. A. (2005). Ephrin-As and neural activity are required for eye-specific patterning during retinogeniculate mapping. *Nat. Neurosci.* 8:1022–1027.

Pfeiffenberger, C., Yamada, J., and Feldheim, D. A. (2006). Ephrin-As and patterned retinal activity act together in the development of topographic maps in the primary visual system. *J. Neurosci.* 26:12873–12884.

Rafols, J. A., and Valverde, F. (1973). The structure of the dorsal lateral geniculate nucleus in the mouse: A Golgi and electron microscopic study. *J. Comp. Neurol.* 150:303–332.

Rakic, P. (1976). Prenatal genesis of connections subserving ocular dominance in the rhesus monkey. *Nature* 261:467–471.

Ramoa, A. S., and McCormick, D. A. (1994). Enhanced activation of NMDA receptor responses at the immature retinogeniculate synapse. *J. Neurosci.* 14:2098–2105.

Rhoades, R. W., and Chalupa, L. M. (1978). Receptive field characteristics of superior colliculus neurons and visually guided behavior in dark-reared hamsters. *J. Comp. Neurol.* 177:17–32.

Salt, T. E. (1986). Mediation of thalamic sensory input by both NMDA receptors and non-NMDA receptors. *Nature* 322:263–265.

Sawtell, N. B., Frenkel, M. Y., Philpot, B. D., Nakazawa, K., Tonegawa, S., and Bear, M. F. (2003). NMDA receptor-dependent ocular dominance plasticity in adult visual cortex. *Neuron* 38:977–985.

Shapley, R., Kaplan, E., and Soodak, R. (1981). Spatial summation and contrast sensitivity of X and Y cells in the lateral geniculate nucleus of the macaque. *Nature* 292:543–545.

Shatz, C. J. (1983). The prenatal development of the cat's retinogeniculate pathway. *J. Neurosci.* 3:482–499.

Shatz, C. J., and Kirkwood, P. A. (1984). Prenatal development of functional connections in the cat's retinogeniculate pathway. *J. Neurosci.* 4:1378–1397.

Shatz, C. J., and Stryker, M. P. (1988). Prenatal tetrodotoxin infusion blocks segregation of retinogeniculate afferents. *Science* 242:87–89.

Sretavan, D., and Shatz, C. J. (1984). Prenatal development of individual retinogeniculate axons during the period of segregation. *Nature* 308:845–848.

Sretavan, D. W., and Shatz, C. J. (1986). Prenatal development of retinal ganglion cell axons: Segregation into eye-specific layers within the cat's lateral geniculate nucleus. *J. Neurosci.* 6:234–251.

Steriade, M., Jones, E. G., and McCormick, D. A. (1997). *Thalamus*. Oxford: Elsevier.

Syken, J., Grandpre, T., Kanold, P. O., and Shatz, C. J. (2006). PirB restricts ocular-dominance plasticity in visual cortex. *Science* 313:1795–1800.

Szentagothai, J. (1963). The structure of the synapse in the lateral geniculate body. *Acta Anat.* (*Basel*) 55:166–185.

Tagawa, Y., Kanold, P. O., Majdan, M., and Shatz, C. J. (2005). Multiple periods of functional ocular dominance plasticity in mouse visual cortex. *Nat. Neurosci.* 8:380–388.

Tavazoie, S. F., and Reid, R. C. (2000). Diverse receptive fields in the lateral geniculate nucleus during thalamocortical development. *Nat. Neurosci.* 3:608–616.

Tian, N., and Copenhagen, D. R. (2003). Visual stimulation is required for refinement of ON and OFF pathways in postnatal retina. *Neuron* 39:85–96.

Torborg, C. L., Hansen, K. A., and Feller, M. B. (2005). High frequency, synchronized bursting drives eye-specific segregation of retinogeniculate projections. *Nat. Neurosci.* 8:72–78.

Tropea, D., Kreiman, G., Lyckman, A., Mukherjee, S., Yu, H., Horng, S., and Sur, M. (2006). Gene expression changes and molecular pathways mediating activity-dependent plasticity in visual cortex. *Nat. Neurosci.* 9:660–668.

Upton, A. L., Ravary, A., Salichon, N., Moessner, R., Lesch, K. P., Hen, R., Seif, I., and Gaspar, P. (2002). Lack of 5-HT(1B) receptor and of serotonin transporter have different effects on the segregation of retinal axons in the lateral geniculate nucleus compared to the superior colliculus. *Neuroscience* 111:597–610.

Upton, A. L., Salichon, N., Lebrand, C., Ravary, A., Blakely, R., Seif, I., and Gaspar, P. (1999). Excess of serotonin (5-HT) alters the segregation of ipsilateral and contralateral retinal projections in monoamine oxidase A knock-out mice: Possible role of 5-HT uptake in retinal ganglion cells during development. *J. Neurosci.* 19:7007–7024.

Vicini, S., Wang, J. F., Li, J. H., Zhu, W. J., Wang, Y. H., Luo, J. H., Wolfe, B. B., and Grayson, D. R. (1998). Functional and pharmacological differences between recombinant *N*-methyl-D-aspartate receptors. *J. Neurophysiol.* 79:555–566.

Wiesel, T. N., and Hübel, D. H. (1963a). Effects of visual deprivation on morphology and physiology of cells in the cat's lateral geniculate body. *J. Neurophysiol.* 26:978–993.

Wiesel, T. N., and Hübel, D. H. (1963b). Single-cell responses in striate cortex of kittens deprived of vision in one eye. *J. Neurophysiol.* 26:1003–1017.

Wiesel, T. N., and Hübel, D. H. (1965). Comparison of the effects of unilateral and bilateral eye closure on cortical unit responses in kittens. *J. Neurophysiol.* 28:1029–1040.

Wilson, J. R., Friedlander, M. J., and Sherman, S. M. (1984). Fine structural morphology of identified X- and Y-cells in the cat's lateral geniculate nucleus. *Pro. R. Soc. Lond. B Biol. Sci.* 221:411–436.

Wong, R. O., Meister, M., and Shatz, C. J. (1993). Transient period of correlated bursting activity during development of the mammalian retina. *Neuron* 11:923–938.

Yamadori, T., Nakamura, T., and Takami, K. (1989). A study on retinal ganglion cell which has an uncrossed bifurcating axon in the albino rat. *Brain Res.* 488:143–148.

Ziburkus, J., and Guido, W. (2006). Loss of binocular responses and reduced retinal convergence during the period of retinogeniculate axon segregation. *J. Neurophysiol.* 96:2775–2784.

36 Ocular Dominance Plasticity

MARK HÜBENER, SONJA B. HOFER, AND THOMAS D. MRSIC-FLOGEL

Plasticity of circuits in the visual cortex has traditionally been studied in several groups of higher mammals with an elaborate visual system. More recently, the mouse has been adopted by a number of researchers in the field. This trend is in part due to the ease of genetic interventions in this species, but there are other practical advantages to studying cortical plasticity in mice, such as their small size and fast generation time, as well as the fact that their genome has been completely sequenced. Moreover, recent experiments show that various aspects of mouse visual system function and plasticity can be readily assessed using behavioral tests (Prusky et al., 2000).

Several standard paradigms have been used to alter the sensory inputs to the visual cortex and thus induce plasticity, among them stripe rearing, squint induction, and focal retinal lesions. By far the most widely used manipulation is monocular deprivation (MD), the temporary closure of one eye. MD results in an overall strengthening of the open eye's and a weakening of the closed eye's representation in the visual cortex. In higher mammals, which possess ocular dominance (OD) columns, the effects of MD can be conveniently read out by observing, either with anatomical or with functional methods, the widening or shrinking of the open and closed eye columns, respectively (Shatz and Stryker, 1978; Hata and Stryker, 1994; Kind et al., 2002). Because mice do not have OD columns, the effects of MD must be assessed by other techniques. In the first part of this chapter we describe the various techniques that have been developed to determine OD in mouse visual cortex. We then focus on a specific aspect of OD plasticity in the mouse that has recently become overt, namely that the adult mouse visual cortex also shows considerable plasticity. Finally, we discuss recent results from our laboratory which show that the potency for plastic changes in mouse visual cortex can be strongly increased by prior episodes of plasticity.

Methods to assess ocular dominance plasticity in mouse visual cortex

Single-Unit Recordings Extracellular single-cell recordings are the most widely used method to determine OD, as well as other response properties of neurons in mouse visual cortex (Dräger, 1978; Gordon and Stryker, 1996; Hensch et al., 1998). They provide an unequivocal measure (the number of spikes) of a neuron's response to stimulation of either eye, which can be used to calculate a response bias for each individual cell. Provided that spikes from multiple units are reliably separated, this method also allows determining the exact proportion of binocular versus monocular neurons, which changes in a characteristic fashion after certain manipulations such as squint induction or alternating reverse occlusion (Gordon and Stryker, 1996). Moreover, the location of recorded cells in the visual cortex can be determined to a good extent, such that layer-specific differences in the degree of plasticity can be assessed (Gordon and Stryker, 1996).

A potential source of error in single-cell recordings is that they are prone to sampling biases. This is of particular concern when small numbers of cells are recorded from an area with a nonrandom distribution of response properties. This is the case in mouse visual cortex, since its binocular region is relatively small, with a rather smooth transition to monocular visual cortex. Thus, the extent of the binocular cortex must be mapped first to ensure that recordings are confined to this part. Another major disadvantage of single-cell recordings is that it is hard to make statements about absolute levels of response strength. The main reason is that typically, the visual stimuli used to determine OD are not optimized in every respect for a given cell, resulting in a large variation in total spike count between cells. This wide variation in overall apparent response strength, in combination with a limited number of recorded cells, makes statistical comparisons difficult. Consequently, in most single-cell recording studies from mouse visual cortex, OD is always expressed as the ratio between contralateral and ipsilateral eye responses (but see Gordon and Stryker, 1996).

Visually Evoked Potentials A number of studies have employed recordings of visually evoked potentials (VEPs) to determine function and plasticity in mouse visual cortex (Huang et al., 1999; Porciatti et al., 1999; Sawtell et al., 2003; Frenkel and Bear, 2004). VEP recordings allow the rapid measurement of basic parameters of mouse visual system, such as grating acuity and contrast response function, which were found to be in good agreement with behavioral or single-cell data (Porciatti et al., 1999). OD can be readily assessed with VEPs, and, unlike single-cell recordings, VEPs provide a reliable measure of the absolute response amplitudes elicited by stimulation of either eye (Sawtell et al., 2003; Frenkel and Bear, 2004). Moreover, VEPs can be recorded relatively easily in awake mice (Sawtell et al., 2003; Frenkel and Bear, 2004), an advantage that turned out to be crucial for the discovery of OD plasticity in adult mice, which seems to be occluded by certain anesthetics. Because VEPs constitute a population signal from many neurons, however, they have a limited spatial resolution, and they do not permit the determination of receptive field (RF) parameters of individual neurons, such as orientation selectivity.

Optical Imaging Several recent studies have used optical imaging to obtain an overall measure of the strength of the representation of both eyes in mouse visual cortex (Cang et al., 2005; Hofer et al., 2006; Heimel et al., 2007). Optical imaging of intrinsic signals is based on a small decrease in light reflectance of neuronal tissue after its activation, which is in part caused by changes in blood oxygenation level and blood volume. It is ideally suited for the rapid mapping of topography in mouse visual cortex (Schuett et al., 2002; Kalatsky and Stryker, 2003) and thus can be used to determine the exact location of the binocular visual cortex in individual mice (figure 36.1). With this technique, we were able to demonstrate strong and fully reversible OD shifts in adult mouse visual cortex, as well as a priming effect of prior MD episodes on later plasticity (Hofer et al., 2006). In juvenile mice, we employed optical imaging to systematically assess the effect of MD duration on the magnitude of the OD shift (figure 36.2). Optical imaging allows repeated measurements to be made in the same animal over extended periods of time (more than a year), such that the responses of individual mice to multiple epochs of MD-induced shifts and recovery can be followed. Long-term imaging in mice is greatly facilitated by the fact that the skull is sufficiently thin and transparent to allow recording of high-quality signals through the closed skull, which minimizes perturbation of cortical tissue. Of note, the reflectance changes measured with optical imaging provide an absolute measure of the activity evoked by each eye, which turns out to be highly reproducible between acutely imaged animals (Hofer et al., 2006).

Levelt and colleagues (Heimel et al., 2007) have recently described several improvements for optical imaging of MD-induced shifts in mouse visual cortex. By introducing a "reset" stimulus in a different part of the visual field between

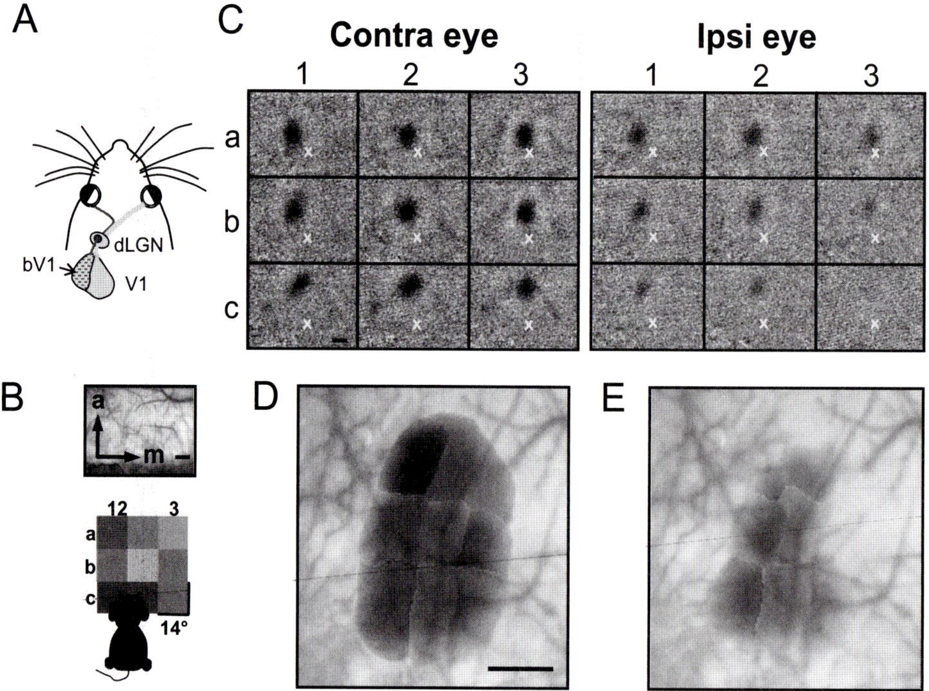

Figure 36.1 Retinotopic mapping of mouse binocular visual cortex using optical imaging of intrinsic signals. *A*, Schematic illustration of primary visual pathway in the mouse, depicting the location of the dorsal lateral geniculate nucleus (dLGN) and the primary visual cortex (V1), with the binocular zone (bV1) located laterally. *B*, *Top*, Cortical blood vessel pattern as imaged through the skull. *Bottom*, Arrangement of grating stimuli used to map the central visual field. Color denotes stimulus position. *C*, Individual activity maps displaying responses to the 3 × 3 stimulus grid depicted in *B* are presented separately to the two eyes. The coordinates of the cross are fixed in each map. *D* and *E*, Color-coded maps of the combined responses to contralateral (*D*) and ipsilateral (*E*) eye stimulation superimposed on the cortical blood vessel pattern, revealing the extent of the binocular zone. Color indicates stimulus position eliciting the strongest response at each pixel. Scale bars = 0.5 mm. See color plate 25.

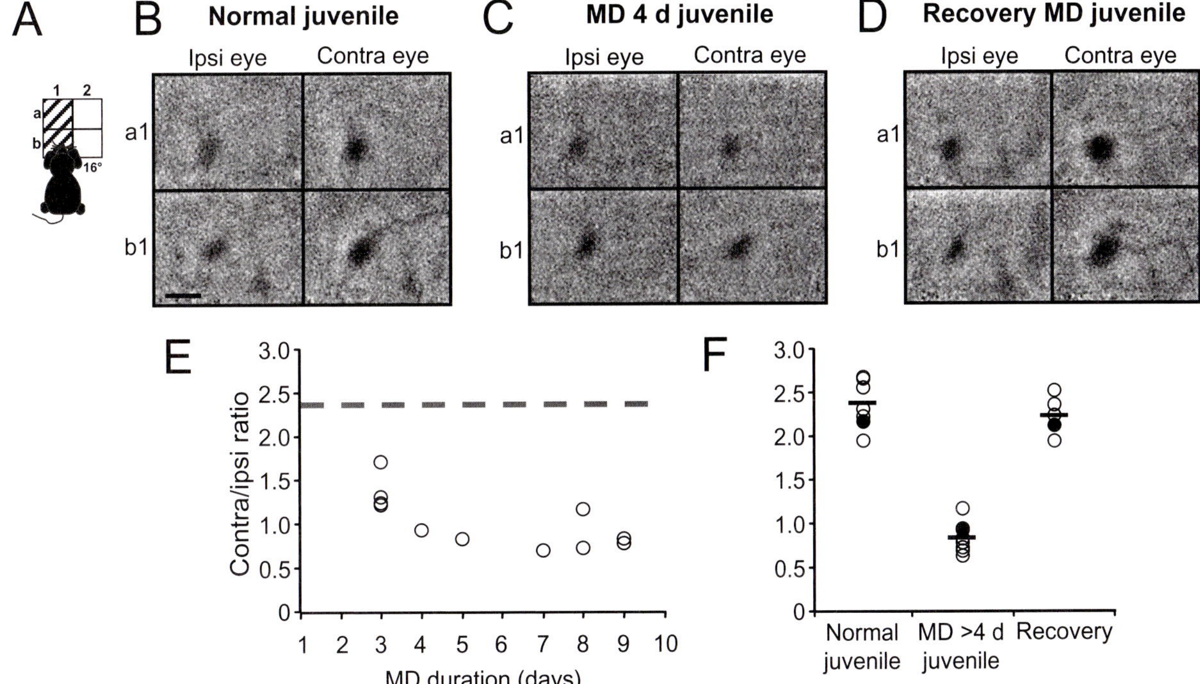

FIGURE 36.2 Optical imaging of MD-induced OD plasticity during the critical period. *A*, Schematic of stimulus arrangement. *B–D*, Ipsilateral (*left*) and contralateral (*right*) eye responses from the central region of the binocular visual cortex to stimuli shown in *A* from a normal P35 mouse (*B*), following MD (P26–P30) of the contralateral eye (*C*), and 46 days after a 4-day MD (*D*). Scale bar = 1 mm. *E*, OD shifts after MD (starting at P26–P28) shown as the ratio of contralateral to ipsilateral eye responses from individual animals (*circles*) plotted against MD duration. *Dashed line* shows average from nondeprived controls. *F*, Contralateral/ipsilateral ratio values for normal juvenile mice, after 4–10 days of MD, and 4–7 weeks after a 4- to 5-day MD. *Horizontal lines* indicate mean group values. *Solid symbols* are data points from the experiments shown in *B*, *C*, and *D*.

subsequent data acquisition trials, they were able to shorten the overall data acquisition time. In addition, normalizing visually evoked reflectance changes to a reference region outside the visual cortex greatly reduced the variability of responses, resulting in a reduction in the number of repetitions needed to obtain a reliable response.

The previously mentioned studies (Hofer et al., 2006; Heimel et al., 2007) employed a standard optical imaging paradigm, which consists of repeated brief (seconds) episodes of visual stimulation and data acquisition, each followed by a short interval without stimulation, during which the optical signal relaxes. An alternative method for optical imaging data acquisition has been introduced by Kalatsky and Stryker (2003). In this method, images from the visual cortex are continuously acquired as a bar is repeatedly swept across the visual field at a certain frequency. Fourier decomposition of the signal time course is then used to determine for each cortical region the power of the stimulation frequency, which is a measure of the activity evoked by the stimulus. Cang et al. (2005) have demonstrated that this optical imaging paradigm can be conveniently used to measure OD plasticity in mice.

In addition to overall reflectance changes, neuronal activity also results in an increased endogenous fluorescence of flavoproteins (Shibuki et al., 2003), which has been used to measure OD plasticity in the mouse (Tohmi et al., 2006). Similar to reflectance-based optical imaging, flavoprotein imaging allows measuring absolute response levels, as well as obtaining multiple recordings from the same animal.

As with VEPs, optical imaging is a population measure and thus has the disadvantage that it cannot be used to determine single-cell properties.

CALCIUM IMAGING WITH TWO-PHOTON MICROSCOPY A method that combines the advantages of single-cell recordings with those of population measures such as VEPs or optical imaging is two-photon-based calcium imaging (Regehr and Tank, 1991; Stosiek et al., 2003; Ohki et al., 2005). After bulk injection of a membrane-permeable calcium indicator dye into the visual cortex, the labeled cell bodies of hundreds of individual neurons can be visualized by two-photon microscopy. Upon activation by a visual stimulus, intracellular calcium levels rise, and the indicator dye glows brighter (figure 36.3). We have used this method to study MD effects in mouse visual cortex and have found that shifts in OD can be reliably detected (Mrsic-Flogel et al., 2007). The magnitudes of the OD shifts observed in juvenile mice were very similar to the ones obtained with electrical single-cell

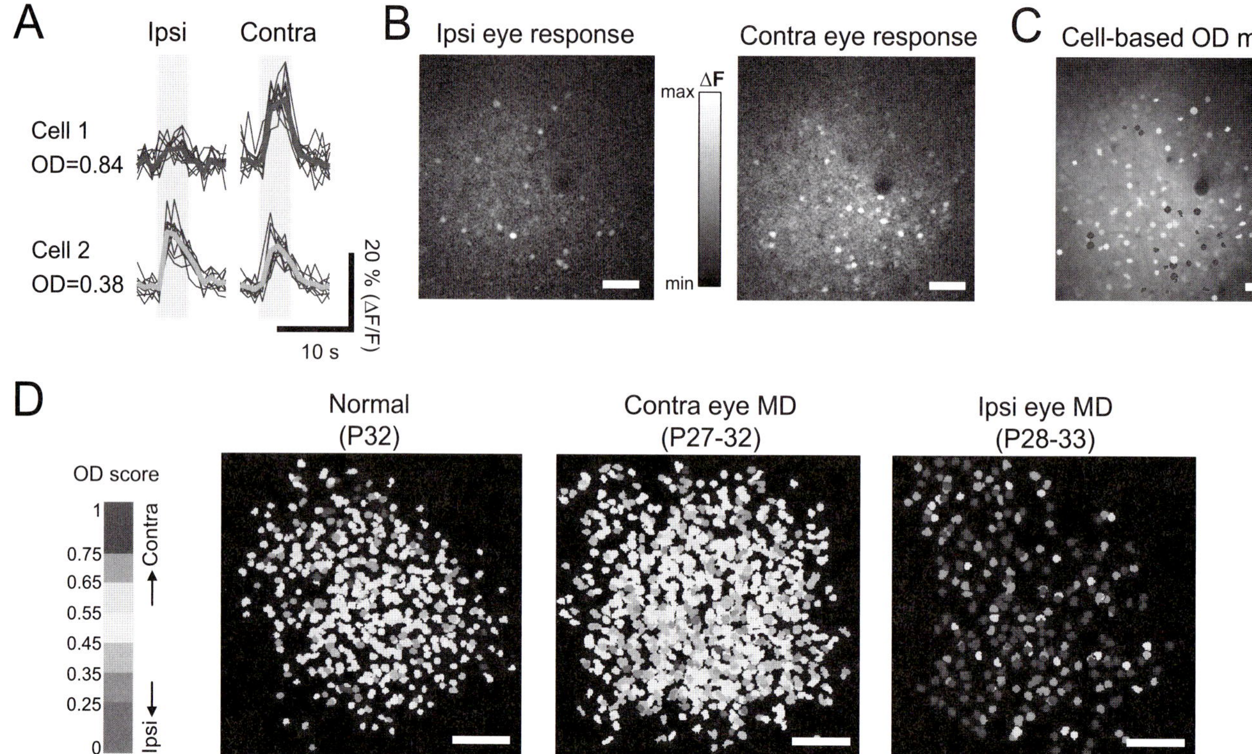

FIGURE 36.3 Mapping OD in mouse binocular visual cortex by two-photon calcium imaging. *A*, Examples of visually evoked calcium transients (fluorescent change, ΔF/F) recorded from two different neurons in the binocular visual cortex loaded with the calcium indicator dye OGB-1AM. *Thin traces* show individual responses to stimulation of each eye; *thick traces* are average responses to eight stimulus presentations. Stimulation periods are indicated by gray bars. *B*, Response maps (ΔF) for the contralateral (*left panel*) and ipsilateral (*right panel*) eye 230 μm below the pial surface in a normal mouse. *C*, A cell-based OD map computed from the single-eye response maps in *B*. Individual neurons are color coded by the OD score, as indicated by the labels in *D*. OD score of 1 or 0 denotes exclusive response to contralateral or ipsilateral eye stimulation, respectively, and a value of 0.5 indicates an equal response to both eyes. *D*, Overlay of cell-based OD maps at different depths for a normal mouse (*left*, four depths, 190–290 μm), after a 5-day contralateral MD (*center*, six depths, 195–410 μm), and after a 5-day ipsilateral MD (*right*, two depths, 200 and 225 μm). Note weak clustering of cells with similar OD values in the normal mouse. Scale bars = 50 μm. See color plate 26.

recordings. Because of the very large number of recorded cells (several thousands from a small number of mice), we were able to determine absolute response levels for each eye in normal as well as MD mice. Of note, two-photon calcium imaging also allows the exact spatial localization of each imaged neuron in the visual cortex such that detailed maps of response properties at cellular resolution can be generated (Ohki et al., 2005, 2006). Figure 36.3 shows examples of color-coded OD maps from normal and MD mice. In line with previous studies (Dräger, 1975; Schuett et al., 2002), there is no obvious, strong organization for OD in mouse visual cortex. Closer inspection of such maps reveals, however, that in most mice there is a weak tendency for a clustering of cells dominated by the same eye (figure 36.3*D*).

So far we have not succeeded in imaging calcium signals repeatedly from the same mouse. This drawback might be overcome once genetically encoded calcium indicators with high signal-to-noise ratios become available for routine use in mammals (Griesbeck, 2004). Another disadvantage of two-photon calcium imaging is that the changes in calcium concentration occur relatively slowly, which makes it difficult, though not impossible (Kerr et al., 2005), to extract the exact number of action potentials from these signals. It follows that great care must be taken to isolate the fluorescence signals of individual cell bodies from changes of the surrounding neuropil, which might otherwise obscure a neuron's specific response characteristics.

GENE EXPRESSION In addition to the functional methods in the previous section, MD effects have also been studied by mapping the expression of activity-related genes, such as Arc (Tagawa et al., 2005) or c-fos (Pham et al., 2004), in histological sections. Although this approach is limited by the fact that in a given mouse, only one stimulus parameter can be tested, it has the advantage that MD-induced changes in activity levels can be assessed in all regions of the cortex, in different cortical layers, and in other parts of the brain, for example the lateral geniculate nucleus (LGN). A variety of additional genes have recently been described that are specifically induced by deprivation paradigms and thus could potentially be used to visualize OD shifts (Majdan and Shatz, 2006; Tropea et al., 2006).

Adult ocular dominance plasticity

The classic studies of MD in kittens by Wiesel and Hübel (1963) led to the notion of the critical period for OD plasticity in the visual cortex, which ends around the onset of adolescence. In line with this, in their quantitative assessment of MD effects in mice using single-unit recordings under barbiturate anesthesia, Gordon and Stryker (1996) described a critical period for OD plasticity that peaks around 4 weeks of age and terminates soon after. However, a large body of literature supports the fact that in principle, the neocortex maintains its capacity for plasticity throughout life. Studies in the visual, auditory, and somatosensory cortex have demonstrated robust experience-dependent reconfiguration of neuronal response properties in adult animals after a variety of manipulations of sensory inputs (Fox and Wong, 2005). This is probably best exemplified by the dramatic reorganization of RFs and synaptic connections in the visual cortex after restricted retinal lesions (Kaas et al., 1990; Darian-Smith and Gilbert, 1994; Giannikopoulos and Eysel, 2006). The recent finding of strong OD plasticity in adult mice well beyond the traditional critical period is therefore not entirely unexpected (Sawtell et al., 2003; Pham et al., 2004; Tagawa et al., 2005; Frenkel et al., 2006; Hofer et al., 2006). Adult OD plasticity was first shown by Sawtell and colleagues (2003) in awake adult mice using VEP recordings. Subsequently, adult OD shifts were also demonstrated in anesthetized mice with several other methods, including extracellular microelectrode recordings (figure 36.4; Hofer et al., 2006), optical imaging of intrinsic signals (see figure 36.4; Hofer et al., 2006; Heimel et al., 2007) and VEP recordings (Pham et al., 2004). A study using the activity reporter gene Arc to assess functional eye representation in mouse visual cortex additionally showed MD effects before and after the traditional critical period (Tagawa et al., 2005). Taken together, these results show that OD shifts in mice occur well into adulthood.

OD plasticity in adult mice, however, is different from that in juvenile animals in that it requires longer MD durations, since MD periods of 4 days or less are not especially effective in shifting OD in adults (Fagiolini and Hensch, 2000; McGee et al., 2005; Hofer et al., 2006; Tohmi et al., 2006). Although there is some debate as to why some studies have not reported robust OD plasticity in adult animals, these differences might be attributed either to the use of MD durations that are too brief (≤4 days; e.g., Tohmi et al., 2006) or to different anesthesia regimens (Pham et al., 2004; Heimel et al., 2007). Interestingly, barbiturate anesthesia, which normally boosts GABAergic transmission, may obscure the expression of OD plasticity specifically in adults. This point is underscored by another study in adult mice showing a masking effect of fentanyl-based anesthesia on OD plasticity (Heimel et al., 2007). Considering that different anesthetics act differentially on various neurotransmitter systems in the brain, these results support the view that distinct mechanisms may underlie OD shifts in juvenile and adult animals.

Thus far, robust adult OD plasticity has been observed only in mice, a species that lacks OD columns. In rats, which have a visual system similarly organized to that of mice, single-unit recordings have not demonstrated adult OD plasticity after 7 days or more of deprivation (Pizzorusso et al., 2002). However, partial OD shifts are nonetheless possible in rats beyond 7 weeks of age (Guire et al., 1999; He et al., 2006). In cats, OD shifts can be induced up to a year of age, but with deprivation periods lasting 3 months (Daw et al., 1992). The clear results demonstrating strong adult OD plasticity in mice should prompt a reexamination of the degree of adult plasticity in these species with different MD durations and anesthetic regimens.

Mechanisms of juvenile and adult ocular dominance plasticity

In juvenile mice, OD shifts are mediated both by an early loss of deprived-eye responsiveness and a delayed gain of open-eye responsiveness (Frenkel and Bear, 2004). Deprived-eye response depression in juvenile mice likely results from the weakening of intracortical synaptic connections serving the deprived eye (Rittenhouse et al., 1999; Heynen et al., 2003; Frenkel and Bear, 2004; Mataga et al., 2004) and may rely on *N*-methyl-D-aspartate (NMDA) receptor-dependent long-term depression (LTD) of excitatory synapses (Heynen et al., 2003) or on long-term potentiation (LTP) of local inhibitory transmission (Maffei et al., 2006), the maturation of which is important for triggering OD plasticity (Hensch, 2005).

The gain of visual drive from the nondeprived eye could be mediated equally well by LTP of intracortical excitatory connections (Abraham and Bear, 1996) or by non-Hebbian, homeostatic mechanisms (Miller, 1996; Turrigiano and Nelson, 2004). It has been proposed that strengthening of nondeprived-eye synapses could be facilitated by promoting the induction of LTP in favor of LTD (Kirkwood et al., 1996), as specified by the Bienenstock-Cooper-Munro theory, which entails a sliding synaptic modification threshold based on the history of postsynaptic activity (Bienenstock et al., 1982; Abraham and Bear, 1996). In support of this LTP-based model, OD plasticity is partially blocked in adult NMDA receptor knockout mice (Sawtell et al., 2003). Although this suggests that MD-induced strengthen-

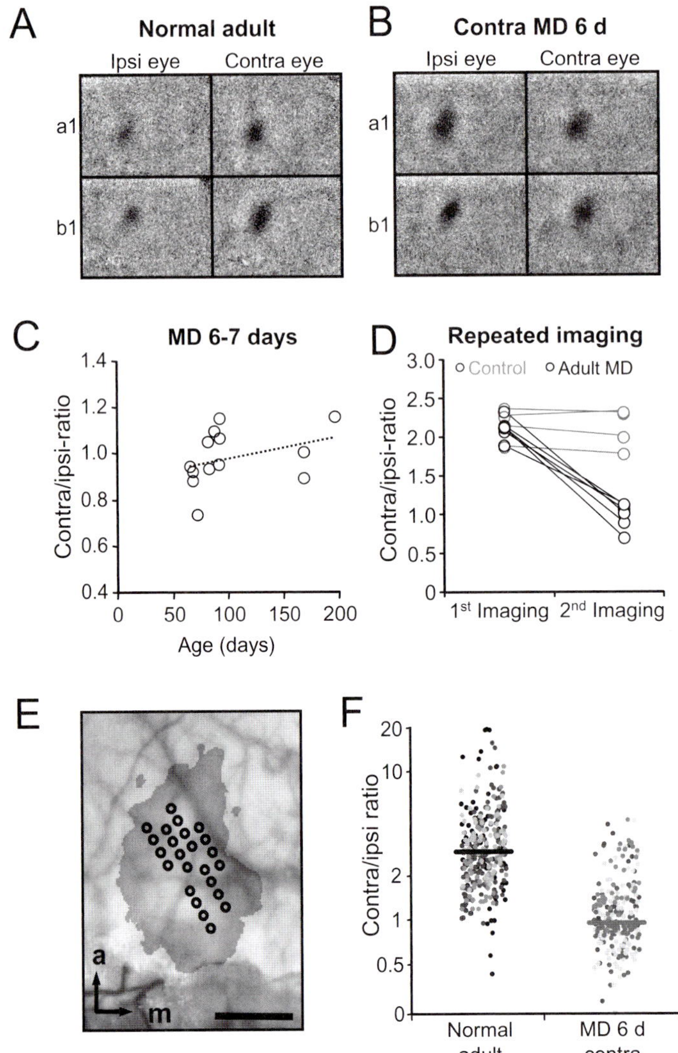

FIGURE 36.4 OD plasticity in adult visual cortex assessed with intrinsic signal imaging and multielectrode recordings. *A* and *B*, Ipsilateral and contralateral eye responses in the same mouse before (*A*, P80, contralateral/ipsilateral ratio = 2.21) and after 6 days of MD (*B*, P92, contralateral/ipsilateral ratio = 1.09). Stimulus arrangement as in figure 36.2*A*. *C*, Ratio of contralateral to ipsilateral eye response strength after 6–7 days of MD in normal adult mice plotted against age shows no significant correlation. $R^2 = 0.12$, $P = 0.24$. *D*, Contralateral/ipsilateral ratio values from repeated experiments in adult control animals (gray, interimaging period 1–3 weeks) and in deprived adult animals before and after 6 days of MD in the contralateral eye (black). *E*, Functional map of the binocular region (green corresponds to the ipsilateral eye representation), used for targeting electrode penetrations (*circles*). Scale bar = 0.5 mm. *F*, Distribution of contralateral/ipsilateral ratio values from all recording sites in adult control (2.99 ± 0.28, mean ± SEM, 324 recording sites, 4 mice) and deprived (1.05 ± 0.12, 260 recording sites, 5 mice) animals, showing strong OD shifts in response to MD. Each color represents a different animal. *Horizontal lines* indicate mean group values. See color plate 27.

ing of open-eye responses may be Hebbian in nature, more work is needed to forge a causal link between LTP and open-eye response potentiation.

In principle, open-eye responses could also be strengthened through homeostatic mechanisms. The concept of homeostatic plasticity is founded on the assumption that neurons engage mechanisms that maintain their responsiveness within a certain range in response to global alterations of neuronal activity levels (Burrone and Murthy, 2003; Turrigiano and Nelson, 2004). Consistent with this notion, visual deprivation increases the strength of excitatory synapses and the excitability of neurons in rodent monocular cortex (Desai et al., 2002; Maffei et al., 2004), where no interocular interactions occur. In principle, such changes are well suited to counteract the chronic reduction of visual drive by increasing neuronal responsiveness. In fact, using two-photon calcium imaging and electrical multi-unit recordings, we found direct in vivo evidence for homeostasis of visually evoked responses in monocular and binocular visual cortex after MD (Mrsic-Flogel et al., 2007). Specifically, the responses of monocular neurons responding exclusively to the deprived eye after MD were larger than those of monocular neurons in nondeprived animals.

Although robust OD shifts in the adult visual cortex occur after longer MD durations, adult OD plasticity is not equivalent to that of juvenile animals (Sawtell et al., 2003; Lickey et al., 2004; Pham et al., 2004; Tagawa et al., 2005; Frenkel et al., 2006; Hofer et al., 2006). For example, not all studies have reported a significant loss of deprived-eye responsiveness in the hemisphere contralateral to the deprived eye (Hofer et al., 2006). The reasons for this difference are unclear. The lack of response depression could be explained by differences in recording methods or anesthetic regimens. Alternatively, it may reflect an age-related decline in the capacity of visual cortex to express LTD at excitatory synapses (Kirkwood et al., 1997; Heynen and Bear, 2001). Consistent with this idea, the loss of spines on layer 2/3 pyramidal neurons in juvenile mice after 4 days of MD does not occur in adults (Mataga et al., 2004).

Prior experience enhances adult ocular dominance plasticity

What are the long-term consequences of OD plasticity in the visual cortex? In mice and other species, restoration of normal binocular vision after a period of MD functionally restores normal binocular responses (Mitchell et al., 1977; Kind et al., 2002; Liao et al., 2004; Hofer et al., 2006). We recently tested whether an OD shift earlier in life affects the capacity of the visual cortex for subsequent plasticity (Hofer et al., 2006). In naive adult mice, 3 days of contralateral eye MD was not sufficient to induce measurable OD plasticity (figure 36.5). However, the same duration of MD resulted in a marked shift of OD in mice that had experienced MD of the same eye up to 2 months earlier (figure 36.5). Notably, this apparent enhancement of adult plasticity occurred irrespective of whether the first deprivation occurred in juvenility or in adulthood. Moreover, OD shifts induced by a second MD episode persisted longer after reopening of the eye. These results indicate that prior MD leaves a lasting mark in the binocular visual cortex such that subsequent OD shifts emerge faster and last longer. The capacity for plasticity in the mammalian cortex can therefore be enhanced by past experience.

In principle, two types of mechanisms could account for the facilitation of OD plasticity just described. Prior MD experience could lead either to a general increase in cortical plasticity or to specific changes in the circuits or synapses affected by the initial deprivation. We found that the enhancement of plasticity was apparent only after repeated deprivation of the same eye, since MD of the other eye 3–4 weeks later did not lead to an improved OD shift, and in fact entirely abolished its occurrence after longer deprivation periods (figure 36.6). These findings indicate that prior deprivation does not increase cortical plasticity in general to any input, as has been observed after dark rearing (Cynader and Mitchell, 1980) or after pharmacological manipulations (Pizzorusso et al., 2002). Instead, they provide evidence for specific changes in cortical circuitry that support the facilitation of OD shifts only in the same direction as experienced earlier in life, while rendering shifts in the opposite direction less effective.

These results argue for a specific trace that is laid down in visual cortex during the first period of plasticity. This trace is not functionally apparent in the intervening period of several weeks but rather requires a second MD to be disclosed. What is the nature of this trace? Prior MD experience could establish changes in the form of lasting biochemical or structural modifications that are (re)activated on the second MD. For instance, activity-dependent changes in visual cortex associated with the initial MD episode could lead to the generation of new synapses that might be disabled functionally during the recovery, which would subsequently facilitate future circuit adaptations.

The view that structural changes might form the basis for the facilitation of OD plasticity is supported by closely related observations in the barn owl's auditory localization system (Knudsen, 1998). Here, the capacity for plasticity of auditory midbrain neurons in response to a prism-induced visual field displacement was extended into adulthood if the owls had a similar prism experience as juveniles. The shifts of auditory

A

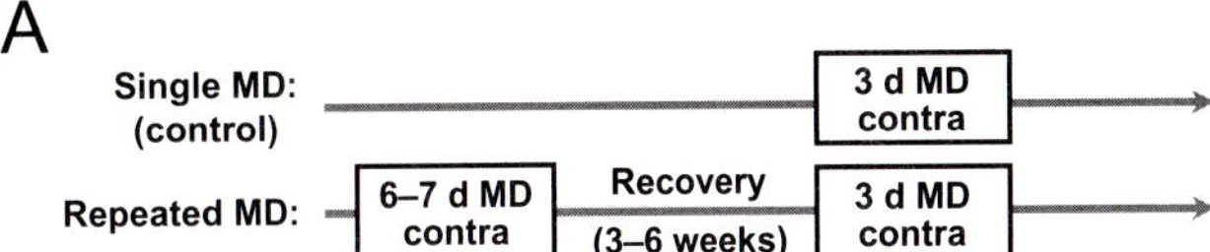

B

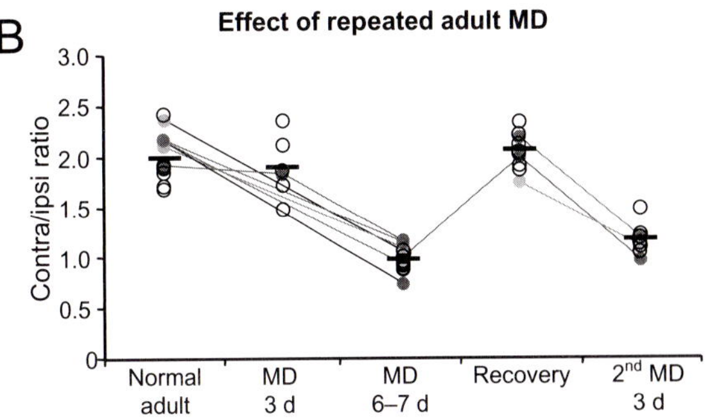

Figure 36.5 Prior MD in adult mice facilitates subsequent OD plasticity. *A*, Experimental timelines for assessing the effect of repeated adult MD in the contralateral eye. *B*, Strong OD shifts after 6–7 days of MD in adult mice recover completely with restored binocular vision (imaged 8–30 days after eye reopening). Reclosure of the eye results in strong OD shifts even after 3 days, unlike in naive mice ($P < 0.001$). *Horizontal lines* indicate mean group values. Lines connect data points from mice imaged repeatedly.

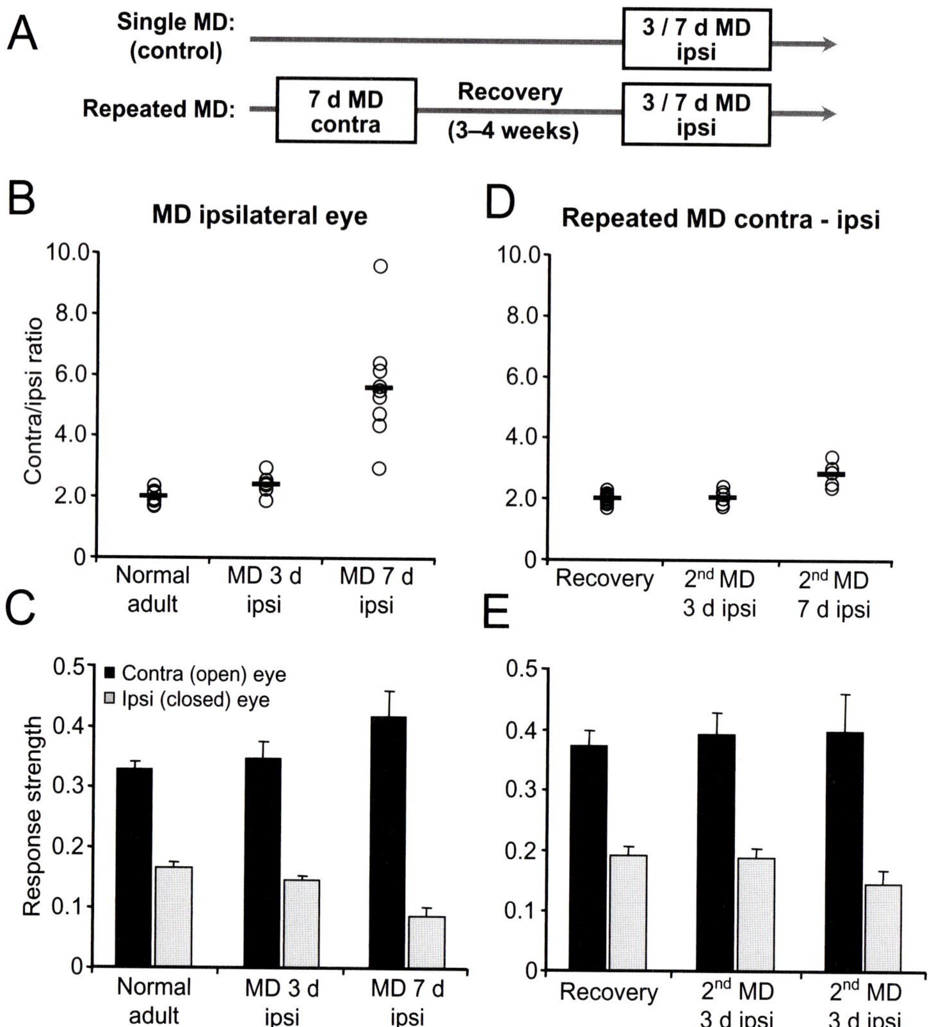

FIGURE 36.6 Facilitatory effect of repeated MD is eye specific. *A*, Experimental timelines for successive MD of opposite eyes. *B*, In naive adult mice, contralateral/ipsilateral ratio values increased marginally after 3 days of MD and strongly after 7 days of MD of the ipsilateral eye. *C*, Response strength of each eye for the same conditions as in *B*. *D*, Previous 7-day MD of the contralateral eye and subsequent recovery did not accelerate plasticity in response to a 3-day ipsilateral eye closure. In contrast, prior deprivation impaired OD plasticity induced by a 7-day ipsilateral MD. *Open circles* denote data from individual animals; *horizontal lines* indicate mean values. *E*, Response strength of each eye for the same conditions as in *D*. Error bars indicate SEM.

space fields in adult owls is explained by the formation of new axonal connections during initial prism rearing (DeBello et al., 2001) that are physically maintained but functionally disabled after removal of the prisms and the shifting back of auditory space fields (Linkenhoker et al., 2005). In mouse visual cortex, too, MD can result in anatomical changes, which have been observed at both the presynaptic level (Antonini et al., 1999) and the postsynaptic level (Mataga et al., 2004; Oray et al., 2004). It is therefore tempting to speculate that these structural changes might outlast the first MD, facilitating the OD shift induced by the second episode of MD.

This idea can be tested experimentally. In vivo two-photon imaging of synaptic structures could be used to test whether spines that are gained during the first MD episode are maintained after reopening of the eye, forming a structural memory of the altered sensory input. The second MD episode might consequently result in only a small increase in newly formed spines. This scenario further raises the question of how these persistent contacts are functionally suppressed after recovery from the first MD. In principle, this could be brought about by specific inhibition of these connections. Alternatively, they could be rendered ineffective by converting them into silent synapses by the removal of AMPA receptors (Malenka and Nicoll, 1997), which could be tested by comparing the ratio of AMPA to NMDA currents in neurons obtained from normal and previously deprived mice.

Behavioral correlates

Changes in cortical circuitry following MD are important for visual behavior in rodents. An imbalance in binocular inputs early in postnatal life can lead to the development of poor visual acuity (Muir and Mitchell, 1973; Prusky and Douglas, 2003), which primarily affects the deprived eye (Iny et al., 2006). Longer deprivation periods in rats and MD in adult mice can lead to improvement in the spatial acuity of the spared eye (Iny et al., 2006; Prusky et al., 2006). Interestingly, the onset and persistence of the enhancement of spatial vision can be further improved after repeated MD in adult mice (Prusky et al., 2006), a result consistent with the effects of prior MD on subsequent OD plasticity (Hofer et al., 2006). These behavioral findings are in close keeping with the loss of deprived-eye function and the gain of nondeprived-eye function in the contralateral visual cortex after juvenile and adult MD, respectively. The MD paradigm in mice, therefore, provides a useful general model for studying the mechanisms underlying plasticity of cortical circuits and related behaviors.

REFERENCES

Abraham, W. C., and Bear, M. F. (1996). Metaplasticity: The plasticity of synaptic plasticity. *Trends Neurosci.* 19:126–130.

Antonini, A., Fagiolini, M., and Stryker, M. P. (1999). Anatomical correlates of functional plasticity in mouse visual cortex. *J. Neurosci.* 19:4388–4406.

Bienenstock, E. L., Cooper, L. N., and Munro, P. W. (1982). Theory for the development of neuron selectivity: Orientation specificity and binocular interaction in visual cortex. *J. Neurosci.* 2:32–48.

Burrone, J., and Murthy, V. N. (2003). Synaptic gain control and homeostasis. *Curr. Opin. Neurobiol.* 13:560–567.

Cang, J. H., Kalatsky, V. A., Lowel, S., and Stryker, M. P. (2005). Optical imaging of the intrinsic signal as a measure of cortical plasticity in the mouse. *Vis. Neurosci.* 22:685–691.

Cynader, M., and Mitchell, D. E. (1980). Prolonged sensitivity to monocular deprivation in dark-reared cats. *J. Neurophysiol.* 43:1026–1040.

Darian-Smith, C., and Gilbert, C. D. (1994). Axonal sprouting accompanies functional reorganization in adult cat striate cortex. *Nature* 368:737–740.

Daw, N. W., Fox, K., Sato, H., and Czepita, D. (1992). Critical period for monocular deprivation in the cat visual cortex. *J. Neurophysiol.* 67:197–202.

DeBello, W. M., Feldman, D. E., and Knudsen, E. I. (2001). Adaptive axonal remodeling in the midbrain auditory space map. *J. Neurosci.* 21:3161–3174.

Desai, N. S., Cudmore, R. H., Nelson, S. B., and Turrigiano, G. G. (2002). Critical periods for experience-dependent synaptic scaling in visual cortex. *Nat. Neurosci.* 5:783–789.

Dräger, U. C. (1975). Receptive fields of single cells and topography in mouse visual cortex. *J. Comp. Neurol.* 160:269–290.

Dräger, U. C. (1978). Observations on monocular deprivation in mice. *J. Neurophysiol.* 41:28–42.

Fagiolini, M., and Hensch, T. K. (2000). Inhibitory threshold for critical-period activation in primary visual cortex. *Nature* 404:183–186.

Fox, K., and Wong, R. O. (2005). A comparison of experience-dependent plasticity in the visual and somatosensory systems. *Neuron* 48:465–477.

Frenkel, M. Y., and Bear, M. F. (2004). How monocular deprivation shifts ocular dominance in visual cortex of young mice. *Neuron* 44:917–923.

Frenkel, M. Y., Sawtell, N. B., Diogo, A. C., Yoon, B., Neve, R. L., and Bear, M. F. (2006). Instructive effect of visual experience in mouse visual cortex. *Neuron* 51:339–349.

Giannikopoulos, D. V., and Eysel, U. T. (2006). Dynamics and specificity of cortical map reorganization after retinal lesions. *Proc. Natl. Acad. Sci. U.S.A.* 103:10805–10810.

Gordon, J. A., and Stryker, M. P. (1996). Experience-dependent plasticity of binocular responses in the primary visual cortex of the mouse. *J. Neurosci.* 16:3274–3286.

Griesbeck, O. (2004). Fluorescent proteins as sensors for cellular functions. *Curr. Opin. Neurobiol.* 14:636–641.

Guire, E. S., Lickey, M. E., and Gordon, B. (1999). Critical period for the monocular deprivation effect in rats: Assessment with sweep visually evoked potentials. *J. Neurophysiol.* 81: 121–128.

Hata, Y., and Stryker, M. P. (1994). Control of thalamocortical afferent rearrangement by postsynaptic activity in developing visual cortex. *Science* 265:1732–1735.

He, H. Y., Hodos, W., and Quinlan, E. M. (2006). Visual deprivation reactivates rapid ocular dominance plasticity in adult visual cortex. *J. Neurosci.* 26:2951–2955.

Heimel, J. A., Hartman, R. J., Hermans, J. M., and Levelt, C. N. (2007). Screening mouse vision with intrinsic signal optical imaging. *Eur. J. Neurosci.* 125:795–804.

Hensch, T. K. (2005). Critical period plasticity in local cortical circuits. *Nat. Rev. Neurosci.* 6:877–888.

Hensch, T. K., Fagiolini, M., Mataga, N., Stryker, M. P., Baekkeskov, S., and Kash, S. F. (1998). Local GABA circuit control of experience-dependent plasticity in developing visual cortex. *Science* 282:1504–1508.

Heynen, A. J., and Bear, M. F. (2001). Long-term potentiation of thalamocortical transmission in the adult visual cortex in vivo. *J. Neurosci.* 21:9801–9813.

Heynen, A. J., Yoon, B. J., Liu, C. H., Chung, H. J., Huganir, R. L., and Bear, M. F. (2003). Molecular mechanism for loss of visual cortical responsiveness following brief monocular deprivation. *Nat. Neurosci.* 6:854–862.

Hofer, S. B., Mrsic-Flogel, T. D., Bonhoeffer, T., and Hübener, M. (2006). Prior experience enhances plasticity in adult visual cortex. *Nat. Neurosci.* 9:127–132.

Huang, Z. J., Kirkwood, A., Pizzorusso, T., Porciatti, V., Morales, B., Bear, M. F., Maffei, L., and Tonegawa, S. (1999). BDNF regulates the maturation of inhibition and the critical period of plasticity in mouse visual cortex. *Cell* 98:739–755.

Iny, K., Heynen, A. J., Sklar, E., and Bear, M. F. (2006). Bidirectional modifications of visual acuity induced by monocular deprivation in juvenile and adult rats. *J. Neurosci.* 26:7368–7374.

Kaas, J. H., Krubitzer, L. A., Chino, Y. M., Langston, A. L., Polley, E. H., and Blair, N. (1990). Reorganization of retinotopic cortical maps in adult mammals after lesions of the retina. *Science* 248:229–231.

Kalatsky, V. A., and Stryker, M. P. (2003). New paradigm for optical imaging: Temporally encoded maps of intrinsic signal. *Neuron* 38:529–545.

Kerr, J. N., Greenberg, D., and Helmchen, F. (2005). Imaging input and output of neocortical networks in vivo. *Proc. Natl. Acad. Sci. U.S.A.* 102:14063–14068.

Kind, P. C., Mitchell, D. E., Ahmed, B., Blakemore, C., Bonhoeffer, T., and Sengpiel, F. (2002). Correlated binocular activity guides recovery from monocular deprivation. *Nature* 416:430–433.

Kirkwood, A., Rioult, M. C., and Bear, M. F. (1996). Experience-dependent modification of synaptic plasticity in visual cortex. *Nature* 381:526–528.

Kirkwood, A., Silva, A., and Bear, M. F. (1997). Age-dependent decrease of synaptic plasticity in the neocortex of alphaCaMKII mutant mice. *Proc. Natl. Acad. Sci. U.S.A.* 94:3380–3383.

Knudsen, E. I. (1998). Capacity for plasticity in the adult owl auditory system expanded by juvenile experience. *Science* 279: 1531–1533.

Liao, D. S., Krahe, T. E., Prusky, G. T., Medina, A. E., and Ramoa, A. S. (2004). Recovery of cortical binocularity and orientation selectivity after the critical period for ocular dominance plasticity. *J. Neurophysiol.* 92:2113–2121.

Lickey, M. E., Pham, T. A., and Gordon, B. (2004). Swept contrast visual evoked potentials and their plasticity following monocular deprivation in mice. *Vision Res.* 44:3381–3387.

Linkenhoker, B. A., der Ohe, C. G., and Knudsen, E. I. (2005). Anatomical traces of juvenile learning in the auditory system of adult barn owls. *Nat. Neurosci.* 8:93–98.

Maffei, A., Nataraj, K., Nelson, S. B., and Turrigiano, G. G. (2006). Potentiation of cortical inhibition by visual deprivation. *Nature* 443:81–84.

Maffei, A., Nelson, S. B., and Turrigiano, G. G. (2004). Selective reconfiguration of layer 4 visual cortical circuitry by visual deprivation. *Nat. Neurosci.* 7:1353–1359.

Majdan, M., and Shatz, C. J. (2006). Effects of visual experience on activity-dependent gene regulation in cortex. *Nat. Neurosci.* 9:650–659.

Malenka, R. C., and Nicoll, R. A. (1997). Silent synapses speak up. *Neuron* 19:473–476.

Mataga, N., Mizuguchi, Y., and Hensch, T. K. (2004). Experience-dependent pruning of dendritic spines in visual cortex by tissue plasminogen activator. *Neuron* 44:1031–1041.

McGee, A. W., Yang, Y., Fischer, Q. S., Daw, N. W., and Strittmatter, S. M. (2005). Experience-driven plasticity of visual cortex limited by myelin and Nogo receptor. *Science* 309: 2222–2226.

Miller, K. D. (1996). Synaptic economics: Competition and cooperation in synaptic plasticity. *Neuron* 17:371–374.

Mitchell, D. E., Cynader, M., and Movshon, J. A. (1977). Recovery from the effects of monocular deprivation in kittens. *J. Comp. Neurol.* 176:53–63.

Mrsic-Flogel, T. D., Hofer, S. B., Ohki, K., Reid, R. C., Bonhoeffer, T., and Hübener, M. (2007). Homeostatic regulation of eye-specific responses in visual cortex during ocular dominance plasticity. *Neuron* 54:961–972.

Muir, D. W., and Mitchell, D. E. (1973). Visual resolution and experience: Acuity deficits in cats following early selective visual deprivation. *Science* 180:420–422.

Ohki, K., Chung, S., Ch'ng, Y. H., Kara, P., and Reid, R. C. (2005). Functional imaging with cellular resolution reveals precise micro-architecture in visual cortex. *Nature* 433:597–603.

Ohki, K., Chung, S. Y., Kara, P., Hübener, M., Bonhoeffer, T., and Reid, R. C. (2006). Highly ordered arrangement of single neurons in orientation pinwheels. *Nature* 442:925–928.

Oray, S., Majewska, A., and Sur, M. (2004). Dendritic spine dynamics are regulated by monocular deprivation and extracellular matrix degradation. *Neuron* 44:1021–1030.

Pham, T. A., Graham, S. J., Suzuki, S., Barco, A., Kandel, E. R., Gordon, B., and Lickey, M. E. (2004). A semi-persistent adult ocular dominance plasticity in visual cortex is stabilized by activated CREB. *Learn. Mem.* 11:738–747.

Pizzorusso, T., Medini, P., Berardi, N., Chierzi, S., Fawcett, J. W., and Maffei, L. (2002). Reactivation of ocular dominance plasticity in the adult visual cortex. *Science* 298:1248–1251.

Porciatti, V., Pizzorusso, T., and Maffei, L. (1999). The visual physiology of the wild type mouse determined with pattern VEPs. *Vision Res.* 39:3071–3081.

Prusky, G. T., Alam, N. M., and Douglas, R. M. (2006). Enhancement of vision by monocular deprivation in adult mice. *J. Neurosci.* 26:11554–11561.

Prusky, G. T., and Douglas, R. M. (2003). Developmental plasticity of mouse visual acuity. *Eur. J. Neurosci.* 17:167–173.

Prusky, G. T., West, P. W. R., and Douglas, R. M. (2000). Behavioral assessment of visual acuity in mice and rats. *Vision Res.* 40:2201–2209.

Regehr, W. G., and Tank, D. W. (1991). Selective fura-2 loading of presynaptic terminals and nerve cell processes by local perfusion in mammalian brain slice. *J. Neurosci. Methods* 37:111–119.

Rittenhouse, C. D., Shouval, H. Z., Paradiso, M. A., and Bear, M. F. (1999). Monocular deprivation induces homosynaptic long-term depression in visual cortex. *Nature* 397:347–350.

Sawtell, N. B., Frenkel, M. Y., Philpot, B. D., Nakazawa, K., Tonegawa, S., and Bear, M. F. (2003). NMDA receptor-dependent ocular dominance plasticity in adult visual cortex. *Neuron* 38:977–985.

Schuett, S., Bonhoeffer, T., and Hübener, M. (2002). Mapping retinotopic structure in mouse visual cortex with optical imaging. *J. Neurosci.* 22:6549–6559.

Shatz, C. J., and Stryker, M. P. (1978). Ocular dominance in layer IV of the cat's visual cortex and the effects of monocular deprivation. *J. Physiol.* 281:267–283.

Shibuki, K., Hishida, R., Murakami, H., Kudoh, M., Kawaguchi, T., Watanabe, M., Watanabe, S., Kouuchi, T., and Tanaka, R. (2003). Dynamic imaging of somatosensory cortical activity in the rat visualized by flavoprotein autofluorescence. *J. Physiol. (Lond.)* 549:919–927.

Stosiek, C., Garaschuk, O., Holthoff, K., and Konnerth, A. (2003). In vivo two-photon calcium imaging of neuronal networks. *Proc. Natl. Acad. Sci. U.S.A.* 100:7319–7324.

Tagawa, Y., Kanold, P. O., Majdan, M., and Shatz, C. J. (2005). Multiple periods of functional ocular dominance plasticity in mouse visual cortex. *Nat. Neurosci.* 8:380–388.

Tohmi, M., Kitaura, H., Komagata, S., Kudoh, M., and Shibuki, K. (2006). Enduring critical period plasticity visualized by transcranial flavoprotein imaging in mouse primary visual cortex. *J. Neurosci.* 26:11775–11785.

Tropea, D., Kreiman, G., Lyckman, A., Mukherjee, S., Yu, H., Horng, S., and Sur, M. (2006). Gene expression changes and molecular pathways mediating activity-dependent plasticity in visual cortex. *Nat. Neurosci.* 9:660–668.

Turrigiano, G. G., and Nelson, S. B. (2004). Homeostatic plasticity in the developing nervous system. *Nat. Rev. Neurosci.* 5:97–107.

Wiesel, T. N., and Hubel, D. H. (1963). Single cell responses in striate cortex of kittens deprived of vision in one eye. *J. Neurophysiol.* 26:1003–1017.

37 Environmental Enrichment and Visual System Plasticity

ALESSANDRO SALE, NICOLETTA BERARDI, AND LAMBERTO MAFFEI

The development of neural circuits and of behavior is regulated by the interaction between genetically coded innate programs and experience. The prevailing consensus that genes and the environment work in concert in shaping brain development is the result of the nature versus nurture debate (for a review, see Krubitzer and Kahn, 2003), in which genetic and environmental influences have long been considered mutually exclusive in regulating mammalian brain development. This position has mostly resulted from the relatively recent (1960s) ability to quantify and measure environment-induced changes in the brain. Beginning in the early 1960s, brain development ceased to be considered an experience-independent process, and its mature structure has proved not to be immutable.

The mouse is used as a privileged model for studies aimed at investigating the influence of the environment on brain and behavior, thanks to the detailed knowledge available on its central nervous system (CNS) functions and the remarkable possibility afforded by the application of genetic engineering techniques in this species, allowing targeting of specific molecules in various transgenic lines. Considerable advances in this field have been obtained with the environmental enrichment (EE) paradigm.

Environmental enrichment was first defined by Rosenzweig et al. (1978) as "a combination of complex inanimate and social stimulation." It is a relative concept: an environmental setting is enriched with respect to other environmental settings. In studies on rodents under laboratory conditions, animals receiving EE are reared in large groups (8–12 individuals per cage) and in cages of large dimensions, with a variety of toys, tunnels, nesting material, and staircases available and changed frequently. In addition to the exploratory activity promoted by the presence of new objects, an essential component of EE is the opportunity for animals to attain high levels of voluntary physical activity on running wheels. For comparison, in the standard laboratory condition, animals are reared in small groups of 3–5 individuals in small cages where no particular items other than nesting material and food and water are present. At the opposite end of an ideal continuum of enrichment is the impoverished condition, in which even normal social interactions are prevented because animals are reared alone in separate cages.

It has often been suggested that EE in laboratory conditions is simply a way of rearing the animals in a setting more similar to the conditions in the wild, where animals explore the environment to find food, engage in physical activity both while foraging and while escaping predators, and cope with several challenges. However, observation of mice and rats that play in the EE and choose when and how much to run on the wheel, explore, and interact with the new objects suggests a different idea, namely, that EE is not just a way to reproduce more natural life conditions. Rather, EE animals are voluntarily exploring a rich environment without having to face the challenges present in the wild. One could speculate that the activity of mice and rats in the wild is mostly driven by necessity, whereas in an EE it is driven by curiosity (and perhaps pleasure). It is as if the ingenuity stimulated by challenge were exchanged for ingenuity stimulated by play.

Rosenzweig and colleagues originally showed that the morphology, chemistry, and physiology of the brain can be altered by exposure to EE (Rosenzweig, 1966; Rosenzweig and Bennett, 1969). Since then, a number of studies have been performed showing that EE can elicit various plastic responses in the brain at molecular, anatomical, and functional levels (for reviews, see Rosenzweig and Bennett, 1996; van Praag et al., 2000; Diamond, 2001).

The use of mice in these studies has made it possible to advance our knowledge of the processes underlying brain responses to the external world, and of the molecules involved. One field that has particularly benefited from studying mice in EE paradigms is visual system plasticity. The visual system is classically considered to be a paradigmatic model for the experience-dependent development and plasticity of the brain, and for the analysis of factors restricting environmental influence to specific developmental time windows, known as critical periods (Wiesel, 1982; Berardi et al., 2003; Hensch, 2005). The fields of visual cortical plasticity and EE, until recently separated, have been combined in the novel approach of investigating the effects of enhanced sensorimotor stimulation on the processes governing experience-dependent development in the visual system. In this analysis, visual system development serves as a model to study the effects of environment on brain development and plasticity, allowing researchers to uncover previously unknown effects of environmental experience on neural circuit development. At the same time, EE turned out to be a useful tool for probing visual circuit plasticity and for discovering previously unknown aspects of developmental visual plasticity. Use of the mouse in such experiments has often led to a characterization of the underlying molecular factors.

This chapter first surveys the vast literature on the effects of EE on the brain at anatomical, molecular, and behavioral levels. We have highlighted those studies in which the analysis particularly benefited from use of the mouse model. We then discuss the influence of early polysensorial stimulation on neural and behavioral development by reviewing data on the effects of maternal care and precocious novelty exposure in rodents. Finally, we present studies ongoing in our laboratory on the influence of EE on the development and plasticity of the visual system.

Influence of environment on brain and behavior: Neural consequences of environmental enrichment

Environmental enrichment has a variety of effects on the brain, and these effects have been found in several species of mammals, from mice and rats to gerbils, ground squirrels, cats, and monkeys (Rosenzweig and Bennett, 1969). At the anatomical level, which was the first to be investigated, exposure to an enriched living condition leads to a robust increase in cortical thickness and weight compared with those same parameters in animals reared under standard laboratory conditions (Rosenzweig et al., 1964). These changes occur in the entire dorsal cortex, including frontal, parietal, and occipital cortex. Since this initial finding was published, many studies have reported various anatomical changes associated with enriched living conditions, including an increase in soma size and in the size of nerve cell nucleus (Diamond, 1988), increased dendritic arborization (Holloway, 1966; Globus et al., 1973; Greenough et al., 1973), increased length of dendritic spines and increased synaptic size and number (Mollgaard et al., 1971; Turner and Greenough, 1985; Black et al., 1990), increased postsynaptic thickening (Diamond et al., 1964), and gliogenesis (Diamond et al., 1966). Recent studies have shown that exposure to an EE increases hippocampal neurogenesis (Kempermann et al., 1997) and reduces apoptotic cell death (Young et al., 1999).

One of the most striking properties of EE is the capacity to modify behavior, with the general rule that the best characterized effects are seen on tasks involving superior cognitive functions, mostly learning and memory (for a review, see Renner and Rosenzweig, 1987). EE enhances spatial learning and memory on the Morris water maze (Pacteau et al., 1989; Tees et al., 1990; Falkenberg et al., 1992; Paylor et al., 1992; Moser et al., 1997; Van Praag et al., 1999; Tees, 1999; Williams et al., 2001), reducing the cognitive decline in spatial memory typically associated with aging (for a review, see Winocur, 1998). The effects of EE on learning and memory are not limited to spatial abilities but extend to visual recognition memory and to classic conditioning, as shown by Rampon et al. (2000b).

Efforts aimed at understanding possible molecular mechanisms underlying the reported changes operated by EE on brain and behavior started very precociously, prompted by an interest in finding molecules that could be manipulated to reproduce the beneficial effects of the enriched experience. Early studies by Rosenzweig et al. (1962, 1967) found an increase in acetylcholinesterase activity, suggesting an effect on the cholinergic system, with subsequent studies confirming and extending this initial observation to the other neurotransmitter systems that have diffuse projections to the entire brain, such as the serotoninergic system (Rasmuson et al., 1998) and the noradrenergic system (Escorihuela et al., 1995; Naka et al., 2002). A large number of genes were found to change their expression levels in response to EE, most of them in functional classes linked to neuronal structure, synaptic transmission and plasticity, neuronal excitability, and neuroprotection (Rampon et al., 2000a; Keyvani et al., 2004). One group of molecules particularly sensitive to environmental stimuli and exerting potent effects on the nervous system are the neurotrophins, a class of neurotrophic factors promoting neuronal development and survival, comprising nerve growth factor (NGF), brain-derived neurotrophic factor (BDNF), neurotrophin-3 (NT-3), and neurotrophin-4 (NT-4). Neurotrophins are strongly implicated in regulating structural and functional plasticity both during development and in the adult (reviewed in Bonhoeffer, 1996; Cellerino and Maffei, 1996; Berardi and Maffei, 1999; Thoenen, 2000; Berardi et al., 2003). EE increases neurotrophic factor expression (reviewed in Pham et al., 2002) in the visual cortex and hippocampus (Torasdotter et al., 1996, 1998). In addition, EE can promote brain uptake of physiologically relevant trophic factors, such as insulin-like growth factor I (IGF-I), levels of which are sensitive to the amount of voluntary physical exercise (Carro et al., 2000, 2001; Koopmans et al., 2006).

Effects of early-life stimulation on neuronal and behavioral development

Experiences acquired between birth and weaning age are essential in promoting and regulating neural development and behavioral traits in the newborn of most mammalian species (Fleming et al., 1999). During this critical period of high developmental plasticity, maternal influence is one of the most important sources of sensory experience for the developing subject (Hofer, 1984; Ronca et al., 1993;

Liu et al., 2000), directly regulating physical growth and promoting neural maturation of brain structures involved in cognitive functions (Fleming et al., 1999). This issue has been intensively studied in laboratory rodents, in which the maternal behavior consists of stereotyped modules that can be easily investigated and manipulated in controlled experimental conditions.

One of the best characterized effects of precocious maternal influence is that on the stress responses exhibited by the offspring when they become adult (for a review, see Francis and Meaney, 1999). It has been repeatedly demonstrated that the offspring of mothers exhibiting high levels of maternal care show reduced behavioral fearfulness and stress levels as adults, compared with the offspring of less active caregivers. These differences extend beyond the system underlying the stress response to involve systems known to mediate cognitive processing. In particular, the offspring of mothers that show high levels of maternal care have enhanced spatial learning and memory when tested as adults in the Morris water maze (Liu et al., 2000). Furthermore, the same animals show increased expression of NMDA receptor subunits and BDNF mRNA in the hippocampus (Liu et al., 2000). Recently it has been shown that mice that received enhanced levels of maternal care owing to the presence of more than one dam in the cage displayed (once adult) a higher propensity to interact socially, achieved more promptly the behavioral profile of either dominant or subordinate male, and had higher NGF and BDNF levels (Branchi and Alleva, 2006).

The reported differences in stress response between the offspring of mothers exhibiting high and low levels of maternal care were found to depend on differences in DNA methylation of the glucocorticoid receptor (GR) gene promoter at the hippocampal level (Weaver et al., 2004). DNA methylation is a stable epigenetic mark of gene regulatory sequences, strongly affecting levels of gene transcription, with hypomethylation being associated with active chromatin structure and transcriptional activity (Keshet et al., 1985; Razin, 1998). In offspring of mothers providing high levels of care, the promoter region of the GR gene in hippocampal neurons undergoes a selective demethylation (Weaver et al., 2004). This difference in DNA methylation is long-lasting, remaining consistent through adulthood. The reduced methylation levels of the GR gene promoter render this sequence more accessible to transcription factor binding, thus resulting in increased GR gene expression. The ensuing higher efficiency of the feedback for circulating stress hormones is enhanced in rats that have experienced intensive maternal care levels during infancy, which explains the typical phenotype of reduced stress response exhibited by these animals (Weaver et al., 2004).

These new results strongly demonstrate that early environmental experiences can profoundly affect the adult phenotype through epigenetic processes affecting structure and function of the chromatin.

Despite the large amount of data obtained from enriched adult animals, the possibility that an enhanced sensorimotor stimulation provided by EE early in life could induce neural and behavioral changes has been little investigated. The scant interest in early-life EE studies can be partially attributed to the fact that preweaning enrichment is characterized by very little voluntary physical exercise, as the pups are simply too small and inert to engage in sustained activities. Since early enrichment provides increased levels of polysensorial stimulation during a period of high anatomical and functional rearrangement of the cerebral cortex, however, it might be expected to elicit brain changes through experience-dependent plasticity processes. This supposition has been confirmed by a handful of reports in the literature. Indeed, more complex dendritic branching has been found in cortical pyramidal cells following EE occurring either in the postnatal day 10 (P10)–P24 period (Venable et al., 1989) or starting post-weaning (Kolb, 1995), and EE attenuates the effects of an early lesion of the motor cortex (Kolb and Gibb, 2001).

A significant increase in neuronal cytodifferentiation has also been found in the motor cortex of rats reared under EE conditions during the early period of P5–P21, with EE animals consistently performing better on many measures of behavioral adaptive responses, as measured in open field, narrow path crossing, hind limb support, and rope climbing (Pascual and Figueroa, 1996).

Environmental enrichment and visual system development and plasticity

Despite the vast literature on the effects of EE on the brain, until recently little was known about the influence exerted by the early environment on the development, physiology, and plasticity of sensory systems. Indeed, in statements such as "the development of visual functions is experience dependent," experience generally refs to visual experience. Only recently has evidence been forthcoming that enhanced levels of sensorimotor stimulation in very young animals, such as that provided by an EE, affect the developmental plasticity of the visual system.

The most striking effect elicited by an EE paradigm starting at birth on visual system development is that it causes a marked acceleration in the maturation of visual acuity, a very sensitive and predictive index of the entire visual system development. Visual acuity development has been assessed in rats reared under EE conditions or in a standard laboratory cage (EE and non-EE rats) using electrophysiological recordings of visual evoked potentials (VEPs) from the binocular portion of the primary visual cortex (Landi et al., 2007b). A pronounced acceleration of visual acuity maturation due to exposure to EE has been replicated in the mouse at the behavioral level, using the visual water box task (Cancedda et al., 2004). The effect of EE on visual acuity maturation is illustrated in figure 37.1*A* (see also color plate 28). The acceleration in visual acuity development elicited by EE is a robust and surprising effect. When the time course for visual acuity development in the rat is rescaled to human development (see Berardi et al., 2000), it is as a child reached his or her final visual acuity at around 3 years of age, about 2 years before the age at which children's acuity development normally ends.

The ability of EE to profoundly affect the time course of visual function development underscores the importance of windows of high experience-dependent plasticity in the maturation of the cerebral cortex (Berardi et al., 2000). These early sensitive phases, known as critical periods, are normally well fitted with the maturational necessities of the developing organism, allowing, for instance, auditory neural circuitries to compensate for progressive enlargement of distances between sensory detectors at the periphery. The very high plasticity of developing neural circuits serves the purpose of allowing experience to guide the maturation of neural connections. As experience promotes the maturation of a set of neural circuits and the corresponding neural function, circuits and function become progressively less modifiable by experience, and plasticity declines.

Not surprisingly, the effects of early EE on visual acuity development are paralleled by a profound influence on the time course of developmental visual cortical plasticity. First,

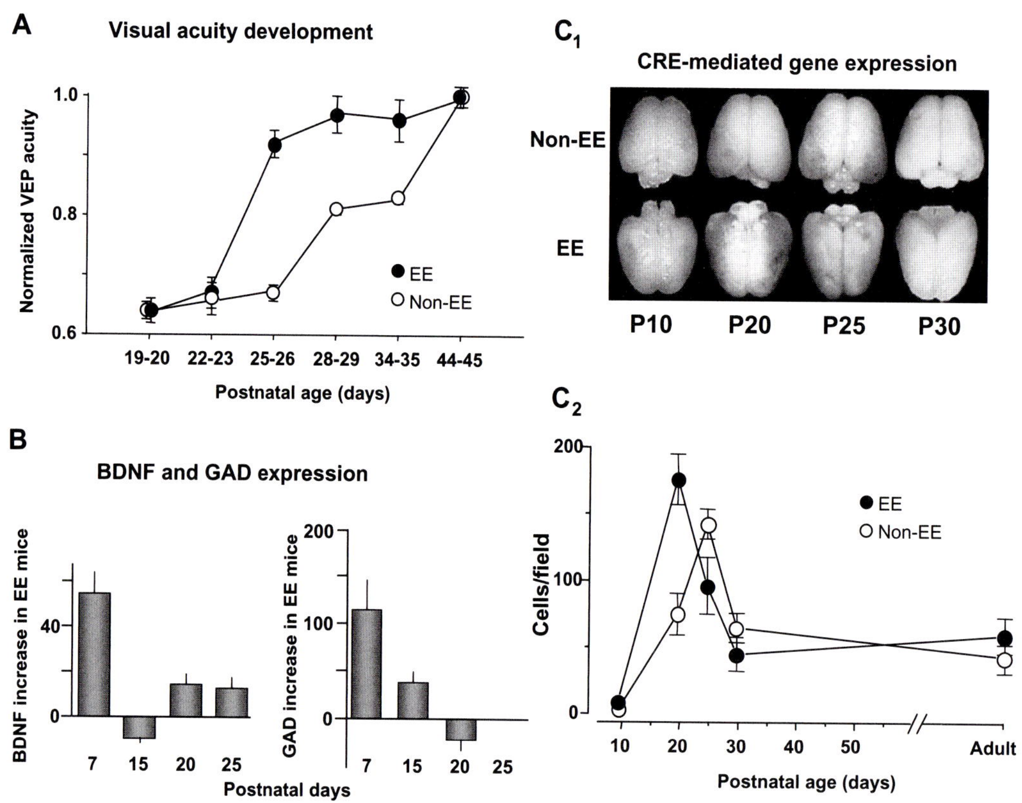

FIGURE 37.1 Acceleration of visual system development by environmental enrichment. *A*, EE accelerates the maturation of visual acuity. Visual acuity of non-EE (white) and EE (black) rats has been assessed by means of visual evoked potentials (VEPs) recorded from the binocular portion of the visual cortex at different ages during postnatal development. VEP acuity is normalized to the acuity value at P44–P45 and is plotted as a function of age for each experimental group to show the leftward shift of the curve for EE animals. *B*, Higher levels of BDNF and GAD65/67 expression in EE pups. ELISA and Western blot analysis have been used to measure, respectively, BDNF and GAD65/67 protein levels in the visual cortex of EE and non-EE animals at different postnatal ages. Data are plotted as percentage of variation between the two groups, with positive values indicating higher levels in EE mice. *C*, Accelerated CRE-mediated gene expression development in the visual cortex of EE mice. C_1, Examples of brains at different ages (P10–P30) from CRE-lacZ transgenic mice reared in non-EE or EE conditions. X-gal histochemistry has been used to reveal the occurrence of CRE-mediated gene expression (black staining). C_2, Quantification of the density of X-gal-positive cells for non-EE (white) and EE (black) mice at the indicated ages. Fields were chosen to sample layers II–VI of the binocular visual cortex. CRE-mediated gene expression is developmentally regulated in both groups, but its peak is accelerated in EE mice. See color plate 28. (*A*, Modified from Landi et al., 2007b. *B* and *C*, Modified from Cancedda et al., 2004.)

EE mice have an accelerated developmental decline of the long-term potentiation (LTP) of layer II/III field potentials induced by theta burst stimulation from the white matter (WM-layer II/III LTP) in their visual cortex. This kind of LTP is a well-established in vitro model of developmental plasticity (Kirkwood et al., 1995; Huang et al., 1999), since the susceptibility to potentiation of layer II/III synaptic responses after stimulation of the white matter is present only during a critical period in the early life of rodents, being absent in adult animals. Although at a very early age, substantial WM-layer II/III LTP is found in both EE and non-EE mice, the developmental decline in LTP magnitude is much faster under EE conditions (Cancedda et al., 2004). Second, EE rats have a precocious closure of the critical period for ocular dominance (OD) plasticity in response to monocular deprivation (MD) (Medini et al., 2008), a classic measure of developmental experience-dependent plasticity in the visual cortex. Therefore, it seems that the quality and intensity of environmental-dependent experience powerfully sculpt the development of the visual system, regulating the interplay between its critical period time course and the maturation of visual functional abilities.

Which molecular factors underly the effects of EE on visual plasticity and development? One important observation is that the acceleration of visual system development in EE mice closely resembles that previously reported in mice engineered to overexpress in their forebrain the neurotrophin BDNF. These mice also exhibit a pronounced acceleration in both the maturation of their visual acuity and in the time course of visual cortical synaptic plasticity (Huang et al., 1999). One possible model put forward to explain the accelerated visual acuity development and visual cortical plasticity decline in BDNF-overexpressing mice (Huang et al., 1999) is that higher BDNF levels would accelerate the development of the inhibitory GABAergic system, which, by affecting receptive field (RF) development and synaptic plasticity, could explain both the faster maturation of visual acuity and the precocious decline of cortical plasticity. Interestingly, the same model turned out to be valid in the case of EE mice. Mice reared from birth in an EE have higher levels of the BDNF protein in their visual cortex at P7 (figure 37.1*B* and color plate 28), an effect accompanied by increased expression of the GABA biosynthetic enzymes, GAD65/67, at both P7 and P15 (See figure 37.1*B* and color plate 28). Therefore, an important mediator of environmentally dependent BDNF action could be intracortical inhibition (Cancedda et al., 2004; Sale et al., 2004). Downstream in the BDNF signaling pathway, an effective role in the acceleration of visual cortical development has been reported for the cAMP/CREB system, which is known to be an important hub in the development and plasticity of sensory systems (Impey et al., 1996; Pham et al., 1999; Barth et al., 2000; Mower et al., 2002; Cancedda et al., 2003). Transgenic mice carrying the lacZ reporter gene under the control of the CRE promoter (CRE-LacZ mice; Impey et al., 1996) offer the possibility to visualize the neural cells in which CRE-mediated gene expression occurs. In these animals the lacZ gene product, β-galactosidase, can be visualized as a blue precipitate using X-gal histochemistry. CRE-mediated gene expression is developmentally regulated in the mouse visual cortex, peaking at around P25 under normal rearing conditions (Cancedda et al., 2004). Notably, this peak of gene expression is markedly accelerated in EE subjects (Cancedda et al., 2004) (figure 37.1C_1 and C_2 and color plate 28). That this change in the time course of CRE-mediated gene expression is involved in the acceleration of visual system maturation found at the physiological level is demonstrated by an experiment in which this molecular pathway was pharmacologically enhanced through injections of rolipram (Cancedda et al., 2004), a specific inhibitor of the high-affinity phosphodiesterase type IV that activates the cAMP system via inhibition of cAMP breakdown, resulting in an increased phosphorylation of the transcription factor CREB (Tohda et al., 1996; Kato et al., 1998; Nakagawa et al., 2002). Mice injected with rolipram from P7 until P21 have accelerated development of visual acuity that mimics, at least in part, that found in EE mice (Cancedda et al., 2004).

These studies show that the environment sculpts the development of the visual system not only through changes in the levels of visual stimulation but also through factors activated even in the absence of vision. This is suggested by the observation that the increased cortical BDNF expression and the accelerated maturation of intracortical inhibition in EE animals are observed at very early ages, before eye opening, and by experiments that have used a temporally restricted EE protocol in which pups are maintained under enriched conditions only until P12, when they are transferred to a normal standard cage. In these animals, exposed to EE up to eye opening, there is a "priming" of visual acuity development: when tested at P25, they show a higher visual acuity than non-EE animals, although the effect is smaller that that found in animals left in EE up to P25 (Baldini et al., 2007). Thus, exposure to EE before eye opening can affect the much later occurring visual acuity development.

This raises the possibility that visual cortical development can be influenced by EE even in the complete absence of vision. This important issue has been addressed in the investigation of EE effects in dark-reared (DR) animals performed by Bartoletti et al. (2004).

Lack of visual experience from birth prevents maturation of the visual cortical circuits. In particular, visual connections do not consolidate, remaining plastic well after the end of the critical period, and visual acuity does not develop (Cynader and Mitchell, 1980; Mower, 1991; Fagiolini et al., 1994; Berardi et al., 2000). All these effects can be completely counteracted by providing DR animals with the opportunity to experience high sensorimotor stimulation in an EE while in the dark (Bartoletti et al., 2004). DR rats exposed to EE show normal closure of the critical period for OD plasticity and normal visual acuity development. In particular, by assessing the effectiveness of MD in shifting the OD of visual cortical neurons after P50, it has been found that MD (1 week) was still effective in shifting the OD of visual cortical neurons in favor of the ipsilateral non-deprived eye in DR-non-EE rats, as expected (figure 37.2*B* and *C*, and color plate 29). However, MD from P50 was ineffective in DR-EE littermates of DR-non-EE rats placed in EE at P18, as is the case for rats with normal visual experience (see figure 37.2*B* and *C* and color plate 29).

The EE effect in this case is also very similar to that found in BDNF-overexpressing mice, where a rescue of DR effects on visual acuity development and the critical period for OD plasticity has been reported (Gianfranceschi et al., 2003). The similarity between the effects obtained using either genetic engineering techniques to increase neurotrophin expression or conditions of increased environmental complexity offers a clear view of the interaction between nature and nurture during the development of sensory systems.

It is known that DR prevents the developmental organization into perineuronal nets of chondroitin sulfate proteoglycans (CSPGs), components of the extracellular matrix that have recently been shown to be important nonpermissive factors for visual cortical plasticity (Lander et al., 1997; Pizzorusso et al., 2002); indeed, removal of CSPGs restores OD plasticity to the adult visual cortex (Pizzorusso et al., 2002, 2006). Interestingly, EE greatly reduces the effects of

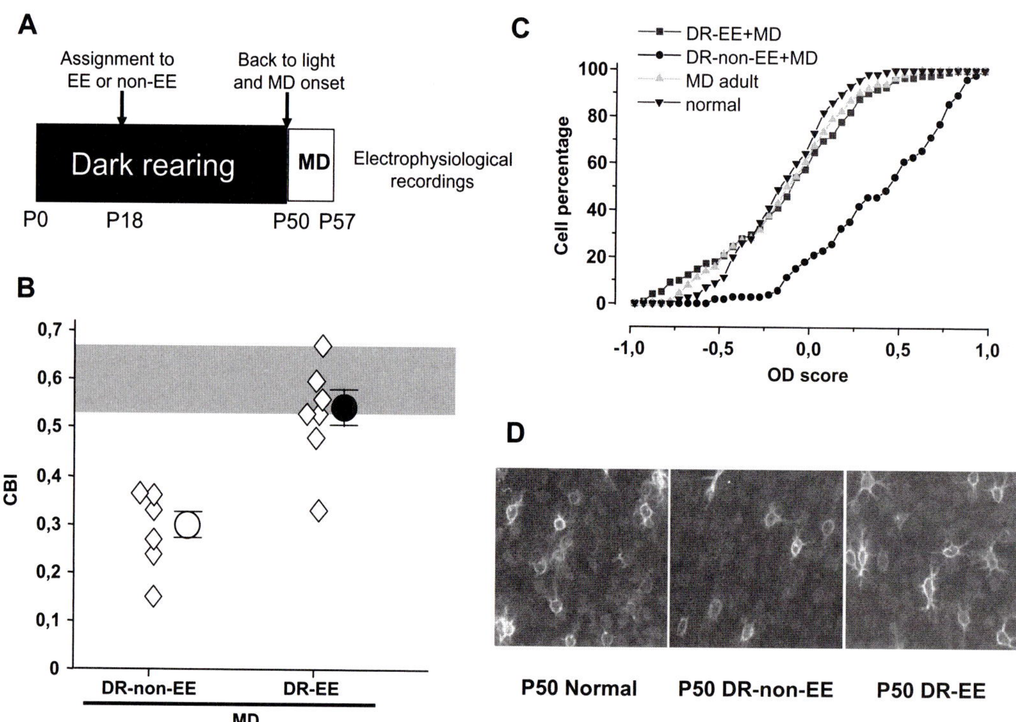

FIGURE 37.2 Environmental enrichment promotes consolidation of visual cortical connections in dark-reared rats. *A*, Schematic diagram of the dark-rearing (DR) protocol combined with EE. Newborn rats were reared in complete darkness from P0 until P50. Together with DR, they were maintained, starting from P18, in either non-EE or EE conditions. Rats were then subjected to 1 week of MD, in normal light conditions. *B* and *C*, Normal closure of the critical period for MD in EE rats. *B*, Summary of MD effects in all DR animals. The OD distribution of each animal has been summarized with the contralateral bias index (CBI = {[N(1) − N(7)] + 1/2[N(2/3) − N(5/6)] + N(Tot)}/2N(Tot), where N(tot) is the total number of recorded cells and N(i) is the number of cells in class (i) (*open diamonds* denote individual data; *circles* denote mean of the group ± SE). CBI scores in DR-non-EE + MD rats differ from those in DR-EE + MD rats, which do not differ from those in normal adults (*shaded rectangle*). *C*, Cumulative fractions for OD scores. For each cell, an OD score was computed as {[Peak(ipsi) − baseline(ipsi)] − [Peak(contra) − baseline(contra)]}/{[Peak(ipsi) − baseline(ipsi)] + [Peak(contra) − baseline(contra)]} (Rittenhouse et al., 1999). This score is −1 for class 1 cells, +1 for class 7 cells, and around 0 for class 4 cells. Only the curve for DR + non-EE MD animals significantly differs from that in normal rats. *D*, Examples of staining for Wisteria floribunda agglutinin, which labels perineural nets, in Oc1B of a normal rat, a DR-non-EE rat, and a DR-EE rat at P50. The decrease caused by DR in the number of perineural net–surrounded neurons is reduced in EE-DR animals. Calibration bar = 100 μm. See color plate 29. (Modified from Bartoletti et al., 2004.)

DR on the development of perineuronal nets (figure 37.2*D* and color plate 29). Bartoletti et al. (2004) also examined the effects of EE on the status of cortical inhibition, as there is growing evidence that the maturation of inhibition in the visual cortex is an important determinant of the critical period (Hensch, 2005). The expression of GAD65 in the presynaptic boutons of GABAergic interneurons around the soma of the target neurons is decreased by DR, as is already known for other markers of GABAergic function (Benevento et al., 1995). In DR-EE animals, however, GAD65 expression was normal.

The observation that EE promotes the development of visual acuity, closure of the critical period for OD plasticity, and the development of crucial determinants of developmental visual cortical plasticity (as perineuronal nets and intracortical inhibition in DR rats) shows that it is possible to modulate the outcome of visual deprivation by varying the environmental conditions in a mammalian species. This confirms the hypothesis, prompted by the precociousness of the molecular effects elicited by EE in the visual cortex, that factors not under the exclusive control of visual experience may contribute to visual cortical development. The possibility of affecting visual cortical development in the complete absence of vision underscores the importance of the interactions between distinct sensory experiences for the maturation of neural circuits.

Which kind of nonvisual experience, then, acts on pups reared in EE? The first 2 weeks of life in rodents are characterized by a general absence of interaction between the newborn and the environment; pups remain in the nest, totally dependent on the mother, which can be considered the most important source of sensory experience for the developing pup (Hofer, 1984; Liu et al., 2000). It has therefore been suggested (Cancedda et al., 2004) that during the first 2 weeks of life, enriched stimuli present in the environment affect pup visual system development through maternal behavior: different levels of maternal care received by pups in different environmental conditions could act as an indirect mediator of the earliest effects of EE on visual system development. Indeed, a detailed quantitative analysis of maternal care behavior in either EE or standard condition showed that enriched pups receive higher levels of maternal care than those reared in the standard condition (Sale et al., 2004). In particular, EE pups experience continuous physical contact owing to the presence of adult females in the nest (figure 37.3*A*) and also receive higher levels of licking (figure 37.3*B*), two of the most critical maternal behaviors for the development of the newborn, which have been associated with hormonal regulation of growth and with the expression of neuroendocrine and behavioral responses to stress (Liu et al., 1997). It is likely that this sustained tactile stimulation can affect pup neural development, providing a source for the earliest changes observed in EE mice. This conclusion is supported by data showing that variations in maternal care can affect BDNF levels and the neural development of offspring (Liu et al., 2000).

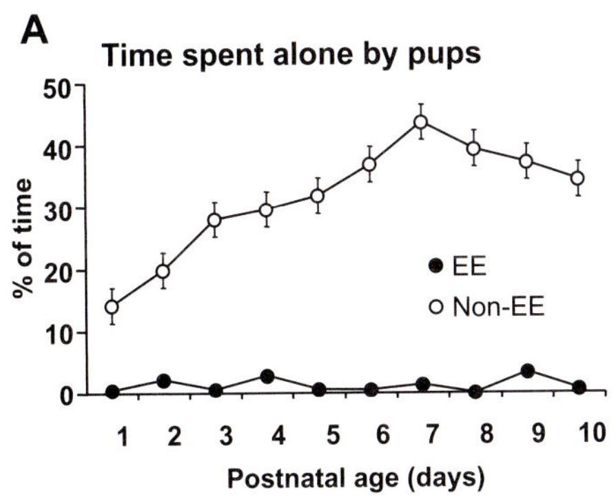

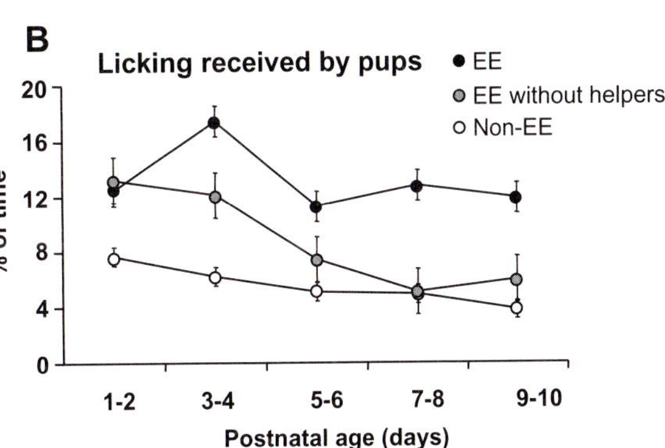

Figure 37.3 Maternal care in EE mice. Maternal care behavior was scored during six daily observation sessions of 75 minutes each for the first 10 days postpartum. The observation sessions occurred at 6:45 a.m., 9:00 a.m., 12:00 a.m., 3:00 p.m., 6:00 p.m., and 9:00 p.m.; the first and last sessions were during dark phase of the daily cycle and were performed under dim red light illumination. During each session the behavior of each adult female was scored every 3 minutes, recording whether or not a target behavior was present. *A*, Frequency of "pups alone" recordings during the first 10 days postpartum in non-EE (white) and EE (black) mice. The percentage of time spent by pups alone in the nest is dramatically lower in EE than in non-EE mice. Indeed, EE pups are virtually never alone in the nest, since when the mother is absent, she is always replaced by another adult female. *B*, Frequency of "licking" recordings during the first 10 days postpartum in non-EE (white), EE (black), and EE in a simplified condition where no adult females other than the mother are present (EE without helpers, gray). In the EE condition, maternal and nonmaternal licking have been summed. EE pups receive the highest levels of licking, followed by pups in the EE without helper condition and then by non-EE pups. Interestingly, an analysis of licking behavior exhibited only by dams (excluding the contribution of helper females) shows that mothers in the EE without helper condition exhibit significantly more licking than both non-EE and EE mothers. (Modified from Sale et al., 2004.)

One protocol particularly informative of the effects of maternal care on pup growth entails maternal separation: pups are removed from the dam some times a day for a total of 3–6 hours during the first 2 weeks of postnatal age. This treatment has many detrimental consequences for newborn development. For instance, just 1 hour of maternal separation in the rat results in a decrease in the activity of ornithine decarboxylase (Wang et al., 1996) and growth hormone, both substances essential for normal somatic and neural development. This effect can be completely prevented through artificial tactile stimulation applied to separated pups with a brush at a frequency resembling that of maternal licking (Pauk et al., 1986). Artificial tactile stimulation during the first 10 days of life also attenuates the effects of a perinatal lesion of the motor cortex (Kolb and Gibb, 2001), reproducing the effects of EE.

If the enhanced tactile stimulation provided to the pups in EE is a crucial part of the "nonvisual experience" that has been shown to act on visual development, it might be possible to induce an acceleration in visual acuity development by providing artificial tactile stimulation to pups reared in a nonenriched condition. This hypothesis has been tested by applying to developing rats a stimulation that combines gentle stroking with a wet brush and a manual massage applied on the pup's trunk and limbs from P1 to P12. These two treatments mimic maternal licking and grooming. The results show that this artificial tactile stimulation is quite effective in "priming" visual acuity development: when tested at P25 and P28 (both electrophysiologically and behaviorally), treated pups showed a higher visual acuity than control rats (Baldini et al., 2007). The acceleration produced by this treatment is less than that shown in age-matched subjects receiving continuous EE from birth to the day of testing but is equal to that obtained using the temporally restricted EE protocol in which pups are maintained under enriched conditions only until P12. These results point toward maternal stimulation as the fundamental factor mediating the effects of EE on visual system development at very early ages, when pups do not engage in direct exploration of the surrounding environment (Sale et al., 2004). It would be important to know whether a similar cross-modal effect of tactile stimulation on visual development could be documented in human newborns. Results obtained in premature infants, in collaboration with the Department of Developmental Neuroscience, Stella Maris, Pisa, and the Neonatology Unit, Dipartimento di Medicina della Procreazione e dell'Età Evolutiva, Pisa University, go in this direction.

In sum, the available evidence has dissipated the mystery that once surrounded the remarkable ability of EE to strongly affect the brain—a phenomenon that in turn has caused EE to be viewed with mistrust as a scientific protocol for studying brain-environment interactions. EE acts during visual system development by modulating well-known factors involved in controlling developmental cortical plasticity. Some of them, such as BDNF and the maturation of intracortical inhibitory circuitry, are precociously affected by EE through the different levels of maternal care experienced by EE pups; others, such as the CRE-CREB system and the perineural nets, are affected later in development and can therefore be modulated both by the direct interactions of pups with the EE and by events triggered by the early factors.

Besides confirming the role of already well known players in the development and plasticity of the rodent visual system, EE has allowed the identification of a new player. There is indeed one molecule whose critical role in mediating the influence of the environment on the development of the visual system has emerged through studies using the EE paradigm, insuline-like growth factor-I (IGF-I). IGF-I crosses the blood-brain barrier and, acting on neurons bearing its receptors, increases their electrical activity, inducing the production of other factors important for visual cortical plasticity, such as BDNF (Thoenen and Sendtner, 2002). IGF-I receptors are expressed in the occipital cortex (Frolich et al., 1998). Recent data suggest that IGF-I might be an important mediator of EE action on the development of the visual cortex. IGF-I is increased postnatally in the visual cortex of EE rats, and after weaning, administration of IGF-I in this structure through osmotic minipumps mimics EE effects on visual acuity maturation, leading to a marked acceleration that is particularly evident at P25 (Ciucci et al., 2007). Furthermore, blocking IGF-I action in the visual cortex of developing EE subjects through infusion of the IGF-I antagonist JB1 completely prevents EE effects on visual acuity development. Interestingly, a role for IGF-I in visual cortical plasticity was recently suggested following a complex genetic screening for factors controlled by visual experience during development: Tropea et al. (2006) demonstrated that MD increases the expression of IGF-I-binding protein and affects several genes in the IGF-I pathway, and that exogenous application of IGF-I prevents the physiological effect of MD on OD plasticity in vivo.

One important issue that has recently begun to be addressed is whether the influence of the environment during development is restricted to the visual cortex or whether structures considered less plastic than the visual cortex, such as the retina, can be affected by EE. It is commonly assumed that retinal development is independent of sensory inputs, leading to the notion that the retina is less plastic than the cortex or hippocampus, the very site of experience-dependent plasticity. For instance, visual deprivation such as MD or DR that are known to dramatically affect visual cortical acuity are virtually ineffective on retinal acuity in cat, rat, and humans (Baro et al., 1990; Fagiolini et al., 1994; Fine et al., 2003). However, it has recently been shown that

DR alters inner retinal development in mice (Tian and Copenhagen, 2001, 2003), preventing the segregation of ON and OFF pathways, at both electrophysiological and anatomical level. EE, which so powerfully affects visual cortical development, seemed a paradigm suitable for probing the actual sensitivity of retinal development to experience, and to gain insight into the factors involved.

To understand whether retinal functional development is a target of EE and to compare EE effects on cortical and retinal development, the development of retinal responses was assessed using pattern electroretinogram (P-ERG) (Landi et al., 2007a). P-ERG is a sensitive measure of the function of retinal ganglion cells (RGCs), the very output of retinal circuitry (Maffei and Fiorentini, 1981). The results show that retinal acuity development is sensitive to EE on the same time scale as cortical acuity. In particular, retinal acuity development is strongly accelerated in EE rats compared with non-EE rats starting from P25, and this accelerated retinal development in EE animals is also found in rats exposed to EE for only the first 10 days of life, that is, before eye opening (figure 37.4*A* and *B*; Landi et al., 2007b). These experiments suggest that factors influenced by EE and sufficient to trigger the much later occurring retinal acuity development are affected during the first 10 days of life. One crucial factor in this process is BDNF: EE causes a precocious increase in BDNF expression in the RGC layer, and

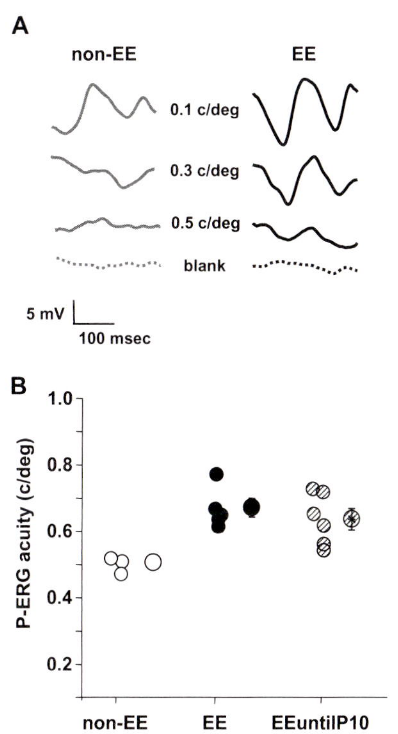

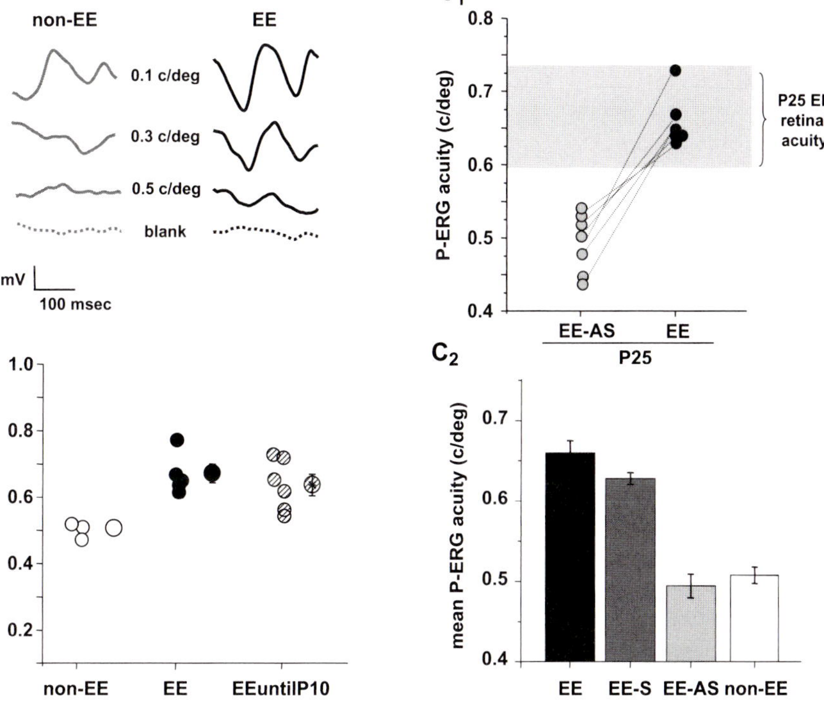

FIGURE 37.4 Retinal functional development is sensitive to environmental enrichment. *A*, Examples of steady-state pattern electroretinogram (P-ERG) signals recorded at P25 in response to visual stimulation with gratings of three different spatial frequencies in one non-EE (*gray traces*) and one EE (*black traces*) rat. The gratings were sinusoidally modulated at a temporal frequency of 4 Hz (period of 250 ms), and the principal component of the P-ERG response is on a temporal frequency twice the temporal frequency of the stimulus. A P-ERG recorded in response to a blank field is reported to show the noise level. A response to a pattern of 0.5 c/deg is still present in the EE rat but not in the non-EE rat. *B*, Acceleration of retinal acuity maturation in EE rats. Retinal acuity values were assessed at P25–P26 (*small symbols* denote individual data; larger symbols denote mean of the group) in non-EE rats (white), in rats enriched until P25 (EE, black), and in rats enriched until P10 (striped). Retinal acuity is higher in EE than in non-EE animals, and, interestingly, retinal acuity of EE-until-P10 rats does not differ from that in EE rats. This suggests that 10 days' enrichment is sufficient to trigger EE effects on retinal functional development. *C*, BDNF is necessary for EE effects on retinal functional development. C_1, Injections of BDNF antisense oligonucleotides block the accelerated maturation of retinal acuity observed in EE animals. Retinal acuity has been determined at P25 for both eyes in EE animals that are treated with BDNF antisense oligos in one eye and are left untreated in the other eye; for each animal, the retinal acuity of the treated and of the untreated eye are reported, joined by a *dotted line*. The acuity of the BDNF antisense-treated eye is significantly lower than that of the fellow eye in all animals. C_2, Mean retinal acuity in EE, EE treated intraocularly with BDNF sense oligos (EE-S, control treatment), EE treated with antisense oligos (EE-AS), and non-EE rats. The EE and non-EE groups are as described in *B*. The retinal acuity of EE-AS rats differs from that of EE animals but not from that of non-EE animals, while the retinal acuity in EE-S rats differs from that of non-EE rats but not from that of EE rats. (Modified from Landi et al., 2007b.)

blocking BDNF expression in the retina during this window of enhanced expression by means of antisense oligonucleotides counteracts the precocious development of retinal acuity in EE animals (figure 37.4C_1 and C_2; Landi et al., 2007b). EE, acting through BDNF, also has a strong effect on the developmental segregation of RGC dendrites into the ON and OFF sublaminae, crucial for the emergence of the ON and OFF pathways: in EE rats, RGC dendrite segregation is accelerated and the effects of DR on this process are prevented. Blocking retinal BDNF by means of antisense oligonucleotides blocks EE effects (Landi et al., 2007b).

Since visual development is strongly affected by manipulations occurring before eye opening and in the absence of visual input, provided that adequate levels of critical molecular factors are available to the developing circuitries, then, pushing the reasoning to the extreme, it should also be possible to manipulate the system during very early stages of maturation, in the prenatal life.

Maternal influence on offspring development occurs not only in the form of maternal care provided to pups during the first postnatal weeks but also in the form of supplying of nutrients, hormones, and respiratory gases to the fetus during pregnancy, through placental exchanges (for a review, see Anthony et al., 1995). The extent to which different environmental conditions experienced by the mother affect fetal development is still debated. Most experimental evidence is concerned with the deleterious effects of prenatal stress on fetal development, which include delayed somatic growth (Barlow et al., 1978, Benesova and Pavlik, 1989), delayed motor development (Gramsbergen and Mulder, 1998), and cognitive and behavioral abnormalities (Shiota and Kayamura, 1989; Schneider, 1992; Poltyrev et al., 1996; Lordi et al., 1997; Weinstock, 1997; Szuran et al., 2000; Kofman, 2002), which also occur in humans (Kofman, 2002; Mulder et al. 2002). Some of these effects on offspring development can be rescued by putting stressed mother and the pups into an EE just after delivery (Koo et al., 2003). Very little is known, on the other hand, regarding the possible beneficial effects on embryonic development that might be derived from maternal exposure to increased social and sensorimotor activities. Recent data show that the environment has a strong influence on the developing visual system during fetal life. Maternal EE extended for the entirety of the pregnancy results in a marked acceleration of retinal anatomical development in the rat embryos, with faster dynamics of programmed cell death in RGCs (Sale et al., 2007a). These effects are under the control of IGF-I: its levels, higher in EE pregnant rats and in their milk, are increased as well in the retina of embryos. Neutralization of IGF-I abolishes the action of maternal enrichment on retinal development, and chronic IGF-I injection given to non-EE dams mimics the effects of EE in the fetuses (Sale et al., 2007a).

Taken together, the results of various studies point to at least three distinct temporal phases during pup development that are controlled by the richness of the environment, through different mechanisms (figure 37.5 and color plate 30). In the first phase, maternal enrichment during pregnancy may affect the expression of factors such as IGF-I in the offspring, determining a faster development. An example is the increased IGF-I expression in the RGC layer, which results in an accelerated completion of the process of natural RGC death.

In the second phase, enhanced maternal care levels in EE rats trigger a precocious maturation of retinal acuity and visual cortical functions in the offspring, providing the developing subject with a robust tactile stimulation that could be responsible for the higher levels of IGF-I and BDNF in both the RGC layer and the visual cortex. Precocious expression of BDNF then leads to a precocious development of intracortical inhibition (Huang et al., 1999); in the retina, the precocious increase in BDNF in EE pups is necessary for the accelerated retinal development caused by EE (Landi et al., 2007b).

Finally, in the third phase, when pups begin to actively explore their surroundings, the complex sensorimotor stimulation provided by EE may directly influence their visual system development through IGF-I and possibly BDNF, and the maturation of perineural nets and intracortical inhibition, further accelerating the maturation of visual acuity, determining a faster closure of the critical period for OD plasticity, and preventing DR effects.

The changes documented for these three phases occur sequentially, but it is conceivable they are causally linked. In other words, each phase might act as a trigger for the successive ones. An example is the triggering effect of exposure to EE up to P10 on retinal acuity development (Landi et al., 2007b). It may also be possible that acceleration of developmental CRE-mediated gene expression in the visual cortex might be triggered by the early increase in BDNF expression, although a direct effect of pup exploratory activity is also likely, given the well-known effects of EE exposure on the CREB pathway and on other plasticity genes impinging on it (Molteni et al., 2002).

The effects of EE on visual cortical plasticity are not limited to the developmental period but seem to be present in the adult as well. Recent data show that exposing adult rats to EE strongly increases visual cortical plasticity to the point that it favors recovery from visual pathologies, such as amblyopia. Amblyopia is characterized by a loss of visual acuity in the eye deprived during the critical period. In all species tested so far, recovery from amblyopia is very limited in the adult because of the decline in visual cortical plasticity that occurs with critical period closure. EE control on adult visual cortical plasticity is achieved by modulating critical period determinants such as the intracortical inhibitory

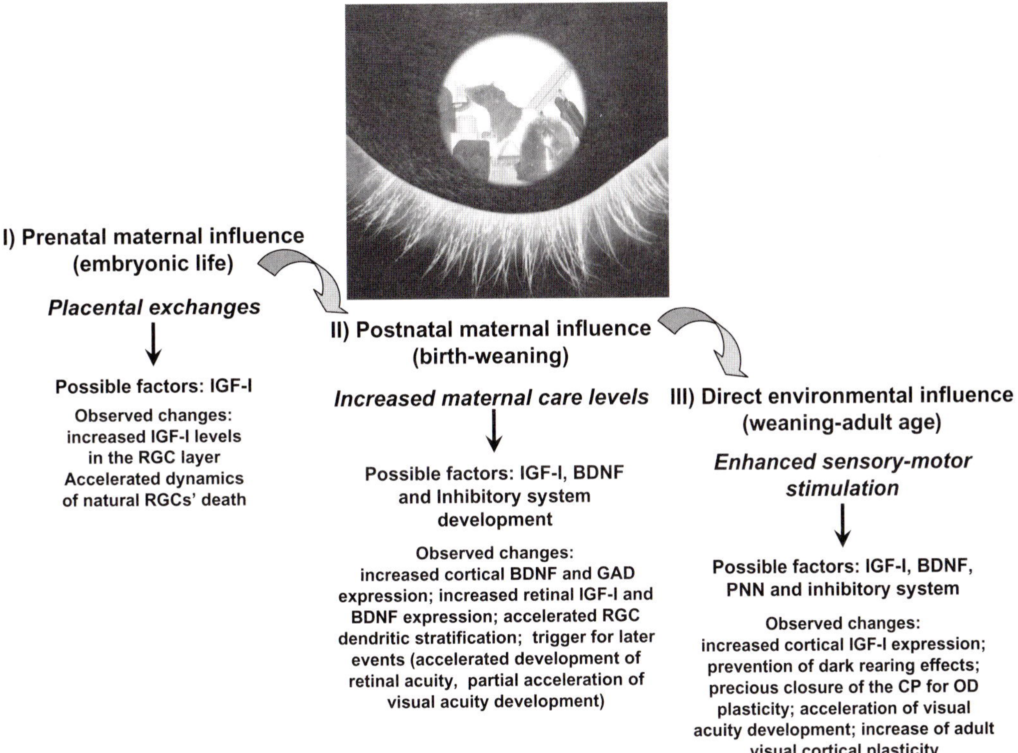
EE and visual system development: A three-phase interpretive model
I) Prenatal maternal influence
(embryonic life)
Placental exchanges
Possible factors: IGF-I
Observed changes:
increased IGF-I levels
in the RGC layer
Accelerated dynamics
of natural RGCs' death
II) Postnatal maternal influence
(birth-weaning)
Increased maternal care levels
Possible factors: IGF-I, BDNF
and Inhibitory system
development
Observed changes:
increased cortical BDNF and GAD
expression; increased retinal IGF-I and
BDNF expression; accelerated RGC
dendritic stratification; trigger for later
events (accelerated development of
retinal acuity, partial acceleration of
visual acuity development)
III) Direct environmental influence
(weaning-adult age)
Enhanced sensory-motor
stimulation
Possible factors: IGF-I, BDNF,
PNN and inhibitory system
Observed changes:
increased cortical IGF-I expression;
prevention of dark rearing effects;
precious closure of the CP for OD
plasticity; acceleration of visual
acuity development; increase of adult
visual cortical plasticity

Figure 37.5 Model of environmental enrichment effects on visual system development and plasticity. Shown is an interpretive framework for understanding the data on EE influence on the developing visual system. The effects elicited by EE on visual system development and plasticity are due not only to changes in the levels of sensory visual stimulation but also to very early factors activated even in the absence of vision. The available data support a model in which three distinct temporal phases during pup development are differently controlled by the richness of the environment: a prenatal phase in which the mother mediates the influence of the environment through placental exchanges with the fetus, an early postnatal phase in which higher levels of maternal care in EE stimulate the expression of experience-dependent factors in the visual system, and a third (and final) phase in which the autonomous interaction of the developing pup with the enriched environment further promotes the maturation of visual functions (see the text for details). See color plate 30.

system, extracellular matrix components, and BDNF (Sale et al., 2007b).

Conclusion

We began this chapter with the statement that each individual is the result of interactions between genes and the environment. Given the nature of the stimulation provided by EE, we think it unlikely that its effects are limited to visual system development. Rather, we think that EE effects on developmental visual cortical plasticity are indicative of the profound control exerted by the environment on sensory systems and more generally on brain development, a control that up to now has been underestimated.

Among the most surprising results are that environmental conditions start affecting neural circuit development during intrauterine life and that, even if restricted to short time windows in development, they set in motion, through specific factors, events that lead to changes in the maturational time course of neural responses that take place weeks later (years later in human terms). This is strongly reminiscent of the longlasting effects of level of maternal care on stress responses in offspring. Maternal care levels appear to be one of the crucial mediators of EE effects on visual system development.

It is good to know that while we are cuddling our infants, in addition to building a love bond we may be contributing to their visual system development.

ACKNOWLEDGMENT Work was supported by MIUR COFIN.

REFERENCES

Anthony, R. V., Pratt, S. L., Liang, R., and Holland, M. D. (1995). Placental-fetal hormonal interactions: impact on fetal growth. *J. Anim. Sci.* 73:1861–1871.

Baldini, S., Sale, A., Baroncelli, L., Putignano, E., Ciucci, F., Berardi, N., and Maffei, L. (2007). Increased tactile stimulation accelerates visual development in rats. *Soc. Neurosci. Abstr.* 346.18. Online.

Barlow, S. M., Knight, A. F., and Sullivan, F. M. (1978). Delay in postnatal growth and development of offspring produced by maternal restraint stress during pregnancy in the rat. *Teratology* 18:211–218.

Baro, J. A., Lehmkuhle, S., and Kratz, K. E. (1990). Electroretinograms and visual evoked potentials in long-term monocularly deprived cats. *Invest. Ophthalmol. Vis. Sci.* 31:1405–1409.

Barth, A. L., McKenna, M., Glazewski, S., Hill, P., Impey, S., Storm, D., and Fox, K. (2000). Upregulation of cAMP response element-mediated gene expression during experience-dependent plasticity in adult neocortex. *J. Neurosci.* 20:4206–4216.

Bartoletti, A., Medini, P., Berardi, N., and Maffei, L. (2004). Environmental enrichment prevents effects of dark-rearing in the rat visual cortex. *Nat. Neurosci.* 7:215–216.

Benesova, O., and Pavlik, A. (1989). Perinatal treatment with glucocorticoids and the risk of maldevelopment of the brain. *Neuropharmacology* 28:89–97.

Benevento, L. A., Bakkum, B. W., and Cohen, R. S. (1995). gamma-Aminobutyric acid and somatostatin immunoreactivity in the visual cortex of normal and dark-reared rats. *Brain Res.* 2:172–182.

Berardi, N., and Maffei, L. (1999). From visual experience to visual function: Roles of neurotrophins. *J. Neurobiol.* 41:119–126.

Berardi, N., Pizzorusso, T., and Maffei, L. (2000). Critical periods during sensory development. *Curr. Opin. Neurobiol.* 10:138–145.

Berardi, N., Pizzorusso, T., Ratto, G. M., and Maffei, L. (2003). Molecular basis of plasticity in the visual cortex. *Trends Neurosci.* 26:369–378.

Black, J. E., Isaacs, K. R., Anderson, B. J., Alcantara, A. A., and Greenough, W. T. (1990). Learning causes synaptogenesis, whereas motor activity causes angiogenesis, in cerebellar cortex of adult rats. *Proc. Natl. Acad. Sci. U.S.A.* 87:5568–5572.

Bonhoeffer, T. (1996). Neurotrophins and activity-dependent development of the neocortex. *Curr. Opin. Neurobiol.* 6:119–126.

Branchi, I., and Alleva, E. (2006). Communal nesting, an early social enrichment, increases the adult anxiety-like response and shapes the role of social context in modulating the emotional behavior. *Behav. Brain Res.* 172:299–306.

Cancedda, L., Putignano, E., Impey, S., Maffei, L., Ratto, G. M., and Pizzorusso, T. (2003). Patterned vision causes CRE-mediated gene expression in the visual cortex through PKA and ERK. *J. Neurosci.* 23:7012–7020.

Cancedda, L., Putignano, E., Sale, A., Viegi, A., Berardi, N., and Maffei, L. (2004). Acceleration of visual system development by environmental enrichment. *J. Neurosci.* 24:4840–4848.

Carro, E., Nunez, A., Busiguina, S., and Torres-Aleman, I. (2000). Circulating insulin-like growth factor I mediates effects of exercise on the brain. *J. Neurosci.* 20:2926–2933.

Carro, E., Trejo, J. L., Busiguina, S., and Torres-Aleman, I. (2001). Circulating insulin-like growth factor I mediates the protective effects of physical exercise against brain insults of different etiology and anatomy. *J. Neurosci.* 21:5678–5684.

Cellerino, A., and Maffei, L. (1996). The action of neurotrophins in the development and plasticity of the visual cortex. *Prog. Neurobiol.* 49:53–71.

Ciucci, F., Putignano, E., Baroncelli, L., Landi, S., Berardi, N., and Maffei, L. (2007). Insulin-like growth factor 1 (IGF-1) mediates the effects of enriched environment (EE) on visual cortical development. *PLoS ONE* 2(5):e475.

Cynader, M., and Mitchell, D. E. (1980). Prolonged sensitivity to monocular deprivation in dark-reared cats. *J. Neurophysiol.* 43:1026–1040.

Diamond, M. C. (1988). *Enriching heredity*. New York: Free Press.

Diamond, M. C. (2001). Response of the brain to enrichment. *An. Acad. Bras. Cienc.* 73:211–220.

Diamond, M. C., Krech, D., and Rosenzweig, M. R. (1964). The effects of an enriched environment on the histology of the rat cerebral cortex. *J. Comp. Neurol.* 123:111–120.

Diamond, M. C., Law, F., Rhodes, H., Lindner, B., Rosenzweig, M. R., Krech, D., and Bennett, E. L. (1966). Increases in cortical depth and glia numbers in rats subjected to enriched environment. *J. Comp. Neurol.* 128:117–126.

Escorihuela, R. M., Fernandez-Teruel, A., Tobena, A., Vivas, N. M., Marmol, F., Badia, A., and Dierssen, M. (1995). Early environmental stimulation produces long-lasting changes on beta-adrenoceptor transduction system. *Neurobiol. Learn. Mem.* 64:49–57.

Fagiolini, M., Pizzorusso, T., Berardi, N., Domenici, L., and Maffei, L. (1994). Functional postnatal development of the rat primary visual cortex and the role of visual experience: Dark rearing and monocular deprivation. *Vision Res.* 34:709–720.

Falkenberg, T., Mohammed, A. K., Henriksson, B., Persson, H., Winblad, B., and Lindefors, N. (1992). Increased expression of brain-derived neurotrophic factor mRNA in rat hippocampus is associated with improved spatial memory and enriched environment. *Neurosci. Lett.* 138:153–156.

Fine, I., Wade, A. R., Brewer, A. A., May, M. G., Goodman, D. F., Boynton, G. M., Wandell, B. A., and MacLeod, D. I. (2003). Long-term deprivation affects visual perception and cortex. *Nat. Neurosci.* 6:915–916.

Fleming, A. S., O'Day, D. H., and Kraemer, G. W. (1999). Neurobiology of mother-infant interactions: Experience and central nervous system plasticity across development and generations. *Neurosci. Biobehav. Rev.* 23:673–685.

Francis, D. D., and Meaney, M. J. (1999). Maternal care and the development of stress responses. *Curr. Opin. Neurobiol.* 9:128–134.

Frolich, L., Blum-Degen, D., Bernstein, H. G., Engelsberger, S., Humrich, J., Laufer, S., Muschner, D., Thalheimer, A., Turk, A., Hoyer, S., et al. (1998). Brain insulin and insulin receptors in aging and sporadic Alzheimer's disease. *J. Neural Transm.* 105:423–438.

Gianfranceschi, L., Siciliano, R., Walls, J., Morales, B., Kirkwood, A., Huang, Z. J., Tonegawa, S., and Maffei, L. (2003). Visual cortex is rescued from the effects of dark rearing by overexpression of BDNF. *Proc. Natl. Acad. Sci. U.S.A.* 100:12486–12491.

Globus, A., Rosenzweig, M. R., Bennett, E. L., and Diamond, M. C. (1973). Effects of differential experience on dendritic spine counts in rat cerebral cortex. *J. Comp. Physiol. Psychol.* 82:175–181.

Gramsbergen, A., and Mulder, E. J. (1998). The influence of betamethasone and dexamethasone on motor development in young rats. *Pediatr. Res.* 44:105–110.

Greenough, W. T., Volkmar, F. R., and Juraska, J. M. (1973). Effects of rearing complexity on dendritic branching in frontolateral and temporal cortex of the rat. *Exp. Neurol.* 41:371–378.

Hensch, T. K. (2005). Critical period plasticity in local cortical circuits. *Nat. Rev. Neurosci.* 6:877–888.

HOFER, M. A. (1984). Relationships as regulators: A psychobiologic perspective on bereavement. *Psychosom. Med.* 46:183–197.

HOLLOWAY, R. L., JR. (1966). Dendritic branching: Some preliminary results of training and complexity in rat visual cortex. *Brain Res.* 2:393–396.

HUANG, Z. J., KIRKWOOD, A., PIZZORUSSO, T., PORCIATTI, V., MORALES, B., BEAR, M. F., MAFFEI, L., and TONEGAWA, S. (1999). BDNF regulates the maturation of inhibition and the critical period of plasticity in mouse visual cortex. *Cell* 98:739–755.

IMPEY, S., MARK, M., VILLACRES, E. C., POSER, S., CHAVKIN, C., and STORM, D. R. (1996). Induction of CRE-mediated gene expression by stimuli that generate long-lasting LTP in area CA1 of the hippocampus. *Neuron* 16:973–982.

KATO, H., ARAKI, T., CHEN, T., ITOYAMA, Y., and KOGURE, K. (1998). Effect of rolipram on age-related changes in cyclic AMP-selective phosphodiesterase in the rat brain: an autoradiographic study. *Methods Find. Exp. Clin. Pharmacol.* 20:403–408.

KEMPERMANN, G., KUHN, H. G., and GAGE, F. H. (1997). More hippocampal neurons in adult mice living in an enriched environment. *Nature* 386:493–495.

KESHET, I., YISRAELI, J., and CEDAR, H. (1985). Effect of regional DNA methylation on gene expression. *Proc. Natl. Acad. Sci. U.S.A.* 82:2560–2564.

KEYVANI, K., SACHSER, N., WITTE, O. W., and PAULUS, W. (2004). Gene expression profiling in the intact and injured brain following environmental enrichment. *J. Neuropathol. Exp. Neurol.* 63: 598–609.

KIRKWOOD, A., LEE, H. K., and BEAR, M. F. (1995). Co-regulation of long-term potentiation and experience-dependent synaptic plasticity in visual cortex by age and experience. *Nature* 375: 328–331.

KOFMAN, O. (2002). The role of prenatal stress in the etiology of developmental behavioral disorders. *Neurosci. Biobehav. Rev.* 26: 457–470.

KOLB, B. (1995). *Brain plasticity and behavior.* Mahwah, NJ: Erlbaum.

KOLB, B., and GIBB, R. (2001). Early brain injuries, plasticity and behavior. In C. A. Nelson and M. Luciana (Eds.), *Handbook of developmental cognitive neuroscience* (pp. 175–190). Cambridge, MA: MIT Press.

KOO, J. W., PARK, C. H., CHOI, S. H., KIM, N. J., KIM, H. S., CHOE, J. C., and SUH, Y. H. (2003). The postnatal environment can counteract prenatal effects on cognitive ability, cell proliferation, and synaptic protein expression. *FASEB J.* 17:1556–1558.

KOOPMANS, G. C., BRANS, M., GOMEZ-PINILLA, F., DUIS, S., GISPEN, W. H., TORRES-ALEMAN, I., JOOSTEN, E. A., and HAMERS, F. P. (2006). Circulating insulin-like growth factor I and functional recovery from spinal cord injury under enriched housing conditions. *Eur. J. Neurosci.* 23:1035–1046.

KRUBITZER, L., and KAHN, D. M. (2003). Nature versus nurture revisited: An old idea with a new twist. *Prog. Neurobiol.* 70: 33–52.

LANDER, C., KIND, P., MALESKI, M., and HOCKFIELD, S. (1997). A family of activity-dependent neuronal cell-surface chondroitin sulfate proteoglycans in cat visual cortex. *J. Neurosci.* 17: 1928–1939.

LANDI, S., CENNI, M. C., BERARDI, N., and MAFFEI, L. (2007a). Environmental enrichment effects on development of retinal ganglion cell dendrite stratification requires retinal BDNF. Neuroscience Meeting Planner. Atlanta, GA: Society for Neuroscience. Online.

LANDI, S., SALE, A., BERARDI, N., VIEGI, A., MAFFEI, L., and CENNI, M. C. (2007). Retinal functional development is sensitive to environmental enrichment: a role for BDNF. *FASEB J.* 21(1):130–139.

LIU, D., DIORIO, J., DAY, J. C., FRANCIS, D. D., and MEANEY, M. J. (2000). Maternal care, hippocampal synaptogenesis and cognitive development in rats. *Nat. Neurosci.* 3:799–806.

LIU, D., DIORIO, J., TANNENBAUM, B., CALDJI, C., FRANCIS, D., FREEDMAN, A., SHARMA, S., PEARSON, D., PLOTSKY, P. M., and MEANEY, M. J. (1997). Maternal care, hippocampal glucocorticoid receptors, and hypothalamic-pituitary-adrenal responses to stress. *Science* 277:1659–1662.

LORDI, B., PROTAIS, P., MELLIER, D., and CASTON, J. (1997). Acute stress in pregnant rats: effects on growth rate, learning, and memory capabilities of the offspring. *Physiol. Behav.* 62:1087–1092.

MAFFEI, L., and FIORENTINI, A. (1981). Electroretinographic responses to alternating gratings before and after section of the optic nerve. *Science* 211:953–955.

MEDINI, P., BARTOLETTI, A., BERARDI, N., and MAFFEI, L. (2008). [Effects of EE on visual cortical development and plasticity.] Unpublished data.

MOLLGAARD, K., DIAMOND, M. C., BENNETT, E. L., ROSENZWEIG, M. R., and LINDNER, B. (1971). Quantitative synaptic changes with differential experience in rat brain. *Int. J. Neurosci.* 2: 113–127.

MOLTENI, R., YING, Z., and GOMEZ-PINILLA, F. (2002). Differential effects of acute and chronic exercise on plasticity-related genes in the rat hippocampus revealed by microarray. *Eur. J. Neurosci.* 16:1107–1116.

MOSER, M. B., TROMMALD, M., EGELAND, T., and ANDERSEN, P. (1997). Spatial training in a complex environment and isolation alter the spine distribution differently in rat CA1 pyramidal cells. *J. Comp. Neurol.* 380:373–381.

MOWER, G. D. (1991). The effect of dark rearing on the time course of the critical period in cat visual cortex. *Brain Res. Dev. Brain Res.* 58:151–158.

MOWER, A. F., LIAO, D. S., NESTLER, E. J., NEVE, R. L., and RAMOA, A. S. (2002). cAMP/Ca^{2+} response element-binding protein function is essential for ocular dominance plasticity. *J. Neurosci.* 22:2237–2245.

MULDER, E. J., ROBLES DE MEDINA, P. G., HUIZINK, A. C., VAN DEN BERGH, B. R., BUITELAAR, J. K., and VISSER, G. H. (2002). Prenatal maternal stress: Effects on pregnancy and the (unborn) child. *Early Hum. Dev.* 70:3–14.

NAKA, F., SHIGA, T., YAGUCHI, M., and OKADO, N. (2002). An enriched environment increases noradrenaline concentration in the mouse brain. *Brain Res.* 924:124–126.

NAKAGAWA, S., KIM, J. E., LEE, R., MALBERG, J. E., CHEN, J., STEFFEN, C., ZHANG, Y. J., NESTLER, E. J., and DUMAN, R. S. (2002). Regulation of neurogenesis in adult mouse hippocampus by cAMP and the cAMP response element-binding protein. *J. Neurosci.* 22:3673–3682.

PACTEAU, C., EINON, D., and SINDEN, J. (1989). Early rearing environment and dorsal hippocampal ibotenic acid lesions: Long-term influences on spatial learning and alternation in the rat. *Behav. Brain Res.* 34:79–96.

PASCUAL, R., and FIGUEROA, H. (1996). Effects of preweaning sensorimotor stimulation on behavioral and neuronal development in motor and visual cortex of the rat. *Biol. Neonate* 69:399–404.

PAUK, J., KUHN, C. M., FIELD, T. M., and SCHANBERG, S. M. (1986). Positive effects of tactile versus kinesthetic or vestibular stimulation on neuroendocrine and ODC activity in maternally-deprived rat pups. *Life Sci.* 39:2081–2087.

PAYLOR, R., MORRISON, S. K., RUDY, J. W., WALTRIP, L. T., and WEHNER, J. M. (1992). Brief exposure to an enriched environment improves performance on the Morris water task and increases hippocampal cytosolic protein kinase C activity in young rats. *Behav. Brain Res.* 52:49–59.

PHAM, T. A., IMPEY, S., STORM, D. R., and STRYKER, M. P. (1999). CRE-mediated gene transcription in neocortical neuronal plasticity during the developmental critical period. *Neuron* 22:63–72.

PHAM, T. M. WINBLAD, B., GRANHOLM, A. C., and MOHAMMED, A. H. (2002). Environmental influences on brain neurotrophins in rats. *Pharmacol. Biochem. Behav.* 73:167–175.

PIZZORUSSO, T., MEDINI, P., BERARDI, N., CHIERZI, S., FAWCETT, J. W., and MAFFEI, L. (2002). Reactivation of ocular dominance plasticity in the adult visual cortex. *Science* 298:1248–1251.

PIZZORUSSO, T., MEDINI, P., LANDI, S., BALDINI, S., BERARDI, N., and MAFFEI, L. (2006). Structural and functional recovery from early monocular deprivation in adult rats. *Proc. Natl. Acad. Sci. U.S.A.* 103:8517–8522.

POLTYREV, T., KESHET, G. I., KAY, G., and WEINSTOCK, M. (1996). Role of experimental conditions in determining differences in exploratory behavior of prenatally stressed rats. *Dev. Psychobiol.* 29:453–462.

RAMPON, C., JIANG, C. H., DONG, H., TANG, Y. P., LOCKHART, D. J., SCHULTZ, P. G., TSIEN, J. Z., and HU, Y. (2000a). Effects of environmental enrichment on gene expression in the brain. *Proc. Natl. Acad. Sci. U.S.A.* 97:12880–12884.

RAMPON, C., TANG, Y. P., GOODHOUSE, J., SHIMIZU, E., KYIN, M., and TSIEN, J. Z. (2000b). Enrichment induces structural changes and recovery from nonspatial memory deficits in CA1 NMDAR1-knockout mice. *Nat. Neurosci.* 3:238–244.

RASMUSON, S., OLSSON, T., HENRIKSSON, B. G., KELLY, P. A., HOLMES, M. C., SECKL, J. R., and MOHAMMED, A. H. (1998). Environmental enrichment selectively increases 5-HT1A receptor mRNA expression and binding in the rat hippocampus. *Brain Res. Mol. Brain Res.* 53:285–290.

RAZIN, A. (1998). CpG methylation, chromatin structure and gene silencing: A three-way connection. *EMBO J.* 17:4905–4908.

RENNER, M. J., and ROSENZWEIG, M. R. (1987). *Enriched and impoverished environments. Effects on brain and behavior.* New York: Springer-Verlag.

RITTENHOUSE, C. D., SHOUVAL, H. Z., PARADISO, M. A., and BEAR, M. F. (1999). Monocular deprivation induces homosynaptic long-term depression in visual cortex. *Nature* 397:347–350.

RONCA, A. E., LAMKIN, C. A., and ALBERTS, J. R. (1993). Maternal contributions to sensory experience in the fetal and newborn rat (*Rattus norvegicus*). *J. Comp. Psychol.* 107:61–74.

ROSENZWEIG, M. R. (1966). Environmental complexity, cerebral change, and behavior. *Am. Psychol.* 21:321–332.

ROSENZWEIG, M. R., and BENNETT, E. L. (1969). Effects of differential environments on brain weights and enzyme activities in gerbils, rats, and mice. *Dev. Psychobiol.* 2:87–95.

ROSENZWEIG, M. R., and BENNETT, E. L. (1996). Psychobiology of plasticity: Effects of training and experience on brain and behavior. *Behav. Brain Res.* 78:57–65.

ROSENZWEIG, M. R., BENNETT, E. L., and DIAMOND, M. C. (1967). Effects of differential environments on brain anatomy and brain chemistry. In *Proceedings of the Annual Meeting of the American Psychopathology Association* 56:45–56.

ROSENZWEIG, M. R., BENNETT, E. L., HEBERT, M., and MORIMOTO, H. (1978). Social grouping cannot account for cerebral effects of enriched environments. *Brain Res.* 153:563–576.

ROSENZWEIG, M. R., BENNETT, E. L., and KRECH, D. (1964). Cerebral effects of environmental complexity and training among adult rats. *J. Comp. Physiol. Psychol.* 57:438–439.

ROSENZWEIG, M. R., KRECH, D., BENNETT, E. L., and DIAMOND, M. C. (1962). Effects of environmental complexity and training on brain chemistry and anatomy: a replication and extension. *J. Comp. Physiol. Psychol.* 55:429–437.

SALE, A., CENNI, M. C., CIUCCI, F., PUTIGNANO, E., CHIERZI, S., and MAFFEI, L. (2007a). Maternal enrichment during pregnancy accelerates retinal development of the fetus. *PLoS ONE* 2(11): e1160.

SALE, A., MAYA VETENCOURT, J. F., MEDINI, P., CENNI, M. C., BARONCELLI, L., DE PASQUALE, R., and MAFFEI, L. (2007b). Environmental enrichment in adulthood promotes amblyopia recovery through a reduction of intracortical inhibition. *Nat. Neurosci.* 10:679–681.

SALE, A., PUTIGNANO, E., CANCEDDA, L., LANDI, S., CIRULLI, F., BERARDI, N., and MAFFEI, L. (2004). Enriched environment and acceleration of visual system development. *Neuropharmacology* 47:649–660.

SCHNEIDER, M. L. (1992). Prenatal stress exposure alters postnatal behavioral expression under conditions of novelty challenge in rhesus monkey infants. *Dev. Psychobiol.* 25:529–540.

SHIOTA, K., and KAYAMURA, T. (1989). Effects of prenatal heat stress on postnatal growth, behavior and learning capacity in mice. *Biol. Neonate* 56:6–14.

SZURAN, T. F., PLISKA, V., POKORNY, J., and WELZL, H. (2000). Prenatal stress in rats: Effects on plasma corticosterone, hippocampal glucocorticoid receptors, and maze performance. *Physiol. Behav.* 71:353–362.

TEES, R. C. (1999). The influences of rearing environment and neonatal choline dietary supplementation on spatial learning and memory in adult rats. *Behav. Brain Res.* 105:173–188.

TEES, R. C., BUHRMANN, K., and HANLEY, J. (1990). The effect of early experience on water maze spatial learning and memory in rats. *Dev. Psychobiol.* 23:427–439.

THOENEN, H. (2000). Neurotrophins and activity-dependent plasticity. *Prog. Brain Res.* 128:183–191.

THOENEN, H., and SENDTNER, M. (2002). Neurotrophins: From enthusiastic expectations through sobering experiences to rational therapeutic approaches. *Nat. Neurosci.* 5(Suppl.):1046–1050.

TIAN, N., and COPENHAGEN, D. R. (2001). Visual deprivation alters development of synaptic function in inner retina after eye opening. *Neuron* 32:439–449.

TIAN, N., and COPENHAGEN, D. R. (2003). Visual stimulation is required for refinement of ON and OFF pathways in postnatal retina. *Neuron* 39:85–96.

TOHDA, M., MURAYAMA, T., NOGIRI, S., and NOMURA, Y. (1996). Influence of aging on rolipram-sensitive phosphodiesterase activity and [3H]rolipram binding in the rat brain. *Biol. Pharm. Bull.* 19:300–302.

TORASDOTTER, M., METSIS, M., HENRIKSSON, B. G., WINBLAD, B., and MOHAMMED, A. H. (1996). Expression of neurotrophin-3 mRNA in the rat visual cortex and hippocampus is influenced by environmental conditions. *Neurosci. Lett.* 218:107–110.

TORASDOTTER, M., METSIS, M., HENRIKSSON, B. G., WINBLAD, B., and MOHAMMED, A. H. (1998). Environmental enrichment results in higher levels of nerve growth factor mRNA in the rat visual cortex and hippocampus. *Behav. Brain Res.* 93:83–90.

Tropea, D., Kreiman, G., Lyckman, A., Mukherjee, S., Yu, H., Horng, S., and Sur, M. (2006). Gene expression changes and molecular pathways mediating activity-dependent plasticity in visual cortex. *Nat. Neurosci.* 5:660–668.

Turner, A. M., and Greenough, W. T. (1985). Differential rearing effects on rat visual cortex synapses. I. Synaptic and neuronal density and synapses per neuron. *Brain Res.* 329:195–203.

van Praag, H., Christie, B. R., Sejnowski, T. J., and Gage, F. H. (1999). Running enhances neurogenesis, learning, and long-term potentiation in mice. *Proc. Natl. Acad. Sci. U.S.A.* 96: 13427–13431.

van Praag, H., Kempermann, G., and Gage, F. H. (2000). Neural consequences of environmental enrichment. *Nat. Rev. Neurosci.* 1:191–198.

Venable, N., Fernandez, V., Diaz, E., and Pinto-Hamuy, T. (1989). Effects of preweaning environmental enrichment on basilar dendrites of pyramidal neurons in occipital cortex: A Golgi study. *Brain Res. Dev. Brain Res.* 49:140–144.

Wang, S., Bartolome, J. V., and Schanberg, S. M. (1996). Neonatal deprivation of maternal touch may suppress ornithine decarboxylase via downregulation of the proto-oncogenes c-*myc* and *max*. *J. Neurosci.* 16:836–842.

Weaver, I. C., Cervoni, N., Champagne, F. A., D'Alessio, A. C., Sharma, S., Seckl, J. R., Dymov, S., Szyf, M., and Meaney, M. J. (2004). Epigenetic programming by maternal behavior. *Nat. Neurosci.* 7:847–854.

Weinstock, M. (1997). Does prenatal stress impair coping and regulation of hypothalamic-pituitary-adrenal axis? *Neurosci. Biobehav. Rev.* 21:1–10.

Wiesel, T. N. (1982). Postnatal development of the visual cortex and the influence of environment. *Nature* 299:583–591.

Williams, B. M., Luo, Y., Ward, C., Redd, K., Gibson, R., Kuczaj, S. A., and McCoy, J. G. (2001). Environmental enrichment: Effects on spatial memory and hippocampal CREB immunoreactivity. *Physiol. Behav.* 73:649–658.

Winocur, G. (1998). Environmental influences on cognitive decline in aged rats. *Neurobiol. Aging* 19:589–597.

Young, D., Lawlor, P. A., Leone, P., Dragunow, M., and During, M. J. (1999). Environmental enrichment inhibits spontaneous apoptosis, prevents seizures and is neuroprotective. *Nat. Med.* 5:448–453.

38 Bidirectional Experience-Dependent Plasticity in Primary Visual Cortex

MIKHAIL Y. FRENKEL AND MARK F. BEAR

The response properties of neurons in the visual cortex can be persistently modified following changes in the visual environment. Such modifications reflect changes in synaptic transmission that shape neuronal circuits and presumably store information. A leading model to study experience-dependent plasticity is the deprivation-induced ocular dominance (OD) shift observed early in postnatal development. Pioneering research by Hübel and Wiesel more than four decades ago demonstrated that if one eye was deprived of vision early in a kitten's life, a dramatic shift in cell responsiveness occurred. The majority of neurons in the primary visual cortex no longer responded to stimuli presented to the deprived eye; these cells were driven by the open eye only (Wiesel and Hübel, 1963). However, in contrast to the profound effects observed in young animals, monocular deprivation (MD) in adult cats had virtually no effect (Hübel and Wiesel, 1970). Thus emerged the notion of a critical period for experience-dependent plasticity—a period of heightened brain plasticity during which experience could produce permanent, large-scale changes in neuronal circuits.

The significance of understanding the synaptic and molecular bases of OD plasticity cannot be overstated. First, although the depth of insight has increased sharply over the past decade with important discoveries about how synaptic transmission and plasticity are mediated in the cerebral cortex, we remain largely ignorant about the molecular basis of OD plasticity, despite more than 40 years of research. Second, the processes revealed by OD plasticity are likely to be the same as those that refine cortical circuitry in response to the qualities of sensory experience during development, and thus determine the capabilities of and limitations to visual performance in adults. Third, rapid OD plasticity is an example of cortical receptive field (RF) plasticity, the most common cellular correlate of memory in the brain. It is therefore likely that understanding the mechanisms of OD plasticity will yield insight into the molecular basis of learning and memory. Fourth, a detailed understanding of how synaptic connections are weakened by sensory deprivation may lead to strategies to reverse such changes, and possibly overcome amblyopia. Finally, a detailed understanding of how synaptic connections are strengthened by experience is expected to lead to strategies to augment such changes and promote recovery of function after brain injury.

The phenomenon of OD plasticity has been studied in great detail in cats and primates. However, it may be a common feature among sighted mammals, as MD has been shown to alter the binocularity of visual cortical neurons in a number of diverse species (Dräger, 1978; Emerson et al., 1982; Issa et al., 1999; Maffei et al., 1992; Van Sluyters and Stewart, 1974). In many respects, mouse visual cortex is ideal for the mechanistic dissection of OD plasticity. First, mice display rapid and robust OD plasticity in response to MD. The kinetics and behavioral consequences of OD plasticity are very similar to those observed in other species, such as the cat. Second, the property of binocularity is established early in cortical processing by the convergence of thalamic inputs onto layer 4 neurons (there are no, or very few, neurons in mouse visual cortex that are activated exclusively by the ipsilateral eye), potentially simplifying analysis of the underlying synaptic changes. Third, mice are genetically homogeneous, easily obtained, and relatively inexpensive, enabling rapid progress using coordinated biochemical and electrophysiological studies in vitro and in vivo. Fourth, the absence of a columnar organization and other cortical anisotropy makes feasible extended duration recordings in awake animals. Fifth, genes can be delivered or deleted in mouse visual cortex by pronuclear injection, targeted insertion into embryonic stem cells, or viral infection. Finally, mice have emerged as valuable genetic models of human developmental disorders (e.g., fragile X syndrome), offering the opportunity to use the powerful paradigm of OD plasticity to understand how experience-dependent cortical development can go awry in genetic disorders and, hopefully, develop targeted treatments for these disorders.

It is worth drawing a distinction between OD plasticity, a phenomenon that appears to be expressed universally in sighted mammals, and OD *column* plasticity. OD columns, also discovered by Hübel and Wiesel, reflect the segregation of lateral geniculate nucleus (LGN) axon terminals into regularly spaced bands or stripes in visual cortex. Although OD columns exist in some carnivores (e.g., cat and ferret) and some primates (e.g., macaque and human), they are not a feature of visual cortex in most mammals. In squirrel monkeys, for example, some individual animals express columns while others lack them or have them only in parts of primary visual cortex (Adams and Horton, 2003). Other species with excellent vision lack columns altogether (Van Hooser et al., 2005), leading some authors to refer to cortical columns as a "structure without a function" (Horton and Adams, 2005). Although the species traditionally used to study OD plasticity—the cat and macaque monkey—do have columns that can rearrange following MD, it is important to recognize that these species diverged very early in mammalian evolution (95 million years ago), 10 million years before the divergence of modern primates and rodents (Murphy et al., 2004). Columns and their modification by experience may arise from very different mechanisms in these divergent species. In any case, the key point is that the absence of columns in mice has no bearing on their value as a model to study the modification of binocular vision as a function of experience.

This chapter reviews recent progress made in the field of mouse visual cortical plasticity. In particular, the effects of changing an animal's visual environment during the classically defined critical period and beyond are discussed in detail. Emphasis is on the use of an extended duration visually evoked potential (VEP) recording technique and its advantages for studying various forms of cortical plasticity, among them deprivation-induced depression, activity-dependent potentiation, and stimulus-selective response potentiation.

Visually evoked potential recording technique

To gain the most from the numerous advantages of using the mouse visual cortex for mechanistic studies, it is necessary to understand the response changes that contribute to OD plasticity in mice. We chose a well-established technique of recording VEPs to monitor population neuronal activity. This technique has been pioneered and successfully used in rodents by Lamberto Maffei's laboratory (Pizzorusso et al., 1997; Porciatti et al., 1999). VEPs are a form of local field potential (LFP) evoked by a visual stimulus. The magnitude of the cortical LFP reflects the extent and geometry of dendrites in the neocortex. The pyramidal cells with their apical dendrites running parallel to each other and perpendicular to the pial surface form an ideal open field arrangement and contribute maximally to the LFPs. Other cortical neurons that are oriented horizontally contribute to a much lesser degree to the sum of potentials (Logothetis, 2003). For many years, VEP recording has been a powerful tool in clinical applications such as the estimation of refractive errors, visual acuity, binocular function, and the prognostic assessment of amblyopia (Sherman, 1979). The high correlation between VEPs and visual acuity testing makes VEP recordings a perfect tool for assessing the functional integrity of the visual system (Sokol, 1976).

Averaged over many stimulus presentations, the amplitude of the VEP waveform provides a quantitative measure of cortical input from the deprived versus nondeprived eye. By comparing VEP amplitudes across deprived and nondeprived eyes within a particular experimental group, it is possible to ascertain whether a change in OD is due to a decrease in the deprived-eye response (synaptic weakening) or an increase in the nondeprived-eye response (synaptic strengthening). In the field of visual cortical plasticity, most electrophysiological data have been derived from acute single-unit recordings that represent the ratio of deprived-eye to nondeprived-eye input. As a population signal, the VEP method avoids the problem of sampling bias due to a limited or skewed sample that is inherent in the single-unit approach. Furthermore, VEPs yield a more rapid assessment of OD than single-unit recordings and are potentially a high-throughput method to screen genetic mutants for visual cortical plasticity phenotypes. In addition, VEP recordings allow a comprehensive evaluation of visual system function. VEPs can be used both to obtain a measure of visual capabilities (spatial resolution, contrast threshold, response timing) that have a counterpart in behavioral capabilities (visual acuity, contrast sensitivity, reaction time) and to probe for information about cortical processing (retinotopy, laminar analysis). The ability to quickly screen numerous aspects of visual system function is critically important in the analysis of visual phenotypes in mutant mice. Finally, the VEP recording technique can be easily adapted to an extended duration recording situation in which the visual responses of a single animal can be followed over time, before and after visual deprivation.

We have developed an extended duration recording preparation in mice to better understand when and how OD is altered by MD. Figure 38.1*A* shows a mouse placed in a restraint apparatus designed in our laboratory. Perhaps the greatest advantage of the extended duration VEP recording technique is that visual activity can be monitored in the same experimental subjects over a prolonged period of time. There are additional benefits to this approach: (1) extended duration recordings can be made without the confounds of anesthesia, (2) the same animals can serve as their own controls, and (3) both absolute and relative changes in visual responsiveness can be measured.

Because chronic VEP recordings had not been attempted previously in mice, we first analyzed the laminar pattern of cortical activation in awake animals by performing current source density (CSD) analysis to better understand the

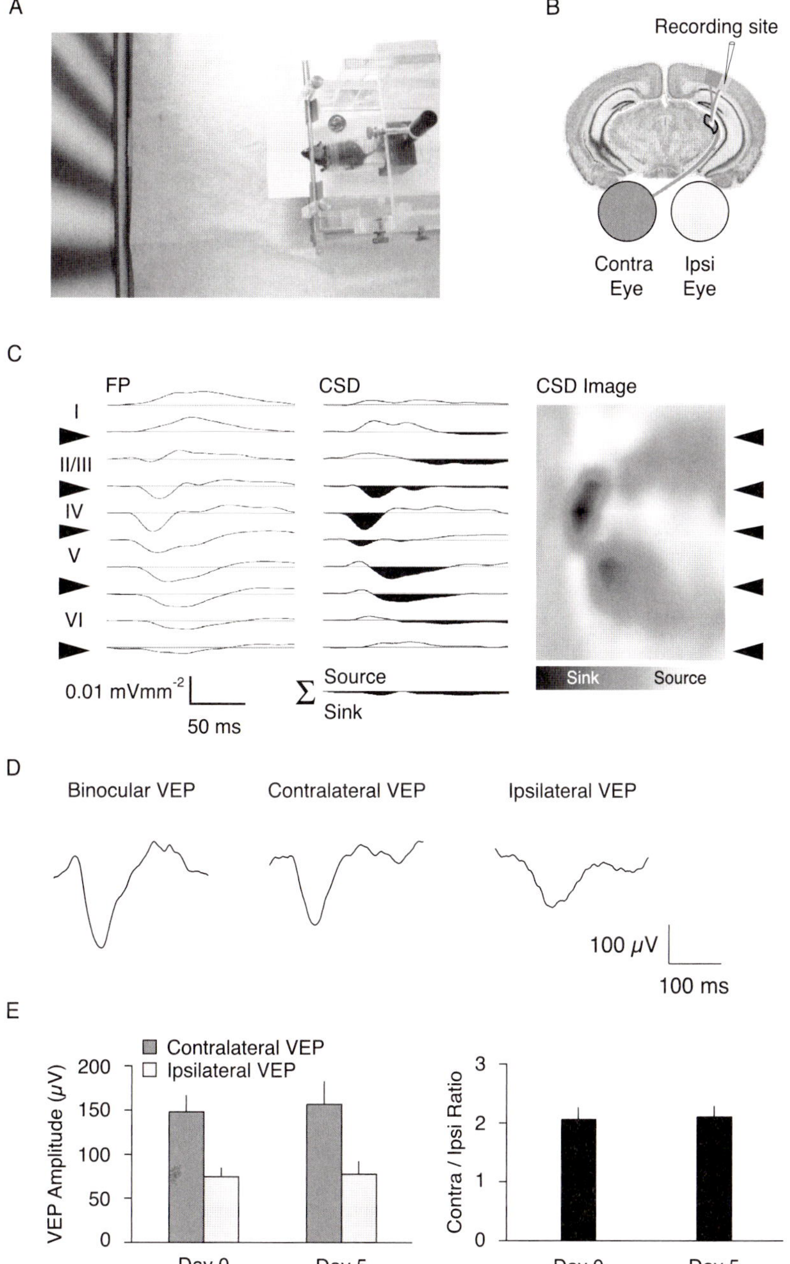

FIGURE 38.1 The extended duration VEP recording technique is a reliable method to assess OD plasticity in mice. *A*, Representation of VEP recording setup. A mouse previously implanted with recording electrodes in Oc1 is placed in a restraint apparatus in front of a computer monitor displaying visual stimuli. Mice are fully awake and alert during all recording sessions. *B*, Schematic diagram of the mouse visual system. Input from the stronger contralateral eye arrives via the LGN to the monocular and binocular zones of V1, whereas input from the weaker ipsilateral eye projects only to the small binocular zone. *C*, Current source density profile of VEPs for an adult mouse. Binocular VEP depth profile is shown in the *left panel*, with the corresponding cortical layers designated by *arrowheads*. *Middle panel* shows the CSD profile. Current sinks are negative-going and shaded black. The color image plot in the *right panel* is an interpolation of CSD traces. The earliest latency current sink is observed in layer 4, followed by longer latency sinks in layers 2/3 and 5. Cold and warm colors represent current sinks and sources, respectively. *D*, Typical VEP responses obtained during the three viewing conditions used in all experiments. Each trace is an average of 100 presentations of a reversing (1 Hz) sinusoidal grating. *E*, VEPs recorded from awake mice are stable over several days. Displayed in the *left panel* are the average VEP amplitude (n = 6 mice) in response to contralateral eye (*blue bars*) and ipsilateral eye (*yellow bars*) stimulation at baseline (day 0) and after 5 days of normal visual experience. *Right panel* shows the stability of contralateral/ipsilateral ratios over days. See color plate 31.

synaptic events responsible for generating the VEP waveform (Mitzdorf, 1985). A recording electrode was tracked radially through primary visual cortex (V1) in 100 μm steps from the pial surface to below the white matter. After each 100 μm advancement of the electrode, at least 200 VEPs were collected in response to a binocularly presented high-contrast sinusoidal grating (0.05 c/deg), pattern reversing at 1 Hz. A representative example of the average VEP recorded at each depth is presented in the *left column* of figure 38.1*C*. VEP waveforms recorded through the depth of the cortex were typically composed of an initial negativity followed by a more variable positivity. These components correspond roughly to those described in the primate (Schroeder et al., 1991). The VEP waveform with the maximum negativity and shortest latency was recorded at a depth corresponding to layer 4 (ca. 450 μm ventral from the pial surface). Based on CSD analyses performed in juvenile and adult mice, recording electrodes were implanted in V1 at a site yielding maximum binocular responsiveness and at a depth yielding the maximum negative-going VEP (figure 38.1*B*), which reflects a synaptic current sink in layer 4 (Huang et al., 1999; Sawtell et al., 2003), likely resulting from activity in thalamocortical inputs to this layer (see figure 38.1*C*, *middle* and *right column*).

OD refers to the relative contribution of the two eyes to visually evoked responses in visual cortex. It is well known from both single-unit and VEP recordings that in mice, there is a substantial bias toward the contralateral eye (Gordon and Stryker, 1996; Hanover et al., 1999; Huang et al., 1999). In the awake mouse preparation, the VEP elicited by contralateral eye stimulation is normally about two to three times greater than that elicited by ipsilateral eye stimulation (figure 38.1*D* and *E*). To assess the stability of the extended duration recording preparation, we tracked changes in this ratio and the absolute VEP amplitude over time in normally reared mice. Under conditions of normal visual experience, the amplitude of the responses evoked by the two eyes and their ratio remained stable for many days (see figure 38.1*E*).

Effects of monocular deprivation in juvenile mice

VEP responses are altered substantially if the contralateral eyelid is sutured (figure 38.2*A*). Although 1 day of MD causes variable changes in OD (figure 38.2A_2), 3 days of MD reliably causes a substantial and significant depression of deprived-eye VEPs (*solid bars* in figure 38.2A_3). Interestingly, nondeprived (ipsilateral)-eye VEPs remained unchanged after 3 days of MD (*open bars* in figure 38.2A_3) but were potentiated after a longer period of MD (*open bars* in figure 38.2A_4 to A_5). Thus, the OD shift observed following MD is initially accounted for entirely by rapid deprivation-induced response depression (figure 38.2A_6). With longer periods of MD, there is a compensatory increase in the response to stimulation of the nondeprived eye (figure 38.2A_7). Had we analyzed contralateral/ipsilateral ratios only, we would not have been able to discern these phases of the OD shift, since the contralateral/ipsilateral ratio is the same after 3 days of MD as it is after 7 days of MD.

This bidirectional plasticity is also reflected in experiments in which binocular VEPs are collected from both hemispheres before and after MD of varying duration (figure 38.3). The VEPs in both hemispheres are equivalent in amplitude before MD (day 0 in figure 38.3*B*). However, after 3 days of MD, there is a dramatic drop in binocular VEP amplitude in the hemisphere contralateral to the deprived eye, reflecting massive synaptic weakening of the dominant input to this hemisphere. Such interhemispheric asymmetry is no longer observed after longer periods of MD (5 days), however. Early depression of deprived (contralateral)-eye responses can account for decreases in binocular VEPs at 3 days, and late potentiation of the open-eye response can explain the "renormalization" of binocular VEPs after 5 days of MD.

Mechanisms of the ocular dominance shift in mice

The synaptic mechanisms for cortical plasticity still remain largely unknown. A common hypothesis is that Hebbian synaptic plasticity, which is implemented in vivo by long-term potentiation (LTP) and long-term depression (LTD), drives rapid components of map plasticity (Malenka and Bear, 2004), whereas a slower anatomical rearrangement of synapses drives later components (Antonini and Stryker, 1996, 1998).

Our experiments show that MD in mice during the preadolescent critical period causes (1) rapid, deprivation-induced response depression and (2) delayed, deprivation-enabled response potentiation. These two responses to MD are mechanistically distinct because they are affected differently by reducing activity in the deprived eye. Depression of deprived-eye responses is eliminated by intraocular injection of tetrodotoxin (TTX), suggesting that this early response to lid closure is triggered by activity originating in the deprived retina (Frenkel and Bear, 2004). On the other hand, potentiation of nondeprived ipsilateral eye responses is promoted by inactivation of the dominant contralateral eye, suggesting that this response to MD is enabled by reducing postsynaptic activity in visual cortex.

Some insight into the mechanisms of the early, deprivation-induced response depression have come from recent studies performed in rats. However, these studies have also revealed some important species-specific differences: (1) the OD shift in rats occurs more rapidly than in mice (after only 1 day of MD; Heynen et al., 2003), and (2) unlike in mice (see figure 38.2*B*) and kittens (Sherman and Wilson, 1975),

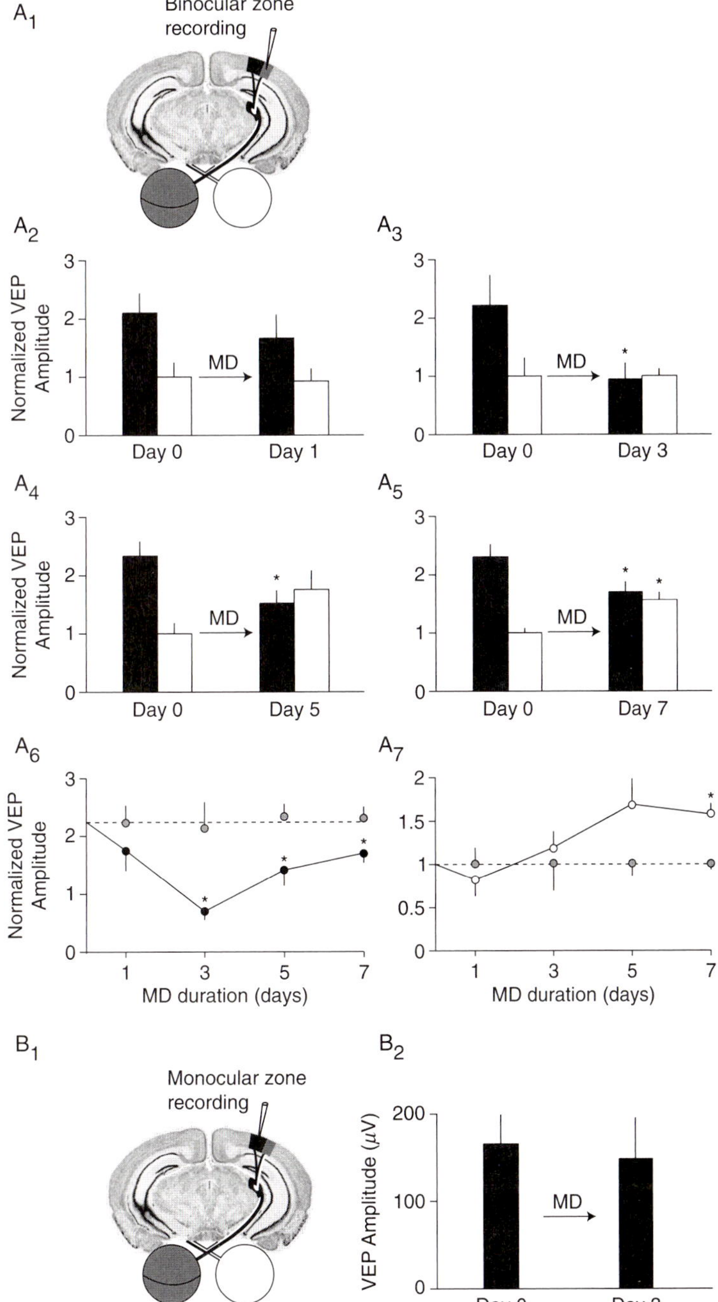

FIGURE 38.2 Effects of MD on visual cortical responsiveness. A_1, Schematic diagram of visual information flow from the retina to the cortex. A recording electrode is implanted in the binocular zone of V1. A_2–A_5, Effects of 1, 3, 5, and 7 days of MD on contralateral and ipsilateral eye responses. A_6 and A_7, Summary of data shown in A_2 to A_5. Deprived-eye responses (A_6, *black symbols*) decrease significantly after 3 days of monocular deprivation (A_3) and stay depressed during longer MD periods (A_4 to A_5). Open-eye responses (A_7, *open symbols*) increase after 5 days of MD (A_4) and reach statistical significance following 7 days of MD (A_5). *Gray symbols* in both panels represent VEP responses obtained on day 0. B_1 and B_2, A brief period of MD that is sufficient to maximally depress responses in the binocular zone has no effect on VEP amplitude in the monocular segment of Oc1.

there is a substantial effect of deprivation on responses in the monocular segment of visual cortex, where there is no substrate for binocular competition (Sherman and Wilson, 1975). With these caveats in mind, we briefly review what the rat studies have revealed about potential mechanisms.

It is well established that at many excitatory synapses in the brain, weak activation of postsynaptic NMDA receptor can induce long-term synaptic depression (Malenka and Bear, 2004). Although the mechanisms vary, depending on location, there is good evidence both in visual cortex and in

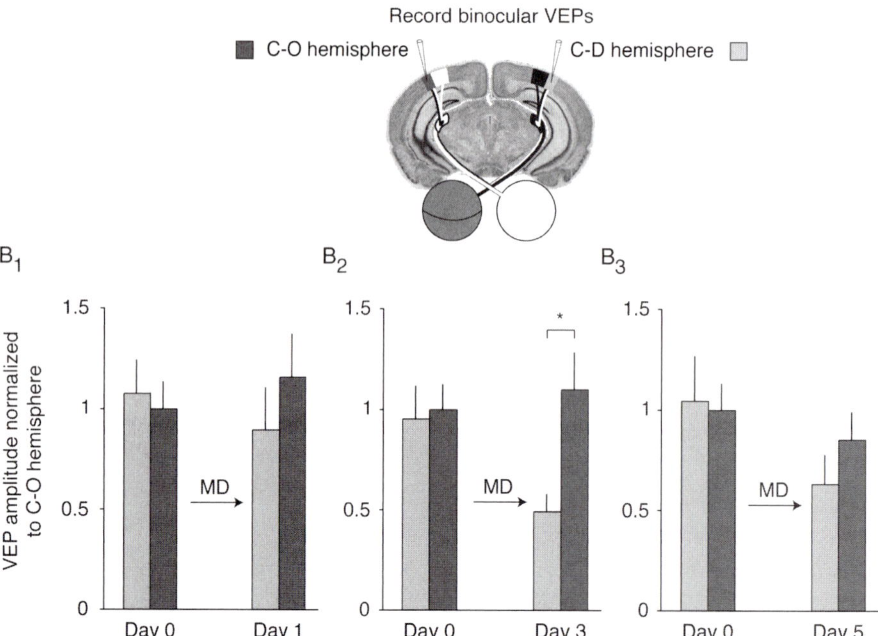

FIGURE 38.3 Three days of MD result in an interhemispheric asymmetry of binocularly elicited VEPs. *A*, Recording electrodes were implanted bilaterally in the binocular zone of V1. *B*, VEPs in response to binocular visual stimulation are identical in amplitude in both hemispheres prior to MD (day 0, B_1 to B_3). B_2, After 3 days of MD, however, binocular VEPs in the hemisphere contralateral to the deprived eye are significantly depressed, which is accounted for by the deprivation-induced depression of the deprived-eye responses. This binocular response depression is not observed after 1 day of MD (B_1) or after a longer period of MD (B_3) due to the delayed potentiation of open-eye responses.

hippocampus that a prominent form of LTD is mediated by the modification and removal of postsynaptic AMPA receptors. Heynen et al. tested the hypothesis that MD in rats induces synaptic depression by the same mechanism as LTD. They showed in rats that monocular lid closure for 24 hours precisely mimics LTD with respect to altered AMPA receptor phosphorylation and decreased surface expression, and that synaptic depression by MD occludes LTD in slices of visual cortex. Moreover, these effects of MD failed to occur if NMDA receptors were blocked or if TTX was injected into the deprived eye. These data provide very strong evidence that MD induces LTD in rat visual cortex (McAllister and Usrey, 2003). Moreover, induction of LTD in visual cortex by electrical stimulation of the LGN caused a depression of VEPs indistinguishable from that caused by MD (Heynen et al., 2003).

A second "noncompetitive" mechanism for response depression in rat visual cortex involves changes in inhibition. Compelling evidence was recently provided that MD induces LTP of inhibitory connections from fast-spiking basket cells onto layer 4 pyramidal neurons in the monocular segment of rat Oc1 (Maffei et al., 2006). This mechanism likely contributes significantly to the depression of VEPs that has been observed in the monocular segment of rats after MD (Heynen et al., 2003). However, it remains to be determined if the same changes occur in the binocular segment. Further, these findings may not apply to mice or cats, since the monocular segment responses are not affected by deprivation in the absence of binocular competition (see figure 38.2*B*).

Although the question of whether the strengthening of inhibition is a basis for response depression in the mouse remains open, there is some evidence that mechanisms of LTD do contribute. However, a recent study of LTD in mouse visual cortex revealed unexpected mechanistic divergence downstream from NMDA receptor activation, depending on the layer. Whereas layer 4 LTD appears to be identical to that observed in area CA1 of the hippocampus, and clearly involves AMPA receptor endocytosis, layer 3 LTD appears to involve a different mechanism that requires endocannabinoid signaling (Crozier et al., 2007). Both types of LTD were occluded by 3 days of MD in vivo, suggesting that both mechanisms can account for response depression in mouse visual cortex. However, the relative extent to which these mechanisms are responsible for the depression of VEPs remains to be determined.

With longer periods of MD, we observe potentiation of responses to the nondeprived eye. The fact that some recovery of deprived-eye responses also occurs at these time points raises the possibility that this potentiation reflects a homeostatic scaling of VEPs following a period of relative cortical inactivity. However, arguing against scaling as an explanation is our finding that binocular deprivation fails to change VEP amplitude. We favor the hypothesis that reducing cortical activity by closing the contralateral eyelid causes a change in the threshold level of activation required to potentiate the nondeprived-eye synapses. This hypothesis is supported by the fact that open-eye potentiation is accelerated when the contralateral eye is inactivated with TTX (Frenkel and Bear, 2004).

The functional significance of electrophysiological findings in deprivation experiments can only be determined by performing behavioral studies. A considerable amount of research has been done to show the functional consequences of MD on deprived-eye acuity using various behavioral assays (Dews and Wiesel, 1970; Mitchell and MacKinnon, 2002). For many years, however, little attention was paid to determining the effects of MD on open-eye acuity. A recent study from our laboratory, utilizing a method developed to assess rodent visual acuity (Prusky and Douglas, 2003), documented an enhancement of acuity in the nondeprived eye of long-term MD rats (Iny et al., 2006). Although it remains to be shown whether the same is true in mice, a new study using a virtual optokinetic system showed a different form of interocular plasticity in adult mice, in which MD leads to an enhancement of the optokinetic response selectively through the nondeprived eye (Prusky et al., 2006).

A well-known mechanism for synaptic potentiation is revealed by the study of LTP. In the hippocampus, where it has been studied most extensively, LTP is associated with the delivery of AMPA receptors to synapses. Delivery of AMPA receptors following strong NMDA receptor activation requires molecular interactions with the long carboxy tails of AMPA receptor subunits, particularly GluR1. Viral overexpression of the C-terminal domain of GluR1 (GluR1-CT) competes with this interaction and blocks LTP (Malinow et al., 2000). LTP with properties similar to those observed in CA1 in hippocampus can also be elicited in visual cortex both in vivo and in vitro (Heynen and Bear, 2001; Kirkwood and Bear, 1994). Consistent with the notion that conserved mechanisms of LTP might be important for cortical plasticity, recent work in barrel cortex showed that GluR1-containing AMPA receptors are delivered to synapses in response to sensory stimulation, and this response was also blocked by overexpression of GluR1-CT (Takahashi et al., 2003). Furthermore, it is now well established that, like the threshold for naturally occurring response potentiation, the LTP threshold is lowered by a period of cortical inactivity (Kirkwood et al., 1996; Philpot et al., 2003).

LTP of potentials evoked by external sensory stimuli has been demonstrated in vivo in the visual cortex of rats (Heynen and Bear, 2001). In that study, the potentiating stimulus was electrical stimulation of the thalamocortical pathway, which resulted in an enhancement of visual potentials evoked by natural visual stimuli. Repetitive noninvasive visual sensory stimulation has also been shown to result in LTP-like enhancements in the visual system of the developing tadpole. Using in vivo whole-cell recordings from the tectum of *Xenopus* tadpoles, Zhang et al. (2000) showed that repetitive dimming-light stimulation (0.3 Hz) applied to the contralateral eye resulted in persistent enhancement of glutamatergic inputs. Recently, Teyler et al. observed LTP in the visual cortex of adult humans by measuring the amplitude of event-related potentials recorded from the scalp before and after a visual conditioning protocol (checkerboard stimulation presented at an average rate of approximately 1 Hz) (Clapp et al., 2006; Teyler et al., 2005).

Thus, there is much indirect support for the general notion that deprivation-enabled potentiation of the open-eye response uses the mechanisms of LTP. How is this modulated by the history of cortical activity? A hypothesis for which there is considerable evidence is that the LTP threshold is set by the number and type of NMDA receptors, which in turn are modified by deprivation. Specifically, it has been shown in both rats and mice that the period of deprivation required to lower the LTP threshold also changes the ratio of NR2A and NR2B subunits in native NMDA receptors (Chen and Bear, 2007; Quinlan et al., 1999). The switch from 2A to 2B lowers the LTP threshold (Barria and Malinow, 2005), and, we speculate, this change enables potentiation of open-eye responses.

Stimulus-selective response potentiation

Although it seems clear that neural activity is necessary for the development of appropriate brain circuits, it is less clear whether it simply allows predetermined growth to move forward or whether it plays an instructive role in determining brain circuitry. One of the classic paradigms for studying whether activity plays a permissive or an instructive role in shaping cortical responses is stripe rearing, or rearing an animal in an environment where only a single orientation is present (Blakemore and Cooper, 1970; Hirsch and Spinelli, 1970). In this situation, a permissive role for activity would imply that, from a starting point where roughly equal numbers of neurons respond to all possible orientations, only those receiving adequate stimulation from the environment will survive and mature, while others will lose responsiveness and may eventually disappear. An instructive role for activity would mean that previously nonselective cells acquire a preference for the orientation present in the environment, or that cells shift their orientation preference toward the experienced orientation, while maintaining normal responsiveness. In other words, a cell's RF would change.

In both juvenile and adult mice we discovered that repeated daily exposure to a sinusoidal grating stimulus of a particular orientation, pattern reversing at 1 Hz, resulted in a gradual and saturable increase in VEP amplitude that was specific to that orientation (Frenkel et al., 2006). Once daily exposure to 200 stimuli gradually increased the response, which saturated after 5 days of exposure (figure 38.4*A*). We tested various parameters to characterize this stimulus-selective response potentiation (SRP). Varying the number of stimuli per session, the intersession interval, and the temporal frequency of visual stimulation did not result in a significant change in SRP expression. Varying the contrast, however, did have an effect on SRP expression: at low stimulus contrast, SRP did not occur. A consolidation period was required for SRP expression, as it does not occur within a single recording session. Interestingly, we failed to observe interocular transfer of SRP (figure 38.4*B*). This finding, along with the fact that specific cortical manipulations of NMDA and AMPA receptors disrupt SRP, strongly suggests that SRP reflects modification of excitatory LGN synapses in layer 4.

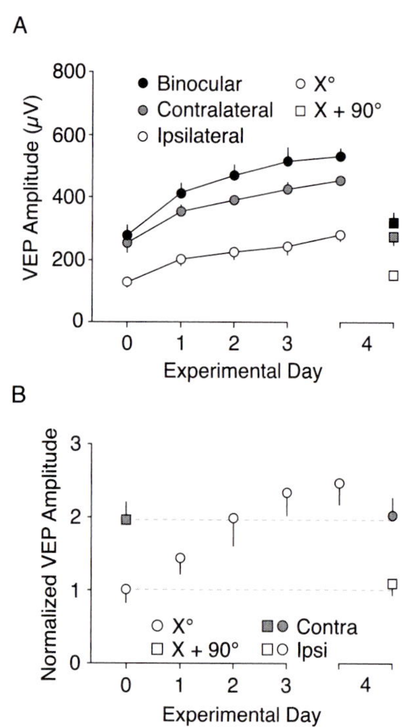

FIGURE 38.4 Characterization of stimulus-selective response potentiation (SRP). *A*, Brief daily exposure to a grating stimulus of a single orientation selectively potentiates the amplitude of VEPs to stimuli of that orientation. VEP amplitude elicited during ipsilateral eye (*open symbols*), contralateral eye (*gray symbols*), and binocular (*black symbols*) viewing conditions increase in response to visual stimuli of a single orientation until it reaches saturation after 4 days of exposure. When stimuli of a novel orientation are also presented on day 4, the amplitude of this new orientation is comparable to the preexposed orientation on day 0. *B*, SRP is eye-specific. SRP elicited to presentations of stimuli of orientation X° to the ipsilateral eye (*open circles*) is not accompanied by SRP in the contralateral eye (*solid circle*). *Squares* indicate VEPs in response to X + 90°; *circles* indicate VEPs in response to X°. VEP amplitudes are normalized to the ipsilateral response elicited on day 1.

Since LTP is a leading model for experience-dependent plasticity as well as for some forms of learning (Rioult-Pedotti et al., 1998, 2000; Whitlock et al., 2006), we hypothesized that SRP and LTP may share common mechanisms. We successfully tested and confirmed this hypothesis by demonstrating that blocking NMDA receptors both pharmacologically and genetically, and disrupting AMPA receptor trafficking, prevents SRP expression. We believe that LTP-like synaptic strengthening is an underlying mechanism for SRP.

Our data reveal a novel form of experience-dependent plasticity in mouse visual cortex. This form of plasticity is not restricted to an early developmental age, as it occurs in animals well beyond the classically defined critical period (P33). SRP is a rapidly induced and robust phenomenon. Moreover, once the response to the experienced orientation increases, the VEP amplitudes remain elevated despite several days in which no testing is performed. This suggests that the mechanisms of SRP may contribute to certain forms of perceptual learning. Based on properties observed in humans, Karni and Sagi (1991) suggested a reductionist model for perceptual learning, involving Hebbian increases in synaptic strength in V1 that require a consolidation period to become manifest. The leading experimental paradigm for Hebbian modifications is LTP, and the key properties of LTP nicely match those of SRP, including input specificity, cooperativity, and persistence. Moreover, at many cortical synapses, induction of LTP requires strong activation of NMDA receptors, and expression of LTP requires the delivery of AMPA receptors. Our experiments reveal that SRP shares identical molecular requirements.

In light of these findings it is especially important to consider that the diverse effects of sensory experience in shaping the nervous system may be mediated by a diversity of cellular and molecular mechanisms. Of particular interest are changes in neural activity that reflect particular qualities of sensory experience. Such changes are likely to be involved in perceptual learning in adults (Ghose, 2004) and may also occur as a result of selective experience during development (Movshon and Van Sluyters, 1981). Little is known regarding the mechanisms underlying such stimulus-specific changes in cortical responses. Our SRP findings lend further support to the idea that diverse effects of sensory experience in shaping the brain may be mediated by common elementary mechanisms of synaptic plasticity.

Adult ocular dominance plasticity

The idea that primary sensory cortex remains plastic beyond the traditionally defined critical period is quite new. It was long assumed that cells in V1 had fixed properties, passing along the product of a stereotyped operation to the next stage in the visual pathway. Any plasticity dependent on visual experience was thought to be restricted to a critical period. It has become clear, however, that the critical period applies to a limited set of properties and connections, each property being subject to its own critical period. Other properties remain mutable throughout life. Therefore, it is very important to study adult cortical plasticity, since it may underlie perceptual learning and participate in recovery of function after brain injury.

Recent evidence suggests that most critical periods do not close abruptly and absolutely but gradually and often incompletely. For example, the capacity for rapid plasticity in somatosensory (S1) cortex declines sharply in some cortical layers soon after birth, but persists in other layers into adulthood (Diamond et al., 1994; Glazewski and Fox, 1996), and a similar pattern has been observed for OD plasticity in some species (Daw et al., 1992). Correspondingly, sensory deprivation or behavioral training can induce substantial plasticity even in adults (Buonomano and Merzenich, 1998; Hofer et al., 2006a; Karmarkar and Dan, 2006; Shuler and Bear, 2006). Whether critical period plasticity and adult plasticity share common cellular and molecular mechanisms is unclear.

Our understanding of visual plasticity in the adult mouse was previously based primarily on single-unit extracellular recordings from cortical neurons, in which the relative balance of inputs representing each eye is assessed within the binocular zone. These studies suggested that brief periods (3–4 days) of MD cause OD plasticity only within a well-defined critical period ending at P35 (Gordon and Stryker, 1996). We reexamined the critical period for OD plasticity in the mouse, initially using an anesthetized preparation, and were surprised to find that 5 days of MD shifted OD in adult mice—a time well beyond the classically defined critical period. The basis for this remarkable adult plasticity was further studied by daily VEP recordings using chronically implanted electrodes in awake animals, which allowed OD and the strength of right eye and left eye inputs to be tracked over time at the same sites. As in anesthetized mice, 5 days of adult MD caused a large OD shift in the hemisphere contralateral to the deprived eye, whereas 3 days of adult MD elicited no significant plasticity. Our data suggested that the adult OD shift was due almost exclusively to an increase in absolute amplitude of ipsilateral (open) eye VEPs rather than to a decrease in the amplitude of contralateral (closed) eye VEPs. Our interpretation was that adult OD plasticity was due to the active strengthening of initially weak ipsilateral inputs in response to closure of the contralateral, dominant eye. Strengthening of ipsilateral inputs developed gradually over the first 3–6 days of MD, explaining why briefer periods of MD failed to elicit OD changes in adult mice. In our study (Sawtell et al., 2003), we demonstrated for the first time that OD plasticity occurs in adult mice, and suggested that it uses different mechanisms than plasticity observed during the classically defined critical period.

This original study (Sawtell et al., 2003) was performed prior to our discovery of SRP, and in these experiments, stimuli of the same orientation were used across multiple days of testing. In the light of our recent discovery of SRP (Frenkel et al., 2006), we reconsidered our prior interpretation of OD plasticity in the adult mouse. In those experiments, the manifestation of deprived-eye weakening could have been easily masked by naturally occurring experience-dependent strengthening of visual responsiveness (SRP). Since we were likely inducing SRP, the experience-dependent strengthening that occurred as a result of baseline VEP measurements may have obscured deprivation-induced weakening of the deprived eye (Sawtell et al., 2003). When we redesigned the experimental protocol to minimize the recording session time and avoided any prolonged patterned visual stimulation with stimuli of the same orientation, we were able to unmask a depression of the deprived-eye response after 7 days of MD (figure 38.5A_2). Thus, the visual cortex of the adult mouse is not immune to synaptic weakening. In fact, the only difference we are able to detect between juvenile and adult OD plasticity is the time scale of the shift: there is no OD shift after 3 days of MD in adult mice (figure 38.5A_1), whereas in juveniles the same manipulation results in a very dramatic shift in juvenile animals (see figure 38.5B_1).

Other laboratories have recently confirmed that rapid experience-dependent plasticity exists in the mature V1 of mice using a variety of measures, including single-unit recordings (Hofer et al., 2006b; Pham et al., 2004; Tagawa et al., 2005). Thus, the finding of adult OD plasticity is robust to assays of input strength (e.g., VEPs in layer 4) and postsynaptic spiking (e.g., single units in all layers). So the question arises: does a mouse have a critical period? Or, put slightly differently, is the mouse a good experimental model in which to study the critical period for OD plasticity? Many laboratories have devoted their resources to studies of the mechanisms underlying the opening and closure of the critical period (Hensch, 2004) and, despite recent findings, it may be premature to dismiss the mouse as a species of choice for studying this question. Nonetheless, it is abundantly clear that the mouse visual cortex is capable of OD plasticity both during early postnatal development and in adulthood, and that many experiments need to be reevaluated in this light. Uncovering the underlying cellular and molecular mechanisms of OD plasticity will require additional experiments that take into account not only age and the length of MD but also laminar and spatial location within the cortex.

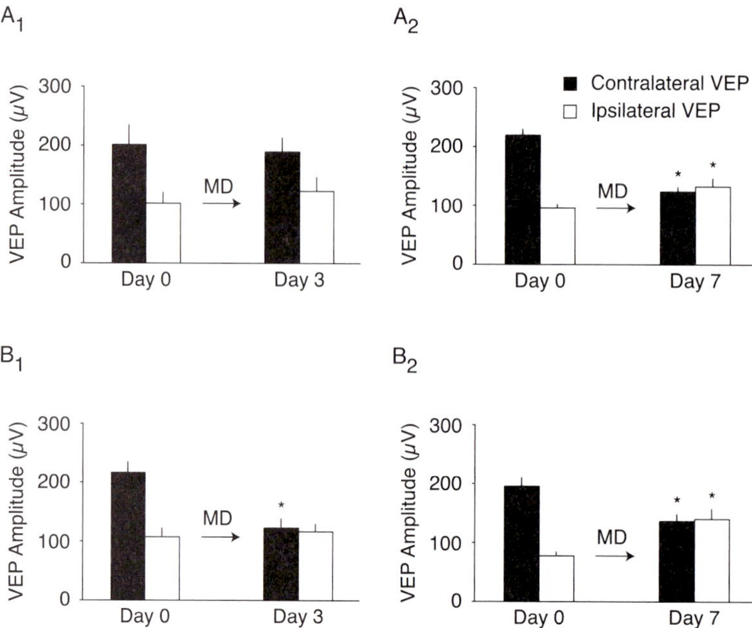

FIGURE 38.5 Juvenile form of OD plasticity is observed in adult mice following longer periods of MD. A_1 to A_2, Effects of 3 and 7 days of MD on OD plasticity in adult mice (P60). B_1 to B_2, Effects of 3 and 7 days of MD on OD plasticity in juvenile mice (P28). Three days of MD had no effect on deprived- and nondeprived-eye VEP amplitude in adult mice (A_1), whereas it resulted in a dramatic shift in juvenile mice (B_1). Longer periods of MD shift ocular dominance in adult mice (A_2). Open-eye responses increase and deprived-eye responses depress following MD. The shift after 7 days of MD is quantitatively the same as in juvenile mice (B_2).

ACKNOWLEDGMENTS Work was supported by grants from the National Eye Institute, the National Institute for Mental Health, and the Howard Hughes Medical Institute. We thank Dr. Arnold Heynen for his valuable comments and help with this chapter.

REFERENCES

ADAMS, D. L., and HORTON, J. C. (2003). Capricious expression of cortical columns in the primate brain. *Nat. Neurosci.* 6:113–114.

ANTONINI, A., and STRYKER, M. P. (1996). Plasticity of geniculocortical afferents following brief or prolonged monocular occlusion in the cat. *J. Comp. Neurol.* 369:64–82.

ANTONINI, A., and STRYKER, M. P. (1998). Effect of sensory disuse on geniculate afferents to cat visual cortex. *Vis. Neurosci.* 15:401–409.

BARRIA, A., and MALINOW, R. (2005). NMDA receptor subunit composition controls synaptic plasticity by regulating binding to CaMKII. *Neuron* 48:289–301.

BLAKEMORE, C., and COOPER, G. F. (1970). Development of the brain depends on the visual environment. *Nature* 228:477–478.

BUONOMANO, D. V., and MERZENICH, M. M. (1998). Cortical plasticity: From synapses to maps. *Annu. Rev. Neurosci.* 21:149–186.

CHEN, W. S., and BEAR, M. F. (2007). Activity-dependent regulation of NR2B translation contributes to metaplasticity in mouse visual cortex. *Neuropharmacology* 52(1):200–214.

CLAPP, W. C., ECKERT, M. J., TEYLER, T. J., and ABRAHAM, W. C. (2006). Rapid visual stimulation induces *N*-methyl-D-aspartate receptor-dependent sensory long-term potentiation in the rat cortex. *Neuroreport* 17:511–515.

CROZIER, R. A., WANG, Y., LIU, C.-H., and BEAR, M. F. (2007). Deprivation-induced synaptic depression via distinct mechanisms in different layers of mouse visual cortex. *Proc. Natl. Acad. Sci. U.S.A.* 104(4):1383–1388.

DAW, N. W., FOX, K., SATO, H., and CZEPITA, D. (1992). Critical period for monocular deprivation in the cat visual cortex. *J. Neurophysiol.* 67:197–202.

DEWS, P. B., and WIESEL, T. N. (1970). Consequences of monocular deprivation on visual behaviour in kittens. *J. Physiol.* 206:437–455.

DIAMOND, M. E., HUANG, W., and EBNER, F. F. (1994). Laminar comparison of somatosensory cortical plasticity. *Science* 265: 1885–1888.

DRÄGER, U. C. (1978). Observations on monocular deprivation in mice. *J. Neurophysiol.* 41:28–42.

EMERSON, V. F., CHALUPA, L. M., THOMPSON, I. D., and TALBOT, R. J. (1982). Behavioural, physiological, and anatomical consequences of monocular deprivation in the golden hamster (*Mesocricetus auratus*). *Exp. Brain Res.* 45(1–2):168–178.

FRENKEL, M. Y., and BEAR, M. F. (2004). How monocular deprivation shifts ocular dominance in visual cortex of young mice. *Neuron* 44:917–923.

FRENKEL, M. Y., SAWTELL, N. B., DIOGO, A. C., YOON, B., NEVE, R. L., and BEAR, M. F. (2006). Instructive effect of visual experience in mouse visual cortex. *Neuron* 51:339–349.

GHOSE, G. M. (2004). Learning in mammalian sensory cortex. *Curr. Opin. Neurobiol.* 14:513–518.

GLAZEWSKI, S., and FOX, K. (1996). Time course of experience-dependent synaptic potentiation and depression in barrel cortex of adolescent rats. *J. Neurophysiol.* 75:1714–1729.

GORDON, J. A., and STRYKER, M. P. (1996). Experience-dependent plasticity of binocular responses in the primary visual cortex of the mouse. *J. Neurosci.* 16:3274–3286.

Hanover, J. L., Huang, Z. J., Tonegawa, S., and Stryker, M. P. (1999). Brain-derived neurotrophic factor overexpression induces precocious critical period in mouse visual cortex. *J. Neurosci.* 19: RC40.

Hensch, T. K. (2004). Critical period regulation. *Annu. Rev. Neurosci.* 27:549–579.

Heynen, A. J., and Bear, M. F. (2001). Long-term potentiation of thalamocortical transmission in the adult visual cortex in vivo. *J. Neurosci.* 21:9801–9813.

Heynen, A. J., Yoon, B. J., Liu, C. H., Chung, H. J., Huganir, R. L., and Bear, M. F. (2003). Molecular mechanism for loss of visual cortical responsiveness following brief monocular deprivation. *Nat. Neurosci.* 6:854–862.

Hirsch, H. V., and Spinelli, D. N. (1970). Visual experience modifies distribution of horizontally and vertically oriented receptive fields in cats. *Science* 168:869–871.

Hofer, S. B., Mrsic-Flogel, T. D., Bonhoeffer, T., and Hübener, M. (2006a). Lifelong learning: Ocular dominance plasticity in mouse visual cortex. *Curr. Opin. Neurobiol.* 16:451–459.

Hofer, S. B., Mrsic-Flogel, T. D., Bonhoeffer, T., and Hübener, M. (2006b). Prior experience enhances plasticity in adult visual cortex. *Nat. Neurosci.* 9:127–132.

Horton, J. C., and Adams, D. L. (2005). The cortical column: A structure without a function. *Philos. Trans. R. Soc. Lond. B. Biol. Sci.* 360:837–862.

Huang, Z. J., Kirkwood, A., Pizzorusso, T., Porciatti, V., Morales, B., Bear, M. F., Maffei, L., and Tonegawa, S. (1999). BDNF regulates the maturation of inhibition and the critical period of plasticity in mouse visual cortex. *Cell* 98: 739–755.

Hübel, D. H., and Wiesel, T. N. (1970). The period of susceptibility to the physiological effects of unilateral eye closure in kittens. *J. Physiol.* 206:419–436.

Iny, K., Heynen, A. J., Sklar, E., and Bear, M. F. (2006). Bidirectional modifications of visual acuity induced by monocular deprivation in juvenile and adult rats. *J. Neurosci.* 26:7368–7374.

Issa, N. P., Trachtenberg, J. T., Chapman, B., Zahs, K. R., and Stryker, M. P. (1999). The critical period for ocular dominance plasticity in the ferret's visual cortex. *J. Neurosci.* 19:6965–6978.

Karmarkar, U. R., and Dan, Y. (2006). Experience-dependent plasticity in adult visual cortex. *Neuron* 52:577–585.

Karni, A., and Sagi, D. (1991). Where practice makes perfect in texture discrimination: Evidence for primary visual cortex plasticity. *Proc. Natl. Acad. Sci. U.S.A.* 88:4966–4970.

Kirkwood, A., and Bear, M. F. (1994). Hebbian synapses in visual cortex. *J. Neurosci.* 14:1634–1645.

Kirkwood, A., Rioult, M. C., and Bear, M. F. (1996). Experience-dependent modification of synaptic plasticity in visual cortex. *Nature* 381:526–528.

Logothetis, N. K. (2003). The underpinnings of the BOLD functional magnetic resonance imaging signal. *J. Neurosci.* 23: 3963–3971.

Maffei, A., Nataraj, K., Nelson, S. B., and Turrigiano, G. G. (2006). Potentiation of cortical inhibition by visual deprivation. *Nature* 443:81–84.

Maffei, L., Berardi, N., Domenici, L., Parisi, V., and Pizzorusso, T. (1992). Nerve growth factor (NGF) prevents the shift in ocular dominance distribution of visual cortical neurons in monocularly deprived rats. *J. Neurosci.* 12:4651–4662.

Malenka, R. C., and Bear, M. F. (2004). LTP and LTD: An embarrassment of riches. *Neuron* 44:5–21.

Malinow, R., Mainen, Z. F., and Hayashi, Y. (2000). LTP mechanisms: From silence to four-lane traffic. *Curr. Opin. Neurobiol.* 10:352–357.

McAllister, A. K., and Usrey, W. M. (2003). Depressed from deprivation? Look to the molecules. *Nat. Neurosci.* 6:787–788.

Mitchell, D. E., and MacKinnon, S. (2002). The present and potential impact of research on animal models for clinical treatment of stimulus deprivation amblyopia. *Clin. Exp. Optom.* 85: 5–18.

Mitzdorf, U. (1985). Current source-density method and application in cat cerebral cortex: Investigation of evoked potentials and EEG phenomena. *Physiol. Rev.* 65:37–100.

Movshon, J. A., and Van Sluyters, R. C. (1981). Visual neural development. *Annu. Rev. Psychol.* 32:477–522.

Murphy, W. J., Pevzner, P. A., and O'Brien, S. J. (2004). Mammalian phylogenomics comes of age. *Trends. Genet.* 20:631–639.

Pham, T. A., Graham, S. J., Suzuki, S., Barco, A., Kandel, E. R., Gordon, B., and Lickey, M. E. (2004). A semi-persistent adult ocular dominance plasticity in visual cortex is stabilized by activated CREB. *Learn. Mem.* 11:738–747.

Philpot, B. D., Espinosa, J. S., and Bear, M. F. (2003). Evidence for altered NMDA receptor function as a basis for metaplasticity in visual cortex. *J. Neurosci.* 23:5583–5588.

Pizzorusso, T., Fagiolini, M., Porciatti, V., and Maffei, L. (1997). Temporal aspects of contrast visual evoked potentials in the pigmented rat: Effect of dark rearing. *Vision. Res.* 37:389–395.

Porciatti, V., Pizzorusso, T., and Maffei, L. (1999). The visual physiology of the wild-type mouse determined with pattern VEPs. *Vision. Res.* 39:3071–3081.

Prusky, G. T., Alam, N. M., and Douglas, R. M. (2006). Enhancement of vision by monocular deprivation in adult mice. *J. Neurosci.* 26:11554–11561.

Prusky, G. T., and Douglas, R. M. (2003). Developmental plasticity of mouse visual acuity. *Eur. J. Neurosci.* 17:167–173.

Quinlan, E. M., Olstein, D. H., and Bear, M. F. (1999). Bidirectional, experience-dependent regulation of *N*-methyl-D-aspartate receptor subunit composition in the rat visual cortex during postnatal development. *Proc. Natl. Acad. Sci. U.S.A.* 96:12876–12880.

Rioult-Pedotti, M. S., Friedman, D., and Donoghue, J. P. (2000). Learning-induced LTP in neocortex. *Science* 290:533–536.

Rioult-Pedotti, M. S., Friedman, D., Hess, G., and Donoghue, J. P. (1998). Strengthening of horizontal cortical connections following skill learning. *Nat. Neurosci.* 1:230–234.

Sawtell, N. B., Frenkel, M. Y., Philpot, B. D., Nakazawa, K., Tonegawa, S., and Bear, M. F. (2003). NMDA receptor-dependent ocular dominance plasticity in adult visual cortex. *Neuron* 38:977–985.

Schroeder, C. E., Tenke, C. E., Givre, S. J., Arezzo, J. C., and Vaughan, H. G., Jr. (1991). Striate cortical contribution to the surface-recorded pattern-reversal VEP in the alert monkey. *Vision Res.* 31:1143–1157.

Sherman, J. (1979). Visual evoked potential (VEP): Basic concepts and clinical applications. *J. Am. Optom. Assoc.* 50:19–30.

Sherman, S. M., and Wilson, J. R. (1975). Behavioral and morphological evidence for binocular competition in the postnatal development of the dog's visual system. *J. Comp. Neurol.* 161: 183–195.

Shuler, M. G., and Bear, M. F. (2006). Reward timing in the primary visual cortex. *Science* 311:1606–1609.

Sokol, S. (1976). Visually evoked potentials: theory, techniques and clinical applications. *Surv. Ophthalmol.* 21:18–44.

Tagawa, Y., Kanold, P. O., Majdan, M., and Shatz, C. J. (2005). Multiple periods of functional ocular dominance plasticity in mouse visual cortex. *Nat. Neurosci.* 8:380–388.

Takahashi, T., Svoboda, K., and Malinow, R. (2003). Experience strengthening transmission by driving AMPA receptors into synapses. *Science* 299:1585–1588.

Teyler, T. J., Hamm, J. P., Clapp, W. C., Johnson, B. W., Corballis, M. C., and Kirk, I. J. (2005). Long-term potentiation of human visual evoked responses. *Eur. J. Neurosci.* 21:2045–2050.

Van Hooser, S. D., Heimel, J. A., Chung, S., Nelson, S. B., and Toth, L. J. (2005). Orientation selectivity without orientation maps in visual cortex of a highly visual mammal. *J. Neurosci.* 25:19–28.

Van Sluyters, R. C., and Stewart, D. L. (1974). Binocular neurons of the rabbit's visual cortex: Effects of monocular sensory deprivation. *Exp. Brain Res.* 19:196–204.

Whitlock, J. R., Heynen, A. J., Shuler, M. G., and Bear, M. F. (2006). Learning induces long-term potentiation in the hippocampus. *Science* 313:1093–1097.

Wiesel, T. N., and Hübel, D. H. (1963). Single-cell responses in striate cortex of kittens deprived of vision in one eye. *J. Neurophysiol.* 26:1003–1017.

Zhang, L. I., Tao, H. W., and Poo, M. (2000). Visual input induces long-term potentiation of developing retinotectal synapses. *Nat. Neurosci.* 3:708–715.

VI MOUSE MODELS OF HUMAN EYE DISEASE

39 Mouse Models: A Key System in Revolutionizing the Understanding of Glaucoma

GARETH R. HOWELL, JEFFREY K. MARCHANT, AND SIMON W. M. JOHN

In this chapter, we highlight important advances that have been made using mouse models to understand the pathogenesis of glaucoma. We also provide insights into how findings in the mouse are likely to affect both our understanding of glaucoma and the development of new therapies. Comprehensive reviews relevant to glaucoma studies in mice are available elsewhere (John et al., 1999; Goldblum and Mittag, 2002; Gould, Smith, et al., 2004; John, 2005; Libby et al., 2005b; Lindsey and Weinreb, 2005; Weinreb and Lindsey, 2005).

An introduction to glaucoma

Glaucoma is a group of genetically heterogeneous diseases characterized by the death of retinal ganglion cells (RGCs), specific visual field deficits, and optic nerve atrophy. It is a major cause of blindness worldwide, with an estimated 70 million people affected (Quigley, 1996). Glaucoma is frequently associated with elevated intraocular pressure (IOP) (Ritch et al., 1996). High IOP and increasing age are strong risk factors for developing the disease. Nevertheless, high IOP is neither necessary to cause glaucoma—some individuals develop glaucoma despite IOPs in the normal range (Ritch et al., 1996)—nor, by itself, sufficient to cause glaucoma. Many individuals with high IOP do not develop glaucomatous visual loss (Leske, 1983). There are profound interpatient differences in the rate of glaucoma progression and the response to treatment. This phenomenon points to the existence of individual susceptibility factors that determine both the magnitude of IOP that is harmful to each individual and the ultimate severity and speed of visual damage (Libby et al., 2005b).

Many forms of glaucoma have a genetic component. Although a number of glaucoma genes have been identified, we are far from understanding the genetic or molecular etiology of glaucoma susceptibility (John, 2005; Libby et al., 2005b). Characterizing the genetic factors that contribute to glaucoma should facilitate the early identification of individuals who are at increased risk for disease and should be monitored closely. Understanding the molecular mechanisms that kill RGCs and the role elevated IOP and other risk factors play in these processes is important for designing new treatments to prevent vision loss.

The mouse as a model system in which to study glaucoma

The mouse is an ideal mammalian model for deciphering the complex genetic interactions that underlie human glaucoma susceptibility (John et al., 1999). Glaucomatous mouse strains often develop glaucoma with a similar age-related progression as people do, and they do so in a relatively short span of time (within 1–2 years). It is possible to generate new models by mutating mouse orthologues of human glaucoma genes or by introducing known human mutant alleles into mice. This facility allows functional studies to be conducted in a highly controlled experimental setting. The burgeoning array of existing transgenic and gene-targeted alleles can also be exploited to study mechanisms of glaucoma. Studies in mice allow strain-specific genetic modifiers of the disease to be characterized. Last, mutagenesis screens can be performed to identify new genes and mechanisms that cause glaucoma. With the development of reliable means of measuring IOP and the availabily of models of both experimentally induced and inherited glaucoma, the mouse glaucoma model is poised to be a key player in revolutionizing our understanding of the molecular and cellular mechanisms of glaucoma susceptibility, initiation, and progression.

Humans and mice have comparable glaucoma-relevant structures

The aqueous drainage (outflow) structures of the eye play an important role in IOP elevation. Careful analysis of the aqueous humor drainage pathway and its role in controlling IOP is a major goal for glaucoma research. The mouse is well suited to these studies because its aqueous drainage structures are similar to those in humans. The two types of outflow pathways present in humans, conventional and uveoscleral, exist in mice (see John et al., 1999; Lindsey and Weinreb, 2002). Both species have an endothelial-lined canal of Schlemm and a trabecular meshwork (TM) consisting of layers of well-organized trabecular beams covered with endothelial-like trabecular cells. The organizational similarity extends to drainage structure development and the genes that influence it (Gould, Smith, et al., 2004). The biggest anatomical difference between mice and humans is that mice have a poorly developed ciliary muscle. Nevertheless, the prostaglandin analogue Latanaprost (which decreases ciliary muscle–mediated resistance to outflow) lowers mouse IOP as it does in humans, and the effects of adenosine receptors on IOP are similar in the two species. The documented similarities between mice and humans in drainage structure anatomy, in functional responses to drugs that inhibit aqueous production and facilitate outflow, and in values for various outflow parameters indicate that mice represent very suitable models for studying IOP and its glaucoma-associated elevation.

The neural retina is the most complex structure of the eye and is considered to be an extension of the brain. Humans and mice have essentially the same neural retinal structures. The human eye has approximately 1.2–1.5 million RGCs, as opposed to 40,000–80,000 in mice (Strom and Williams, 1998). The common denominator in human glaucomas is the loss of RGCs along with their axons in the optic nerve and a specific pattern of optic nerve atrophy called excavation (Shields, 1997), and these same changes occur in the mouse.

Accurate intraocular pressure measurements can be generated in mice

Measuring IOP accurately and precisely is fundamental to the study of glaucoma. In humans, IOP is measured by a noninvasive technique known as tonometry. The mouse eye is only 3 mm in diameter (eight times smaller than the human eye), and this makes it more challenging to measure IOP. Noninvasive tonometric devices are available for use in mouse eyes, and two newer tonometric methods have recently been assessed (Filippopoulos et al., 2006). The impact-rebound (I/R) tonometer functions on the dynamic principle of probe deceleration following contact with the cornea (Danias et al., 2003a). In contrast, optical interferometry tonometry (OIT) is based on a static principle whereby an applied force applanates a specific area of the cornea (Ahmed et al., 2003). Only the OIT and I/R tonometers have been directly compared with a more accurate, invasive measuring method in the same eye in vivo (Filippopoulos et al., 2006; Morris et al., 2006), and so these are the best validated instruments. We and others could not obtain accurate or reliable readings using the Tono-Pen tonometer (John et al., 1997; Reitsamer et al., 2004; Dalke et al., 2005; Pease et al., 2006). A commercial version of the I/R tonometer recently became available and gives accurate group means (Wang et al., 2005) but awaits direct in vivo comparison with an invasive method. Noninvasive methods have the advantage of allowing many repeated measurements but are not as accurate as invasive methods (even on human eyes), and must be used with great care. Differences in user technique, differences in normal corneal properties between mouse strains, and the presence of any corneal abnormalities alter the measured IOP. These factors can render these instruments substantially inaccurate. Thus, it is worth mentioning that the commonly used glaucomatous mouse strain (DBA/2J) has keratopathy at a young age and develops corneal calcification with increasing age.

Invasive methods for measuring IOP in the mouse entail inserting a cannula into the eye. They are widely accepted to be the only true measure of IOP in mice and other species. In one system, a very fine fluid-filled glass microneedle is inserted into the anterior chamber. The needle is connected to a pressure transducer and the pressure reading is monitored on a computer (John et al., 1997; Savinova et al., 2001). Since we developed this method, it has been successfully adopted by other groups. Another system available is an adaptation of the servo-null micropipette system (SNMS), which was developed for measuring pressure in structures smaller than 25 μm (Avila et al., 2001). Cannulation methods have the disadvantage of penetrating the eye, and thus limiting the number of reasonable longitudinal readings. Nevertheless, because large numbers of genetically identical mice of different ages can be evaluated, an accurate record of IOP for a given population or strain can be achieved. It is also possible to study the variability of response and the effects of systematic manipulations. Invasive methods require general anesthesia, which can alter IOP. With appropriate care and attention to anesthetic mix, dose, and environment, however, anesthetic effects can be avoided (Savinova et al., 2001).

Mouse models of glaucoma

Mouse models relevant to high IOP and glaucoma can be divided into two classes, experimentally induced and inherited. Experimentally induced models have the advantage that IOP can be elevated conveniently and experiments can be conducted over a short time frame, and these models are therefore a valuable resource. However, they may have at least some mechanistic differences from inherited glaucoma. IOP-independent toxic effects on RGCs induced by the IOP-elevating procedure have not been carefully controlled in most cases. Not all investigators have readily reproduced reliably or consistently elevations in IOP, and so consultation on technical details with the appropriate groups is advised. Although experiments involving inherited forms of glaucoma are more time-consuming, the outcomes are more likely to accurately model human glaucoma, which has a strong genetic component. Optic nerve head excavation, a hallmark of human glaucoma, is reported only for the inherited models.

EXPERIMENTALLY INDUCED GLAUCOMA Translimbal laser photocoagulation is used to damage the drainage structures themselves or the blood vessels into which they drain. The net effect is to reduce aqueous outflow and induce ocular hypertension. Single-session treatments are reported to elevate IOP for up to 12 weeks. Although some studies have shown laser treatment alone to be sufficient to increase IOP (Gross et al., 2003), others have coupled laser treatment with preflattening of the anterior chamber (by aqueous aspiration) to appose the cornea, iris, and drainage structures during laser use (Aihara et al., 2003a).

Evaluation of retinas following sustained IOP elevation (4–12 weeks) has indicated increased RGC apoptosis (Gross et al., 2003; Grozdanic et al., 2003), decreased optic nerve cross-sectional area and axonal density (Gross et al., 2003; Grozdanic et al., 2003), preferential loss of superior axons in the optic nerve (Mabuchi et al., 2004), and sustained ERG deficits (Grozdanic et al., 2003). A number of complications from these procedures do occur, such as corneal edema and opacity, hyphema, and cataracts, but these appear to be short-lived.

The injection of hyperosmotic saline into the limbus is an alternative means of increasing aqueous outflow resistance and hence IOP. This is an established method for use in the rat (Morrison et al., 1997) but is only preliminarily reported (in abstract form) in the mouse (McKinnon et al., 2003). Eight weeks after injection of 2.0M NaCl into the limbus of C57BL/6 mice, IOP was elevated and an average of 20% RGC axonal loss was observed. In this initial study, the animal numbers were low, so, although the results are promising, further testing is needed. The real benefit of these experimentally induced glaucoma models is the ability to induce chronic elevated IOP in genetically manipulated mice at will. As more mouse mutants become available, these models should help shed light on the risk factors that predispose to RGC death following sustained chronic ocular hypertension.

MODELS OF INHERITED GLAUCOMA Because glaucoma represents a set of heterogeneous disorders, in this section different inherited glaucoma models are discussed in relation to pertinent types of human glaucoma.

Primary open-angle glaucoma. Primary open-angle glaucoma (POAG) is the most common clinically defined subset of glaucoma. The term open-angle is used because the angle and drainage routes are clinically observed to be unimpeded. Based on existing genetic mapping studies, there are at least 10 loci implicated in initiating POAG, and several genes known to contribute to the disease have been identified (see Libby et al., 2005a). The two best characterized are myocilin (*GLC1A*) and optineurin (*GLC1E*).

Myocilin (*MYOC*) was the first identified POAG gene. Mutations exist in approximately 3%–5% of late-onset POAG patients and up to 30% of juvenile open-angle glaucoma patients (JOAG, an earlier and more severe form of POAG). Myocilin is found in many ocular tissues, including the aqueous humor, TM, ciliary body, and RGCs. Despite its discovery nearly 10 years ago, its function is still unclear. Most of the 70 *MYOC* mutations so far identified in human glaucoma patients occur in a region with homology to the extracellular matrix protein olfactomedin (Kanagavalli et al., 2004).

The disease-causing mutations are believed to act through a gain-of-function mechanism. In both people and mice with null alleles, glaucoma does not develop (Kim et al., 2001). In addition, neither 15-fold overexpression of mouse MYOC (Gould, Miceli-Libby, et al., 2004) nor elevated expression of human MYOC from the mouse lens (Zillig et al., 2005) leads to glaucoma in mice. In experiments using cultured human TM cells, MYOC containing a Pro370Leu mutation accumulates in cells and stimulates the unfolded protein response, ER stress, and cell death when cells are grown at normal body temperature. However, when cells are grown at a lower temperature that promotes protein folding and secretion, the cells survive (Liu and Vollrath, 2004). These data strongly suggest that the accumulation of misfolded proteins is pathogenic.

In one in vivo mouse study by Gould et al. (2006), expression of a *Myoc* allele (Tyr423His), equivalent to a severe disease-associated human mutation (Tyr437His), led to the accumulation of mutant protein within the iridocorneal angle of the eye but did not activate ER stress or lead to elevated IOP and glaucoma. Several mouse strains were used, including CBA/CaJ, AKR/J, BALB/cJ, and C57BL/6J, and all demonstrated consistent, nonpathological phenotypes. In humans, the equivalent mutation is associated with the development of aggressive glaucoma, so the lack of disease progression in the mouse is surprising. There is just 82% identity between the mouse and human MYOC protein. The mouse protein may contain sequences that make it unable to induce the unfolded protein response and ER stress. Alternatively, activation of the unfolded protein response may not occur in vivo in mice or in humans. Abnormally accumulating mutant proteins that form insoluble polymeric aggregates do not always activate the unfolded protein response, and to date, activation of the response by mutant MYOC has been observed only in vitro. The production of mice that express the mutant version of the human protein in the iridocorneal angle should provide a useful means of testing these possibilities.

In a separate in vivo study by Senatorov et al. (2006), the same Tyr423His mutation also led to MYOC accumulation in the TM. In this study, a modest increase (2 mm Hg) in IOP was observed, and apoptotic RGC loss and axonal degeneration occurred with age. Optic nerve head excavation was not demonstrated, however. Additionally, the reported elevation of IOP was minor, far below the typical values induced by glaucomatous *MYOC* mutations. Thus, it remains unclear whether the mice truly had a form of glaucoma or whether the transgene insertion site or the level of transgene expression directly induced the RGC death. The slightly elevated IOP in this study may also reflect a greater expression level of the mutant *Myoc* than in the study by Gould et al., which used a knock-in strategy to introduce the mutation into the endogenous *Myoc* gene. Also, it is possible that the divergent results from these two studies may relate to genetic background. Senatorov et al. used a C57BL/6Hsd background rather than C57BL/6J background that was used in the study by Gould et al. RGC loss has been reported in the parental nontransgenic Hsd substrain beginning at 12–15 months, and to be as high as 46% by 18 months of age (Danias et al., 2003b).

Several potential modifier genes have been identified that may affect MYOC function. In one study, a specific MYOC mutation was associated with POAG, but the age at onset was substantially younger when patients were also heterozygous for a mutation in another glaucoma gene, *CYP1B1* (Vincent et al., 2002). The *CYP1B1* allele was suggested to modify the glaucoma phenotype. It is not clear, however, whether heterozygosity for the mutation truly affects the phenotype or whether it simply acts as a marker for a linked modifier gene. Similarly, an allele of optineurin was proposed to exacerbate *MYOC*-associated phenotypes, (Willoughby et al., 2004), but further examination is needed. These studies highlight the complexity of POAG and suggest that phenotypic differences observed between patients may be affected by modifier genes. The future analysis of mouse models with mutations in the human MYOC gene may facilitate the characterization of modifier genes relevant to the severity of glaucoma in different patients.

Optineurin (*OPTN*) has been associated with POAG and normal-tension glaucoma (NTG). Mutations in *OPTN* have been shown to cause a dominant NTG in humans (Rezaie et al., 2002). OPTN is expressed throughout the eye, including the TM, canal of Schlemm, ciliary epithelium, retina, and optic nerve. It is also expressed in neuronal and glial cells of the retina and optic nerve. Although the function of OPTN is unclear, it has been shown in vitro to interfere with TNFα-mediated apoptosis and thus could directly affect RGC survival. In a recent in vivo study, however, OPTN ectopically expressed in lens cells of transgenic mice was unable to modulate apoptosis (Kroeber et al., 2006). This study also provided evidence for a cytoplasmic localization for OPTN rather than extracellular as reported by Rezaie et al. (2002). Thus, further characterization studies of this protein and its functions are clearly needed.

A number of *OPTN* sequence variants have been identified in glaucoma patients. Although the majority of these are associated with NTG, a significant number appear to be associated with POAG. However, a clear role in glaucoma has not been definitively proved for many of the alleles reported. Many of the known *OPTN* variants identified in glaucoma patients are also found in controls. Either these alleles are not important for glaucoma or other factors must interact with them to induce disease (Libby et al., 2005b). One possibility is that *OPTN* mutations do not induce glaucoma unless the genetic context is permissive; this would explain why mutations are also present in controls. This complexity can confound genotype to phenotype associations and makes it difficult to define alleles that truly contribute to disease. For these reasons, animal experiments are needed as an important complement to human studies. For instance, it will be useful to generate mice with the E50K mutation, which is clearly a disease-associated allele and leads to a severe form of NTG. A potentially useful mouse resource exists since the *OPTN* orthologue (*Optn*) of strain C57BL/6J has a glutamine (Q) at residue 552 and a lysine (K) at residue 98 (orthologous to the POAG-associated variants R545Q and M98K, respectively). Although we have not found age-related glaucoma in C57BL/6J mice, a related mouse strain, C57BL/6Hsd, is reported to lose almost 50% of its RGCs during aging but does not appear to have elevated IOP (Danias et al., 2003b). This suggests that C57BL/Hsd may be a useful model for studying NTG.

Collagen I. Although the iridocorneal angle remains open in POAG, extracellular alterations that develop coincident with disease progression are commonly reported. It has long been suggested that extracellular matrix (ECM) components of the ocular drainage pathways are crucial determinants of resistance to aqueous humor outflow (Scott and Wirtz, 1996). It is of interest that mice harboring a targeted mutation in the α1 subunit of collagen I (COL1A1) develop elevated IOP and that by 1 year of age lose almost 25% of their RGC axons (Aihara et al., 2003b). This mutation substitutes 5 amino acids adjacent to the MMP-1 cleavage site and completely blocks MMP-1 hydrolysis (Wu et al., 1990). These results implicate an association between fibrillar collagen turnover and IOP regulation. We have not reproduced these findings in our laboratory, however, and so environmental differences or genetic complexity must affect the phenotype. With further characterization, this will be an exciting new model with relevance to IOP elevation and RGC loss in POAG.

Developmental glaucoma. Developmental glaucoma refers to the subset of glaucomas associated with anterior segment dysgenesis. Many relevant genes have been described (see Gould, Smith, et al., 2004). Although the phenotypes often exhibit autosomal dominant or recessive inheritance, variable expressivity and incomplete penetrance point to a multifactorial etiology (see Gould and John, 2002). Many of the conditions involve obvious dysgenesis of readily visible anterior chamber structures such as the iris and pupil. In others (primary congenital glaucoma), the defects are subtle, involving abnormal development of canal of Schlemm and TM drainage structures of the iridocorneal angle.

Primary congenital glaucoma. Primary congenital glaucoma (PCG) is a severe form of early-onset glaucoma. Many PCG cases are caused by recessive mutations in the *CYP1B1* gene (Libby et al., 2005b). Striking phenotypic differences exist between individuals with *CYP1B1* mutations, suggesting the involvement of modifier gene(s). Consistent with this human phenotypic variability, *Cyp1b1* mutant mice have focal angle abnormalities similar to those observed in PCG patients but do not develop high IOP or glaucoma. Motivated by these observations, studies have identified a modifier gene that alters the phenotype in *Cyp1b1* mutant mice (Libby et al., 2003). A null allele of the tyrosinase gene (*Tyr*) was identified as an enhancer of angle dysgenesis. *Cyp1b1*-deficient mice that are also deficient for *Tyr* have more severe angle malformations than do mice carrying the *Cyp1b1* mutation alone (Libby et al., 2003). *Tyr* also modified the phenotype of *Foxc1*-deficient mice, another gene whose orthologue causes human glaucoma. Tyrosinase produces levodopa, and it was demonstrated that administration of levodopa in the drinking water of pregnant mice deficient in both CYP1B1 and tyrosinase substantially alleviated the developmental abnormalities (Libby et al., 2003).

These experiments raise the possibility that mutations in multiple genes contributing to developmental glaucomas affect dopa levels. Dopa levels may be altered in the neural crest cells from which the angle structures and iris stroma derive. Tyrosine hydroxylase (TH) is the major enzyme responsible for producing dopa from tyrosine. Remarkably, a number of the genes that are known to cause anterior segment dysgenesis and glaucoma in humans or mice are known to promote either TH-expression or the proliferation of TH-expressing neural crest cells during development (Gould, Smith, et al., 2004). These findings demonstrate the utility of mice for defining multifactorial genetic interactions and for defining new pathways that are relevant to glaucoma.

Pigmentary glaucoma. Pigment dispersion syndrome (PDS) is a common condition that often progresses to pigmentary glaucoma. PDS involves focal iris pigment epithelial atrophy and dispersal of liberated pigment onto anterior chamber structures and into the ocular drainage structures. Clinically, there is a radial slit-like pattern of iris transillumination. Various mechanisms have been suggested to account for the pigment dispersion, including iris rubbing against the zonules or lens, developmental defects, inherited disease of the pigment epithelium, and hypovascularity of the iris (Ritch et al., 1996; Shields, 1997), but the molecular mechanisms of pigment dispersion are not conclusively established. Although autosomal dominant inheritance has been reported, the majority of PDS cases do not exhibit clear Mendelian inheritance and likely have a multifactorial etiology.

DBA/2J mice develop a pigmentary form of glaucoma characterized by a pigment liberating iris disease, increased IOP, and optic nerve degeneration. The degree of pigment dispersion and iris destruction in DBA/2J mice is much greater than that observed in human PDS patients. This is likely explained by the discovery that DBA/2J mice are mutant for two genes that can independently cause disease but when inherited together interact to cause the severe DBA/2J phenotype (John et al., 1998). The DBA/2J disease is induced by the *b* allele of tyrosinase-related protein 1 gene ($Tyrp1^{b}$) and a stop codon mutation in the glycoprotein (transmembrane) *nmb* gene ($Gpnmb^{R150X}$). While mice homozygous for both $Tyrp1^{b}$ and $Gpnmb^{R150X}$ develop severe iris disease, single homozygotes are more mildly affected and have distinct phenotypes (figure 39.1) (Chang et al., 1999; Anderson et al., 2002). Mice homozygous for $Tyrp1^{b}$ develop an iris stromal atrophy phenotype, whereas mice homozygous for $Gpnmb^{R150X}$ develop an iris pigment dispersion phenotype involving deterioration of the iris pigment epithelium.

The etiology of DBA/2J pigment dispersion lies with dysfunction of pigmented iris cells. Under normal conditions, potentially toxic intermediates generated during melanin production are sequestered inside melanosomes. The *Gpnmb* and *Tyrp1* gene products are melanosome components, and their mutations perturb melanosome structure and appear to allow these toxic molecules to escape, damaging the cells that contain them (Chang et al., 1999; Anderson et al., 2002, 2006; Libby et al., 2005b).

In addition to being present in iris cells, *Gpnmb* is also present in dendritic cells. Insofar as dendritic cells are normally present in the iris and ocular outflow pathway (McMenamin, 1999; McMenamin and Holthouse, 1992), the *Gpnmb* mutation may alter dendritic cell function(s) and promote iris disease through ocular immune abnormalities. DBA/2J eyes have deficiencies in some aspects of immune privilege before overt pigment dispersion (Mo et al., 2003). For example, they are deficient in anterior chamber–associated immune deviation (ACAID), an active physiological process that acts to suppress pro-inflammatory responses to antigens that are first detected in the eye (Mo et al., 2003). Although

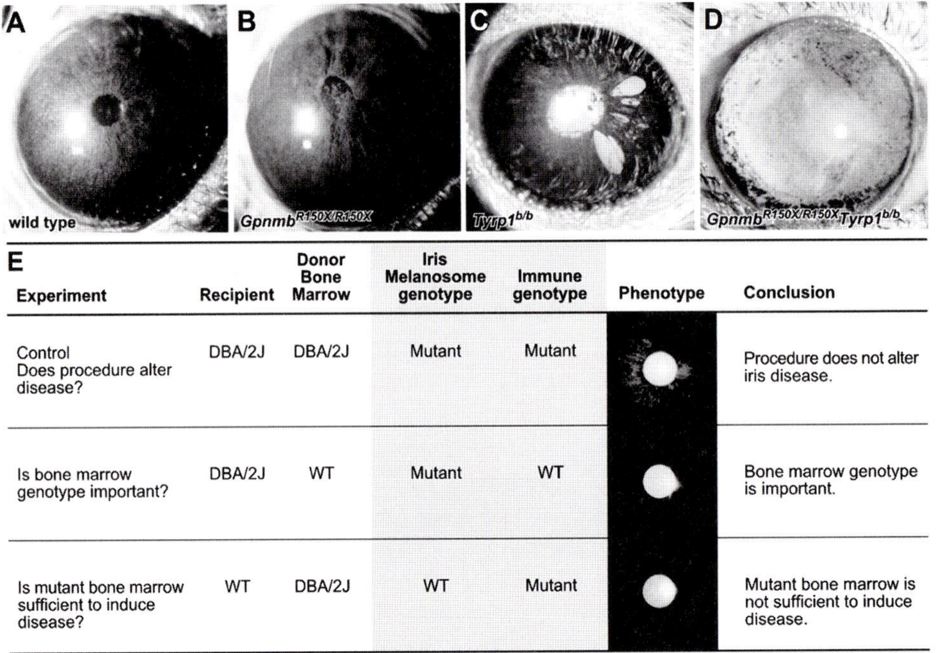

Experiment	Recipient	Donor Bone Marrow	Iris Melanosome genotype	Immune genotype	Phenotype	Conclusion
Control Does procedure alter disease?	DBA/2J	DBA/2J	Mutant	Mutant		Procedure does not alter iris disease.
Is bone marrow genotype important?	DBA/2J	WT	Mutant	WT		Bone marrow genotype is important.
Is mutant bone marrow sufficient to induce disease?	WT	DBA/2J	WT	Mutant		Mutant bone marrow is not sufficient to induce disease.

FIGURE 39.1 Melanosomes contribute to DBA/2J pigment dispersion. *A–D*, Mutations in genes encoding the melanosomal proteins TYRP1 and GPNMB cause iris disease. DBA/2J mice that are homozygous mutant for both genes have the most severe disease (*D*). All images are from 24-month-old mice. *E*, Evidence of an immune contribution to DBA/2J pigment dispersion. Bone marrow genotype has an important effect on the phenotype. See color plate 32. (Modified from John, 2005. *A–D*, Reproduced from Mo et al., 2003 [*Journal of Experimental Medicine*, 2003, 197:1335–1344. Copyright 2003, Rockefeller University Press]. *E*, Reproduced from John, 2005 [*Investigative Ophthalmology and Visual Science*, 2005, 46:2650–2661. Copyright 2005, Association for Research in Vision and Ophthalmology].)

DBA/2J eyes lack clinical signs of overt inflammation, a chronic but mild form of inflammation does attack the iris (Mo et al., 2003). Furthermore, reconstituting the immune system of DBA/2J mice with cells that express wild-type *Gpnmb* (through bone marrow transfer) substantially alleviates the pigment dispersion (Mo et al., 2003) (figure 39.1*E*). Of note, a *Gpnmb* mutant immune system is not sufficient to induce the disease in otherwise wild-type mice (Mo et al., 2003). Overall, these experiments suggest that DBA/2J iris damage is initiated by melanosome toxicity and that inadequate immune suppression resulting from a susceptible immune genotype then allows an inflammatory response to propagate the disease.

In many human cases, PDS progresses to high IOP and causes pigmentary glaucoma. However, a significant number of PDS patients do not progress to high IOP. This implies that factors in addition to direct obstruction of the drainage structures by pigment are necessary to cause sustained IOP elevation. It is likely that a genetic susceptibility of the drainage tissues to a pigment/cell debris–induced pathology is needed for glaucoma progression. Mouse experiments provide strong evidence for such inherited susceptibility. The DBA/2J mutations have now been introduced into a genetically different strain background, C57BL/6J. On this new background these mutations induce the iris disease, but there is rarely progression to high IOP or glaucoma (Anderson et al., 2006). This strongly suggests that genetic susceptibility factors determine the likelihood of pigment dispersion progressing to elevated IOP. The DBA/2J and double mutant C57BL/6J strains represent powerful tools for understanding the pathways conferring susceptibility or resistance to IOP elevation.

TM alteration in DBA/2J. By the time of overt pigment liberation, large aggregates of the protein cochlin have accumulated in the TM of DBA/2J mice (Bhattacharya et al., 2005a). Interestingly, cochlin is reported to progressively accumulate in the TM of human POAG patients as well. In one study, Western analyses detected cochlin in 20 out of 20 TM samples from patients with POAG (irrespective of source, fresh trabeculectomy or cadaver glaucomatous tissue) and in 0 out of 20 TM samples from normal control tissue donors (Bhattacharya et al., 2005b). In both mice and humans, cochlin accumulates as large aggregates in acellular regions and is often associated with mucopolysaccharide deposits. Cochlin is the major noncollagenous ECM protein in the inner ear, and mutations in the cochlin gene (*Coch*) are pathogenic for the sensorineurial deafness and vestibular disorder, DFNA9. Although its function in the ear is still unknown, cochlin aggregates may alter ECM function or turnover in the TM. Cochlin possesses two von Willebrand factor A (vWFA)-like domains, and as cochlin accumulates, these domains may interfere with similar vWFA-like domains that are abundant in ECM proteins present in the TM. Interestingly, both DBA/2J mice and human POAG patients show a concomitant decrease in type II collagen in parallel with cochlin accumulation. Currently, a cochlin knockout allele is being crossed to DBA/2J, and this mouse model should help determine if cochlin has a role in the IOP elevation of these mice; it may shed light on a possible role in human POAG as well (Bhattacharya et al., 2005a).

Glaucoma and neurodegeneration

The mechanisms leading to RGC death in glaucoma in response to an IOP insult are not clearly understood. Proposed theories include ischemia, excitotoxicity, autoimmunity, axonal injury, and glial activation (figure 39.2) (see Libby et al., 2005b). A combination of these insults may be active in any one patient. The relative significance of each insult likely varies between patients depending on the kinetics and magnitude of IOP elevation, the individual constellation of risk factors in the optic nerve and retina, and the effects of environment and lifestyle.

In this section we describe how the DBA/2J model is being used to understand the mechanisms involved in glaucomatous optic neuropathy. DBA/2J glaucoma shows hallmarks of human glaucoma, including age-related variable progression of optic nerve atrophy in response to elevated IOP, asynchrony, and optic nerve excavation. (A second substrain of DBA/2, DBA/2NNia, has also been used, and in terms of glaucoma progression is considered essentially the same as DBA/2J.)

Regional Patterns of Retinal Ganglion Cell Death A diagnostic feature of human glaucoma is the occurrence of focal visual defects due to region-specific loss or impairment of RGCs. The most reliable of these are arcuate defects or scotomas measured on visual field tests (Shields, 1997). The arcuate nerve fibers originate in the temporal region of the retina and arch above or below the fovea to the optic nerve head. The molecular mechanisms inducing these defects are not well defined. In the mouse, the RGC axons do not curve across the retinal surface but radiate straight toward the optic nerve. For this reason, equivalent regional damage occurs in mice. In DBA/2 retinas with glaucoma, RGCs and their axons are lost in fan-shaped or patchy regions (figure 39.3) (Danias et al., 2003b; Jakobs et al., 2005; Schlamp et al., 2006). These fan-shaped regions of axon loss are likely to be analogous to the arcuate scotomas seen in human glaucoma.

Understanding regional patterns of retinal ganglion cell death

The link between a generalized insult, high IOP, and specific, regional deficits of RGCs in many patients is unclear. The lamina cribrosa (LC) has long been considered an important site of early damage in glaucoma (Quigley et al., 1983). In primates and humans, the LC consists of fenestrated plates of ECM covered with astrocytes. The LC is located in the optic nerve and the RGC axons pass through

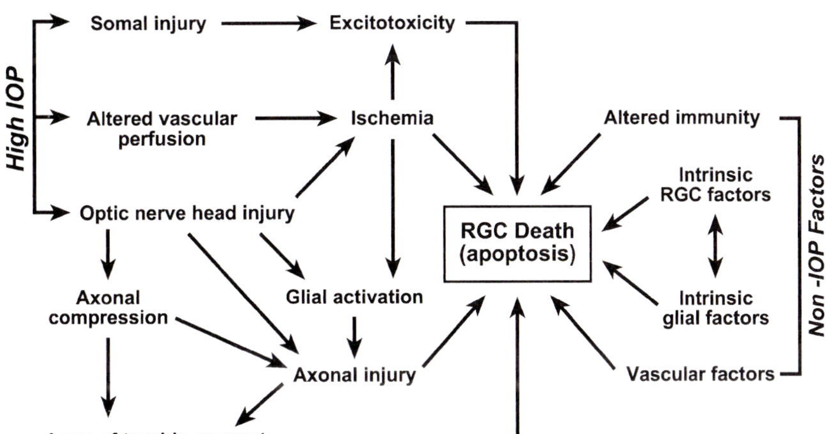

Figure 39.2 Diverse insults may contribute to retinal ganglion cell (RGC) death in glaucoma. A number of commonly proposed damaging factors are shown. An array of these factors may conspire to cause glaucoma in an individual, and genetic differences will determine susceptibility or resistance to each damaging mechanism. The relative importance of specific damaging processes may differ between patients. (Reproduced from Libby et al., 2005b. Reprinted with permission from the *Annual Review of Genomics and Human Genetics*, vol. 6, copyright © 2005 by Annual Reviews, www.annualreviews.org.)

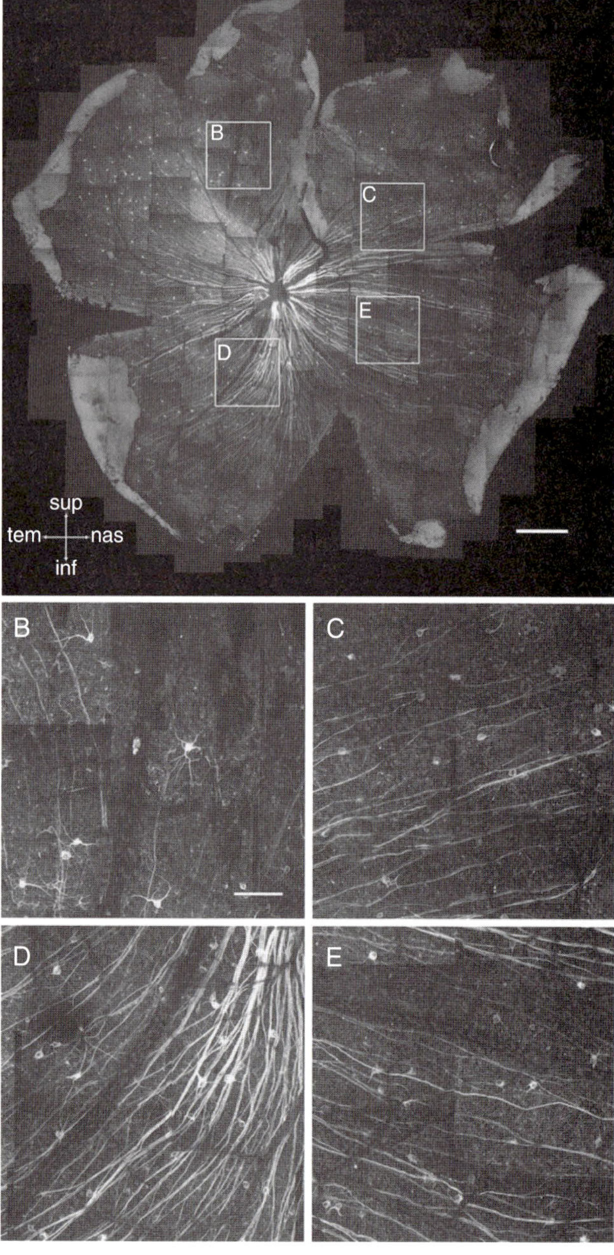

FIGURE 39.3 Whole-mounted glaucomatous retina showing fan-shaped patterns of RGC loss and survival. *A*, High-resolution survey of a whole-mounted retina from a moderately affected eye stained for axons (green, Smi32) and amacrine cells (red, ChAT) and nuclei counterstained with TOPRO (blue). The axon bundles entering the optic nerve head are markedly reduced and show sectors of relatively high axon densities alternating with sectors with almost no persisting axons. Scale bar = 500 μm. *B–E*, High-power views of the boxed areas outlined in *A*. Scale bar = 100 μm. See color plate 33. (Reproduced from Jakobs et al., 2005 [*Journal of Cell Biology*, 2005, 171:313–325. Copyright © 2005, Rockefeller University Press].)

the spaces in the plates as they exit the eye. Mechanical distortion of the ECM plates of the lamina by high IOP is suggested to locally damage RGC axons in glaucoma (Quigley et al., 1983). Local damage of axon bundles would explain the regional patterns of RGC dysfunction and loss.

Although an attractive hypothesis, mechanical injury of axons by the ECM plates of the lamina is not proved. Evidence supporting this mechanical hypothesis includes reports of the first identified site of RGC damage as the axon segment in the LC (shown in both human glaucoma and primate models) (Quigley, 1995). However, identifying the first part of a neuron to degenerate does not necessarily implicate that region as the site of primary insult to the neuron. A primary insult to one region of a neuron may result in degeneration of a secondary region, especially if the secondary region has greater metabolic needs or has greater sensitivity to damage. Additionally, it is debatable whether the sometimes small pressure increases in some glaucoma patients are sufficient to cause mechanical distortion of the LC; furthermore, high IOP is not detected in all glaucoma patients. Since mice develop glaucoma but are suggested to lack a lamina with robust ECM plates (May and Lutjen-Drecoll, 2002), further studies evaluating the role of the LC are needed. Evidence is growing to suggest that mice do not have an ECM-based LC but instead have a cellular lamina (John, 2005) formed by astrocytes (May and Lutjen-Drecoll, 2002; Petros et al., 2006; Schlamp et al., 2006). Nevertheless, some mouse studies suggest that the RGC axons are damaged early, prior to the death of RGCs (Jakobs et al., 2005; Schlamp et al., 2006; May and Mittag, 2006).

Evidence from experiments with DBA/2 supports the theory that the optic nerve is a site of early damage in glaucoma. Semithin sections through the optic nerve head region of DBA/2NNia mice with mild glaucoma revealed focal degeneration around the entrance of the central retinal artery into the eye at the optic nerve head, close to the retinal side of the cellular lamina. It was concluded that axons in this region may be preferentially at risk from early axon damage in glaucoma (May and Mittag, 2006). In contrast, a second study using DBA/2J mice showed that degeneration was first observed in axons proximal (with respect to the brain) to the cellular lamina and continued in a retrograde direction toward the cell body (Schlamp et al., 2006). More experiments are needed to resolve these differences and to establish the role specific components of the lamina may have in glaucoma.

Retinal ganglion cell soma death and axon degeneration

Although the distinctions are not always clear-cut, neurons can degenerate through different processes, including apoptosis, necrosis, and autophagy. It is also clear that within a single neuron, degeneration can occur by different mechanisms in separate compartments (e.g., soma and axon) (see John, 2005). RGCs die by apoptosis in experimentally induced and inherited models of glaucoma (Huang et al., 2005; Reichstein et al., 2007). Huang et al. showed that calcineurin, a Ca^{2+} calmodulin-dependent protein phosphatase, participates in the molecular events leading to apoptosis of RGCs after experimentally induced IOP elevation (Huang et al., 2005). Of note, genetically ablating the function of BAX, a proapoptotic molecule, in DBA/2J mice prevents the death of essentially all RGC somata (figure 39.4) (Libby et al., 2005c). The axons in these mice still degenerate but at a slower rate than axons in DBA/2J mice that retain BAX function. This study uncoupled RGC soma death (completely BAX dependent) from axon degeneration (occurs without BAX). Interestingly, survival of RGC soma was seen in DBA/2J mice with only one functioning copy of *Bax* (D2. *Bax*$^{+/-}$). This heterozygous deficiency mimics the quantitative variation of BAX levels that are known to occur in the human population (see Libby et al., 2005c). Thus, these data suggest that BAX is a reasonable candidate gene to assess as a modulator of susceptibility of RGC death in human glaucoma.

Future prospects for new glaucoma therapies

Now that mouse studies have uncovered mechanisms involved in the pathogenesis of glaucoma, an important goal is to apply this knowledge to the development of new therapies to treat glaucoma in humans. Most available treatments endeavor to reduce IOP levels. However, glaucoma can occur without an elevated IOP, and symptoms may become evident only after RGC death is well under way. New treatments need to be developed that directly target RGC death and optic nerve degeneration.

Neuroprotection Many groups are now using inherited and induced models to study neuroprotection relevant to glaucoma. Over the next several years, we anticipate many important advances. Because of disease complexity, it is important to use large numbers of mice when using the inherited models (see Libby et al., 2005b). Here we highlight two of our studies in DBA/2J mice that had a large effect on disease outcome.

The protective effect of BAX deficiency in DBA/2J mice raises the possibility that BAX inhibitors may have a similar protective effect in humans. One can imagine that such treatments might block or delay RGC soma death until regenerative treatments can be developed to regrow axons. Alternatively, combination therapies may be developed involving both BAX inhibitors and drugs that target axon degeneration. These ideas can be tested first in mice.

A radiation-based neuroprotective treatment has been discovered that completely prevents glaucomatous damage in DBA/2J mice. This treatment, discovered serendipitously, entails administering a dose of lethal radiation to mice in combination with a syngeneic bone marrow transplant (figure 39.5) (Anderson et al., 2005). The treatment is administered to young mice and remains protective until old age. This protection appears to exist in humans as well, since the incidence of glaucoma is lower in populations exposed to

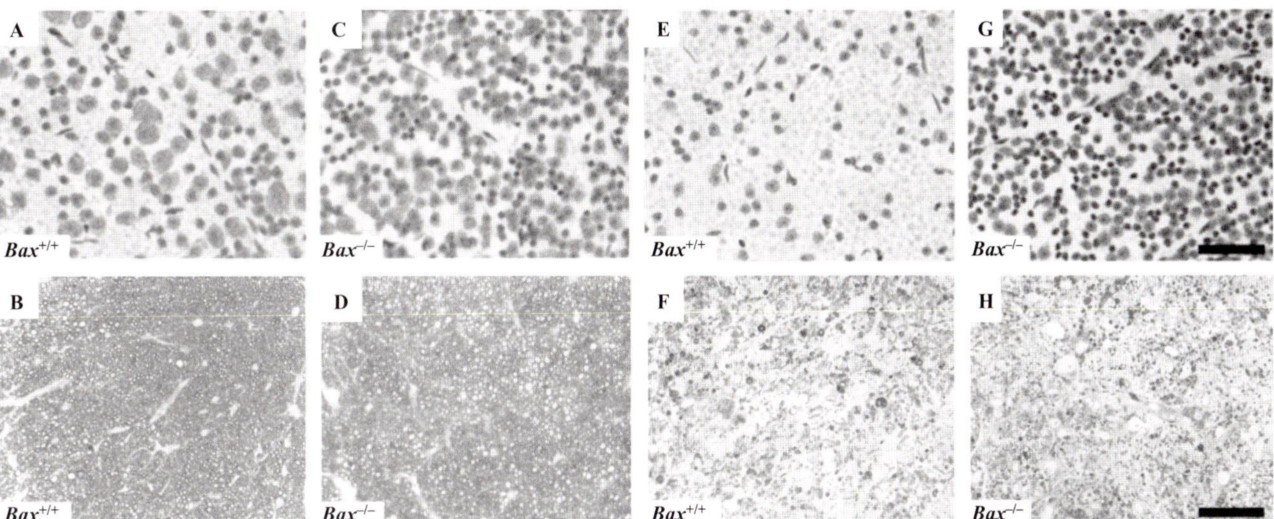

Figure 39.4 *Bax* deficiency prevents glaucomatous RGC death but is not required for optic nerve degeneration. RGC layers (*A*, *C*, *E*, and *G*) and optic nerves (*B*, *D*, *F*, and *H*) were analyzed in *Bax*-sufficient and *Bax*-deficient DBA/2J mice (genotype indicated). Mice were analyzed at preglaucomatous (*A–D*) and severe glaucomatous (*E–H*) stages. *Bax*-deficient DBA/2J mice had severe optic nerve damage but no RGC death. See color plate 34. (Modified from Libby et al., 2005c.)

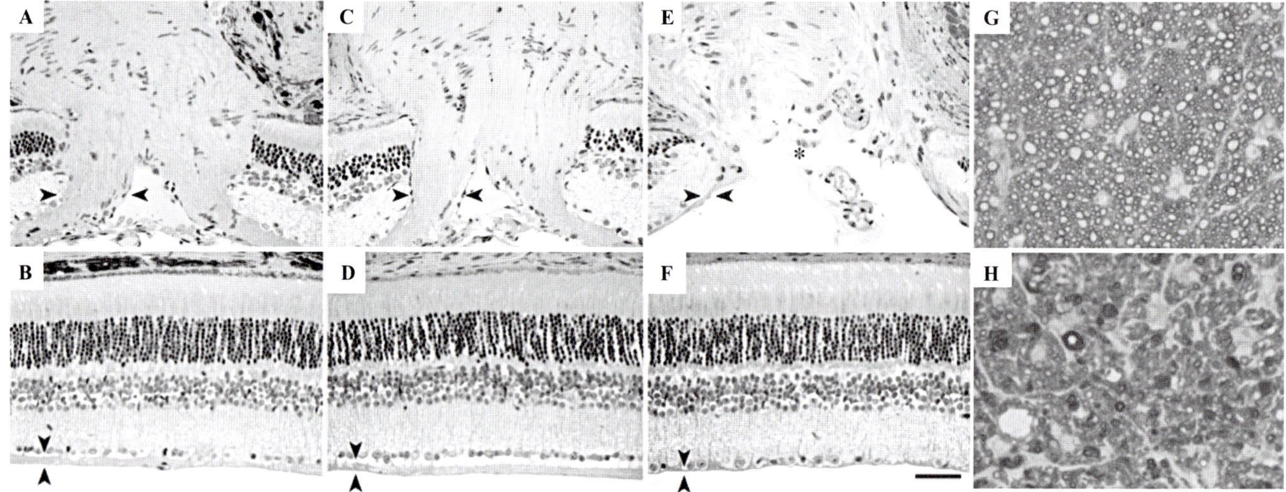

FIGURE 39.5 Radiation treatment prevents glaucomatous optic nerve excavation. *A–F*, Hematoxylin-eosin-stained sections of untreated and treated DBA/2J mouse eyes (*A* and *B*). Optic nerve head (ONH) (*A*) and retina (*B*) from nonglaucomatous DBA/2J mice showing large numbers of axons as evidenced by a thick nerve fiber layer (NFL) (*arrowheads*). ONH (*C*) and retina (*D*) of a treated DBA/2J mouse (14 months old) is indistinguishable from nonglaucomatous controls. *E* and *F*, In contrast, untreated DBA/2J mice show severe excavation of ONH (*) and no NFL. Cross sections of the optic nerve from treated (*G*) and untreated (*H*) DBA/2J mice stained with PPD, a stain that labels myelin sheath and sick or dying axons. The severe axon loss and scarring in the untreated eye are absent in the treated eye. The vast majority (>96%) of eyes from radiation-treated DBA/2J mice were completely rescued from glaucoma. See color plate 35. (Modified from Anderson et al., 2005. Reproduced from *Proceedings of the National Academy of Sciences of the USA*, 2005, 102:4566–4571. Copyright © 2005 National Academy of Sciences.)

radiation (such as atomic bomb survivors; Anderson et al., 2005). At this time, the mechanisms of neuroprotection are not known, and in its current form the treatment is not directly transferable to humans. Further studies designed, to elucidate the processes involved in radiation-induced neuroprotection have great potential for the development of powerful neuroprotective human therapies.

GENOMICS AND PROTEOMICS To improve our understanding of glaucoma and develop novel therapies, it is essential that the genes, proteins, and pathways involved in IOP elevation and glaucomatous optic nerve degeneration be identified. The human and mouse genome sequences are now available, and in functionally conserved units, such as protein-coding genes, they are more than 90% similar at the sequence level (Lander et al., 2001; Waterston et al., 2002). The majority of human genes have a mouse counterpart, and therefore the identification of genes that play a role in glaucoma in mice may provide important insight into mechanisms involved in human glaucoma.

Microarray-based technologies enable glaucoma-relevant tissues to be probed for genes that change in response to IOP elevation and those involved in RGC death and axon degeneration. In the first study of its kind in DBA/2J mice, microarray data have provided insight into pathways likely to be activated downstream of IOP elevation. RNA isolated from retinas from 8-month-old DBA/2J mice that had received a pressure insult was compared with RNA from 3-month-old control retinas. Sixty-eight genes showed differences in their expression, including genes involved in glial activation (e.g., ceruloplasmin and glial fibrillary acidic protein) and immune responses (e.g., lipocalin) (Steele et al., 2006). These findings are in general agreement with experiments carried out in the rat, but further work is needed to determine whether these are primary causes or a consequence of an earlier glaucomatous insult.

As a complement to microarray-based approaches, proteomic analyses are uncovering proteins and pathways involved in glaucoma. Peptidyl arginine deiminase (PAD2), an enzyme that converts protein arginine to citrulline, was found only in samples taken from human POAG patients, and not in samples from unaffected individuals (Bhattacharya et al., 2006). This difference suggests a role for citrullination and structural disruption of myelination in glaucoma and can be interrogated further using mouse models.

Mutagenesis and new models

Glaucoma in humans is a complex multifactorial disease. DBA/2J is currently the most utilized mouse model of glaucoma and has many of the hallmarks of human glaucoma, including a multifactorial and complex etiology. Nevertheless, because glaucoma is a manifestation of a heterogeneous group of complex processes, it is important to develop alternative models of other forms of inherited glaucoma and on strains with distinct genetic backgrounds. POAG is the most common form of glaucoma, and models with altered genes shown to cause POAG in humans have been made (e.g., MYOC, discussed earlier). However, no convincing mouse model of POAG, with IOP elevation and optic nerve excavation, has been reported. An important strategy for producing such models involves the random mutagenesis of the mouse genome. Since the genes underlying these new models can be identified, this approach simultaneously provides valuable resources for identifying new causative pathways of IOP elevation. Commonly, the genomes of founder males are mutagenized with chemical agents such as ethyl nitrosourea, and breeding and screening strategies are developed to uncover phenotypes of interest (Thaung et al., 2002). This type of strategy has proved successful in other complex diseases and is crucial for full exploitation of the strengths of the mouse system to understand the diverse causes of glaucoma.

Conclusion

The genetic networks that determine glaucoma susceptibility are still largely undefined. Many components remain to be identified, and the ways in which known genes interact with other genes are not well characterized. Genetic studies in the mouse have yielded fundamental insights into glaucoma. Aggressive use of model systems and new advances in genomics, proteomics, and genetic analysis will make mouse models even more valuable. Mouse studies are an important complement to those in humans and other species. Only by integrating information from diverse sources will we gain an in-depth understanding of the pathogenesis of glaucoma and begin to develop improved glaucoma therapies.

REFERENCES

Ahmed, E., Ma, J., Rigas, I., Hafezi-Moghadam, N., Iliaki, E., Gragoudas, E. S., Miller, J. W., and Adamis, A. P. (2003). Non-invasive tonometry in the mouse. *Invest. Opthalmol. Vis. Sci.* 44:3336.

Aihara, M., Lindsey, J. D., and Weinreb, R. N. (2003a). Experimental mouse ocular hypertension: Establishment of the model. *Invest. Ophthalmol. Vis. Sci.* 44(10):4314–4320.

Aihara, M., Lindsey, J. D., and Weinreb, R. N. (2003b). Ocular hypertension in mice with a targeted type I collagen mutation. *Invest. Ophthalmol. Vis. Sci.* 44(4):1581–1585.

Anderson, M. G., Libby, R. T., Gould, D. B., Smith, R. S., and John, S. W. (2005). High-dose radiation with bone marrow transfer prevents neurodegeneration in an inherited glaucoma. *Proc. Nat. Acad. Sci. U.S.A.* 102(12):4566–4571.

Anderson, M. G., Libby, R. T., Mao, M., Cosma, I. M., Wilson, L. A., Smith, R. S., and John, S. W. (2006). Genetic context determines susceptibility to intraocular pressure elevation in a mouse pigmentary glaucoma. *BMC Biol.* 4:20.

Anderson, M. G., Smith, R. S., Hawes, N. L., Zabaleta, A., Chang, B., Wiggs, J. L., and John, S. W. (2002). Mutations in genes encoding melanosomal proteins cause pigmentary glaucoma in DBA/2J mice. *Nat. Gen.* 30(1):81–85.

Avila, M. Y., Carre, D. A., Stone, R. A., and Civan, M. M. (2001). Reliable measurement of mouse intraocular pressure by a servo-null micropipette system. *Invest. Ophthalmol. Vis. Sci.* 42 (8):1841–1846.

Bhattacharya, S. K., Crabb, J. S., Bonilha, V. L., Gu, X., Takahara, H., and Crabb, J. W. (2006). Proteomics implicates peptidyl arginine deiminase 2 and optic nerve citrullination in glaucoma pathogenesis. *Invest. Ophthalmol. Vis. Sci.* 47(6):2508–2514.

Bhattacharya, S. K., Peachey, N. S., and Crabb, J. W. (2005a). Cochlin and glaucoma: A mini-review. *Vis. Neurosci.* 22(5):605–613.

Bhattacharya, S. K., Rockwood, E. J., Smith, S. D., Bonilha, V. L., Crabb, J. S., Kuchtey, R. W., Robertson, N. G., Peachey, N. S., Morton, C. C., et al. (2005b). Proteomics reveal cochlin deposits associated with glaucomatous trabecular meshwork. *J. Biol. Chem.* 280(7):6080–6084.

Chang, B., Smith, R. S., Hawes, N. L., Anderson, M. G., Zabaleta, A., Savinova, O., Roderick, T. H., Heckenlively, J. R., Davisson, M. T., et al. (1999). Interacting loci cause severe iris atrophy and glaucoma in DBA/2J mice. *Nat. Genet.* 21(4): 405–409.

Dalke, C., Pleyer, U., and Graw, J. (2005). On the use of Tono-Pen XL for the measurement of intraocular pressure in mice. *Exp. Eye Res.* 80(2):295–296.

Danias, J., Kontiola, A. I., Filippopoulos, T., and Mittag, T. (2003a). Method for the noninvasive measurement of intraocular pressure in mice. *Invest. Ophthalmol. Vis. Sci.* 44(3):1138–1141.

Danias, J., Lee, K. C., Zamora, M. F., Chen, B., Shen, F., Filippopoulos, T., Su, Y., Goldblum, D., Podos, S. M., et al. (2003b). Quantitative analysis of retinal ganglion cell (RGC) loss in aging DBA/2NNia glaucomatous mice: Comparison with RGC loss in aging C57/BL6 mice. *Invest. Ophthalmol. Vis. Sci.* 44(12):5151–5162.

Filippopoulos, T., Matsubara, A., Danias, J., Huang, W., Dobberfuhl, A., Ren, L., Mittag, T., Miller, J. W., and Grosskreutz, C. L. (2006). Predictability and limitations of non-invasive murine tonometry: Comparison of two devices. *Exp. Eye Res.* 83(1):194–201.

Goldblum, D., and Mittag, T. (2002). Prospects for relevant glaucoma models with retinal ganglion cell damage in the rodent eye. *Vision Res.* 42(4):471–478.

Gould, D. B., and John, S. W. (2002). Anterior segment dysgenesis and the developmental glaucomas are complex traits. *Hum. Mol. Genet.* 11(10):1185–1193.

Gould, D. B., Miceli-Libby, L., Savinova, O. V., Torrado, M., Tomarev, S. I., Smith, R. S., and John, S. W. (2004). Genetically increasing Myoc expression supports a necessary pathologic role of abnormal proteins in glaucoma. *Mol. Cell. Biol.* 24(20): 9019–9025.

Gould, D. B., Reedy, M., Wilson, L. A., Smith, R. S., Johnson, R. L., and John, S. W. (2006). Mutant myocilin nonsecretion in vivo is not sufficient to cause glaucoma. *Mol. Cell. Biol.* 26(22):8427–8436.

Gould, D. B., Smith, R. S., and John, S. W. (2004). Anterior segment development relevant to glaucoma. *Int. J. Dev. Biol.* 48(8–9):1015–1029.

Gross, R. L., Ji, J., Chang, P., Pennesi, M. E., Yang, Z., Zhang, J., and Wu, S. M. (2003). A mouse model of elevated intraocular pressure: Retina and optic nerve findings. *Trans. Am. Ophthalmol. Soc.* 101:163–169 [discussion 169–171].

Grozdanic, S. D., Betts, D. M., Sakaguchi, D. S., Allbaugh, R. A., Kwon, Y. H., and Kardon, R. H. (2003) Laser-induced mouse model of chronic ocular hypertension. *Invest. Ophthalmol. Vis. Sci.* 44(10):4337–4346.

Huang, W., Fileta, J. B., Dobberfuhl, A., Filippopolous, T., Guo, Y., Kwon, G., and Grosskreutz, C. L. (2005). Calcineurin cleavage is triggered by elevated intraocular pressure, and calcineurin inhibition blocks retinal ganglion cell death in experimental glaucoma. *Proc. Nat. Acad. Sci. U.S.A.* 102(34):12242–12247.

Jakobs, T. C., Libby, R. T., Ben, Y., John, S. W., and Masland, R. H. (2005). Retinal ganglion cell degeneration is topological but not cell type specific in DBA/2J mice. *J. Cell. Biol.* 171 (2):313–325.

John, S. W. (2005). Mechanistic insights into glaucoma provided by experimental genetics. The Cogan Lecture. *Invest. Ophthalmol. Vis. Sci.* 46(8):2650–2661.

John, S. W., Anderson, M. G., and Smith, R. S. (1999). Mouse genetics: A tool to help unlock the mechanisms of glaucoma. *J. Glaucoma* 8(6):400–412.

John, S. W., Hagaman, J. R., MacTaggart, T. E., Peng, L., and Smithes, O. (1997). Intraocular pressure in inbred mouse strains. *Invest. Ophthalmol. Vis. Sci.* 38(1):249–253.

John, S. W., Smith, R. S., Savinova, O. V., Hawes, N. L., Chang, B., Turnbull, D., Davisson, M., Roderick, T. H., and Heckenlively, J. R. (1998). Essential iris atrophy, pigment dispersion, and glaucoma in DBA/2J mice. *Invest. Ophthalmol. Vis. Sci.* 39(6):951–962.

Kanagavalli, J., Pandaranayaka, E., Krishnadas, S. R., Krishnaswamy, S., and Sundaresan, P. (2004). A review of genetic and structural understanding of the role of myocilin in primary open angle glaucoma. *Ind. J. Ophthalmol.* 52(4):271–280.

Kim, B. S., Savinova, O. V., Reedy, M. V., Martin, J., Lun, Y., Gan, L., Smith, R. S., Tomarev, S. I., John, S. W., et al. (2001). Targeted disruption of the myocilin gene (Myoc) suggests that human glaucoma-causing mutations are gain of function. *Mol. Cell. Biol.* 21(22):7707–7713.

Kroeber, M., Ohlmann, A., Russell, P., and Tamm, E. R. (2006). Transgenic studies on the role of optineurin in the mouse eye. *Exp. Eye Res.* 82(6):1075–1085.

Lander, E. S., Linton, L. M., Birren, B., Nusbaum, C., Zody, M. C., Baldwin, J., Devon, K., Dewar, K., Doyle, M., et al. (2001). Initial sequencing and analysis of the human genome. *Nature* 409(6822):860–921.

Leske, M. C. (1983). The epidemiology of open-angle glaucoma: A review. *Am. J. Epidemiol.* 118(2):166–191.

Libby, R. T., Anderson, M. G., Pang, I. H., Robinson, Z. H., Savinova, O. V., Cosma, I. M., Snow, A., Wilson, L. A., Smith, R. S., et al. (2005a). Inherited glaucoma in DBA/2J mice: Pertinent disease features for studying the neurodegeneration. *Vis. Neurosci.* 22(5):637–648.

Libby, R. T., Gould, D. B., Anderson, M. G., and John, S. W. (2005b). Complex genetics of glaucoma susceptibility. *Annu. Rev. Genom. Hum. Genet.* 6:15–44.

Libby, R. T., Li, Y., Savinova, O. V., Barter, J., Smith, R. S., Nickells, R. W., and John, S. W. (2005c). Susceptibility to neurodegeneration in a glaucoma is modified by Bax gene dosage. *PLoS Genet.* 1(1):17–26.

Libby, R. T., Smith, R. S., Savinova, O. V., Zabaleta, A., Martin, J. E., Gonzalez, F. J., and John, S. W. (2003). Modification of ocular defects in mouse developmental glaucoma models by tyrosinase. *Science* 299(5612):1578–1581.

Lindsey, J. D., and Weinreb, R. N. (2002). Identification of the mouse uveoscleral outflow pathway using fluorescent dextran. *Invest. Ophthalmol. Vis. Sci.* 43(7):2201–2205.

Lindsey, J. D., and Weinreb, R. N. (2005). Elevated intraocular pressure and transgenic applications in the mouse. *J. Glaucoma* 14(4):318–320.

Liu, Y., and Vollrath, D. (2004). Reversal of mutant myocilin non-secretion and cell killing: Implications for glaucoma. *Hum. Mol. Gene.* 13(11):1193–1204.

Mabuchi, F., Aihara, M., Mackey, M. R., Lindsey, J. D., and Weinreb, R. N. (2004). Regional optic nerve damage in experimental mouse glaucoma. *Invest. Ophthalmol. Vis. Sci.* 45(12): 4352–4358.

May, C. A., and Lutjen-Drecoll, E. (2002). Morphology of the murine optic nerve. *Invest. Ophthalmol. Vis. Sci.* 43(7):2206–2212.

May, C. A., and Mittag, T. (2006). Optic nerve degeneration in the DBA/2NNia mouse: Is the lamina cribrosa important in the development of glaucomatous optic neuropathy? *Acta Neuropathol.* 111(2):158–167.

McKinnon, S. J., Reitsamer, H. A., Ransom, N. L., Caldwell, M., Harrison, J. M., and Kiel, J. W. (2003). Induction and TonoPen measurement of ocular hypertension in C57BL/6 Mice. ARVO Abstract.

McMenamin, P. G. (1999). Dendritic cells and macrophages in the uveal tract of the normal mouse eye. *Br. J. Ophthalmol.* 83(5): 598–604.

McMenamin, P. G., and Holthouse, I. (1992). Immunohistochemical characterization of dendritic cells and macrophages in the aqueous outflow pathways of the rat eye. *Exp. Eye Res.* 55 (2):315–324.

Mo, J. S., Anderson, M. G., Gregory, M., Smith, R. S., Savinova, O. V., Serreze, D. V., Ksander, B. R., Streilein, J. W., and John, S. W. (2003). By altering ocular immune privilege, bone marrow-derived cells pathogenically contribute to DBA/2J pigmentary glaucoma. *J. Exp. Med.* 197(10):1335–1344.

Morris, C. A., Crowston, J. G., Lindsey, J. D., Danias, J., and Weinreb, R. N. (2006). Comparison of invasive and non-invasive tonometry in the mouse. *Exp. Eye Res.* 82(6):1094–1099.

Morrison, J. C., Moore, C. G., Deppmeier, L. M., Gold, B. G., Meshul, C. K., and Johnson, E. C. (1997). A rat model of chronic pressure-induced optic nerve damage. *Exp. Eye Res.* 64(1):85–96.

Pease, M. E., Hammond, J. C., and Quigley, H. A. (2006). Manometric calibration and comparison of TonoLab and TonoPen tonometers in rats with experimental glaucoma and in normal mice. *J. Glaucoma* 15(6):512–519.

Petros, T. J., Williams, S. E., and Mason, C. A. (2006). Temporal regulation of EphA4 in astroglia during murine retinal and optic nerve development. *Mol. Cell. Neurosci.* 32(1–2):49–66.

Quigley, H. A. (1995). Ganglion cell death in glaucoma: Pathology recapitulates ontogeny. *Aust. N.Z. J. Ophthalmol.* 23(2):85–91.

Quigley, H. A. (1996). Number of people with glaucoma worldwide. *Br. J. Ophthalmol.* 80(5):389–393.

Quigley, H. A., Hohman, R. M., Addicks, E. M., Massof, R. W., and Green, W. R. (1983). Morphologic changes in the lamina cribrosa correlated with neural loss in open-angle glaucoma. *Am. J. Ophthalmol.* 95(5):673–691.

Reichstein, D., Ren, L., Filippopoulos, T., Mittag, T., and Danias, J. (2007). Apoptotic retinal ganglion cell death in the DBA/2 mouse model of glaucoma. *Exp. Eye Res.* 84(1): 13–21.

Reitsamer, H. A., Kiel, J. W., Harrison, J. M., Ransom, N. L., and McKinnon, S. J. (2004). TonoPen measurement of intraocular pressure in mice. *Exp. Eye Res.* 78(4):799–804.

Rezaie, T., Child, A., Hitchings, R., Brice, G., Miller, L., Coca-Prados, M., Heon, E., Krupin, T., Ritch, R., et al. (2002). Adult-onset primary open-angle glaucoma caused by mutations in optineurin. *Science* 295(5557):1077–1079.

Ritch, R., Shields, M. B., and Krupin, T. (1996). *The glaucomas: Clinical science*, 2nd ed. St Louis: Mosby–Year Book.

Savinova, O. V., Sugiyama, F., Martin, J. E., Tomarev, S. I., Paigen, B. J., Smith, R. S., and John, S. W. (2001). Intraocular pressure in genetically distinct mice: An update and strain survey. *BMC Genet.* 2:12.

Schlamp, C. L., Li, Y., Dietz, J. A., Janssen, K. T., and Nickells, R. W. (2006). Progressive ganglion cell loss and optic nerve degeneration in DBA/2J mice is variable and asymmetric. *BMC Neurosci.* 7:66.

Scott, T. S., and Wirtz, M. K. (1996). Biochemistry of aqueous outflow. In R. Ritch, M. B. Shields, and T. Krupin (Eds.), *The glaucomas*, 2nd ed. (vol. 1, pp. 281–305). St Louis: Mosby.

Senatorov, V., Malyukova, I., Fariss, R., Wawrousek, E. F., Swaminathan, S., Sharan, S. K., and Tomarev, S. (2006). Expression of mutated mouse myocilin induces open-angle glaucoma in transgenic mice. *J. Neurosci.* 26(46):11903–11914.

Shields, M. B. (1997). *Shields' textbook of glaucoma*, 4th ed. Baltimore: Williams and Wilkins.

Steele, M. R., Inman, D. M., Calkins, D. J., Horner, P. J., and Vetter, M. L. (2006). Microarray analysis of retinal gene expression in the DBA/2J model of glaucoma. *Invest. Ophthalmol. Vis. Sci.* 47(3):977–985.

Strom, R. C., and Williams, R. W. (1998). Cell production and cell death in the generation of variation in neuron number. *J. Neurosci.* 18(23):9948–9953.

Thaung, C., West, K., Clark, B. J., McKie, L., Morgan, J. E., Arnold, K., Nolan, P. M., Peters, J., Hunter, A. J., et al. (2002). Novel ENU-induced eye mutations in the mouse: Models for human eye disease. *Hum. Mol. Genet.* 11(7):755–767.

Vincent, A. L., Billingsley, G., Buys, Y., Levin, A. V., Priston, M., Trope, G., Williams-Lyn, D., and Heon, E. (2002). Digenic inheritance of early-onset glaucoma: CYP1B1, a potential modifier gene. *Am. J. Hum. Genet.* 70(2):448–460.

Wang, W. H., Millar, J. C., Pang, I. H., Wax, M. B., and Clark, A. F. (2005). Noninvasive measurement of rodent intraocular pressure with a rebound tonometer. *Invest. Ophthalmol. Vis. Sci.* 46(12):4617–4621.

Waterston, R. H., Lindblad-Toh, K., Birney, E., Rogers, J., Abril, J. F., Agarwal, P., Agarwala, R., Ainscough, R., Alexandersson, M., et al. (2002). Initial sequencing and comparative analysis of the mouse genome. *Nature* 420(6915): 520–562.

Weinreb, R. N., and Lindsey, J. D. (2005). The importance of models in glaucoma research. *J. Glaucoma* 14(4):302–304.

Willoughby, C. E., Chan, L. L., Herd, S., Billingsley, G., Noordeh, N., Levin, A. V., Buys, Y., Trope, G., Sarfarazi, M., et al. (2004). Defining the pathogenicity of optineurin in juvenile open-angle glaucoma. *Invest. Ophthalmol. Vis. Sci.* 45(9): 3122–3130.

Wu, H., Byrne, M. H., Stacey, A., Goldring, M. B., Birkhead, J. R., Jaenisch, R., and Krane, S. M. (1990). Generation of collagenase-resistant collagen by site-directed mutagenesis of murine pro alpha 1(I) collagen gene. *Proc. Nat. Acad. Sci. U.S.A.* 87(15):5888–5892.

Zillig, M., Wurm, A., Grehn, F. J., Russell, P., and Tamm, E. R. (2005). Overexpression and properties of wild-type and Tyr437His mutated myocilin in the eyes of transgenic mice. *Invest. Ophthalmol. Vis. Sci.* 46(1):223–234.

40 Cataract Genetics

JOCHEN GRAW

Cataracts as lens opacities are associated with a group of well-known diseases that are particularly common in the elderly population. In contrast to age-related forms of cataract, congenital cataracts, or cataracts that develop in early childhood, are rather rare and occur in developed countries with a frequency of around 30 cases per 100,000 births, with another 10 cases being diagnosed by the age of 15 years (mainly as dominant forms). Rates are likely to be higher in developing countries because of rubella infections and consanguinity (for the recessive forms; Gibert et al., 2003).

In recent years, mice have proved to be excellent models for ophthalmologists, because the clinical phenotypes are quite similar to human conditions. The first systematic evaluation of large mouse populations for mutations affecting the eye lens at birth was initiated in 1979, when Kratochvilova and Ehling described screening for murine dominant cataract mutants in the F_1 generation after paternal radiation treatment. Systematic screening for eye mutants was extended to the use of ethylnitrosourea (ENU) as a mutagenic agent (Ehling et al., 1985), and to the targeted inactivation of genes. In this chapter, I review mutant mouse strains in which the lens is affected early in embryonic development or later in life, resulting in senile cataracts. Because lens development and the developmental genetics of the eye and retina are treated elsewhere in this book (see chapters 22 and 24), only the most important aspects are discussed here. The large number of transgenic mice strains that overexpress various genes in the lens also are excluded from this chapter's discussion because the ectopic expression of a gene in the lens frequently leads to cataracts. The interested reader is directed to previously published reviews with many original citations (Graw, 2003, 2004). The chromosomal position of genes and their corresponding mutations can be found at the Web site of the Jackson Laboratory (www.informatics.jax.org/; menu, "Genes and Markers").

Mutations at early stages of lens development

Pax6 and *Pitx3* One of the central genes in eye development is the paired-box gene *Pax6*, which was recognized as being affected in the mouse *small eye* (*Sey*) mutants (Hill et al., 1991). *Pax6* maps at mouse chromosome 2; the actual list of the Jackson Laboratory (January 2008) contains 28 alleles in the mouse, of which four are targeted mutations. In the classic *Sey* mutant, the failure in lens development is attributed to a defect in the inductive interaction between the optic vesicle and the overlying ectoderm, since these tissues fail to make discrete contacts. A typical example is shown in figure 40.1*A*. Homozygotes die around the time of birth because of breathing problems.

The expressivity of heterozygous *Pax6* mutations is variable, with mutants expressing a range of phenotypes from small anterior polar cataracts to the more extreme phenotype of anterior polar opacity, corneal adhesions, iris abnormalities, and microphthalmia. The morphological alterations correspond to the expression pattern of *Pax6*. *Pax6* transcripts are first detected in the presumptive fore- and hindbrain of 8-day-old mouse embryos; at E8.5 it is present in the optic sulcus, the lateral evagination at the basis of the forebrain. Later, at E9.5, *Pax6* is expressed in the optic vesicle, the optic stalk, and the surface ectoderm, which will give rise to the lens. Between E10 and E12, *Pax6* is observed in the inner layer of the optic cup, in the lens, and in the surface ectoderm, which at this stage gives rise to the future cornea. In the elongating primary fiber cells, *Pax6* has a posterior localization. At E15.5, *Pax6* is expressed in the two layers of the neural retina, the anterior epithelium of the cornea, and the lens. Besides the eye, *Pax6* occurs in specific regions of the brain, the olfactory epithelium, and the pancreas (for a review, see Graw, 2004). In particular, mouse *Pax6* mutants exhibit changes in neurogenesis, cell proliferation, and patterning in the brain (Haubst et al., 2004; Graw et al., 2005).

The second interesting gene in the context of early lens development is *Pitx3*. In the mouse mutant *aphakia* (*ak*), the promoter of the *Pitx3* gene is affected by two deletions (Semina et al., 2000; Rieger et al., 2001). The phenotype is characterized at early stages of development by a small lens vesicle with a stable contact to the cornea, the lens stalk. In later stages the lens vesicle is degraded, which leads to the formation of a lensless eye, giving this mutant its name. This feature is shown in figure 40.1*B*. Another mutant line, *Cat4*^{a}, shares one aspect with the *aphakia* mutant, the inhibition of the separation of the lens vesicle from the surface ectoderm (Grimes et al., 1998). However, *Cat4*^{a} is mapped to mouse chromosome 8, suggesting that it is different from *Pitx3*.

The phenotype of the mouse mutant correlates well with the expression pattern of the affected gene *Pitx3*. It is strongly expressed in the developing lens vesicle starting at E11, but later also throughout the lens, particularly in the anterior

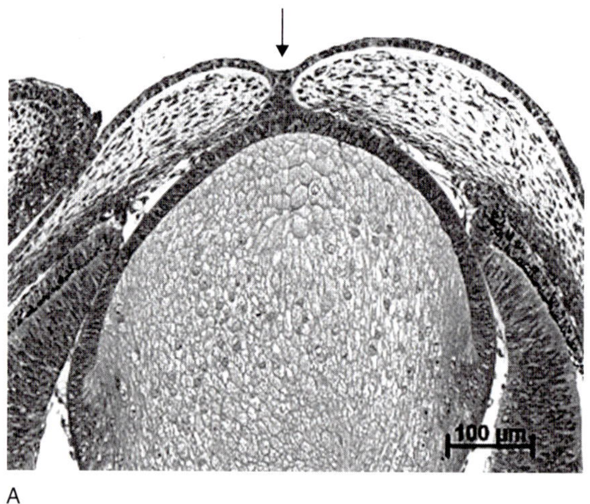

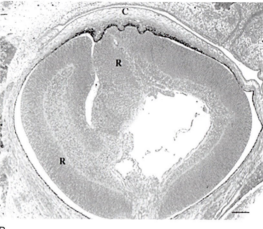

FIGURE 40.1 Mutations in transcription factors and their effect on lens development. *A*, Histological section through a developing eye of a Pax6 mutant (*Pax6*^{Aey11}; E17.5) clearly demonstrates the persisting lens stalk (*arrow*), the connection between the lens and the cornea. *B*, Histological section of the developing eye of the *aphakia* mouse (deletions in the *Pitx3* promoter) shows absence of the lens at E18.5; the eyeball is filled with retinal derivatives. C, cornea; R, retina. See color plate 36. (*A*, From Graw et al., 2005. *B*, From Semina et al., 2000.)

epithelium and equator region. Moreover, there are recent reports that *Pitx3* is also expressed in the dopaminergic neurons of the substantia nigra in the brain. It is not surprising, then, that *aphakia* mice also exhibit a selective loss of these particular neurons (Hwang et al., 2003) and a malformation of the mesencephalic dopamine system (Smidt et al., 2004).

MAF, FOX, AND *SOX* Other genes coding for transcription factors important for eye and lens development include *Maf, Sox1, Sox2, FoxC1,* and *FoxE3.* In particular, *Maf* and *Sox1* act as transcription factors on the promoters of the γ-crystallin-encoding genes (*Cryg*).

The Fox transcription factors are characterized by a 110-amino acid motif originally defined as a DNA-binding domain in the *Drosophila* transcription factor forkhead (Fox: forkhead box). A mutation in *FoxE3* was shown to cause the phenotype in the mouse mutant *dysgenic lens* (*dyl*), first published in 1979. In this mutant, the lens vesicle fails to separate from the ectoderm, causing the lens and the cornea to fuse; the *dyl* phenotype includes loss of lens epithelium; a small, cataractous lens; and malformations of most tissues of the anterior segment (iris, cornea, ciliary body, and trabecular meshwork; Blixt et al., 2006). Moreover, a mutation in the mouse *Foxc1* mutant led to a similar phenotype with additional glaucoma (Hong et al., 1999).

The Maf family of basic region leucine zipper (bZIP) transcription factors was first identified through the *v-maf* oncogene, an avian retrovirus-transforming gene. The targeted deletion of *c-Maf* in the mouse leads to a stop of lens primary fiber cell elongation at the lens vesicle stage (Ring et al., 2000); the same feature was published for a mild pulverulent cataract mutant in mouse (opaque flecks in the lens, *Opj*; Lyon et al., 2003). The point mutation affects the basic region of the DNA-binding domain. In general, Maf binds as homo- or heterodimer to so-called Maf-responsive elements (MAREs). MAREs are found in the promoters of the crystallin-encoding genes; *Maf* itself is upregulated by *Pax6* (Civil et al., 2002).

The Sox family of transcription factors has an HMG domain (high mobility group) in common; the founder of this family is the *Sry* gene (sex-determining region of Y chromosome). The genes *Sox1, Sox2,* and *Sox3* are expressed in the mouse in the CNS and in the sensory placodes. In particular, *Sox2* is expressed during early eye development in the lens placode in the portion of the ectoderm that is in contact with the optic cup and invaginates to form the lens vesicle. This invagination coincides with the onset of *Sox1* expression in the mouse lens placode. At later stages, *Sox2* is downregulated and *Sox1* is upregulated (Kamachi et al., 2000).

A targeted deletion of *Sox1* in mice causes microphthalmia and cataract. Mutant lens fiber cells fail to elongate, probably as a result of an almost complete absence of *Cryg* transcripts (Nishiguchi et al., 1998). The phenotype of the homozygous *Sox1* deletion mutant is very similar to the most severe *Cryg* mutation, *Cryge*^{t}. In contrast to *Sox1*, mutations in the human *SOX2* gene cause anophthalmia (without cataract; Fantes et al., 2003), however, the heterozygous knockout mice of *Sox2* appeared normal, but the homozygous mutants are peri-implantationally lethal (Avilion et al., 2003).

Miscellaneous Several other genes (e.g., *Shh*, *rx/eyeless*, *Lhx*, *Bmp4*, *Bmp7*) are known to be expressed at these early stages; however, the phenotypes of the corresponding knockout or null mutants manifest mainly with anophthalmia (loss of the entire ocular structure) or microphthalmia (small eye), but no cataracts. For a further discussion of these genes, readers may refer to previous reviews and references therein (e.g., Graw, 2003; see also chapter 22, this volume).

After the lens placode stage, the next important step is the formation of the lens vesicle. Its key role is addressed by some mouse mutants, such as *extra toes* ($Gli3^{Xt}$: Franz and Besecke, 1991), *eye lens aplasia* (*elap*: Aso et al., 2001), and some "blebbing" mutants (*bl*, *my*, *eb*, *heb*). All these mouse models have in common a microphthalmic phenotype with major disturbances in most of the ocular tissues. The lens is frequently missing; correspondingly, these mutations are not associated with cataracts. The blebbing mutants are characterized by mutations in genes affecting extracellular matrix proteins (Kiyozumi et al., 2006). For the *Gli3* mutant, an interesting increase in the penetrance of the ocular phenotype (including lens defects) was reported if it was crossed with a $Pax6^{+/-}$ background (Zaki et al., 2006).

Mutations affecting the lens membranes

As discussed earlier, in only a few cases are cataracts formed at the early stages of eye development. However, one might assume that more and diverse phenotypes of cataracts would occur if stages are affected when the lens vesicle is already formed. This section describes mutants that show defects in the lens cell membrane.

Aquaporin/Mip One of the first detected cataract mutations was the *Fraser cataract* (Cat^{Fr}; Fraser and Schabtach, 1962). In this mutant, the cell nuclei in the deep cortex become abnormally pyknotic (beginning at E14); degeneration of cytoplasm and destruction of the lenticular nucleus follow. Cat^{Fr} was shown to be allelic with another mouse mutant, referred to as *lens opacity* (*Lop*). The two alleles, Cat^{Lop} and Cat^{Fr}, were mapped 20 cM distal to *steel* (*Sl*) on chromosome 10. A candidate gene for the *Cat* locus encodes the membrane intrinsic protein (gene symbol: *Mip*), and sequence analysis finally revealed that the Cat^{Fr} mutation is due to a transposon-induced splicing error leading to a truncated form of *Mip* transcripts. The other allele, Cat^{Lop} (G151C), leads to a single amino acid substitution (Ala51Pro), which inhibits targeting of Mip to the cell membrane (Shiels and Bassnett, 1996). In total, seven phenotypic alleles have been reported (MGI database, December 2006); in general, homozygous mutants have microphthalmia and lens opacity. Other defects may include degeneration of lens fiber cells, vacuolization of lens fibers, and a reduced γ- to α-crystallin ratio. Heterozygotes have less severe forms of lens cataract and microphthalmia.

Mip forms specialized junctions between the fiber cells and can be first detected in the primary fiber cells of the early lens vesicle. In situ hybridization demonstrated that *Mip* expression is highest in the elongating fiber cells in the bow region of the lens; Mip antiserum specifically decorates fiber cell membranes, highlighting their regular anterior to posterior organization. Mip is also referred to aquaporin-0; a review on the role of aquaporin water channels in eye function was published a few years ago (Verkman, 2003). Recently, an *Aqp1*-knockout mutation was reported. These mice do not exhibit lens opacification; however, if these mutants are treated first with 3-methylcholantrene and later with acetaminophen, all mice tested develop cataract, indicating a complex interaction of environmental factors (chemical treatment) and genetic constitution (Ruiz-Ederra and Verkman, 2006).

Lim2 The *total opacity* (*To3*) gene mutation is placed on chromosome 7; mice heterozygous or homozygous for the *To3* mutation exhibit a total opacity of the lens with a dense cataract. Additionally, homozygotes exhibit microphthalmia and abnormally small eyes. Histological analysis revealed vacuolization of the lens and gross disorganization of the fibers; posterior lens rupture can be observed only in homozygotes. The *To3* mutation was characterized as a single G→T transversion within the first exon of the *Lim2* gene coding for a lens-specific integral membrane protein, MP19. It was predicted that this DNA change would result in a nonconservative substitution (Gly15Val; Steele et al., 1997). In the mutants, MP19 is not transported to the lens fiber cell membranes but appears to be trapped in a subcellular compartment within the cells (Chen et al., 2002).

Connexins in the Lens Lens fiber cells are coupled by intercellular gap junction channels, particularly by the connexins 46 and 50 (also known as MP70). Since they are referred to as α3 or α8 subunits, their gene symbols are *Gja3* and *Gja8*, respectively. Connexins have four transmembrane domains with three intracellular regions (the N-terminus, a cytoplasmatic loop, and the C-terminus) and two extracellular loops. Six connexin subunits oligomerize to form one hemichannel; the entire channel is formed by the docking of extracellular loops of two opposing hemichannels. The presence of two types of subunits in a cell allows the formation of a broad variety of channels.

Gja3 is mapped to mouse chromosome 14; a knockout mutation of *Gja3* exhibits nuclear cataract, which was associated with the proteolysis of crystallins. Obviously, there is no influence on the early stages of lens formation (Gong et al., 1997). No other mouse *Gja3* mutation has been described to date. A mutation in the human *GJA3* gene results in an amino acid substitution in the first transmembrane region of connexin 46. The mutation was shown to be causative of a congenital nuclear pulverulent cataract (Jiang et al., 2003); however, a few years ago, Rees et al. (2000) and Mackay et al. (1999) showed that mutations in the human *GJA3* gene also led to zonular pulverulent cataracts. The phenotypic differences might be explained by the fact that they affect different parts of the protein (the extracellular and intracellular domain).

In contrast to *Gja3*, actually seven cataract-causing alleles of the *Gja8* gene are reported. *Gja8* maps to mouse chromosome 3 and was demonstrated to be affected by a single A→C transversion within codon 47 of the *No2* (nuclear opacity 2) mouse cataract. The sequence alteration is predicted to result in the nonconserved substitution of Ala for the normally encoded Asp (Steele et al., 1998). A similar phenotype (microphthalmia and nuclear cataract) was observed in *Cx50* null mice (White et al., 1998). Typical examples of isolated lenses from *Gja8* mutant mice are shown in figure 40.2*A*. A recent article on *Gja3* and *Gja8* mutations discusses in detail the role of the corresponding connexins during lens fiber cell formation (Xia et al., 2006b).

Mutations affecting the structural proteins of the lens

Up to 90% of the soluble protein in the postmitotic lens cells consists of proteins, which are referred to as α-, β-, and γ-crystallins (Mörner, 1893). The α-crystallins form high-molecular-weight aggregates formed by both, αA- and αB-crystallins. These large complexes have chaperone activity and belong to the family of the small heat shock proteins. In contrast to αB-crystallin (gene symbol: *Cryab*), which is ubiquitously expressed, the αA-crystallin (gene symbol: *Cryaa*) occurs mainly in the lens. The β/γ-crystallin superfamily exhibits a characteristic protein motif, the so-called Greek key motif, in a quadruple organization. It is considered to be essential for the extremely high protein concentration in the lens (for a review, see Piatigorsky, 2003). Moreover, because of the unique morphology of the lens fiber cells, it is not surprising that certain cytoskeletal proteins are also expressed preferentially in the lens (for a review, see Perng and Quinlan, 2005).

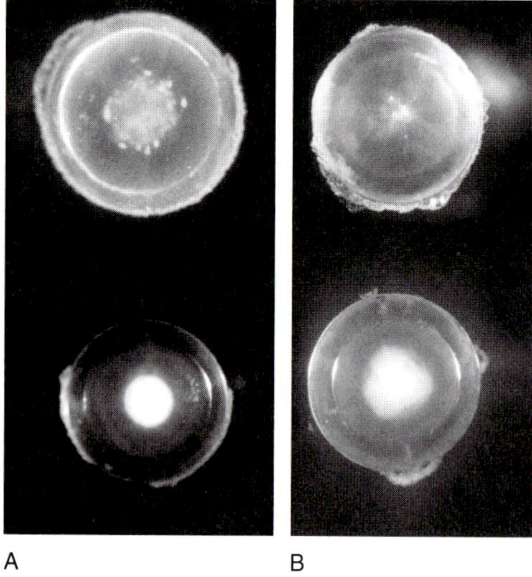

FIGURE 40.2 Mutations in *Gja8* and *Cryaa*. Gross appearance of lenses of the $Gja8^{Aey5}$ mutant mouse (*A*) compared with lenses from a $Cryaa^{Aey7}$ mutant mouse (*B*). The upper row indicates the phenotype for the heterozygotes and the lower row that for the homozygous mutants. In both cases, a gene dose effect can be observed. See color plate 37.

THE α-CRYSTALLINS AND HEAT SHOCK TRANSCRIPTION FACTOR When the *Cryaa* knockout was published (Brady et al., 1997), researchers were surprised that it led to a recessive phenotype and that cataracts became visible only in the homozygous mutants. The opacification starts in the nucleus and progresses to a general opacification with age. Cataract formation ultimately results from insolubility of the αB-crystallin. *Cryaa* is mapped to mouse chromosome 17; cataract-causing mutations are recessive ($Cryaa^{lop18}$: Chang et al., 1999; $Cryaa^{2J}$: Xia et al., 2006b) or dominant ($Cryaa^{Aey7}$: Graw et al., 2001a; $Cryaa^{L1N}$: Xia et al., 2006a); an example of a dominant phenotype is given in figure 40.2*B*. The two recessive mutations both affect the Arg54 residue: in the case of the *lop18* mutation, it is changed to a His, whereas the $Cryaa^{2J}$ allele is translated at codon 54 into a Cys. In contrast, the dominant mutations affect the C-terminal part of the protein (*Aey7*: V124E; *L1N*: Y118D). Similarly, both dominant and recessive *CRYAA* mutations have been reported in humans: the dominant cataract-causing alleles are R21L, R49C, and R116C (Litt et al., 1998; Mackay et al., 2003; Graw et al., 2006), whereas the nonsense mutation W9X leads to a recessive cataract in an inbred Jewish Persian family (Pras et al., 2000).

Cryab knockout mice (missing αB-crystallin) are cataract-free, but they die prematurely because of myopathy and other organ defects (Brady et al., 2001). *Cryab* is mapped to mouse chromosome 9; no other *Cryab* mutation has been reported. In contrast to this finding in the mouse, in humans two different cataract-causing mutations have been described in *CRYAB*, a dominant myopathy associated with cataract (R120G; Vicart et al., 1998) and a deletion mutation in exon 3 of *CRYAB* that resulted in a frameshift in codon 150 and an aberrant protein consisting of 184 residues (Berry et al., 2001).

Since the α-crystallins belong to the family of small heat shock proteins, it might be interesting to note that a null mutation in the mouse *Hsf4* gene (located on chromosome 8 and coding for heat shock transcription factor 4) causes cataract formation with abnormal lens fiber cells containing inclusion-like structures (probably due to decreased expression of γ-crystallins; see Fujimoto et al., 2004, and Min et al., 2004). Similarly, a mutation in the human *HSF4* gene is associated with a dominant, lamellar cataract (Bu et al., 2002a).

The β-Crystallins The first cataract mutation characterized at a molecular level was the so-called *Philly* mouse. It was demonstrated to be caused by an in-frame deletion of 12 bp in the βB2-crystallin encoding gene (*Crybb2*), resulting in a loss of four amino acids (Chambers and Russell, 1991). The region in which the deletion occurs is close to the carboxy-terminus and essential for the formation of the tertiary structure of the βB2-crystallin. The increasing severity of the phenotype is temporally correlated with the expression of the *Crybb2* gene; *Crybb2* is mapped to mouse chromosome 5. After the first postnatal week, the characteristic bow configuration of the nuclei in the lens cortex was replaced by a fan-shaped configuration, and swelling of the lens fibers occurred. Faint anterior opacities seen at P15 are followed by sutural cataracts at P25, nuclear cataract at P30, lamellar perinuclear opacities at P35, and total nuclear with anterior and posterior polar cataracts at P45. Cataractogenesis is associated with an intralenticular increase in water, sodium, and calcium and a decrease in potassium, reduced glutathione, and ATP. Altered membrane permeability is the cause of an increased outward leak (for a review, see Graw, 2004). A similar phenotype (referred to as *Aey2*) was also shown to be caused by a mutation affecting the fourth Greek key motif in the βB2-crystallin; however, in this case it was just an amino acid exchange (V187E; Graw et al., 2001b).

Similar to mutations in other crystallin-encoding genes, mutations in the human *CRYBB2* gene lead to cataract, too. However, three of the independent human *CRYBB2* mutations are caused by gene conversion between *CRYBB2* and its closely linked pseudogene, leading to a chain-termination mutation (Vanita et al., 2001). The *CRYBB2* pseudogene is specific for the human lineage and does not exist in the mouse genome. A fourth but different *CRYBB2* mutation was described recently (W151C in exon 6; Santhiya et al., 2004).

Among the β-crystallin-encoding genes, *Cryba1* is the second *Cryb* gene affected by cataract-causing mutations. It codes for two β-crystallins, βA1- and βA3-crystallin, which differ by the length of their N-terminal extension (Peterson and Piatigorsky, 1986). In the mouse, one *Cryba1* mutation has been described (*progressive opacity*, *Po1*), which has a similar phenotype to the murine *Crybb2* mutations cited earlier. It is characterized by a splicing defect at the end of intron 5, which leads to two distinct mRNA products and therefore to different predicted proteins: the Trp at position 168 is either deleted or changed into an Arg (Graw et al., 1999).

Similarly, in humans, two independent mutations affect the same 5′ (donor) splice site of intron 3. However, there is usually no access to human lens cDNA, and the novel splice product could not be characterized (for a review, see Graw, 2003). The third mutation was reported as a G91 deletion, causing a lamellar cataract with variable severity (Reddy et al., 2004). In humans, additional cataract-causing mutations in *CRYB* genes have been described in *CRYBB1* (Mackay et al., 2002) and *CRYBA4* (Billingsley, 2006); however, in the mouse, the other *Cryb* genes are not yet reported to be targeted by a mutation.

The γ-Crystallins An intermediate member of the β/γ-crystallin superfamily is γS-crystallin, previously also referred to as βS-crystallin. The corresponding gene *Crygs* maps to mouse chromosome 16, and two dominant mutations have been shown to be associated with *Crygs*: the ENU-induced, dominant mutation *Opj* (*opacity due to poor junctions*) was shown to have a mutation coding for a key residue in the core of the N-terminal domain of the protein (Phe9Ser; Sinha et al., 2001). In contrast, the spontaneous recessive mutation in mouse *Crygs* is characterized by a stop codon leading to a truncated protein missing 16 amino acids at the C-terminus of the mouse *Crygs* gene (Bu et al., 2002b).

The other six *Cryg* genes are organized as a cluster of very similar genes (*Cryga*→*Crygf*) within approximately 50 kb on mouse chromosome 1. In mice, mutations have been characterized affecting all six genes; however, it is apparent that *Cryge* has the highest mutation frequency. An overview of about 20 characterized mouse mutants has been published recently (Graw et al., 2004). Two very different phenotypes are presented in figure 40.3. The first *Cryg* mutant to be identified was the *Elo* mutant (*eye lens obsolescence*); it was characterized by a single nucleotide deletion in the *Cryge* gene. The mutation destroys the reading frame of the gene, and at the protein level one of the Greek key motifs is affected (Cartier et al., 1992). One of the cataract mutants most characterized among this group was originally referred to as *Nop* (*nuclear opacity*). It was of spontaneous origin and shown to be caused by a small deletion of 11 bp and an insertion of 4 bp in the third exon of the *Crygb* gene (allele symbol: *Crygb*^{nop}). It leads to a frameshift and ultimately creates a new stop codon; the corresponding γB-crystallin protein is predicted to be truncated after 144 amino acids; the last six amino acids are different from the wild-type γB-crystallin. Western blot analysis demonstrated stable expression of the wrong protein (Klopp et al., 1998). An additional, ENU-induced *Crygb* mutation (I4F) was described recently by Liu et al. (2005). The authors discuss a higher affinity to α-crystallin as the major cause of cataract formation in this particular mutant.

All these *Cryg* mutations affect only the lens cells and no other part of the eye; however, the size of the entire eye is

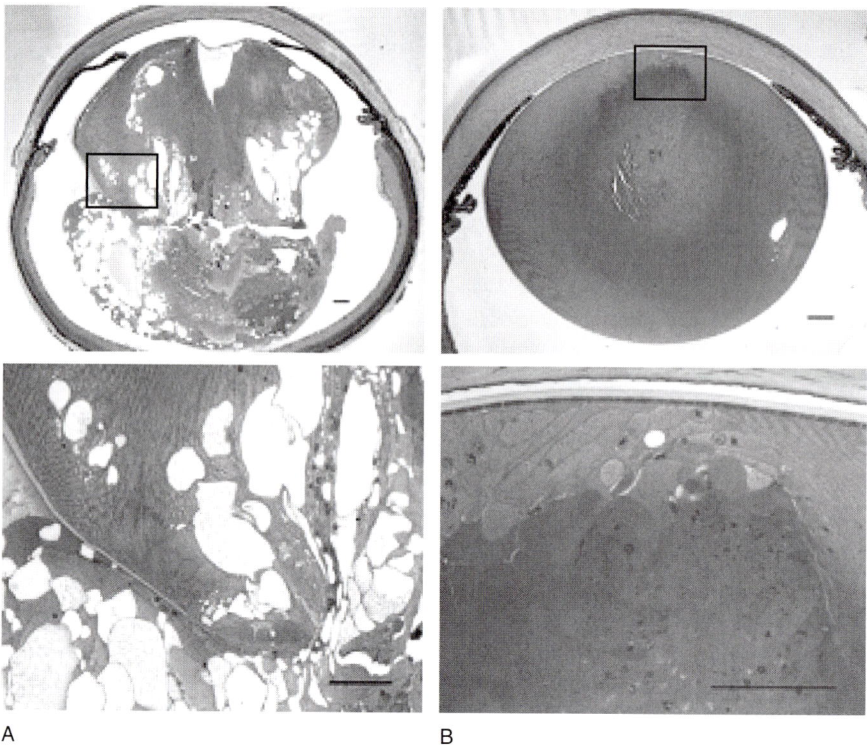

FIGURE 40.3 Mutations in *Cryg*. Histological sections of cataractous lenses from two different mutant lines are shown. The mutations have been induced by ENU in the *Cryga* gene (*A*) or in the *Crygd* gene (*B*). Inset in the overview marks the magnification, which is given below. The differences in severity are apparent. Bars = 100 μm. See color plate 38. (From Graw et al., 2004.)

always smaller than in the wild type. With the aid of in situ hybridization techniques with a probe detecting all *Cryg* transcripts in embryonic sections, a lower extent of *Cryg* transcripts was detected in the $Crygb^{nop}$ mutants beginning from E13.5. The first morphological abnormality in the mutant lenses was observed as a swelling of lens fibers at E15.5 (Santhiya et al., 1995). A common feature in three *Cryg* mutants investigated (including $Crygb^{nop}$) was inhibition of a Mg^{2+}-dependent DNase in the lens. The decrease of DNase activity followed the same directionality ($Cryge^{ns}$ > $Crygb^{nop}$ > $Cryge^{t}$) as the decrease in the relative content of water-soluble lens protein, which might be used as a rough indicator of the severity of cataractogenesis (Graw and Liebstein, 1993). Although *Cryg* mutation-mediated mechanisms of cataract formation are not fully understood, it is known that the mutations interfere with the breakdown of the lens fiber cell nuclei during terminal differentiation. The alteration of this process was demonstrated for three mouse *Cryg* mutants ($Crygb^{nop}$, $Cryge^{elo}$, $Cryge^{t}$); in these mutants, it was shown that the mutant γ-crystallins contributed to the formation of amyloid-like fibers in the lens fiber cell nuclei (Sandilands et al., 2002).

Some of the inherited cataracts in humans are also related to mutations in the γ-crystallin-encoding genes. In humans, two of the six *CRYG* genes on chromosome 2 are pseudogenes, but mutations associated with a clinical phenotype have been found up to now only in *CRYGC* and *CRYGD*. Surprisingly, the *CRYGD*-P23T mutation was observed in five independent families from different continents and reported to be causative for phenotypically diverse cataractous features. In all cases, the wild-type sequence CCAC <u>C</u>CCAA changes to CCAC<u>A</u>CCAA. Moreover, one of the dominant human *CRYGD* mutations (W156X) is identical to the dominant mouse *Lop12* mutation; the common single base-pair exchange is G→A, which cannot be explained by a slippage mechanism during DNA replication. Consequently, in mouse and human, 18 amino acids are missing at the C-terminus, leading to a dominant phenotype (in contrast to the 16 amino acids that are missing in the recessive mouse *Crygs* mutation).

CYTOSKELETAL PROTEINS There are three major lens cytoskeletal proteins, filensin (CP94 or beaded filament structural protein 1; gene symbol *Bfsp1*), phakinin (also referred to as CP49 or beaded filament structural protein 2; gene symbol *Bfsp2*), and vimentin. Since vimentin knockout mutants do not show an ocular phenotype, the two *Bfsp* genes are important for lens transparency. CP49 and filensin, together with α-crystallins, have been localized at unique cytoskeletal structures within the lens fiber cells known as beaded filaments. They are considered to be important in facilitating the chaperone activity of α-crystallin assemblies. Mutations in these two genes lead to cataract formation.

Disruption of the *Bfsp1* gene reduced levels of filensin's assembly partner CP49 and prevented the assembly of beaded filaments. These knockouts began to show evidence of light scattering by 2 months and worsened with age. Heterozygous animals exhibited an intermediate phenotype, showing a moderate light scattering at 5 months (Alizadeh et al., 2003).

However, the knockout of the *Bfsp2* gene does not lead to cataracts, even if the absence of CP49 causes a subtle loss of optical clarity in the lens (Alizadeh et al., 2002; Sandilands et al., 2003). Moreover, a deletion of the splice-acceptor site in exon 2 of the mouse *Bfsp2* results in a splicing of exon 1 to exon 3 and causes a frameshift in the reading frame as well as the introduction of a stop codon at position 2 of exon 3 in the *Bfsp2* transcript. The phenotype of this mutation is also subtle, as described for the knockout of the entire gene. Since this mutation is present in several mouse strains (129, 101, and CBA), it might interfere with other mutations or targeted deletions, and therefore it might have important implications for lens studies using these strains (Sandilands et al., 2004). Mutations in CP49-encoding gene *BFSP2* were shown to be responsible for dominant cataracts in humans (Conley et al., 2000; Jakobs et al., 2000); their phenotypes, however, seem to be variable ranging from congenital nuclear, sutural, or stellate cataracts to juvenile-onset cataracts.

Another protein, one associated with the lens cytoskeleton, is the Nhs1 protein, which is affected in the human Nance-Horan syndrome (NHS). Recently, a large insertion between exon 1 and exon 2 of the mouse *Nhs1* gene was shown to underlie the X-linked dominant cataract *Xcat*, which was recovered after parental irradiation. Histological analysis during embryonic development revealed that in the affected embryos, the primary fiber cells are irregularly arranged and show small foci of cellular disintegration; the fibers progressively degenerate. Molecularly, the insertion inhibits the expression of the *Nhs1* isoform containing exon 1 and results in exclusive expression of the alternative isoform containing exon 1A. The presence of *Nhs1* exon 1 is critical for localization of the protein to the cytoplasm, whereas proteins lacking Nhs1 exon 1 are predominantly nuclear. These results indicate that the first exon of *Nhs1* contains crucial information required for the proper expression and localization of Nhs1 protein (Huang et al., 2006).

Mouse models for metabolic cataracts

Sugar-Induced Cataracts in the Mouse Inborn errors in the galactose pathway and diabetes are known risk factors for the development of cataracts in humans. Sugar is converted to the corresponding sugar alcohol, which accumulates in the lens and creates osmotic problems, eventually leading to cataract.

For a long time, appropriate mouse models were missing. One hypothesis was that the enzyme aldose reductase (responsible for the conversion of sugar to its alcohol) has a very low activity in the mouse compared to human. Therefore, it was not surprising that the galactokinase (*Glk1*) knockout in the mouse does not suffer from cataracts at all. However, the introduction of a human aldose reductase transgene into a *Glk1*-deficient background resulted in cataract formation within the first postnatal day (Ai et al., 2000). This result highlights the importance of aldose reductase in sugar-dependent cataract formation.

Another candidate for cataract formation under diabetic conditions came from investigation of the bifunctional protein DCoH (dimerizing cofactor for HNF1). It acts as an enzyme in intermediary metabolism (gene symbol *Pcbd1*: pterin 4α-carbinolamine dehydratase) and as a binding partner of the HNF1 family of transcriptional activators. Knockout mutants of *Pcbd1* are viable and fertile but display hyperphenylalaninemia and a predisposition to cataracts. Lens opacities were visually detectable in about 20% of the *Pcbd1* null mice, if maintained on the outbred CD1 genetic background. The age at onset varied widely, with the earliest detection at 12 days; most of the affected animals had developed cataracts by the age of 24 weeks. The incidence of cataract formation was reduced in the C57BL/6J inbred genetic background (Bayle et al., 2002).

Protein-Bound Carbohydrates and Cataract Besides the free sugars of the intermediate metabolic pathways, sugar residues are present in a variety of glycoproteins. One of the corresponding enzymes is the α(1,3)-galactosyltransferase, which catalyzes the addition of galactose in an α(1,3) configuration to particular glycoproteins. Therefore, it is also referred to as glycoprotein galactosyltransferase α1,3 (gene symbol *Ggta1*); the corresponding gene is mapped to chromosome 2. The transfer of galactose to particular glycoproteins creates a highly immunogenic epitope that is present in all mammals except humans, apes, and Old World monkeys. *Ggta1* knockout mice have impaired glucose tolerance and decreased insulin sensitivity, and develop cataracts. A white pinhead opacity was observed in one eye at an average age of 36–37 days and in the second eye 1–2 days later. Rapid progression to full opacities occurred on average within 7–8 days. Early nuclear and posterior cortical changes, as well as fiber folds and swollen sutures, have been observed (see Dahl et al., 2006, and references therein).

Another interesting mouse model for congenital cataracts was characterized by targeting the gene coding for perlecan (*Hspg2*, mapped to chromosome 4). Perlecan is a large, multidomain, heparan sulfate proteoglycan found in all basement membranes; besides type IV collagen and laminin, it is a core protein of the lens capsule. Therefore it is not surprising that the homozygous deletion of the exon 3 by gene targeting leads to leakage of cellular material through the lens capsule and degeneration of the lens within 3 weeks after birth. In detail, loss of exon 3 removes the attachment sites for three heparan sulfate side chains composed of linear polysaccharides. It is speculated that this deletion might also change the affinity of perlecan for basic fibroblast growth factor. The cataractogenic potential of deletion within the *Hspg2* gene is dramatically enhanced in double knockouts, including both *Hspg2* and *Col18a1*; the *Col18a1* knockouts do not have any eye phenotype (Rossi et al., 2003).

Cholesterol Metabolism and Cataract One of the "old" syndromic, dominant mouse cataract mutants is the X-linked *bare patches* (*Bpa*). Whereas hemizygous males die before birth, heterozygous females have patches of bare skin. Lens cortical "frost figure" opacities are present. Molecular analysis showed that mutations in the gene *Nsdhl* (encoding an NAD(P)H steroid dehydrogenase-like protein) are responsible for the phenotype in two independent *Bpa* and three independent striated (*Str*) alleles (Liu et al., 1999). At the time it was published, it was the first mammalian locus associated with an X-linked dominant, male-lethal phenotype. In total, 10 alleles are reported (three spontaneous, two chemically induced, and five irradiation induced). It is also the first cataract phenotype shown to be related to the cholesterol pathway.

Mouse models for senile cataracts

The Emory mouse is a well-characterized genetic model for age-onset cataract. Emory mice develop cataracts at 5–6 months (early cataract strain) or 6–8 months (late cataract strain). Emory mouse cataracts increase in severity with age and first develop in the anterior superficial cortex region of the lens. They eventually progress into the anterior deep cortex region and ultimately result in complete lens opacification. Emory mouse cataracts are also associated with changes in numerous biochemical parameters and gene expression levels in the lens (see Sheets et al., 2002, and references therein). The first unpublished results from our laboratory concerning the mapping of the underlying mutation strongly suggest that the late Emory cataract (gene symbol *Em*) is a complex genetic disease that results from mutations in several genes, which must interact to produce this particular type of cataract.

Another genetic mouse model for senile cataracts is the senescence-accelerated mouse (SAM), which was identified at Kyoto University in 1970 on an AKR/J background strain. There are eight senescence-prone (SAM-P) strains, which are characterized by an earlier onset and more rapid advancement of senescence resulting from a significantly shorter life span. Cataracts have been found in the SAM-P/1 and SAM-P/9 strains. The earliest change was the appearance of a ripple mark body at about 3 months of age. The number of rippled rings increased with age. These changes later induced refractive distortion of retinal vessels. Whole-mount flat preparations of the epithelium showed that the number of cells was markedly decreased in advanced stages of cataract. In the late stages of life, the lens cortex became liquefied and developed into a mature cataract (Nishimoto et al., 1993). The mode of inheritance and the linkage to a particular chromosome still remain to be investigated.

Recently, the phenotypic characterization of a conditional knockout of the murine *Nbn* gene (encoding nibrin) was reported. The *Nbn* gene is the mouse homologue for the human Nijmegen breakage syndrome gene. All *Nbn*-deficient lenses develop cataracts at an early age due to altered lens fiber cell differentiation, including disruption of normal lens epithelial and fiber cell architecture and incomplete denucleation of fiber cells. In addition, *Nbn*-deficient lenses show dysregulated transcription of various crystalline genes. These features implicate a function of *Nbn* in terminal differentiation of the lens fiber cells and cataractogenesis (Yang et al., 2006). The encoded protein nibrin has a role in DNA double-strand-break sensing in response to DNA damage and repair. Since defects in DNA damage repair are frequently associated with premature aging processes, the mutation in the *Nbn* gene might be a first hint at the participation of the corresponding repair and cell cycle control proteins in the formation of age-related cataracts.

Open questions and conclusions

Database searches indicate additional mouse mutants exhibiting diverse forms of cataract that have not yet been characterized with respect to their mutations. One of them is *Tim* (translocation-induced circling mutation), which is associated with a reciprocal chromosomal translocation between chromosomes 4 and 17. Affected mice develop an anterior subcapsular cataract that appears after birth and is progressive and accompanied by abnormal head tossing and circling behavior. The most likely explanation for the phenotype is that the translocation breakpoint disrupted a gene or its regulation; this breakpoint remains to be determined (Smith et al., 1999). Other mutants include the following (details and references are available on the Web site of the Jackson Laboratory [www.informatics.jax.org]):

- The mutation *vacuolated lens* (*vl*) is mapped to mouse chromosome 1 and leads to opaque white lenses. Additionally, the mutants are characterized by a white belly spot and spina bifida. Small lens vacuoles are present at birth.

• The mutant *blind-sterile* (*bs*) is characterized by bilateral nuclear cataracts, microphthalmia, and glossy coats. The cataracts are detectable at E16. Females are fertile, but males are sterile. The mutation was mapped to mouse chromosome 2.

• The *Tcm* mutation (total cataract with microphthalmia), a cataract with iris dysplasia and coloboma, and the *Ccw* mutation, *cataract and curly whiskers*, are localized to mouse chromosome 4.

• The *nuclear posterior polar opacity* (*Npp*) maps to chromosome 5.

• *Cat5* (previously *To2*), a total opacity, is located close to the centromer on chromosome 10.

• Two alleles of *Cat3* ($Cat3^{vl}$, vacuolated lens; $Cat3^{vao}$, cataract with anterior opacity) arose independently in the F_1 generation after paternal γ-irradiation and map to the central region of chromosome 10.

• The so-called *rupture of lens cataract* (*rlc*) was mapped to chromosome 14; a similar form, *lr2* (*lens rupture 2*), was mapped to a close position. The opacity in the *rlc/rlc* mice becomes apparent at 35–60 days of age; there are no developmental changes reported.

• Finally, a form of cataract that forms postnatally without observed developmental alterations is the *Nakano cataract* (*nct*). The mutation was mapped to chromosome 16.

A more detailed analysis of these mutants should allow a more precise description of the mechanisms leading to cataracts. The list of already characterized mutants and the list of not yet characterized mutants (which is still increasing, owing to ongoing mutagenesis screens and improved phenotyping strategies) underline the power of this particular genetic system.

REFERENCES

Ai, Y., Zheng, Z., O'Brien-Jenkins, A., Bernard, D. J., Wynshaw-Boris, T., Ning, C., Reynolds, R., Segal, S., Huang, K., et al. (2000). A mouse model of galactose-induced cataracts. *Hum. Mol. Genet.* 12:1821–1827.

Alizadeh, A., Clark, J., Seeberger, T., Hess, J., Blankenship, T., and FitzGerald, P. G. (2003). Targeted deletion of the lens fiber cell-specific intermediate filament protein filensin. *Invest. Ophthalmol. Vis. Sci.* 44:5252–5258.

Alizadeh, A., Clark, J. I., Seeberger, T., Hess, J., Blankenship, T., Spicer, A., and FitzGerald, P. G. (2002). Targeted genomic deletion of the lens-specific intermediate filament protein CP49. *Invest. Ophthalmol. Vis. Sci.* 43:3722–3727.

Aso, S., Ishikawa, A., Wakana, S., Baba, R., Fujita, M., and Namikawa, T. (2001). The eye lens aplasia (*elap*) maps to mouse chromosome 2. *Exp. Anim.* 50:97–98.

Avilion, A. A., Nicolis, S. K., Pevny, L. H., Perez, L., Vivian, N., and Lovell-Badge, R. (2003). Multipotent cell lineages in early mouse development depend on SOX2 function. *Genes. Dev.* 17:126–140.

Bayle, J. H., Randazzo, F., Johnen, G., Kaufman, S., Nagy, A., Rossant, J., and Crabtree, G. R. (2002). Hyperphenylalaninemia and impaired glucose tolerance in mice lacking the bifunctional DCoH gene. *J. Biol. Chem.* 277:28884–28891.

Berry, V., Francis, P., Reddy, M. A., Collyer, D., Vithana, E., MacKay, I., Dawson, G., Carey, A. H., Moore, A., et al. (2001). Alpha-B crystallin gene (*CRYAB*) mutation causes dominant congenital posterior polar cataract in humans. *Am. J. Hum. Genet.* 69:1141–1145.

Billingsley, G., Santhiya, S. T., Paterson, A. D., Ogata, K., Wodak, S., Hosseini, S. M., Manisastry, S. M., Vijayalakshmi, P., Gopinath, P. M., et al. (2006). *CRYBA4*, a novel cataract gene, is also involved in microphthalmia. *Am. J. Hum. Genet.* 79:702–709.

Blixt, Å., Landgren, H., Johansson, B. R., and Carlsson, P. (2006). *Foxe3* is required for morphogenesis and differentiation of the anterior segment of the eye and is sensitive to *Pax6* gene dosage. *Dev. Biol.* doi:10.1016/j.ydbio.2006.09.021.

Brady, J. P., Garland, D., Duglas-Tabor, Y., Robison, W. G., Jr., Groome, A., and Wawrousek, E. F. (1997). Targeted disruption of the mouse αA-crystallin gene induces cataract and cytoplasmic inclusion bodies containing the small heat shock protein αB-crystallin. *Proc. Natl. Acad. Sci. U.S.A.* 94:884–889.

Brady, J. P., Garland, D. L., Green, D. E., Tamm, E. R., Giblin, F. J., and Wawrousek, E. F. (2001). αB-crystallin in lens development and muscle integrity: A gene knockout approach. *Invest. Ophthalmol. Vis. Sci.* 42:2924–2934.

Bu, L., Jin, Y., Shi, Y., Chu, R., Ban, A., Eiberg, H., Andres, L., Jiang, H., Zheng, G., et al. (2002a). Mutant DNA-binding domain of HSF4 is associated with autosomal dominant lamellar and Marner cataract. *Nat. Genet.* 31:276–278.

Bu, L., Yan, S., Jin, M., Jin, Y., Yu, C., Xiao, S., Xie, Q., Hu, L., Xie, Y., et al. (2002b). The γS-crystallin gene is mutated in autosomal recessive cataract in mouse. *Genomics* 80:38–44.

Cartier, M., Breitman, M. L., and Tsui, L. C. (1992). A frameshift mutation in the γE-crystallin gene of the *Elo* mouse. *Nat. Genet.* 2:42–45.

Chambers, C., and Russell, P. (1991). Deletion mutation in an eye lens β-crystallin. *J. Biol. Chem.* 266:6742–6746.

Chang, B., Hawes, N. L., Roderick, T. H., Smith, R. S., Heckenlively, J. R., Horwitz, J., and Davisson, M. T. (1999). Identification of a missense mutation in the αA-crystallin gene of the *lop18* mouse. *Mol. Vis.* 5:21.

Chen, T., Li, X. L., Yang, Y., and Church, R. L. (2002). Localization of lens intrinsic membrane protein MP19 and mutant protein $MP19^{To3}$ using fluorescent expression vectors. *Mol. Vis.* 8:372–388.

Civil, A., van Genesen, S. T., and Lubsen, N. H. (2002). C-Maf, the γD-crystallin Maf-responsive element and growth factor regulation. *Nucl. Acid Res.* 30:975–982.

Conley, Y. P., Erturk, D., Keverline, A., Mah, T. S., Keravala, A., Barnes, L. R., Bruchis, A., Hess, J. F., FitzGerald, P. G., et al. (2000). A juvenile-onset, progressive cataract locus on chromosome 3q21–q22 is associated with a missense mutation in the beaded filament structural protein-2. *Am. J. Hum. Genet.* 66: 1426–1431.

Dahl, K., Buschard, K., Gram, D. X., d'Apice, A. J. F., and Hansen, A. K. (2006). Glucose intolerance in a xenotransplantation model: Studies in alpha-gal knockout mice. *APMIS* 114: 805–811.

Ehling, U. H., Charles, D. J., Favor, J., Graw, J., Kratochvilova, J., Neuhäuser-Klaus, A., and Pretsch, W. (1985). Induction of gene mutations in mice: The multiple endpoint approach. *Mutat. Res.* 150:393–401.

Fantes, J., Ragge, N. K., Lynch, S. A., McGill, N. I., Collin, J. R. O., Howard-Peebles, P. N., Hayward, C., Vivian, A. J., Williamson, K., et al. (2003). Mutations in *SOX2* cause anophthalmia. *Nat. Genet.* 33:1–2.

Franz, T., and Besecke, A. (1991). The development of the eye in homozygotes of the mouse mutant Extra-toes. *Anat. Embryol.* 184:355–361.

Fraser, F. C., and Schabtach, G. (1962). "shrivelled": A hereditary degeneration of the lens in the house mouse. *Genet. Res. Camb.* 3:383–387.

Fujimoto, M., Izu, H., Seki, K., Fukuda, K., Nishida, T., Yamada, S., Kato, K., Yonemura, S., Inouye, S., et al. (2004). HSF4 is required for normal cell growth and differentiation during mouse lens development. *EMBO J.* 23:4297–4306.

Gilbert, C., Rahi, J. S., and Quinn, G. E. (2003). Visual impairment and blindness in children. In G. J. Johnson, D. C. Minassian, R. A. Weale, and S. K. West (Eds.), *The epidemiology of eye disease* (pp. 260–286). London: Arnold.

Gong, X., Li, E., Klier, G., Huang, Q., Wu, Y., Lei, H., Kumar, N. M., Horwitz, J., and Gilula, N. B. (1997). Disruption of *α3 connexin* gene leads to proteolysis and cataractogenesis in mice. *Cell* 91:833–843.

Graw, J. (2003). The genetic and molecular basis of congenital eye defects. *Nat. Rev. Genet.* 4:877–888.

Graw, J. (2004). Congenital hereditary cataracts. *Int. J. Dev. Biol.* 48:1031–1044.

Graw, J., Jung, M., Löster, J., Klopp, N., Soewarto, D., Fella, C., Fuchs, H., Reis, A., Wolf, E., et al. (1999). Mutation in the βA3/A1-crystallin encoding gene *Cryba1* causes a dominant cataract in the mouse. *Genomics* 62:67–73.

Graw, J., Klopp, N., Illig, T., Preising, M. N., and Lorenz, B. (2006). Congenital cataract and macular hypoplasia in humans associated with a de novo mutation in CRYAA and compound heterozygous mutations in P. *Graefes Arch. Clin. Exp. Ophthalmol.* 244:912–919.

Graw, J., and Liebstein, A. (1993). DNase activity in murine lenses: Implications for cataractogenesis. *Graefes Arch. Clin. Exp. Ophthalmol.* 231:354–358.

Graw, J., Löster, J., Puk, O., Münster, D., Haubst, N., Soewarto, D., Fuchs, H., Meyer, B., Nürnberg, P., et al. (2005). Three novel *Pax6* alleles in the mouse leading to the same small-eye phenotype caused by different consequences at target promoters. *Invest. Ophthalmol. Vis. Sci.* 46:4671–4683.

Graw, J., Löster, J., Soewarto, D., Fuchs, H., Meyer, B., Reis, A., Wolf, E., Balling, R., and Hrabé de Angelis, M. (2001a). Characterization of a new, dominant V124E mutation in the mouse αA-crystallin encoding gene. *Invest. Ophthalmol. Vis. Sci.* 42:2909–2915.

Graw, J., Löster, J., Soewarto, D., Fuchs, H., Reis, A., Wolf, E., Balling, R., and Hrabé de Angelis, M. (2001b). *Aey2*, a new mutation in the βB2-crystallin encoding gene in the mouse. *Invest. Ophthalmol. Vis. Sci.* 42:1574–1580.

Graw, J., Neuhäuser-Klaus, A., Klopp, N., Selby, P. B., Löster, J., and Favor, J. (2004). Genetic and allelic heterogeneity of *Cryg* mutations in eight distinct forms of dominant cataract in the mouse. *Invest. Ophthalmol. Vis. Sci.* 45:1202–1213.

Grimes, P. A., Koeberlein, B., Favor, J., Neuhäuser-Klaus, A., and Stambolian, D. (1998). Abnormal eye development associated with *Cat4a*, a dominant mouse cataract mutation on chromosome 8. *Invest. Ophthalmol. Vis. Sci.* 39:1863–1869.

Haubst, N., Berger, J., Radjendirane, V., Graw, J., Favor, J., Saunders, G. F., Stoykova, A., and Götz, M. (2004). Molecular dissection of *Pax6* function: the specific roles of the paired domain and homeodomain in brain development. *Development* 131: 6131–6140.

Hill, R. E., Favor, J., Hogan, B. L. M., Ton, C. C. T., Saunders, G. F., Hanson, I. M., Prosser, J., Jordan, T., Hastie, N. D., et al. (1991). Mouse *Small eye* results from mutations in a paired-like homeobox-containing gene. *Nature* 354:522–525.

Hong, H. K., Lass, J. H., and Chakravarti, A. (1999). Pleiotropic skeletal and ocular phenotypes of the mouse mutation congenital hydrocephalus (*ch/Mf1*) arise from a winged helix/forkhead transcription factor gene. *Hum. Mol. Genet.* 8:625–637.

Huang, K. M., Wu, J., Duncan, M. K., Moy, C., Dutra, A., Favor, J., Da, T., and Stambolian, D. (2006). *Xcat*, a novel mouse model for Nance-Horan syndrome inhibits expression of the cytoplasmic-targeted *Nhs1* isoform. *Hum. Mol. Genet.* 15: 319–327.

Hwang, D. Y., Ardayfio, P., Kang, U. J., Semina, E. V., and Kim, K. S. (2003). Selective loss of dopaminergic neurons in the substantia nigra of Pitx3-deficient aphakia mice. *Mol. Brain. Res.* 114:123–131.

Jakobs, P. M., Hess, J. F., FitzGerald, P. G., Kramer, P., Weleber, R. G., and Litt, M. (2000). Autosomal-dominant congenital cataract associated with a deletion mutation in the human beaded filament protein BFSP2. *Am. J. Hum. Genet.* 66:1432–1436.

Jiang, H., Jin, Y., Bu, L., Zhang, W., Liu, J., Cui, B., Kong, X., and Hu, L. (2003). A novel mutation in *GJA3* (connexin46) for autosomal dominant congenital nuclear pulverulent cataract. *Mol. Vis.* 9:579–583.

Johnson, G. J., and Foster, A. (2004). Prevalence, incidence and distribution of visual impairment. In G. J. Johnson, D. C. Minassian, R. A. Weale, and S. K. West (Eds.), *The epidemiology of eye disease* (pp. 3–28). London: Arnold.

Kamachi, Y., Uchikawa, M., and Kondoh, H. (2000). Pairing SOX off with partners in the regulation of embryonic development. *Trends Genet.* 16:182–187.

Kiyozumi, D., Sugimoto, N., and Sekiguchi, K. (2006). Breakdown of the reciprocal stabilization of QBRICK/Frem1, Fras1, and Frem2 at the basement membrane provokes Fraser syndrome-like defects. *Proc. Natl. Acad. Sci. U.S.A.* 103:11981–11986.

Klopp, N., Favor, J., Löster, J., Lutz, R. B., Neuhäuser-Klaus, A., Prescott, A., Pretsch, W., Quinlan, R. A., Sandilands, A., et al. (1998). Three murine cataract mutants (*Cat2*) are defective in different γ-crystallin genes. *Genomics* 52:152–158.

Kratochvilova, J., and Ehling, U. H. (1979). Dominant cataract mutations induced by γ-irradiation of male mice. *Mutat. Res.* 63:221–223.

Litt, M., Kramer, P., LaMorticella, D. M., Murphey, W., Lovrien, E. W., and Weleber, R. G. (1998). Autosomal-dominant congenital cataract associated with a missense mutation in the human alpha-crystallin gene *CRYAA*. *Hum. Mol. Genet.* 7:471–474.

Liu, H., Du, X., Wang, M., Huang, Q., Ding, L., McDonald, H. W., Yates, J. R., III, Beutler, B., Horwitz, J., et al. (2005). Crystallin γB-I4F mutant protein binds to α-crystallin and affects lens transparency. *J. Biol. Chem.* 280:25071–25078.

Liu, X. Y., Dangel, A. W., Kelley, R. I., Zhao, W., Denny, P., Botcherby, M., Cattanach, B., Peters, J., Hunsicker, P. R., et al. (1999). The gene mutated in bare patches and sdtriated mice encodes a novel 3β-hydroxysteroid dehydrogenase. *Nat. Genet.* 22:182–187.

Lyon, M. F., Jamieson, R. V., Perveen, R., Glenister, P. H., Griffiths, R., Boyd, Y., Glimcher, L. H., Favor, J., Munier,

F. L., et al. (2003). A dominant mutation within the DNA-binding domain of the bZIP transcription factor Maf causes murine cataract and results in selective alteration in DNA binding. *Hum. Mol. Genet.* 12:585–594.

Mackay, D. S., Andley, U. P., and Shiels, A. (2003). Cell death triggered by a novel mutation in the αA-crystallin gene underlies autosomal dominant cataract linked to chromosome 21q. *Eur. J. Hum. Genet.* 11:784–793.

Mackay, D. S., Boskovska, O. B., Knopf, H. L. S., Lampi, K. J., and Shiels, A. (2002). A nonsense mutation in *CRYBB1* associated with autosomal dominant cataract linked to human chromosome 22q. *Am. J. Hum. Genet.* 71:1216–1221.

Mackay, D., Ionides, A., Kibar, Z., Rouleau, G., Berry, V., Moore, A., Shiels, A., and Bhattacharya, S. (1999). Connexin46 mutations in autosomal dominant congenital cataract. *Am. J. Hum. Genet.* 64:1357–1364.

Min, J. N., Zhang, Y., Mosykophidis, D., and Mivechi, N. F. (2004). Unique contribution of heat shock transcription factor 4 in ocular lens development and fiber cell differentiation. *Genesis* 40:205–217.

Mörner, C. T. (1893). Untersuchungen der Proteinsubstanzen in den lichtbrechenden Medien des Auges. *Z. Physiol. Chem.* 18: 61–106.

Nishiguchi, S., Wood, H., Kondoh, H., Lovell-Badge, R., and Episkopou, V. (1998). *Sox1* directly regulates the γ-crystallin gene and is essential for lens development in mice. *Genes Dev.* 12: 776–781.

Nishimoto, H., Uga, S., Miyata, M., Ishikawa, S., and Yamashita, K. (1993). Morphological study of the cataractous lens of the senescence accelerated mouse. *Graefes Arch. Clin. Exp. Ophthalmol.* 231:722–728

Perng, M. D., and Quinlan, R. A. (2005). Seeing is believing! The optical properties of the eye lens are dependent upon functional intermediate filament cytoskeleton. *Exp. Cell. Res.* 305: 1–9.

Peterson, C. A., and Piatigorsky, J. (1986). Preferential conservation of the globular domains of the βA3/A1-crystallin polypeptide of the chicken eye lens. *Gene* 45:139–147.

Piatigorsky, J. (2003). Crystallin genes: Specialization by changes in gene regulation may precede gene duplication. *J. Struct. Funct. Genomics* 3:131–137.

Pras, E., Frydman, M., Levy-Nissenbaum, E., Bakhan, T., Raz, J., Assia, E. I., Goldman, B., and Pras, E. (2000). A nonsense mutation (W9X) in *CRYAA* causes autosomal recessive cataract in an inbred Jewish Persian family. *Invest. Ophthalmol. Vis. Sci.* 41:3511–3515.

Reddy, M. A., Bateman, O. A., Chakarova, C., Ferris, J., Berry, V., Lomas, E., Sarra, R., Smith, M. A., Moore, A. T., et al. (2004). Characterization of the G91del CRYBA1/3-crystallin protein: A cause of human inherited cataract. *Hum. Mol. Genet.* 13:945–953.

Rees, M. I., Watts, P., Fenton, I., Clarke, A., Snell, R. G., Owen, M. J., and Gray, J. (2000). Further evidence of autosomal dominant congenital zonular pulverulent cataracts linked to 13q11 (*CZP3*) and a novel mutation in connexin 46 (*GJA3*). *Hum. Genet.* 106:206–209.

Rieger, D. K., Reichenberger, E., McLean, W., Sidow, A., and Olsen, B. R. (2001). A double-deletion mutation in the *Pitx3* gene causes arrested lens development in *aphakia* mice. *Genomics* 72:61–72.

Ring, B. Z., Cordes, S. P., Overbeek, P. A., and Barsh, G. S. (2000). Regulation of mouse lens fiber cell development and differentiation by the Maf gene. *Development* 127:307–317.

Rossi, M., Morita, H., Sormunen, R., Airenne, S., Kreivi, M., Wang, L., Fukai, N., Olsen, B. R., Tryggvason, K., et al. (2003). Heparan sulfate chains of perlecan are indispensable in the lens capsule but not in the kidney. *EMBO J.* 22:236–245.

Ruiz-Ederra, J., and Verkman, A. S. (2006). Accelerated cataract formation and reduced lens epithelial water permeability in aquaporin-1-deficient mice. *Invest. Ophthalmol. Vis. Sci.* 47: 3960–3967.

Sandilands, A., Hutcheson, A. M., Long, H. A., Prescott, A. R., Vrensen, G., Löster, J., Klopp, N., Lutz, R. B., Graw, J., et al. (2002). Altered aggregation properties of mutant γ-crystallins cause inherited cataract. *EMBO J.* 21:6005–6014.

Sandilands, A., Prescott, A. R., Wegener, A., Zoltoski, R. K., Hutcheson, A. M., Masaki, S., Kuszak, J. R., and Quinlan, R. A. (2003). Knockout of the intermediate filament protein CP49 destabilises the lens fibre cytoskeleton and decreases lens optical quality, but does not induce cataract. *Exp. Eye Res.* 76:385–391.

Sandilands, A., Wang, X., Hutcheson, A. M., James, J., Prescott, A. R., Wegener, A., Pekny, M., Gong, X., and Quinlan, R. A. (2004). *Bfsp2* mutation found in mouse 129 strains causes the loss of CP49′ and induces vimentin-dependent changes in the lens fibre cell cytoskeleton. *Exp. Eye Res.* 78:875–889.

Santhiya, S. T., Abd-Alla, S. M., Löster, J., and Graw, J. (1995). Reduced levels of γ-crystallin transcripts during embryonic development of murine *Cat2^nop^* mutant lenses. *Graefes Arch. Clin. Exp. Ophthalmol.* 233:795–800.

Santhiya, S. T., Manisastry, S. M., Rawlley, D., Malathi, R., Anishetty, S., Gopinath, P. M., Vijayalakshmi, P., Namperumalsamy, P., Adamski, J., et al. (2004). Mutation analysis of congenital cataracts in Indian families: Identification of SNPs and a new causative allele in *CRYBB2* gene. *Invest. Ophthalmol. Vis. Sci.* 45:3599–3607.

Semina, E., Murray, J. C., Reiter, R., Hrstka, R. F., and Graw, J. (2000). Deletion in the promoter region and altered expression of *Pitx3* homeobox gene in *aphakia* mice. *Hum. Mol. Genet.* 9: 1575–1585.

Sheets, N. L., Chauhan, B. K., Wawrousek, E., Hejtmancik, J. F., Cvekl, A., and Kantorow, M. (2002). Cataract- and lens-specific upregulation of ARK receptor tyrosine kinase in Emory mouse cataract. *Invest. Ophthalmol. Vis. Sci.* 43:1870–1875.

Shiels, A., and Bassnett, S. (1996). Mutations in the founder of the MIP gene family underlie cataract development in the mouse. *Nat. Genet.* 12:212–215.

Sinha, D., Wyatt, M. K., Sarra, R., Jaworski, C., Slingsby, C., Thaung, C., Pannell, L., Robison, W. G., Favor, J., et al. (2001). A temperature-sensitive mutation of *Crygs* in the murine *Opj* cataract. *J. Biol. Chem.* 276:9308–9315.

Smidt, M. P., Smits, S. M., Bouwmeester, H., Hamers, F. P., van der Linden, A. J., Hellemons, A. J., Graw, J., and Burbach, J. P. (2004). Early developmental failure of substantia nigra dopamine neurons in mice lacking the homeodomain gene *Pitx3*. *Development* 131:1145–1155.

Smith, R. S., Johnson, K. R., Hawes, N. L., Harris, B. S., Sundberg, J. P., and Davisson, M. T. (1999). Lens epithelial proliferation cataract in segmental trisomy involving mouse chromosomes 4 and 7. *Mamm. Genome* 10:102–106.

Steele, E. C., Jr., Kerscher, S., Lyon, M. F., Glenister, P. H., Favor, J., Wang, J., and Church, R. L. (1997). Identification of a mutation in the MP19 gene, *Lim2*, in the cataractous mouse mutant *To3*. *Mol. Vis.* 3:5.

Steele, E. C., Jr., Lyon, M. F., Favor, J., Guillot, P. V., Boyd, Y., and Church, R. L. (1998). A mutation in the *connexin 50* (*Cx50*) gene is a candidate for the *No2* mouse cataract. *Curr. Eye Res.* 17:883–889.

Vanita, Sarhad, V., Reis, A., Jung, M., Singh, D., Sperling, K., Singh, J. R., and Burger, J. (2001). A unique form of autosomal dominant cataract explained by gene conversion between β-crystallin B2 and its pseudogene. *J. Med. Genet.* 38:392–396.

Verkman, A. S. (2003). Role of aquaporin water channels in eye function. *Exp. Eye Res.* 76:137–143.

Vicart, P., Caron, A., Guicheney, P., Li, Z., Prévost, M. C., Faure, A., Chateau, D., Chapon, F., Tomé, F., et al. (1998). A missense mutation in the αB-crystallin chaperone gene causes a desmin-related myopathy. *Nat. Genet.* 20:92–95.

White, T. W., Goodenough, D. A., and Paul, D. L. (1998). Targeted ablation of connexin50 in mice results in microphthalmia and zonular pulverulent cataracts. *J. Cell. Biol.* 143:815–825.

Xia, C., Liu, H., Chang, B., Cheng, C., Cheung, D., Wang, M., Huang, Q., Horwitz, J., and Gong, X. (2006a). Arginine 54 and tyrosine 118 residues of αA-crystallin are crucial for lens formation and transparency. *Invest. Ophthalmol. Vis. Sci.* 47:3004–3010.

Xia, C., Liu, H., Cheung, D., Cheng, C., Wang, M., Du, X., Beutler, B., Lo, W. K., and Gong, X. (2006b). Diverse gap junctions modulate distinct mechanism for fiber cell formation during lens development and cataractogenesis. *Development* 133:2033–2040.

Yang, Y. G., Frappart, P. O., Frappart, L., Wang, Z. Q., and Tong, W. M. (2006). A novel function of DNA repair molecule Nbs1 in terminal differentiation of the lens fibre cells and cataractogenesis. *DNA Repair* 5:885–893.

Zaki, P. A., Collinson, J. M., Toraiwa, J., Simpson, T. I., Price, D. J., and Quinn, J. C. (2006). Penetrance of eye defects in mice heterozygous for mutation of *Gli3* is enhanced by heterozygous mutation of *Pax6*. *BMC Dev. Biol.* 6:46; doi:10.1186/1471-213X-6-46.

41 Mouse Models of Infectious Eye Diseases

LINDA D. HAZLETT

The pathogenesis of ocular infectious disease is determined by the virulence of the microorganism, the host immune response, and the anatomical features of the site of infection. In the eye, the cornea is unique anatomically, as it must remain optically clear and avascular, yet able to respond rapidly to microbial insult, protecting itself and the interior structures of the eye, such as the retina, from sight-threatening microbially initiated damage. Understanding innate and acquired immune response mechanisms during viral, bacterial, fungal, and parasitic eye infections remains fundamental to the rational design of therapeutic strategies to eliminate the microorganisms, control inflammatory responses, and minimize the action of their virulence factors, thus preventing permanent structural damage to the cornea and interior ocular structures, which would render them optically dysfunctional.

Numerous animal models have provided much information about immune system responses to infection. Among them, the mouse is often regarded as a model of choice. Mice are susceptible to a similar range of microbial infections as humans, and marked differences between inbred strains can be exploited to analyze the genetic basis of infections. In addition, the genetic tools that are available for use in the laboratory mouse, and new techniques to monitor the expression of genes (e.g., bacterial) in vivo, make the mouse the principal experimental animal model for studying mechanisms of infection and immunity (Buer and Balling, 2003).

Herpetic infections of the cornea

Herpetic viral infection of the cornea caused by herpes simplex virus (HSV) is a leading nontraumatic cause of blindness, despite the availability of both immunosuppressive and antiviral drugs (O'Brien and Hazlett, 1996). Acute infection of the corneal surface is a manifestation of virus-induced cytolysis. The corneal stroma may also be involved as a result of recurring infections associated with reactivation from latency. Stromal inflammation reflects an immunopathological process that often leads to corneal scarring, neovascularization, permanent endothelial dysfunction, and vision impairment. HSV also may be causative in dermatitis, blepharitis, conjunctivitis, iridiocyclitis, and retinitis.

The mouse model has greatly furthered our understanding of the role of the immune response in tissue damage. Mice are experimentally infected with certain strains of HSV and develop keratitis. Wounding of the cornea is usually required, and not all mouse strains are susceptible. Herpes stromal keratitis (HSK) in the mouse is a model of disciform nonnecrotizing keratitis in which the inflammation may be dominated eventually by lymphocytes and other mononuclear cells (O'Brien and Hazlett, 1996). HSK is T cell mediated, and in BALB/c mice infected with HSV-1, tissue-destructive inflammation in the cornea (HSK) and other periocular lesions develop about 7 days after viral infection. CD4+ T cells and T helper 1 (Th1)-type cytokines contribute both to the immunopathology in the cornea and to the eradication of viral replication in the skin. Studies in CD4+ T cell–deficient mice showed that these cells preferentially mediate HSK, but in their absence, a high infectious dose of HSV-1 can induce histologically similar but transient HSK that is mediated by CD8+ T cells (Lepisto et al., 2006). Disruption of CD40/154 signaling does not affect the initial expansion of CD4+ T cells in the draining lymph nodes but dramatically reduces the persistence and Th1 polarization of these cells. It was concluded that CD154 signaling is required during the inductive but not the effector phase of the Th1 immune response in the infected cornea, and therefore local disruption of this signaling pathway would not likely be a useful therapy for HSK (Xu et al., 2004). In contrast, others have used mice to show that CD86, a member of the costimulatory family of molecules, is important in the development of cytotoxic T cells and in reducing viral replication in the eyes of HSV-1-infected mice (Osorio et al., 2005). In mice, low delayed-type hypersensitivity (DTH) responses were found to be associated with less severe disease, while high DTH responsive mice exhibited worse disease. IL-10 knockout mice also had worsened disease, while mice given recombinant (r) IL-10 protein by ocular and intraperitoneal routes had less severe lesions (Keadle and Stuart, 2005).

Recurrent HSV-1 usually results from reactivation of latent virus in sensory neurons, followed by transmission to peripheral sites (Liu et al., 2000). The mechanism of this has been extensively studied in mouse models. It was shown that CD8+ T cells that are present in the trigeminal ganglion at the time of its excision can maintain HSV-1 in a latent state in sensory neurons in ex vivo trigeminal ganglion cultures (Liu et al., 2000). The use of T cell transgenic mice with severe combined immunodeficiency syndrome (SCID) or mice on a recombinase-activating gene–deficient background lacking both T and B lymphocytes also suggests that CD8+ T cell control is expressed in the trigeminal ganglion, serving to curtail the source of the virus to the cornea (Banerjee et al., 2004).

The pathogenesis of corneal scarring and vascularization in HSK is uncertain but appears to reflect a complex interaction of various cytokines, chemokines, and growth factors brought in by inflammatory cells or produced locally in the cornea in response to HSV-1 infection. Evidence suggests that HSV-1 infection disrupts the normal equilibrium between angiogenic and antiangiogenic stimuli, leading to vascularization of the normally avascular cornea. Thrombospondin 1 and 2, matrix proteins involved in wound healing, are potent antiangiogenic factors and may be among the critical players involved. It has been suggested that elucidating their role in corneal scarring and vascularization may lead to improved therapies for HSK (Kaye and Choudhary, 2006).

In this regard, matrix metalloproteinase-9 (MMP-9), a type IV collagenase, has been shown to contribute to corneal neovascularization in the mouse corneal stroma infected with HSV. Neutrophils (PMNs), which invade the cornea soon after infection, were considered a likely source of the matrix-degrading enzyme, since using a PMN-specific monoclonal antibody (mAb) diminished MMP-9 expression, as well as the extent of angiogenesis. MMP-9 knockout mice also had diminished disease, while use of tissue inhibitor of metalloproteinase-1 (TIMP-1), a specific MMP-9 inhibitor, reduced disease in wild-type mice. These data suggest that targeting MMP-9 for inhibition may improve therapy for HSK (Lee et al., 2002). Rapid improvement of HSV-1-induced keratitis also was noted after amniotic membrane transplantation onto the cornea. It was postulated that this was caused by reduced expression of MMP-8 and -9 and increased expression of TIMP-1 (Heiligenhaus et al., 2005). Others have shown that in the virus-infected cornea, interleukin-6 (IL-6) promotes corneal infection by acting in an autocrine-paracrine fashion to induce resident corneal cells to make macrophage inhibitory protein-2 (MIP-2) and macrophage inflammatory protein-1α (MIP-1α/CCL3), which in turn recruit PMNs to the virus infection site in the murine cornea (Fenton et al., 2002). Use of a transgenic mouse that overexpresses the IL-1 receptor antagonist (IL-1ra) protein revealed that these mice were markedly resistant to HSK, compared with IL-1ra knockout and C57BL/6 WT control mice. Resistance was the consequence of reduced expression of molecules such as IL-6 and MIP-2, as well as vascular endothelial growth factor (VEGF) production, normally upregulated directly or indirectly by IL-1. These mice also had a marked reduction in angiogenesis, an essential step in HSK pathogenesis (Biswas et al., 2004a). Mice receiving IL-1ra protein also had diminished disease severity (Biswas et al., 2004b). A better understanding of the role of VEGF in induction of angiogenesis and in the pathogenesis of HSK was derived from experiments in which mice were injected with the VEGF inhibitor mFlt(1-3)-immune globulin G. These mice had diminished angiogenesis, and the severity of lesions after HSV infection was less (Zheng et al., 2001). Administration of a cyclooxygenase 2 (COX-2) selective inhibitor also was tested and was found to decrease PMN infiltration into the HSV-infected cornea and diminished corneal VEGF levels, likely accounting for the reduced angiogenic response noted in these mice (Biswas et al., 2005). In another study, application of plasmid DNA encoding IL-18 to the cornea of mice before HSV-1 ocular infection also reduced angiogenesis and diminished HSK lesions (Kim et al., 2005). Systemic injection of VEGF pathway-specific silencing (si) RNAs before infection was another confirmation of the role of VEGF in disease, as knocking down the gene for VEGF inhibited ocular angiogenesis induced by HSV (Kim et al., 2004). The absence of the chemokine receptor CCR5, a shared receptor for the beta chemokines CCL3 and CCL5, appeared to play a role in regulating leukocyte trafficking and control of virus burden, but was not critical to prevent mortality after corneal HSV-1 infection (Carr et al., 2006).

Findings from mouse studies have also suggested that HSK may be the result of either molecular mimicry or bystander activation phenomenon (Wickham and Carr, 2004). Molecular mimicry has been difficult to prove and is based on the tenet that causative viruses express epitopes that cross-react with a host protein and that the initial immune response to viruses carries over to include antihost reactivity. Bystander activation represents a complex that could include the release of normally sequestered antigens from damaged cells that have become immunogenic, alteration of host protein structure, and the subversion of host cells, causing pro-inflammatory mediator production or the synthesis of abnormal products such as autoantibodies (Wickham and Carr, 2004).

Bacterial infections and keratitis

Pseudomonas aeruginosa is a gram-negative opportunistic pathogen that rapidly induces bacterial keratitis, a disease often associated with extended-wear contact lens use (O'Brien and Hazlett, 1996). The host innate immune response to this pathogen includes local PMN recruitment, which is essential to control bacterial replication, bacterial spread, and host survival. Nonetheless, PMN persistence in the cornea is also associated with destructive pathology, including stromal scarring and perforation, potentially requiring corneal transplantation (Steuhl et al., 1987; Hazlett, 2004). PMN infiltration into inflamed tissue is largely controlled by local production of inflammatory mediators. In the mouse, two members of the C-X-C family of chemokines, MIP-2 (functional homologue of human IL-8) and KC, are potent chemoattractants and activators of PMN. In corneal infections, MIP-2 was shown to be the major chemokine that attracts PMNs into the *P. aeruginosa*-infected cornea, and the persistence of PMNs in the cornea of susceptible (cornea perforates) C57BL/6 versus resistant BALB/c (no corneal perforation) mice was found to correlate with higher MIP-2 chemokine levels (both mRNA and protein) (Kernacki et al., 2000). IL-1, produced by macrophages, monocytes, and resident corneal cells (Niederkorn et al., 1989; Dinarello, 1996), also influences PMN infiltration into tissues (Dinarello and Wolff, 1993). When tested, levels of IL-1α and IL-1β (mRNA and protein) were elevated in the infected cornea of C57BL/6 (susceptible) over BALB/c (resistant) mice. Neutralization of IL-1β in infected C57BL/6 mice (Rudner et al., 2000) reduced disease severity, as evidenced by a reduction in PMNs in the cornea (MPO assay), a decreased bacterial load, and decreased levels of MIP-2 at both the mRNA and protein levels. The use of caspase-1 inhibitor treatment in C57BL/6 mice confirmed these data, even when inhibitor treatment was initiated after disease onset. In addition, improvement was augmented when the caspase-1 inhibitor was given after infection together with the antibiotic ciprofloxacin (Thakur et al., 2004). A live attenuated *P. aeruginosa* vaccine has also been tested and been found to elicit outer membrane protein-specific active and passive protection against corneal infection (Zaidi et al., 2006).

The role of T cells in *P. aeruginosa* corneal infection was first studied in inbred C57BL/6 WT and CD8+ T-deficient, β2-microglobulin knockout mice (on the C57BL/6 background) (Kwon and Hazlett, 1997). Corneas of both groups of mice perforated by 7 days post infection and the histopathology was similar, with infiltration of PMNs within 24 hours post infection. In contrast, corneas of wild-type mice antibody depleted of CD4+ T cells and infected with *P. aeruginosa* did not perforate at 7 days post infection, versus mice depleted of CD8+ T cells or treated with an irrelevant antibody. Antibody neutralization of IFN-γ before infecting C57BL/6 mice also prevented corneal perforation and was associated with a lower DTH response when compared with C57BL/6 mice similarly treated with an irrelevant antibody. These data support that a CD4+ T cell (Th1)–dominant response following *P. aeruginosa* infection is associated with genetic susceptibility and corneal perforation in C57BL/6 mice (Kwon and Hazlett, 1997) and provided the first evidence that CD4+ T cells are important in the development of keratitis. In addition, the use of gene array studies confirmed a Th1 versus Th2 bias of C57BL/6 versus BALB/c mice to infection with *Pseudomonas* (Huang and Hazlett, 2003). Other studies investigated whether IL-12 (IL-12 p40) was associated with IFN-γ production and the susceptibility response of C57BL/6 mice after *P. aeruginosa* challenge. IL-12 p40 knockout mice (C57BL/6 background) versus wild-type mice were tested to examine disease progression in the endogenous absence of the cytokine. When tested, both groups of mice were susceptible to corneal challenge with *P. aeruginosa*, with corneal perforation observed 5–7 days post infection. Semiquantitative RT-PCR and ELISA analyses confirmed that IL-12 p40 message and protein levels were elevated after infection in the wild-type mice over the expected absence of IL-12 p40 in the knockout mouse cornea. Immunostaining for IL-12 in wild-type C57BL/6 mice revealed that stromal PMNs were at least one source of the cytokine (Hazlett et al., 2002).

The role of IL-18 and IFN-γ production in the resistance response of the predominantly Th2 responding BALB/c mouse was also tested. Semiquantitative RT-PCR detected IFN-γ mRNA expression levels in the cornea of infected mice at 1–7 days post infection. Cytokine levels were significantly upregulated when compared with control, uninfected normal mouse corneas (Huang et al., 2002). With RT-PCR, IL-18 mRNA expression was detected constitutively in the normal, uninfected cornea, but levels were significantly elevated 1–7 days post infection. To test whether IL-18 regulated IFN-γ production, BALB/c mice were injected with an anti-IL-18 mAb. Treatment decreased corneal IFN-γ mRNA (Huang et al., 2002) levels, and both bacterial load and disease severity increased when compared with IgG-injected control mice. These data provide evidence that IL-18 is critical to the resistance response of BALB/c mice by induction of IFN-γ and that IFN-γ is required for bacterial killing or stasis in the cornea (Hazlett, 2002; Hazlett et al., 2005). Another study showed that the killing effect of IFN-γ was indirect, through regulation of nitric oxide levels (McClellan et al., 2006).

Further study of the resistance response in BALB/c mice examined the role of the pro-inflammatory neuropeptide, substance P (SP), in IFN-γ production. Natural killer cells were required to produce IFN-γ; the cells expressed the neurokinin-1 receptor (a major SP receptor) and directly regulated IFN-γ production through interaction with this receptor (Lighvani et al., 2005), suggesting a unique link between the nervous system and the development of innate immunity in the cornea.

Staphylococcus aureus is a gram-positive organism that is seen in patients with epithelial defect, especially those on prolonged corticosteroid treatment (O'Brien and Hazlett, 1996). The disease progresses gradually and induces stromal opacity. A mouse model of the disease has been developed (Girgis et al., 2003) that should be usable in a large range of studies that were not feasible in a rabbit keratitis model, particularly those requiring a genetically altered host or specific immunologic reagents. It was reported that different strains of mice had disparate cytokine responses correlated with disease severity (Hume et al., 2005). Aged mice also were more susceptible to disease than young mice (Girgis et al., 2004), and bacterial toxins, especially α-toxin, could mediate corneal disease in mice (Girgis et al., 2005). Differences in severity of the keratitis in aged versus young mice correlated with their susceptibility to α-toxin. In the mouse model of *S. aureus*-induced endophthalmitis (a serious and potentially blinding ocular infection usually associated with recent intraocular surgery), it was shown that Fas ligand, but not complement, is critical for control of the disease (Engelbert and Gilmore, 2005).

The mouse has also been used as a model to study conjunctival infection. Immune responses in mice after conjunctival exposure to *Chlamydia trachomatis* have been examined (Barsoum et al., 1988). *Chlamydia* was consistently isolated from the conjunctiva and draining lymph node at 1 and 7 days after conjunctival exposure, but by about 5 weeks, blastogenic responsiveness was very low, perhaps reflecting a state of immunosuppression (Barsoum et al., 1988).

The introduction of *Listeria monocytogenes* into the anterior chamber of mice was used to test whether immune privilege (anterior chamber–associated immune deviation, ACAID) of the anterior chamber, resulting in reduced DTH, extended to this bacterial pathogen (Li and Niederkorn, 1997). The results showed that immune privilege is not extended to all foreign antigens that enter the anterior chamber, and as a result, some intraocular antigens can provoke a strong systemic DTH response.

Mouse eye infection models have also been used to study the role of Toll receptors in disease. The Toll family of receptors (TLR), conserved throughout evolution from flies to humans, is central in initiating innate immune responses. This family of receptors, composed of transmembrane molecules, links the extracellular compartment where contact and recognition of microbial pathogens occur, and the intracellular compartment, where signaling cascades leading to cellular responses are initiated. Gene array data showed that the expression of TLRs and related molecules, including CD14, soluble IL-1ra, TLR6, and IL-18R-accessory protein, were significantly elevated in susceptible (C57BL/6) versus resistant (BALB/c) mice following challenge with *P. aeruginosa* (Huang and Hazlett, 2003). In a sterile keratitis model (Khatri et al., 2002), when C3H/HeJ (TLR4 point mutation) and control mice were treated with lipopolysaccharide from *P. aeruginosa*, a significant increase in stromal thickness and haze was seen in the cornea of control mice but not in TLR4 mutant mice, and the severity of the disease coincided with PMN stromal infiltration. Another study showed that the corneal epithelium has functional TLR2 and TLR9, and that TLR2, TLR4, and TLR9 signal through myeloid differentiation factor 88 (MyD88) (Johnson et al., 2005). Recent evidence showed that a single Ig IL-1R related molecule (SIGIRR) is differentially expressed in BALB/c (resistant) compared to B6 (susceptible) mice and that this Toll receptor is critical in resistance to *P. aeruginosa* infection in BALB/c animals, functioning to downregulate type 1 immunity and negatively regulating IL-1 and TLR4 signaling (Huang et al., 2006). siRNA treatment to knockdown TLR9 was also found to influence bacterial keratitis, leading to reduced inflammation but also decreased bacterial killing (Huang et al., 2005). Modulation of bacterial factors has also been shown to reduce ocular virulence (Zolfaghar et al., 2006; Parks and Hobden, 2005).

Mouse models of fungal infection

Compared with bacterial infections, there are relatively few studies on the pathogenesis of oculomycoses, and a complete understanding of appropriate therapy is lacking. A murine model of keratomycosis has been established, despite mice being innately resistant to the fungal pathogen, *Candida albicans*. Moderate to severe keratomycosis was established using immunocompromised mice and a route of corneal scarification (Wu et al., 2003). A mouse model of corneal fusariosis by infection with the fungal pathogen *Fusarium solani* has also been established and permits evaluation of fungal infection and pathogenesis. Immunosuppression and surface scarification were also needed for this model to establish infection (Wu et al., 2004).

Mouse models of parasitic infection

Parasitic infections of the eye are a leading cause of blindness in many parts of the world. Inflammation of the corneal stroma is a serious complication of infection with the nematode parasite, *Onchocerca volvulus* (Pearlmann et al., 1996), a cause of river blindness in humans. An essential role for PMNs and eosinophils, as well antibody, has been shown for their recruitment (Pearlman et al., 1998; Hall et al., 1999). Further studies showed that disease is exacerbated in BALB/c IL-4 knockout mice and that both IL-4 and Th2 cells were required for disease development (Pearlman et al., 1995). Use of this mouse model of river blindness in which soluble extracts of filarial nematodes were injected into the corneal stroma also made it possible to demonstrate that the predominant inflammatory response in the cornea was due to a species of endosymbiotic *Wolbachia* bacteria and that the inflammatory response induced was dependent on Toll-like 4 receptors on host cells (Saint Andre et al., 2002), as well as signaling through MyD88 (Gillette-Ferguson et al., 2006).

Critical to infection with another parasite genus, *Acanthamoeba*, small, free-living protozoa that are widely distributed in nature, is the ability of the parasite to bind to the corneal surface. Epidemiological studies have shown that contact lens wear is the most significant risk factor, while trauma is the second most significant factor. Poor lens hygiene is frequently encountered in association with tap water rinsing of the lens (O'Brien and Hazlett, 1996). Eleven host species of *Acanthamoeba* were tested, and parasites failed to bind to or damage intact epithelium in the mouse cornea. Results indicate that *A. castellani*, the species tested, exercises rigid host specificity at the host cell surface (Niederkorn et al., 1992). Intracorneal inoculation of nude, athymic (lacking T cells) mice with *A. hatchetti*, however, was capable of inducing keratitis (Paniagua-Crespo et al., 1989).

Mouse models of retinal infection

Herpes simplex may be a cause of viral retinitis or encephalitis in immunologically competent and incompetent adults (O'Brien and Hazlett, 1996). The full-thickness necrotizing retinitis presents as diffuse retinal opacification and edema with perivascular inflammation. In AIDS patients, selected rampant cases of cytomegalovirus retinopathy and encephalitis have also been documented to be coinfected with HSV (O'Brien and Hazlett, 1996). Herpetic retinitis in humans is characterized by a high frequency of bilateral localization. The mouse has been used to examine HSV-1 retinitis after anterior chamber inoculation. Modulation of disease by CD4+ T cells was detected in the uninoculated eye (Azumi et al., 1994); natural killer cells prevented direct anterior-posterior spread of virus (Tanigawa et al., 2000), and spread of HSV-2 to the suprachiasmatic nuclei and retina was detected in T cell–depleted mice (Matsubara and Atherton, 1997). The observation that in the inoculated eye, T cells arrive in the sensory retina at the onset of retinal necrosis and not during acute retinitis and the peak of viral replication, suggests that T cells play a role in the development of retinal necrosis; they may also have a role in resolution of the disease, as they were observed as late as 63 days post infection in the uninoculated eye (Azumi and Atherton, 1998). Injection of HSV-1 into the vitreous of BALB/c mice was also used to examine the occurrence of contralateral virus spread, and the data suggested that spread was mediated by local (nonsynaptic) transfer in the optic chiasm from infected to uninjected axons in the optic nerves (Labetoulle et al., 2000). Nectin-1, a member of the immune globulin superfamily, has been shown to be a receptor for HSV, and this molecule was found widely expressed in murine ocular tissues (Valyi-Nagy et al., 2004).

Murine cytomegalovirus infections (MCMV) (AIDS-related in human retinitis) were examined in the mouse, and the virus was found to spread to and replicate in the retina after LPS-induced disruption of the blood-retinal barrier in immunosuppressed mice (Zhang et al., 2005a). Apoptosis in the retina was detected in uninfected retinal cells in this model (Bigger et al., 2000). The mouse has served to allow detection of ocular reactivation of MCMV after immunosuppression of latently infected mice (Zhang et al., 2005b). Therapy for MCMV used a SCID mouse model, and the efficacy of therapy with cidofovir was successfully monitored with electroretinography (Garneau et al., 2003). MCMV retinitis in the mouse was examined in retrovirus-induced immunodeficiency (MAIDS) in mice, and loss of the perforin cytotoxic pathway appeared to predispose mice to retinitis (Dix et al., 2003); susceptibility also correlated with intraocular levels of TNF-α and IFN-γ (Dix and Cousins, 2004).

Murine coronavirus, mouse hepatitis virus (MHV), JHM strain, induces disease in mice, and a genetic predisposition to disease induction of the retina has been shown (Wang et al., 1996). Intraocular coronavirus injection results in a biphasic retinal disease in susceptible BALB/c mice characterized by acute inflammation and retinal degeneration associated with autoimmune reactivity. Resistant CD-1 mice develop only the early phase of the disease (Vinores et al., 2001). Retinal apoptosis may be one of the host mechanisms contributing to limiting this retinal infection (Wang et al., 2000).

Toxoplasma gondii, a protozoan parasite, can cause severe, life-threatening disease, especially in newborns and immunosuppressed (e.g., HIV-infected) patients. The active phase of retinal disease is self-limited, but it can recur, and the destructive nature of the infection places patients at risk for blindness if tissues critical for vision, such as the optic nerve or macula, are involved (O'Brien and Hazlett, 1996). Toxoplasmosis, caused by an obligate intracellular parasite, is established in mice by either an intravitreal or an instillation route of infection using *T. gondii* Me-49 strain. The route of inoculation influences the inflammatory pattern and the instillation route was preferred, as it avoids extensive needle damage in a small animal (Tedesco et al., 2005). The effects of sulfamethoxazole treatment have been assessed using other toxoplasmosis strains in IFN-γ knockout mice. This model allowed the quantitative assessment of treatment effects (Norose et al., 2006).

Summary

The mouse provides a valuable animal model for infectious disease studies in the eye. The ability to manipulate genetically based experimental systems because of the availability of numerous inbred strains, the wealth of gene knockout and transgenic animals, and the easy availability of immunological and molecular reagents are only a few of the reasons that this is the case.

ACKNOWLEDGMENTS Work was supported by NIH grant nos. R01EY02986, R01EY016058, and P30EY04068 and by a grant from Ciba-Vision.

REFERENCES

Arend, W. P., Malyak, M., Guthridge, C. J., and Gabay, C. (1998). Interleukin-1 receptor antagonist: Role in biology. *Annu. Rev. Immunol.* 16:27–32.

Azumi, A., and Atherton, S. S. (1998). T cells in the uninjected eye after anterior chamber inoculation of herpes simplex virus type 1. *Invest. Ophthalmol. Vis. Sci.* 39:78–83.

Azumi, A., Cousins, S. W., Kanter, M. Y., and Atherton, S. S. (1994). Modulation of murine herpes simplex virus type 1 retinitis in the uninoculated eye by CD4+ T lymphocytes. *Invest. Ophthalmol. Vis. Sci.* 35:54–63.

Banerjee, K., Biswas, P. S., Kumaraguru, U., Schoenberger, S. P., and Rouse, B. T. (2004). Protective and pathological roles of virus-specific and bystander CD8+ T cells in herpetic stromal keratitis. *J. Immunol.* 173:7575–7583.

Barsoum, I. S., Hardin, L. K., and Colley, D. G. (1988). Immune responses after conjunctiva exposure to *Chlamydia trachomatis* serovar A. *Med. Microbiol. Immunol. (Berl.)* 177:349–356.

Bigger, J. E., Tanigawa, M., Zhang, M., and Atherton, S. S. (2000). Murine cytomegalovirus infection causes apoptosis of uninfected retinal cells. *Invest. Ophthalmol. Vis. Sci.* 41:2248–2254.

Biswas, P. S., Banerjee, K., Kim, B., Kinchington, P. R., and Rouse, B. T. (2005). Role of inflammatory cytokine-induced cyclooxygenase 2 in the ocular immunopathologic disease herpetic stromal keratitis. *J. Virol.* 79:10589–10600.

Biswas, P. S., Banerjee, K., Kim, B., and Rouse, B. T. (2004a). Mice transgenic for IL-1 receptor antagonist protein are resistant to herpetic stromal keratitis: Possible role for IL-1 in herpetic stromal keratitis pathogenesis. *J. Immunol.* 172:3736–3744.

Biswas, P. S., Banerjee, K., Zheng, M., and Rouse, B. T. (2004b). Counteracting corneal immunoinflammatory lesion with interleukin-1 receptor antagonist protein. *J. Leukoc. Biol.* 76:868–875.

Buer, J., and Balling, R. (2003). Mice, microbes and models of infection. *Nat. Rev. Genet.* 4:195–205.

Carr, D. J., Ash, J., Lane, T. E., and Kuziel, W. A. (2006). Abnormal immune response of CCR5-deficient mice to ocular infection with herpes simplex virus type 1. *J. Gen. Virol.* 87:489–499.

Dinarello, C. A. (1996). Biological basis for interleukin-1 in disease. *Blood* 87:2095–2147.

Dinarello, C. A., and Wolff, S. M. (1993). The role of interleukin-1 in disease. *N. Engl. J. Med.* 328:106–113.

Dix, R. D., and Cousins, S. W. (2004). Susceptibility to murine cytomegalovirus retinitis during progression of MAIDS: Correlation with intraocular levels of tumor necrosis factor-alpha and interferon gamma. *Curr. Eye Res.* 29:173–180.

Dix, R. D., Podack, E. R., and Cousins, S. W. (2003). Loss of the perforin cytotoxic pathway predisposes mice to experimental cytomegalovirus retinitis. *J. Virol.* 77:3402–3408.

Engelbert, M., and Gilmore, M. S. (2005). Fas ligand but not complement is critical for control of experimental *Staphylococcus aureus* endophthalmitis. *Invest. Ophthalmol. Vis. Sci.* 46:2479–2486.

Fenton, R. R., Molesworth-Kenyon, S., Oakes, J. E., and Lausch, R. N. (2002). Linkage of IL-6 with neutrophil chemoattractant expression in virus-induced ocular inflammation. *Invest. Ophthalmol. Vis. Sci.* 43:737–743.

Garneau, M., Bolger, G. T., Bousquet, C., Kibler, P., Tremblay, F., and Cordingley, M. G. (2003). HPMC therapy of MCMV-induced retinal disease in the SCID mouse measured by electroretinography, a non-invasive technique. *Antiviral Res.* 59:193–200.

Gillette-Ferguson, I., Hise, A. G., Sun, Y., Diaconu, E., McGarry, H. F., Taylor, M. J., and Pearlman, E. (2006). *Wolbachia-* and *Onchocerca volvulus*-induced keratitis (river blindness) is dependent on myeloid differentiation factor 88. *Infect. Immun.* 74:2442–2445.

Girgis, D. O., Sloop, G. D., Reed, J. M., and O'Callaghan, R. J. (2003). A new topical model of *Staphylococcus* corneal infection in the mouse. *Invest. Ophthalmol. Vis. Sci.* 44:1591–1597.

Girgis, D. O., Sloop, G. D., Reed, J. M., and O'Callaghan, R. J. (2004). Susceptibility of aged mice to *Staphylococcus aureus* keratitis. *Curr. Eye Res.* 29:269–275.

Girgis, D. O., Sloop, G. D., Reed, J. M., and O'Callaghan, R. J. (2005). Effects of toxin production in a murine model of *Staphylococcus aureus* keratitis. *Invest. Ophthalmol. Vis. Sci.* 46:2064–2070.

Hall, L. R., Lass, J. H., Diaconu, E., Strine, E. R., and Pearlman, E. (1999). An essential role for antibody in neutrophil and eosinophil recruitment to the cornea: B cell-deficient (microMT) mice fail to develop Th2-dependent, helminth mediated keratitis. *J. Immunol.* 163:4970–4975.

Hazlett, L. D. (2002). Pathogenic mechanisms of *P. aeruginosa* keratitis: A review of the role of T cells, Langerhans cells, PMN, and cytokines. *DNA Cell Biol.* 21:383–390.

Hazlett, L. D. (2004). The corneal response to *Pseudomonas aeruginosa* infection. *Prog. Retin. Eye Res.* 23(1):1–30.

Hazlett, L. D., McClellan, S., and Goshgarian, C. (2005). The role of nitric oxide in resistance to *P. aeruginosa* ocular infection. *Ocul. Immunol. Inflamm.* 13:279–288.

Hazlett, L. D., Rudner, X. L., McClellan, S. A., Barrett, R. P., and Lighvani, S. S. (2002). Role of IL-12 and IFN-γ in *Pseudomonas aeruginosa* corneal infection. *Invest. Ophthalmol. Vis. Sci.* 43:419–424.

Heiligenhaus, A., Li, H. F., Yang, Y., Wasmuth, S., Bauer, D., and Steuhl, K. P. (2005). Transplantation of amniotic membrane in murine herpes stromal keratitis modulates matrix metalloproteinases in the cornea. *Invest. Ophthalmol. Vis. Sci.* 46:4079–4085.

Huang, X., Barrett, R. P., McClellan, S. A., and Hazlett, L. D. (2005). Silencing Toll-like receptor-9 in *Pseudomonas aeruginosa* keratitis. *Invest. Ophthalmol. Vis. Sci.* 46:4209–4216.

Huang, X., and Hazlett, L. D. (2003). Analysis of *Pseudomonas aeruginosa* corneal infection using oligonucleotide microarray. *Invest. Ophthalmol. Vis. Sci.* 44:3409–3416.

Huang, X., Hazlett, L. D., Du, W., and Barrett, R. P. (2006). SIGIRR promotes resistance against *Pseudomonas aeruginosa* keratitis by down-regulating type-1 immunity and IL-1R1 and TLR4 signaling. *J. Immunol.* 177:548–556.

Huang, X., McClellan, S. A., Barrett, R. P., and Hazlett, L. D. (2002). IL-18 contributes to host resistance against infection with *Pseudomonas aeruginosa* through induction of IFN-gamma production. *J. Immunol.* 68:5756–5763.

Hume, E. B., Cole, N., Khan, S., Garthwaite, L. L., Aliwarga, Y., Schubert, T. L., and Willcox, M. D. (2005). A *Staphylococcus aureus* mouse keratitis topical infection model: Cytokine balance in different strains of mice. *Immunol. Cell Biol.* 83:294–300.

Johnson, A. C., Heinzel, F. P., Diaconu, E., Sun, Y., Hise, A. G., Golenbock, D., Lass, J. H., and Pearlman, E. (2005). Activation of Toll-like receptor (TLR)2, TLR4, and TLR9 in the mammalian cornea induces MyD88-dependent corneal inflammation. *Invest. Ophthalmol. Vis. Sci.* 46:589–595.

Kaye, S., and Choudhary, A. (2006). Herpes simplex keratitis. *Prog. Retin. Eye Res.* 25:355–380.

Keadle, T. L., and Stuart, P. M. (2005). Interleukin-10 (IL-10) ameliorates corneal disease in a mouse model of recurrent herpetic keratitis. *Microb. Pathog.* 38:13–21.

Kernacki, K. A., Barrett, R. P., Hobden, J. A., and Hazlett, L. D. (2000). MIP-2 is a mediator of PMN influx in ocular bacterial infection. *J. Immunol.* 164:1037–1045.

Khatri, S., Lass, J. H., Heinzel, F. P., Petroll, W. M., Gomez, J., Diaconu, E., Kalsow, C. W., and Pearlman, E. (2002). Regulation of endotoxin-induced keratitis by PECAM-1, MIP-2, and Toll-like receptor 4. *Invest. Ophthalmol. Vis. Sci.* 43:2278–2284.

Kim, B., Lee, S., Suvas, S., and Rouse, B. T. (2005). Application of plasmid DNA encoding IL-18 diminishes development of herpetic stromal keratitis by antiangiogenic effects. *J. Immunol.* 175:509–516.

Kim, B., Tang, Q., Biswas, P. S., Xu, J., Schiffelers, R. M., Xie, F. Y., Ansari, A. M., Scarla, P. V., Woodle, M. C., Lu, P., and Rouse, B. T. (2004). Inhibition of ocular angiogenesis by siRNA targeting vascular endothelial growth factor pathway genes: Therapeutic strategy for herpetic stromal keratitis. *Am. J. Pathol.* 165:2177–1285.

Kwon, B., and Hazlett, L. D. (1997). Association of CD4+ T cell-dependent keratitis with genetic susceptibility to *Pseudomonas aeruginosa* ocular infection. *J. Immunol.* 159:6283–6290.

Labetoulle, M., Kucera, P., Ugolini, G., Lafay, F., Frau, E., Offret, H., and Flamand, A. (2000). Neuronal pathways for the propagation of herpes simplex virus type 1 from one retina to the other in a murine model. *J. Gen. Virol.* 81:1201–1210.

Lee, S., Zheng, M., Kim, B., and Rouse, B. T. (2002). Role of matrix metalloproteinase-9 in angiogenesis caused by ocular infection with herpes simplex virus. *J. Clin. Invest.* 110:1105–1111.

Lepisto, A. J., Frank, G. M., Xu, M., Stuart, P. M., and Hendricks, R. L. (2006). CD8 T cells mediate transient herpes stromal keratitis in CD4 deficient mice. *Invest. Ophthalmol. Vis. Sci.* 47:3400–3409.

Li, X. Y., and Niederkorn, J. Y. (1997). Immune privilege in the anterior chamber of the eye is not extended to intraocular *Listeria monocytogenes*. *Ocul. Immunol. Inflamm.* 5:245–257.

Lighvani, S., Huang, X., Trivedi, P. P., Swanborg, R. H., and Hazlett, L. D. (2005). Substance P regulates NK cell IFN-γ production and resistance to *Pseudomonas aeruginosa* infection. *Eur. J. Immunol.* 35:1567–1575.

Liu, T., Khanna, K. M., Chen, X., Fink, D. J., and Hendricks, R. L. (2000). CD8(+) T cells can block herpes simplex virus type 1 (HSV-1) reactivation from latency in sensory neurons. *J. Exp. Med.* 191:1459–1466.

Matsubara, S., and Atherton, S. S. (1997). Spread of HSV-1 to the suprachiasmatic nuclei and retina in T cell depleted BALB/c mice. *J. Neuroimmunol.* 75:51–58.

McClellan, S. A., Lighvani, S., and Hazlett, L. D. (2006). IFN-gamma: Regulation of nitric oxide in the *P. aeruginosa*-infected cornea. *Ocul. Immunol. Inflamm.* 14:21–28.

Niederkorn, J. Y., Peeler, J. S., and Mellon, J. (1989). Phagocytosis of particulate antigen by corneal epithelial cells stimulates interleukin-1 secretion and migration of Langerhans cells into the central cornea. *Reg. Immunol.* 2:83–90.

Niederkorn, J. Y., Ubelaker, J. E., McCulley, J. P., Stewart, G. L., Meyer, D. R., Mellon, J. A., Silvany, R. E., He, Y. G., Pidherney, M., et al. (1992). Susceptibility of corneas from various animal species to in vitro binding and invasion by *Acanthamoeba castellanii*. *Invest. Ophthalmol. Vis. Sci.* 33:104–112.

Norose, K., Aosai, F., Mun, H. S., and Yano, A. (2006). Effects of sulfamethoxazole on murine ocular toxoplasmosis in interferon-gamma knockout mice. *Invest. Ophthalmol. Vis. Sci.* 47: 265–271.

O'Brien, T. P., and Hazlett, L. D. (1996). Pathogenesis of ocular infection. In Jay S. Pepose, Gary N. Holland, and Kirk R. Wilhelmus (Eds.), *Ocular infection and immunity* (pp. 200–214). St. Louis: Mosby.

Osorio, Y., Cai, S., and Ghiasi, H. (2005). Treatment of mice with anti-CD86 reduces CD8+ T cell mediated CTL activity and enhances ocular viral replication in HSV-1 infected mice. *Ocul. Immunol. Inflamm.* 13:159–167.

Paniagua-Crespo, E., Hasle, D. P., Humphrey-Smith, I., Bellon, C., and Simitzis, A. M. (1989). Value of nu/nu mice in the production of experimental amoebic keratitis with Acanthamoeba. *CR Acad. Sci. III* 309:499–503.

Parks, Q. M., and Hobden, J. A. (2005). Polyphosphate kinase 1 and the ocular virulence of *Pseudomonas aeruginosa*. *Invest. Ophthalmol. Vis. Sci.* 46:248–251.

Pearlman, E., Hall, L. R., Higgins, L. W., Bardenstein, D. S., Diaconu, E., Hazlett, F. E., Albright, J., Kazura, J. W., and Lass, J. H. (1998). The role of eosinophils and neutrophils in helminth-induced keratitis. *Invest. Ophthalmol. Vis. Sci.* 39:1176–1182.

Pearlman, E., Lass, J. H., Bardenstein, D. S., Diaconu, E., Hazlett, F. E., Albright, J., Higgins, A. W., and Kazura, J. W. (1996). *Onchocerca volvulus*-mediated keratitis: Cytokine production by IL-4 deficient mice. *Exp. Parasitol.* 84:274–281.

Pearlman, E., Lass, J. H., Bardenstein, D. S., Kopf, M., Hazlett, F. E., Diaconu, E., and Kazura, J. W. (1995). Interleukin 4 and T helper type 2 cells are required for development of experimental onchocercal keratitis (river blindness). *J. Exp. Med.* 182:931–941.

Rudner, X. L., Kernacki, K. A., Barrett, R. P., and Hazlett, L. D. (2000). Prolonged elevation of IL-1 in *Pseudomonas aeruginosa* ocular infection regulates macrophage inflammatory protein-2 production, polymorphonuclear neutrophil persistence, and corneal perforation. *J. Immunol.* 164:6576–6582.

Saint Andre, A., Blackwell, N. M., Hall, L. R., Hoerauf, A., Brattig, N. W., Volkmann, L., Taylor, M. J., Ford, L., Hise, A. G., et al. (2002). The role of endosymbiotic Wolbachia bacteria in the pathogenesis of river blindness. *Science* 295: 1892–1895.

Steuhl, K. P., Doring, G., Henni, A., Thiel, H. J., and Botzenhart, K. (1987). Relevance of host-derived and bacterial factors in *Pseudomonas aeruginosa* corneal infection. *Invest. Ophthalmol. Vis. Sci.* 28:1559–1568.

Tanigawa, M., Bigger, J. E., Kanter, M. Y., and Atherton, S. S. (2000). Natural killer cells prevent direct anterior-to-posterior spread of herpes simplex virus type 1 in the eye. *Invest. Ophthalmol. Vis. Sci.* 41:132–137.

Tedesco, E. C., Smith, R. L., Corte-Real, S., and Calabrese, K. S. (2005). Ocular toxoplasmosis in mice: Comparison of two routes of infection. *Parasitology* 131:303–307.

Thakur, A., Barrett, R. P., Hobden, J. A., and Hazlett, L. D. (2004). Caspase-1 inhibitor reduces severity of *Pseudomonas aeruginosa* keratitis in mice. *Invest. Ophthalmol. Vis. Sci.* 45:3177–3184.

Valyi-Nagy, T., Sheth, V., Clement, C., Tiwari, V., Scanlan, P., Kavouras, J. H., Leach, L., Guzman-Hartman, G., Dermody, T. S., et al. (2004). Herpes simplex virus entry receptor nectin-1 is widely expressed in the murine eye. *Curr. Eye Res.* 29:303–309.

VINORES, S. A., WANY, Y., VINORES, M. A., DERERJANIK, N. L., SHI, A., KLEIN, D. A., DETRICK, B., and HOOKS, J. J. (2001). Blood-retinal barrier breakdown in experimental coronavirus retinopathy: Association with viral antigen, inflammation, and VEGF in sensitive and resistant strains. *J. Neuroimmunol.* 119: 175–182.

WANG, Y., BURNIER, M., DETRICK, B., and HOOKS, J. J. (1996). Genetic predisposition to coronavirus-induced retinal disease. *Invest. Ophthalmol. Vis. Sci.* 37:250–254.

WANG, Y., DETRICK, B., YU, Z. X., ZHANG, J., CHESKY, L., and HOOKS, J. J. (2000). The role of apoptosis within the retina of coronavirus-infected mice. *Invest. Ophthalmol. Vis. Sci.* 41:3011–3018.

WICKHAM, S., and CARR, D. J. (2004). Molecular mimicry versus bystander activation: Herpetic stromal keratitis. *Autoimmunity* 37:393–397.

WU, T. G., KEASLER, V. V., MITCHELL, B. M., and WILHELMUS, K. R. (2004). Immunosuppression affects the severity of experimental *Fusarium solani* keratitis. *J. Infect. Dis.* 190:192–198.

WU, T. G., WILHELMUS, K. R., and MITCHELL, B. M. (2003). Experimental keratomycosis in a mouse model. *Invest. Ophthalmol. Vis. Sci.* 44:210–216.

XU, M., LEPISTO, A. J., and HENDRICKS, R. L. (2004). CD154 signaling regulates the Th1 response to herpes simplex virus-1 and inflammation in infected corneas. *J. Immunol.* 173:1232–1239.

ZAIDI, T. S., PRIEBE, G. P., and PIER, G. B. (2006). A live-attenuated *Pseudomonas aeruginosa* vaccine elicits outer membrane protein-specific active and passive protection against corneal infection. *Infect. Immun.* 74:975–983.

ZHANG, M., XIN, H., and ATHERTON, S. S. (2005a). Murine cytomegalovirus (MCMV) spreads to and replicates in the retina after endotoxin-induced disruption of the blood-retinal barrier of immunosuppressed BALB/c mice. *J. Neurovirol.* 11:365–375.

ZHANG, M., XIN, H., DUAN, Y., and ATHERTON, S. S. (2005b). Ocular reactivation of MCMV after immunosuppression of latently infected BALB/c mice. *Invest. Ophthalmol. Vis. Sci.* 46:252–258.

ZHENG, M., DESHPANDE, S., LEE, S., FERARA, N., and ROUSE, B. T. (2001). Contribution of vascular endothelial growth factor in the neovascularization process during the pathogenesis of herpetic stromal keratitis. *J. Virol.* 75:9828–9835.

ZOLFAGHAR, I., EVANS, D. J., RONAGHI, R., and FLEISZIG, S. M. (2006). Type III secretion-dependent modulation of innate immunity as one of multiple factors regulated by *Pseudomonas aeruginosa* RetS. *Infect. Immun.* 3880–3889.

42 Mouse Models of Autoimmune and Immune-Mediated Uveitis

RACHEL R. CASPI

Uveitis, or inflammation of the uvea, is a generic term that denotes ocular inflammation. The condition may be of infectious or noninfectious origin. Infectious uveitis is discussed in chapter 41. Noninfectious uveitis, the subject of this chapter, was initially referred to as idiopathic but is now known to be of autoimmune or immune system–mediated etiology in many cases. Several human diseases typically characterized by detectable responses to protein antigens found in the retina and uvea fall in this category (Body et al., 2001; Nussenblatt and Whitcup, 2004). Some of these diseases are part of a generalized systemic syndrome in which the eye is only one of the organs involved. Examples of such diseases are anterior uveitis associated with juvenile rheumatoid arthritis or with ankylosing spondylitis (HLA-B27 related), and uveitides involving the posterior pole, such as Behçet's disease, Vogt-Koyanagi-Harada disease, and ocular sarcoidosis. Other types of uveitis target primarily the eye, with no signs of disease observed in other organs. Examples are sympathetic ophthalmia and birdshot retinochoroidopathy.

Traditionally, the rat (particularly the Lewis strain) served as a model for these diseases, but in the past two decades, mouse models of anterior and posterior uveitis have been developed and have given a tremendous push to basic studies of disease mechanisms. Models of uveitis can be divided into autoimmune, where a particular self antigen is known to be the target of an immunological attack, as opposed to immune-mediated, where inflammation is not driven by a response to a particular antigen. Autoimmune models can be further subdivided into induced models, with disease being precipitated by immunization with a retinal or uveal protein, and "spontaneous," which occur in genetically or surgically altered animals that have not, however, been actively immunized. A graphical representation of mechanistic relationships in rodent models of uveitis is shown in figure 42.1. The various uveitis models are reviewed by Caspi (2006a). This chapter concentrates on mouse models of experimental autoimmune uveitis (uveoretinitis) (EAU), induced and spontaneous, and also mentions endotoxin-induced uveitis (EIU), an important nonautoimmune model of anterior segment inflammation.

Although there are differences in the structure and composition of the retina between human and mouse, in the case of immune-mediated uveitis, anatomical interspecies differences are thought to be secondary. Of primary importance is the relationship between the eye and the immune system, which is believed to be similar in both species. This permits extrapolation from mouse models to the human in terms of immunological mechanisms involved in the pathogenesis and resolution of ocular autoimmune and inflammatory disease. The following discussion addresses the rapidly expanding uveitis research exploiting mouse models, its contribution to the understanding of fundamental mechanisms driving the disease, and the translational potential of using mouse models in terms of approaches to therapy.

Endotoxin-induced uveitis: Nonautoimmune anterior uveitis

Endotoxin-induced uveitis (EIU) is a model of anterior uveitis induced by peripheral injection of bacterial endotoxin (lipopolysaccharide, LPS), with primary involvement of the innate immune response elements, such as resident ocular macrophages that secrete cytokines and chemokines (Smith et al., 1998). EIU, initially developed in rats (Rosenbaum et al., 1980), was first reported in endotoxin-sensitive C3H/HeN mice by Kogiso et al. in 1992, and subsequently C3H/SW and FVB/N were also found to be susceptible (Li et al., 1995). EIU typically develops and peaks within 24 hours of a peripheral injection of endotoxin. A second peak of disease has been described 5 days after the first (Kozhich et al., 2000).

Although the EIU model is very robust, its limitation is that it may be "a model in search of a disease." Namely, there is some debate over which human disease it should represent. There may be parallels to anterior uveitis without systemic disease. It has also been used to represent anterior uveitis associated with rheumatic disease; however, LPS uveitis is of short duration and self-limiting, unlike anterior uveitis associated with rheumatic syndromes. A human equivalent to EIU that is not usually considered may be what is known as toxic anterior chamber syndrome, a sterile inflammation seen occasionally after intraocular surgery (e.g., cataract extraction) that is usually transient and is

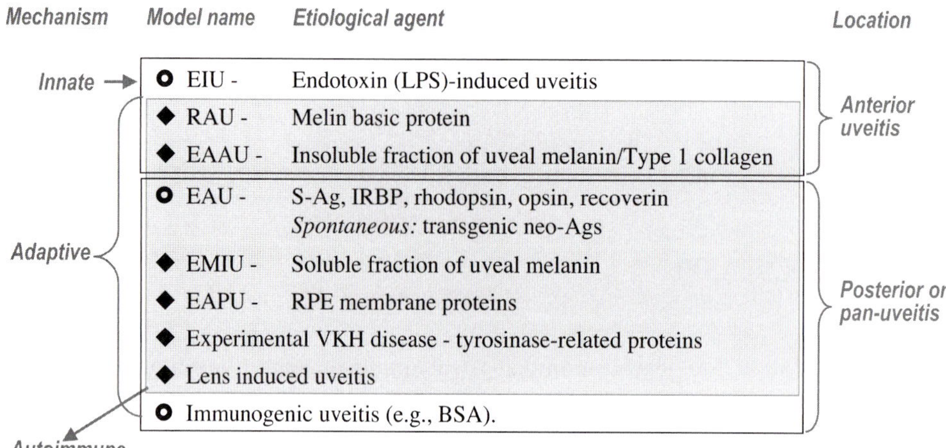

Mechanism
Model name
Etiological agent
Location
Innate
EIU - Endotoxin (LPS)-induced uveitis
RAU - Melin basic protein
EAAU - Insoluble fraction of uveal melanin/Type 1 collagen
Anterior uveitis
Adaptive
EAU - S-Ag, IRBP, rhodopsin, opsin, recoverin
Spontaneous: transgenic neo-Ags
EMIU - Soluble fraction of uveal melanin
EAPU - RPE membrane proteins
Experimental VKH disease - tyrosinase-related proteins
Lens induced uveitis
Immunogenic uveitis (e.g., BSA).
Posterior or pan-uveitis
Autoimmune

FIGURE 42.1 Inflammatory and autoimmune animal models of uveitis. Except as noted, all models are induced (endotoxin or immunization with the specified antigen). ◆, disease inducible in Lewis rats; **O**, disease inducible in both mice and rats. BSA, bovine serum albumin; EAAU, experimental autoimmune anterior uveitis; EAPU, experimental autoimmune posterior uveitis; EIU, endotoxin-induced uveitis; EMIU, experimental melanin-protein induced uveitis; RAU, recurrent anterior uveitis; VKH, Vogt-Koyanagi-Harada syndrome.

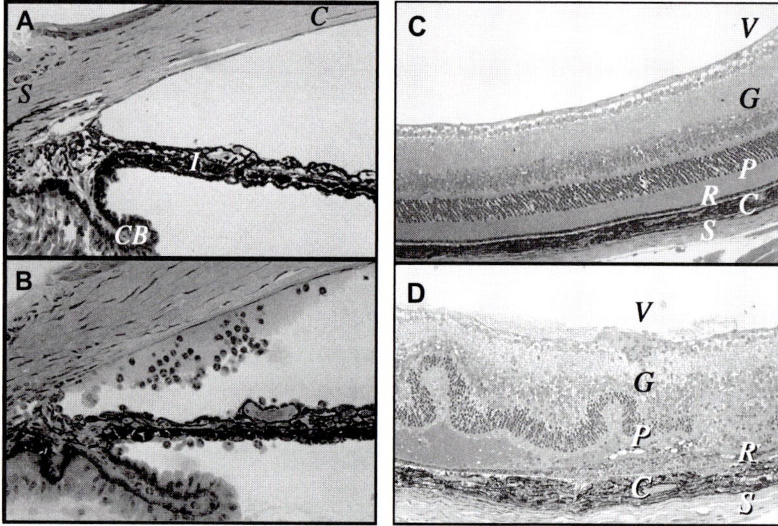

FIGURE 42.2 Typical histology of EIU and EAU in the mouse. Healthy compared to diseased eye tissue in EIU (*A* and *B*) and in EAU (*C* and *D*). *A*, Healthy anterior chamber. Shown is the angle where the iris and ciliary body connect to the sclera. C, cornea; CB, ciliary body; I, iris; S, sclera. *B*, EIU in a C3H mouse induced by subcutaneous injection of LPS. Note infiltration of inflammatory cells in the angle and around the iris and ciliary processes. Original magnification ×1200. *C*, Healthy mouse retina. C, choroid; G, ganglion cell layer; P, photoreceptor cell layer; R, retinal pigment epithelium; S, sclera; V, vitreous. *D*, EAU in the B10.RIII mouse induced by immunization with IRBP. Note structural disorganization and loss of nuclei in the ganglion and photoreceptor cell layers, retinal folds, subretinal exudate, vasculitis, damage to the retinal pigment epithelium, and choroid inflammation. Original magnification ×1000. See color plate 39. (Photomicrographs courtesy of Dr. Chi-Chao Chan, NEI, NIH.)

attributed to improper composition of surgical solutions (nonphysiologic or containing an irritant) or inadequate sterilization (endotoxin contamination) of solutions and instruments (Mamalis et al., 2006; Holland et al., 2007). It seems that a variety of noxious stimuli, not just LPS, can precipitate this syndrome. The release of pro-inflammatory cytokines could conceivably be triggered by a variety of noxious stimuli that cause tissue damage and constitute endogenous "danger" signals. In this scenario, endotoxin would be a model of a spectrum of causes having in common the triggering of local cytokine and chemokine release from innate immune and resident ocular cells. Irrespective of its exact human parallel, EIU continues to provide a useful model for the study of mechanisms of inflammation and inflammatory cell recruitment into the eye. Typical histological appearance of EIU in a C3H mouse can be seen in figure 42.2*B*.

A limitation to using the mouse as a model of anterior uveitis is that no autoimmune model of anterior uveitis in mice has yet been developed. Experimental autoimmune anterior uveitis (EAAU) or experimental melanin-induced uveitis (EMIU), two closely related models of anterior uveitis induced by melanin-associated antigens, so far are inducible only in rats. EAAU/EMIU is felt to be a more relevant model of human anterior uveitis than EIU because of its autoimmune etiology and recurrent nature (Smith et al., 1998). A robust model of mouse anterior uveitis on an autoimmune basis is needed.

Experimental autoimmune uveoretinitis and related models

EAU is autoimmune in nature and is thought to be a reasonably accurate representation of those (mainly posterior) uveitic diseases in which patients exhibit responses to retinal or uveal antigens. Although no single animal model can reproduce the complexity of human uveitis, there are now a number of EAU variants that may be useful for studying distinct aspects of uveitis or that provide unique insights into basic mechanisms of pathogenesis. The target antigen in EAU is usually a retinal antigen; therefore, it manifests as a uveoretinitis. However, the terms uveitis and uveoretinitis are used here interchangeably.

Experimental Autoimmune Uveoretinitis Induced by Active Immunization with Retinal Antigen Most patients who respond to retinal antigen, respond to a limited number of fragments (epitopes) of the retinal soluble antigen (S-Ag, retinal arrestin), although in advanced disease, additional specificities may be recognized (de Smet et al., 2001). This may suggest that S-Ag has a primary involvement and that responses to other antigens are secondary, resulting from autoimmunization to tissue breakdown products. EAU can be elicited in rats by immunization with S-Ag injected in emulsion with complete Freund's adjuvant (CFA) and has served for many years as a model of human uveitis. Unfortunately, and not for lack of trying by many laboratories, immunization with S-Ag has failed to reliably induce EAU in the commonly available strains of laboratory mice. A compounding difficulty was that many strains of laboratory mice carry the *rd* gene and have no photoreceptor cells by weaning time, eliminating them from evaluation. Among these are strains such as SJL/J and PL/J, which are susceptible to related autoimmune diseases, such as experimental autoimmune encephalomyelitis (EAE). In 1987 it was found that another retinal antigen, interphotoreceptor retinoid-binding protein (IRBP), is uveitogenic in rats (Gery et al., 1986), and subsequently we found that it also induces uveitis in several strains of mice (Caspi et al., 1988, 1990). As in rats, EAU in mice is induced by active immunization with IRBP in CFA, and a coinjection of pertussis toxin (PT) as additional adjuvant is usually needed. An exception is the B10.RIII strain (Jax strain B10.RIII-H2r H2-T18b/(71NS)SnJ; stock no. 000457), the most susceptible mouse strain currently known, which develops severe EAU after immunization with IRBP in CFA without the need for PT (Silver et al., 1999). Antibodies are produced as a result of immunization and have an amplifying role (Pennesi et al., 2003). Typical pathology of EAU in a B10.RIII mouse can be seen in figure 42.2*D*.

Because it is induced by immunization with a soluble protein, the EAU model as described earlier is MHC class II restricted; that is, the antigenic fragments of IRBP are presented by class II (mouse I-A and/or I-E) molecules and recognized by CD4+ T lymphocytes. The uveitogenic fragments of IRBP that induce disease in mice of the H-2^r, H-2^b, and H-2^a haplotypes have been identified, and disease can be induced by immunization with the synthetic peptides or by transfer of cells from donors immunized with the peptides, obviating the need to purify IRBP from natural sources or to produce it recombinantly. Table 42.1 summarizes the uveitogenic fragments of IRBP defined to date.

Experimental Autoimmune Uveoretinitis Induced by Adoptive Transfer of Antigen-Specific T Cells EAU is a cell-mediated response with central involvement of T lymphocytes with specificity for the immunizing retinal antigen. The full-blown disease can be induced by transferring T cells from donors immunized for induction of uveitis to genetically compatible recipients (Tarrant et al., 1998). Antigen-specific T cells can be propagated in vitro as long-term antigen-specific T cell lines (Silver et al., 1995). The adoptively transferred model is useful to represent the efferent (effector) phase of disease without any confounding effects of a continuing induction (priming) phase or effects of CFA.

Experimental Autoimmune Uveoretinitis in Mice Expressing a Transgenic Target Antigen in the Retina A variation on the theme of traditional EAU is the use of transgenic mice that are genetically engineered to express a foreign protein under control of a retina-specific promoter. Mice have been created that express β-galactosidase (β-gal) under the arrestin promoter, or that express hen egg lysozyme (HEL) under the rhodopsin promoter (Gregerson et al., 1999; Ham et al., 2004). This neo-self antigen can serve as an antigenic target for uveitis induced by active immunization or by adoptive transfer of the specific T cells, similarly to the native target IRBP. The advantages of such neo-antigen-driven EAU models are that they can permit more sophisticated approaches and questions that cannot be addressed in the more traditional EAU models, for example, by combining use of such mice with mice expressing a transgenic T cell receptor (TCR) specific for the retinal

Table 42.1

Uveitogenic peptides of IRBP

Strain	Class II Haplotype	Peptide Position and Amino Acid Sequence	Reference
B10.RIII	r	51–70: QTLASVLTAGVQSSLNDPRL	Cortes et al. (in press)
		161–180: SGIPYIISYLHPGNTILHVD	Silver et al., 1995
		541–560: SLGWATLVGEITAGNLLHTR	Cortes et al. (in press)
C57BL/6	b	1–20: GPTHLFQPSLVLDMAKVLLD	Avichezer et al., 2000
		461–480: LRHNPGGPSSAVPLLLSYFQ	Cortes et al. (in press)
		651–670: LAQGAYRTAVDLESLASQLT	Cortes et al. (in press)
		681–700: RLLVFHSPGELWEEAPPPP	Cortes et al. (in press)
B10.A, B10.BR	k	201–216: ADKDVVVLTSSRTGGV	Namba et al., 1998

neo-self antigen. A disadvantage of the use of neo-self antigen transgenic models is that expression of transgenic antigens is subject to integration effects, potentially resulting in unexpected expression patterns and artifacts. Transgenic mice expressing IRBP-specific TCRs are under development (Caspi et al., 2008).

Experimental Autoimmune Uveoretinitis Induced by Injection of Antigen-Pulsed Dendritic Cells An alternative model of IRBP-EAU that has recently been developed is elicited by adoptive transfer of in vitro matured dendritic cells (DCs) pulsed with the uveitogenic 161–180 peptide of IRBP (Tang et al., 2007). DCs have been identified as the most important antigen-presenting cells and are believed to be the only antigen-presenting cells that prime naive T cells that respond to their antigen for the first time. Understanding the requirements to prime a T cell for effector function versus regulatory function is of paramount importance. It is of interest that the disease induced by matured and antigen-pulsed DCs has a different clinical course and appearance and is also associated with a different type of effector response. The limitation of this model is the requirement for large numbers of DCs that have to be administered twice to elicit good disease scores (Tang et al., 2007). Its special advantage is that it provides an alternative model of EAU with unique characteristics and permits direct manipulation of DCs to study requirements for uveitogenic antigen presentation and possibly for tolerogenic presentation to already primed cells.

"Humanized" Experimental Autoimmune Uveoretinitis Model in Human Lymphocyte Antigen Transgenic Mice Although animal models can teach us about pathogenesis of disease, they cannot serve as templates for dissecting the antigenic specificity of the response, for the simple reason that they recognize different antigens, and different regions in the same antigens. This necessarily follows from the fact that their MHC molecules, which bind and present antigenic fragments to T lymphocytes, are different from those of humans. To address this issue, a number of laboratories have generated genetically engineered mice that transgenically express human MHC molecules (human lymphocyte antigen, HLA) in lieu of mouse MHC molecules (known as H-2). We examined susceptibility to EAU of single-transgenic mice expressing HLA-DR3, HLA-DR2, HLA-DQ6, or HLA-DQ8 (Pennesi et al., 2003). The HLA-Tg mice, similarly to wild-type mice, developed EAU after immunization with IRBP. Interestingly, HLA-DR3 Tg mice, and to a lesser extent other HLA transgenic mice, developed EAU with S-Ag, to which the parental wild-type strains are resistant. As mentioned earlier, S-Ag is the retinal antigen to which human patients most often exhibit lymphocyte responses. Interestingly, double-transgenic mice carrying a DR and a DQ molecule, which more closely mimics the situation in humans, exhibited changes in epitope recognition and enhanced susceptibility compared to the single transgenic counterparts (Mattapallil and Caspi, 2008). Thus, the "humanized" EAU model may help to identify the antigenic molecules and their critical regions that might be involved in driving human uveitis, and can help dissect the epistatic effects of HLA antigens on disease susceptibility and epitope recognition.

Spontaneous Experimental Autoimmune Uveoretinitis–Like Models of Uveitis Several models of spontaneous uveitis have been described. They differ from the induced models by not requiring active immunization or transfer of immune cells to trigger the disease, although they develop only in mice that have been genetically or surgically manipulated.

In humans, a type of uveitis known as birdshot retinochoroidopathy is highly associated with HLA-A29. Relative risks between 50 and 249 have been reported in different ethnic groups in various studies (Nussenblatt and Whitcup, 2004). Szpak et al. (2001) made an HLA-A29 Tg mouse and found that it spontaneously develops a posterior uveitis that closely resembles birdshot retinochoroidopathy. The target antigen has not been identified, but, owing to association with HLA-A29, an MHC class I molecule, it is expected to be an epitope(s) recognized by CD8+ effector T cells.

Two other spontaneous models, although developing in a very different way, probably share an underlying etiology, namely, spontaneous development of responsiveness to IRBP. (1) Ichikawa and collaborators (1991) reported that nude mice implanted with a neonatal rat thymus, which are known to develop a variety of autoimmune diseases, also develop spontaneous uveitis accompanied by humoral and cellular responses to IRBP. (2) A similar situation exists in mice deficient in the gene encoding the AIRE protein (Auto-Immune REgulator). AIRE is a molecule that controls ectopic expression of tissue antigens in the thymus, including several retinal antigens. As they age, AIRE knockout mice develop spontaneous uveitis also associated with responses to IRBP (Anderson et al., 2002; Devoss et al., 2006). The insights into basic mechanisms of uveitic disease gained from these models are discussed later in the chapter.

Uveitis Associated with Antitumor Response to Melanoma Antigen Gp100 (*Si*) is an antigen associated with melanin pigment that serves as a vaccination target for immunotherapy of melanoma. The antitumor effector cells induced by the vaccination regimen are CD8+ cytotoxic lymphocytes specific to gp100. Successful eradication of experimental melanoma in mouse models as well as in ongoing clinical trials of human melanoma immunotherapy is typically associated with autoimmune vitiligo (Kawakami and Rosenberg, 1997; Overwijk et al., 2003). It has recently been appreciated that these mice, in addition to generalized vitiligo, also develop a uveitis that can be quite severe (D. Palmer and N. P. Restifo, pers. comm., 2007). Of note, some melanoma patients given cellular immunotherapy targeting gp100 also were observed to develop uveitis (Robinson et al., 2004). This condition is reminiscent of Vogt-Koyanagi-Harada disease, in which patients develop vitiligo and uveitis and exhibit responses to melanin-related antigens (Boyd et al., 2001).

Basic mechanisms involved in uveitic disease as revealed by mouse models

Over the years, the various EAU models have provided invaluable insights into the fundamental mechanisms involved in acquisition of self tolerance to ocular antigens, its breakdown, the subsequent events that result in pathology, and the processes involved in resolution (figure 42.3). Based on combined evidence from many studies, the following discussion presents a putative scenario of the pathogenesis of uveitis. In a nutshell, retina-specific T cells that escape negative selection in the thymus cannot be efficiently tolerized in the periphery, owing to relative inaccessibility of retinal antigens, thus leaving a circulating pool of potentially uveitogenic T cells. “Natural” thymic-derived T-regulatory cells keep them under control, but upon encountering antigen-specific signals in the context of innate immune stimuli (“danger” signals), they can differentiate to an auto-aggressive Th1 or Th17 effector phenotype. When they reach the eye and recognize their specific antigen there, they initiate a cascade of recruitment and amplification that culminates in characteristic EAU. Ocular antigens released from inflamed tissue subsequently induce antigen-specific

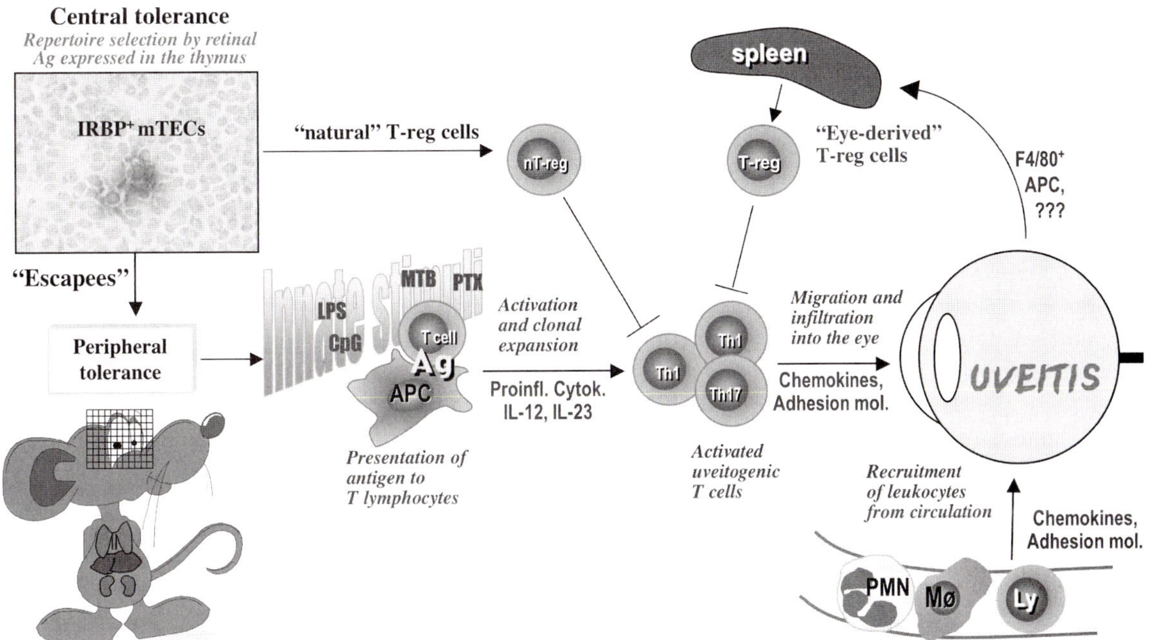

Figure 42.3 Critical checkpoints in EAU pathogenesis. Schematic representation of critical events and checkpoints in the pathogenesis of EAU as revealed by studies in mouse models. See color plate 40. (This figure was previously published in Caspi, 2006. Copyright does not apply.)

T-regulatory cells in a process requiring the spleen, which helps to reestablish homeostasis and limits recurrence of disease (reviewed in Caspi 2006b).

Susceptibility to Experimental Autoimmune Uveoretinitis Starts from Defects in T Cell Repertoire Selection

Self tolerance to tissue antigens, including uveitogenic retinal antigens such as S-Ag and IRBP, is first established through thymic selection (Kyewski and Klein, 2006). Lymphocytes passing through the thymus during their natural maturation process are selected for survival or death according to their ability to recognize self molecules. Many if not most tissue-specific antigens, including the retinal antigens S-Ag and IRBP, are expressed by specialized thymic epithelial cells. Immature lymphocytes that fail to recognize any self antigens undergo death "by neglect"; lymphocytes that recognize self with low affinity are selected for survival (positive selection), and lymphocytes possessing high-affinity antigen receptors for a self antigen are eliminated or tolerized (negative selection). Egwuagu et al. (1997) demonstrated that mice express relatively high levels of S-Ag in the thymus but low levels of IRBP, which correlates with their relative resistance to uveitis induced by S-Ag and susceptibility to IRBP-induced EAU. The lowest expression of IRBP was seen in B10.RIII mice, the mouse strain most susceptible to IRBP-induced EAU. These findings support the notion that inefficient thymic elimination of uveitogenic cells due to low expression of the selecting antigen predisposes to uveitis. (However, this does not explain the susceptibility to S-Ag-EAU of HLA-DR3 transgenic mice, unless their thymic expression of S-Ag is in some way altered by expression of human, instead of mouse, class II MHC molecules!)

Direct evidence that insufficient thymic elimination of retinal antigen-specific cells predisposes to autoimmune uveitis comes from the observation that T cells originating from IRBP-deficient mice are much more highly uveitogenic than T cells from wild-type mice, suggesting that a repertoire that has not been properly depleted of IRBP-reactive T cells indeed predisposes to autoimmunity (Avichezer et al., 2003). The two models of spontaneous uveitis described in the previous section lend further support to this notion (it should be noted that these models develop also other tissue-specific autoimmune manifestations, which are disregarded for the purposes of this discussion). Antiretina antibodies and cellular responses develop in mice deficient in the AIRE molecule, a transcription factor controlling ectopic expression of tissue antigens in the thymus. These mice fail to express retinal antigens in the thymus, and therefore, similarly to IRBP knockouts, cannot cull their lymphocyte repertoire of high-affinity uveitogenic T cells (Anderson et al., 2002; Devoss et al., 2006). This is reminiscent of the spontaneous uveitis that develops in athymic (nude) mice implanted with neonatal rat thymus. Although there is proper expression of retinal antigens in the thymus, they apparently cannot be presented to the mouse T cells because of an incompatibility between the participating thymic elements of the donor and the immune system of the recipient (Ichikawa et al., 1991).

Of note, in both these spontaneous models the antiretina response that develops targets IRBP, even though negative selection fails to other retinal antigens as well. Even in the absence of IRBP (double knockouts for AIRE and for IRBP), no other retinal antigens are recognized as surrogate targets for autoimmunity. This supports the concept of a species-specific primary autoantigen, which may help to explain why S-Ag is by far the most frequent antigen recognized by uveitis patients.

The thymus also selects "natural" regulatory T cells, which characteristically coexpress the molecules CD4 and CD25 (IL-2Rα chain, gene symbol *Il2ra*), which have a role in raising the threshold of susceptibility to EAU by keeping the potentially uveitogenic T cells in check (Avichezer et al., 2003; Grajewski et al., 2006). Interestingly, although IRBP expression in the thymus is required to select natural T-regulatory cells specific to IRBP, "polyclonal" T-regulatory cells specific to other antigens can also be harnessed to inhibit induction of uveitogenic effector T cells by innate stimuli (Grajewski et al., 2006), which might overlap with the innate stimuli necessary to trigger the induction of effector T cells.

Deficient Peripheral Tolerance as a Factor in Susceptibility to Experimental Autoimmune Uveoretinitis

Negative selection in the thymus is never fully efficient and, as discussed previously, is affected by the quantitative aspects of self-antigen expression in the thymus. Potentially autoreactive T cells that exit the thymus into the periphery normally have a "second chance" at tolerance as they recirculate through the tissues and encounter self antigens under noninflammatory conditions. However, unlike other organs, the eye becomes separated from the immune system early in ontogeny by an efficient blood-organ barrier that restricts free entry of lymphocytes into the eye, and also limits free exit of antigenic molecules from the eye, especially from the posterior segment. This separation from the immune system results in a circulating pool of uveitogenic lymphocytes that are not truly tolerant but merely "ignorant" of retinal antigens, and that can potentially be triggered into action by an (in)appropriate stimulus.

The notion that inadequate peripheral tolerance contributes to susceptibility is borne out by the finding that if these circulating, potentially uveitogenic lymphocytes are tolerized by expressing the uveitogenic retinal antigen outside of the eye, thus making it accessible to peripheral tolerance mechanisms, such mice become profoundly resistant to

EAU. Mice transgenic for β-gal on the S-Ag (arrestin) promoter express β-gal as a neo-self antigen in the retina, where it can serve as a target for EAU. Mice that also express β-gal in the periphery (ROSA26, JAX strain ID 004847) are tolerant and resist EAU induction by immunization with β-gal (Gregerson et al., 1999). In adult animals, infusion of genetically compatible B cells retrovirally transduced to express a uveitogenic fragment of IRBP also results in resistance to EAU (Agarwal et al., 2000). Peripheral tolerance thus constitutes a "weak link" in homeostasis of tolerance to retinal antigens, which might be successfully targeted therapeutically once the inciting retinal antigens in humans are positively identified.

Antigen Presentation to Uveitogenic Lymphocytes: What, Where, and by Whom? It is believed that the triggering event for uveitis is exposure of the circulating "ignorant" retina-specific T cells to their cognate antigen. A prototypic autoimmune disease of the eye that is believed to be triggered in this way is sympathetic ophthalmia, where a penetrating wound to one eye is followed after weeks or months by a destructive inflammation in the contralateral, "sympathizing" eye, apparently as a result of autoimmunization to retinal or uveal proteins (Boyd et al., 2001). However, for most types of autoimmune uveitis an exposure to antigen originating from the eye cannot be demonstrated, and it is believed that cross-reactive microbial antigens may provide such a stimulus through antigenic mimicry. A number of antigenic substances have been identified that cross-react with retinal S-Ag and induce EAU in rats, supporting the antigenic mimicry hypothesis (Wildner and Diedrichs-Mohring, 2004), but there are no reports as yet of molecular mimics that induce EAU in mice.

Where does the exposure to retinal antigens occur? The retina resides behind an efficient blood-organ barrier that restricts passage of molecules and of cells. Those lymphocytes that do enter the eye encounter a hostile environment composed of a variety of cell-bound and soluble inhibitory factors, as well as a paucity of professional antigen-presenting cells (APCs). Therefore, it is unlikely that priming of errant lymphocytes in the eye could occur and be a cause of uveitis. Rather, it is believed that lymphocyte priming takes place in the periphery, that is, in the lymph nodes, likely in conjunction with an adjuvant effect provided by a concomitant infection. Although the inside of the healthy eye lacks lymphatic drainage, antigen from an injured eye escapes into the subconjunctival, scleral, and periocular space, which is drained by the submandibular and cervical lymph nodes. In support of this notion, Camelo et al. (2006) demonstrated that injected antigen from the anterior chamber of the eye initially travels in a soluble form to secondary lymphoid organs via lymphatic and vascular routes. A microbial mimic antigen encountered through a wound or infection elsewhere in the body would drain to the relevant local lymph node, and would in addition provide its own adjuvant effect.

Who are the antigen-presenting cells? In order to present antigen for acquisition of effector function, the APC must express appropriate costimulatory molecules, which are induced by microbial or endogenous "danger" signals. Hence the need for adjuvant, whose role is discussed in more detail in the next section. In the draining lymph nodes, resident and migrating DCs serve as APCs to naive T cells, and the ability to induce EAU with antigen-pulsed DCs (Tang et al., 2007) is in line with this being a mechanism of priming in EAU. However, experimental evidence indicates that although the uveitogenic cells have been primed in the periphery, they must recognize their antigen within the eye for EAU to be induced (Prendergast et al., 1998; Chen et al., 2004). Although in the healthy eye there are few or no functional APCs in the retina, it is conceivable that those initial effector T cells that infiltrate the eye might induce a microenvironment through local cytokine secretion that would result in "arming" of resident cells such as microglia to acquire APC function. However, resident APCs may not be essential in the case of peripherally primed T cells, as APCs recruited from the circulation are sufficient to support EAU induction with activated retina-specific T cells (Gregerson and Kawashima, 2004).

Interestingly, and arguably of functional relevance to induction of uveitis, retinal antigens may facilitate their own presentation to uveitogenic T and B cells. We recently reported that both S-Ag and IRBP induce migration of immature DCs, as well as T and B lymphocytes, by binding to the chemotactic receptors CXCR3 and CXCR5 (Howard et al., 2005). This would accomplish a dual role, on one hand attracting immunocompetent cells to the site where antigen is present, and on the other hand promoting antigen presentation, as association of antigens with cells' surface receptors strongly enhances their uptake by APCs and their immunogenicity (Biragyn et al., 2004; Bonifaz et al., 2004).

Innate Immune Signals Trigger Autoimmunity: Toll Receptors and Other Danger Signals EAU is elicited by immunization with the retinal antigen in emulsion with CFA. The role of the adjuvant, through its mycobacterial component, is to provide innate immune danger signals to DCs, which then become activated and direct the ensuing adaptive T cell response toward a pro-inflammatory, tissue-destructive, effector phenotype. In the past decade much attention was focused on Toll-like receptors (TLRs) that recognize conserved pathogen-associated molecular patterns (PAMPs) and activate cells of the innate immune system, including macrophages, DCs, and granulocytes, although TLRs are by no means the only receptors that activate innate immune responses. The antigen-pulsed DCs used to elicit EAU in the model described earlier must be activated ("matured") in vitro using LPS (a TLR4 agonist) and at the same time crosslinking the CD40 molecules (costimulatory *tnfsf5*) by a monoclonal antibody, to acquire the ability to prime uveitogenic T cells for effector function (Tang et al., 2007). Antigen-pulsed DCs that have not been matured prime retinal antigen-specific T cells into a nonpathogenic, or even overtly regulatory, phenotype, and protect mice from a uveitogenic challenge with IRBP in CFA, presumably through induction of regulatory T cells (Jiang et al., 2003; Siepmann et al., 2007). It is currently not clear whether such immature DCs could convert to regulatory function T cells that had already acquired effector function, or whether the T-regulatory cells they induce are capable of inhibiting already primed effector cells, which would be important from the clinical point of view.

CFA provides its innate stimulatory effect not only through TLRs. The extent of dependence of EAU induction on TLR stimulation currently appears somewhat contradictory. In a transgenic uveitis model using mice that express HEL in their retina and receive an infusion of TCR transgenic T cells that express a HEL-specific TCR, coinjection of HEL with any one of several TLR ligands is sufficient to induce EAU (Fujimoto et al., 2006). Interestingly, PT, which in addition to being a TLR4 ligand also has other biological activities, was superior to "pure" TLR ligands in supporting induction of disease. In some situations, TLR signaling may be redundant with other innate signals. For example, in EAU induced with IRBP in CFA, single knockout mice deficient in TLR4, TLR9 or TLR2 (as well as double knockout mice lacking any two of these receptors) remain fully susceptible (Su et al., 2005). However, abrogation of IL-1 signaling (which, like the TLRs, also uses the MyD88 signaling pathway) prevented induction of EAU, indicating that whereas IL-1 signaling is necessary and nonredundant for effector T cell generation in EAU, signaling through TLRs may be replaced by other innate stimuli.

Recent data indicate that innate signaling is also important in activating natural T-regulatory cells (nT-regs) that protect from EAU. nT-regs can be activated by mycobacterial components present in CFA (Grajewski et al., 2006) and limit induction of uveitogenic effector T cells, though it is obviously the latter that "win out" when EAU is induced. Preliminary data implicate TLR signaling in nT-reg activation (Grajewski, 2006), but it is currently not clear whether the effect is direct or indirect.

Pathogenic Effectors: Th1 or Th17? Retinal antigen-specific T cells that have encountered a uveitogenic stimulus acquire a pro-inflammatory, tissue-destructive effector phenotype. This depends strictly on the presence of the innate danger signals discussed earlier, many of which are still probably unidentified, that induce appropriate cytokine production and costimulatory molecule expression on APCs. It has long been known that Th1-like cells, which are induced in the presence of IL-12 and whose hallmark is the production of IFN-γ, are a pathogenic effector phenotype (Xu et al., 1997). EAU can be transferred with a few million primary IRBP-specific IFN-γ-producing effector T cells, or less than a million cells from a polarized IRBP-specific Th1 cell line (Silver et al., 1999). IRBP-specific T cells that do not produce IFN-γ and are not pathogenic can be converted in the presence of IL-12 into a pathogenic, IFN-γ-producing phenotype (Tarrant et al., 1998).

Recently a new effector phenotype has been described and shown to be centrally involved in several autoimmune and inflammatory diseases. Its induction and maintenance depend, respectively, on TGF-β + IL-6 and on IL-23, and its hallmark cytokine is IL-17 (Bowman et al., 2006). Some studies have gone so far as to suggest that it is the IL-17-producing "Th17" effectors that are the main players in tissue destructive autoimmunity, and that Th1 cells play at best only a minor role. However, recent data in the EAU model support a distinct role for the Th1 effector phenotype.

In murine EAU, both Th1 and Th17 antigen-specific effectors are induced in mice by uveitogenic immunization with IRBP. Studies aimed at elucidating their relative roles suggest that both participate in pathogenesis, and conceivably complement each other. On one hand, a small number of cells from an IRBP-specific Th1 cell line, which is unable to produce IL-17, elicits severe EAU. This speaks strongly in favor of an important role for Th1 effector T cells. On the other hand, polarized Th17 cell lines unable to produce IFN-γ elicit EAU, and neutralization of IL-17 in IRBP/CFA-immunized hosts aborts EAU even when started 7 days after immunization, implicating IL-17 as an effector cytokine (Luger et al., in press). The question of whether IFN-γ is an effector cytokine or just a hallmark of Th1 cells is more complex to answer, as neutralization of IFN-γ in immunized mice exacerbates EAU, and IFN-γ knockout mice develop severe disease. This appears to be due at least in part to inhibition of Th1 effector cell generation by a feedback effect of IFN-γ in a process involving induction of nitric oxide and apoptosis (Tarrant et al., 1999). However, when EAU is induced by adoptive transfer of polarized IFN-γ-producing Th1 effector lymphocytes, treatment with anti-IFN-γ inhibits disease, suggesting that IFN-γ does have an effector function(s) (Luger et al., in press). Additionally, antigen-pulsed mature DCs from wild-type mice fail to induce EAU in IFN-γ knockout recipients, even though these mice produce large amounts of IL-17, suggesting that an IFN-γ-producing antigen-specific effector is important (Tang et al., 2007). IFN-γ is thus a double-edged sword, and its effects on disease depend on where and when it is produced.

Effector Cell Migration, Infiltration, and Inflammatory Cell Recruitment Activated antigen-specific T cells that had been primed in peripheral lymphoid tissues must migrate and find their way to the eye if uveitis is to occur. Although often we refer to this as "homing" to the eye, the term is probably not correct, as it is unlikely that immune cells are able to detect retinal antigens on the other side of the blood-retinal barrier in a healthy, unmanipulated eye (Gregerson et al., 1999). It is likely that extravasation of antigen-specific T cells primed elsewhere into the eye occurs at random (Prendergast et al., 1998; Caspi, 2006b). Because of the small size of the retina it is possible to retrieve essentially all the cells that have entered the target tissue. By a simple calculation of how many cells were injected versus how many can be retrieved from the retina it appears that only a few such cells (fewer than 15) are needed to trigger the sequence of events leading to EAU (Caspi, 2006b). Release of inflammatory mediators by these initial cells "activates" the vascular endothelium of the retina and uvea, promoting adhesion of passing cells and facilitating recruitment of all types of leukocytes from the circulation. Since the great majority of the infiltrating cells found in a uveitic eye are the recruited leukocytes (Pennesi et al., 2003; Chen et al., 2006), it is clear that this recruitment provides a massive amplification mechanism.

When antigen-specific donor T cells are transferred into a naive host with a healthy eye, there is a period of several days after the initial antigen-specific donor T cells enter the retina when nothing much seems to happen in the eye. However, changes undetectable by current methods must be taking place in the local microenvironment, including changes in the blood-retinal barrier and the production of chemotactic substances in the target tissue, that will facilitate subsequent massive recruitment of leukocytes from the periphery. This is evident from the finding that only transfer of retinal antigen-specific T cells, but not of activated T cells that do not recognize retinal antigens, is followed by a massive entry of additional donor T cells and of recruited host cells into the eye on the fourth day after transfer (Prendergast et al., 1998; Chen et al., 2004, 2006). Studies in a transgenic EAU model showed that during this seemingly quiescent period, the bulk of the uveitogenic T cells accumulate in the recipient's spleen, where they proliferate and activate nonspecific host CD4+ T cells. They also undergo (and induce) changes in chemokine and adhesion molecule expression, which culminates on day 4 in a mass emigration of donor and host cells from the spleen to the eye and EAU induction (Chen et al., 2004, 2006).

Owing to the transparency of ocular media, the eye offers special advantages as a model for analyzing cellular interactions, leukocyte flow, adhesion, and extravasation of cells by intravital microscopy. Unlike in other tissues, intravital microscopy in the eye does not require invasive procedures, which by themselves may modify cellular interactions and behavior. Thus, it is possible to easily visualize sticking, rolling, and extravasation of leukocytes, and to track the T cell infiltration into the eye and the cells' interactions with putative APCs there (Rosenbaum et al., 2002). Similar techniques are being applied to the human eye and should yield important information about the pathogenic processes in human uveitis.

Natural Resolution Mechanisms In humans, uveitis can remit spontaneously even without treatment, and the disease in animal models is self-limiting without necessarily proceeding to destruction of the entire retina and elimination of the source of inciting antigen. The mechanisms that bring about remission are not completely understood. Unraveling natural resolution mechanisms of disease can give us clues to the types of processes that we would wish to promote via immunotherapy.

An important mechanism that is being actively studied in mouse models is regulatory T cells. Several types of T-regulatory cells related to uveitis have been described (Stein-Streilein and Taylor, 2007), but their origin and the relationships between them remain unclear. As mentioned earlier, CD4+CD25+ thymic-derived nT-regs protect from induction of EAU (Grajewski et al., 2006), and although in disease their threshold of protection has obviously been overcome, they may proliferate and constitute a homeostatic mechanism that would help to bring about remission. T-regulatory cells can also be induced or converted from CD25− populations, which also give rise to effector T lymphocytes, and under some conditions functional effectors may also convert to acquire T-regulatory properties. As an example, IRBP-specific T cells may be converted from effectors to regulators by aqueous humor, a phenomenon that has been attributed to the effects of TGF-β and inhibitory neuropeptides (Stein-Streilein and Taylor, 2007). Natural T-regulatory cells as well as some types of induced T-regulatory cells express the transcription factor FoxP3, but although expression of this molecule is generally recognized to be indicative of T-regulatory cell function, it does not follow that the regulatory cells that express it are necessarily descended from CD4+CD25+ nT-regs (Ziegler, 2006).

The uniquely eye-related phenomenon of anterior chamber–associated immune deviation (ACAID) has been well studied. It is induced by injection of antigen into the anterior chamber of the eye and results in development of regulatory CD4+ and CD8+ T cells that inhibit, respectively, the induction and the expression of antigen-specific immune responses (Stein-Streilein and Streilein, 2002). Although elicitation of ACAID to IRBP protects mice from EAU (Hara et al., 1992), it is difficult to conclude that ACAID represents a natural mechanism of protection from autoimmunity used by the intact eye. This is because ACAID results from injection of an antigen into the anterior chamber of the eye, necessarily perturbing its integrity. It is possible, in fact, that such mechanisms come into play as a result of damage to the eye. IRBP-specific T-regulatory cells, though apparently distinct from ACAID-induced T-regulatory cells, are induced as a result of EAU. Such cells are found in mice that have recovered from EAU and limit reinduction of disease (Kitaichi et al., 2005). Interestingly, their induction is dependent on the presence of the eye, indicating that something originating in the eye is crucial to their development. The eye could be necessary as a source of antigen, or of inhibitory factors such as α-MSH, which has been shown to convert primed IRBP-specific T cells to a regulatory phenotype (Stein-Streilein and Taylor, 2007).

Other mechanisms of suppression could conceivably include production of inhibitory cytokines, such as IL-10 and TGF-β, or inhibition by contact-driven mechanisms. IL-10 is detected in the retina of mice recovering from EAU, and can inhibit activation and function of already immune effector T cells, which are impervious to the inhibitory effects of TGF-β (Xu et al., 1997; Rizzo et al., 1998; Xu et al., 2003). They could also include contact with ocular resident cells, such as retinal glial Müller cells, which proliferate during uveitis as part of the process of healing and retinal scar formation, and whose proliferation in vitro is induced by activated lymphocyte/monocyte products (Caspi et al., 1987). Müller cells are able to inhibit activation and function of T cells, even if these T cells have previously been activated, and similar inhibitory effects are exerted by retinal pigment epithelial cells and iris/ciliary body epithelial cells (Caspi et al., 1987; Yoshida et al., 2000). In some cases interaction with ocular resident cells additionally induces conversion of T cells to a regulatory phenotype (Ishida et al., 2003; Sugita et al., 2006). Only some of the molecular interactions involved in these phenomena have been characterized.

Translational potential

Many of critical checkpoints in pathogenesis of uveitis, as defined in mouse models and depicted in figure 42.3, can serve as targets for immunotherapeutic intervention. To mimic the clinical situation in which the patient already has acquired immunity to retinal autoantigens, ideally the experimental approaches should be able not only to prevent but also to reverse disease. However, approaches that target only acquisition of immunity may also be of value, since chronic autoimmunity involves constant priming of new lymphocytes and their entry into the effector pool. This section provides some examples of possible immunotherapeutic approaches, drawing on what we have learned about disease pathogenesis, but it is by no means an exhaustive discussion of the translation of experimental approaches to the clinic.

Deficits in peripheral tolerance could be corrected in the adult animal by expressing the retinal antigen outside the eye in a tolerance-inducing form. Agarwal et al. showed that infusion of B cells, made to express a uveitogenic fragment of IRBP into susceptible mice, resulted in a profound and long-term induction of resistance to EAU, and moreover was able not only to prevent but also to reverse the disease process (Agarwal et al., 2000). Adapting this regimen to autologous human B cells using S-Ag, which appears to be the major retinal antigen recognized by humans, could represent a viable approach to therapy of uveitis, a notion that is supported by the ability of S-Ag-transduced B cells to inhibit EAU in HLA-DR3 transgenic mice (Liang et al., 2006). Another antigen-based approach to prevent EAU that has been successful in animal models is induction of oral tolerance by feeding retinal antigens. In uveitis patients, oral administration of S-Ag showed promise in a double-blind, placebo-controlled Phase I/II clinical trial; however, larger trials are required to establish efficacy (Nussenblatt, 2002).

A limitation of antigen-based therapy is that it requires knowledge of the inciting retinal antigen. Although uveitis-associated antigens are increasingly being identified, there are still many unknowns. Furthermore, the phenomenon of epitope and antigen spreading, which can accompany chronic autoimmune disease, could make identification of the antigen(s) driving pathology at a given time a moving target. Finally, there are concerns about introducing the putative disease-inciting antigen into an already immune individual.

Immunotherapeutic approaches that target common pathways of lymphocyte activation do not require knowledge of the inciting antigen, but are not as selective, and therefore have the potential to also inhibit immunity to pathogens. Several such approaches have been examined in mouse models of uveitis, and some appear to have clinical potential. For example, costimulatory molecule blockade targeting the B7 or CD40 pathways inhibits induction of EAU pathology in mice (Silver et al., 2000; Bagenstose et al., 2005). However, it does not induce long-term tolerance, contrary to reports in transplantation models. Thus, in theory, continuing treatment would be needed to maintain protection. A related approach is blockade of the IL-2 receptors, which are present on all activated T cells. This approach was shown to inhibit EAU in animals, and IL-2 receptor blockade with humanized anti-CD25 antibodies (Daclizumab or Zenapax) showed efficacy in clinical trials (Nussenblatt et al., 1999). Surprisingly, the mechanism of action of this treatment in humans appears to involve CD56-high regulatory natural killer (NK) cells rather than elimination of the CD25+ effector T cells, as had initially been assumed (Li et al., 2005).

Migration and infiltration of recruited cells into the eye, which constitutes a necessary mechanism for disease induction and progression, could be targeted by blockade of adhesion molecules or of chemokines and chemokine receptors. Blockade of the adhesion molecules ICAM-1 and LFA-1 in mice inhibited EAU, presumably by blocking inflammatory cell recruitment (Whitcup et al., 1993), as does blockade of the chemokine receptor CXCR3, which is important for migration of uveitogenic and recruited cells into the eye (Chen et al., 2004).

Finally, the effector cytokines produced by pathogenic T cells and the inflammatory leukocytes recruited by them may serve as targets for inhibition or neutralization. Neutralization of IL-17 by monoclonal antibodies in mice aborts disease even when instituted after the uveitogenic effectors have already been generated (Luger et al., in press). Similarly, TNF-α neutralization, which had been shown in animal models to be protective, is showing efficacy in clinical trials for some types of uveitis (Greiner et al., 2004).

These examples underscore the contribution of research in animal models to understanding the fundamental mechanisms driving ocular autoimmune and inflammatory disease, and their importance in devising novel therapies to combat sight-threatening uveitic diseases.

REFERENCES

Agarwal, R. K., Kang, Y., Zambidis, E., Scott, D. W., Chan, C. C., and Caspi, R. R. (2000). Retroviral gene therapy with an immunoglobulin-antigen fusion construct protects from experimental autoimmune uveitis. *J. Clin. Invest.* 106:245–252.

Anderson, M. S., Venanzi, E. S., Klein, L., Chen, Z., Berzins, S. P., Turley, S. J., von Boehmer, H., Bronson, R., Dierich, A., et al. (2002). Projection of an immunological self shadow within the thymus by the aire protein. *Science* 298:1395–1401.

Avichezer, D., Grajewski, R. S., Chan, C. C., Mattapallil, M. J., Silver, P. B., Raber, J. A., Liou, G. I., Wiggert, B., Lewis, G. M., et al. (2003). An immunologically privileged retinal antigen elicits tolerance: Major role for central selection mechanisms. *J. Exp. Med.* 198:1665–1676.

Avichezer, D., Silver, P. B., Chan, C. C., Wiggert, B., and Caspi, R. R. (2000). Identification of a new epitope of human IRBP that induces autoimmune uveoretinitis in mice of the H-2b haplotype. *Invest. Ophthalmol. Vis. Sci.* 41:127–131.

Bagenstose, L. M., Agarwal, R. K., Silver, P. B., Harlan, D. M., Hoffmann, S. C., Kampen, R. L., Chan, C. C., and Caspi, R. R. (2005). Disruption of CD40/CD40-ligand interactions in a retinal autoimmunity model results in protection without tolerance. *J. Immunol.* 175:124–130.

Biragyn, A., Ruffini, P. A., Coscia, M., Harvey, L. K., Neelapu, S. S., Baskar, S., Wang, J. M., and Kwak, L. W. (2004). Chemokine receptor-mediated delivery directs self-tumor antigen efficiently into the class II processing pathway in vitro and induces protective immunity in vivo. *Blood* 104:1961–1969.

Bonifaz, L. C., Bonnyay, D. P., Charalambous, A., Darguste, D. I., Fujii, S., Soares, H., Brimnes, M. K., Moltedo, B., Moran, T. M., et al. (2004). In vivo targeting of antigens to maturing dendritic cells via the DEC-205 receptor improves T cell vaccination. *J. Exp. Med.* 199:815–824.

Bowman, E. P., Chackerian, A. A., and Cua, D. J. (2006). Rationale and safety of anti-interleukin-23 and anti-interleukin-17A therapy. *Curr. Opin. Infect. Dis.* 19:245–252.

Boyd, S. R., Young, S., and Lightman, S. (2001). Immunopathology of the noninfectious posterior and intermediate uveitides. *Surv. Ophthalmol.* 46:209–233.

Camelo, S., Kezic, J., Shanley, A., Rigby, P., and McMenamin, P. G. (2006). Antigen from the anterior chamber of the eye travels in a soluble form to secondary lymphoid organs via lymphatic and vascular routes. *Invest. Ophthalmol. Vis. Sci.* 47: 1039–1046.

Caspi, R. R. (2006a). Animal models of autoimmune and immune-mediated uveitis (http://dx.doi.org/10.1016/j.ddmod.2006.03.005). *Drug Discov. Today: Dis. Mod.* 3:3–10 (www.sciencedirect.com/science/journal/17406757).

Caspi, R. R. (2006b). Ocular autoimmunity: The price of privilege? *Immunol. Rev.* 213:23–35.

Caspi, R. R. (2008). Unpublished results.

Caspi, R. R., Chan, C. C., Leake, W. C., Higuchi, M., Wiggert, B., and Chader, G. J. (1990). Experimental autoimmune uveoretinitis in mice: Induction by a single eliciting event and dependence on quantitative parameters of immunization. *J. Autoimmun.* 3:237–246.

Caspi, R. R., Roberge, F. G., Chan, C. C., Wiggert, B., Chader, G. J., Rozenszajn, L. A., Lando, Z., and Nussenblatt, R. B. (1988). A new model of autoimmune disease. Experimental autoimmune uveoretinitis induced in mice with two different retinal antigens. *J. Immunol.* 140:1490–1495.

Caspi, R. R., Roberge, F. G., and Nussenblatt, R. B. (1987). Organ-resident, nonlymphoid cells suppress proliferation of autoimmune T-helper lymphocytes. *Science* 237:1029–1032.

Chen, J., Fujimoto, C., Vistica, B. P., Wawrousek, E. F., Kelsall, B., and Gery, I. (2006). Active participation of antigen-nonspecific lymphoid cells in immune-mediated inflammation. *J. Immunol.* 177:3362–3368.

Chen, J., Vistica, B. P., Takase, H., Ham, D. I., Fariss, R. N., Wawrousek, E. F., Chan, C. C., DeMartino, J. A., Farber, J. M., et al. (2004). A unique pattern of up- and down-regulation of chemokine receptor CXCR3 on inflammation-inducing Th1 cells. *Eur. J. Immunol.* 34:2885–2894.

Cortes, L. M., Mattapallil, M. J., Silver, P. B., Donoso, L. A., Liou, G. I., Zhu, W., Chan, C. C., and Caspi, R. R. (in press). Repertoire analysis and new pathogenic epitopes of IRBP in C57BL/6 ($H-2^b$) and B10.RIII ($H-2^r$) mice. *Invest. Ophthalmol. Vis. Sci.*

de Smet, M. D., Bitar, G., Mainigi, S., and Nussenblatt, R. B. (2001). Human S-antigen determinant recognition in uveitis. *Invest. Ophthalmol. Vis. Sci.* 42:3233–3238.

Devoss, J., Hou, Y., Johannes, K., Lu, W., Liou, G. I., Rinn, J., Chang, H., Caspi, R., Fong, L., et al. (2006). Spontaneous autoimmunity prevented by thymic expression of a single self-antigen. *J. Exp. Med.* 203:2727–2735.

Egwuagu, C. E., Charukamnoetkanok, P., and Gery, I. (1997). Thymic expression of autoantigens correlates with resistance to autoimmune disease. *J. Immunol.* 159:3109–3112.

Fujimoto, C., Yu, C. R., Shi, G., Vistica, B. P., Wawrousek, E. F., Klinman, D. M., Chan, C. C., Egwuagu, C. E., and Gery, I. (2006). Pertussis toxin is superior to TLR ligands in enhancing pathogenic autoimmunity, targeted at a neo-self antigen, by triggering robust expansion of Th1 cells and their cytokine production. *J. Immunol.* 177:6896–6903.

Gery, I., Wiggert, B., Redmond, T. M., Kuwabara, T., Crawford, M. A., Vistica, B. P., and Chader, G. J. (1986).

Uveoretinitis and pinealitis induced by immunization with interphotoreceptor retinoid-binding protein. *Invest. Ophthalmol. Vis. Sci.* 27:1296–1300.

Grajewski, R. S. (2006). Unpublished results.

Grajewski, R. S., Silver, P. B., Agarwal, R. K., Su, S. B., Chan, C. C., Liou, G. I., and Caspi, R. R. (2006). Endogenous IRBP can be dispensable for generation of natural CD4+CD25+ regulatory T cells that protect from IRBP-induced retinal autoimmunity. *J. Exp. Med.* 203:851–856.

Gregerson, D. S., and Kawashima, H. (2004). APC derived from donor splenocytes support retinal autoimmune disease in allogeneic recipients. *J. Leukoc. Biol.* 76:383–387.

Gregerson, D. S., Torseth, J. W., McPherson, S. W., Roberts, J. P., Shinohara, T., and Zack, D. J. (1999). Retinal expression of a neo-self antigen, beta-galactosidase, is not tolerogenic and creates a target for autoimmune uveoretinitis. *J. Immunol.* 163: 1073–1080.

Greiner, K., Murphy, C. C., Willermain, F., Duncan, L., Plskova, J., Hale, G., Isaacs, J. D., Forrester, J. V., and Dick, A. D. (2004). Anti-TNFalpha therapy modulates the phenotype of peripheral blood CD4+ T cells in patients with posterior segment intraocular inflammation. *Invest. Ophthalmol. Vis. Sci.* 45:170–176.

Ham, D. I., Kim, S. J., Chen, J., Vistica, B. P., Fariss, R. N., Lee, R. S., Wawrousek, E. F., Takase, H., Yu, C. R., et al. (2004). Central immunotolerance in transgenic mice expressing a foreign antigen under control of the rhodopsin promoter. *Invest. Ophthalmol. Vis. Sci.* 45:857–862.

Hara, Y., Caspi, R. R., Wiggert, B., Chan, C. C., Wilbanks, G. A., and Streilein, J. W. (1992). Suppression of experimental autoimmune uveitis in mice by induction of anterior chamber-associated immune deviation with interphotoreceptor retinoid-binding protein. *J. Immunol.* 148:1685–1692.

Holland, S. P., Morck, D. W., and Lee, T. L. (2007). Update on toxic anterior segment syndrome. *Curr. Opin. Ophthalmol.* 18: 4–8.

Howard, O. M., Dong, H. F., Su, S. B., Caspi, R. R., Chen, X., Plotz, P., and Oppenheim, J. J. (2005). Autoantigens signal through chemokine receptors: Uveitis antigens induce CXCR3- and CXCR5-expressing lymphocytes and immature dendritic cells to migrate. *Blood* 105:4207–4214.

Ichikawa, T., Taguchi, O., Takahashi, T., Ikeda, H., Takeuchi, M., Tanaka, T., Usui, M., and Nishizuka, Y. (1991). Spontaneous development of autoimmune uveoretinitis in nude mice following reconstitution with embryonic rat thymus. *Clin. Exp. Immunol.* 86:112–117.

Ishida, K., Panjwani, N., Cao, Z., and Streilein, J. W. (2003). Participation of pigment epithelium in ocular immune privilege. 3. Epithelia cultured from iris, ciliary body, and retina suppress T-cell activation by partially non-overlapping mechanisms. *Ocul. Immunol. Inflamm.* 11:91–105.

Jiang, H. R., Muckersie, E., Robertson, M., and Forrester, J. V. (2003). Antigen-specific inhibition of experimental autoimmune uveoretinitis by bone marrow-derived immature dendritic cells. *Invest. Ophthalmol. Vis. Sci.* 44:1598–1607.

Kawakami, Y., and Rosenberg, S. A. (1997). Immunobiology of human melanoma antigens MART-1 and gp100 and their use for immuno-gene therapy. *Int. Rev. Immunol.* 14:173–192.

Kitaichi, N., Namba, K., and Taylor, A. W. (2005). Inducible immune regulation following autoimmune disease in the immune-privileged eye. *J. Leukoc. Biol.* 77:496–502.

Kogiso, M., Tanouchi, Y., Mimura, Y., Nagasawa, H., and Himeno, K. (1992). Endotoxin-induced uveitis in mice. 1. Induction of uveitis and role of T lymphocytes. *Jpn. J. Ophthalmol.* 36:281–290.

Kozhich, A. T., Chan, C. C., Gery, I., and Whitcup, S. M. (2000). Recurrent intraocular inflammation in endotoxin-induced uveitis. *Invest. Ophthalmol. Vis. Sci.* 41:1823–1826.

Kyewski, B., and Klein, L. (2006). A central role for central tolerance. *Annu. Rev. Immunol.* 24:571–606.

Li, Q., Peng, B., Whitcup, S. M., Jang, S. U., and Chan, C. C. (1995). Endotoxin induced uveitis in the mouse: Susceptibility and genetic control. *Exp. Eye Res.* 61:629–632.

Li, Z., Lim, W. K., Mahesh, S. P., Liu, B., and Nussenblatt, R. B. (2005). Cutting edge: In vivo blockade of human IL-2 receptor induces expansion of CD56(bright) regulatory NK cells in patients with active uveitis. *J. Immunol.* 174:5187–5191.

Liang, W., Karabekian, Z., Mattapallil, M., Xu, Q., Viley, A. M., Caspi, R., and Scott, D. W. (2006). B-cell delivered gene transfer of human S-Ag-Ig fusion protein protects from experimental autoimmune uveitis. *Clin. Immunol.* 118:35–41.

Luger, D., Silver, P. B., Tang, J., Cua, D., Chen, Z., Iwakura, Y., Bowman, E. P., Sgambellone, N. M., Chan, C. D., et al. (in press). Either a Th17 or a Th1 effector response can drive autoimmunity: Conditions of disease induction affect dominant effector category. *J. Exp. Med.*

Mamalis, N., Edelhauser, H. F., Dawson, D. G., Chew, J., LeBoyer, R. M., and Werner, L. (2006). Toxic anterior segment syndrome. *J. Cataract Refract. Surg.* 32:324–333.

Mattapallil, M. J., and Caspi, R. R. (2008). Unpublished results.

Namba, K., Ogasawara, K., Kitaichi, N., Matsuki, N., Takahashi, A., Sasamoto, Y., Kotake, S., Matsuda, H., Iwabuchi, K., et al. (1998). Identification of a peptide inducing experimental autoimmune uveoretinitis (EAU) in H-2Ak-carrying mice. *Clin. Exp. Immunol.* 111:442–449.

Nussenblatt, R. B. (2002). Bench to bedside: New approaches to the immunotherapy of uveitic disease. *Int. Rev. Immunol.* 21: 273–289.

Nussenblatt, R. B., Fortin, E., Schiffman, R., Rizzo, L., Smith, J., Van Veldhuisen, P., Sran, P., Yaffe, A., Goldman, C. K., et al. (1999). Treatment of noninfectious intermediate and posterior uveitis with the humanized anti-Tac mAb: A phase I/II clinical trial. *Proc. Natl. Acad. Sci. U.S.A.* 96:7462–7466.

Nussenblatt, R. B., and Whitcup, S. M. (2004). *Uveitis: Fundamentals and clinical practice.* Philadelphia: Mosby (Elsevier).

Overwijk, W. W., Theoret, M. R., Finkelstein, S. E., Surman, D. R., de Jong, L. A., Vyth-Dreese, F. A., Dellemijn, T. A., Antony, P. A., Spiess, P. J., et al. (2003). Tumor regression and autoimmunity after reversal of a functionally tolerant state of self-reactive CD8+ T cells. *J. Exp. Med.* 198:569–580.

Pennesi, G., Mattapallil, M. J., Sun, S. H., Avichezer, D., Silver, P. B., Karabekian, Z., David, C. S., Hargrave, P. A., McDowell, J. H., et al. (2003). A humanized model of experimental autoimmune uveitis in HLA class II transgenic mice. *J. Clin. Invest.* 111:1171–1180.

Prendergast, R. A., Iliff, C. E., Coskuncan, N. M., Caspi, R. R., Sartani, G., Tarrant, T. K., Lutty, G. A., and McLeod, D. S. (1998). T cell traffic and the inflammatory response in experimental autoimmune uveoretinitis. *Invest. Ophthalmol. Vis. Sci.* 39:754–762.

Rizzo, L. V., Xu, H., Chan, C. C., Wiggert, B., and Caspi, R. R. (1998). IL-10 has a protective role in experimental autoimmune uveoretinitis. *Int. Immunol.* 10:807–814.

Robinson, M. R., Chan, C. C., Yang, J. C., Rubin, B. I., Gracia, G. J., Sen, H. N., Csaky, K. G., and Rosenberg, S. A. (2004).

Cytotoxic T lymphocyte–associated antigen 4 blockade in patients with metastatic melanoma: A new cause of uveitis. *J. Immunother.* 27:478–479.

Rosenbaum, J. T., McDevitt, H. O., Guss, R. B., and Egbert, P. R. (1980). Endotoxin-induced uveitis in rats as a model for human disease. *Nature* 286:611–613.

Rosenbaum, J. T., Planck, S. R., Martin, T. M., Crane, I., Xu, H., and Forrester, J. V. (2002). Imaging ocular immune responses by intravital microscopy. *Int. Rev. Immunol.* 21:255–272.

Siepmann, K., Biester, S., Plskova, J., Muckersie, E., Duncan, L., and Forrester, J. V. (2007). CD4(+)CD25(+) T regulatory cells induced by LPS-activated bone marrow dendritic cells suppress experimental autoimmune uveoretinitis in vivo. *Graefes. Arch. Clin. Exp. Ophthalmol.* 245:221–229.

Silver, P. B., Chan, C. C., Wiggert, B., and Caspi, R. R. (1999). The requirement for pertussis to induce EAU is strain-dependent: B10.RIII, but not B10.A mice, develop EAU and Th1 responses to IRBP without pertussis treatment. *Invest. Ophthalmol. Vis. Sci.* 40:2898–2905.

Silver, P. B., Hathcock, K. S., Chan, C. C., Wiggert, B., and Caspi, R. R. (2000). Blockade of costimulation through B7/CD28 inhibits experimental autoimmune uveoretinitis, but does not induce long-term tolerance. *J. Immunol.* 165:5041–5047.

Silver, P. B., Rizzo, L. V., Chan, C. C., Donoso, L. A., Wiggert, B., and Caspi, R. R. (1995). Identification of a major pathogenic epitope in the human IRBP molecule recognized by mice of the H-2r haplotype. *Invest. Ophthalmol. Vis. Sci.* 36:946–954.

Smith, J. R., Hart, P. H., and Williams, K. A. (1998). Basic pathogenic mechanisms operating in experimental models of acute anterior uveitis. *Immunol. Cell Biol.* 76:497–512.

Stein-Streilein, J., and Streilein, J. W. (2002). Anterior chamber associated immune deviation (ACAID): Regulation, biological relevance, and implications for therapy. *Int. Rev. Immunol.* 21: 123–152.

Stein-Streilein, J., and Taylor, A. W. (2007). An eye's view of T regulatory cells. *J. Leukoc. Biol.* 81:593–598.

Su, S. B., Silver, P. B., Grajewski, R. S., Agarwal, R. K., Tang, J., Chan, C. C., and Caspi, R. R. (2005). Essential role of the MyD88 pathway, but nonessential roles of TLRs 2, 4, and 9, in the adjuvant effect promoting Th1-mediated autoimmunity. *J. Immunol.* 175:6303–6310.

Sugita, S., Ng, T. F., Lucas, P. J., Gress, R. E., and Streilein, J. W. (2006). B7+ iris pigment epithelium induce CD8+ T regulatory cells; both suppress CTLA-4+ T cells. *J. Immunol.* 176: 118–127.

Szpak, Y., Vieville, J. C., Tabary, T., Naud, M. C., Chopin, M., Edelson, C., Cohen, J. H., Dausset, J., de Kozak, Y., et al. (2001). Spontaneous retinopathy in HLA-A29 transgenic mice. *Proc. Natl. Acad. Sci. U.S.A.* 98:2572–2576.

Tang, J., Zhu, W., Silver, P. B., Su, S.-B., Chan, C.-C., and Caspi, R. R. (2007). Autoimmune uveitis elicited with antigen-pulsed dendritic cells has a distinct clinical signature and is driven by unique effector mechanisms: Initial encounter with autoantigen defines disease phenotype. *J. Immunol.* 178:7072–7080.

Tarrant, T. K., Silver, P. B., Chan, C. C., Wiggert, B., and Caspi, R. R. (1998). Endogenous IL-12 is required for induction and expression of experimental autoimmune uveitis. *J. Immunol.* 161:122–127.

Tarrant, T. K., Silver, P. B., Wahlsten, J. L., Rizzo, L. V., Chan, C. C., Wiggert, B., and Caspi, R. R. (1999). Interleukin 12 protects from a T helper type 1–mediated autoimmune disease, experimental autoimmune uveitis, through a mechanism involving interferon gamma, nitric oxide, and apoptosis. *J. Exp. Med.* 189:219–230.

Whitcup, S. M., DeBarge, L. R., Caspi, R. R., Harning, R., Nussenblatt, R. B., and Chan, C. C. (1993). Monoclonal antibodies against ICAM-1 (CD54) and LFA-1 (CD11a/CD18) inhibit experimental autoimmune uveitis. *Clin. Immunol. Immunopathol.* 67:143–150.

Wildner, G., and Diedrichs-Mohring, M. (2004). Autoimmune uveitis and antigenic mimicry of environmental antigens. *Autoimmun. Rev.* 3:383–387.

Xu, H., Rizzo, L. V., Silver, P. B., and Caspi, R. R. (1997). Uveitogenicity is associated with a Th1-like lymphokine profile: Cytokine-dependent modulation of early and committed effector T cells in experimental autoimmune uveitis. *Cell. Immunol.* 178:69–78.

Xu, H., Silver, P. B., Tarrant, T. K., Chan, C. C., and Caspi, R. R. (2003). Tgf-beta inhibits activation and uveitogenicity of primary but not of fully polarized retinal antigen-specific memory-effector T cells. *Invest. Ophthalmol. Vis. Sci.* 44:4805–4812.

Yoshida, M., Kezuka, T., and Streilein, J. W. (2000). Participation of pigment epithelium of iris and ciliary body in ocular immune privilege. 2. Generation of TGF-beta-producing regulatory T cells. *Invest. Ophthalmol. Vis. Sci.* 41:3862–3870.

Ziegler, S. F. (2006). FOXP3: Of mice and men. *Annu. Rev. Immunol.* 24:209–226.

43 Mouse Models of Norrie Disease

WOLFGANG BERGER

Norrie disease is a severe X-linked recessive trait with the hallmark features of congenital blindness, deafness, and mental retardation. The disorder is caused by mutations in a gene encoding norrin, a small extracellular protein. To characterize the function of norrin and to study the pathophysiology of Norrie disease, a knockout mouse model was generated and examined. The results of these studies showed that abnormal retinal angiogenesis during development is one of the most prominent observations in mice lacking norrin. This causes severe retinal hypoxia, which leads to profound tissue damage. The disease phenotype was rescued by breeding knockout mice with transgenic animals with ectopic norrin expression in the lens. In addition, transgenic lenses induced proliferation of microvascular endothelial cells in coculture. These and other findings identified norrin as a key regulator of angiogenic processes in the retina. Most of the ocular symptoms in human patients may also be attributed to oxygen deficiency during retinal development, and the mouse lines significantly contributed to a better understanding of the primary events of this severe neurological disorder.

Clinical background

Norrie disease was named after Gordon Norrie, a consultant ophthalmologist at the Eye Clinic of the Institute for the Blind in Copenhagen. Norrie was the first to describe this trait as a nosological entity, in the late 1920s (Norrie, 1927). The medical condition was given its name by Mette Warburg, another Danish ophthalmologist, who reported the clinical picture and X-linked inheritance in a comprehensive monograph (Warburg, 1966). She decided to use this eponym in part to avoid a descriptive name that might reflect only secondary clinical features. Norrie realized that the disease was familial and that only boys were affected. Warburg then provided evidence that the disease is inherited in a sex chromosome–linked fashion (Andersen and Warburg, 1961; Warburg et al., 1965). In an X-linked recessive mode of inheritance, only males are affected, but a few exceptions exist (Chen et al., 1993b; Woodruff, et al., 1993; Kellner et al., 1996; Sims et al., 1997; Yamada et al., 2001).

The most prominent clinical finding in affected patients is early-onset bilateral blindness. Soon after birth, leukokoria is observed, a white pupillary reflex due to vascularized retrolental membranes and masses. This is a cardinal symptom but not pathognomonic, as it is present in a number of other eye diseases (Francois, 1978). Additional ocular manifestations consist of vitreoretinal hemorrhages, retinal folding and detachment, bilateral and congenital pseudotumor of the retina (pseudoglioma), and atrophy of the bulbus (phthisis bulbi) late in the disease. The appearance of the vitreal cavity alludes to persistent primary vitreous and hyaloid vessels. The lens becomes cataractous during the first months or years of life. Also, the cornea, iris, ciliary body, and retinal pigment epithelium may be affected by the disease.

The extraocular features of Norrie disease include deafness and mental retardation. The latter also occurs early in childhood in one-third to one-half of patients. The onset of progressive hearing loss was observed in the second or third decade of life. Initially, deafness was reported in about one-third of patients (Warburg, 1966), but recent data suggest an almost 100% occurrence of hearing loss in patients (Halpin et al., 2005). Some histological studies of affected tissues (eye, ear, brain) available in the literature describe advanced stages of the disease. Hypotheses regarding the pathophysiology of Norrie disease involve an early arrest in neuroectodermal development, as well as abnormal vasoproliferative processes (Warburg, 1966; Parsons et al., 1992).

The molecular basis of Norrie disease

With the advent of molecular genetic mapping in humans, the responsible locus has been localized to the short arm of the human X chromosome (Xp11.4). Linkage mapping was consistent with deletions of the same chromosomal segment in affected male patients (L. M. Bleeker-Wagemakers et al., 1985; Gal et al., 1985, 1986; E. M. Bleeker-Wagemakers et al., 1988; Diergaarde et al., 1989). Detailed analysis of the corresponding genetic interval led to the identification of the mutation-carrying gene by positional cloning (Berger, Meindl, et al., 1992; Chen et al., 1992). The official gene symbol is *NDP* (Norrie disease pseudoglioma), and the protein was designated norrin. The human gene spans a genomic region of approximately 25 kb (24,729 bps) and consists of three exons. The length of the transcript is 1,833 nucleotides. It codes for a protein of 133 residues, including a signal peptide of 24 amino acids. The small size of the gene allows rapid diagnostic testing. Around 100 mutations have been described so far. Point mutations in *NDP* represent missense and nonsense mutations, as well as frameshifting and splice site mutations (Berger, van de Pol, et al., 1992; Meindl et al., 1992, 1995). Approximately 20% of patients have complete or partial gene deletions (see Berger, 1998, and references therein).

NDP mutations were also found in the DNA of patients with X-linked recessive familial exudative vitreoretinopathy (XLEVR), or Coats' disease, and were associated with advanced stages of retinopathy of prematurity (Black et al., 1999; Chen et al., 1993a; Shastry et al., 1997). Thus, the clinical expressivity of mutations in the *NDP* gene is highly variable, even within a family, and both genetic and environmental modifiers are likely to influence the disease course (Zaremba et al., 1998). However, all these traits have the common feature of retinal blood vessel malformations. Therefore, a role of norrin in vascular development and homeostasis seems reasonable. It should be noted, however, that only classic Norrie disease is associated with deafness and mental retardation; the allelic traits do not show this pleiotropic effect.

Evolutionary conservation of the NDP *gene and its expression pattern*

Norrin shows high conservation in different species, as revealed by multiple protein sequence alignment (figure 43.1). The human sequence showed 95% identity on the amino acid level with rat, mouse, and dog, and 94% with cow. Lower levels of sequence identity of 87%, 60%, 57%, and 54% were observed with chicken, zebrafish, tetraodon, and fugu, respectively. This high degree of conservation implies an important function of norrin in vertebrates. In particular, the number and positions/spacing of 11 cysteine residues are highly conserved in all the species just mentioned. They form a cystine knot motif, which is a characteristic feature of a structural superfamily of growth factors that includes nerve growth factor (NGF), platelet-derived growth factor-β (PDGF-β), vascular endothelial growth factor (VEGF)-A and -B, placental growth factor (PlGF), and transforming growth factor-β (TGF-β) (McDonald and Hendrickson, 1993). The first cysteine residue occurs at position 39 in the human peptide sequence of norrin. The degree of conservation from this position toward the C-terminus of the protein is conspicuously higher in comparison to the N-terminal part, which contains the signal peptide and shows less conservation (see figure 43.1).

To date, tissue- or cell type–specific expression of the *NDP* gene has been studied only at the transcriptional level. Protein expression by immunohistochemistry has not yet been reported. RNA in situ hybridizations (RISH) detected transcripts of the *NDP* gene in different tissues, including eye, ear, and brain. Thus, the gene is expressed in all tissues or organs that are affected in Norrie disease. In mouse, rabbit, and human retina, norrin mRNA is expressed in the inner nuclear layer (INL) as well as the ganglion cell layer (GCL) (Chen et al., 1995; Berger et al., 1996; Hartzer et al., 1999), and might also be expressed in the outer nuclear layer (ONL) and the choroid (Hartzer et al., 1999). In mouse and rabbit brain, transcripts were detected by RISH in the olfactory bulbus and epithelium, cerebellum, cortex, and hippocampus (Chen et al., 1995; Berger et al., 1996; Hartzer et al., 1999). Transcriptional activity in the ear has been reported in neurons of the spiral ganglion cells and marginal cells of the stria vascularis of the cochlea (Chen et al., 1995; Hartzer et al., 1999). Furthermore, norrin has also been shown to be expressed in the endometrium of pregnant female mice (Luhmann et al., 2005b). In addition to these RISH studies, the more sensitive RT-PCR has also revealed norrin mRNA in other tissues, including several cell lines, as well as mouse endometrium and human placenta (Luhmann et al., 2005b), muscle, liver, and lung (Chen et al., 1995). The expression of norrin in mouse endometrium and human placenta is particularly interesting, because homozygous knockout mice show a characteristic infertility phenotype, as discussed later in the chapter.

Putative norrin function

Computational modeling of the gene product, norrin, revealed a three-dimensional structure very similar to TGF-β (Meitinger et al., 1993). The amino acid sequence contains a cystine knot motif that is present in several other proteins, including several growth factors, as well as in mucins, the *Drosophila* slit protein, von Willebrandt factor, and others. The common feature of the cystine knot in all these proteins is responsible for protein interaction and, most likely, dimerization of the respective molecules.

NDP mutations lead to exudative vitreoretinopathy, a disease characterized by an avascular retinal periphery, leakiness of retinal blood vessels, and vitreoretinal hemorrhages. Similar symptoms are observed in patients with a mutation in the Wnt receptor Frizzled-4 (FZD4) and its coreceptor LRP5 (low-density lipoprotein receptor–related protein 5) (Robitaille et al., 2002; Toomes et al., 2004). This observation and the fact that Frizzled-4 knockout mice show a similar phenotype prompted Xu, Wang, and co-workers to analyze norrin as a ligand for FZD4/LRP5 (Xu et al., 2004). The results of these experiments revealed that norrin is able to activate the canonical Wnt β-catenin pathway and to drive reporter gene transcription in a cell line (HEK293) coexpressing norrin, FZD4/LRP5, and a luciferase reporter gene under the control of transcription factor–binding sites (LEF/TCF). They concluded that norrin is a high-affinity ligand for FZD4/LRP5 and transcriptionally activates downstream target genes. Ligand binding depends on coexpression of both receptor molecules Lrp5 and Fzd4. No significant or very little activation of the Wnt pathway was

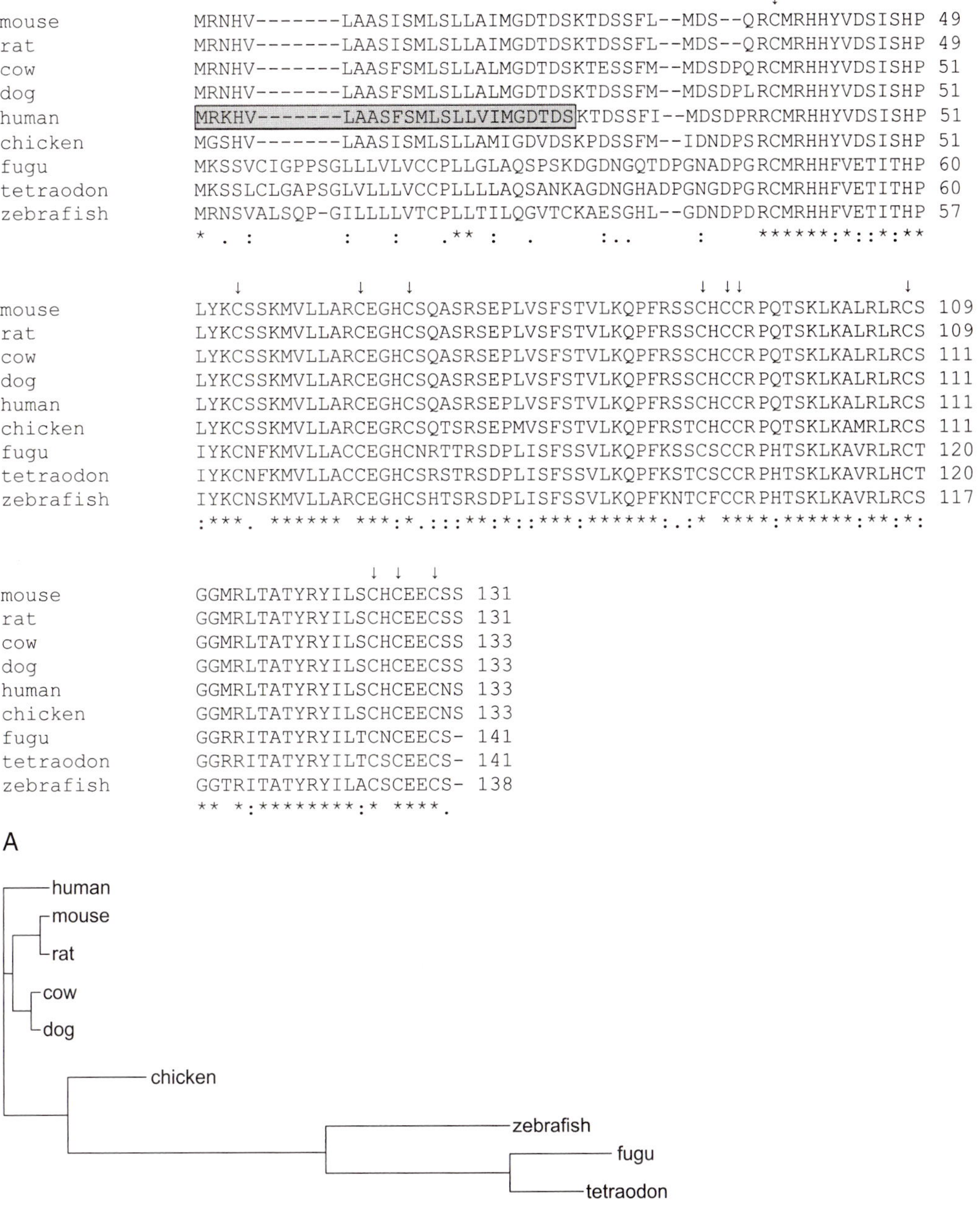

FIGURE 43.1 Multiple norrin protein sequence alignment from different species using the Clustal algorithm (Clustal W [1.83], www.ebi.ac.uk/clustalw). *A*, Alignment of the peptide sequences clearly shows a much higher conservation after the first of 11 cysteine residues (indicated by *arrows* above the mouse sequence of norrin). *Asterisks* in the bottom line indicate identical amino acids; *dots* designate similar properties of the residues. The putative signal peptide is highlighted in gray in the human sequence. *B*, The phylogenetic tree shows the evolutionary relationship of norrin protein sequences in different species. Sequence identity between human, dog, mouse, and rat is 95%. Identity with cow, chicken, zebrafish, tetraodon, and fugu is 94%, 87%, 60%, 57%, and 54%, respectively.

observed when cell lines were transfected with either of the two receptors. Mutations in *LRP5* are also associated with autosomal recessive osteoporosis-pseudoglioma (OPPG) syndrome, which is characterized by congenital or early childhood onset visual loss and bone fragility (Gong et al., 2001; Ai et al., 2005).

Generation of a knockout mouse model for Norrie disease

Given the high conservation between human and mouse and the tissue-specific transcription of the mouse norrin gene (gene symbol: *Ndph*, Norrie disease pseudoglioma homologue) in eye, brain, and ear, the mouse may provide an adequate model for Norrie disease and allelic disorders. Reverse genetics is a powerful tool to establish models for human gene defects and use them to study the pathology at the phenotypic and molecular levels. The gene-targeting approach has been used to generate a knockout mouse model for Norrie disease (Berger et al., 1996). The targeting construct replaced the coding part of exon 2 with a neomycin cassette in opposite transcriptional orientation to *Ndph*. As a consequence of this replacement, the translation start codon, the splice donor site of exon 2 and 55 additional N-terminal amino acids, including the signal peptide for extracellular transport, are removed from the gene. After homologous recombination of this construct in embryonic stem cells, blastocysts were injected to produce chimeric embryos. Chimeric male offspring were crossed to wild-type females to obtain female carriers for the knockout allele. Approximately half of the male offspring were hemizygous for the knockout allele, which is consistent with Mendelian transmission of a viable mutation.

In an initial survey to characterize the corresponding phenotype, the retinal morphology of hemizygous knockout mice (*Ndph*$^{-/Y}$) was compared with that in wild-type (*Ndph*$^{+/Y}$) littermates (Berger et al., 1996). One of the most prominent findings in knockout mice was the presence of fibrous masses containing blood vessels in the vitreous of all nine mice analyzed. This is probably the anatomical correlate to the precipitate-like structures that had been observed on slit lamp biomicroscopy. Likewise, an abnormal organization of nuclei in the GCL had been reported in all *Ndph*$^{-/y}$ mice examined. Occasionally, outer retinal layers, including the ONL and outer segments of photoreceptor cells, also showed a characteristic pattern of disorganization. Heterozygous female carriers (*Ndph*$^{+/-}$) were inconspicuous. These initial data revealed a clear retinal phenotype in *Ndph* knockout mice. Histopathological data from human patients in whom the clinical diagnosis was confirmed by molecular testing are rare. There is one report in the literature in which retinal and vitreal tissues were examined after vitreoretinal surgery in a 6-month-old boy with a frameshift mutation in the *NDP* gene (Schroeder et al., 1997). In this case, a reduction in the number of ganglion cells was observed, along with a largely disarranged INL but otherwise normally differentiated retina. Massive fibrovascular proliferation was present in the vitreous.

Retinal physiology of knockout mice

To examine the consequences of the knockout mutation and the morphological changes on retinal physiology, electroretinography (ERG) was performed. This analysis allows direct measurement of the activity of photoreceptor cells and second-order neurons in the retina as a response to light stimuli. The two major ERG components are the a- and b-waves, which reflect photoreceptor and second-order neuron (bipolar, amacrine, and horizontal cells) activities, respectively. Also, the two photoreceptor systems, rods and cones, can be discriminated by using dark adaptation and excitation with different light intensities. When the retina is dark adapted and the photoreceptors receive light stimuli of low to moderate intensity, the corresponding a-wave mainly represents the response of rod photoreceptors. In the light-adapted state, when bright flashes are utilized to excite photoreceptors, the corresponding a-wave primarily reflects cone photoreceptor activity. Therefore, the ERG is a suitable tool to characterize retinal function.

ERG measurements were performed in hemizygous knockout mice from 7 months of age up (Ruether et al., 1997). Data from hemizygous knockouts were compared with data from a group of heterozygous females and wild-type male litters. Both a- and b-waves were attenuated in hemizygous knockout mice but not in wild-type mice or female carriers. An interesting finding was that the a-waves of the three different genotypes (wild type, hemizygous knockout, heterozygous) were not much different at low intensities but became prominent at higher intensities of light stimuli. Conversely, the b-wave amplitudes were much lower in the group of hemizygous knockout mice at all intensities. Oscillatory potentials, which reflect the response of part of the second-order neurons in the retina, were severely reduced in male mice with the knockout allele. In summary, the ERG recordings revealed a more severe functional effect of the knockout mutation on the inner retina compared to photoreceptor cells. This is in agreement with molecular studies in which a late involvement of photoreceptor cells was found (Lenzner et al., 2002). In this study, the expression of photoreceptor-specific gene transcripts was normal until the age of 12 months in knockout mice and significantly reduced only after 2 years, indicating a rather slow progression of photoreceptor cell degeneration.

Abnormal retinal vascular development in norrin knockout mice

In normal mouse development, three vascular networks, superficial, deep, and intermediate, appear in the retina. The superficial retinal vasculature, located within the GCL/nerve fiber layer, spreads from the entry point of the large artery and vein from the central retina (at the optic nerve head) toward the periphery between days 3 and 17 post partum (P3–P17). Around P7 or P8, the deep retinal vasculature starts forming by angiogenic sprouting from the superficial network. After completion, the deep vascular system will be present in the outer plexiform layer (OPL). From P12, an intermediate vascular system develops between the superficial and deep networks, close to the boundary between inner nuclear and plexiform layers.

Abnormalities and changes in the retinal vasculature in norrin knockout mice have been reported by several authors (Richter et al., 1998; Rehm et al., 2002; Luhmann et al., 2005a). Vascular development between P5 and P21 in knockout mice was studied in detail by Luhmann and co-workers and was correlated with molecular analyses of angiogenic signaling pathways. The outgrowth of the superficial vascular system was temporally retarded and never completed. In wild-type mice, the retina was entirely covered by superficial vessels at P21. The periphery of the retina in hemizygous knockout mice remained avascular, and only three-quarters of the retina was supplied with vessels. The development of the deep capillary network, which normally starts at P7, was completely abolished in norrin-deficient mice (figures 43.2 and 43.3). Although the vascular tubes of the superficial network branched out and tried to initiate angiogenic sprouting, this process was never completed but was entirely blocked at this point, leading to microaneurysm-like capillary lesions. Of note, the astrocytic network, which is important for vessel guidance, seemed to be normal in knockout mice in early disease phases. Rather, a primary effect on endothelial cells has been suggested by Luhmann and co-workers. This view is supported by some molecular findings. The transcript (mRNA) levels of Tie1, Tie2, and Pdgfb, which are involved in angiogenesis and vessel maturation and represent endothelial markers, were significantly lower in norrin-deficient mice at P5 and P10 than in wild-type controls.

The defect in vascular development in norrin knockout mice can be summarized as delayed and incomplete outgrowth of the superficial retinal blood vessels, leading to an avascular retinal periphery. Additionally, the deep and intermediate vessel networks fail to develop, owing to an arrest in sprouting angiogenesis.

Failure in sprouting angiogenesis leads to retinal hypoxia and leakiness of blood vessels, but not retinal neovascularization

As noted, the retinal vasculature in norrin-deficient mice does not develop properly. As a consequence, oxygen deficiency occurs in the inner retina. This hypoxic condition leads to an activation of angiogenic cascades, as shown by the transcriptional upregulation of Vegfa from P10 onward (Luhmann et al., 2005a). At P15, several other factors in the retina are transcriptionally activated: angiopoietin-2 (Agpt2), ephrin-B4 (EphB4), frizzled-4 (Fzd4), integrins α-V and β-III (Itga5, Itgb3), pdgfb and its receptor (pdgfrb), as well as Tie1. All of them also show higher transcript levels at P21 in addition to the Vegf receptors 1 and 2 (Vegfr1/Flt1 and Vegfr2/Flk1). This transcriptional activation of angiogenic factors indicates a response of retinal cells to hypoxia and provides an explanation for microaneurysms and the leakiness of blood vessels, which leads to retinal and vitreal hemorrhages and exudates. Another excellent indicator of hypoxia is the presence of hypoxia-inducible factor 1α (Hif1-α), which is known to be stabilized at the protein level under hypoxic conditions. Indeed, the Hif1-α protein level was increased in norrin knockout mice compared to wild-type litters at P15 and P21, but not at P5 and P10 (Luhmann

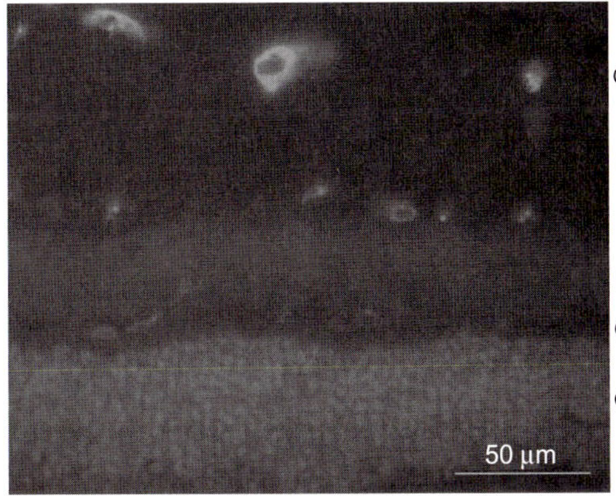

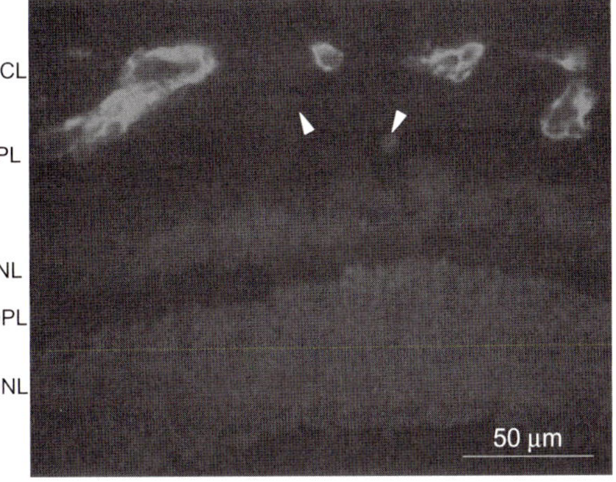

FIGURE 43.2 Sections of the central retina from wild-type and knockout mice at P21 after staining with a collagen IV antibody (red), which detects the extracellular matrix of endothelial cells, and diamidinophenylindol/DAPI (blue), which labels cell nuclei. Blood vessels (red) in wild-type mice are present in three layers, indicating completed development of the superficial (ganglion cell layer [GCL]), deep (outer plexiform layer [OPL]), and intermediate (border between the inner plexiform layer [IPL] and inner nuclear layer [INL]) vessel networks. In contrast, age-matched knockout mice show only enlarged superficial vessels, while the deeper and intermediate networks failed to develop. In addition, the presence of nuclei in the IPL (*white arrowheads*) may reflect the characteristic disorganization in the GCL. See color plate 41. (Images acquired and provided courtesy of Nikolaus Schäfer, Division of Medical Molecular Genetics, Institute of Medical Genetics, University of Zurich, Switzerland.)

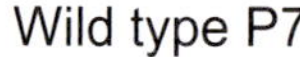

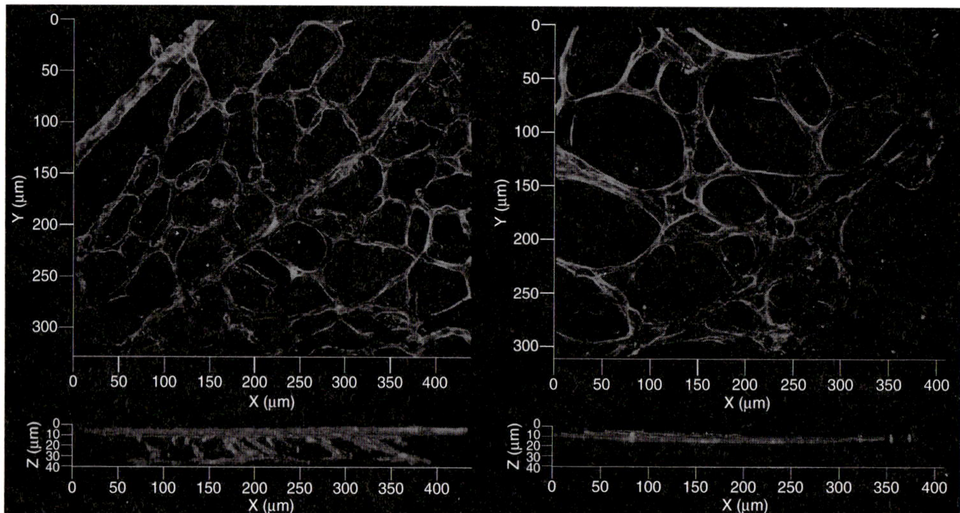

FIGURE 43.3 Three-dimensional microscopy of retinal flat mounts stained with anticollagen IV from wild-type and knockout mice at P7. *Top panels* show an area of approximately 300 × 400 μm from wild-type and knockout mice. Vessels in the knockout are dilated, and the capillary network is less dense than in the wild-type control. *Bottom panels* (*z*-axis) show how blood vessels enter the deeper retinal layers in wild-type mice by angiogenic sprouting. In contrast, this process is abolished in knockout mice, and the vessels do not invade the deeper retinal layers. See color plate 42. (Images acquired using the Zeiss ApoTome technology and provided courtesy of Nikolaus Schäfer, Division of Medical Molecular Genetics, Institute of Medical Genetics, University of Zurich, Switzerland.)

et al., 2005a). Particularly Hif1-α and Vegfa clearly indicate retinal hypoxia, and many aforementioned angiogenic factors are known to be regulated by them, including Pdgfb. Strikingly, reduced Pdgfb, as shown in norrin knockout mice at P10, results in the formation of microaneurysms, as reported previously (Enge et al., 2002).

In many other cases of retinal hypoxia, neovascularization occurs as a result of increased activity of pro-angiogenic signaling cascades. Obviously, this does not apply to norrin-deficient mice. Retinal neovascularization has never been reported, not even in late stages of the disease. Thus, high VEGF-α alone is not sufficient to induce the formation of new blood vessels in the retina if norrin is lacking.

Regression of hyaloid vessels versus angiogenesis of retinal blood vessels

In addition to the characteristic abnormal pattern of retinal vasculature, norrin is required for normal regression of the hyaloid vessels, which is completed by P21 in control mice but heavily delayed in norrin knockout mice (figure 43.4) (Ohlmann et al., 2004; Luhmann et al., 2005a). Nevertheless, these hyaloid vessels are obliterated and most likely nonfunctional in knockout mice, as shown by angiography (Luhmann et al., 2005a). Between P14 and P21, the number and diameter of hyaloid vessels were reduced. This obliteration continued until the age of 6–8 weeks, when most of them became nonfunctional. Occasionally, hyaloid vessels were found to grow into the peripheral retina of knockout mice (Ohlmann et al., 2004; Luhmann et al., 2005a).

There are two alternative hypotheses regarding the primary defect in norrin-deficient mice: (1) Norrin causes persistence of the hyaloid vessels that supply oxygen to the retina, and thus retinal vascular development is dispensable (Ohlmann et al., 2004). (2) Norrin deficiency in the retina results in an arrest of vascular development of the deep capillary networks, which leads to hypoxia and subsequent upregulation of VEGF. This excess of VEGF provides an antiapoptotic signal to the endothelial cells of the hyaloid vasculature and its persistence or extremely delayed regression (Luhmann et al., 2005a).

The second alternative is supported by the fact that hyaloid vessels are obliterated and most likely nonfunctional. Moreover, it has been shown in mice that, by blocking *PGF*, functional hyaloid vessels can persist without significantly affecting retinal vascular development (Feeney et al., 2003).

The two phases of Norrie disease in the eye

Examination of blood vessel development in norrin knockout versus wild-type mice has revealed a delayed outgrowth of the superficial retinal vasculature, an arrest in sprouting angiogenesis that forms the deep and intermediate retinal capillary networks, and a delay in hyaloid regression. According to Luhmann et al. (2005a), there are two phases of

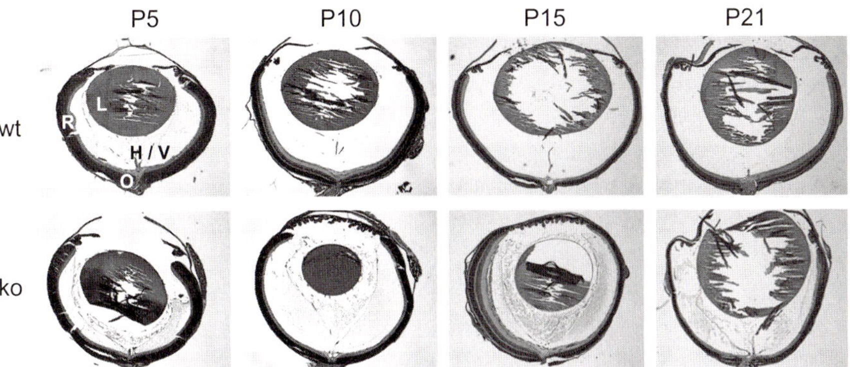

Figure 43.4 Hematoxylin-eosin-stained sections of whole eyes from wild-type (wt) and norrin knockout (ko) mice at P5, P10, P15, and P21. The hyaloid vessel system (H) in the vitreous body (V) is clearly present in wild-type mice at P5 and P10, and remnants are evident at P15. In knockout mice, the hyaloid vasculature persists through P21 and beyond, and regression of this vascular network is profoundly delayed. L, lens; O, optic nerve; R, retina. See color plate 43. (Images acquired and provided courtesy of Dr. Ulrich Luhmann, Division of Medical Molecular Genetics, Institute of Medical Genetics, University of Zurich, Switzerland.)

pathology in knockout mice. The first phase is characterized by the abnormal vascular development and may last until P7 or P8. After this, hypoxia-driven activation of angiogenic signaling cascades lead to severe lesions in the vitreous and retina and the characteristic disease symptoms, which include vitreoretinal hemorrhages and exudates caused by leaky blood vessels in the vitreous and retina, an avascular retinal periphery, and retinal folding and detachment. Very similar symptoms were described in human patients. Thus, the *Ndph* knockout mouse may represent a suitable model not only for the classic form of Norrie disease but also for allelic traits such as exudative vitreoretinopathy or Coats' disease, as well as more common vasoproliferative retinal diseases (retinopathy of prematurity, diabetic retinopathy, age-related macular dystrophy).

Hearing loss and abnormal cochlear vasculature in Ndph *knockout mice*

Because one of the clinical hallmarks of Norrie disease is progressive deafness in human patients, knockout mice were examined with respect to auditory performance. The auditory brainstem response (ABR) test is a useful diagnostic tool for measuring hearing performance. ABR records activities in the auditory centers of the brain in response to sound stimuli of different frequencies (e.g., 5–45 kHz). The test is considered reliable and objective, because it does not depend on subjective feedback as other, more conventional hearing tests do.

ABR test results were compared for hemizygous knockout mice at three ages (3–4, 6.5, and 15 months) and wild-type littermates (Rehm et al., 2002). ABR recordings were correlated with cochlear pathology that had been scored by histological approaches, namely, conventional histology of cochlear structures, including the stria vascularis, spiral ganglion, outer and inner hair cells, and cochlear vasculature. These analyses revealed a progressive hearing loss in hemizygous knockout mice across all frequencies (5–45 kHz). At younger ages (3–4 months), hearing impairment was more severe in the higher frequencies, but it progressed to a profound loss at all frequencies by the age of 15 months.

This functional decline in the auditory system in knockout mice was found to be consistent with morphological changes in the cochlea, which was completely normal at P12 (Rehm et al., 2002). Thus, cochlear structures progressively degenerate over time, while normal development is not affected by the knockout mutation. The most affected structure was the stria vascularis in all three age groups. Vessels were significantly enlarged, particularly in the apical cochlear turn. The loss of outer hair cells progressed consistently, with an increase in auditory threshold. With progression of hearing loss, neurons in the spiral ganglion degenerated. Obviously, the outer hair cells of knockout mice are more susceptible to premature cell death than the inner hair cells, which show significant cell death at 15 months but not in the two groups of animals aged 3–4 months and 6.5 months. In addition, characteristic changes were found in the cochlear vasculature. The average vessel size was larger in knockout mice than in wild-type mice, and the number of vessels decreased significantly over time. Differences in vessel quantity between control animal and knockout mice were marginal at 3–4 months. However, enlarged vessels in the stria vascularis and a sparse capillary network in the spiral ganglion were clearly visible at this age. At 15 months, two-thirds of vessels had disappeared.

To summarize these findings, the stria vascularis might be the primarily affected cochlear structure, followed by the spiral ganglion. Hearing loss is progressive in knockout mice, with only mild symptoms or almost normal hearing present at younger ages, although the expressivity of hearing impairment shows a high degree of interindividual variability even in mice (Rehm et al., 2002). These observations suggest normal development of the auditory system but a defect in its homeostasis, probably resulting from degenerative processes in the cochlear vasculature. This is in contrast to the retina, where part of the vasculature fails to develop properly because of a defect in angiogenic sprouting. Thus, norrin might have different effects in eye and ear. Still, a major role in angiogenesis is reconcilable as the mechanism of angiogenic sprouting is necessary in both processes, development and homeostasis.

Generation and analysis of a transgenic mouse line with norrin overexpression in the lens

The role of norrin in vascular development has also been demonstrated in transgenic mice overexpressing norrin in the lens. The transgenic lines have been established by pronucleus injection of a transgene construct containing the chicken βB1-crystallin promoter in front of the coding region of the mouse norrin cDNA (Ohlmann et al., 2005). In addition, a polyadenylation signal was present downstream of the translation termination codon of the norrin cDNA. Four founder lines were obtained containing 3, 9, 10, and 11 copies of the transgene, respectively. At the transcript and protein level, norrin expression from the transgene construct approximately correlated with the copy number. The line with 3 copies of the transgene showed less norrin mRNA and protein than the transgenic lines with 9–11 copies but more than wild-type littermates. Expression studies also showed that norrin expression in transgenic animals was restricted to the lens; other ocular structures did not express the transgene.

At the morphological level, the lenses and eye bulbs of transgenic mice carrying between 9 and 11 copies were smaller than those of wild-type mice or the line with 3 transgene copies (approximately 30%). The tunica vasculosa lentis, an extensive blood vessel network of capillaries spreading over the posterior and lateral lens surface, in transgenic mice contained significantly more capillaries than in wild-type litters at P0–P2. Ultrastructurally, the capillaries were very similar in wild-type and transgenic mice. They were unfenestrated and surrounded by pericytes. Quantitatively, the number of capillaries was 1.5- to 2-fold higher in transgenic animals with 9–11 gene copies and increased by 20% in the transgenic line with 3 copies of the transgene.

Lenses with overexpression of norrin were also examined with respect to stimulation of growth and proliferation of endothelial cells. Indeed, there was a positive effect of lenses expressing norrin on human dermal microvascular endothelial cells (HDMECs). The presence of norrin resulted in a 66% or 40% increase in proliferation of HDMECs when the culture medium was preconditioned with lenses from transgenic mice at P1 or P7, respectively, which might also suggest a direct effect of norrin on endothelial cells.

Rescue of the knockout phenotype by ectopic norrin expression in the lens

Norrin-deficient mice (Berger et al., 1996) were crossed with transgenic mice carrying 11 copies of the transgene, showing norrin expression at the transcript and protein levels (Ohlmann et al., 2005). Offspring were examined morphologically and electrophysiologically (ERG). These tests showed a rescue of the vascular and ERG phenotype of norrin knockout mice.

The deep and intermediate vascular systems present in the OPL and IPL, respectively, were restored in knockout mice with ectopic norrin expression in the lens at P21 (Ohlmann et al., 2005). Also, disorganization of the GCL, which is seen in knockout animals, disappeared. The ERG pattern of knockout mice, characterized by a reduced b-wave and almost absent oscillatory potentials, was rescued completely, although the amplitudes of the responses were lower than in wild-type litters, probably due to the reduced size of the bulbus. These findings were surprising, since diffusion of norrin from the lens to the retina, a prerequisite for the observed rescue effects, might be limited by the high affinity of norrin for the extracellular matrix (ECM). However, this retarded spatial spreading had been reported for norrin expressed and secreted from COS-7 (African green monkey kidney fibroblasts) cells (Perez-Vilar and Hill, 1997). The differences in ECM composition between cultured cells and in the vitreous body might explain this observation.

Over and above the rescue effects of ectopic norrin, it might have a sort of neurotrophic or neuroprotective effect. Ohlmann and co-workers (2005) observed an increase in thickness of the ONL and INL, as well as an increase in the number of nuclei in the GCL. It is not yet clear whether these observations are mediated by Vegfa, which was shown to be more abundant in the retinas of transgenic mice. Compensation for a smaller eye size in transgenic mice may be another reason for this finding.

Fetal loss in homozygous knockout female mice

Almost complete infertility of female mice homozygous for the knockout allele ($Ndph^{-/-}$) has been reported (Luhmann et al., 2005b). Breeding of $Ndph^{-/-}$ females revealed a mean litter size of 0.3, while the control litters had seven offspring. The number of implantation sites was not different in homozygous knockout females, indicating normal implantation. However, massive bleeding at the implantation sites was reported at all embryonic stages from E9 onward, and occasionally at E7. Embryonic tissues were highly disorganized and surrounded by blood. A normal chorioallantoic placenta was never observed, but yolk sac and trophoblast derivatives were differentiated. However, the spatial pattern of the trophoblast was severely disrupted, and the number of spongiotrophoblast cells was reduced. The labyrinthine area failed to develop and was filled with blood. Implantation of blastocysts and decidual reaction still occurred in homozygous females, but decidualization was compromised, which led to severely reduced fertility. The observed bleeding, which occurred before normal development of the chorioallantois placenta, might be a result of defects in decidual angiogenesis and blood vessel remodeling due to impaired angiogenic processes similar to those observed in the retina. Homozygous Frizzled-4 knockout female mice were also reported to be infertile, but as a result of failure of corpora lutea formation and function, which causes a defect in implantation (Hsieh et al., 2005).

The expression of norrin has also been shown in human placenta at the RNA level (Luhmann et al., 2005b), implicating a role for norrin in human female reproduction. However, because of the low frequency of *NDP* gene mutations, homozygous females have never been described, and the function of this gene in human female reproductive tissues remains elusive. It might be noteworthy in this context that genotypic wild-type (for *NDP*) male and female offspring of *NDP* gene mutation carriers showed abnormal vascular patterns in the peripheral retina reminiscent of mild retinopathy of prematurity (Mintz-Hittner et al., 1996). This might be caused by the expression of norrin in the placenta of female mutation carriers from the mutant allele. The mildness of the phenotype can be explained by the presence of the wild-type allele in the embryos.

Summary

Taken together, the data that have emerged from these knockout and transgenic mouse models indicate that Norrie disease is caused by a primary defect in the inner retina and vitreous. In the retina, the failure of proper blood vessel development leads to oxygen deficiency (hypoxia), which activates angiogenic signaling cascades. Activation of these pathways causes subsequent leakiness of blood vessels, hemorrhages, and fibrovascular membranes. The vitreal phenotype may be caused primarily by a delayed regression of the hyaloid vasculature and leaky blood vessels. The data obtained in mice can explain the leading ocular symptoms in patients with Norrie disease, exudative vitreoretinopathy, Coats' disease, and retinopathy of prematurity, and indicate a role for norrin in vascular development in the eye. In contrast, its function in the auditory system might be vascular maintenance in the stria vascularis and spiral ganglion rather than vascular development in these structures, as shown in the knockout mouse. This is also consistent with the human condition, where auditory function is normal in the beginning and the onset of sensorineural hearing loss or impairment occurs in adolescence.

ACKNOWLEDGMENTS I thank Dr. Ulrich Luhmann and Nikolaus Schäfer for critical reading of the manuscript and helpful comments and suggestions, as well as for providing the images in figures 43.2, 43.3, and 43.4.

REFERENCES

Ai, M., Heeger, S., Bartels, C. F., Schelling, D. K., and the Osteoporosis-Pseudoglioma Collaborative Group. (2005). Clinical and molecular findings in osteoporosis-pseudoglioma syndrome. *Am. J. Hum. Genet.* 77:741–753.

Andersen, S. R., and Warburg, M. (1961). Norrie's disease: Congenital bilateral pseudotumor of the retina with recessive X-chromosomal inheritance. Preliminary report. *Arch. Ophthalmol.* 66:614–618.

Berger, W. (1998). Molecular dissection of Norrie disease. *Acta. Anat. (Basel)* 162:95–100.

Berger, W., Meindl, A., van de Pol, T. J., Cremers, F. P., Ropers, H. H., Doerner, C., Monaco, A., Bergen, A. A., Lebo, R., et al. (1992). Isolation of a candidate gene for Norrie disease by positional cloning. *Nat. Genet.* 1:199–203 [erratum in *Nat. Genet.* 1992; 2:84].

Berger, W., van de Pol, D., Bachner, D., Oerlemans, F., Winkens, H., Hameister, H., Wieringa, B., Hendriks, W., and Ropers, H. H. (1996). An animal model for Norrie disease (ND): Gene targeting of the mouse ND gene. *Hum. Mol. Genet.* 5: 51–59.

Berger, W., van de Pol, D., Warburg, M., Gal, A., Bleeker-Wagemakers, L., de Silva, H., Meindl, A., Meitinger, T., Cremers, F., and Ropers, H. H. (1992). Mutations in the candidate gene for Norrie disease. *Hum. Mol. Genet.* 1:461–465.

Black, G. C., Perveen, R., Bonshek, R., Cahill, M., Clayton-Smith, J., Lloyd, I. C., and McLeod, D. (1999). Coats' disease of the retina (unilateral retinal telangiectasis) caused by somatic mutation in the NDP gene: A role for norrin in retinal angiogenesis. *Hum. Mol. Genet.* 8:2031–2035.

Bleeker-Wagemakers, E. M., Zweije-Hofman, I., and Gal, A. (1988). Norrie disease as part of a complex syndrome explained by a submicroscopic deletion of the X chromosome. *Ophthalmic. Paediatr. Genet.* 9:137–142.

Bleeker-Wagemakers, L. M., Friedrich, U., Gal, A., Wienker, T. F., Warburg, M., and Ropers, H. H. (1985). Close linkage between Norrie disease, a cloned DNA sequence from the proximal short arm, and the centromere of the X chromosome. *Hum. Genet.* 71:211–214.

Chen, Z. Y., Battinelli, E. M., Fielder, A., Bundey, S., Sims, K., Breakefield, X. O., and Craig, I. W. (1993a). A mutation in the Norrie disease gene (NDP) associated with X-linked familial exudative vitreoretinopathy. *Nat. Genet.* 5:180–183.

Chen, Z. Y., Battinelli, E. M., Woodruff, G., Young, I., Breakefield, X. O., and Craig, I. W. (1993b). Characterization of a mutation within the NDP gene in a family with a manifesting female carrier. *Hum. Mol. Genet.* 2:1727–1729.

Chen, Z. Y., Denney, R. M., and Breakefield, X. O. (1995). Norrie disease and MAO genes: Nearest neighbors. *Hum. Mol. Genet.* 4:1729–1737.

Chen, Z. Y., Hendriks, R. W., Jobling, M. A., Powell, J. F., Breakefield, X. O., Sims, K. B., and Craig, I. W. (1992). Isolation and characterization of a candidate gene for Norrie disease. *Nat. Genet.* 1:204–208.

Diergaarde, P. J., Wieringa, B., Bleeker-Wagemakers, E. M., Sims, K. B., Breakefield, X. O., and Ropers, H. H. (1989). Physical fine-mapping of a deletion spanning the Norrie gene. *Hum. Genet.* 84:22–26.

Enge, M., Bjarnegard, M., Gerhardt, H., Gustafsson, E., Kalen, M., Asker, N., Hammes, H. P., Shani, M., Fassler, R., et al. (2002). Endothelium-specific platelet-derived growth factor-B ablation mimics diabetic retinopathy. *EMBO. J.* 21: 4307–4316.

Feeney, S. A., Simpson, D. A., Gardiner, T. A., Boyle, C., Jamison, P., and Stitt, A. W. (2003). Role of vascular endothelial growth factor and placental growth factors during retinal vascular development and hyaloid regression. *Invest. Ophthalmol. Vis. Sci.* 44:839–847.

Francois, J. (1978). Differential diagnosis of leukokoria in children. *Ann. Ophthalmol.* 10:1375–1378.

Gal, A., Stolzenberger, C., Wienker, T., Wieacker, P., Ropers, H. H., Friedrich, U., Bleeker-Wagemakers, L., Pearson, P., and Warburg, M. (1985). Norrie's disease: Close linkage with genetic markers from the proximal short arm of the X chromosome. *Clin. Genet.* 27:282–283.

Gal, A., Wieringa, B., Smeets, D. F., Bleeker-Wagemakers, L., and Ropers, H. H. (1986). Submicroscopic interstitial deletion of the X chromosome explains a complex genetic syndrome dominated by Norrie disease. *Cytogenet. Cell Genet.* 42: 219–224.

Gong, Y., Slee, R. B., Fukai, N., Rawadi, G., Roman-Roman, S., Reginato, A. M., Wang, H., Cundy, T., Glorieux, F. H., et al., the Osteoporosis-Pseudoglioma Syndrome Collaborative Group. (2001). LDL receptor-related protein 5 (LRP5) affects bone accrual and eye development. *Cell* 107:513–523.

Halpin, C., Owen, G., Gutierrez-Espeleta, G. A., Sims, K., and Rehm, H. L. (2005). Audiologic features of Norrie disease. *Ann. Otol. Rhinol. Laryngol.* 114:533–538.

Hartzer, M. K., Cheng, M., Liu, X., and Shastry, B. S. (1999). Localization of the Norrie disease gene mRNA by in situ hybridization. *Brain Res. Bull.* 49:355–358.

Hsieh, M., Boerboom, D., Shimada, M., Lo, Y., Parlow, A. F., Luhmann, U. F., Berger, W., and Richards, J. S. (2005). Mice null for Frizzled4 ($Fzd4^{-/-}$) are infertile and exhibit impaired corpora lutea formation and function. *Biol. Reprod.* 73:1135–1146.

Hutcheson, K. A., Paluru, P. C., Bernstein, S. L., Koh, J., Rappaport, E. F., Leach, R. A., and Young, T. L. (2005). Norrie disease gene sequence variants in an ethnically diverse population with retinopathy of prematurity. *Mol. Vis.* 11:501–508.

Jiao, X., Ventruto, V., Trese, M. T., Shastry, B. S., and Hejtmancik, J. F. (2004). Autosomal recessive familial exudative vitreoretinopathy is associated with mutations in LRP5. *Am. J. Hum. Genet.* 75:878–884.

Kellner, U., Fuchs, S., Bornfeld, N., Foerster, M. H., and Gal, A. (1996). Ocular phenotypes associated with two mutations (R121W, C126X) in the Norrie disease gene. *Ophthalmic. Genet.* 17:67–74.

Lenzner, S., Prietz, S., Feil, S., Nuber, U. A., Ropers, H. H., and Berger, W. (2002). Global gene expression analysis in a mouse model for Norrie disease: Late involvement of photoreceptor cells. *Invest. Ophthalmol. Vis. Sci.* 43:2825–2833.

Luhmann, U. F., Lin, J., Acar, N., Lammel, S., Feil, S., Grimm, C., Seeliger, M. W., Hammes, H. P., and Berger, W. (2005a). Role of the Norrie disease pseudoglioma gene in sprouting angiogenesis during development of the retinal vasculature. *Invest. Ophthalmol. Vis. Sci.* 46:3372–3382.

Luhmann, U. F., Meunier, D., Shi, W., Luttges, A., Pfarrer, C., Fundele, R., and Berger, W. (2005b). Fetal loss in homozygous mutant Norrie disease mice: A new role of norrin in reproduction. *Genesis* 42:253–262.

McDonald, N. Q., and Hendrickson, W. A. (1993). A structural superfamily of growth factors containing a cystine knot motif. *Cell* 73:421–424.

Meindl, A., Berger, W., Meitinger, T., van de Pol, D., Achatz, H., Dorner, C., Haasemann, M., Hellebrand, H., Gal, A., et al. (1992). Norrie disease is caused by mutations in an extracellular protein resembling C-terminal globular domain of mucins. *Nat. Genet.* 2:139–143.

Meindl, A., Lorenz, B., Achatz, H., Hellebrand, H., Schmitz-Valckenberg, P., and Meitinger, T. (1995). Missense mutations in the NDP gene in patients with a less severe course of Norrie disease. *Hum. Mol. Genet.* 4:489–490.

Meitinger, T., Meindl, A., Bork, P., Rost, B., Sander, C., Haasemann, M., and Murken, J. (1993). Molecular modelling of the Norrie disease protein predicts a cystine knot growth factor tertiary structure. *Nat. Genet.* 5:376–380.

Mintz-Hittner, H. A., Ferrell, R. E., Sims, K. B., Fernandez, K. M., Gemmell, B. S., Satriano, D. R., Caster, J., and Kretzer, F. L. (1996). Peripheral retinopathy in offspring of carriers of Norrie disease gene mutations: Possible transplacental effect of abnormal norrin. *Ophthalmology.* 103:2128–2134.

Norrie, G. (1927). Causes of blindness in children. *Acta Ophthalmol.* 76:141–147.

Ohlmann, A. V., Adamek, E., Ohlmann, A., and Lutjen-Drecoll, E. (2004). Norrie gene product is necessary for regression of hyaloid vessels. *Invest. Ophthalmol. Vis. Sci.* 45:2384–2390.

Ohlmann, A., Scholz, M., Goldwich, A., Chauhan, B. K., Hudl, K., Ohlmann, A. V., Zrenner, E., Berger, W., Cvekl, A., et al. (2005). Ectopic norrin induces growth of ocular capillaries and restores normal retinal angiogenesis in Norrie disease mutant mice. *J. Neurosci.* 25:1701–1710.

Parsons, M. A., Curtis, D., Blank, C. E., Hughes, H. N., and McCartney, A. C. (1992). The ocular pathology of Norrie disease in a fetus of 11 weeks' gestational age. *Graefes. Arch. Clin. Exp. Ophthalmol.* 230:248–251.

Perez-Vilar, J., and Hill, R. L. (1997). Norrie disease protein (norrin) forms disulfide-linked oligomers associated with the extracellular matrix. *J. Biol. Chem.* 272:33410–33415.

Rehm, H. L., Gutierrez-Espeleta, G. A., Garcia, R., Jimenez, G., Khetarpal, U., Priest, J. M., Sims, K. B., Keats, B. J., and Morton, C. C. (1997). Norrie disease gene mutation in a large Costa Rican kindred with a novel phenotype including venous insufficiency. *Hum. Mutat.* 9:402–408.

Rehm, H. L., Zhang, D. S., Brown, M. C., Burgess, B., Halpin, C., Berger, W., Morton, C. C., Corey, D. P., and Chen Z. Y. (2002). Vascular defects and sensorineural deafness in a mouse model of Norrie disease. *J. Neurosci.* 22:4286–4292.

Richter, M., Gottanka, J., May, C. A., Welge-Lussen, U., Berger, W., and Lutjen-Drecoll, E. (1998). Retinal vasculature changes in Norrie disease mice. *Invest. Ophthalmol. Vis. Sci.* 39:2450–2457.

Robitaille, J., MacDonald, M. L., Kaykas, A., Sheldahl, L. C., Zeisler, J., Dube, M. P., Zhang, L. H., Singaraja, R. R., Guernsey, D. L., et al. (2002). Mutant frizzled-4 disrupts retinal angiogenesis in familial exudative vitreoretinopathy. *Nat. Genet.* 32:326–330.

Ruether, K., van de Pol, D., Jaissle, G., Berger, W., Tornow, R. P., and Zrenner, E. (1997). Retinoschisislike alterations in the mouse eye caused by gene targeting of the Norrie disease gene. *Invest. Ophthalmol. Vis. Sci.* 38:710–718.

Schroeder, B., Hesse, L., Bruck, W., and Gal, A. (1997). Histopathological and immunohistochemical findings associated with a null mutation in the Norrie disease gene. *Ophthalmic Genet.* 18:71–77.

Shastry, B. S., Pendergast, S. D., Hartzer, M. K., Liu, X., and Trese, M. T. (1997). Identification of missense mutations in the Norrie disease gene associated with advanced retinopathy of prematurity. *Arch. Ophthalmol.* 115:651–655.

Sims, K. B., Irvine, A. R., and Good, W. V. (1997). Norrie disease in a family with a manifesting female carrier. *Arch. Ophthalmol.* 115:517–519.

Toomes, C., Bottomley, H. M., Jackson, R. M., Towns, K. V., Scott, S., Mackey, D. A., Craig, J. E., Jiang, L., et al. (2004). Mutations in LRP5 or FZD4 underlie the common familial exudative vitreoretinopathy locus on chromosome 11q. *Am. J. Hum. Genet.* 74:721–730.

Warburg, M. (1966). Norrie's disease: A congenital progressive oculo-acoustico-cerebral degeneration. *Acta Ophthalmol. (Copenh.)* Suppl. 89:1–47.

Warburg, M., Hauge, M., and Sanger, R. (1965). Norrie's disease and the XG blood group system: Linkage data. *Acta Genet. Stat. Med.* 15:103–115.

Woodruff, G., Newbury-Ecob, R., Plaha, D. S., and Young, I. D. (1993). Manifesting heterozygosity in Norrie's disease? *Br. J. Ophthalmol.* 77(12):813–814.

Xu, Q., Wang, Y., Dabdoub, A., Smallwood, P. M., Williams, J., Woods, C., Kelley, M. W., Jiang, L., Tasman, W., et al. (2004). Vascular development in the retina and inner ear: Control by norrin and frizzled-4, a high-affinity ligand-receptor pair. *Cell* 116:883–895.

Yamada, K., Limprasert, P., Ratanasukon, M., Tengtrisorn, S., Yingchareonpukdee, J., Vasiknanonte, P., Kitaoka, T., Ghadami, M., Niikawa, N., et al. (2001). Two Thai families with Norrie disease (ND): Association of two novel missense mutations with severe ND phenotype, seizures, and a manifesting carrier. *Am. J. Med. Genet.* 100:52–55.

Zaremba, J., Feil, S., Juszko, J., Myga, W., van Duijnhoven, G., and Berger, W. (1998). Intrafamilial variability of the ocular phenotype in a Polish family with a missense mutation (A63D) in the Norrie disease gene. *Ophthalmic Genet.* 19:157–164.

44 The Lipofuscin of Retinal Pigment Epithelial Cells: Learning from Mouse Models of Retinal Disease

JANET R. SPARROW, SO R. KIM, YOUNG P. JANG, AND JILIN ZHOU

Within the visual cycle, 11-*cis*-retinal, the chromophore of visual pigment in photoreceptor cells, absorbs a photon of light, is isomerized to all-*trans*-retinal, and is then regenerated through a series of biochemical reactions within the retinal pigment epithelium (RPE). Not all of the highly reactive all-*trans*-retinal generated by photoisomerization of 11-*cis*-retinal within photoreceptor cells remains within the visual cycle, however; a minor portion inadvertently reacts to form retinoid-derived fluorophores that reside in photoreceptor outer segments until the latter are phagocytosed by RPE cells, whereupon the compounds accumulate as the lipofuscin of RPE (Sparrow and Boulton, 2005). Accordingly, all of the RPE lipofuscin fluorophores that have been isolated to date, including A2E, the A2E photoisomer iso-A2E, minor *cis*-isomers of A2E, and the all-*trans*-retinal dimer-conjugates, all-*trans*-retinal dimer-phosphatidylethanolamine (atRAL-dimer-PE), and all-*trans*-retinal dimer-ethanolamine (atRAL-dimer-E) (figure 44.1), are generated by reactions of all-*trans*-retinal. Because of their unusual structures, including that of a pyridinium bisretinoid in the case of A2E, these pigments cannot be enzymatically degraded, and thus they accumulate. The excessive accumulation of the retinoid-derived nondegradable lipofuscin in RPE cells is considered the primary cause of RPE atrophy in autosomal recessive Stargardt disease (arSTGD), a form of macular degeneration having onset in the early decades of life; RPE lipofuscin may also be a factor contributing to age-related macular degeneration (Sparrow and Boulton, 2005).

Rpe65$^{-/-}$ *mouse: Absence of all-*trans*-retinal-derived fluorophores*

Important insight into the origin of RPE lipofuscin as a by-product of the visual cycle was provided by studies of mice carrying a null mutation in Rpe65 (*Rpe65*$^{-/-}$) (Redmond et al., 1998), an essential protein of the visual cycle that is reported to be the isomerohydrolase responsible for generating 11-*cis*-retinol from all-*trans*-retinyl esters (Jin et al., 2005; Moiseyev et al., 2006). Without Rpe65, the 11-*cis*-retinal chromophore of rhodopsin is not generated, photoisomerization does not occur, and all-*trans*-retinal is not produced. We compared the constituents present in chloroform-methanol extracts of eyecups obtained from 3-month-old wild-type C57BL/6J mice to that from age-matched *Rpe65*$^{-/-}$ mice (figure 44.2), the latter lacking the 11-cisRAL and atRAL chromophores (Redmond et al., 1998). When eluent was monitored for absorbance at 440 nm using a C4 column (figure 44.2*A* and *B*), *Rpe65*$^{-/-}$ samples generated a chromatographic profile of reduced complexity as compared to C57BL/6J mice samples. Representative chromatograms are presented in figure 44.2. By simple visual subtraction analysis it was apparent that there were several peaks in the C57BL/6J profile for which there was no match in chromatograms generated from *Rpe65*$^{-/-}$ mice samples. In particular, peaks in the C57BL/6J profile were attributed to the bisretinoid lipofuscin fluorophores A2E (λ_{max} 335, 437 nm), atRAL dimer-PE (λ_{max} 271, 518 nm), and the A2E precursors, NRPE (λ_{max} 440 nm) and A2PE (λ_{max} 332, 450 nm; 333, 448 nm), all of which were identified by coelution with synthetic standard and all of which we have previously identified. None of these pigments was detectable in *Rpe65*$^{-/-}$ eyes. Further analysis of the eyecup extracts with a reverse phase C18 column (figure 44.2*C* and *D*) revealed peaks corresponding to all-*trans*-retinal (λ_{max} 378 nm), A2E (λ_{max} 335, 439 nm), iso-A2E (λ_{max} 330, 445 nm), and a conjugate of all-*trans*-retinal with ethanolamine (NRE; λ_{max} 440 nm), all of which were absent in *Rpe65*$^{-/-}$ mice. These results are consistent with the observation that lipofuscin-specific autofluorescence in the RPE is reduced by more than 90% in *Rpe65*$^{-/-}$ mice (Katz and Redmond, 2001), and they indicate that chloroform/methanol-soluble RPE lipofuscin fluorophores are derived primarily from retinoid precursors (Sparrow, Fishkin, et al.,

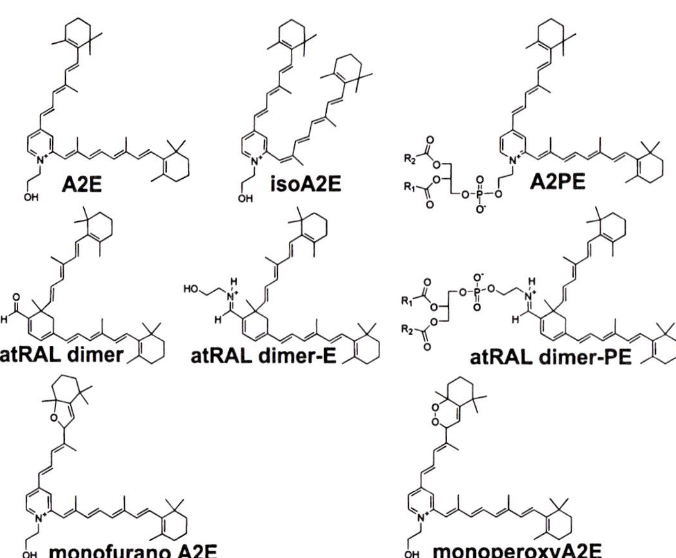

FIGURE 44.1 RPE lipofuscin pigments, precursors, and photo-oxidation products. Shown are the structures of A2E and its photoisomer, iso-A2E, and the precursor of the latter pigments, A2PE, all-*trans*-retinal dimer-phosphatidylethanolamine (atRAL dimer-PE), all-*trans*-retinal dimer-ethanolamine (atRAL dimer-E), and the precursor all-*trans*-retinal dimer (atRAL dimer). Monofurano-A2E and peroxy-A2E are photo-oxidation products of A2E.

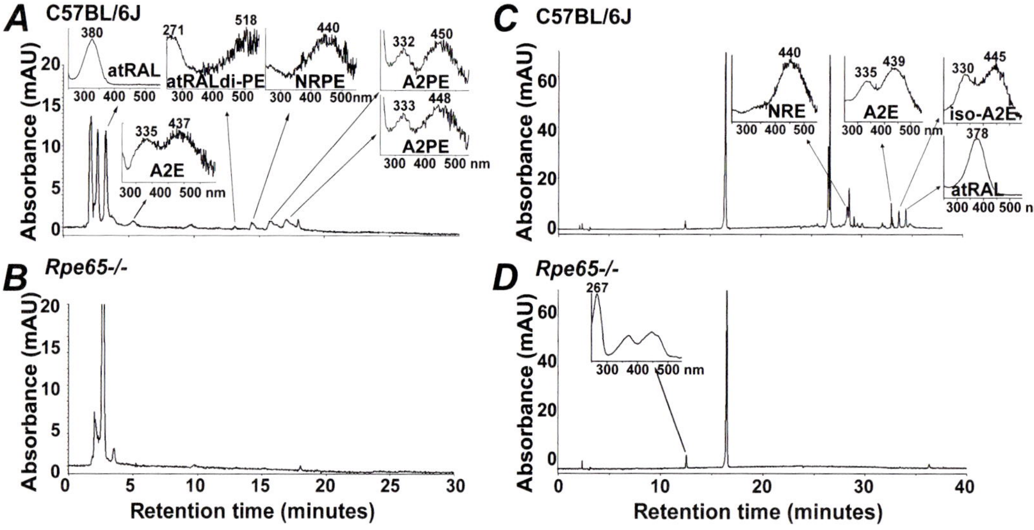

FIGURE 44.2 HPLC detection of RPE lipofuscin pigments in C57BL/6J mouse eyecups and the absence of these compounds in *Rpe65* null mutant mice. Shown are chromatograms generated from hydrophobic extracts of eyecups (6 eyecups per sample) from 3-month-old C57BL/6J (*A* and *C*) and *Rpe65*$^{-/-}$ (*B* and *D*) mice using reverse phase C4 (*A* and *B*) and C18 (*C* and *D*) columns with monitoring at 440 nm. Compounds were identified by UV/visible absorbance and by coinjection of authentic standards. The two peaks attributable to A2PE (*A*) have retention times and UV/visible absorbance that correspond to the synthesized standard dipalmitoyl-A2PE and likely reflect A2PE of varying fatty acid composition. (*Rpe65*$^{-/-}$ mice were a gift from Dr. Michael Redmond, National Eye Institute, Bethesda, MD.)

2003). Indeed, a number of observations over the years have also shown that the deposition of lipofuscin fluorophores in RPE is dependent on vitamin A availability (Katz et al., 1986, 1987). Significantly, in patients with early-onset retinal dystrophy associated with mutations in RPE65, RPE lipofuscin is also lacking (Lorenz et al., 2004).

Stargardt macular degeneration and the Abca4/Abcr *null mutant mice*

The relationship between Stargardt macular degeneration and RPE lipofuscin was elucidated by studies in *Abca4/Abcr* null mutant mice (Weng et al., 1999; Mata et al., 2000, 2001, 2002; Kim et al., 2004) (figure 44.3). ABCA4/ABCR (rim

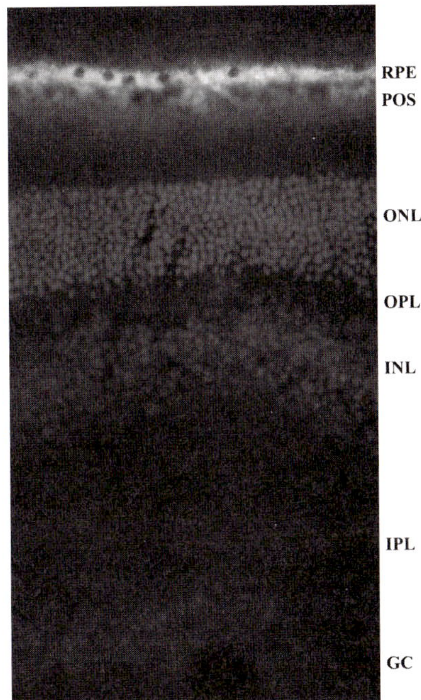

Figure 44.3 Autofluorescence of RPE lipofuscin in *Abca4/Abcr*$^{-/-}$ mouse retina. Cross section of mouse retina viewed by epifluorescence microscopy (excitation 425 ± 45 nm, emission 510 nm long pass). Nuclei are stained with DAPI. The yellow-gold autofluorescence in RPE cells is associated with lipofuscin in RPE cells. The less pronounced autofluorescence in photoreceptor outer segments (POS) is attributable to lipofuscin precursors that form in this location. The albino mouse was 8 months old and homozygous for leucine at amino acid 450 of Rpe65. GC, ganglion cell layer; INL, inner nuclear layer; IPL, inner plexiform layer; ONL, outer nuclear layer; OPL, outer plexiform layer; RPE, retinal pigment epithelium. See color plate 44.

protein) is an ATP-binding-cassette transporter and the protein product of the Stargardt disease gene, *ABCA4/ABCR* (Allikmets et al., 1997). Studies of purified and reconstituted ABCA4/ABCR protein (Sun and Nathans, 1997, 2001a, 2001b; Sun et al., 1999; Ahn et al., 2000; Beharry et al., 2004), together with work in *Abca4/Abcr*$^{-/-}$ mice (Weng et al., 1999), have shown that this photoreceptor-specific protein aids in the movement of all-*trans*-retinal to the cytosolic side of the disc membrane so that it can be reduced to all-*trans*-retinol by retinol dehydrogenase. The ligand recognized by ABCA4/ABCR is probably *N*-retinylidene-phosphatidylethanolamine (NRPE), the conjugate formed by Schiff base reaction between a single all-*trans*-retinal molecule and phosphatidylethanolamine. The reaction of NRPE with a second molecule of all-*trans*-retinal leads to a series of random/nonenzymatic reactions and the formation of an unstable dihydropyridinium (dihydro-A2PE) (Kim et al., 2007a) (see figure 44.1) compound. Simulation by time-dependent density functional theory reveals that dihydro-A2PE exhibits a UV-visible spectrum with two absorbance maxima at approximately 494 and 344 nm. Dihydro-A2PE is an unstable intermediate that automatically undergoes oxidative aromatization to yield A2PE (see figure 44.1), the precursor of A2E detectable in photoreceptor outer segments (Parish et al., 1998; Liu et al., 2000). A2PE is internalized by RPE cells concomitant with outer segment phagocytosis; within RPE cell lysosomes, A2PE subsequently undergoes phosphate cleavage to generate A2E. Due to its unusual pyridinium bisretinoid structure (Sakai et al., 1996), A2E cannot be enzymatically degraded and thus is amassed with age (figure 44.4*A*). Conversely, A2PE does not accumulate with age; this would be expected of a precursor that is continually being cleaved to generate A2E (see figure 44.4*A*).

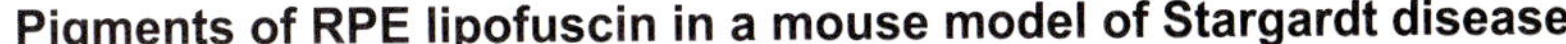

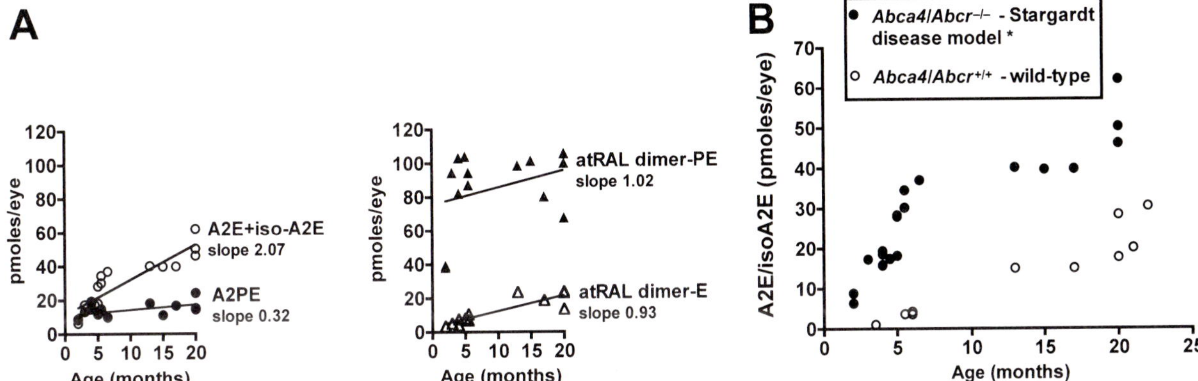

Figure 44.4 RPE lipofuscin pigments in a mouse model of Stargardt disease. *A*, A2E/iso-A2E (*left*) increases with age in *Abca4/Abcr*$^{-/-}$ mice; A2PE, the precursor of A2E in photoreceptor outer segments, does not accrue with age. Compared with A2E/iso-A2E, atRAL dimer-PE and atRAL dimer-E (*right*) exhibit increase with age. *B*, A2E increases with age and is more abundant in *Abca4/Abcr*$^{-/-}$ mice than in wild-type mice (*Abca4/Abcr*$^{+/+}$). Compounds were quantified from HPLC chromatograms and external standards to calibrate analyte peak areas.

Chromatographic studies of extracts of eyecups harvested from *Abca4/Abcr* null mutant mice have consistently demonstrated that the availability of all-*trans*-retinal resulting from a loss of *Abca4/Abcr* activity leads to levels of A2E that are increased manyfold relative to age-matched wild-type eyes (Parish et al., 1998; Mata et al., 2000; Kim et al., 2004, 2006; Fishkin et al., 2005) (figure 44.4*B*). As a model of Stargardt disease, these increases in A2E in *Abca4/Abcr*$^{-/-}$ mice parallel similar increases in individuals diagnosed with Stargardt disease (Delori et al., 1995).

A2E has an amphiphilic structure that is conferred by hydrophobic side-arms extending from a positively charged aromatic head group. A number of different approaches have shown that A2E can perturb cell membrane integrity when present in sufficient concentration (Sparrow et al., 1999, 2006; De and Sakmar, 2002; Sparrow, Fishkin, et al., 2003). This detergent-like behavior may be one means by which lipofuscin constitutents exert adverse effects on RPE cells.

A2E also has an absorbance maximum in the blue range of the visible spectrum (ca. 440 nm). Photosensitization of A2E leads to the generation of singlet oxygen and perhaps other reactive forms of oxygen. In the process, A2E is photo-oxidized along the retinoid-derived side-arms of the molecule, with the result that reactive photolytic products are generated (Sparrow et al., 2000, 2002; Schutt et al., 2000; Ben-Shabat et al., 2002; Sparrow, Vollmer-Snarr, et al., 2003; Dillon et al., 2004; Jang et al., 2006). Studies in *Abca4/Abcr*$^{-/-}$ mice have enabled detection of photo-oxidized forms of A2E. Specifically, analysis of eyecups of *Abca4/Abcr*$^{-/-}$ mice (Jang et al., 2006) by liquid chromatography-mass spectrometry permitted the detection of both monofuran-A2E (Dillon et al., 2004), a product generated by the addition of one atom of oxygen, and monoperoxy-A2E, resulting from the addition of molecular oxygen (O_2) at two carbon-carbon double bonds (see figure 44.1). In vitro studies indicate that the photo-oxidation of A2E can involve the incorporation of as many as nine oxygens into the retinoid-derived side-arms of A2E; thus we anticipate that a complex mixture of oxidized products may form in vivo, with multiple oxygen-containing moieties situated within an A2E molecule. Moreover, mass spectral studies also demonstrate that irradiation-induced oxidation can lead to A2E fragmentation. Evidence indicates that the production of reactive oxidized forms of A2E may account at least in part for the cellular damage ensuing from photochemical mechanisms initiated by blue light excitation of A2E (Sparrow, Vollmer-Snarr, et al., 2003). Indeed, the amount of A2E that undergoes photo-oxidation and cleavage in a lifetime may be significant: high performance liquid chromatography (HPLC) quantitation of A2E and its precursor, A2PE, in posterior eyecups of young mice (9 weeks) revealed that the amounts of A2PE that form are greater than is reflected in the levels of A2E that accumulate, an observation that indicates that some portion of A2E may undergo degradation (Kim et al., 2006), perhaps subsequent to oxidation.

Work in the *Abca4/Abcr*$^{-/-}$ mouse has further served in the detection and characterization of diretinal RPE lipofuscin constituents other than A2E. In particular, we found that condensation reactions between two all-*trans*-retinal leads to the generation of an aldehyde-bearing dimer (all-*trans*-retinal dimer, atRAL dimer), which then forms conjugates with primary amines such as phosphatidylethanolamine via Schiff base linkages (Fishkin et al., 2004, 2005; Kim et al., 2007b) (see figure 44.1). The pigment all-*trans*-retinal dimer-PE that forms through this unique biosynthetic pathway has a structure that is distinct from A2E/isoA2E and an absorbance maximum in the visible spectrum that is red-shifted relative to A2E (A2E/iso-A2E, λ_{max} ca. 435 nm; atRAL dimer-PE, λ_{max} ca. 510 nm). Another ca. 510 nm absorbing dimer-conjugate, atRAL dimer-E, forms by phosphate cleavage of atRAL dimer-PE. Both atRAL dimer-PE and atRAL dimer-E have been identified in the lipofuscin-filled RPE of *Abca4/Abcr*$^{-/-}$ mice and are present at higher levels in the mutant mice than in wild-type mice (see figure 44.4*A*).

The Leu450Met variant in murine Rpe65 is associated with reduced levels of retinal pigment epithelial lipofuscin

As part of our effort to understand factors that modulate RPE lipofuscin formation, we have studied the relationship between the kinetics of the visual cycle and A2E formation. The Rpe65 polymorphism present in inbred strains of mice is such that the amino acid variant at residue 450 is either leucine or methionine (Danciger et al., 2000). From biochemical and electroretinographic studies it was apparent that in C57BL/6J mice that express methionine at codon 450, regeneration of rhodopsin is slowed and photon catch is reduced as compared to BALB/cByJ mice, which have leucine at that position (Wenzel et al., 2001, 2003; Nusinowitz et al., 2003). To determine whether the reduced availability of all-*trans*-retinal is accompanied by a decrease in RPE lipofuscin formation, we relied on quantitative HPLC to measure A2E and iso-A2E levels in mice homozygous for either the Leu-450 or Met-450 allele (Kim et al., 2004) (figure 44.5). Accordingly, whether the comparison was made between C57BL/6J-c^{2J} (Met-450) and BALB/cByJ (Leu-450) mice or between Leu-450 and Met-450 in *Abca4/Abcr*$^{-/-}$ mice, the levels of A2E in the presence of the methionine variant were consistently 25%–30% of that occurring with the leucine variant. The difference in the quantity of A2E associated with the Leu-450 variant versus the Met-450 variant occurred in pigmented and albino mice and in mice of varying ages. It is likely that the reduced flux of all-

trans-retinal that accompanies slowing of the visual cycle is responsible for the decreased formation of A2E in the presence of the methionine variant in C57BL/6J-c^{2J} mice. The slowing of the visual cycle at the stage involving RPE65, a protein that has a rate-determining role in the visual cycle, can clearly provide protection against RPE lipofuscin formation.

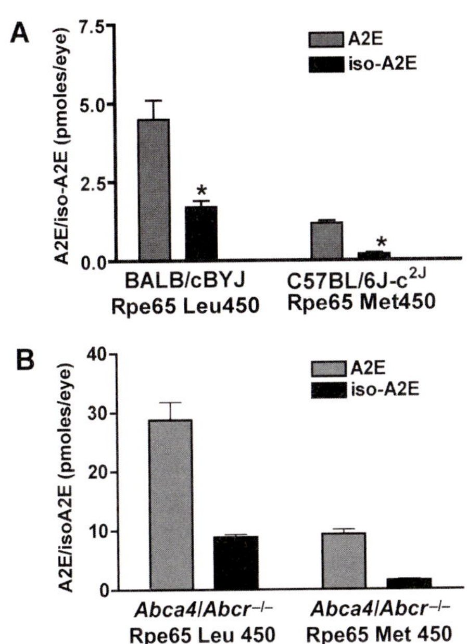

FIGURE 44.5 The levels of A2E and iso-A2E in mouse eyecups varies in relation to the Rpe65 Leu450Met variant. A2E and iso-A2E were measured in wild-type (BALB/cByJ and C57BL/6J-c^{2J}) mice (*A*) and in *Abca4/Abcr*$^{-/-}$ mice expressing either the Leu-450 or Met-450 variant of Rpe65 (*B*). Levels (mean ± SEM) were determined from HPLC chromatograms as integrated peak areas normalized to an external standard of A2E.

Targeting the visual cycle to inhibit the formation of retinal pigment epithelial lipofuscin fluorophores

Given the adverse behavior of the diretinoid pigments that form RPE lipofuscin (Sparrow et al., 1999, 2000; Schutt et al., 2000; De and Sakmar, 2002; Sparrow et al., 2002; Sparrow, Fishkin, et al., 2003; Sparrow, Vollmer-Snarr, et al., 2003; Sparrow et al., 2006), there is considerable interest in retarding A2E formation as a means to prevent vision loss in Stargardt disease and perhaps in age-related macular degeneration. Accordingly, isotretinoin (13-*cis*-retinoic acid), the acne medication that induces night blindness and protects against light damage by retarding 11-*cis*-retinal regeneration (Sieving et al., 2001), can reduce A2E deposition in RPE of *Abca4/Abcr*$^{-/-}$ mice (Radu et al., 2003). Isotretinoin is suggested to act, at least partially, by inhibiting 11-*cis*-retinol dehydrogenase (Sieving et al., 2001). Nonetheless, 13-*cis*-retinoic acid has severe side effects, including teratogenicity (Sparrow, 2003), and thus is not appropriate for long-term therapy.

The evidence garnered from studies of the Rpe65 Leu450Met variant suggested that RPE65 would be an excellent target for therapeutic interventions aimed at reducing A2E formation in arSTGD and other retinal disorders characterized by aberrant RPE lipofuscin accumulation. Thus, in a collaborative effort, we tested nonretinoid isoprenoid compounds for their ability to compete with retinyl esters for binding to RPE65, thereby interfering with visual cycle kinetics (Maiti et al., 2006). Following a single intraperitoneal injection (50 mg/kg) of the compounds TDT (figure 44.6) and TDH (not shown) in mice, recovery of dark-adapted ERG b-wave amplitudes to prebleach levels was delayed and 11-*cis*-retinal regeneration was slowed. Moreover, twice-weekly treatment of *Abca4/Abcr*$^{-/-}$ mice for 1 or 2 months resulted in substantial decreases in A2E accumulation (see figure 44.6). Thus, these nontoxic isoprenoid RPE65

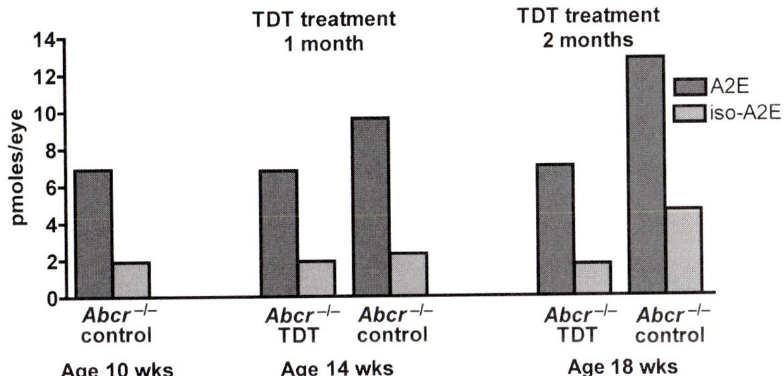

FIGURE 44.6 Nonretinoid RPE65 antagonists suppress A2E/iso-A2E formation in a mouse model of recessive Stargardt disease. Shown is the quantitation of A2E and iso-A2E in eyecups of *Abca4/Abcr*$^{-/-}$ mice. *Abca4/Abcr*$^{-/-}$ mice were treated with TDT (50 mg/kg twice weekly, intraperitoneally) for 1 or 2 months beginning at age 10 weeks, and A2E and iso-A2E levels at the end of treatment (age 14 weeks or 18 weeks) were compared to levels in 10-week-old vehicle-treated (control) mice and 14- or 18-week-old vehicle-treated (control) mice. A2E/iso-A2E levels were determined from HPLC chromatograms by integrating peak areas and normalizing to external standards. Values are expressed as picomoles per eye and are based on single samples obtained by pooling data from four eyes.

antagonists are candidates for the treatment of forms of macular degeneration in which lipofuscin accumulation is an important risk factor.

In an alternative approach, the excessive accumulation of A2E in *Abca4/Abcr*$^{-/-}$ mice has been reduced by daily administration of the retinoic acid analogue *N*-(4-hydroxyphenyl)retinamide (HPR) for 1 month (Radu et al., 2005). As shown by the investigators, HPR acts by competing for binding sites on retinol-binding protein, thus reducing serum retinol levels. As a result, retinol uptake by the eye is reduced and visual cycle retinoids are decreased. The accompanying decrease in atRAL leads to retarded A2E formation.

Future directions

Mouse models of retinal disease have elucidated the relationship between the visual cycle and RPE lipofuscin formation and will continue to be central to the development of gene- and drug-based therapies that can combat vision loss in disorders in which aberrant lipofuscin accumulation threatens RPE cell function and survival. Studies have shown that RPE lipofuscin in ABCR-associated disorders is similar in composition to age-related lipofuscin, although in ABCR-associated disorders the formation and accumulation occur at a faster rate. Work in mice should also clarify mechanisms involved in the higher levels of RPE lipofuscin reported in autosomal dominant Stargardt-like (STGD3) macular degeneration (Karan et al., 2005), an early-onset disorder due to mutations in *ELOVL4* (Zhang et al., 2001; Bernstein et al., 2001; Maugeri et al., 2004), and in Best vitelliform macular dystrophy (BMD), an autosomal dominant form of macular degeneration caused by mutations in *VMD2* (Petrukhin et al., 1998), the gene encoding bestrophin-1 (hBest1), a protein in RPE (Marmorstein et al., 2000).

ACKNOWLEDGMENTS Work was supported by National Institutes of Health grant no. EY 12951, Foundation Fighting Blindness, the American Health Assistance Foundation, the Steinbach Fund, and Research to Prevent Blindness. JRS is a recipient of an Alcon Research Institute Award.

REFERENCES

Ahn, J., Wong, J. T., and Molday, R. S. (2000). The effect of lipid environment and retinoids on the ATPase activity of ABCR, the photoreceptor ABC transporter responsible for Stargardt macular dystrophy. *J. Biol. Chem.* 275:20399–20405.

Allikmets, R., Singh, N., Sun, H., Shroyer, N. F., Hutchinson, A., Chidambaram, A., Gerrard, B., Baird, L., Stauffer, D., et al. (1997). A photoreceptor cell-specific ATP-binding transporter gene (ABCR) is mutated in recessive Stargardt macular dystrophy. *Nat. Genet.* 15:236–246.

Beharry, S., Zhong, M., and Molday, R. S. (2004). *N*-retinylidene-phosphatidylethanolamine is the preferred retinoid substrate for the photoreceptor-specific ABC transporter ABCA4 (ABCR). *J. Biol. Chem.* 279:53972–53979.

Ben-Shabat, S., Itagaki, Y., Jockusch, S., Sparrow, J. R., Turro, N. J., and Nakanishi, K. (2002). Formation of a nona-oxirane from A2E, a lipofuscin fluorophore related to macular degeneration, and evidence of singlet oxygen involvement. *Angew Chem. Int. Ed.* 41:814–817.

Bernstein, P. S., Tammur, J., Singh, N., Hutchinson, A., Dixon, M., Pappas, C. M., Zabriskie, N. A., Zhang, K., Petrukhin, K., et al. (2001). Diverse macular dystrophy phenotype caused by a novel complex mutation in the ELOVL4 gene. *Invest. Ophthalmol. Vis. Sci.* 42:3331–3336.

Danciger, M., Matthes, M. T., Yasamura, D., Akhmedov, N. B., Rickabaugh, T., Gentleman, S., Redmond, T. M., La Vail, M. M., and Farber, D. B. (2000). A QTL on distal chromosome 3 that influences the severity of light-induced damage to mouse photoreceptors. *Mam. Genome.* 11:422–427.

De, S., and Sakmar, T. P. (2002). Interaction of A2E with model membranes: Implications to the pathogenesis of age-related macular degeneration. *J. Gen. Physiol.* 120:147–157.

Delori, F. C., Staurenghi, G., Arend, O., Dorey, C. K., Goger, D. G., and Weiter, J. J. (1995). In vivo measurement of lipofuscin in Stargardt's disease: Fundus flavimaculatus. *Invest. Ophthalmol. Vis. Sci.* 36:2327–2331.

Dillon, J., Wang, Z., Avalle, L. B., and Gaillard, E. R. (2004). The photochemical oxidation of A2E results in the formation of a 5,8,5′,8′-bis-furanoid oxide. *Exp. Eye Res.* 79:537–542.

Fishkin, N., Pescitelli, G., Sparrow, J. R., Nakanishi, K., and Berova, N. (2004). Absolute configurational determination of an all-trans-retinal dimer isolated from photoreceptor outer segments. *Chirality* 16:637–641.

Fishkin, N., Sparrow, J. R., Allikmets, R., and Nakanishi, K. (2005). Isolation and characterization of a retinal pigment epithelial cell fluorophore: An all-trans-retinal dimer conjugate. *Proc. Natl. Acad. Sci. U.S.A.* 102:7091–7096.

Jang, Y. P., Matsuda, H., Itagaki, Y., Nakanishi, K., and Sparrow, J. R. (2006). Characterization of peroxy-A2E and furan-A2E photooxidation products and detection in human and mouse retinal pigment epithelial cells lipofuscin. *J. Biol. Chem.* 280:39732–39739.

Jin, M. L., Li, S., Moghrabi, W. N., Sun, H., and Travis, G. H. (2005). Rpe65 is the retinoid isomerase in bovine retinal pigment epithelium. *Cell* 122:449–459.

Karan, G., Lillo, C., Yang, Z., Cameron, D. J., Locke, K. G., Zhao, Y., Thirumalaichary, S., Li, C., Birch, D. G., et al. (2005). Lipofuscin accumulation, abnormal electrophysiology, and photoreceptor degeneration in mutant ELOVL4 transgenic mice: A model for macular degeneration. *Proc. Natl. Acad. Sci. U.S.A.* 102:4164–4169.

Katz, M. L., Drea, C. M., Robison, W. G., Jr. (1986). Relationship between dietary retinol and lipofuscin in the retinal pigment epithelium. *Mech. Ageing Dev.* 35:291–305.

Katz, M. L., Eldred, G. E., Robison, W. G., Jr. (1987). Lipofuscin autofluorescence: Evidence for vitamin A involvement in the retina. *Mech. Ageing Dev.* 39:81–90.

Katz, M. L., and Redmond, T. M. (2001). Effect of Rpe65 knockout on accumulation of lipofuscin fluorophores in the retinal pigment epithelium. *Invest. Ophthalmol. Vis. Sci.* 42:3023–3030.

Kim, S. R., Fishkin, N., Kong, J., Nakanishi, K., Allikmets, R., and Sparrow, J. R. (2004). The Rpe65 Leu450Met variant is associated with reduced levels of the RPE lipofuscin fluorophores A2E and iso-A2E. *Proc. Natl. Acad. Sci. U.S.A.* 101:11668–11672.

Kim, S. R., He, J., Yanase, E., Jang, Y. P., Berova, N., Sparrow, J. R., and Nakanishi, K. (2007a). Characterization of dihydro-A2PE: An intermediate in the A2E biosynthetic pathway. *Biochem.* 46;10122–10129.

Kim, S. R., Jang, Y. P., Jockusch, S., Fishkin, N. E., Turro, N. J., and Sparrow, J. R. (2007b). The all-*trans*-retinal dimer series of lipofuscin pigments in retinal pigment epithelial cells in a recessive Stargardt disease model. *Proc. Natl. Acad. Sci. U.S.A.* 104:19273–19278.

Kim, S. R., Nakanishi, K., Itagaki, Y., and Sparrow, J. R. (2006). Photooxidation of A2-PE, a photoreceptor outer segment fluorophore, and protection by lutein and zeaxanthin. *Exp. Eye Res.* 82:828–839.

Liu, J., Itagaki, Y., Ben-Shabat, S., Nakanishi, K., and Sparrow, J. R. (2000). The biosynthesis of A2E, a fluorophore of aging retina, involves the formation of the precursor, A2-PE, in the photoreceptor outer segment membrane. *J. Biol. Chem.* 275: 29354–29360.

Lorenz, B., Wabbels, B., Wegscheider, E., Hamel, C. P., Drexler, W., and Presing, M. N. (2004). Lack of fundus autofluorescence to 488 nanometers from childhood on in patients with early-onset severe retinal dystrophy associated with mutations in RPE65. *Ophthalmology* 111:1585–1594.

Maiti, P., Kong, J., Kim, S. R., Sparrow, J. R., Allikmets, R., and Rando, R. R. (2006). Small molecule RPE65 antagonists limit the visual cycle and prevent lipofuscin formation. *J. Biochem.* 45:852–860.

Marmorstein, A. D., Marmorstein, L. Y., Rayborn, M., Wang, X. D., Hollyfield, J. G., and Petrukhin, K. (2000). Bestrophin, the product of the Best vitelliform macular dystrophy gene (VMD2), localizes to the basolateral plasma membrane of the retinal pigment epithelium. *Proc. Natl. Acad. Sci. U.S.A.* 97: 12758–12763.

Mata, N. L., Radu, R. A., Clemmons, R. S., and Travis, G. H. (2002). Isomerization and oxidation of vitamin A in cone-dominant retinas: A novel pathway for visual-pigment regeneration in daylight. *Neuron* 36:69–80.

Mata, N. L., Tzekov, R. T., Liu, X., Weng, J., Birch, D. G., and Travis, G. H. (2001). Delayed dark adaptation and lipofuscin accumulation in $abcr^{+/-}$ mice: Implications for involvement of ABCR in age-related macular degeneration. *Invest. Ophthalmol. Vis. Sci.* 42:1685–1690.

Mata, N. L., Weng, J., and Travis, G. H. (2000). Biosynthesis of a major lipofuscin fluorophore in mice and humans with ABCR-mediated retinal and macular degeneration. *Proc. Natl. Acad. Sci. U.S.A.* 97:7154–7159.

Maugeri, A., Meire, F., Hoyng, C. B., Vink, C., Van Regemorter, N., Karan, G., Yang, Z., Cremers, F. P., and Zhang, K. (2004). A novel mutation in the ELOVL4 gene causes autosomal dominant Stargardt-like macular dystrophy. *Invest. Ophthalmol. Vis. Sci.* 45:4263–4267.

Moiseyev, G., Takahashi, Y., Chen, Y., Gentleman, S., Redmond, T. M., Crouch, R. K., and Ma, J. X. (2006). RPE65 is an iron(II)-dependent isomerohydrolase in the retinoid visual cycle. *J. Biol. Chem.* 281:2835–2840.

Nusinowitz, S., Nguyen, L., Radu, R. A., Kashani, Z., Farber, D. B., and Danciger, M. (2003). Electroretinographic evidence for altered phototransduction gain and slowed recovery from photobleaches in albino mice with a MET450 variant in RPE6. *Exp. Eye Res.* 77:627–638.

Parish, C. A., Hashimoto, M., Nakanishi, K., Dillon, J., and Sparrow, J. R. (1998). Isolation and one-step preparation of A2E and iso-A2E, fluorophores from human retinal pigment epithelium. *Proc. Natl. Acad. Sci. U.S.A.* 95:14609–14613.

Petrukhin, K., Koisti, M. J., Bakall, B., Li, W., Xie, G., Marknell, T., Sandgren, O., Forsman, K., Holmgren, G., et al. (1998). Identification of the gene responsible for Best macular dystrophy. *Nat. Genet.* 19:241–247.

Radu, R. A., Han, Y., Bui, T. V., Nusinowitz, S., Bok, D., Lichter, J., Widder, K., Travis, G. H., and Mata, N. L. (2005). Reductions in serum vitamin A arrest accumulation of toxic retinal fluorophores: A potential therapy for treatment of lipofuscin-based retinal diseases. *Invest. Ophthalmol. Vis. Sci.* 46:4393–4401.

Radu, R. A., Mata, N. L., Nusinowitz, S., Liu, X., Sieving, P. A., and Travis, G. H. (2003). Treatment with isotretinoin inhibits lipofuscin and A2E accumulation in a mouse model of recessive Stargardt's macular degeneration. *Proc. Natl. Acad. Sci. U.S.A.* 100:4742–4747.

Redmond, T. M., Yu, S., Lee, E., Bok, D., Hamasaki, D., Chen, N., Goletz, P., Ma, J.-X., Crouch, R. K., et al. (1998). Rpe65 is necessary for production of 11-*cis*-vitamin A in the retinal visual cycle. *Nat. Genet.* 20:344–351.

Sakai, N., Decatur, J., Nakanishi, K., and Eldred, G. E. (1996). Ocular age pigment "A2E": An unprecedented pyridinium bisretinoid. *J. Am. Chem. Soc.* 118:1559–1560.

Schutt, F., Davies, S., Kopitz, J., Holz, F. G., and Boulton, M. E. (2000). Photodamage to human RPE cells by A2-E, a retinoid component of lipofuscin. *Invest. Ophthalmol. Vis. Sci.* 41:2303–2308.

Sieving, P. A., Chaudhry, P., Kondo, M., Provenzano, M., Wu, D., Carlson, T. J., Bush, R. A., and Thompson, D. A. (2001). Inhibition of the visual cycle in vivo by 13-*cis* retinoic acid protects from light damage and provides a mechanism for night blindness in isotretinoin therapy. *Proc. Natl. Acad. Sci. U.S.A.* 98:1835–1840.

Sparrow, J. R. (2003). Therapy for macular degeneration: Insights from acne. *Proc. Natl. Acad. Sci. U.S.A.* 100:4353–4354.

Sparrow, J. R., and Boulton, M. (2005). RPE lipofuscin and its role in retinal photobiology. *Exp. Eye Res.* 80:595–606.

Sparrow, J. R., Cai, B., Jang, Y. P., Zhou, J., and Nakanishi, K. (2006). A2E, a fluorophore of RPE lipofuscin, can destabilize membrane. *Adv. Exp. Med. Biol.* 572:63–68.

Sparrow, J. R., Fishkin, N., Zhou, J., Cai, B., Jang, Y. P., Krane, S., Itagaki, Y., and Nakanishi, K. (2003). A2E, a byproduct of the visual cycle. *Vision Res.* 43:2983–2990.

Sparrow, J. R., Nakanishi, K., and Parish, C. A. (2000). The lipofuscin fluorophore A2E mediates blue light-induced damage to retinal pigmented epithelial cells. *Invest. Ophthalmol. Vis. Sci.* 41:1981–1989.

Sparrow, J. R., Parish, C. A., Hashimoto, M., and Nakanishi, K. (1999). A2E, a lipofuscin fluorophore, in human retinal pigmented epithelial cells in culture. *Invest. Ophthalmol. Vis. Sci.* 40:2988–2995.

Sparrow, J. R., Vollmer-Snarr, H. R., Zhou, J., Jang, Y. P., Jockusch, S., Itagaki, Y., and Nakanishi, K. (2003). A2E-epoxides damage DNA in retinal pigment epithelial cells. Vitamin E and other antioxidants inhibit A2E-epoxide formation. *J. Biol. Chem.* 278:18207–18213.

Sparrow, J. R., Zhou, J., Ben-Shabat, S., Vollmer, H., Itagaki, Y., and Nakanishi, K. (2002). Involvement of oxidative mechanisms in blue light induced damage to A2E-laden RPE. *Invest. Ophthalmol. Vis. Sci.* 43:1222–1227.

Sun, H., Molday, R. S., and Nathans, J. (1999). Retinal stimulates ATP hydrolysis by purified and reconstituted ABCR, the photoreceptor-specific ATP-binding cassette transporter responsible for Stargardt disease. *J. Biol. Chem.* 274:8269–8281.

Sun, H., and Nathans, J. (1997). Stargardt's ABCR is localized to the disc membrane of retinal rod outer segments. *Nat. Genet.* 17:15–16.

Sun, H., and Nathans, J. (2001a). ABCR, the ATP-binding cassette transporter responsible for Stargardt macular dystrophy, is an efficient target of all-trans retinal-mediated photo-oxidative damage in vitro: Implications for retinal disease. *J. Biol. Chem.* 276:11766–11774.

Sun, H., and Nathans, J. (2001b). Mechanistic studies of ABCR, the ABC transporter in photoreceptor outer segments responsible for autosomal recessive Stargardt disease. *J. Bioenerg. Biomembrane.* 33:523–530.

Weng, J., Mata, N. L., Azarian, S. M., Tzekov, R. T., Birch, D. G., and Travis, G. H. (1999). Insights into the function of Rim protein in photoreceptors and etiology of Stargardt's disease from the phenotype in *Abcr* knockout mice. *Cell* 98:13–23.

Wenzel, A., Grimm, C., Samardzija, M., and Reme, C. E. (2003). The genetic modified Rpe65Leu450: Effect on light damage susceptibility in c-Fos-deficient mice. *Invest. Ophthalmol. Vis. Sci.* 44:2798–2802.

Wenzel, A., Reme, C. E., Williams, T. P., Hafezi, F., and Grimm, C. (2001). The Rpe65 Leu450Met variation increases retinal resistance against light-induced degeneration by slowing rhodopsin regeneration. *J. Neurosci.* 21:53–58.

Zhang, K., Kniazeva, M., Han, M., Li, W., Yu, Z., Yang, Z., Li, Y., Metzker, M. L., Allikmets, R., et al. (2001). A 5-bp deletion in ELOVL4 is associated with two related forms of autosomal dominant macular dystrophy. *Nat. Genet.* 27:89–93.

45 Studies of Diabetic Retinopathy Using Mice

ROSE A. GUBITOSI-KLUG AND TIMOTHY S. KERN

Diabetic retinopathy is a progressive retinal disease that threatens patients with blindness. The retinopathy develops slowly, over decades in humans, making investigation of its pathogenesis challenging. Many animal models have been developed to study the evolution of the retinopathy (Kern and Mohr, 2008). The rate of development of the early stages of the retinopathy seems to vary among species, with at least the early stages of the retinal disease apparently progressing faster in smaller species such as the mouse. The relatively short interval until pathology presents, coupled with the ability to genetically engineer the mouse, has prompted an increased interest in mouse models. This chapter reviews mouse models of diabetic retinopathy, compares pathological changes in the retina of the diabetic mouse with those in humans, and highlights advances made using mice to understand the pathogenesis of the retinopathy.

Diabetic retinopathy in humans

Diabetic retinopathy has classically referred to alterations in the retinal microvasculature visualized on ophthalmoscopic examination (Davis et al., 1997). Over the course of disease progression, two stages of retinal pathology have been defined:

1. Retinal lesions observed clinically in early retinopathy, or the *nonproliferative stage of retinopathy* (previously referred to as background retinopathy), consist of nonperfused capillaries, microaneurysms, retinal hemorrhages, cotton wool spots, exudates, and edema. Each of these lesions is believed to represent local alteration in the microvascular circulation of the retina, which in some cases results in damage to the surrounding retinal cells.

Histological studies using techniques to isolate the retinal vasculature have demonstrated that the vascular histopathology includes capillary microaneurysms, pericyte-deficient capillaries, basement membrane thickening, and degenerate (acellular) capillaries (Aguilar et al., 2003; Cogan and Kuwabara, 1967; Engerman, 1989; Kohner and Henkind, 1970). In addition, histological analysis of the human retina has demonstrated changes in the nonvascular retina as well, including ganglion cell loss (Barber et al., 1998; Bloodworth and Molitor, 1965; Bresnick and Palta, 1987a, 1987b; Lieth et al., 2000). Currently, several different therapies, including intensive insulin therapy and blood pressure medications, are available to inhibit the development of the nonproliferative stage of diabetic retinopathy (The Diabetes Control and Complications Trial Research Group, 1993; Jandeleit-Dahm and Cooper, 2006; Zhang et al., 2001).

2. Subsequently, a *proliferative retinopathy* develops in about 10%–15% of diabetic patients, with marked growth of new blood vessels growing out of the existing retinal vasculature onto the surface of the retina and into the vitreous. These newly formed blood vessels (as well as other blood vessels in the retina) leak, occasionally resulting in vitreous hemorrhages, which can obstruct vision (Cunha-Vaz et al., 1975). In addition, with the development of these new vessels a preretinal fibrovascular membrane can form that also can obstruct vision. The neovascularization, preretinal hemorrhage, and membranes currently can be corrected using photocoagulation or vitrectomy, respectively.

In addition to vitreous hemorrhages, other late retinal changes that lead to visual impairment in diabetic retinopathy include retinal detachments (caused by traction of the fibrovascular membrane associated with new vessel formation) and retinal edema secondary to breakdown of the blood-retinal barrier and leakage of plasma from the microvasculature. The evolution of these stages of diabetic retinopathy in humans occurs over years, with nonproliferative changes first detected at 5–10 years of diabetes and proliferative changes developing later.

Diabetic retinopathy in mice

The desire to investigate the pathogenesis of diabetic retinopathy has driven the development and evaluation of many animal models of diabetic retinopathy. Of course, the better the human disease is replicated, the better the animal model. To date, the diabetic dog is the animal model that best reproduces the nonproliferative stages of diabetic retinopathy, reproducibly developing lesions seen rarely or not at all in rodent models (Engerman, 1989; Engerman and Bloodworth, 1965; Kern and Mohr, 2007). Because retinopathy in the dog requires 3–5 years to develop, however, the associated time and cost make using this model cumbersome.

Moreover, the availability of antibodies and reagents to conduct molecular studies is very limited for dogs. Mice develop degenerate, acellular capillaries in the retina, a critical step in the progression of diabetic retinopathy, as well as some other lesions characteristic of the early stages of retinopathy (Feit-Leichman et al., 2005). The mouse model has a number of advantages over larger models, including lesser space requirements and cost. The mouse also allows genetic manipulation and relatively easy administration of limited pharmacological therapies.

Anatomical differences between the mouse and human retina do exist. The mouse retina has multiple arteries emanating from the optic nerve that feed the different regions of the retina (figure 45.1), whereas the human retina receives its blood supply from one main artery, the ophthalmic artery, which divides only after entering the retina. In addition, retinas from mice (as well as all other nonprimate species) differ from the human retina in that only humans and primates possess a macula (see figure 45.1).

Initial investigations using the mouse as a model of diabetic retinopathy yielded controversial results, but, more recent results have shown the mouse model to reliably develop capillary degeneration, pericyte loss, and capillary basement membrane thickening (Feit-Leichman et al., 2005; Hammes et al., 2002; Joussen et al., 2004; Midena et al., 1989). Diabetes can be induced experimentally using drugs such as streptozotocin and alloxan to disrupt pancreatic beta cells, thus reproducing an insulinopenia like that of type I diabetes. Several strains of mice (including the C57BL/6J-Ins2^{Akita} [Akita], db/db, KK.Cg-A^{y}/J [KKAY], and NOD strains) develop diabetes spontaneously and have microvascular changes of the retina consistent with nonproliferative retinopathy (capillary degeneration, pericyte loss, thickening of capillary basement membrane) over a period of 6–9 months (Barber et al., 2005; Cheung et al., 2005; Feit-Leichman et al., 2005; Naeser and Agren, 1978; Ning et al., 2004; Whetzel et al., 2006). The Akita and NOD strains are models of type I diabetes, and db/db and KKAY strains are models of type II diabetes.

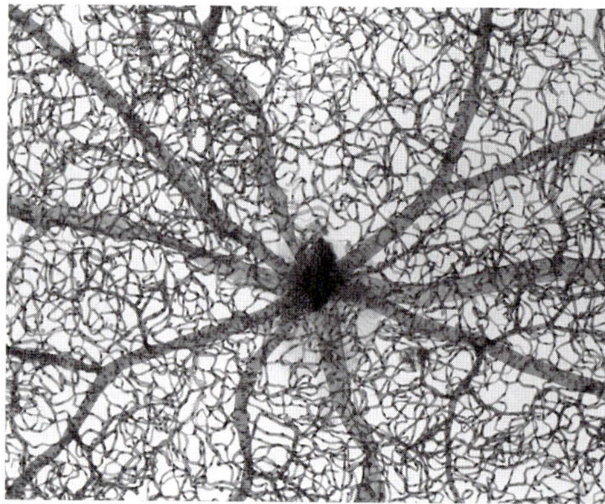

Figure 45.1 The retinal vasculature of the mouse, following isolation by proteolytic digestion of the formalin-fixed retina. See color plate 45.

Retinal function, as demonstrated by the electroretinogram (ERG), becomes impaired in diabetic mice and other models (Barile et al., 2005; Zheng et al., 2007). Whether or not diabetes causes degeneration of retinal neurons in mice is an area of controversy. Some investigators have reported extensive degeneration of retinal ganglion cells (RGCs) in C57BL/6J mice after diabetes duration as little as 14 weeks (Martin et al., 2004), whereas others have not detected retinal neurodegeneration in that strain even after durations of up to 1 year (Feit-Leichman et al., 2005). Retinal neurodegeneration has been detected in a different diabetic mouse strain, the Akita. Whether or not neuronal cell loss plays an important role in diabetic retinopathy and eventual visual impairment remains an open question.

To date, diabetic mice have not been found to develop preretinal neovascularization secondary to diabetes. (Likewise, neither experimentally diabetic dogs, cats, rats, nor other species have been found to develop the proliferative retinopathy; Kern and Mohr, 2007.) The relatively short duration of diabetes in most studies and the resulting modest extent of capillary degeneration in studies of mice are believed to be the reason that neovascularization has not been observed in these models. Advanced proliferative retinopathy similar to that seen in diabetic patients does develop in nondiabetic mice, however, under specific stresses or gene alterations (Lai et al., 2005; Ruberte et al., 2004; Smith et al., 1999). This is discussed further in a later section.

The mouse models used to study the nonproliferative vascular lesions, neurodegenerative changes, and proliferative stages of diabetic retinopathy are detailed in the next section. Each model is evaluated based on the histopathological changes observed and the pathogenic mechanisms tested using these models.

Mouse models of vascular lesions of nonproliferative retinopathy

Chemically Induced Diabetes The C57BL/6J mouse is the strain of mouse most used in studies of diabetic retinopathy. Typically, diabetes is induced as a result of a 3- to 5-day course of streptozotocin (50–75 mg/kg of body weight), although other single-dose regimens exist. Several days after chemical induction, randomly sampled blood glucose levels of 250 mg/dL or higher denote diabetes. Long-term monitoring of glycohemoglobin (HbA1c or GHb) ensures comparable degrees of hyperglycemia among experimental groups. Vascular changes consistent with diabetic retinopathy, including acellular capillaries, pericyte loss, and capillary cell apoptosis, become apparent beginning about 6 months after the onset of diabetes (figure 45.2)

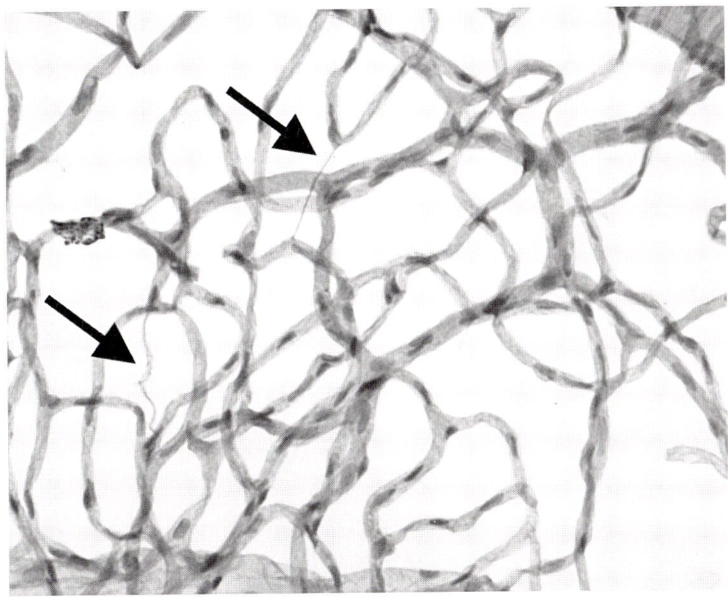

FIGURE 45.2 Degenerate (acellular) capillaries (*arrows*) in the diabetic mouse retina. The degenerate vessels lack vascular cell nuclei and have an irregular or shrunken diameter compared to surrounding healthy capillaries. See color plate 46.

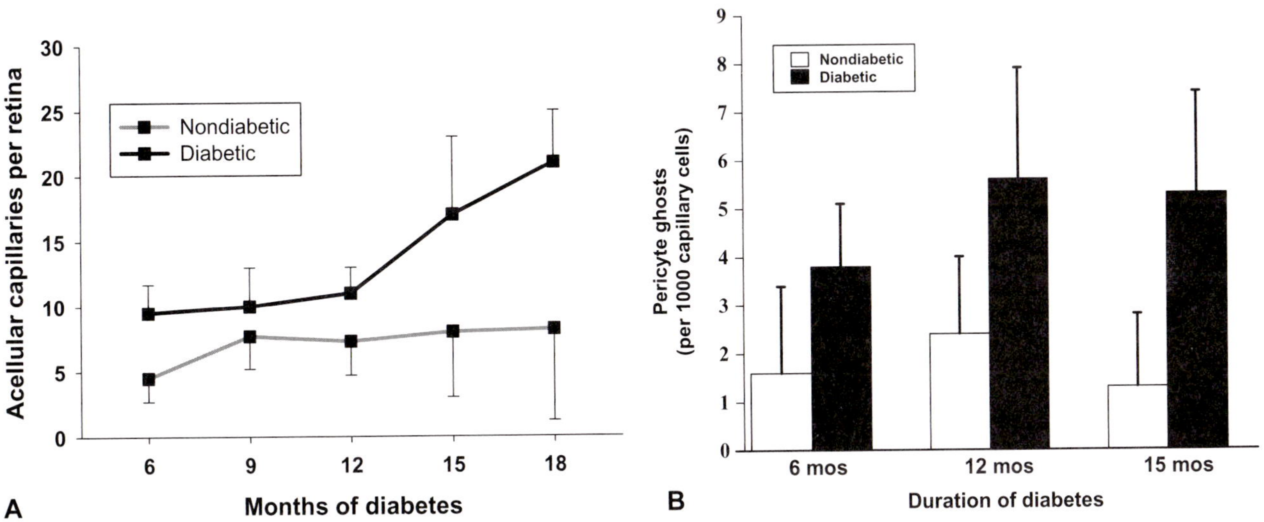

FIGURE 45.3 Frequency of acellular capillaries (*A*) and pericyte loss (*B*) increase with duration of diabetes in the C57BL/6J mouse.

(Feit-Leichman et al., 2005). The number of acellular capillaries and pericyte ghosts increases with diabetes duration (figure 45.3). Maintaining diabetes for 12 months or more is difficult, owing to increasing mortality, but administration of insulin in doses sufficient to prevent body weight loss but not reduce hyperglycemia (0.1–0.2 U; 2–3 times per week) seems to reduce mortality. Several characteristic lesions of early diabetic retinopathy in humans (including microaneurysms and retinal hemorrhages) have not been reproducibly detected in diabetic mice over the 6–12 months that the animals commonly are studied.

SPONTANEOUS DIABETES

Akita mouse. The Akita mouse develops type I diabetes spontaneously due to a dominant point mutation in the insulin 2 gene (Barber et al., 2005). Heterozygote male mice show hyperglycemia and hypoinsulinemia by 4 weeks of age. By 12 weeks of age, the diabetic mice develop increased vascular permeability compared to sibling wild-type mice. Acellular capillary formation and pericyte loss become statistically greater than in nondiabetic animals at about 6 months of diabetes, and increase with longer diabetes duration (Barber et al., 2005).

db/db mouse. The db/db mouse is a genetic model of type II diabetes. A mutation in the leptin receptor gene leads to obesity and subsequent obesity-induced type II diabetes mellitus. These mice have been reported to develop an increased endothelial cell:pericyte ratio (Midena et al., 1989). This was interpreted as a reduction in the number of capillary pericytes, but this ratio could also increase as a result of endothelial cell proliferation (Cuthbertson and Mandel, 1986). Diabetes-induced vessel leakage, degeneration of capillaries, thickening of retinal capillary basement membrane, and increased expression of vascular endothelial growth factor (VEGF, the protein encoded by gene *Vegfa*) and platelet/endothelial cell adhesion molecule-1 (PECAM-1, the protein encoded by gene *Pecam1*) have been detected at 15 months of age (Cheung et al., 2005).

db/db mice were crossed with apolipoprotein E (Apoe)-deficient mice to generate insulin-deficient and hyperlipidemic animals (Barile et al., 2005). The superimposition of hyperlipidemia on diabetes resulted in accelerated development of acellular capillaries and pericyte loss at 6 months of diabetes (Barile et al., 2005). This same hyperglycemic, hyperlipidemic model was used to study the role of advanced glycation end products (AGEs) in the development of diabetic retinopathy. Diabetes-induced capillary degeneration and pericyte loss could be inhibited by the administration of soluble receptors for AGEs (sRAGE) daily from 8 weeks to 6 months of diabetes (Barile et al., 2005), thus suggesting that AGEs play a role in the development of retinal histopathology in this model. Consistent with the conclusions of that study, the diabetes-induced thickening of retinal capillary basement membranes in the outer plexiform layer (OPL) of the retina from diabetic db/db mice was not observed after intraperitoneal injection with antibodies against glycated albumin (Clements et al., 1998). Whether or not this therapeutic approach also had effects on other aspects of the microvascular disease was not determined.

Aldose reductase deficiency in db/db mice, achieved by crossing db/db mice and aldose reductase null mutation mice, resulted in less of the diabetes-induced increase in vascular permeability, VEGF expression, and PECAM-1 expression than that seen in control db/db mice (Cheung et al., 2005). The effect of aldose reductase deficiency on the development of retinal histopathology has not been reported to date in diabetic mice, but results in other species have been mixed (Dagher et al., 2004; Engerman and Kern, 1993).

KKAY mouse. The KKAY mouse develops diabetes mellitus when fed a high fat diet, thus, it is considered a genetic model of type II diabetes mellitus (Siracusa, 1994). Control animals are fed a standard diet. After 3 months of diabetes, KKAY mice demonstrated microvascular changes that included variable basement membrane thickening, mitochondrial swelling, capillary peripheral cell edema and degeneration, and endothelial cell hyperplasia, as detected by transmission electron microscopy (Ning et al., 2004). These animals have not been studied with respect to susceptibility to developing capillary degeneration, microaneurysms, or other characteristic vascular histopathology.

NOD mouse. The nonobese diabetic mouse (NOD) develops diabetes through an autoimmune-mediated destruction of pancreatic beta cells (Leiter et al., 1987). The resulting insulitis leads to spontaneous hyperglycemia, again modeling type I diabetes in humans. Retinas from the NOD mouse have not yet been examined for the development of the characteristic microvascular lesions of diabetic retinopathy.

ob/ob mouse. ob/ob mice are leptin deficient, and phenotypically are obese by 4 weeks of age. Regression of pancreatic islets results in severe diabetes and early death when on the C57BLKS background. In control animals (C57BL/6J background), the mice are only transiently hyperglycemic, blood glucose returning to normal by 14–16 weeks. Retinas from these obese, hyperglycemic mice were morphologically the same as in littermate controls, with a similar endothelial: pericyte ratio and absence of microaneuryms (Naeser and Agren, 1978).

Nondiabetic Mouse Models That Develop Diabetic-Like Retinopathy

Galactose feeding. Feeding nondiabetic mice a high-galactose diet results in systemic elevation of blood galactose levels, but glucose levels remain normal. This model confirms the causative role of elevated hexose in the pathogenesis of diabetic retinopathy, since the other metabolic alterations characteristic of insulin deficiency, including altered lipid metabolism, are not observed (Engerman and Kern, 1984). In mice fed 30% galactose, the retinopathy can be followed for up to 24 months because the animals generally are quite healthy. Mice (C57BL/6J or BALB/cJ) fed 30% galactose develop a diabetic-like retinopathy with acellular capillaries, pericyte ghosts, basement membrane thickening, and occasional saccular microaneurysms (Joussen et al., 2004; Kern and Engerman, 1996). The advantages of this model are that experimental galactosemia is easy to establish and the animals require less care than diabetic animals. A possible deficiency of the model is that galactosemic retinopathy might differ in several ways from that in diabetes (Frank et al., 1997; Kern et al., 2000; Mohr et al., 2002). Moreover, the cost of the galactose diet can be expensive for large experimental groups.

Plasminogen activator inhibitor-1 (PAI-1). PAI-1 regulates serine proteases known as plasminogen activators (PAs). PAs convert plasminogen to plasmin, which then degrades fibrin, as well as basement membrane components such as laminin and fibronectin. A transgenic mouse model was developed with the human PAI-1 gene sequence (*SERPINE1*) under regulation of the metallothionein promoter (Grant et al., 2000). Administration of $ZnSO_4$, which allows for continuous expression of the transgene, resulted in increased PAI-1 immunoreactivity in the retinal capillaries. Electron microscopy demonstrated increased basement membrane thickening in the PAI-1-overexpressing mice compared to control animals. Whole-mount retinal analysis revealed an increased endothelial cell:pericyte ratio (even in the absence of diabetes), suggesting that PAI-1 might contribute to alterations in vascular structure. Degeneration of capillaries in diabetes has not been determined in this model.

Platelet-derived growth factor(PDGF-B). PDGF-B (encoded by gene *Pdgfb*) is an important factor in pericyte recruitment, and studies support a role for pericytes in the formation and stabilization of vessels. Mice that are heterozygous for *Pdgfb* (i.e., with one functional allele) have fewer pericytes and a significant increase in the number of acellular capillaries in their retinas compared to wild-type littermates (Hammes et al., 2002). Under diabetic conditions, the retinopathy of the *Pdgfb* heterozygous mice was worsened, with increased formation of acellular capillaries and lesions regarded as microaneurysms. In addition, studies of nondiabetic mice deficient in endothelium-specific PDGF-B demonstrated pericyte deficiency associated with capillaries of variable diameter, density, and ring structure, as well as microaneurysms (Enge et al., 2002). This suggests an important role for PDGF-B in the development of diabetic retinopathy.

Use of mouse models to study diabetes-induced retinal neurodegeneration

Of the many experimental models of developing retinal microvascular lesions described in the previous section, only a few have been examined for neurodegenerative changes to date. The mouse models evaluated thus far are reviewed in this section. Techniques to quantify neurodegenerative changes in the retina include counting the number of cells in the ganglion cell layer (GCL) per length of retina, quantifying the number of retinal neurons that are immunopositive for activated caspase-3 (encoded by gene *Casp3*) or TUNEL stain, or measuring the thickness of the retina or neuroretinal layers.

C57BL/6J mouse. The C57BL/6J mouse strain has been evaluated for diabetes-induced neurodegeneration in the retina. Some investigators reported a 20%–25% reduction in cells of the GCL of the retina as early as 14 weeks of diabetes (Martin et al., 2004). In contrast, others did not detect any GC loss at diabetes durations of up to 1 year (Feit-Leichman et al., 2005). No explanation for these different conclusions has yet been put forth. Retinal glia cells also have been reported to show signs that suggest cell death in diabetes (Kusner et al., 2004). Translocation of glyceraldehyde-3-phosphate dehydrogenase (GAPDH) to the nucleus, which is strongly associated with cell death in cerebral injury (Tatton et al., 2000), has also been demonstrated in retinal Müller cells of diabetic mice and humans (Kusner et al., 2004).

Akita mouse. In the Akita mouse at 22 weeks of hyperglycemia, neurodegenerative changes detected included a reduction in (1) the thickness of the inner plexiform layer in the central and peripheral portions of the retina, (2) the thickness of the inner nuclear layer, and (3) the number of nuclei in the RGC layer (Barber et al., 2005). Although morphological alterations in the astrocytes and microglia were observed, no changes in glial fibrillary acidic protein (GFAP) immunoreactivity were noted. After 4 weeks of diabetes, caspase-3 immunoreactivity increased, suggesting increased apoptosis of some cells of the neuroglial retina.

db/db mouse. At 15 months of age, db/db mice have been reported to demonstrate accelerated ganglion cell apoptosis and glial cell activation as detected by GFAP staining (Cheung et al., 2005).

At 6 months of diabetes, db/db mice crossed with Apoe-deficient mice had abnormal function of retinal neurons as characterized by abnormal electroretinograms (ERGs) (Barile et al., 2005).

Aldose reductase deficiency in the db/db mouse resulted in a reduction in the number of caspase-3 immunoreactive cells and GFAP-positive cells compared to the wild-type db/db diabetics (Cheung et al., 2005).

KKAY mouse. In this model, neurodegeneration was quantified by the use of TUNEL staining of ultrathin sections of fixed retinas at 1 and 3 months of diabetes (Ning et al., 2004). An increased rate of neuronal cell loss in the ganglion cell in diabetic compared to control animals has been reported. The number of apoptotic cells increased with the duration of diabetes in both the RGC layer and the inner nuclear layer.

Biochemical changes in the mouse retina that contribute to the development of diabetic retinopathy

In both clinical trials and experimental studies of diabetic models, hyperglycemia has been found to be closely associated with the development of the spectrum of lesions regarded as diabetic retinopathy (Engerman and Kern, 1995; Zhang et al., 2001). Diabetes-induced death of retinal capillary and neuroglial cells likely is due to (1) metabolic abnormalities within those cells or (2) extracellular events, such as capillary obstruction by leukocytes, platelets, or erythrocytes, or receptor-mediated processes initiated by binding of AGE or insulin-like growth factor I (IGF-I) (figure 45.4). Oxidative stress, protein kinase C, the sequelae of nonenzymatic glycation, altered metabolism of sugar through glycolysis and the polyol pathways, and inflammatory processes have been postulated to be intracellular abnormalities contributing to the pathogenesis of the retinopathy (Joussen et al., 2004; Kowluru, 2002; Moore et al., 2003; Ruberte et al., 2004; Vlassara, 2001). The respective contributions of these sequelae of hyperglycemia to the pathogenesis of diabetic retinopathy remain under investigation.

A comparison of metabolic abnormalities in the retinas of diabetic mice and rats has demonstrated both similarities and differences. At 2 months' duration of diabetes, diabetes-induced reductions in glutathione and increases in nitric oxide, lipid peroxide, and protein kinase C activity in the mouse retina paralleled results in the rat model (Kowluru, 2002). Another study compared the mouse and rat models using a different panel of biochemical changes at 6 weeks of diabetes (Obrosova et al., 2006). Whereas the rat model showed enhanced VEGF expression, increased poly(ADP-ribosyl)ation, and decreased antioxidant enzyme activities, the mouse model reflected none of these changes. However, documentation of long-term hyperglycemia was not presented in the latter publication, and differences in the severity of hyperglycemia between the studies might have contributed to the differences between the rat and mouse models. Overall, it seems that the biochemical alterations in the mouse model are less severe than in the rat model, although in both models animals develop a similar severity of capillary degeneration at approximately the same duration of diabetes (6–8 months).

The administration of pharmacological therapies that can inhibit a particular biochemical defect or the induction of diabetes in mice having selective gene deficiencies has provided novel insights into the pathogenesis of the early stages of diabetic retinopathy. Several of these areas of investigation are summarized here.

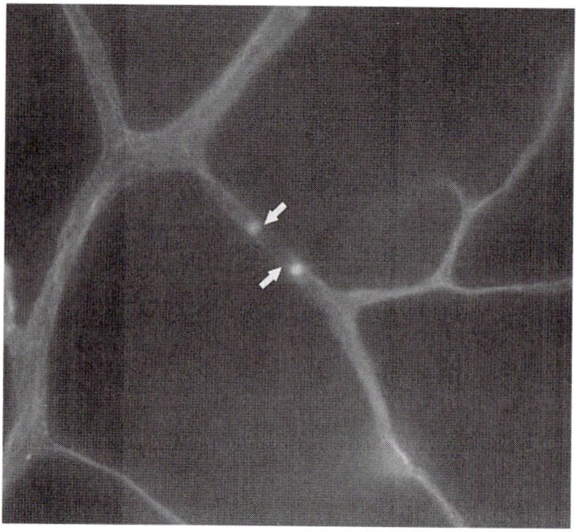

FIGURE 45.4 Leukocyte adherence, or leukostasis (*arrows*), in the retinal microvasculature of the diabetic mouse. See color plate 47.

Advanced glycation end products. AGEs form and accumulate in the retinal microvascular cells of diabetic animals and have been linked to generation of oxidative stress and activation of NFkB, a transcription factor that regulates expression of a variety of pro-inflammatory proteins, including inducible nitric oxide synthase (iNOS, which is encoded by gene *Nos2*) and intracellular adhesion molecule-1 (ICAM-1, the protein encoded by gene *Icam1*) (Goldin et al., 2006; Vlassara, 2001). To assess in vivo the role of AGEs in retinal microvascular disease, nondiabetic C57BL/6J mice received 7 daily intraperitoneal injections of AGE-albumin or albumin alone as control (Moore et al., 2003). The mice receiving AGE-albumin demonstrated a threefold increase in NFkB expression compared to control animals, as well as a significant increase in *Icam1* mRNA, leukocyte adherence, and blood-retinal barrier breakdown. Moreover, hyperlipidemic diabetic mice were protected from capillary degeneration, pericyte loss, and neural dysfunction by administration of sRAGE (a soluble form of the receptor for AGE, which is a therapy that reduces binding of AGEs to cellular receptors) (Barile et al., 2005).

Aldose reductase. Aldose reductase (AR) is the first enzyme in the polyol pathway. During hyperglycemia, excess glucose is converted by AR to sorbitol and then potentially to fructose by sorbitol dehydrogenase. AR activity is increased in diabetes, although more modestly so in the mouse retina than in the rat retina (Kowluru, 2002; Obrosova et al., 2006). Transgenic mice overexpressing human AR (*AKR1B1*) fed a galactose-rich diet for 7 days demonstrated occlusion of the retinochoroidal vessels. AR (encoded by gene *Akr1b3*)-deficient mice crossed with db/db mice were protected from diabetes-associated microvascular and neurodegenerative changes (Cheung et al., 2005).

Angiopoietin. Pericyte loss is heralded as an early morphological change in diabetic retinopathy, in part because pericytes are believed to regulate endothelial proliferation. Evidence indicates that angiopoietin-1 and -2 regulate vessel sprouting and regression through pericyte recruitment. Both angiopoietin-1 and -2 have been evaluated in mouse models for roles in diabetic retinopathy pathogenesis. At 16 weeks of diabetes, mice injected via tail vein with an adenovirus coding for human angiopoietin-1 (gene *ANGPT1*) demonstrated less leukocyte adherence, reduced endothelial cell damage or death (as detected by propidium iodide staining), and inhibition of blood-retinal barrier breakdown (Joussen et al., 2002). Recently, heterozygous deficiency of angiopoietin-2 (mouse gene *Angpt2*) in Ang-2 lacZ knock-in mice prevented loss of pericytes and acellular capillary formation at 26 weeks of diabetes (Hammes et al., 2004). This suggests that angiopoietin-1 and -2 are involved in various proposed pathogenic mechanisms leading to diabetic retinopathy.

Eicosanoids. Eicosanoids, metabolites of arachidonic acid, are known inflammatory mediators. 5-Lipoxygenase (Alox5) products, including leukotriene B_4 and leukotriene C_4/D_4/E_4, function in leukocyte recruitment and vascular permeability, respectively. Over a period of 9 months of diabetes, Alox5 deficiency inhibited the degeneration of retinal capillaries (Gubitosi-Klug and Kern, 2006). In addition, diabetes-induced leukostasis (Gubitosi-Klug and Kern, 2006) and superoxide generation (Gubitosi-Klug and Kern, 2008) in the retina were significantly inhibited in the Alox5-deficient mice compared to diabetic wild-type controls.

Intracellular adhesion molecule-1 and CD18. ICAM-1 (encoded by gene *Icam1*) and its ligand CD18 (encoded by gene *Itgb2*) are involved in the adherence of leukocytes to the vascular endothelium, especially in inflammatory conditions. The role of these molecules and leukostasis in diabetic retinopathy was explored using ICAM-1- and CD18-deficient mice (Joussen et al., 2004). In both the streptozotocin-induced diabetic and galactosemic models, permeability of the retinal vasculature and the number of leukocytes adhering to the retinal vasculature were less in the diabetic ICAM-1- or CD18-deficient mice than in diabetic wild-type controls. Of note, capillary degeneration and pericyte loss also were inhibited in these genetically deficient animals compared to wild-type diabetic controls (Joussen et al., 2004).

Inducible nitric oxide synthase. Nitric oxide (NO) is an important signaling molecule in many physiological processes such as inflammation and cell survival. It is synthesized by two types of nitric oxide synthase, one that is expressed constitutively and another that is regulated or induced (iNOS) by cellular stimuli such as cytokines. After 9 months of diabetes, mice deficient in iNOS (encoded by gene *Nos2*) had developed significantly less degeneration of retinal capillaries than wild-type diabetic control animals (Zheng et al., 2007). Diabetic iNOS-deficient mice had less leukostasis and less production of nitric oxide, PGE2, and superoxide.

Interleukin-1β. IL-1β (encoded by gene *IL1β*) is a proinflammatory cytokine that acts through IL-1β receptors on cells. The role of IL-1β in the development of diabetic retinopathy has been investigated in two mouse models. Inhibition of caspase-1 activity (the enzyme that activates IL-1β) by administration of minocycline inhibited retinal levels of IL-1β and inhibited the degeneration of retinal capillaries in C57BL/6J mice having chemically induced diabetes or galactosemia (Vincent and Mohr, 2007). As a further confirmation of the role of IL-1β in degeneration of retinal capillaries, mice lacking the IL-1β receptor likewise were protected from degeneration of retinal capillaries in diabetes (Vincent and Mohr, 2007).

Superoxide dismutase. It has been demonstrated in rats (Du et al., 2003) and mice (unpublished results) that diabetes induces an increase in superoxide production. Retinal mitochondrial superoxide dismutase activity has been found to be subnormal in diabetic rats (Du et al., 2003), likely contributing to this increase in superoxide. A recent report examined the effect of mitochondrial superoxide dismutase (encoded by gene *Sod2*) overexpression on retinal oxidative and nitrative stress parameters at 7 weeks of diabetes duration (Kowluru et al., 2006). In contrast to wild-type diabetic mice, diabetic mice overexpressing *Sod2* did not show subnormal glutathione levels or elevated nitrotyrosine levels. Possible effects on the development of retinal lesions in diabetes have not been reported to date.

Mouse models of proliferative retinopathy

To date, diabetic mice have not been found to develop proliferative (preretinal neovascularization) retinopathy without the superimposition of some other stress. Thus, studies of retinal neovascularization have relied on other pathological processes that result in new vessel growth in the retina. The nondiabetic models of retinal neovascularization are being used as models of the neovascular process in diabetic proliferative retinopathy. Available evidence suggests that VEGF-mediated neovascularization in diabetes is similar to that underlying other conditions of retinal neovascularization, such as retinopathy of prematurity. Non-VEGF-mediated mechanisms of neovascularization have been identified recently, and the ability of the nondiabetic and acute models to reproduce the complexity of all the stimuli of neovascularization induced by diabetes remains to be learned.

Oxygen-induced retinopathy. This model differs from that of diabetic retinopathy in that the retina in oxygen-induced retinopathy is immature and poorly differentiated. Newborn mice, typically C57BL/6J, are exposed from P7 to P12 to hyperoxic conditions, during which interval vascular development is arrested. The mice then are returned to room air, the retinas thus becoming relatively "hypoxic" as a result of the inadequate vascularization of the retina. Preretinal neovascularization and upregulation of VEGF develop during the subsequent days in room air (Smith et al., 1994).

Using this mouse model, multiple in vivo studies have been done to investigate candidate antiangiogenic drugs. For example, inhibition of neovascularization has been achieved by intravitreal injection of soluble VEGF receptor/IgG fusion proteins, Vegfa antisense oligonucleotides, neutralizing VEGF antibodies, soluble erythropoietin receptor, and intravitreal injection of MAE 87, a receptor tyrosine kinase inhibitor (Agostini et al., 2005; Aiello et al., 1995; Robinson et al., 1996; Sone et al., 1999; Watanabe et al., 2005). In addition, insulin receptor and IGF-I receptor gene deficient mice are protected from hypoxia-induced retinal neovascularization (Kondo et al., 2003). Lentivirus-mediated expression of angiostatin, a derivative of plasminogen, also inhibited this hypoxia-induced retinal neovascularization (Igarashi et al., 2003).

An important role of nitric oxide in the neovascular response and retinal development has been demonstrated in mice lacking iNOS. Oxygen-induced retinopathy induced less apoptosis and thinning in the inner nuclear layer and retina, respectively, of newborn iNOS knockout mice than in wild-type controls (Sennlaub et al., 2002). Fewer TUNEL-positive cells were found in the avascular retina and ONL and GCLs of the retina of these animals. Decreased 3-nitrotyrosine production also was detected in retinas from the iNOS-deficient mice compared to wild-type controls. The iNOS inhibitor 1400W injected intravitreally gave similar results with less apoptosis in the INL and less intravitreal neovascularization.

Increased cyclooxygenase-2 (COX-2) activity also has been implicated in angiogenesis in tumors, and neovascularization in cornea and retina. In the mouse model of oxygen-induced retinopathy, preretinal (intravitreal) neovascularization was inhibited using selective COX-2 inhibitors (Sennlaub et al., 2003). Surprisingly, COX-2 (encoded by gene *Ptgs2*)-deficient mice showed an increased area of retinal nonperfusion, suggesting that COX-2 also might have a vasoprotective effect in the ischemic retina (Cryan et al., 2006). This was not confirmed using the COX-2 inhibitor (Sennlaub et al., 2003).

Endothelial cell interactions with extracellular matrix proteins, such as fibronectin, are a critical step in angiogenesis. This integrin-mediated adhesive interaction can be inhibited by small peptides, such as the α-defensins, which are activated during inflammatory processes. Administration of α-defensins systemically or locally blocked neovascularization in the oxygen-induced retinopathy mouse model (Economopoulou et al., 2005).

ob/ob mice develop less neovascularization than controls in the oxygen-induced retinopathy model. Opposite of these results in leptin-deficient mice, overexpression of leptin in this mouse model worsened neovascularization (Suganami et al., 2004). The role of leptin in the development of diabetes-induced retinal neovascularization remains to be clarified.

VEGF overexpression. VEGF has been implicated in diabetic retinopathy and is a known potent angiogenic factor in normal retinal development (Saint-Geniez and D'Amore, 2004). Intravitreal injection of human VEGF (*VEGFA*) causes severe neovascularization in several animal models (Ozaki et al., 1997; Tolentino et al., 1996; Wong et al., 2001). Transgenic mice in which *VEGFA* expression was under the control of the mouse rhodopsin promoter developed intraretinal and subretinal neovascularization ranging from mild to severe (Lai et al., 2005; Vinores et al., 2000). *VEGFA* expression directed by a lens-specific promoter resulted in some abnormal growth of vessels on the retinal surface but lacked extension of the vessels into the vitreous, which is characteristic of the preretinal neovascularization in diabetes. The more severe phenotype included more extensive subretinal neovascularization with hemorrhages and retinal detachment (Lai et al., 2005).

Insulin-like growth factor-I. IGF-I (encoded by gene *IgfI*) stimulates retinal endothelial cell growth, and IGF-I signaling through the IGF-I receptor leads to increased VEGF levels (Smith et al., 1999). Retinas from nondiabetic mice that overexpress an *IgfI* transgene reportedly demonstrate lesions characteristic of nonproliferative diabetic retinopathy, including pericyte loss, thickened capillary basement membrane, and intraretinal microvascular abnormalities. In addition, these models have been reported to progress to proliferative retinopathy and retinal detachment (Ruberte et al., 2004).

Summary

The use of mice to model diabetic retinopathy has allowed investigators to creatively test the contributions of various mechanisms in the pathogenesis of early, nonproliferative diabetic retinopathy (e.g., the roles of various pro-inflammatory mediators) and more advanced proliferative retinopathy (e.g., VEGF). Studies using pharmacological therapies to inhibit retinopathy have generated considerable excitement, but the lack of absolute specificity of most available pharmacological therapies complicates the interpretation of how they might be acting. Genetically modified mice will continue to be an important tool to further dissect the pathogenesis of retinopathy. Additional studies in the mouse hold the potential of offering new insight into the pathogenesis of diabetic retinopathy, and thus a means to identify new therapeutic approaches to inhibit the retinopathy.

REFERENCES

Agostini, H., Boden, K., Unsold, A., Martin, G., Hansen, L., Fiedler, U., Esser, N., and Marme, D. (2005). A single local injection of recombinant VEGF receptor 2 but not of Tie2 inhibits retinal neovascularization in the mouse. *Curr. Eye Res.* 30(4):249–257.

AGUILAR, E., FRIEDLANDER, M., and GARIANO, R. F. (2003). Endothelial proliferation in diabetic retinal microaneurysms. *Arch. Ophthalmol.* 121(5):740–741.

AIELLO, L. P., PIERCE, E. A., FOLEY, E. D., TAKAGI, H., CHEN, H., RIDDLE, L., N. FERRARA, N., KING, G. L., and SMITH, L. E. (1995). Suppression of retinal neovascularization in vivo by inhibition of vascular endothelial growth factor (VEGF) using soluble VEGF-receptor chimeric proteins. *Proc. Natl. Acad. Sci. U.S.A.* 92(23):10457–10461.

BARBER, A. J., ANTONETTI, D. A., KERN, T. S., REITER, C. E., SOANS, R. S., KRADY, J. K., LEVISON, S. W., GARDNER, T. W., and BRONSON, S. K. (2005). The Ins2Akita mouse as a model of early retinal complications in diabetes. *Invest. Ophthalmol. Vis. Sci.* 46(6):2210–2218.

BARBER, A. J., LIETH, E., KHIN, S. A., ANTONETTI, D. A., BUCHANAN, A. G., and GARDNER, T. W. (1998). Neural apoptosis in the retina during experimental and human diabetes: Early onset and effect of insulin. *J. Clin. Invest.* 102(4):783–791.

BARILE, G. R., PACHYDAKI, S. I., TARI, S. R., LEE, S. E., DONMOYER, C. M., MA, W., RONG, L. L., BUCIARELLI, L. G., WENDT, T., et al. (2005). The RAGE axis in early diabetic retinopathy. *Invest. Ophthalmol. Vis. Sci.* 46(8):2916–2924.

BLOODWORTH, J. M., JR., and MOLITOR, D. L. (1965). Ultrastructural aspects of human and canine diabetic retinopathy. *Invest. Ophthalmol.* 4(6):1037–1048.

BRESNICK, G. H., and PALTA, M. (1987a). Predicting progression to severe proliferative diabetic retinopathy. *Arch. Ophthalmol.* 105 (6):810–814.

BRESNICK, G. H., and PALTA, M. (1987b). Oscillatory potential amplitudes: Relation to severity of diabetic retinopathy. *Arch. Ophthalmol.* 105(7):929–933.

CHEUNG, A. K., FUNG, M. K., LO, A. C., LAM, T., SO, K. F., CHUNG, S. S., and CHUNG, S. K. (2005). Aldose reductase deficiency prevents diabetes-induced blood-retinal barrier breakdown, apoptosis, and glial reactivation in the retina of db/db mice. *Diabetes* 54(11):3119–3125.

CLEMENTS, R. S., JR., ROBISON, W. G., JR., and COHEN, M. P. (1998). Anti-glycated albumin therapy ameliorates early retinal microvascular pathology in db/db mice. *J. Diabetes Complications* 12(1):28–33.

COGAN, D. G., and KUWABARA, T. (1967). The mural cell in perspective. *Arch. Ophthalmol.* 78(2):133–139.

CRYAN, L. M., PIDGEON, G. P., FITZGERALD, D. J., and O'BRIEN, C. J. (2006). COX-2 protects against thrombosis of the retinal vasculature in a mouse model of proliferative retinopathy. *Mol. Vis.* 12:405–414.

CUNHA-VAZ, J., FARIA DE ABREU, J. R., and CAMPOS, A. J. (1975). Early breakdown of the blood-retinal barrier in diabetes. *Br. J. Ophthalmol.* 59(11):649–656.

CUTHBERTSON, R. A., and MANDEL, T. E. (1986). Anatomy of the mouse retina: Endothelial cell-pericyte ratio and capillary distribution. *Invest. Ophthalmol. Vis. Sci.* 27(11):1659–1664.

DAGHER, Z., PARK, Y. S., ASNAGHI, V., HOEHN, T., GERHARDINGER, C., and LORENZI, M. (2004). Studies of rat and human retinas predict a role for the polyol pathway in human diabetic retinopathy. *Diabetes* 53(9):2404–2411.

DAVIS, M., KERN, T., and RAND, L. (1977). Diabetic retinopathy. In P. Zimmet and R. DeFronzo (Eds.), *International textbook of diabetic retinopathy*. New York: John Wiley and Sons.

The Diabetes Control and Complications Trial Research Group. (1993). The effect of intensive treatment of diabetes on the development and progression of long-term complications in insulin-dependent diabetes mellitus. *N. Engl. J. Med.* 329(14):977–986.

DU, Y., MILLER, C. M., and KERN, T. S. (2003). Hyperglycemia increases mitochondrial superoxide in retina and retinal cells. *Free Radic. Biol. Med.* 235(11):1491–1499.

ECONOMOPOULOU, M., BDEIR, K., CINES, D. B., FOGT, F., BDEIR, Y., LUBKOWSKI, J., LU, W., PREISSNER, K. T., HAMMES, H. P., et al. (2005). Inhibition of pathologic retinal neovascularization by alpha-defensins. *Blood* 106(12):3831–3838.

ENGE, M., BJARNEGARD, M., GERHARDT, H., GUSTAFSSON, E., KALEN, M., ASKER, N., HAMMES, H. P., SHANI, M., FASSLER, R., et al. (2002). Endothelium-specific platelet-derived growth factor-B ablation mimics diabetic retinopathy. *EMBO J.* 21(16): 4307–4316.

ENGERMAN, R. L. (1989). Pathogenesis of diabetic retinopathy. *Diabetes* 38(10):1203–1206.

ENGERMAN, R. L., and BLOODWORTH, J. M., JR. (1965). Experimental diabetic retinopathy in dogs. *Arch. Ophthalmol.* 73:205–210.

ENGERMAN, R. L., and KERN, T. S. (1984). Experimental galactosemia produces diabetic-like retinopathy. *Diabetes* 33(1):97–100.

ENGERMAN, R. L., and KERN, T. S. (1993). Aldose reductase inhibition fails to prevent retinopathy in diabetic and galactosemic dogs. *Diabetes* 42(6):820–825.

ENGERMAN, R. L., and KERN, T. S. (1995). Retinopathy in galactosemic dogs continues to progress after cessation of galactosemia. *Arch. Ophthalmol.* 113(3):355–358.

FEIT-LEICHMAN, R. A., KINOUCHI, R., TAKEDA, R. M., FAN, Z., MOHR, S., KERN, T. S., and CHEN, D. F. (2005). Vascular damage in a mouse model of diabetic retinopathy: Relation to neuronal and glial changes. *Invest. Ophthalmol. Vis. Sci.* 46(11):4281–4287.

FRANK, R. N., et al. (1997). An aldose reductase inhibitor and aminoguanidine prevent vascular endothelial growth factor expression in rats with long-term galactosemia. *Arch. Ophthalmol.* 115(8):1036–1047.

GOLDIN, A., AMIN, R., KENNEDY, A., and HOHMAN, T. C. (2006). Advanced glycation end products: Sparking the development of diabetic vascular injury. *Circulation* 114(6):597–605.

GRANT, M. B., SPOERRI, P. E., PLAYER, D. W. D., BUSH, M., ELLIS, E. A., CABALLERO, S., and ROBISON, W. G. (2000). Plasminogen activator inhibitor (PAI)-1 overexpression in retinal microvessels of PAI-1 transgenic mice. *Invest. Ophthalmol. Vis. Sci.* 41(8):2296–2302.

GUBITOSI-KLUG, R., and KERN, T. (2006). A role for 5-Lipoxygenase in diabetic retinopathy. Presented at the annual meeting of the ADA, Washington, DC.

GUBITOSI-KLUG, R., and KERN, T. (2008). [5-Lipoxygenase, but not 12/5-lipoxygenase, contributes to degeneration of retinal capillaries in a mouse model of diabetic retinopathy.] Unpublished results.

HAMMES, H. P., LIN, J., RENNER, O., SHANI, M., LUNDQVIST, A., BETSHOLTZ, C., BROWNLEE, M., and DEUTSCH, U. (2002). Pericytes and the pathogenesis of diabetic retinopathy. *Diabetes* 51(10):3107–3112.

HAMMES, H. P., LIN, J., WAGNER, P., FENG, Y., VOM HAGEN, F., KRZIZOK, T., RENNER, O., BREIER, G., BROWNLEE, M., et al. (2004). Angiopoietin-2 causes pericyte dropout in the normal retina: Evidence for involvement in diabetic retinopathy. *Diabetes* 53(4):1104–1110.

IGARASHI, T., MIYAKE, K., KATO, K., WATANABE, A., ISHIZAKI, M., OHARA, K., and SHIMADA, T. (2003). Lentivirus-mediated expression of angiostatin efficiently inhibits neovascularization in a murine proliferative retinopathy model. *Gene Ther.* 10(3):219–226.

Jandeleit-Dahm, K., and Cooper, M. E. (2006). Hypertension and diabetes: Role of the renin-angiotensin system. *Endocrinol. Metab. Clin. North Am.* 35(3):469–490, vii.

Joussen, A. M., Poulaki, V., Le, M. L., Koizumi, K., Esser, C., Janicki, H., Schraermeyer, U., Kociok, N., Fauser, S., et al. (2004). A central role for inflammation in the pathogenesis of diabetic retinopathy. *FASEB J.* 18(12):1450–1452.

Joussen, A. M., Poulaki, V., Tsujikawa, A., Qin, W., Qaum, T., Xu, W., Moromizato, Y., Bursell, S. E., Wiegand, S. J., et al. (2002). Suppression of diabetic retinopathy with angiopoietin-1. *Am. J. Pathol.* 160(5):1683–1693.

Kern, T. S., and Engerman, R. L. (1996). A mouse model of diabetic retinopathy. *Arch. Ophthalmol.* 114(8):986–990.

Kern, T. S., and Mohr, S. (2007). Nonproliferative diabetic retinopathy. In A. M. Joussen, T. W. Gardner, B. Kirchhof, and S. J. Ryan (Eds.), *Ratinal vascular disease.* Heidelberg: Springer.

Kern, T. S., Tang, J., Mizutani, M., Kowluru, R. A., Nagaraj, R. H., Romeo, G., Podesta, F., and Lorenzi, M. (2000). Response of capillary cell death to aminoguanidine predicts the development of retinopathy: Comparison of diabetes and galactosemia. *Invest. Ophthalmol. Vis. Sci.* 41(12):3972–3978.

Kohner, E. M., and Henkind, P. (1970). Correlation of fluorescein angiogram and retinal digest in diabetic retinopathy. *Am. J. Ophthalmol.* 69(3):403–414.

Kondo, T., Vicent, D., Suzuma, K., Yanagisawa, M., King, G. L., Holzenberger, M., and Kahn, C. R. (2003). Knockout of insulin and IGF-1 receptors on vascular endothelial cells protects against retinal neovascularization. *J. Clin. Invest.* 111(12): 1835–1842.

Kowluru, R. A. (2002). Retinal metabolic abnormalities in diabetic mouse: Comparison with diabetic rat. *Curr. Eye Res.* 24(2):123–128.

Kowluru, R. A., Kowluru, V., Xiong, Y., and Ho, Y. S. (2006). Overexpression of mitochondrial superoxide dismutase in mice protects the retina from diabetes-induced oxidative stress. *Free Radic. Biol. Med.* 41(8):1191–1196.

Kusner, L. L., Sarthy, V. P., and Mohr, S. (2004). Nuclear translocation of glyceraldehyde-3-phosphate dehydrogenase: A role in high glucose-induced apoptosis in retinal Müller cells. *Invest. Ophthalmol. Vis. Sci.* 45(5):1553–1561.

Lai, C. M., Dunlop, S. A., May, L. A., Gorbatov, M., Brankov, M., Shen, W. Y., Binz, N., Lai, Y. K., Graham, C. E., et al. (2005). Generation of transgenic mice with mild and severe retinal neovascularisation. *Br. J. Ophthalmol.* 89(7):911–916.

Leiter, E. H., Prochazka, M., and Coleman, D. L. (1987). The non-obese diabetic (NOD) mouse. *Am. J. Pathol.* 128(2):380–383.

Lieth, E., Gardner, T. W., Barber, A. J., and Antonetti, D. A. (2000). Retinal neurodegeneration: Early pathology in diabetes. *Clin. Exp. Ophthalmol.* 28(1):3–8.

Martin, P. M., Roon, P., Van Ells, T. K., Ganapathy, V., and Smith, S. B. (2004). Death of retinal neurons in streptozotocin-induced diabetic mice. *Invest. Ophthalmol. Vis. Sci.* 45(9):3330–3336.

Midena, E., Segato, T., Radin, S., di Giorgio, G., Meneghini, F., Piermarocchi, S., and Belloni, A. S. (1989). Studies on the retina of the diabetic db/db mouse. I. Endothelial cell-pericyte ratio. *Ophthalmic Res.* 21(2):106–111.

Mohr, S., Xi, X., Tang, J., and Kern, T. S. (2002). Caspase activation in retinas of diabetic and galactosemic mice and diabetic patients. *Diabetes* 51(4):1172–1179.

Moore, T. C., Moore, J. E., Kaji, Y., Frizzell, N., Usui, T., Poulaki, V., Campbell, I. L., Stitt, A. W., Gardiner, T. A., et al. (2003). The role of advanced glycation end products in retinal microvascular leukostasis. *Invest. Ophthalmol. Vis. Sci.* 44 (10):4457–4464.

Naeser, P., and Agren, A. (1978). Morphology and enzyme activities of the retinal capillaries in mice with the obese-hyperglycaemic syndrome (gene symbol ob). *Acta. Ophthalmol. (Copenh.)* 56 (4):607–616.

Ning, X., Baoyu, Q., Yuzhen, L., Shuli, S., Reed, E., and Li, Q. Q. (2004). Neuro-optic cell apoptosis and microangiopathy in KKAY mouse retina. *Int. J. Mol. Med.* 13(1):87–92.

Obrosova, I. G., Drel, V. R., Kumagai, A. K., Szabo, C., Pacher, P., and Steven, M. J. (2006). Early diabetes-induced biochemical changes in the retina: Comparison of rat and mouse models. *Diabetologia* 49:2525–2233.

Ozaki, H., Hayashi, H., Vinores, S. A., Moromizato, Y., Campochiaro, P. A., and Oshima, K. (1997). Intravitreal sustained release of VEGF causes retinal neovascularization in rabbits and breakdown of the blood-retinal barrier in rabbits and primates. *Exp. Eye Res.* 64(4):505–517.

Robinson, G. S., Pierce, E. A., Rook, S. L., Foley, E., Webb, R., and Smith, L. E. (1996). Oligodeoxynucleotides inhibit retinal neovascularization in a murine model of proliferative retinopathy. *Proc. Natl. Acad. Sci. U.S.A.* 93(10):4851–4856.

Ruberte, J., Ayuso, E., Navarro, M., Carretero, A., Nacher, V., Haurigot, V., George, M., Llombart, C., Casellas, A., et al. (2004). Increased ocular levels of IGF-1 in transgenic mice lead to diabetes-like eye disease. *J. Clin. Invest.* 113(8):1149–1157.

Saint-Geniez, M., and D'Amore, P. A. (2004). Development and pathology of the hyaloid, choroidal and retinal vasculature. *Int. J. Dev. Biol.* 48(8–9):1045–1058.

Sennlaub, F., Courtois, Y., and Goureau, O. (2002). Inducible nitric oxide synthase mediates retinal apoptosis in ischemic proliferative retinopathy. *J. Neurosci.* 22(10):3987–3993.

Sennlaub, F., Valamanesh, F., Vazquez-Tello, A., El-Asrar, A. M., Checchin, D., Brault, S., Gobeil, F., Beauchamp, M. H., Mwaikambo, B., et al. (2003). Cyclooxygenase-2 in human and experimental ischemic proliferative retinopathy. *Circulation* 108(2):198–204.

Siracusa, L. D. (1994). The agouti gene: Turned on to yellow. *Trends Genet.* 10(12):423–428.

Smith, L. E., Shen, W., Perruzzi, C., Soker, S., Kinose, F., Xu, X., Robinson, G., Driver, S., Bischoff, J., et al. (1999). Regulation of vascular endothelial growth factor-dependent retinal neovascularization by insulin-like growth factor-1 receptor. *Nat. Med.* 5(12):1390–1395.

Smith, L. E., Wesolowski, E., McLellan, A., Kostyk, S. K., D'Amato, R., Sullivan, R., and D'Amore, P. A. (1994). Oxygen-induced retinopathy in the mouse. *Invest. Ophthalmol. Vis. Sci.* 35(1):101–111.

Sone, H., Kawakami, Y., Segawa, T., Okuda, Y., Sekine, Y., Honmura, S., Segawa, T., Suzuki, H., Yamashita, K., et al. (1999). Effects of intraocular or systemic administration of neutralizing antibody against vascular endothelial growth factor on the murine experimental model of retinopathy. *Life Sci.* 65(24):2573–2580.

Suganami, E., Takagi, H., Ohashi, H., Suzuma, K., Suzuma, I., Oh, H., Watanabe, D., Ojima, T., Suganami, T., et al. (2004). Leptin stimulates ischemia-induced retinal neovascularization: possible role of vascular endothelial growth factor expressed in retinal endothelial cells. *Diabetes* 53(9):2443–2448.

Tatton, W. G., Chalmers-Redman, R. M., Elstner, M., Leesch, W., Jagodzinski, F. B., Stupak, D. P., Sugrue, M. M., and

Tatton, N. A. (2000). Glyceraldehyde-3-phosphate dehydrogenase in neurodegeneration and apoptosis signaling. *J. Neural Transm. Suppl.* 2000(60):77–100.

Tolentino, M. J., Miller, J. W., Gragoudas, E. S., Jakobiec, F. A., Flynn, E., Chatzistefanou, K., Ferrara, N., and Adamis, A. P. (1996). Intravitreous injections of vascular endothelial growth factor produce retinal ischemia and microangiopathy in an adult primate. *Ophthalmology* 103(11):1820–1828.

Vincent, J. A., and Mohr, S. (2007). Inhibition of caspase-1/interleukin-1β signaling prevents degeneration of retinal capillaries in diabetes and galactosemia. *Diabetes* 56(1):224–230.

Vinores, S. A., Seo, M. S., Okamoto, N., Ash, J. D., Wawrousek, E. F., Xiao, W. H., Hudish, T., Derevjanik, N. L., and Campochiaro, P. A. (2000). Experimental models of growth factor-mediated angiogenesis and blood-retinal barrier breakdown. *Gen. Pharmacol.* 35(5):233–239.

Vlassara, H. (2001). The AGE-receptor in the pathogenesis of diabetic complications. *Diabetes Metab. Res. Rev.* 17(6):436–443.

Watanabe, D., Suzuma, K., Matsui, S., Kurimoto, M., Kiryu, J., Kita, M., Suzuma, I., Ohashi, H., Ojima, T., et al. (2005). Erythropoietin as a retinal angiogenic factor in proliferative diabetic retinopathy. *N. Engl. J. Med.* 353(8):782–792.

Whetzel, A. M., Bolick, D. T., Srinivasan, S., Macdonald, T. M., Morris, M. A., Ley, K., and Hedrick, C. C. (2006). Sphingosine-1 phosphate prevents monocyte/endothelial interactions in type 1 diabetic NOD mice through activation of the S1P1 receptor. *Circ. Res.* 99(7):731–739.

Wong, C. G., Rich, K. A., Liaw, L. H., Hsu, H. T., and Berns, M. W. (2001). Intravitreal VEGF and bFGF produce florid retinal neovascularization and hemorrhage in the rabbit. *Curr. Eye Res.* 22(2):140–147.

Yamaoka, T., Nishimura, C., Yamashita, K., Itakura, M., Yamada, T., Fujimoto, J., and Kokai, Y. (1995). Acute onset of diabetic pathological changes in transgenic mice with human aldose reductase cDNA. *Diabetologia* 38(3):255–261.

Zhang, L., Krzentowski, G., Albert, A., and Lefebvre, P. J. (2001). Risk of developing retinopathy in Diabetes Control and Complications Trial type 1 diabetic patients with good or poor metabolic control. *Diabetes Care* 24(7):1275–1279.

Zheng, L., Du, Y., Miller, C., Gubitosi-Klug, R. A., Kern, T. S., Ball, S., and Berkowitz, R. A. (2007). Critical role of inducible nitric oxide synthase in degeneration of retinal capillaries in mice with streptozotocin-induced diabetes. *Diabetologia* 50(9):1987–1996.

46 Roles of Oxygen in the Stability of Photoreceptors: Evidence from Mouse and Other Models of Human Disease

JONATHAN STONE AND KRISZTINA VALTER

Photoreceptors are the most fragile of retinal neurons in the face of genetic and environmental stress, and oxygen and oxidative stress are emerging as major environmental factors affecting their stability and contributing to retinal degeneration. This chapter addresses the question of why photoreceptors are vulnerable to a wider range of mutations than any other neuron class of the retina or brain. Increasing evidence suggests that this fragility results in great part from environmental factors such as tissue oxygen levels. Although studies of the mouse retina have been prominent in the growing literature on the subject, this chapter also considers relevant findings from other species, including humans.

Photoreceptors are selectively vulnerable not only to genetic mutations but also to a range of environmental stresses, metabolic toxins (Eells et al., 2003; Graymore and Tansley, 1959), hypoxia and hyperoxia (Wellard et al., 2005), trauma such as retinal detachment (Fisher et al., 2001; Mervin et al., 1999), and the cumulative stresses of aging (Gao and Hollyfield, 1992; Jackson et al., 2002). Genetic mutations act on a background of stress to and degeneration of photoreceptors. The phenotypes that emerge—the many forms of retinitis pigmentosa, the normal aging of the retina, the edge-specific degeneration that begins in childhood, the collapse of the macula with age—occur on a normal background. Appropriate therapy requires knowledge of both the normal and mutation-driven degeneration of photoreceptors and of the interaction between environmental and genetically induced stress.

In this chapter, we focus on the delivery of oxygen to the retina, the regulation and dysregulation of that delivery, and the consumption of oxygen by photoreceptors. Clinically, there are two reasons for this focus. First, tissue oxygen levels affect the stability of the normal retina, from neonatal life to advanced age. Second, the role of environmental stress in genetically driven degeneration has long gone unrecognized and provides an unexplored avenue for therapy of the degenerating retina.

The delivery of oxygen to the retina

The mouse retina has a retinal vasculature, like the human and many other mammalian retinas. Oxygen is delivered from two sources, the retinal and choroidal circulations. These circulations have distinct properties, and the interaction between them is critical in determining oxygen levels across the retina, and therefore the stability of photoreceptors.

THE RETINAL CIRCULATION The retinal circulation is a conventional system of arteries, capillaries, and veins. It forms developmentally from the hyaloid artery, which forms to supply the lens vesicle well before the retina requires its own circulation. At birth in the rat (Cairns, 1959), the retina is almost avascular, but the hyaloid artery passes from the optic disc to the developing lens. Over the first 10 days of postnatal life, the hyaloid circulation regresses and the retinal circulation forms by growth from the hyaloid vessels, following a template of astrocytes that spread from the optic disc across the retinal surface (Chan-Ling et al., 1990; Stone et al., 1995), expressing potent angiogenic factors (reviewed in Stone and Maslim, 1997). In the mouse, the retinal circulation begins to form before birth (Connolly et al., 1988) and also forms along a preexisting astrocyte template (Dorrell et al., 2002). Once the branches of the hyaloid vessels that supply the lens have regressed, the stem vessels are termed retinal vessels, and supply the inner layers of the retina.

In the adult retina, arteries radiate from the optic disc across the inner surface of the retina and branch to form to arterioles and capillaries, which spread through the inner half of the retina. The capillaries space themselves through the inner layers of the retina and are described as concentrating in three layers, in the ganglion cell layer (GCL) and at the inner and outer surfaces of the inner nuclear layer (INL). Capillaries drain to venules, and these in turn drain to veins, which converge on the optic disc, to leave the eye.

Physiologically, arterial and venous oxygen levels have been measured in the human (Alm, 1992) and cat (Alm and Bill, 1970, 1972a, 1972b). The consistent outcome is that oxygen extraction from the retinal circulation is 30%–40%, a level of oxygen extraction similar to that in the cerebral circulation.

Rates of blood flow through retinal tissue have been estimated for a range of animals (reviewed in Paques et al., 2003), including rodents and primates. The rate of capillary flow in the mouse retinal circulation was estimated by Paques and colleagues at 1.26 mm/s, within the range reported for cat, rat, and monkey but higher than in other rodent tissues, including the rat brain (0.7 mm/s). Paques et al. note that the relatively high flow rate would be advantageous for oxygen delivery. Retinal vessels show blood-brain barrier properties, induced by their contact with neuroglial cells (Chan-Ling and Stone, 1992; Janzer and Raff, 1987; Tout et al., 1993; reviewed in Stone and Maslim, 1997).

Further, the capillaries of the retinal circulation show the conventional property of autoregulation (Alm and Bill, 1970, 1972a, 1972b; Eperon et al., 1975); that is, they constrict, reducing flow, when oxygen levels in the tissue they supply rise, and dilate when oxygen levels fall. The mechanism of constriction is believed to lie in muscular control of arteriolar diameter, or in the control of capillary flow by pericytes (Peppiatt et al., 2006). Paques and colleagues (2003) note that the architecture of the mouse retinal circulation (which may be representative of mammalian retinal circulations) has features that favor control of capillary flow by local tissue conditions. Some superficial capillaries, for example, connect directly to large veins, and could provide a shunt past the deeper capillary beds.

The one distinctive feature of the retinal circulation is that its capillaries reach only halfway across the thickness of the retina. From arteries at the inner surface of the retina, capillaries extend radially as far as the outer plexiform layer (OPL), and never (normally) into the outer nuclear layer (ONL). Their growth into that layer is robustly inhibited by a mechanism that has been explored in the mouse. The development of the retinal circulation is severely disturbed by antibodies to R-cadherin (Dorrell et al., 2002; reviewed in Stone et al., 2006), which presumably prevent the normal adherence of vessels to cells that express cadherin. Cadherin is strongly expressed in the OPL of the mouse, and Dorrell and colleagues suggest that vessels growing radially outward in the retina are diverted to follow this line of expression, along the OPL. Vessels grow past the OPL into the ONL only if this barrier is disturbed (by masking cadherin with antibodies) or overcome by an abnormal expression of angiogenic factors by cells of the ONL (Tobe et al., 1998). As a consequence, the ONL and the layers of inner and outer segments—effectively, the photoreceptors—are normally avascular, the only avascular parts of the CNS. Oxygen diffuses to the photoreceptors from the deepest capillaries of the retinal circulation, but the major oxygen supply to photoreceptors reaches them from the external surface of the retina, by diffusion (Yu and Cringle, 2001). This dual supply of oxygen to photoreceptors is distinctive and an important factor in their relative fragility.

The Choroidal Circulation In all vertebrates, a rich vascular bed forms just external to the neural retina. Known as the choroidal circulation, this vascular bed is highly distinctive structurally and functionally. Anatomically, the choroidal circulation is a rich vascular bed that forms the tunica vasculosa of the eyeball, between the retina (tunica nervosa) and sclera (tunica fibrosa). The capillaries of the choroidal circulation (the choriocapillaris) are coarse and profuse and form a lake of blood at the outer surface of the retina. The choriocapillaris abuts the outer surface of the basement membrane of the retinal pigmented epithelium (RPE) (Bruch's membrane), and oxygen diffuses across Bruch's membrane, across the RPE and subretinal space to reach the mitochondria of the inner segments.

The capillaries of the choriocapillaris do not have barrier properties but are highly fenestrated and permeable (Bill et al., 1980). Further, the rates of blood flow through the choroidal circulation are very high. When expressed in milliliters per minute per gram of tissue supplied, the choroidal blood flow is several times higher than in other high-rate tissues, such as the cortex of the kidney, cardiac muscle, the inner retina, and cerebral cortex (see Alm, 1992, fig. 6.15 therein). Veins converge into distinctively convoluted vortex veins, which emerge from the eyeball near its equator and join orbital veins.

As a result of the very high rates of blood flow through the choroidal circulation, the partial pressure of oxygen in vortex vein blood is only 3%–4% below arterial levels (Alm, 1992; Bill et al., 1983); that is, the level of oxygen extraction is much lower than in retinal and cerebral circulations. As a consequence, the capillary bed of the choroidal circulation (the choriocapillaris) forms a lake of near-arterial blood around the outer surface of the retina, which is the main source of oxygen to photoreceptors.

An important feature of the anatomy of the choroidal circulation is that its capillaries do not lie in the tissue they supply and do not respond to conditions in that tissue. Choroidal blood flow shows some evidence of regulation, in response, for example, to experimental increases in arterial pressure (Riva et al., 1997), but is not responsive to oxygen or metabolite levels in the outer retina, the tissue it supplies. As a consequence, oxygen levels in the outer retina can fluctuate more widely than in any other retinal layer, and this fluctuation underlies the pathogenesis of a range of retinal diseases, among them retinopathy of prematurity, retinopathy of detachment, and retinitis pigmentosa.

Finally, the choroid develops early, well before the neural differentiation of the retina. Choroidal development has been described in most detail for the human (Allende et al., 2006). It shows a centroperipheral pattern of formation and forms well before the photoreceptors (which in the normal adult retina consume all the oxygen delivered by the choroid) have begun to function. The development of the retinal circulation occurs much later, in the mouse in the first 2 weeks of postnatal life (Connolly et al., 1988), well after vessels invade the cerebral cortex (in midgestation; Stone and Maslim, 1997), and is strongly influenced by oxygen reaching the retina from the choroid.

Oxygen consumption in the retina

Oxygen Consumption in the Adult The consumption of oxygen by the retina has been scrutinized with a range of technologies. For the mouse, the most direct and recent data are oxygen tension measurements obtained in vivo with oxygen-sensitive electrodes. These data (figure 46.1*A*) demonstrate that in the mouse (Yu and Cringle, 2006), as in the rat, cat, and monkey (reviewed by Yu and Cringle, 2001), oxygen flows into the retina from two sources, one in inner retina and corresponding to the retinal circulation and the other at the outer surface of the retina and corresponding to the choriocapillaris.

Oxygen is consumed in the retina at locations corresponding to the sites of mitochondria. Most of the oxygen flowing from the choriocapillaris is consumed by the dense concentration of mitochondria in the inner segment. In the dark-adapted retina, the oxygen tension in the ONL is near zero; oxygen from the choriocapillaris does not reach beyond the inner segments. The oxygen sinks of the inner retina are more distributed, in ganglion cells, in the IPL and OPL.

As already noted, the flow of blood through the choriocapillaris and the level of oxygen in choroidal blood do not vary with the level of oxygen in the tissue being supplied. As a consequence, oxygen flows from the choroid to the outer

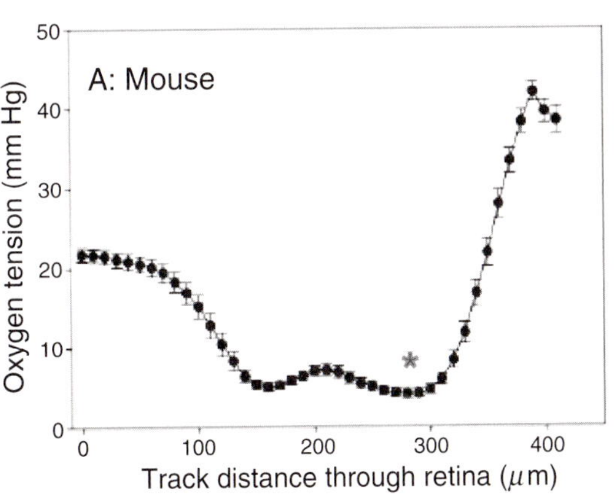

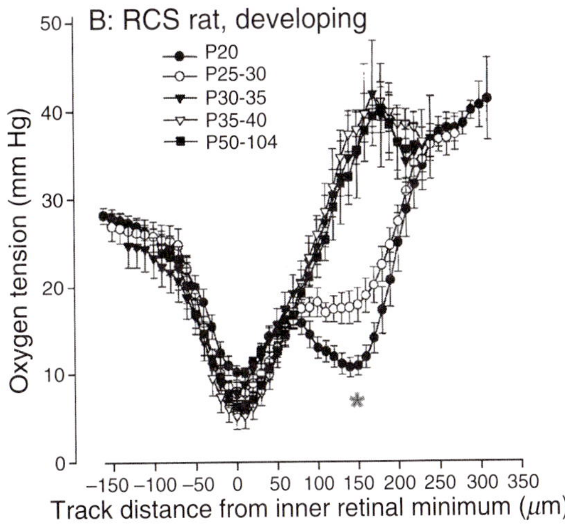

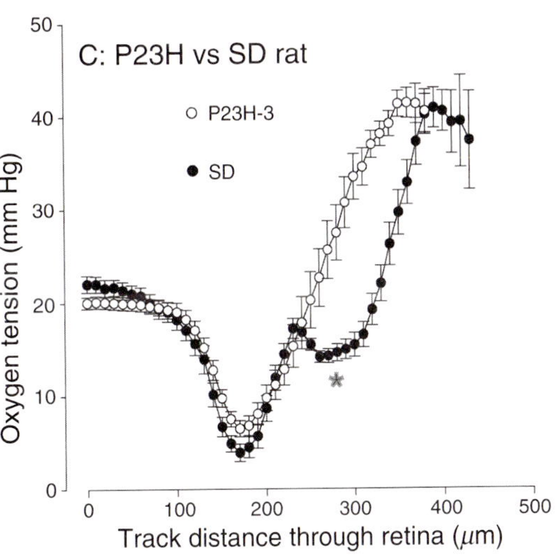

Figure 46.1 Oxygen levels within the retina, measured with oxygen-sensitive electrodes stepped through the retina, and the effect of depletion. In all three graphs the inner surface of the retina is at *left*, and the outer (choroidal) surface is at *right*. *A*, In the mouse, oxygen levels are maximal at the outer surface, close to the choriocapillaris. A second area of increased oxygen level is apparent at the inner surface, representing oxygen delivered by the retinal circulation. *Asterisk* marks a minimum in the region of the ONL; the sharp fall in tissue oxygen tension between the choroidal maximum and this minimum results from intense oxygen consumption by photoreceptor inner segments. *B*, Corresponding measurements in the naturally degenerative RCS rat. This is a developmental series. The minimum produced by photoreceptor oxygen consumption is evident in the youngest age studied (P20) but disappears as the animals age and the photoreceptor population is exhausted. *C*, Comparison of oxygen tension profiles obtained from a nondegenerative Sprague-Dawley (SD) rat and the degenerative P23H-3 transgenic strain. The minimum produced by photoreceptor consumption of oxygen is absent from the P23H-3 strain. (*A*, From Yu and Cringle, 2006. *B*, From Yu et al., 2000. *C*, From Yu et al., 2004.)

retina (i.e., to photoreceptors) following physical gradients; there is no mechanism to regulate that flow in response to the needs of photoreceptors.

The Developmental Onset of Oxygen Consumption The onset of oxygen consumption by photoreceptors has been well documented in rodents. Graymore (1959, 1960, 1963) used as a measure of metabolism the retina's production of lactic acid, an end product of glycolysis. He showed that the retina's production of lactate is low at birth and increases dramatically, in the rat between P15 and P20. This period corresponds to the onset of several measures of photoreceptor function, including the development of the electroretinogram (Fulton et al., 1995), the growth of the inner and outer segments of photoreceptors (Weidman and Kuwabara, 1968), the onset of oxygen consumption by the photoreceptors (Cringle et al., 2006), and the onset of a period of physiological hypoxia (Chan-Ling et al., 1995a), which induces the expression of angiogenic factors in glial templates on which the retinal blood vessels form (Dorrell et al., 2002; Stone et al., 1995).

The development of the retinal vasculature is thus driven by the development of photoreceptor function (reviewed in Stone and Maslim, 1997). The mechanism that links photoreceptor function to vascular development is hypoxia; the onset of photoreceptor function and oxygen consumption reduces the flow of choroidal oxygen to the inner retina, and the resulting hypoxia serves as a signal for vasogenesis.

Neuroglobin: An Oxygen-Binding Globin Prominent in the Retina Neuroglobin is a member of the globins, heme proteins found in plants, bacteria, fungi, and animals, with the property of reversibly binding oxygen. Neuroglobin was first described in the mouse and human (Burmester and Hankeln, 2004) and was named for its specific location in brain tissue (Burmester and Hankeln, 2004; Sun et al., 2001); it is a candidate protein for providing an oxygen store in brain tissue, as hemoglobin does in blood. Neuroglobin expression is upregulated in hypoxia (Sun et al., 2001) and is expressed roughly 100 times more strongly in the retina than in brain tissue (Schmidt et al., 2003), arguably reflecting the high oxygen utilization of the retina. The distribution of neuroglobin in the retina, in the IPL and OPL, and in the inner segments of photoreceptors correlates with the distribution of mitochondria, the organelles in which oxygen is recruited in the energy-producing mechanisms of oxidative phosphorylation (Schmidt et al., 2003). Correspondingly, neuroglobin levels are low in the inner retina of the guinea pig (Bentmann et al., 2005), in which species a retinal vasculature is lacking and oxygen metabolism cannot be detected (Yu and Cringle, 2001). The cellular and laminar distribution of neuroglobin in humans (Rajendram and Rao, 2007) and dogs (Ostojic et al., 2006) is similar to that observed in mice, and its amino acid sequence is highly conserved within mammals (Zhang et al., 2002).

Consequences of lack of regulation of oxygen supply to the outer retina

As we have argued previously (Chan-Ling and Stone, 1993; Lewis et al., 1999; Stone and Maslim, 1997; Stone et al., 1999), the inability of the choroidal circulation to regulate its delivery of oxygen to the retina underlies the pathogenesis of several retinal diseases, including retinopathy of prematurity, retinopathy of detachment, and the photoreceptor degenerations. The following sections trace the underlying mechanisms.

Inhaled Oxygen Reaches the Retina Selectively The lack of regulation of the choroidal circulation is evident in the effect that raising oxygen levels in inhaled air has on body tissues. The two body tissues most directly affected by hyperoxia are the epithelium of the lung (where hyperoxia induces a dysplasia; Barazzone et al., 1998; O'Brodovich and Mellins, 1985) and the retina, where effects include a narrowing of retinal vessels and the death of photoreceptors. Other tissues appear to be protected from hyperoxia by autoregulatory mechanisms induced by the hyperoxia. The contrast between autoregulation and the lack of it is evident in studies of the effect of hyperoxia on tissue oxygen levels across the retina, where there is a retinal circulation (Yu and Cringle, 2001; figure 46.2). As the level of oxygen in inhaled air is increased, oxygen levels rise throughout the retina, but much more so in the outer retina.

The flow of higher than normal levels of oxygen from the choroid to the retina has two spectacular effects on the structure of the retina. It causes the death of photoreceptors, and it causes the constriction and in some circumstances the closure of vessels of the retinal circulation.

Inhaled oxygen kills photoreceptors. Because inhaled oxygen reaches the outer retina from the choroid, simply breathing oxygen-enriched air can kill photoreceptors. The first evidence of this toxicity came from Noell's brief report in 1955 that inhalation of 100% oxygen causes the total degeneration of photoreceptors in the rabbit retina within 3 days. The inner retinal layers appeared unaffected. The selective vulnerability of photoreceptors was subsequently confirmed in the mouse (Walsh, Bravo-Nuevo, et al., 2004; Yamada et al., 2001) and rat (Geller et al., 2006; Wellard et al., 2005) (figure 46.3). The effect takes longer (2 weeks) in rodents than in the rabbit, but it is also highly specific to photoreceptors and is accompanied by an upregulation of stress-inducible proteins (fibroblast growth factor-2 [FGF-2], glial fibrillary acidic protein [GFAP]). Wellard et al. (2005) reported that the vulnerability of photoreceptors to hyperoxia is part

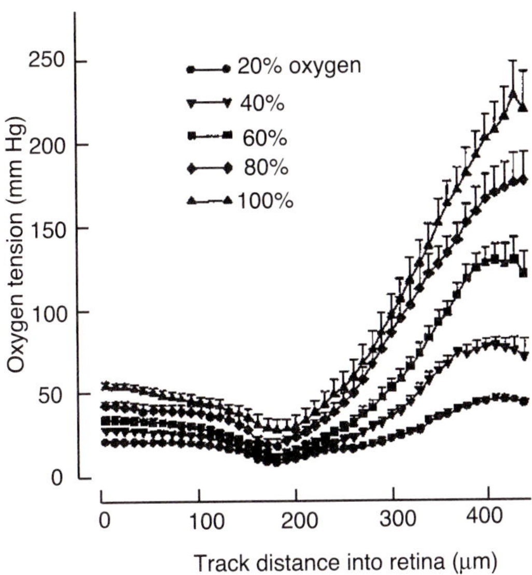

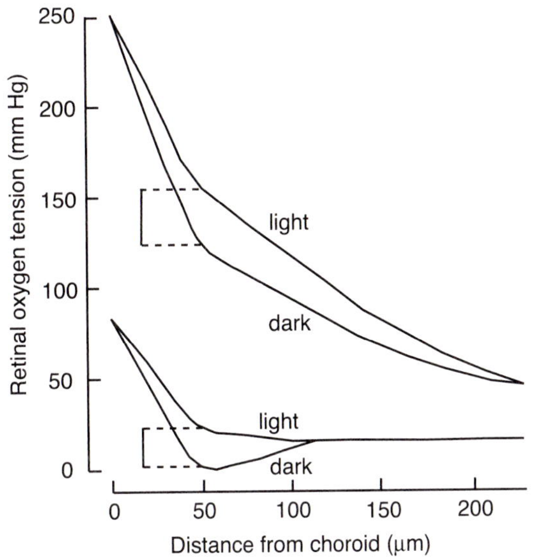

FIGURE 46.2 Effects of inhaled oxygen and light on intraretinal oxygen, measured in the eye of the rat (*left*) and cat (*right*). *Left*, The lower-most curve is equivalent to the SD data in figure 46.1*C*, the oxygen tension profile across the retina, in normoxia. As the proportion of oxygen in the air inhaled increases, oxygen levels rise all across the retina. The rise is much greater near the choriocapillaris (at *right*) than in the inner retina; this greater rise results from the lack of regulation of the choroidal circulation (From Cringle et al., 2002). *Right*, The lower pair of curves shows the oxygen tension profiles across the cat retina, in normoxic conditions, light- and dark-adapted. The dark-adapted curve shows the same general features as reported for other mammals (see figure 46.1); in this graph the choroidal side of the retina is to the *right*. Light adaptation causes a rise (shown by the *bracket*) in tissue oxygen tension in the outer retina, the result of a light-induced reduction in the consumption of oxygen by photoreceptors. The upper pair of curves shows the oxygen tension profiles obtained when the animal breathed oxygen-enriched air. Oxygen tension is raised all across the retina, but again more markedly so at the choroidal side, and light adaptation increases tissue oxygen tension further (*bracketed area*). That is, the effects of hyperoxia and light on oxygen tension are additive. (From Linsenmeier and Yancey, 1989.)

of a wider pattern in which photoreceptors are maximally stable at 21% oxygen (room air) and are destabilized (i.e., the rate of their death is increased) by both hypoxia and hyperoxia.

Finally on this point, it has been reported that in mice, the vulnerability of photoreceptors to oxygen is strain dependent (Walsh et al., 2004a), being less in the Balb/c strain than in the C57BL/6 strain. These strain differences are currently being used in our laboratory to identify genes that regulate the oxygen vulnerability of photoreceptors.

Inhaled oxygen blocks vasogenesis and thins or obliterates formed vessels. The impact of choroidal oxygen on the retinal vasculature was first detected in the analysis of the causes of retinopathy of prematurity, a neovascularizing disease of the infant retina associated with the use of oxygen to relieve respiratory difficulties in prematurely born infants (reviewed in Chan-Ling and Stone, 1993). Work in mouse (Browning et al., 1997; Smith et al., 1994), rat (Penn et al., 1994), and cat (Chan-Ling and Stone, 1992, 1993; Chan-Ling et al., 1992; Stone et al., 1996) models established that oxygen flowing from the choroid in the neonatal retina inhibits the normal development of retinal vessels and causes the thinning or obliteration of vessels already formed. When the baby or pup or kitten is returned to room air, the inner retina, lacking its normal complement of vessels, becomes abnormally hypoxic, triggering the death of astrocytes (the cells that normally express angiogenic factors such as vascular endothelial growth factor, VEGF) and upregulation of the same factors by neurons (Stone et al., 1996). The resulting rapid growth of vessels in the absence of astrocytes, which both induce barrier properties in new vessels and form part of the inner limiting membrane, results in the formation of leaky vessels, which grow into the vitreous humor. The use of supplemental oxygen to allow the late, nearly normal growth of vasculature has been explored (Chan-Ling et al., 1995b). In recent decades, the incidence of retinopathy of prematurity has been greatly reduced with the careful monitoring of arterial oxygen levels.

Vessels in the developing retina are particularly vulnerable to oxygen. In the rat, molecular events associated with the spread of pericytes at the end of the first postnatal month make adult vessels resistant to obliteration (Benjamin et al., 1998).

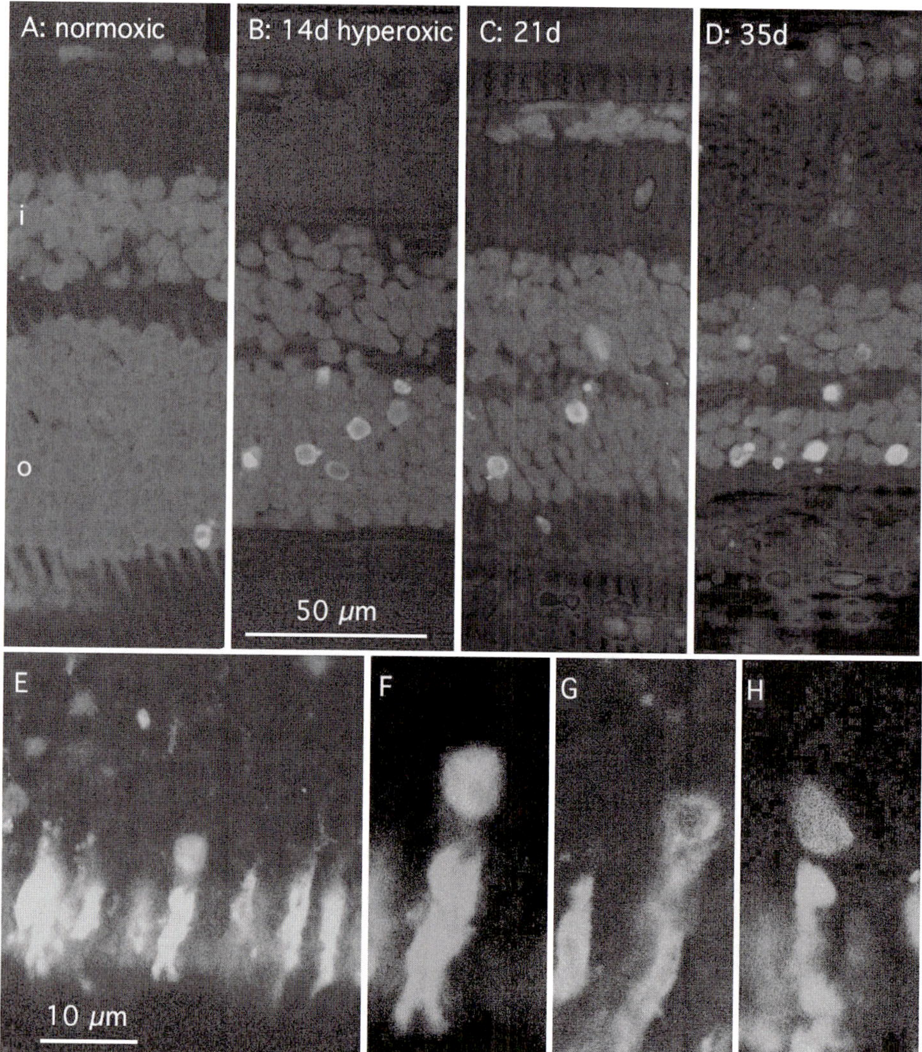

FIGURE 46.3 Oxygen is selectively toxic to photoreceptors. *A–D*, Sections across the retina of C57BL/6 mice exposed to high oxygen levels in inhaled air. Before exposure, dying (red, TUNEL-labeled) cells were rare. Exposure to hyperoxia for 14–35 days (*B–D*) increased the frequency of dying cells, selectively in the ONL (o). By 35 days, the ONL had thinned and TUNEL+ debris appeared in the inner nuclear layer (i), probably ingested by Müller cells. The blue dye is a DNA label (bisbenzamide). *E* and *F*, When the sheaths of cones were labeled with PNA lectin, the nuclei of some were TUNEL labeled (red), indicating that cones as well as rods were oxygen sensitive. See color plate 48. (From Geller et al., 2006.)

RETINAL DETACHMENT CAUSES INTENSE HYPOXIA OF THE OUTER RETINA: THE USE OF OXYGEN RELIEVES THE RETINOPATHY OF DETACHMENT The viability of the retina is threatened when it becomes detached from the outer walls of the eyeball. This detachment can be spontaneous or trauma induced; typically the neural retina detaches from the RPE, separating photoreceptors from their major source of oxygen. The results of detachment have been well studied (Fisher et al., 2001) and include photoreceptor death and proliferation and hypertrophy of neuroglia, which in humans can result in the total loss of retinal function.

The effects of detachment are greatly reduced by giving supplemental oxygen (i.e., enriching the inhaled air with oxygen). Photoreceptor death is reduced (Mervin et al., 1999), glial proliferation and hypertrophy are limited (Lewis et al., 1999), and the neurochemistry of the retina is less disturbed. This indicates that hypoxia plays a major role in inducing the pathological changes, and that hypoxic damage occurs because the choroid has no mechanism to detect or respond to abnormal hypoxia in the outer layers of the detached (or attached) retina.

A REDUCTION IN PHOTORECEPTOR METABOLISM RAISES OXYGEN LEVELS IN THE OUTER RETINA Once it is accepted that the flow of oxygen from the choroid to the outer retina is unregulated, it follows that any reduction in the oxidative metabolism of photoreceptors will, because the choroidal circulation cannot autoregulate, lead to an increase in the oxygen reaching the retina (Stone et al., 1999). This prediction was formalized in models of oxygen supply and consumption in the retina developed from the laminar analysis of oxygen distribution in the retina (Haugh et al., 1990; Yu and Cringle, 2001). These models include a major oxygen sink at the inner segments of photoreceptors. If that sink weakens in intensity, then, the models predict, oxygen from the choroid will flow into the cellular layers of the retina. Further, the thinning of the outer retina caused when photoreceptors degenerate will reduce the required diffusion path and add to this effect.

Experimentally, light raises oxygen levels in the outer retina. Photoreceptors generate an electrical response to light (beginning the coding of vision) by reducing their dark current. Molecules generated when rhodopsin absorbs light sequester cyclic guanosine monophosphate (cGMP) from the cytoplasm, closing cGMP-gated Na^+ channels, and reducing the need for Na^+ pumps in the inner segment to expel Na^+ from the cell. These pumps utilize adenosine triphosphate (ATP), so that light reduces the photoreceptors' requirement of ATP, and therefore for oxygen, which is used in oxidative phosphorylation to produce ATP.

As a consequence, a maintained increase in light absorbed by photoreceptors causes a maintained increase in oxygen tension in the outer retina (reviewed in Wangsa-Wirawan and Linsenmeier, 2003; see figure 46.2). The rise is reversible; decreasing light falling on the retina decreases retinal oxygen tension. The dynamics of the oxygen change are relatively rapid; oxygen levels rise and fall with increases and decreases in light, with a time constant of seconds with dim light, and of minutes with bright (photopic) levels of light (see Linsenmeier, 1986, fig. 46.4 therein).

Experimentally, photoreceptor depletion raises oxygen levels in the outer retina. A sustained rise in oxygen tension in the outer (photoreceptor) layers of retina has now been demonstrated in three animal models of photoreceptor degeneration, the RCS rat (Yu et al., 2000) (see figure 46.1*B*), P23H-3 rat (Yu et al., 2004) (see figure 46.1*C*), and Abyssinian cat (Padnick-Silver et al., 2006). These degenerations are all genetic in origin, but the mutations are diverse. In the RCS rat, a mutation in the receptor tyrosine kinase *Mertk* is associated with failure of the RPE to phagocytose the discarded membrane of photoreceptors (D'Cruz et al., 2000); in the P23H-3 rat, a transgene generates rhodopsin with a single amino acid substitution (Machida et al., 2000). The mutation in the Abyssinian cat (Ehinger et al., 1991) remains unidentified but appears not to involve rhodopsin (Gould and Sargan, 2002). All these studies relate the rise in oxygen levels in the outer retina to a decrease in oxygen consumption by photoreceptors.

Clinically, photoreceptor degeneration protects against retinal neovascularization. Confirmation of the idea that, when photoreceptors degenerate, oxygen from the choroidal circulation reaches the inner layers of retina comes from reports that retinal degeneration is protective against hypoxic neovascularizing diseases of the retina, in particular diabetic retinopathy (Arden, 2001; Sternberg et al., 1984). The protective effect has been confirmed (Lahdenranta et al., 2001) in a mouse model of photoreceptor degeneration; these authors noted that the normal hypoxia-induced expression of the angiogenic factor VEGF during development, which is critical for vessel formation, does not occur in the degenerative mouse retina.

Clinically, laser burns limit retinal neovascularization. The still current use of laser burns to peripheral retina to protect central retina from neovascularization, particularly in diabetic retinopathy, provides further evidence that photoreceptor depletion results in increased oxygen levels in the retina. Laser treatment was developed initially without a theory of its mechanism (reviewed in Benson et al., 1988). Several authors (Stefansson et al., 1981, 1986; Stone and Maslim, 1997) have argued that the well-established protective effects of laser treatment arise from depletion of the photoreceptor layer at the site of the burn and a consequent flow of oxygen from the choroid to the inner retina. This oxygen counteracts the hypoxia caused in diabetic retinopathy by capillary closure, reducing or delaying the damaging neovascularization. The recent study of Yu and colleagues (2005) addressed this question, demonstrating that partial laser burns at the level of the RPE and outer segments in rabbit retina caused increased retinal oxygen levels internal to the lesions.

Depletion-Induced Hyperoxia Is Inhibitory to Vessels and May Be Toxic to Rods and Cones If the increases in retinal oxygen levels known to be induced by photoreceptor depletion are sufficient to influence the cell biology of the retina, then effects similar to those induced by inhaling oxygen (the death of photoreceptors and the thinning of vessels) should be apparent.

Retinal vessels are thinned. Evidence of depletion-induced thinning of retinal vessels is substantial. Clinicians had long noted that vessels in the degenerating human retina are abnormally thin (Heckenlively, 1988), and thinning of the retinal vessels has been documented in several animal models of photoreceptor degeneration, including the rd mouse (Blanks and Johnson, 1986), the P23H-3 mouse (Penn et al., 2000), and the Abyssinian cat (Nilsson et al., 2001). Penn and colleagues noted that the effect was reduced by hypoxia, confirming that the thinning is caused by hyperoxia. Nilsson and colleagues noted further that as the degeneration of photoreceptors progresses in the Abyssinian cat, the volume of blood passing through the retinal circulation decreases markedly, while the choroidal circulation continues without reduction.

Cones are damaged by rod dysfunction. Evidence that the depletion of rods can damage surviving photoreceptors is clearest in the rod-cone dystrophies, in which photoreceptor death occurs first among rods, perhaps owing to mutations in a protein expressed only in rods (e.g., rhodopsin), and later involves cones. Arguably, the tendency of macular degeneration to follow relatively severe loss of rod function in normal human retina (Curcio et al., 2000; Jackson et al., 2002) represents a form of rod-cone dystrophy.

Two explanations, one specific and one general, have been developed to explain the impact of rod loss on cone viability. The specific explanation is that rods produce a cone survival factor (Hicks and Sahel, 1999; Mohand-Said et al., 1998), for want of which cones die when rods are depleted. The more general explanation is the oxygen toxicity hypothesis (Stone et al., 1999), namely, that the depletion-induced hyperoxia will damage all surviving photoreceptors, rods, and cones. These two mechanisms are not exclusive.

Shen and colleagues (2005) reported evidence, from a rod-degenerative pig model, that surviving cones are subject to oxidative stress, which they related to the depletion of rods, giving support to the idea that hyperoxia may be the factor linking rod death to cone damage. There is no reason, moreover, to expect surviving rods to be immune to the oxidative stress caused by rod depletion, and evidence is available to demonstrate that rods surviving in a rod-specific mutant degeneration, such as the P23H-3 rat, are damaged. Comparing nondegenerative (Sprague-Dawley) and P23H-3 retinas raised in identical conditions, Walsh and colleagues (2004b) showed that the P23H-3 photoreceptors have shorter, more disorganized outer segments, with a higher rate of cell death and a smaller a-wave. Evidence that this damage to P23H-3 photoreceptors is at least partly due to an environmental factor came from the demonstration that, when the ambient light to which the retina is exposed was raised, damage to surviving rods increased, and the damage could be reversed by reducing ambient illumination (Jozwick et al., 2006).

Light Accelerates Many Forms of Photoreceptor Degeneration The effect of light experience on the progress of retinal degenerations varies with the underlying mutations. Light exposure has been known for many years to accelerate retinal degenerations in the RCS rat (Dowling and Sidman, 1962; Kaitz and Auerbach, 1978, 1979), in the P23H-3 mouse (Naash et al., 1996), and in the P23H-3 rat (Walsh et al., 2004b). Evidence in the human is limited but suggests that light restriction may slow degenerations in some cases (reviewed in Stone et al., 1999). The variability in the human response to light exposure has yet to be related to the underlying genetic defect. In animal rodent models as in humans, light either exacerbates the degeneration or has no effect (Paskowitz et al., 2006); there appear to be no reports of light being protective to photoreceptors.

As Paskowitz and colleagues note, the effect of light is now well understood in a number of animal models, down to the molecular level. This evidence (which is beyond our present scope) makes clear how photoreceptor signaling is disturbed by mutations in proteins related to phototransduction, but the link between the disturbed signaling and cell death remains elusive.

Recent analyses of the P23H-3 rat model, which is light sensitive (Jozwick et al., 2006; Walsh et al., 2004b), showed that the damaging effect of light can occur quickly (within a week) and in response to very modest increases in just the daylight part of the day-night cycle. Further, the effects were reversible; within 2–5 weeks of a reduction in ambient light, the P23H-3 photoreceptors rebuilt their outer segments and partially (30%–40%) regained their sensitivity to light. We have recently demonstrated (Chrysostomou et al., 2008) that the same modest rise in ambient illumination that caused severe rod damage in the P23H-3 retina also damaged cones, and the damage to cones was also reversible. Since the transgene is in rhodopsin and cones do not express rhodopsin, the toxic factors that damaged cones must all have been environmental. One possibility, as we argued when proposing the idea of oxygen toxicity in 1999 (Stone et al., 1999), is that the toxic effect of increased ambient light on both rods and cones is mediated by a rise in oxygen tension in the outer retina induced by light.

The Edge of the Normal Retina Degenerates The normal (wild-type) retina degenerates at its edge. The degeneration has been shown in rodent models to begin as soon as photoreceptors begin to function (Mervin and Stone, 2002b; reviewed in Stone et al., 2005) (figure 46.4). In humans, a cystoid degeneration of the edge of the retina becomes evident in childhood and progresses with age until it involves the peripheral several millimeters of retina (Bell and Stenstrom, 1983).

There is considerable evidence that this "normal" degeneration of the edge of the retina is driven by hyperoxia. The structural factors that control retinal oxygen levels in the retina are perturbed at the edge of the retina by the sharp discontinuity of the retina itself. Specifically, the choroidal circulation extends past the edge, and as a result, oxygen can be predicted to reach the edge of the retina by diffusing around the edge. Working with the C57BL/6 mouse, Mervin (Mervin and Stone, 2002a, 2002b) demonstrated that the adult mouse retina shows an edge-specific degeneration. Retinal layers are thinned at the edge; photoreceptor mor-

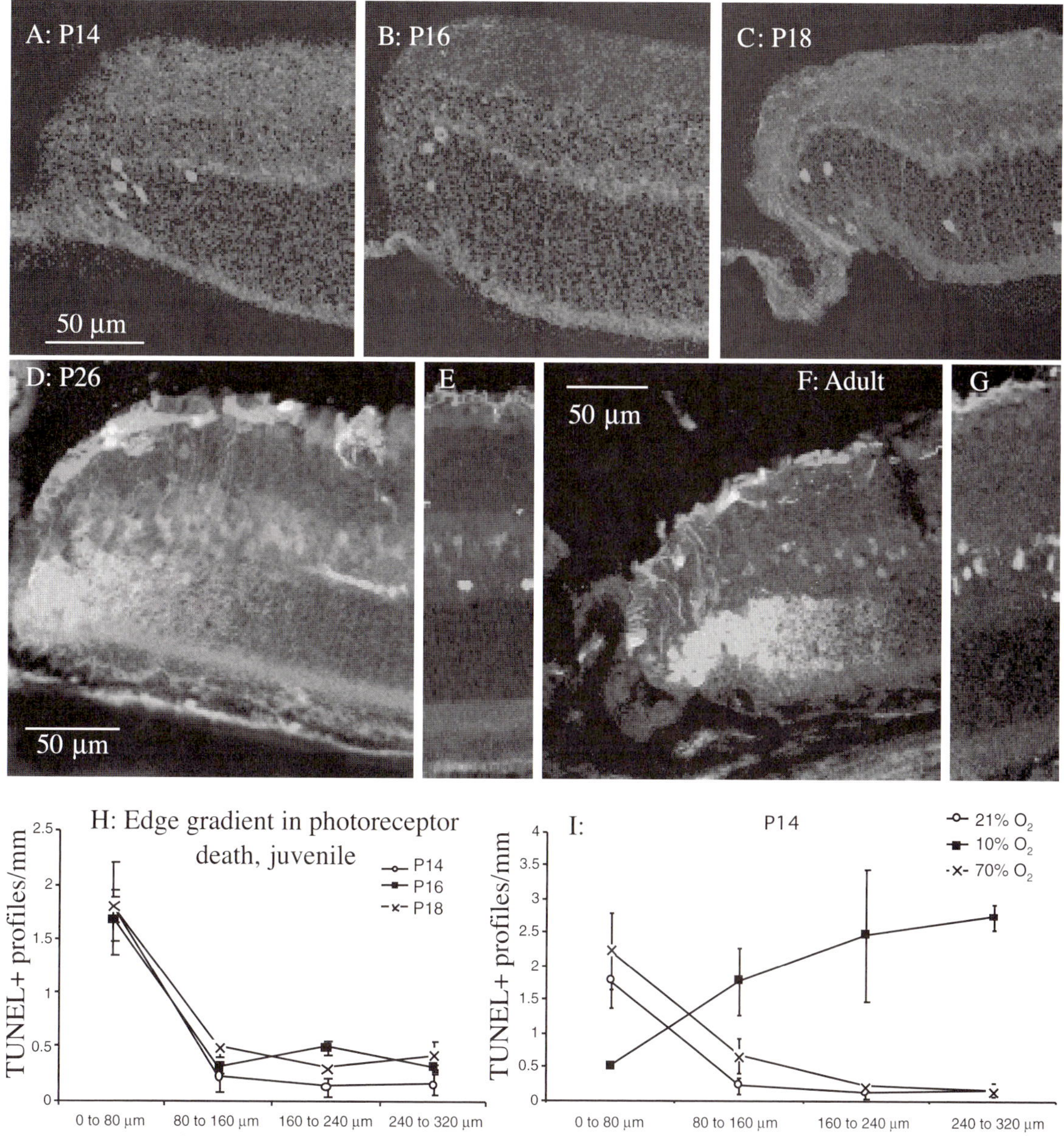

FIGURE 46.4 Photoreceptors at the most peripheral margin of the retina are subject to stress from early postnatal life. *A–C*, The edge of the retina of C57BL/6 mouse retina, with dying cells (bright red, TUNEL labeled) clustering at the edge of P14, P16, and P18. All are in the ONL. *D* and *E*, This cluster of dying cells colocalizes with the upregulation of two stress-induced proteins. GFAP is normally expressed (red) only at the inner surface of the retina, by astrocytes (*E* and *G*). At the edge, GFAP is upregulated also in Müller cells. FGF-2 is strongly upregulated (green) in photoreceptors, in a gradient that is maximal at the end. *H*, Quantification of the frequency of dying cells in the peripheral-most 100 µm of retina. *I*, Oxygen influences this distribution of dying cells at the edge of the early postnatal retina. Hypoxia increases photoreceptor death throughout most of the retina; at the edge, however, hyperoxia reduces death, suggesting that the edge-related death is driven by oxygen stress (see the text). Hyperoxia causes a small increase in the frequency of dying cells at the edge of the retina. See color plate 49. (From Mervin and Stone, 2002a, 2002b.)

phology is disturbed, and stress-sensitive proteins (FGF-2, GFAP) are sharply upregulated (figures 46.4*D–G*). Second, a focus of accelerated photoreceptor death was detected at the edge, occurring in early postnatal life, between P12 and P20, as photoreceptors start to function. Third, the acceleration was slowed by hypoxia, indicating that it is caused by hyperoxia. Throughout the rest of the retina, by contrast, hypoxia increased the rate of photoreceptor death. The oxygen status of the most peripheral 100 µm of the retina is distinctive, however; the region is degenerative and the degeneration is progressive, and related to high levels of oxygen.

Edge-related degeneration is evident in all species in which it has been studied (rats, mice, and humans; reviewed in Stone et al., 2005). In humans, the edge of the retina is eroded throughout life by a process called cystoid degeneration (Bell and Stenstrom, 1983; Vrabec, 1967). The degeneration is most severe at the edge of the retina, where the layered structure of the retina breaks down; cysts form within the retina, and eventually, pigmented cells invade from the RPE. This invasion mimics the pigmentation of the prematurely degenerating retina, which led to the term retinitis pigmentosa.

In the area of degeneration, vessels are absent, a symptom of raised oxygen levels. Central to the cystoid degeneration, extending some millimeters toward the center of the retina, the layered structure of the retina is intact, but vessels are absent or reduced, and the morphology of photoreceptors is degraded (Stone et al., 2005). More centrally, the morphology of photoreceptors and their content, the metabolic enzyme cytochrome oxidase, and the retinal circulation are normal. This grading of the degeneration from the edge of the retina suggests that the source of stress is at the edge. Further, the extent of the degeneration increases with age (Stone et al., 2005), indicating, as we originally suggested, that the normal retina is unstable under hyperoxic stress and the degeneration is progressive.

Oxygen stress during development: The concept of a critical period in photoreceptor development

The relationship between photoreceptor stability and retinal oxygen levels described in the previous section—that photoreceptors are maximally stable in normoxia and are destabilized by both hypoxia and hyperoxia—is true for the adult. Different relationships hold during development, however. In early postnatal life in mouse (Mervin and Stone, 2002a) and rat (Maslim et al., 1997), a period of accelerated photoreceptor death has been described. This "critical period" of development (P15–P20 in the mouse, P15–P25 in the rat) coincides with a period of physiological hypoxia caused by a rapid increase in photoreceptor metabolism (Graymore, 1960). This period of physiological hypoxia (Chan-Ling et al., 1995a) is critical in inducing angiogenesis of the retinal circulation.

Testing whether the death of photoreceptors in the developing retina is driven by hypoxia, Maslim and colleagues (1997) demonstrated that the rate is sharply increased by hypoxia and decreased by hyperoxia. Mervin and Stone (2002) extended these observations to the C57BL/6 mouse. After about P30 in both species, the effects of oxygen levels on photoreceptor death shift subtly but significantly, in two ways. First, photoreceptors become relatively resistant to variations in oxygen levels; some still unidentified stabilizing factor ends the developmental period of high naturally occurring death rates. Second, the sign of the effect of hyperoxia changes. During the critical period, hyperoxia is protective; in the adult, hyperoxia is toxic.

Finally, it has become clear that many forms of mutation-induced retinal degeneration accelerate during the critical period, suggesting an interaction between environmental or cell biological factors (the critical period) and the gene mutation (RCS rat: Valter et al., 1998; P23H-3 rat: Walsh et al., 2004b; the *rd* mouse: Hafezi et al., 1998).

In our original (1999) review, we speculated on the teleological significance of a period of development during which photoreceptors are hypoxia sensitive. We suggested that, like most classes of retinal cells, photoreceptors are overproduced during development and then culled to adult populations by a process of cell death. In photoreceptors but not other retinal cells, the culling is driven by the supply of oxygen to the retina, with the effect (we suggested) of matching the photoreceptor population to the supply of oxygen available.

Implications for the retinal degenerations

The analysis just developed draws attention to environmental factors, such as tissue oxygen levels, that influence the course of retinal degenerations. How powerful is this influence? Can purely environmental factors precipitate degenerations? Can they provide effective therapy?

Evidence that environmental factors can precipitate degenerations has come from two sources. Earlier we referred to evidence that age-related macular degeneration may be preceded by significant loss of rods. Curcio and colleagues (2000) suggest that the rod loss follows age-related changes in the recycling of retinoids, that rod loss contributes somehow to the degeneration of the cone-rich macula, and that improving rod survival could be the key to the stability of the macula. Considering the possibility of significant environmentally induced photoreceptor degeneration early in life, we (Stone et al., 2001) examined a cohort of cases of retinal degeneration, separating them into groups in which a familial pattern could and could not be detected. Our working hypothesis was that perinatal stress, which is associated with a wide range of adult-onset diseases, might also contribute to retinal degenerations, perhaps by precipitating degeneration in the developing photoreceptor population. A history of perinatal stress was significantly more common in the nonfamilial group, suggesting that in a proportion of nonfamilial cases, perinatal stress (which includes hypoxic stress) contributes to the cause of photoreceptor degenerations.

We have mentioned the ability of light restriction not only to slow photoreceptor loss in a degenerative model, the P23H-3 rat, but also to restore photoreceptor structure and function. This recovery of function stems from a capacity of individual cells to repair their outer segments and restore their functional organization. Obviously, this self-repair capacity has therapeutic potential; but is it special to this model? In normal (wild-type) retina, photoreceptors also respond to sustained (over weeks) increases in ambient light by decreasing the length of their outer segments. The result is a drop in rhodopsin levels in the retina and a reduction in the dark current and a-wave. The effects are reversible, and the effect and its reversal have been summarized in the principle of photostasis (reviewed in Williams, 1998), which states that the retina regulates the amount of active rhodopsin deployed to keep the daily quantum catch constant.

The effect of light on wild-type outer segments goes beyond shortening and lengthening, however. Reports of the effect of ambient light on normal photoreceptors (Kuwabara, 1970; Penn and Anderson, 1991) describe significant disorganization of the outer segment membrane, very like that seen in the P23H-3 model. This damage is also reversed, as the cell replaces its outer segment membrane. It thus seems likely that the ability of photoreceptors to self-repair is general, and likely to be available in any retina.

These examples of environmentally induced damage, degeneration, and recovery of photoreceptors are unlikely to be all oxygen mediated. The level of oxygen in the outer retina is only one measure of the impact of light, photoreceptor depletion, and age-related factors such as the recycling of retinoids on the stability of photoreceptors. Nevertheless, oxidative stress is prominent in many recent ideas of the mechanisms that precipitate photoreceptor death. Photoreceptors produce reactive oxygen species when exposed to light (especially blue light; Yang et al., 2003), and their production follows the activation of rhodopsin, before the downstream events of visual transduction (Demontis et al., 2002). Thus, oxidative stress may be intrinsically linked to the absorption of visible light by rhodopsin, and photoreceptors are rich in antioxidant molecules, such as docosahexaenoic acid (Rotstein et al., 2003). As a consequence, measures such as light restriction, filtering out just blue light (Margrain et al., 2004), dietary supplementation with antioxidants (Militante and Lombardini, 2004), and infrared radiation to repair oxidatively damaged mitochondria (Eells et al., 2003) are being debated and studied. As emphasized in this chapter, environmental factors can add significantly to the stresses that cause photoreceptor degeneration, and consequently, management of these factors can be valuable therapeutically.

REFERENCES

Allende, A., Madigan, M. C., and Provis, J. M. (2006). Endothelial cell proliferation in the choriocapillaris during human retinal differentiation. *Br. J. Ophthalmol.* 90:1046–1051.

Alm, A. (1992). Ocular circulation. In *Adler's Physiology of the eye: Clinical application* (pp. 198–227). St. Louis: Mosby-Year Book.

Alm, A., and Bill, A. (1970). Blood flow and oxygen extraction in the cat uvea at normal and high intraocular pressures. *Acta Physiol. Scand.* 80:19–28.

Alm, A., and Bill, A. (1972a). The oxygen supply to the retina. I. Effects of changes in intraocular and arterial blood pressures, and in arterial PO_2 and PCO_2 on the oxygen tension in the vitreous body of the cat. *Acta Physiol. Scand.* 84:261–274.

Alm, A., and Bill, A. (1972b). The oxygen supply to the retina. II. Effects of high intra-ocular pressure and of increased arterial carbon dioxide tension on uveal and retinal blood flow in cats. *Acta Physiol. Scand.* 84:306–319.

Arden, G. B. (2001). The absence of diabetic retinopathy in patients with retinitis pigmentosa: Implications for pathophysiology and possible treatment. *Br. J. Ophthalmol.* 85:366–370.

Barazzone, C., Horowitz, S., Donati, Y. R., Rodriguez, I., and Piguet, P. F. (1998). Oxygen toxicity in mouse lung: Pathways to cell death. *Am. J. Respir. Cell. Mol. Biol.* 19:573–581.

Bell, F. C., and Stenstrom, W. J. (1983). *Atlas of the peripheral retina.* Philadelphia: W. B. Saunders.

Benjamin, L., Hemo, I., and Keshet, E. (1998). A plasticity window for blood vessel remodelling is defined by pericyte coverage of the preformed endothelial network and is regulated by PDGF-B and VEGF. *Development* 125:1591–1598.

Benson, W. E., Brown, G. C., and Tasman, W. (1988). Treatment of neovascularization of the retina and the iris. In *Diabetes and Its Ocular Complications* (pp. 128–143). Philadelphia: W. B. Saunders.

Bentmann, A., Schmidt, M., Reuss, S., Wolfrum, U., Hankeln, T., and Burmester, T. (2005). Divergent distribution in vascular and avascular mammalian retinae links neuroglobin to cellular respiration. *J. Biol. Chem.* 280:20660–20665.

Bill, A., Sperber, G., and Ujiie, K. (1983). Physiology of the choroidal vascular bed. *Int. Ophthalmol.* 6:101–107.

Bill, A., Törnquist, P., and Alm, A. (1980). Permeability of the intraocular blood vessels. *Trans. Ophthalmol. Soc. U.K.* 100:332–336.

Blanks, J. C., and Johnson, L. V. (1986). Vascular atrophy in the retinal degenerative rd mouse. *J. Comp. Neurol.* 254:543–553.

Browning, J., Wylie, C., and Cole, G. (1997). Quantification of oxygen-induced retinopathy in the mouse. *Invest. Opthalmol. Vis. Sci.* 38:1168–1174.

Burmester, T., and Hankeln, T. (2004). Neuroglobin: A respiratory protein of the nervous system. *News Physiol. Sci.* 19:110–113.

Cairns, J. E. (1959). Normal development of the hyaloid and retinal vessels in the rat. *Br. J. Ophthalmol.* 43:385–393.

Chan-Ling, T., Gock, B., and Stone, J. (1995a). The effect of oxygen on vasoformative cell division: Evidence that "physiological hypoxia" is the stimulus for normal retinal vasculogenesis. *Invest. Ophthalmol. Vis. Sci.* 36:1201–1214.

Chan-Ling, T., Gock, B., and Stone, J. (1995b). Supplemental oxygen therapy: Basis for noninvasive treatment of retinopathy of prematurity. *Invest. Ophthalmol. Vis. Sci.* 36:1215–1230.

Chan-Ling, T., Halasz, P., and Stone, J. (1990). Development of retinal vasculature in the cat: Processes and mechanisms. *Curr. Eye Res.* 9:459–478.

Chan-Ling, T., and Stone, J. (1992). Degeneration of astrocytes in feline retinopathy of prematurity causes failure of the blood-retinal barrier. *Invest. Ophthalmol. Vis. Sci.* 33:2148–2159.

Chan-Ling, T., and Stone, J. (1993). Retinopathy of prematurity: Origins in the architecture of the retina. *Prog. Retin. Res.* 12:155–176.

Chan-Ling, T., Tout, S., Holländer, H., and Stone, J. (1992). Vascular changes and their mechanisms in the feline model of retinopathy of prematurity. *Invest. Ophthalmol. Vis. Sci.* 33:2128–2147.

Chrysostomou, V., Stone, J., Barnett, N., Valter, K. (2008). The status of cones in the rhodopsin-mutant P23H-3 retina: Light-regulated damage and repair in parallel with rods. *Invest. Ophthalmol. Vis. Sci.* 49:DoI:10.1167/iovs.07-1158.

Connolly, S., Hores, T. A., Smith, L. E., and D'Amore, P. A. (1988). Characterization of vascular development in the mouse retina. *Microvasc. Res.* 36:275–290.

Cringle, S. J., Yu, P. K., Su, E. N., and Yu, D. Y. (2006). Oxygen distribution and consumption in the developing rat retina. *Invest. Ophthalmol. Vis. Sci.* 47:4072–4076.

Cringle, S. J., Yu, D. Y., Yu, P. K., and Su, E. N. (2002). Intraretinal oxygen consumption in the rat in vivo. *Invest. Ophthalmol. Vis. Sci.* 43:1922–1927.

Curcio, C. A., Owsley, C., and Jackson, G. R. (2000). Spare the rods, save the cones in aging and age-related maculopathy. *Invest. Ophthalmol. Vis. Sci.* 41:2015–2018.

D'Cruz, P. M., Yasumura, D., Weir, J., Matthes, M. T., Abderrahim, H., LaVail, M. M., and Vollrath, D. (2000). Mutation of the receptor tyrosine kinase gene Mertk in the retinal dystrophic RCS rat. *Hum. Mol. Genet.* 9:645–651.

Demontis, G. C., Longoni, B., and Marchiafava, P. L. (2002). Molecular steps involved in light-induced oxidative damage to retinal rods. *Invest. Ophthalmol.* 43:2421–2427.

Dorrell, M., Aguilar, E., and Friedlander, M. (2002). Retinal vascular development is mediated by endothelial filopodia, a preexisting astrocytic template and specific R-cadherin adhesion. *Invest. Ophthalmol. Vis. Sci.* 43:3500–3510.

Dowling, J., and Sidman, R. (1962). Inherited retinal dystrophy in the rat. *J. Cell Biol.* 14:73–109.

Eells, J., Henry, M. M., Summerfelt, P., Wong-Riley, M. T., Buchmann, E. V., Kane, M., Whelan, N. T., and Whelan, H. T. (2003). Therapeutic photobiomodulation for methanol-induced retinal toxicity. *Proc. Natl. Acad. Sci. U.S.A.* 100:3439–3444.

Ehinger, B., Narfström, K., Nilsson, S. E., and Van Veen, T. (1991). Photoreceptor degeneration and loss of immunoreactive GABA in the Abyssinian cat retina. *Exp. Eye Res.* 52:17–25.

Eperon, G., Johnson, M., and David, N. J. (1975). The effect of arterial PO_2 on relative retinal blood flow in monkeys. *Invest. Ophthalmol.* 14:342–352.

Fisher, S. K., Stone, J., Rex, T. S., Linberg, K. A., and Lewis, G. P. (2001). Experimental retinal detachment: A paradigm for understanding the effects of induced photoreceptor degeneration. *Prog. Brain Res.* 131:679–698.

Fulton, A. B., Hansen, R. M., and Findl, O. (1995). The development of the rod photoresponse from dark-adapted rats. *Invest. Ophthalmol. Vis. Sci.* 36:1038–1045.

Gao, H., and Hollyfield, J. G. (1992). Aging of the human retina: Differential loss of neurons and retinal pigment epithelial cells. *Invest. Ophthalmol. Vis. Sci.* 33:1–17.

Geller, S., Krowka, R., Valter, K., and Stone, J. (2006). Toxicity of hyperoxia to the retina: Evidence from the mouse. *Adv. Exp. Med. Biol.* 572:425–437.

Gould, D. J., and Sargan, D. R. (2002). Autosomal dominant retinal dystrophy (Rdy) in Abyssinian cats: Exclusion of PDE6G and ROM1 and likely exclusion of Rhodopsin as candidate genes. *Anim. Genet.* 33:436–440.

Graymore, C. (1959). Metabolism of the developing retina. *Br. J. Ophthalmol.* 43:34–39.

Graymore, C. (1960). Metabolism of the developing retina: Respiration in the developing normal rat retina and the effect of an inherited degeneration of the retinal neuro-epithelium. *Br. J. Ophthalmol.* 44:363–369.

Graymore, C. (1963). Metabolism of the developing retina: Lactic dehydrogenase isoenzyme in the normal and degenerating retina. A preliminary communication. *Exp. Eye Res.* 3:5–8.

Graymore, C., and Tansley, K. (1959). Iodoacetate poisoning of the rat retina. *Br. J. Ophthalmol.* 43:486–493.

Hafezi, F., Abegg, M., Grimm, C., Wenzel, A., Munz, K., Sturmer, J., Farber, D. B., and Reme, C. E. (1998). Retinal degeneration in the rd mouse in the absence of c-fos. *Invest. Ophthalmol. Vis. Sci.* 39:2239–2244.

Haugh, L., Linsenmeier, R., and Goldstick, T. (1990). Mathematical models of the spatial distribution of retinal oxygen tension and consumption, including changes upon illumination. *Ann. Biomed. Engin.* 18:19–36.

Heckenlively, J. (1988). *Retinitis pigmentosa.* Philadelphia: Lippincott.

Hicks, D., and Sahel, J. (1999). The implications of rod-dependent cone survival for basic and clinical research. *Invest. Ophthalmol. Vis. Sci.* 40:3071–3074.

Jackson, G. R., Owsley, C., and Curcio, C. A. (2002). Photoreceptor degeneration and dysfunction in aging and age-related maculopathy. *Ageing Res. Rev.* 1:381–396.

Janzer, R. C., and Raff, M. C. (1987). Astrocytes induce blood-brain barrier properties in endothelial cells. *Nature* 325:253–257.

Jozwick, C., Valter, K., and Stone, J. (2006). Reversal of functional loss in the P23H-3 rat retina by management of ambient light. *Exp. Eye Res.* 83:1074–1080.

Kaitz, M., and Auerbach, E. (1978). Action spectrum for light-induced retinal degeneration in dystrophic rats. *Vision Res.* 19:1041–1044.

Kaitz, M., and Auerbach, E. (1979). Retinal degeneration in RCS rats raised under ambient light levels. *Vision Res.* 19:79–81.

Kuwabara, T. (1970). Retinal recovery from exposure to light. *Am. J. Ophthalmol.* 70:187–198.

Lahdenranta, J., Pasqualini, R., Schlingemann, R. O., Hagedorn, M., Stallcup, W. B., Bucana, C. D., Sidman, R. L., and Arap, W. (2001). An anti-angiogenic state in mice and humans with retinal photoreceptor cell degeneration. *Proc. Natl. Acad. Sci. U.S.A.* 98:10368–10373.

Lewis, G., Mervin, K., Valter, K., Maslim, J., Kappel, P., Stone, J., and Fisher, S. (1999). Limiting the proliferation and reactivity of retinal müller cells during detachment: The value of oxygen supplementation. *Am. J. Ophthalmol.* 128:165–172.

Linsenmeier, R. A. (1986). Effects of light and dark on oxygen distribution and consumption in the cat retina. *J. Gen. Physiol.* 88:521–542.

Linsenmeier, R., and Yancey, C. (1989). Effects of hyperoxia on the oxygen distribution in the intact cat retina. *Invest. Ophthalmol. Vis. Sci.* 30:612–618.

Machida, S., Kondo, M., Jamison, J. A., Khan, N. W., Kononen, L. T., Sugawara, T., Bush, R. A., and Sieving, P. A. (2000). P23H rhodopsin transgenic rat: Correlation of retinal function with histopathology. *Invest. Ophthalmol. Vis. Sci.* 41:3200–3209.

Margrain, T. H., Boulton, M., Marshall, J., and Sliney, D. H. (2004). Do blue light filters confer protection against age-related macular degeneration? *Prog. Retin. Eye Res.* 23:523–531.

Maslim, J., Valter, K., Egensperger, R., Hollander, H., and Stone, J. (1997). Tissue oxygen during a critical developmental period controls the death and survival of photoreceptors. *Invest. Ophthalmol. Vis. Sci.* 38:1667–1677.

Mervin, K., and Stone, J. (2002a). Developmental death of photoreceptors in the C57BL/6J mouse: Association with retinal function and self-protection. *Exp. Eye Res.* 75:703–713.

Mervin, K., and Stone, J. (2002b). Regulation by oxygen of photoreceptor death in the developing and adult C57BL/6J mouse. *Exp. Eye Res.* 75:715–722.

Mervin, K., Valter, K., Maslim, J., Lewis, G., Fisher, S., and Stone, J. (1999). Limiting photoreceptor death and deconstruction during experimental retinal detachment: The value of oxygen supplementation. *Am. J. Ophthalmol.* 128:155–164.

Militante, J., and Lombardini, J. B. (2004). Age-related retinal degeneration in animal models of aging: Possible involvement of taurine deficiency and oxidative stress. *Neurochem. Res.* 29:151–160.

Mohand-Said, S., Deudon-Combe, A., Hicks, D., Simonutti, M., Forster, V., Fintz, A. C., Leveillard, T., Dreyfus, H., and Sahel, J. A. (1998). Normal retina releases a diffusible factor stimulating cone survival in the retinal degeneration mouse. *Proc. Natl. Acad. Sci. U.S.A.* 95:8357–8362.

Naash, M., Peachey, N., Yi Li, Z., Gryczan, C., Goto, Y., Blanks, J., Milam, A., and Ripps, H. (1996). Light-induced acceleration of photoreceptor degeneration in transgenic mice expressing mutant rhodopsin. *Invest. Ophthalmol. Vis. Sci.* 37:775–782.

Nilsson, S. F., Maepea, O., Alm, A., and Narfstrom, K. (2001). Ocular blood flow and retinal metabolism in Abyssinian cats with hereditary retinal degeneration. *Invest. Ophthalmol. Vis. Sci.* 42:1038–1044.

Noell, W. K. (1955). Visual cell effects of high oxygen pressures. *Am. Physiol. Soc. Fed. Proc.* 14:107–108.

O'Brodovich, H., and Mellins, R. (1985). Bronchopulmonary dysplasia: Unresolved neonatal acute lung injury. *Am. Rev. Respir. Dis.* 132:694–709.

Ostojic, J., Sakaguchi, D. S., de Lathouder, Y., Hargrove, M. S., Trent, J. T. III, Kwon, Y. H., Kardon, R. H., Kuehn, M. H., Betts, D. M., et al. (2006). Neuroglobin and cytoglobin: Oxygen-binding proteins in retinal neurons. *Invest. Ophthalmol. Vis. Sci.* 47:1016–1023.

Padnick-Silver, L., Derwent, J. J., Giuliano, E., Narfstrom, K., and Linsenmeier, R. A. (2006). Retinal oxygenation and oxygen metabolism in Abyssinian cats with a hereditary retinal degeneration. *Invest. Ophthalmol. Vis. Sci.* 47:3683–3689.

Paques, M., Tadayoni, R., Sercombe, R., Laurent, P., Genevois, O., Gaudric, A., and Vacaut, E. (2003). Structural and hemodynamic analysis of the mouse retinal microcirculation. *Invest. Ophthalmol. Vis. Sci.* 44:4960–4967.

Paskowitz, D. M., LaVail, M. M., and Duncan, J. L. (2006). Light and inherited retinal degeneration. *Br. J. Ophthalmol.* 90:1060–1066.

Penn, J., and Anderson, R. (1991). Effects of light history on the rat retina. *Prog. Retin. Res.* 11:75–98.

Penn, J. S., Li, S., and Naash, M. I. (2000). Ambient hypoxia reverses retinal vascular attenuation in a transgenic mouse model of autosomal dominant retinitis pigmentosa. *Invest. Ophthalmol. Vis. Sci.* 41:4007–4013.

Penn, J. S., Tolman, B. L., and Henry, M. M. (1994). Oxygen-induced retinopathy in the rat: Relationship of retinal nonperfusion to subsequent neovascularization. *Invest. Ophthalmol. Vis. Sci.* 35:3429–3435.

Peppiatt, C. M., Howarth, C., Mobbs, P., and Attwell, D. (2006). Bidirectional control of CNS capillary diameter by pericytes. *Nature* 443:700–704.

Rajendram, R., and Rao, N. A. (2007). Neuroglobin in normal retina and retina from eyes with advanced glaucoma. *Br. J. Ophthalmol.* 91:663–666.

Riva, C., Titze, P., Hero, M., and Petrig, B. L. (1997). Effect of acute decreases of perfusion pressure on choroidal blood flow in humans. *Invest. Ophthalmol. Vis. Sci.* 38:1752–1760.

Rotstein, N. P., Politi, L. E., German, O. L., and Girotti, R. (2003). Protective effect of docosahexaenoic acid on oxidative stress-induced apoptosis of retina photoreceptors. *Invest. Ophthalmol. Vis. Sci.* 44:2252–2259.

Schmidt, M., Giessl, A., Laufs, T., Hankeln, T., Wolfrum, U., and Burmester, T. (2003). How does the eye breathe? Evidence for neuroglobin-mediated oxygen supply in the mammalian retina. *J. Biol. Chem.* 278:1932–1935.

Shen, J., Yang, X., Dong, A., Petters, R., Peng, Y.-W., Wong, F., and Campochiaro, P. (2005). Oxidative damage is a potential cause of cone cell death in retinitis pigmentosa. *J. Cell. Physiol.* 203:457–464.

Smith, L. E. H., Wesolowski, E., McLellan, A., Kostyk, S. K., D'Amato, R., Sullivan, R., and D'Amore, P. A. (1994). Oxygen-induced retinopathy in the mouse. *Invest. Ophthalmol. Vis. Sci.* 35:101–111.

Stefansson, E., Hatchell, D. L., Fisher, B. L., Sutherland, F. S., and Machemer, R. (1986). Panretinal photocoagulation and retinal oxygenation in normal and diabetic cats. *Am. J. Ophthalmol.* 101:657–664.

Stefansson, E., Landers, M. B., and Wolbarsht, M. L. (1981). Increased retinal oxygen supply following pan-retinal photocoagulation and vitrectomy and lensectomy. *Trans. Am. Ophthalmol. Soc.* 74:307–334.

Sternberg, P. M., Landers, M. I. M., and Wolbarsht, M. P. (1984). The negative coincidence of retinitis pigmentosa and proliferative diabetic retinopathy. *Am. J. Ophthalmol.* 97:788–789.

Stone, J., Chan-Ling, T., Pe'er, J., Itin, A., Gnessin, H., and Keshet, E. (1996). Roles of vascular endothelial growth factor and astrocyte degeneration in the genesis of retinopathy of prematurity. *Invest. Ophthalmol. Vis. Sci.* 37:290–299.

Stone, J., Itin, A., Alon, T., Pe'er, J., Gnessin, H., Chan-Ling, T., and Keshet, E. (1995). Development of retinal vasculature is mediated by hypoxia-induced vascular endothelial growth factor (VEGF) expression by neuroglia. *J. Neurosci.* 15:4738–4747.

Stone, J., and Maslim, J. (1997). Mechanisms of retinal angiogenesis. *Prog. Ret. Eye. Res.* 16:157–181.

Stone, J., Maslim, J., Fawsi, A., Lancaster, P., and Heckenlively, J. (2001). The role of perinatal stress in retinitis pigmentosa: Evidence from surveys in Australia and the USA. *Can. J. Ophthalmol.* 36:315–322.

Stone, J., Maslim, J., Valter-Kocsi, K., Mervin, K., Bowers, F., Chu, Y., Barnett, N., Provis, J., Lewis, G., et al. (1999). Mechanisms of photoreceptor death and survival in mammalian retina. *Prog. Retin. Eye Res.* 18:689–735.

Stone, J., Mervin, K., Walsh, N., Valter, K., Provis, J., and Penfold, P. (2005). Photoreceptor stability and degeneration in mammalian retina: Lessons from the edge. In P. Penfold and J. Provis (Eds.), *Macular degeneration: Science and medicine in practice* (pp. 149–165). New York: Springer-Verlag.

Stone, J., Sandercoe, T. M., and Provis, J. (2006). Mechanisms of the formation and stability of retinal blood vessels. In J. Tombran-Tink and C. Barnstable (Eds.), *Ocular angiogenesis: Diseases, mechanisms and therapeutics* (pp. 101–126). Totowa, NJ: Humana Press.

Sun, Y., Jin, K., Mao, X. O., Zhu, Y., and Greenberg, D. A. (2001). Neuroglobin is up-regulated by and protects neurons from hypoxic-ischemic injury. *Proc. Natl. Acad. Sci. U.S.A.* 98: 15306–15311.

Tobe, T., Okamoto, N., Vinores, M., Derevjanik, N., Vinores, S., Zack, D., and Campochiaro, P. (1998). Evolution of neovascularization in mice with overexpression of vascular endothelial growth factor in photoreceptors. *Invest. Ophthalmol. Vis. Sci.* 39: 180–188.

Tout, S., Chan-Ling, T., Hollander, H., and Stone, J. (1993). The role of Müller cells in the formation of the blood-retinal barrier. *Neuroscience* 55:291–301.

Valter, K., Maslim, J., Bowers, F., and Stone, J. (1998). Photoreceptor dystrophy in the RCS rat: Roles of oxygen, debris and bFGF. *Invest. Ophthalmol. Vis. Sci.* 39:2427–2442.

Vrabec, F. (1967). Neurohistology of cystoid degeneration of the peripheral human retina. *Am. J. Ophthalmol.* 64:90–99.

Walsh, N., Bravo-Nuevo, A., Geller, S., and Stone, J. (2004a). Resistance of photoreceptors in the C57BL/6-c2J, C57BL/6J, and BALBB/cj mouse strains to oxygen stress: Evidence of an oxygen phenotype. *Curr. Eye Res.* 29:441–448.

Walsh, N., Van Driel, D., Lee, D., and Stone, J. (2004b). Multiple vulnerability of photoreceptors to mesopic ambient light in the P23H transgenic rat. *Brain Res.* 1013:197–203.

Wangsa-Wirawan, N. D., and Linsenmeier, R. A. (2003). Retinal oxygen: Fundamental and clinical aspects. *Arch. Ophthalmol.* 121:547–557.

Weidman, T. A., and Kuwabara, T. (1968). Postnatal development of the rat retina. An electron microscopic study. *Arch. Ophthalmol.* 79:470–484.

Wellard, J., Lee, D., Valter, K., and Stone, J. (2005). Photoreceptors in the rat retina are specifically vulnerable to both hypoxia and hyperoxia. *Vis. Neurosci.* 22:501–507.

Williams, T. P. (1998). Light history and photostastis. In *Photostasis and related phenomena* (pp. 17–32). New York: Plenum Press.

Yamada, H., Yamada, E., Ando, A., Esumi, N., Bora, N., Saikia, J., Sung, C. H., Zack, D. J., and Campochiaro, P. A. (2001). Fibroblast growth factor-2 decreases hyperoxia-induced photoreceptor cell death in mice. *Am. J. Pathol.* 159:1113–1120.

Yang, J. H., Basinger, S. F., Gross, R. L., and Wu, S. M. (2003). Blue light-induced generation of reactive oxygen species in photoreceptor ellipsoids requires mitochondrial electron transport. *Invest. Ophthalmol. Vis. Sci.* 44:1312–1319.

Yu, D., and Cringle, S. (2001). Oxygen distribution and consumption within the retina in vascularised and avascular retinas and in animal models of retinal disease. *Prog. Retin. Eye Res.* 20: 175–208.

Yu, D., and Cringle, S. (2006). Oxygen distribution in the mouse retina. *Invest. Ophthalmol. Vis. Sci.* 47:1109–1112.

Yu, D., Cringle, S., Su, E., and Yu, P. K. (2000). Intraretinal oxygen levels before and after photoreceptor loss in the RCS Rat. *Invest. Ophthalmol. Vis. Sci.* 41:3999–4006.

Yu, D., Cringle, S., Su, E., Yu, P. K., Humayun, M. S., and Dorin, G. (2005). Laser-induced changes in intraretinal oxygen distribution in pigmented rabbits. *Invest. Ophthalmol. Vis. Sci.* 46:988–999.

Yu, D. Y., Cringle, S., Valter, K., Walsh, N., Lee, D., and Stone J. (2004). Photoreceptor death, trophic factor expression, retinal oxygen status, and photoreceptor function in the P23H rat. *Invest. Ophthalmol. Vis. Sci.* 45:2013–2019.

Zhang, C., Wang, C., Deng, M., Li, L., Wang, H., Fan, M., Xu, W., Meng, F., Qian, L., et al. (2002). Full-length cDNA cloning of human neuroglobin and tissue expression of rat neuroglobin. *Biochem. Biophys. Res. Commun.* 290:1411–1419.

47 Complex Genetics of Photoreceptor Light Damage

MICHAEL DANCIGER

The understanding of music is in the understanding of a single note.
—Unknown

Retinal degeneration (RD) can be caused by a number of different factors: gene mutations, such as those responsible for retinitis pigmentosa (RP) or other forms of RD; environmental exposures, such as toxic levels of light; and a combination of environmental factors and genetic tendencies, such as those producing age-related macular degeneration (AMD). Regardless of cause, the end stage is loss of photoreceptors due to apoptosis. Therefore, RD in experimental animals (in this case, mice) caused by toxic levels of light is a good model in which to study photoreceptor death because it is easy to manage in the laboratory. In addition, patients with some retinal diseases who are exposed to high levels of light for extended periods, such as fishermen or skiers, may have their disease course worsened (Taylor et al., 1990; Cruickshanks et al., 1993; Simons, 1993; Cideciyan et al., 1998; Mata et al., 2000). Supporting this is the fact that in some animal models of inherited RD, the disease process is accelerated by light exposures (Sanyal and Hawkins, 1986; Wang et al., 1997; LaVail et al., 1999; Organisciak et al., 1999). Therefore, it is not surprising that there has been a tremendous amount of work on light damage to the retina in many different fields. In this chapter, we cover work on the complex genetics of light-induced RD in the mouse model.

In the late 1980s, LaVail and colleagues published two studies on photoreceptor (PR) light damage of albino mice (LaVail et al., 1987a, 1987c). Several albino strains were exposed to constant light at about 115–130 foot-candles (ft-c) (1,265–1,400 lux) for 2 weeks. After exposure, the PR outer nuclear layer (ONL) was measured and used as an indicator of PR loss. Compared to unexposed control mouse retinal ONLs, the B6(Cg)-Tyr^{c-2J}/J albino (B6alb) still had 80% of the PR ONL, while the other strains (NZWLacJ, A/J, BALB/c, AKR, Ma/My, RF/J, RIIIs/J) had only 40% or less (LaVail et al., 1987a, 1987c). The B6alb strain is co-isogenic with the standard pigmented C57BL/6J strain; the only genetic difference is the homozygous mutation in the tyrosinase gene carried by B6alb, causing it to be albino. (*Co-isogenic* or *congenic* refers to nearly identical strains of an organism that vary at only a single locus.) Why were B6alb PRs so much more resistant to light insult than those of the other strains? Insofar as the mice were all raised and maintained under the same circumstances, the answer had to be genetics. Of course, this is what the LaVail group thought and demonstrated in a second study in which they performed the same type of light damage protocol on B6alb, BALB/c (C), and F_1 mice (in this case, F_1 = progeny of a B6alb × C cross). The results confirmed the substantial and significant difference in loss of PRs to light insult between the B6alb and C strains, with an intermediate response from the F_1s (skewed a bit toward the C phenotype), demonstrating the genetic influence on the trait (LaVail et al., 1987b). We became interested in this work and set up a collaboration with Dr. LaVail (Beckman Research Center, University of California–San Francisco) to try to identify the gene (or genes) and alleles responsible for this remarkable difference in light-induced PR loss between the C and B6alb strains.

Identification and verification of a gene modifier that has a strong influence on photoreceptor light damage

We started with the simplest explanation: a single gene is responsible for the difference in phenotype between the strains. The B6alb allele protects the PRs from light insult, and the C allele makes them more sensitive. We performed a backcross with the B6alb and C strains and attempted to score the ONL of the progeny after the same constant light exposure as before. The term *backcross* refers to a cross of the F_1 of two strains (for example, strains A and B) with one of the original strains. Thus, F_1(A × B) × B or F_1(A × B) × A, or, in our case, F_1(B6alb × C) × B6alb. If one gene was responsible for the difference, there should have been only two phenotypes, resistant (B6alb/B6alb) and sensitive (B6alb/C). Linkage analysis with genetic markers evenly spanning the genome at regular intervals of ≤30 centimorgans (cM) within chromosomes and ≤15 cM from the telomere or centromere (mouse chromosomes are acrocentric—they have the centromere at one end) should have revealed the chromosomal location of the gene. It did not work. First, it was difficult in many individual cases to score the light damage phenotype as resistant or sensitive, and second, no marker cosegregated with the phenotype; that is, no marker was B6alb/B6alb for all mice with the resistant phenotype and B6alb/C for all mice with the sensitive phenotype (data not published). Therefore, we hypothesized that PR damage in response to constant light exposure is a complex trait.

The definition of a complex trait in the circumstance in which the environment is controlled—that is, it is not a differentiating factor—is a trait or phenotype that is governed by two or more genes. Since the number of genes that govern the trait is unknown at the outset, the number of phenotypes is unknown as well. For example, one gene governing a trait with alleles that are additive would produce three phenotypes. *Additive* means that the alleles are not dominant or recessive but instead, when both are present, the phenotype is intermediate. Two additive genes would produce nine phenotypes, three genes 27 phenotypes, and so on. Therefore, the phenotype is measured or quantified. In this case, the phenotype was the average of 54 measurements of the ONL thickness along a central retinal section running far superior through the optic nerve head to far inferior. To do the experiment, we used the same backcross protocol and light exposure as before, but instead of linkage analysis, quantitative genetics analysis was performed, using the Map Manager QTX program (Manly et al., 2001). This software identifies quantitative trait loci (QTL) by regression analysis. Thus, it computes the degree of significance for the association of a marker with the phenotype by evaluating the genotype of all markers comprising a genome-wide scan in all progeny animals and comparing that with the phenotypes of all progeny animals. Significance is identified when a high proportion of progeny with a particular genotype for a marker (for example, B6alb/B6alb) tend to have a particular phenotype, and at the same time when the genotype is different for that marker (B6alb/C, in this case) the phenotype tends to be opposite. In this way, utilizing the Map Manager program, we identified several QTL that influenced PR light damage in this cross. The most significant of these was on distal chromosome 3, which accounted for nearly 50% of the genetic effect and had a probability of 10^{-19} of being a random, chance phenomenon (LOD score was ca. 19) (Danciger et al., 2000).

When we examined that locus on the gene map for candidates, we found the *Rpe65* gene, a gene present in the retinal pigmented epithelium (RPE) but known to be involved in the response of the PR cell to light. When we sequenced the *Rpe65* cDNA, we found an A for the first nucleotide of codon 450 in B6alb and a C in the BALB/c strain, predicting a methionine for B6alb and a leucine for the BALB/c. Since both methionine and leucine are nonpolar amino acids, the change from one to the other is conservative and would not predict the normal function of RPE65 to be affected. This was supported by studies showing normal responses of B6alb mice in water mazes and by studies showing normal electrophysiological responses of B6alb retinas (Balkema and Dräger, 1991; Hayes and Balkema, 1993; Nusisnovitz et al., 2003). Our hypothesis was that under the oxidative conditions of constant light, however, the methionine would be susceptible to oxidation to methionine sulfoxide, rendering the RPE65 protein more susceptible to degradation, while the leucine 450 would not be. Oxidation of key methionines in other proteins has been shown to disrupt function (Vogt, 1995). Lower levels of RPE65 would decrease the cycles of rhodopsin regeneration and thereby protect the PRs by slowing down the vision transduction process and its concomitant hyperpolarization and depolarization cycling. The PR response to light involves the stimulation of rhodopsin involving the conversion of 11-*cis*-retinal to all-*trans*-retinal and separation from the opsin protein. The activated protein interacts with the G protein transducin as the first step in a biochemical pathway resulting in the hyperpolarization of the PR cell with a concomitant alteration in neurotransmission to the next level of neurons in the retina. To stop the process, both rhodopsin kinase and arrestin interact with rhodopsin, stopping its interaction with transducin and preparing it for ligation with 11-*cis*-retinal. 11-*cis*-retinal is recycled by a pathway that involves RPE65 in the RPE cells and appropriate transport from and to the PRs (for reviews, see Chabre and Deterre, 1989; Chen, 2005).

Support for our hypothesis came from two publications demonstrating the same PR sensitivity to perturbations in the visual transduction process under different circumstances. In one case, PRs were protected from intense light exposures by the absence of RPE65 protein in the corresponding knockout mice (Grimm et al., 2000), and in the other, PRs degenerated even in the presence of dim light, owing to the absence of rhodopsin kinase (*Grk1*) in the corresponding knockout mice (Chen et al., 1999a). In the first case, the cycling of rhodopsin and the hyperpolarization and depolarization cycles of PRs were stopped, and in the second case the PRs were overstimulated because activated rhodopsin could not be shut off in a timely way. Verification of the hypothesis and a more precise explanation of the protective effect of the RPE65 met450 variant were demonstrated in studies by Wenzel et al. (2001b, 2003). The sum of the two studies (done on wild-type and c-*FOS* −/− backgrounds) was severalfold. Mice homozygous for RPE65 leu450, for met450, or heterozygous were exposed to intense light after dilation of their pupils producing a bleach of a high number of PRs (a high percentage of the retinal rhodopsin) and then held in the dark. At various time points the amount of rhodopsin regenerated was measured spectrophotometrically and compared to the baseline before the bleach application. The presence of the met450 variant significantly slowed the regeneration of rhodopsin. The speed of regeneration was directly correlated to the amount of RPE65 protein present in the RPE measured by Western blot and to the PR damage to the retina measured in stained histological sections. Thus, mice homozygous for RPE65 met450 had lower levels of RPE65 protein in their RPE, slower regeneration of rhodopsin, and less PR loss after intense light exposure (Wenzel et al., 2001b, 2003). The amount of *Rpe65* mRNA, however, was the same in eyes with RPE65 met450 and RPE65 leu450 (Danciger et al., 2000; Wenzel et al., 2001b, 2003).

An additional piece of information was the fact that the protective effect of the met/met genotype was not great enough to account for the resistance of B6 mice to damage following toxic light exposure (Wenzel et al., 2001b). This substantiated the original quantitative genetics study demonstrating the presence of several other B6alb gene alleles that also protect against light-induced damage (Danciger et al., 2000). In addition, several other QTL were identified in a light damage study of an F_1 intercross of the BALB/c and 129S1/SvImJ strains (Danciger et al., 2004). These QTL were on chromosomes 1, 4, 6, and 2, representing a completely different set of QTL than in the original light damage study of BALB/c and B6alb. However, in the earlier study the mice were exposed to 2 weeks of constant light at an intensity of approximately 115–130 ft-c (1,265–1,400 lux) and sacrificed immediately after exposure. In the 129 × BALB/c study the mice were exposed (with dilated pupils) to 1 hour of 15,000 lux, allowed to stay in the dark for 16 hours, and then kept in dim cyclic light for about 12 days before evaluation of retinal damage by measurement of the amount of rhodopsin remaining (Danciger et al., 2004).

To evaluate the argument that the visual transduction response was slowed in the PRs of mice carrying the RPE65 met450 variant at the physiological level, an electroretinogram study was carried out as follows: BALB/c and B6alb mice were exposed to a bleaching light and then placed in the dark. At various time points, the mice were tested for the rod response to light and compared to normal. For both the a-wave and b-wave, the BALB/c retinas recovered significantly sooner than those of B6alb (Nusinowitz et al., 2003). The slower physiological recovery of the response to light in B6alb mice compared to BALB/c mice corresponded perfectly to results of the previous biochemical studies showing a slower regeneration of rhodopsin (Wenzel et al., 2001b). A further substantiation of the RPE65 met/leu450 variant as a modifier of PR light damage was demonstrated when RPE65 protein activity and concentration were measured in the eyes of various breeding combinations of BALB/c, B6 and RPE65−/− (knockout) mice (the knockout mice were on a mixed background of 129S1/SvImJ and B6). The order of concentration of RPE65 in the eye from highest to lowest was BALB/c (leu/leu) > (BALB/c × B6)F_1 (leu/met) > BALB × KO (leu/−) > B6alb (met/met) > B6alb × KO (met/−). The rate of rhodopsin regeneration matched that order, but the rate of rhodopsin regeneration per unit RPE65 protein was not influenced by the leu/met variant; it was the different amount of RPE65 protein present (Lyubarsky et al., 2005). This same conclusion can be extracted from two very recent cell expression studies. In the first case, it took 5–10 × met450 cDNA to express the same amount of RPE65 protein as leu450 cDNA in 293T-LC cells, but both RPE65 proteins had the same activity (Jin et al., 2006). In the second case, amounts of RPE65 protein expressed by cell transfection of cDNA were directly related to the presence of the met450 or leu450 variant, whether it was in cDNA from mouse or from dog. Based on predicted protein structure, the authors of this work hypothesized that the RPE65 met450 variant made the protein much less stable than the leu450 variant (Redmond et al., 2007).

The evidence cited so far demonstrated that the met450 variant of RPE65 reduced the amount of RPE65 protein present in the eye relative to the leu450 variant. This reduction protected the PRs from light-induced damage by slowing the recycling of rhodopsin, and therefore slowing the recovery of the capability to respond to light physiologically. There was, however, a fly in the ointment (something inconsistent). The met450 variant of RPE65 is rare (figure 47.1). However, the albino NZW/LacJ mouse (NZW) carries the met variant yet is almost as sensitive to light-induced retinal damage as BALB/c mice, and far more sensitive than B6alb mice (LaVail et al., 1987a, 1987c; Danciger et al., 2005). We could think of three explanations for this: (1) The met450 variant of RPE65 is not responsible for the retinal light damage resistance found in B6alb. It is instead a nonfunctional sequence variant that segregates with the actual nearby gene responsible for the effect. The protective allele of this gene is present in B6alb and the sensitive allele in BALB/c and NZW. (2) There is a second change in the NZW *Rpe65* gene or a nearby sequence that suppresses the protective effect of RPE65 met450. (3) There are other NZW susceptibility gene alleles that overcome the protective effect of the met450 variant.

To evaluate these possibilities, we repeated the constant light–induced retinal damage protocol on a small test cross between B6alb and NZW. If the first or second explanation was true, we would expect a strong and highly significant QTL at distal chromosome 3 with a B6alb protective allele because the NZW allele of the gene in this QTL would not be present either because met450 was suppressed or because the allele of the true gene responsible for the QTL was not present. We found no such distal chromosome 3 QTL and did find other QTL supporting the third explanation (Danciger et al., 2005). In addition, we bred the met450 variant from NZW to BALB/c to the N8 generation and tested it under the same conditions of light exposure and by

Mouse Strains - From the MGI mouse SNP database

(http://www.informatics.jax.org/javawi2/servlet/WIFetch?page=snpQF)

Inbred

	AA residue	
C57BL/6J (AA residue)	#450	GLNHFVPDKLCK**M**NVKTKE
NZW/LacJ	450	GLNHFVPDKLCK**M**NVKTKE
129S1/SvImJ	450	GLNHFVPDKLCK**L**NVKTKE
A/J	450	GLNHFVPDKLCK**L**NVKTKE
AKR/J	450	GLNHFVPDKLCK**L**NVKTKE
BALB/cByJ	450	GLNHFVPDKLCK**L**NVKTKE
BTBR <+> tf	450	GLNHFVPDKLCK**L**NVKTKE
C3H/HeJ	450	GLNHFVPDKLCK**L**NVKTKE
DBA/2J	450	GLNHFVPDKLCK**L**NVKTKE
FVB/NJ	450	GLNHFVPDKLCK**L**NVKTKE
KK/HIJ	450	GLNHFVPDKLCK**L**NVKTKE
NOD/LtJ	450	GLNHFVPDKLCK**L**NVKTKE

Wild

	AA residue	
MOLF/EiJ	450	GLNHFVPDKLCK**M**NVKTKE
CAST/EiJ	450	GLNHFVPDKLCK**L**NVKTKE
WSB/EiJ	450	GLNHFVPDKLCK**L**NVKTKE

Animal species - From NCBI (http://www.ncbi.nlm.nih.gov/)

Species	AA residue	Sequence
C57-mouse	450	GLNHFVPDKLCK**M**NVKTKE
Rat	450	GLNHFVPDKLCK**L**NVKTKE
Dog	450	GLNHFVPDRLCK**L**NVKTKE
Human	450	GLNHFVPDRLCK**L**NVKTKE
Rhesus Monkey	450	GLNHFVPDRLCK**L**NVKTKE
Vervet monkey	450	GLNHFVPDRLCK**L**NVKTKE
Cow	450	GLNHFVPDRLCK**L**NVKTKE
Gray Opossum	791	GLNHFVPDRLCK**L**NVKTKE
Chicken	450	GLNHFVPDRLCK**L**NVKTKE
Japanese Firebelly Newt	450	GLNHFVPDRLSK**L**NVKTKE
Chimpanzee	467	GLNHFVPDRLCK**L**NVKTKE
Tiger Salamander	450	GLNHFVPDRLSK**L**NVKTKE
Aquatic frog	450	GLNHFVPDRLTK**L**NVKTKE
Zebrafish	450	GLNHFVPDRICK**L**NVKSKE
Pufferfish	451	GLNHFIPDRICK**L**NVKTKE

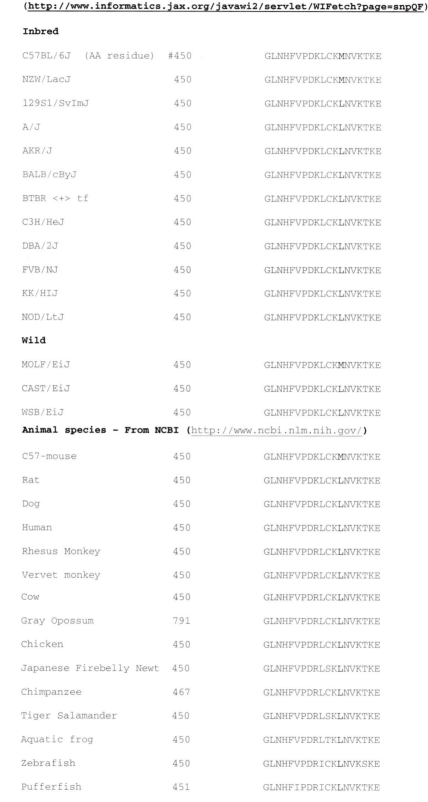

FIGURE 47.1 The RPE65 met/leu450 variant in wild and inbred strains of mice and from other animal species.

the same ONL thickness measurements described earlier in the text. Figure 47.2 shows that the RPE65 met450 coming from NZW and operating in the BALB/c background now protected the PRs from light-induced damage. To make the N8 generation, BALB/c mice were crossed with NZW. The offspring (F_1) were crossed into BALB/c mice to produce N2 mice. Tail DNAs from these mice were tested for the presence of the met450 variant by PCR, and those that were positive (RPE65 heterozygous met/leu450) were bred to BALB/c again to produce N3 offspring. The same process was repeated until N8. N refers to the number of generations of one strain (in this case BALB/c) bred into the F_1 such that the higher the N, the greater the percentage of the mouse that is BALB/c while still carrying the selected allele—in this case, around 99.6% BALB/c background and heterozygous for met/leu450. The N8, BALB/c, RPE65 met/leu450 mice were intercrossed to produce mice homozygous for leu450, homozygous for met450, and heterozygous.

Glazier et al. (2002) recently published a set of criteria that must be demonstrated to establish that a gene is responsible for a QTL (quantitative trait gene, or QTG). These include: (1) the demonstration of a linkage or association between the locus of the gene and the trait; (2) a significant sequence variant in the QTG between two strains with different phenotypes; (3) functional tests of the candidate QTG variants; and (4) an explanation of any complicating or confounding factors. A QTL on distal mouse chromosome 3, the locus of the *Rpe65* gene, was demonstrated to be associated with differences in a retinal light damage phenotype between the BALB/c and B6alb albino mouse strains (point 1). The BALB/c sequence of the *Rpe65* gene has the CTG code for leucine at residue 450, while the B6alb sequence has ATG for methionine (point 2). There is less RPE65 protein when met450 is present (demonstrated by Western blot), resulting in a slower recovery of the visual transduction response of the PR demonstrated physiologically, a slower regeneration of rhodopsin after bleach demonstrated biochemically, and a decreased level of PR damage after light insult demonstrated histologically (point 3). The presence of the "protective" met450 variant of RPE65 in the NZW strain that is relatively sensitive to light insult was explained by the presence of other QTL genes that negate the protective effect (point 4). The types and quality of data cited in this review match or exceed the criteria for establishing a variant gene to be one QTG or one modifier of several comprising the genetic portion of the complex trait of PR light damage.

Some genes identified in microarray expression studies and studies of single genes are candidates for light damage quantitative trait loci

Differential or comparative studies of mRNA expression and studies of individual genes bring much information about the light damage process in their own right, and also provide candidates for QTL based on chromosomal map locations. In the first approach, the upregulation (or downregulation) of retinal mRNAs in response to damaging levels of light is determined by comparing expression before and after light exposure, generally using microarray chips. The second approach involves measuring the effect on light damage of an increase or decrease or elimination of the expression of a gene or genes. The point of these studies is to identify the genes that govern the response to light insult, the protective defensive response, and the pathophysiological process of PR death. Three quantitative genetics studies designed to identify the chromosomal loci of genes that are involved in the retinal light damage process have been carried out, and, along with the chromosome 3 QTL (shown to be the *Rpe65*

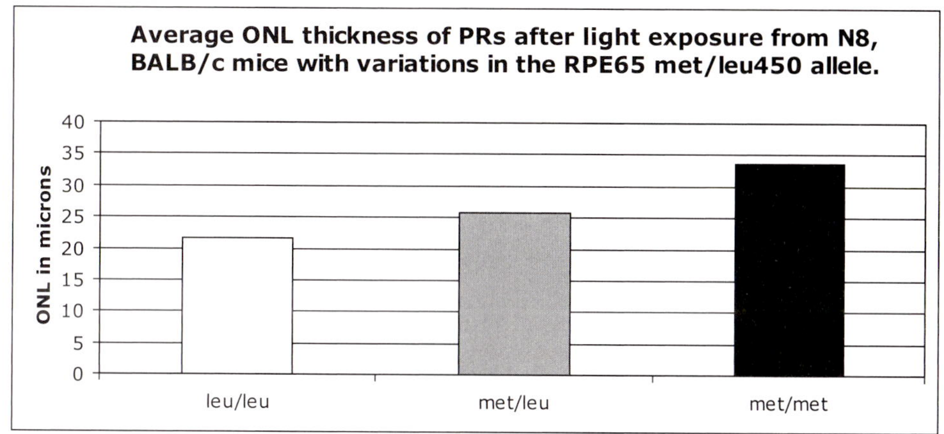

FIGURE 47.2 The number of mice measured for ONL was 15 for leu/leu, 18 for met/leu, and 5 for met/met. Probabilities derived from the student's unpaired *t*-test were 0.03 between leu/leu and met/met, 0.31 between leu/leu and met/leu, and 0.01 between met/leu and met/met.

gene), 11 other QTL have been described (Danciger et al., 2000, 2004, 2005). Are any of the genes implicated in light damage and discovered by microarray or single-gene studies located in the loci of these 11 QTL?

Three parallel studies asked what changes occur in levels of mRNA after a toxic light exposure (Chen et al., 2004; Roca et al., 2004; Rattner and Nathans, 2005). The BALB/c albino was the mouse strain, the retina was the source of the mRNA, and a comprehensive Affymetrix (Santa Clara, Calif.) genome chip was used for mRNA probe hybridization in all three studies. The conditions before and after light exposure and the intensity and duration of light differed. Dark adaptation ranged from 24 hours (Chen et al., 2004) to 1–2 weeks (Rattner and Nathans, 2005) to rearing in the dark (Roca et al., 2004). Light exposures ranged from 1,500–2,000 lux for 3 hours to 6,000 lux for 6 hours to 10,000 lux for 7 hours. Mice were sacrificed immediately (Chen et al., 2004; Roca et al., 2004) or kept in the dark for 24 hours first (Rattner and Nathans, 2005). Despite differences in the light exposure protocol, many genes were upregulated in common, particularly in the category of transcription factors. Many of the genes most highly upregulated appeared to be induced in Müller cells, even though light damage occurs primarily in PRs (Rattner and Nathans, 2005). At least part of the function of retinal Müller cells is thought to be to help maintain PRs and protect them from stress. The total number of upregulated genes in the three studies was greater than 300. Searching among 300 genes for those that are located in any of 11 chromosomal QTL loci would certainly provide candidate genes just by chance. In one of the studies, only 15 genes were upregulated (Roca et al., 2004); in another study, well over 200 were (Rattner and Nathans, 2005), and in the third study, about 70 genes were upregulated (Chen et al., 2004). The first study had more stringent criteria for considering a gene upregulated. Therefore, we considered the 15 genes most highly upregulated (the only 15 genes, in one case) from each study. Of the 45 genes, 6 were upregulated in more than one study and 12 were located within the loci of retinal light damage QTL. One gene (*Cebpd*) was shown to be upregulated in all three microarray reports. This gene was located in a QTL from one retinal light damage study. Two more upregulated genes were each located in QTL present in two light damage studies (table 47.1).

Examples of single-gene studies show that many genes influence retinal light damage. *Bax* and *Bak1* double knockout mice were protected from intense light exposure (Hahn et al., 2004). *Bax* and *Bak1* are pro-apoptotic genes of the bcl-2 family. Inhibition of the apoptotic factor AP-1 also protected PR cells from light-induced damage (Wenzel et al., 2001a). AP-1 is either a heterodimer of any of several Fos and Jun proteins or a homodimer of any of several Jun proteins (Curran and Franza, 1988). The absence of the antioxidant glutathione peroxidase-1 (*Gpx1*) in knockout mice left the retinas more sensitive to light-induced damage (Gosbell et al., 2006). The absence of the apoptotic regulator p53 (*Trp53*) or the absence of the Müller cell neurotrophin receptor p75 (*Ngfr*) in knockout mice had no effect on retinal light damage (Marti et al., 1998; Rohrer et al., 2003). Overexpression of erythropoietin (*Epo*) by hypoxic preconditioning protected the retina (Grimm et al., 2004), while overexpression of the EAT/mcl-1 gene (*Mcl1*), another member of the bcl-2 family, worsened light damage to the retina (Shinoda et al., 2001). These examples are apoptotic or other genes that are widely expressed and have a function that is not specific to the retina. On the other hand, the mouse orthologue of human *RDH12* (*Rdh12*), a gene involved

Table 47.1

Upregulated genes after damaging light exposure that map to retinal light damage QTL

Retinal Light Damage Study	Gene Symbol	Gene Name	QTL
B6alb × BALB/c	*Klf10*	Kruppel-like factor 10—TGF-β-inducible early growth response	12 proximal
B6alb × NZW	*Ifi204*	Interferon-γ-inducible gene 204	1 distal
	Atf3	Activating transcription factor 3	1 distal
	Ctgf	Fibroblast-inducible secreted protein	10 proximal
	Cebpd	CCAAT/enhancer-binding protein δ	16 proximal
129 × BALB/c	*Edn2*	Endothelin 2	4 distal
	Egr1	Early growth response 1	4 distal
	Pdpn	Podoplanin; glycoprotein 38	4 distal
	Lcn2	Lipocalin 2	2 proximal
	Mthfd2	Methylenetetrahydrofolate dehydrogenase (NAD+ dependent)	6 middle
B6alb × BALB/c and B6alb × NZW	*Ednrb*	Endothelin receptor type B	14 distal
129 × BALB/c and B6alb × NZW	*Chi3l1*	Chitinase 3-like 1	1 middle

in the specific retinal function of visual transduction, particularly in the vitamin A recycling system (Thomson et al., 2005), protected the mouse retina from light-induced damage (Maeda et al., 2006). Specifically, the absence of mouse *Rdh12* did not cause RD in the mouse, but it did make the mouse retina more sensitive to intense light. The absence of *Rdh12* caused 11-*cis*-retinal to be regenerated more rapidly under excessive light (Maeda et al., 2006), increasing the cycles of rhodopsin regeneration and increasing the levels of all-*trans*-retinaldehyde in the inner segments. The increased levels of all-*trans*-retinal made PRs more sensitive to light. On the other hand, an opposite mechanism was involved when RPE65 protein was removed (Grimm et al., 2000) or decreased due to the met450 variant (Danciger et al., 2000; Wenzel et al., 2001b, 2003) with opposite effect. As mentioned earlier, mice homozygous for RPE65 met450 or with no RPE65 had lower or no levels of RPE65 protein in their RPE, slower regeneration of rhodopsin, and less PR loss after intense light exposure (Danciger et al., 2000; Grimm et al., 2000; Wenzel et al., 2001b, 2003).

In summary, quantitative genetics studies have demonstrated the presence of many genes that affect light damage by the discovery of QTL. Microarray studies show the upregulation of many genes after damaging light exposure. Some of these genes are located in QTL and may be considered light damage effector gene candidates. Not surprisingly, single-gene knockout or enhanced gene expression studies have implicated apoptotic genes in PR light damage. Such genes are involved in cell death initiated in many other tissues as well. So far, only one specific eye gene expressed in the RPE, *Rpe65*, has been shown to be a naturally occurring complex trait gene or gene modifier. The influence of the met450 variant of RPE65 is to protect PRs from light damage by slowing down the visual cycle (Wenzel et al., 2001b, 2003). However, this same mechanism is in play in several genetically modified mice. The absence of *Rdh12* speeds up regeneration of rhodopsin during intense light exposure, exacerbating PR damage (Thompson et al., 2005). Absence of the α -subunit of transducin (*Gnat1*) protects PRs from light damage under some circumstances (Hao et al., 2002). α-Transducin is an integral part of the visual cycle, and without it there is no hyperpolarization-depolarization cycle. The absence of either rhodopsin kinase (*Grk1*) (Chen et al., 1999a) or arrestin (*Sag*) (Chen et al., 1999b), both needed to shut off rhodopsin, brings about RD even in dim cyclic light because the visual cycle is kept on. Therefore, one component of the complex trait of light damage to PRs is perturbation of the very biochemical-physiological cycle that mediates vision under normal circumstances. Thus, in the retina of a mouse expressing the naturally occurring but rare RPE65 met450 modifier, damage is modulated under the stressed conditions of toxic light, while under nonstressed conditions the retina is normal. This is a very nice example of an allele or gene variant that perturbs a system only under abnormal conditions and thereby modifies the effect of the abnormal conditions.

REFERENCES

Balkema, G. W., and Dräger, U. C. (1991). Impaired visual thresholds in hypopigmented animals. *Vis. Neurosci.* 6:577–585.

Chabre, M., and Deterre, P. (1989). Molecular mechanism of visual transduction. *Eur. J. Biochem.* 179:255–266.

Chen, C. K. (2005). The vertebrate phototransduction cascade: Amplification and termination mechanisms. *Rev. Physiol. Biochem. Pharmacol.* 154:101–121.

Chen, C. K., Burns, M. E., Spencer, M., Niemi, G. A., Chen, J., Hurley, J. B., Baylor, D. A., and Simon, M. I. (1999a). Abnormal photoresponses and light-induced apoptosis in rods lacking rhodopsin kinase. *Proc. Natl. Acad. Sci. U.S.A.* 96:3718–3722.

Chen, J., Simon, M. I., Matthes, M. T., Yasumura, D., and LaVail, M. M. (1999b). Increased susceptibility to light damage in an arrestin knockout mouse model of Oguchi disease (stationary night blindness). *Invest. Ophthalmol. Vis. Sci.* 40:2978–2982.

Chen, L., Wu, W., Dentchev, T., Zeng, Y., Wang, J., Tsui, I., Tobias, J. W., Bennett, J., Baldwin, D., et al. (2004). Light damage induced changes in mouse retinal gene expression. *Exp. Eye Res.* 79:239–247.

Cideciyan, A. V., Hood, D. C., Huang, Y., Banin, E., Li, Z. Y., Stone, E. M., Milam, A. H., and Jacobson, S. G. (1998). Disease sequence from mutant rhodopsin allele to rod and cone photoreceptor degeneration in man. *Proc. Natl. Acad. Sci. U.S.A.* 95: 7103–7108.

Cruickshanks, K. J., Klein, R., and Klein, B. E. (1993). Sunlight and age-related macular degeneration: The Beaver Dam Eye Study. *Arch. Ophthalmol.* 111:514–518.

Curran, T., and Franza, B. R., Jr. (1988). Fos and Jun: The AP-1 connection. *Cell* 55:395–397.

Danciger, M., Lyon, J., Worrill, D., Hoffman, S., Lem, J., Reme, C. E., Wenzel, A., and Grimm, C. (2004). New retinal light damage QTL in mice with the light-sensitive RPE65 LEU variant. *Mamm. Genome* 15:277–283.

Danciger, M., Matthes, M. T., Yasamura, D., Akhmedov, N. B., Rickabaugh, T., Gentleman, S., Redmond, T. M., LaVail, M. M., and Farber, D. B. (2000). A QTL on distal chromosome 3 that influences the severity of light-induced damage to mouse photoreceptors. *Mamm. Genome* 11:422–427.

Danciger, M., Yang, H., Handschumacher, L., and LaVail, M. M. (2005). Constant light-induced retinal damage and the RPE65-MET450 variant: Assessment of the NZW/LacJ mouse. *Mol. Vis.* 11:374–379.

Glazier, A. M., Nadeau, J. H., and Aitman, T. J. (2002). Finding genes that underlie complex traits. *Science* 298:2345–2349.

Gosbell, A. D., Stefanovic, N., Scurr, L. L., Pete, J., Kola, I., Favilla, I., and de Haan, J. B. (2006). Retinal light damage: Structural and functional effects of the antioxidant glutathione peroxidase-1. *Invest. Ophthalmol. Vis. Sci.* 47:2613–2622.

Grimm, C., Wenzel, A., Hafezi, F., Yu, S., Redmond, T. M., and Reme, C. E. (2000). Protection of Rpe65-deficient mice identifies rhodopsin as a mediator of light-induced retinal degeneration. *Nat. Genet.* 25:63–66.

Grimm, C., Wenzel, A., Stanescu, D., Samardzija, M., Hotop, S., Groszer, M., Naash, M., Gassmann, M., and Reme, C.

(2004). Constitutive overexpression of human erythropoietin protects the mouse retina against induced but not inherited retinal degeneration. *J. Neurosci.* 24:5651–5658.

Hahn, P., Lindsten, T., Lyubarsky, A., Ying, G. S., Pugh, E. N., Jr., Thompson, C. B., and Dunaief, J. L. (2004). Deficiency of Bax and Bak protects photoreceptors from light damage in vivo. *Cell Death Differ.* 11:1192–1197.

Hao, W., Wenzel, A., Obin, M. S., Chen, C. K., Brill, E., Krasnoperova, N. V., Eversole-Cire, P., Kleyner, Y., Taylor, A., et al. (2002). Evidence for two apoptotic pathways in light-induced retinal degeneration. *Nat. Genet.* 32:254–260.

Hayes, J. M., and Balkema, G. W. (1993). Visual thresholds in mice: Comparison of retinal light damage and hypopigmentation. *Vis. Neurosci.* 10:931–938.

Jin, M., Li, S., Moghrabi, W. N., Philp, A. R., and Travis, G. H. (2006). Mutational analysis to determine key residues essential for activity and membrane association of Rpe65 isomerohydrolase. ARVO Abstract.

LaVail, M. M., Gorrin, G. M., and Repaci, M. A. (1987a). Strain differences in sensitivity to light-induced photoreceptor degeneration in albino mice. *Curr. Eye Res.* 6:825–834.

LaVail, M. M., Gorrin, G. M., Repaci, M. A., Thomas, L. A., and Ginsberg, H. M. (1987b). Genetic regulation of light damage to photoreceptors. *Invest. Ophthalmol. Vis. Sci.* 28:1043–1048.

LaVail, M. M., Gorrin, G. M., Repaci, M. A., and Yasumura, D. (1987c). Light-induced retinal degeneration in albino mice and rats: Strain and species differences. *Prog. Clin. Biol. Res.* 247: 439–454.

LaVail, M. M., Gorrin, G. M., Yasumura, D., and Matthes, M. T. (1999). Increased susceptibility to constant light in nr and pcd mice with inherited retinal degenerations. *Invest. Ophthalmol. Vis. Sci.* 40:1020–1024.

Lyubarsky, A. L., Savchenko, A. B., Morocco, S. B., Daniele, L. L., Redmond, T. M., and Pugh, E. N., Jr. (2005). Mole quantity of RPE65 and its productivity in the generation of 11-*cis*-retinal from retinyl esters in the living mouse eye. *Biochemistry* 44:9880–9888.

Maeda, A., Maeda, T., Imanishi, Y., Sun, W., Jastrzebska, B., Hatala, D. A., Winkens, H. J., Hofmann, K. P., Janssen, J. J., et al. (2006). Retinol dehydrogenase (RDH12) protects photoreceptors from light-induced degeneration in mice. *J. Biol. Chem.* 281:37697–37704.

Manly, K. F., Cudmore, R. H., Jr., and Meer, J. M. (2001). Map Manager QTX, cross-platform software for genetic mapping. *Mamm. Genome* 12:930–932.

Marti, A., Hafezi, F., Lansel, N., Hegi, M. E., Wenzel, A., Grimm, C., Niemeyer, G., and Reme, C. E. (1998). Light-induced cell death of retinal photoreceptors in the absence of p53. *Invest. Ophthalmol. Vis. Sci.* 39:846–849.

Mata, N. L., Weng, J., and Travis, G. H. (2000). Biosynthesis of a major lipofuscin fluorophore in mice and humans with ABCR-mediated retinal and macular degeneration. *Proc. Natl. Acad. Sci. U.S.A.* 97:7154–7159.

Nusinowitz, S., Nguyen, L., Radu, R., Kashani, Z., Farber, D., and Danciger, M. (2003). Electroretinographic evidence for altered phototransduction gain and slowed recovery from photobleaches in albino mice with a MET450 variant in RPE65. *Exp. Eye Res.* 77:627–638.

Organisciak, D. T., Li, M., Darrow, R. M., and Farber, D. B. (1999). Photoreceptor cell damage by light in young Royal College of Surgeons rats. *Curr. Eye Res.* 19:188–196.

Rattner, A., and Nathans, J. (2005). The genomic response to retinal disease and injury: Evidence for endothelin signaling from photoreceptors to glia. *J. Neurosci.* 25:4540–4549.

Redmond, T. M., Weber, C. H., Poliakov, E., Yu, S. S., and Gentleman, S. (2007). Effect of leu/met variation at residue 450 on isomerase activity and protein expression of RPE65 and its modulation by variation at other residues. *Mol. Vis.* 13:1813–1821.

Roca, A., Shin, K. J., Liu, X., Simon, M. I., and Chen, J. (2004). Comparative analysis of transcriptional profiles between two apoptotic pathways of light-induced retinal degeneration. *Neuroscience* 129:779–790.

Rohrer, B., Matthes, M. T., LaVail, M. M., and Reichardt, L. F. (2003). Lack of p75 receptor does not protect photoreceptors from light-induced cell death. *Exp. Eye Res.* 76:125–129.

Sanyal, S., and Hawkins, R. K. (1986). Development and degeneration of retina in rds mutant mice: Effects of light on the rate of degeneration in albino and pigmented homozygous and heterozygous mutant and normal mice. *Vision Res.* 26:1177–1185.

Shinoda, K., Nakamura, Y., Matsushita, K., Shimoda, K., Okita, H., Fukuma, M., Yamada, T., Ohde, H., Oguchi, Y., et al. (2001). Light induced apoptosis is accelerated in transgenic retina overexpressing human EAT/mcl-1, an anti-apoptotic bcl-2 related gene. *Br. J. Ophthalmol.* 85:1237–1243.

Simons, K. (1993). Artificial light and early-life exposure in age-related macular degeneration and in cataractogenic phototoxicity. *Arch. Ophthalmol.* 111:297–298.

Taylor, H. R., Munoz, B., West, S., Bressler, N. M., Bressler, S. B., and Rosenthal, F. S. (1990). Visible light and risk of age-related macular degeneration. *Trans. Am. Ophthalmol. Soc.* 88:163–173 [discussion 173–178].

Thompson, D. A., Janecke, A. R., Lange, J., Feathers, K. L., Hubner, C. A., McHenry, C. L., Stockton, D. W., Rammesmayer, G., Lupski, J. R., et al. (2005). Retinal degeneration associated with RDH12 mutations results from decreased 11-*cis* retinal synthesis due to disruption of the visual cycle. *Hum. Mol. Genet.* 14:3865–3875.

Vogt, W. (1995). Oxidation of methionyl residues in proteins: Tools, targets, and reversal. *Free Radic. Biol. Med.* 18:93–105.

Wang, M., Lam, T. T., Tso, M. O., and Naash, M. I. (1997). Expression of a mutant opsin gene increases the susceptibility of the retina to light damage. *Vis. Neurosci.* 14:55–62.

Wenzel, A., Grimm, C., Samardzija, M., and Reme, C. E. (2003). The genetic modifier Rpe65Leu(450): Effect on light damage susceptibility in c-Fos-deficient mice. *Invest. Ophthalmol. Vis. Sci.* 44:2798–2802.

Wenzel, A., Grimm, C., Seeliger, M. W., Jaissle, G., Hafezi, F., Kretschmer, R., Zrenner, E., and Reme, C. E. (2001a). Prevention of photoreceptor apoptosis by activation of the glucocorticoid receptor. *Invest. Ophthalmol. Vis. Sci.* 42:1653–1659.

Wenzel, A., Reme, C. E., Williams, T. P., Hafezi, F., and Grimm, C. (2001b). The Rpe65 Leu450Met variation increases retinal resistance against light-induced degeneration by slowing rhodopsin regeneration. *J. Neurosci.* 21:53–58.

48 Age-Related Eye Diseases

BO CHANG

Age-related eye diseases are the leading causes of vision impairment and blindness throughout the world. With the world's population of senior citizens growing rapidly, the issue of vision loss in the older population is of paramount importance. Age-related eye diseases are costly to treat, threaten the ability of older adults to live independently, and increase the risk for accidents and falls. Of the age-related eye diseases, age-related macular degeneration (AMD) increases dramatically with age in men and women and is the most important cause of irreversible visual loss in the elderly. Cataracts are the leading cause of blindness in the world, affecting nearly 20.5 million Americans age 40 and older (Congdon et al., 2004; Blindness and visual impairment [editorial], 2004).

From the available data, it appears that age-related eye diseases are caused by environmental factors triggering disease in genetically susceptible subjects. Identifying the genetic factors would contribute to understanding the pathogenesis. If those at risk could be identified, it might be possible to modify lifestyle or develop novel therapies in the presymptomatic stage to prevent disease or decrease severity. However, direct research on human ocular conditions is impeded by the poor availability of tissues and the impossibility of performing genetic manipulation in humans. Human eye tissue (including biopsy material) in most ocular diseases is seldom available, because it is difficult to obtain eye tissue samples without the risk of damaging the patient's vision. Since genetic and biochemical experiments in human patients are not possible, animal models serve an important and unique role. Historically, mouse models have been especially useful in determining biochemical mechanisms in human ocular diseases. In this chapter, I focus on mouse age-related retinal degeneration disorders as possible models for human AMD and mouse age-related cataract mutants as models for human cataracts.

Mice as models for human age-related eye diseases

The mouse lens and retina are remarkably similar in structure to the human lens and retina, and both species experience similar ocular disorders (Chang et al., 2005). Not only are developmental and invasive studies possible in mice, but the mouse's accelerated life span and generation time (one mouse year equals about 30 human years, based on a ratio of average life span for each species) make it possible to follow the natural progression of eye diseases in a relatively brief period. Studying aging diseases in mice has many advantages: typically mice live 2 years and thus age quickly, and they are relatively inexpensive and easy to maintain. The availability of inbred strains provides a population that is genetically the same from one mouse to the rest; each inbred strain is like an infinite set of monozygotic or identical twins. All mice of the same inbred strain generally can be expected to have the same phenotype. By contrast, differing environmental factors combined with many genetic variations between affected and unaffected individuals make it difficult to identify specific genes responsible for age-related eye diseases in humans. Environmental factors can play an especially strong confounding role in the etiology of late-onset eye diseases in humans because of the long period of life with exposure to different variables before any age-related eye diseases are detected. In the mouse, environmental factors can be controlled to a high degree by raising mice in standard conditions of diet, light-dark cycle, cage-changing schedules, experienced animal handlers, and constant and clean air exchange in the mouse rooms, and with a high standard of disease prevention and animal health care. With environmental variance controlled, researchers can focus on the underlying genetic causes. Genetically homogeneous inbred mice, accessible at any age, offer an opportunity to study the histopathological and biochemical changes that occur during age-related eye disease formation and permit controlled study of single gene variations in a constant genetic background. The high level of homology between mouse and human genomes (>95% of genes are conserved) means that similar disease manifestations are often identified in mice and humans. Preservation of gene function is the reason that mice are often useful in studies of disease mechanisms in humans (Davisson et al., 1991; Nadeau et al., 1992; Quiring et al., 1994). Thus, the high degree of conservation between human and mouse chromosomes makes the mouse a powerful research tool with which to identify human genes, which can then be used in presymptomatic testing and for developing preventive treatment.

The search for age-related eye diseases in mice

The Jackson Laboratory (TJL), having the world's largest collection of mouse mutant stocks and genetically diverse inbred strains—more than 3,000 strains in 2006—is an ideal place to discover genetically determined eye variations and disorders. While screening mouse strains and stocks at TJL for genetic mouse models of human ocular disorders, we have identified numerous spontaneous or naturally occurring mutations (table 48.1). However, the search for late-onset eye disease has never been done, and the best place to do this is at TJL. TJL has the best collection of genetically unrelated inbred strains available anywhere. For clinical characterization, a primary search for gross eye abnormalities has been done by examining the eyelids, globe, cornea, and iris, first with visual inspection and then using a Nikon biomicroscope (slit lamp). The cornea is checked for clarity, size (bupthalmos vs. microcornea), surface texture, and vascularization. The iris is examined for pupil size, constriction, reflected luminescence, and synechiae. The eye is then dilated with 1% atropine and the lens is examined for cataracts. Finally, an indirect ophthalmoscope is used to examine the fundus for signs of retinal degeneration. In mice, the typical changes are retinal vessel constriction or retinal pigment epithelial disturbance, drusen, or other retinal deposits. Mice with a suspected abnormality are followed up with a secondary examination that includes electroretinography (ERG) and histological investigation. For genetic characterization, an initial genetic analysis to determine the mode of inheritance is carried out by making outcrosses and backcrosses or intercrosses. Once an eye disorder has been shown to be due to a new mutation, a linkage cross is set up to determine the mutant gene's chromosomal location by doing a genome scan of DNA markers using PCR analysis. Mice with age-related eye diseases often are past the breeding age. Because all mice in an inbred strain are genetically identical, this can be overcome by doing the genetic crosses with young mice from the same strain, because they will acquire the same eye disease. Dominant and semidominant mutations are mapped by backcrosses or outcrosses to wild-type (+/+) mice. Recessive mutations are mapped using intercrosses, which are more efficient, because each F_2 mouse obtains two potentially recombinant chromosomes, one from each parent. Modifying genes often can be detected in the initial cross by finding more than one chromosomal region associated with the disease phenotype. Polygenic traits are recognized by phenotype loss in outcrosses. If a disease turns out to be polygenic—that is, influenced by more genes than can be identified in standard genetic crosses—mice of the strain are still histologically and clinically characterized to provide a model for clinically similar human ocular disorders.

Age-related retinal degenerations in human and mouse eyes

For many people, retirement means more time to read, watch television, sew, play cards, or drive to places they have always longed to visit. Yet by the time they reach age 65, many retirees find they no longer have those options because they have lost much of their vision to age-related eye disorders, such as age-related macular degeneration (AMD) and many forms of late-onset retinal degeneration, the most common uncorrectable causes of vision loss in the elderly. Although mice do not have a macula, mice do have homologues of genes that are associated with human AMD, and mutations in such genes in mice likely cause age-related retinal degeneration (ARRD). For example, partial loss of the ABCA4 or rim protein is sufficient to cause a phenotype in mice similar to recessive Stargardt disease and AMD, a common cause of visual loss in the human elderly (Mata et al., 2001). In the *Abca4^{tm1Ght}* homozygous mouse model, the presence of A2E and lipofuscin granules is seen, along with shortening of the photoreceptor outer segments (Weng et al., 1999; Mata et al., 2000; Radu et al., 2004). Another example is that the *ELOVL4* gene is associated with two related forms of human autosomal dominant macular dystrophy, and in situ hybridization on mouse retinal sections shows a strong uniform signal in the photoreceptor layer, particularly in the region corresponding to the photoreceptor inner segments (Zhang et al., 2001). Mutant mice carrying an *Elovl4* transgene demonstrate an accumulation of A2E and lipofuscin-like material, but they also show photoreceptor outer segment disc disorganization and geographic atrophy (Karan et al., 2005). Mice with a 5 bp deletion knock-in of *Elovl4* develop progressive photoreceptor degeneration (Vasireddy et al., 2006). Recently, a known polymorphism in human complement factor H (CFH), T → C substitution in exon 9, which resulted in the substitution of an uncharged tyrosine with a positively charged histidine (Y402H), was shown to be associated with increased risk for AMD (Edwards et al., 2005; Hageman et al., 2005; Haines et al., 2005; Klein et al., 2005; Zareparsi et al., 2005). The human and mouse CFH proteins contain 20 repetitive units of 60 amino acids, referred to as the short consensus repeat or the complement control protein module, arranged in a continuous fashion like a string of 20 beads (Rodriguez de Cordoba et al., 2004). In human and mouse, the *CFH* expression pattern was found to be similar, with the highest level of expression in the liver. In ocular tissue, CFH was detected in the distalmost optic nerve (3 mm) cut from the scleral surface of the eyeball, sclera, RPE-choroid, retina, lens, and ciliary body. In mouse, *Cfh* expression was observed from early embryonic stages, and in the eye, its expression increased with age (Mandal and Ayyagari, 2006).

Historically, mouse models have been especially useful in determining biochemical mechanisms in retinal diseases. For example, invaluable information about the molecular and pathological basis of some of these diseases has been provided by the discoveries of gene mutations in several mouse retinal degeneration models. Discovery of the mouse

Table 48.1

Mouse models of ocular disease for which chromosomal locations have been established

Gene (or Strain)	Location	Phenotype Description
Retinal Models		
rd3	Chr 1	Retinal degeneration 3
$Cln8^{mnd}$	Chr 8	Retinal degeneration discovered in *mnd* mice
Rd4	Chr 4	Retinal degeneration 4
Tub^{tub}	Chr 7	Retinal degeneration 5 discovered in *tub* mice
$Mfrp^{rd6}$	Chr 9	Retinal degeneration 6
$Nr2e3^{rd7}$	Chr 9	Retinal degeneration 7
$Cln6^{nclf}$	Chr 9	Retinal degeneration discovered in *nclf* mice
$Crb1^{rd8}$	Chr 1	Retinal degeneration 8
Rd9	Chr X	Retinal degeneration 9
$Pde6b^{rd10}$	Chr 5	Retinal degeneration 10
rd11	Chr 13	Retinal degeneration 11
$Rpe65^{rd12}$	Chr 3	Retinal degeneration 12
rd13	Chr 15	Retinal degeneration discovered in *nmf5* mice
rd14	Chr 18	Retinal degeneration 14
rd15	Chr 7	Retinal degeneration 15
rd16	Chr 10	Retinal degeneration 16
rd17	Chr 9	No ERG a-wave and retinal degeneration 17
B6-$Trp53^{tm}$	Chr 11	Abnormal retinal layers, extra tissue and vessels in posterior chamber
B6-$Nr2e1^{frc}$	Chr 10	No retinal vessels and bad ERG response
$Col2a1^{sed}$	Chr 15	Retinoschisis
nob2	Chr X	Missing retinal outer plexiform layer (OPL) and no ERG b-wave 2
lvi	Chr 18	Light-induced visual impairment and missing retinal OPL
nob3	Chr 11	No ERG b-wave 3
cpfl1	Chr 19	Cone photoreceptor function loss 1
Cpfl2	Chr 3	White retinal spots with cone photoreceptor function loss 2
cpfl3	Chr 3	Cone photoreceptor function loss 3
Cpfl4	Chr 17	White retinal spots with cone photoreceptor function loss 4
cpfl5	Chr 1	Cone photoreceptor function loss 5
cpfl6	Chr 13	Cone photoreceptor function loss 6
cpfl7	Chr 19	Cone photoreceptor function loss 7
$Vldlr^{tm1Her}$	Chr 19	Develop retinal spots and subretinal neovascularization
Nm2621*	Chr 6	Severe retinal pigment loss, it is allelic to $Mitf^{mi}$
Nm2641	Chr 19	Dominant optic nerve coloboma
nm3344	Chr 13	Recessive retinal degeneration
Rico	Chr 13	Retina and iris coloboma
Cataract Models		
$Gja8^{Lop10}$	Chr 3	Homozygous mice are microphthalmic with dense white cataracts
lop11	Chr 8	Recessive, vacuolated cataract
$Crygd^{Lop12}$	Chr 1	Dominant, nuclear lumpy irregular cataract
lop13	Chr 15	Early white cataract (former name *nuc*)
lop14	Chr 14	Extruded lens cataract
Nm1853	Chr 1	Dominant cataract
lop16	Chr 10	Muscle paresis and cataract, mutants die at 1 month of age
$Cryaa^{lop18}$	Chr 17	Recessive cataract
$Dstn^{corn1}$	Chr 2	Corneal epithelial dystrophy and white cataract
$Dstn^{corn1\text{-}2J}$	Chr 2	Mild corneal epithelial dystrophy and white cataract

Continued

Table 48.1

Mouse models of ocular disease for which chromosomal locations have been established (continued)

Gene (or Strain)	Location	Phenotype Description
bs2	Chr 2	Blind-sterile-2 with microphthalmia and cataract
lop20	Chr 1	Cataract with variable expression
Lop21	Chr 16	Transgenic cataract
Nm2249	Chr 3	Fetal cataract with microphthalmia
Nm2520	Chr 5	Cataract and coloboma
Nm2541	Chr 5	Dominant cataract
Nm2620	Chr 10	Dominant cataract
nm2897	Chr 2	Recessive cataract
Nm3062	Chr 1	Dominant cataract
nm3347	Chr 5	Recessive cataract starts at 1 month of age
nm3364	Chr 2	Recessive cataract
nm3365	Chr 17	Recessive cataract
Glaucoma Models		
Gpnmb^{ipd}	Chr 6	Iris pigment dispersion
Tryp1^{isa}	Chr 4	Iris stromal atrophy
Nm2702	Chr 11	Swollen eyes, inner retina loss, and optic nerve cupping
Other Eye Disease Models		
Lse	Chr 7	Low-set ear, vascular hazy cornea; homozygotes have cataracts
wa3	Chr 12	Wavy coat, eyelids fail to develop, enlarged heart and esophagus
eyeless	Chr 3	Anophthalmos in 80% of offspring; mice with intact globes have microophthalmia and frequently congenital corneal perforations, with collapse of the anterior chamber
A/J	Chr X	Crystal deposits in iris
nm1863	Chr 12	Cataract, abnormal iris and cornea
nm2619	Chr 9	Mouse model for persistant hyperplastic primary vitreous
Nm2557	Chr X	X-linked model for aniridia: heterozygous females have a small iris, homozygous females and males have a cataract
Nm3408	Chr 2	Eyeless, lens-cornea synechiae
JR4326	Chr 2	Eyeless, lens-cornea synechiae

*New mutation (NM, Nm or nm) numbers are assigned in TJL's program as temporary unique identifiers until sufficient information is available to name the mutant allele or the mutated gene is identified.

retinal degeneration 1 (*rd1*) mutation in the gene for the β-subunit of cGMP-phosphodiesterase (*Pde6b*) (Bowes et al., 1990) led to the identification of mutations in the human homologue (*PDE6B*) in similar human disorders (McLaughlin et al., 1993), and identification of the tubby (*tub*) mouse gene family (Noben-Trauth et al., 1996) led to the finding of tubby-like protein 1 (TULP1) alterations in individuals affected with autosomal recessive RP (Hagstrom et al., 1998; Banerjee et al., 1998). Similarly, discovery of the mutations *Rds* (retinal degeneration slow) in the peripherin 2 (*Prph2*) (Travis et al., 1989) and shaker 1 (*sh1*) in the myosin 7A (*Myo7a*) (Gibson et al., 1995) mouse genes paved the way for the identification of defects in the RDS-peripherin gene in patients with autosomal dominant RP, and various cone, cone-rod, and macular dystrophies (Keen and Inglehearn, 1996) and in *MYO7A* in patients with Usher's syndrome type 1b (Weil et al., 1995).

Discovery of 15 Strains of Mice with Age-Related Retinal Degeneration At TJL we have a productive screening and evaluation program for identifying new mouse models of ocular diseases. A component of this program, the study of age-related genetic eye diseases in mice, was funded by the Foundation Fighting Blindness. We aged 10 mice from each of 35 different inbred strains and screened them from 6 months to 2 years of age and up for late-onset retinal disorders. The 35 strains listed in table 48.2 have known abnormalities (low ERG, iris atrophy, cataracts) as strain characteristcs or are wild-derived strains that have not been characterized for age-related eye diseases.

Table 48.2
Eye disorders in aged 35 inbred strains

Laboratory Strains	
C57BL/6J	Cataract* and normal retina at 30 months old
A/J	ARRD at 26 months old and iris calcium deposits at 6 months old, normal lens† at 26 months old
RIII/DmMobJ	Subcapsular cataract‡ and ARRD at 24 months old
129 P3/J	ARRD and normal lens† at 23 months old
DBA/1J	Pigment in angle, thin iris, cataract§ and normal retina at 25 months old
BALB/cByJ	ARRD and normal lens† at 25 months old
BALB/cJ	ARRD and normal lens† at 25 months old
LP/J	ARRD and cataract§ at 25 months old
NZW/LacJ	ARRD and normal lens† at 25 months old
SJL/J	*Pdeb*^{rd1} and normal lens† at 24 months old
YBR/EiJ	Cornea opacity (dystrophy), normal lens† and ARRD at about 24 months old
CE/J	Subcapsular cataract§ and normal retina at 24 months old
RF/J	Normal lens† and retina at about 18 months old
SWR/J	*Pdeb*^{rd1}, normal lens† at 24 months old
CBA/CaJ	Nuclear cataract‡ and normal retina at 26 months old
C57BR/cdJ	Iris transillumination, cataract,* and normal retina at 26 months old
Wild-Derived Strains	
CASA/RkJ *(M.m. castaneus)*	Subcapsular cataract‡ and normal retina at 23 months old
CAST/EiJ *(M.m. castaneus)*	Subcapsular cataract‡ and normal retina at 25 months old
CZECHII/EiJ (*Mus musculus*)	Cataract* and ARRD at 23 months old
AU/SsJ	Pupils don't fully dilate, cataract* and normal retina at 24 months old
LEWES/EiJ *(Mus domesticus)*	Nuclear cataract‡ and ARRD at 30 months old
MOLC/RkJ *(M.m. molossinus)*	Cataract* and normal retina at 24 months old
MOLD/RkJ *(M.m. molossinus)*	Iris holes, *Pdeb*^{rd1} and subcapsular cataract* at 24 months old
MOLF/EiJ *(M.m. molossinus)*	*Pdeb*^{rd1} and normal lens† at 24 months old
Mus caroli/EiJ	Areas of disrupted ONL and RPE, normal lens† and ARRD at 28 months old
PANCEVO/EiJ *(Mus hortulanus)*	Posterior cataract§ and normal retina at 26 months old
PERA/EiJ *(Peru-Atteck)*	Cortical cataract‡ and ARRD at 24 months old
PERC/EiJ *(Peru-Coppock)*	Cataract* and ARRD at 24 months old
SF/CamEiJ *(San Francisco)*	*Pdeb*^{rd1}, normal lens† at 30 months old
SKIVE/EiJ*(Mus musculus/domesticus)*	Cataract* and normal retina at 24 months old
SPRET/EiJ *(Mus spretus, Spain)*	Cortical cataract§ and normal retina at 24 months old
TIRANO/EiJ *(Mus domesticus)*	Cortical cataract‡ and normal retina at 26 months old
WSB/EiJ *(Mus domesticus)*	Subcapsular cataract§ and ARRD at 30 months old
WMP/PasDnJ *(Mus domesticus)*	Cornea spots, normal lens† and ARRD at 30 months old
ZALENDE/EiJ *(Mus domesticus)*	Retinal cupping and detachment, normal lens† at about 20 months old

*Cataract starting at 14 months of age.
†Clear lenses throughout their lives.
‡Lens opacity starting at 8 months of age.
§Mild lens opacity starting at 22 months of age.
ARRD, age-related retinal degeneration.

We have discovered 15 strains in which all mice screened had ARRD (late-onset retinal degeneration). Seven of these were wild-derived strains (PERA/EiJ, PERC/EiJ, CZECHII/EiJ, LEWES/EiJ, *Mus Caroli*/EiJ, WSB/EiJ, WMP/PasDnJ) and eight were laboratory strains (A/J, 129P3/J, BALB/cJ, BALB/cByJ, RIII/DmMobJ, LP/J, YBR/EiJ, NZW/LacJ) (see table 48.2). Wild-derived strains have been inbred from mice captured in natural populations and are expected to harbor different mutations from those found in long-inbred laboratory strains. Mice from three of the 15 strains in which ARRD was found were blind at 2 years of age as confirmed by ERG (no response) and histology (no outer nuclear layer, ONL), and mice of the other 12 strains experienced slow retinal degeneration with very poor vision, as confirmed by low ERG response and reduced ONL (2–6 layers compared to the normal 10 layers of ONL) at 2 years of age. The data presented here document the disease phenotype in seven wild-derived ARRD strains with retinal degeneration (figure 48.1) and eight laboratory ARRD strains of mice with ONL cell loss (figure 48.2). In six of these laboratory strains the retinal degeneration may be caused by light damage during aging, because these six strains of mice are albino and lack a pigmented iris to protect the retina from light during the daily 14 hours of light in the

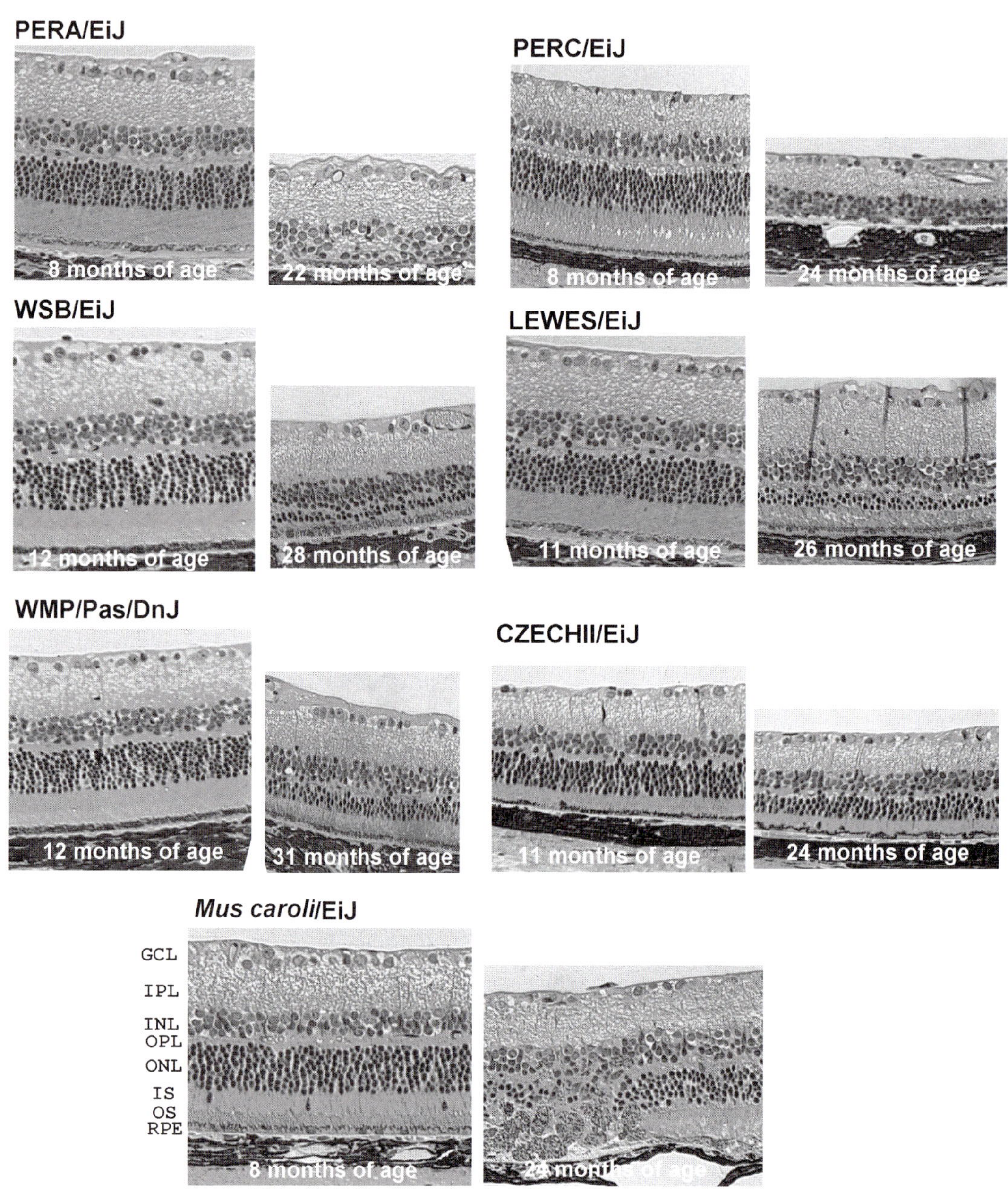

Figure 48.1 Retinal histological sections in seven wild-derived ARRD strains showing relatively normal retinal structure at relatively younger ages and retinal degeneration at older ages. The strain names are labeled at the top and the ages are labeled within each retinal section. GCL, ganglion cell layer; INL, inner nuclear layer; IPL, inner plexiform layer; IS, photoreceptor inner segments; ONL, outer nuclear layer; OPL, outer plexiform layer; OS, photoreceptor outer segments; RPE, retinal pigment epithelial cells.

light-dark cycle of the mouse room. Retinal degeneration can be induced by exposure to excessive doses of light and is used as a model to study photoreceptor apoptosis, the common final pathway of cell loss in human AMD and some forms of inherited retinal degenerations (Rome et al., 1998).

Genetic factors reducing the light damage susceptibility (LDS) of retinal photoreceptors in C57BL/6J mice were postulated in 1987 (LaVail et al., 1987); however, the underlying molecular mechanisms have not yet been identified. Recently, by comparing progeny from a cross between

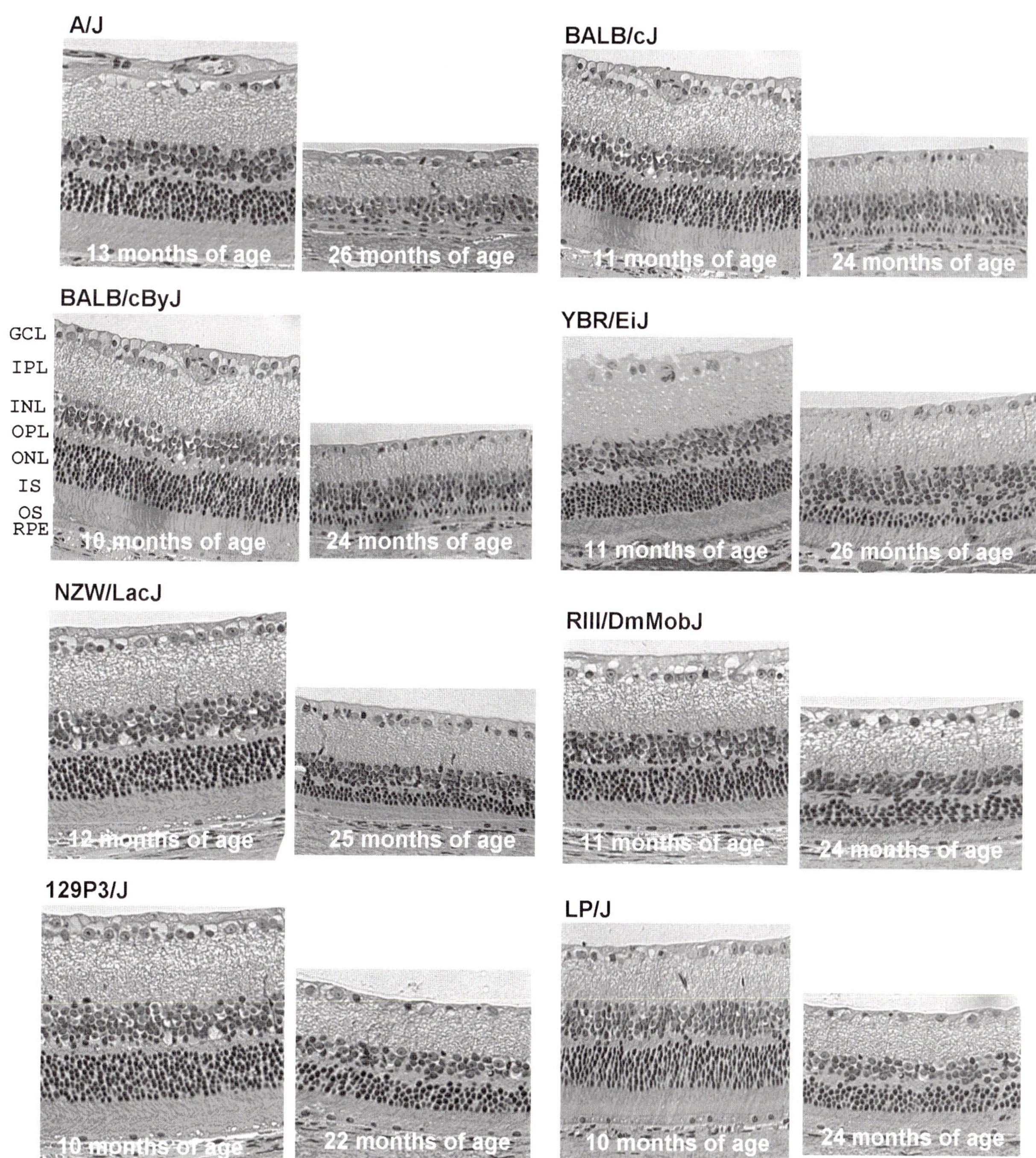

Figure 48.2 Retinal histological sections in eight laboratory ARRD strains showing relatively normal retinal structure at relatively younger ages and retinal degeneration at older ages. The strain names are labeled at the top and the ages are labeled within each retinal section. GCL, ganglion cell layer; INL, inner nuclear layer; IPL, inner plexiform layer; IS, photoreceptor inner segments; ONL, outer nuclear layer; OPL, outer plexiform layer; OS, photoreceptor outer segments; RPE, retinal pigment epithelial cells.

BALB/cJ and C57BL/6J mice, a sequence variation in the *Rpe65* gene cosegregated with the low LDS of C57BL/6J mice (Danciger et al., 2000). We have typed the six albino strains of mice with ARRD identified in our screening study for sequence variation in the *Rpe65* gene and found that two of them (RIII/DmMobJ and NZW/LacJ) have the same *Rpe65* genotype as C57BL/6J. The other four carry the susceptibility allele.

Cataracts in human and mouse eyes

Early in life the lens is transparent, and incoming light encounters no difficulty in its passage through the eye. With aging, the lens becomes less clear, incoming light is scattered to an increasing degree, and, if loss of lens clarity is severe enough, vision is affected. When clouding of the lens impairs vision, a clinically significant cataract is present. More than half of Americans over age 65 have a cataract (Jacques et al., 1997). Cataracts account for 42% of all vision loss, making the disorder the leading cause of blindness worldwide (National Eye Institute report, *Vision Research: A National Plan: 1999–2003*). Based on our preliminary studies, age-related cataracts are also very common in mice. At TJL, when we screened aged mice from 35 strains for models of human age-related ocular diseases, we identified 21 strains with a high incidence of late-onset cataracts. Onset ranged from 8 to 22 months, and 14 strains of mice had clear lenses throughout their lives (see table 48.2).

There is increasing epidemiological evidence that age-related cataracts are a multifactorial disease, with environmental and genetic components interacting (West and Valmadrid, 1995). Epidemiological studies also suggest a major inherited genetic component in the etiology of both anterior cortical and nuclear cataracts (Heiba et al., 1993, 1995), and twin studies suggest that 50% of age-related cataracts can be accounted for by inheritance (Hammond et al., 2000). Inheritance is already known to be the major contributor to congenital cataract occurring in childhood, and several mutated genes causing human congenital cataracts have already been identified (Francis et al., 2000).

Because cataracts are easily detected by external clinical examination, the number of described mouse cataract models has grown rapidly. A 1982 review listed 18 spontaneous and induced mutations that cause cataracts as part of the resulting phenotype (Foster et al., 1982). By 1997 the number had grown to 46 (Smith et al., 1997). Research by our group at TJL has identified the spontaneous mutation *lop18* in the mouse *Cryaa* (α-crystallin) gene (Chang et al., 1999), the spontaneous mutation *Lop12* in the *Crygd* (γD-crystallin) gene (Smith et al., 2000), and the spontaneous mutation *Lop10* in the *Gja8* (connexin 50) gene (Chang et al., 2002). Currently, human mutations have been identified in the genes encoding some lens-specific crystallins, connexins, aquaporin, and beaded filament protein, BFSP2 (Sheils et al., 1998; Heon et al., 1999; Mackay et al., 1999; Berry et al., 2000; Jakobs et al., 2000; Rees et al., 2000). In most cases the genetic mutations causing cataracts have been identified using a candidate gene approach once the chromosomal location of the mutation has been determined. It has been estimated that there might be as many as 40 genes contributing to congenital cataracts in the mouse, and it would be reasonable to assume a similar number in humans (Hejtmancik and Kantorow, 2004). Thus, the concept of genetic mechanisms causing early-onset cataracts is well established, but to date, very little is known concerning the identity of genes that, either alone or together with environmental factors, confer susceptibility to age-related cataracts.

Discovery of Age-Related Cataracts in Mouse In our search for late-onset ocular diseases in mice, we have found that the majority of eye diseases occur in aged mice, just as they do in humans. In the study described earlier in which we evaluated aged mice of 35 selected, genetically diverse inbred strains at greater than 2 years of age for age-related eye disorders, we also screened for lens opacity. As part of this program, we have found seven strains of mice with lens opacity starting at eight months of age (RIII/DmMobJ, CBA/CaJ, CASA/RkJ, CAST/EiJ, LEWES/EiJ, PERA/EiJ, TIRANO/EiJ), eight strains of mice with cataract starting at 14 months of age (C57BL/6J, C57BR/cdJ, AU/SsJ, CZECHII/EiJ, MOLC/RkJ, MOLD/RkJ, PERC/EiJ, SKIVE/EiJ), and six strains of mice with a mild lens opacity starting at 22 months of age (DBA/1J, LP/J, CE/J, PANCEVO/EiJ, SPRET/EiJ, WSB/EiJ). Mice of another 14 strains have clear lenses throughout their lives (see table 48.2).

Summary

Because the 35 strains of mice in our age-related vision loss study were all inbred, the individuals in a strain are genetically identical (like monozygotic twins), and all mice were maintained in the same standard environment, our findings demonstrate that genetic mechanisms contribute to the etiology and pathogenesis of ARRD and cataracts. No matter what the mode of inheritance or number of genes involved, the strains themselves provide reproducible models for research on similar human eye disorders.

acknowledgments Work was supported by the Foundation Fighting Blindness. I am grateful to Norm Hawes, Ron Hurd, Jieping Wang, Muriel Davisson, Tom Roderick, and John Heckenlively for their excellent help on the mouse aging project, and Melissa Berry for her critical reading of the manuscript.

REFERENCES

Banerjee, P., Kleyn, P. W., Knowles, J. A., Lewis, C. A., Ross, B. M., Parano, E., Kovats, S. G., Lee, J. J., Penchaszadeh, G. K., et al. (1998). TULP1 mutation in two extended Dominican kindreds with autosomal recessive retinitis pigmentosa. *Nat. Genet.* 18:177–179.

Berry, V., Francis, P., Haushal, S., Moore, A., and Bhattacharya, S. (2000). Missense mutations in MIP underlie autosomal dominant "polymorphic" and lamellar cataracts linked to 12q. *Nat. Genet.* 25:15–17.

[No Author] (2004). Blindness and visual impairment: A public health issue for the future as well as today (editorial). *Arch. Ophthalmol.* 122:451–452.

Bowes, C., Li, T., Danciger, M., Baxter, L. C., Applebury, M. L., and Farber, D. B. (1990). Retinal degeneration in the rd mouse is caused by a defect in the beta subunit of rod cGMP-phosphodiesterase. *Nature* 347:677–680.

Chang, B., Hawes, N. L., Hurd, R. E., Wang, J., Howell, D., Davisson, M. T., Roderick, T. H., Nusinowitz, S., and Heckenlively, J. R. (2005). Mouse models of ocular diseases. *Vis. Neurosci.* 22:587–593.

Chang, B., Hawes, N. L., Roderick, T. H., Smith, R. S., Heckenlively, J. R., Horwitz, J., and Davisson, M. T. (1999). Identification of a missense mutation in the A-crystallin gene in the lop18 mouse. *Mol. Vis.* 5:21.

Chang, B., Wang, X., Hawes, N. L., Ojakian, R., Davisson, M. T., Lo, W., and Gong, X. (2002). A Gja8 (Cx50) point mutation causes an alteration of alpha 3 connexin (Cx46) in semi-dominant cataracts of *Lop10* mice. *Hum. Mol. Genet.* 11:507–513.

Congdon, N., O'Colmain, B., Klaver, C. C., Klein, R., Munoz, B., Friedman, D. S., Kempen, J., Taylor, H. R., and Mitchell, P, for the Eye Diseases Prevalence Research Group. (2004). Causes and prevalence of visual impairment among adults in the United States. *Arch. Ophthalmol.* 122:477–485.

Danciger, M., Matthes, M. T., Yasamura, D., Akhmedov, N. B., Rickabaugh, T., Gentleman, S., Redmond, T. M., LaVail, M. M., and Farber, D. B. (2000). A QTL on distal chromosome 3 that influences the severity of light-induced damage to mouse photoreceptors. *Mamm. Genome* 11:422–427.

Davisson, M. T., Lalley, P. A., Peters, J., Doolittle, D. P., Hillyard, A. L., and Searle, A. G. (1991). Report of the Comparative Subcommittee for Human, Mouse, and Other Rodents (HGM11). *Cytogenet. Cell Genet.* 58:1152–1159.

Edwards, A. O., Ritter, R., III, Abel, K. J., Manning, A., Panhuysen, C., and Farrer, L. A. (2005). Complement factor H polymorphism and age-related macular degeneration. *Science* 308:421–424.

Foster, H. L., Small, J. D., and Fox, J. G. (Eds.). (1982). *The mouse in biomedical research.* New York: Academic Press.

Francis, P. J., Berry, V., Bhattachaya, S. S., and Moore, A. T. (2000). The genetics of childhood cataract. *J. Med. Genet.* 37: 481–488.

Gibson, F., Walsh, J., Mburu, P., Varela, A., Brown, K. A., Antonio, M., Beisel, K. W., Steel, K. P., and Brown, S. D. (1995). A type VII myosin encoded by the mouse deafness gene *shaker*-1. *Nature* 374:62–64.

Hageman, G. S., Anderson, D. H., Johnson, L. V., Hancox, L. S., Taiber, A. J., Hardisty, L. I., Hageman, J. L., Stockman, H. A., Borchardt, J. D., et al. (2005). A common haplotype in the complement regulatory gene factor H (HF1/CFH) predisposes individuals to age-related macular degeneration. *Proc. Natl. Acad. Sci. U.S.A.* 102:7227–7232.

Hagstrom, S. A., North, M. A., Nishina, P. L., Berson, E. L., and Dryja, T. P. (1998). Recessive mutations in the gene encoding the tubby-like protein TULP1 in patients with retinitis pigmentosa. *Nat. Genet.* 18:174–176.

Haines, J. L., Hauser, M. A., Schmidt, S., Scott, W. K., Olson, L. M., Gallins, P., Spencer, K. L., Kwan, S. Y., Noureddine, M., et al. (2005). Complement factor H variant increases the risk of age-related macular degeneration. *Science* 308:419–421.

Hammond, G. J., Sneider, H., Spector, T. D., and Gilbert, G. E. (2000). Genetic and environmental factors in age-related nuclear cataracts in monozygotic and dizygotic twins. *N. Engl. J. Med.* 342:1786–1790.

Heiba, I. M., Elston, R. C., Klein, B. E., and Klein, R. (1993). Genetic etiology of nuclear cataract: Evidence for a major gene. *Am. J. Med. Genet.* 47:1208–1214.

Heiba, I. M., Elston, R. C., Klein, B. E., and Klein, R. (1995). Evidence for a major gene for cortical cataract. *Invest. Ophthalmol. Vis. Sci.* 36:227–235.

Hejtmancik, J. F., and Kantorow, M. (2004). Molecular genetics of age-related cataract. *Exp. Eye Res.* 79(1):3–9.

Heon, E., Priston, M., Schorederet, D., Billingsley, G., Girard, P., Lubsen, N., and Munier, F. L. (1999). The gamma crystallins and human cataracts: A puzzle made clearer. *Am. J. Hum. Genet.* 65:1261–1267.

Jacques, P. F., Taylor, A., Hankinson, S. E., Willett, W. C., Mahnken, B., Lee, Y., Vaid, K., and Lahav, M. (1997). Long-term vitamin C supplement use and prevalence of early age-related lens opacities. *Am. J. Clin. Nutr.* 66:911–916.

Jakobs, P. M., Hess, J. F., Fitzgerald, P. G., Kramer, P., Weleber, R. G., and Litt, M. (2000). Autosomal dominant congenital cataract associated with a deletion mutation in the human beaded filament protein gene BFSP2. *Am. J. Hum. Genet.* 66: 1432–1436.

Karan, G., Lillo, C., Yang, Z., Cameron, D. J., Locke, K. G., Zhao, Y., Thirumalaichary, S., Li, C., Birch, D. G., et al. (2005). Lipofuscin accumulation, abnormal electrophysiology and photoreceptor degeneration in mutant ELOVL4 transgenic mice: A model for macular degeneration. *Proc. Natl. Acad. Sci. U.S.A.* 102:4164–4169.

Keen, T. J., and Inglehearn, C. F. (1996). Mutations and polymorphisms in the human peripherin-RDS gene and their involvement in inherited retinal degeneration. *Hum. Mutat.* 8: 297–303.

Klein, R. J., Zeiss, C., Chew, E. Y., Tsai, J. Y., Sackler, R. S., Haynes, C., Henning, A. K., San Giovanni, J. P., Mane, S. M., et al. (2005). Complement factor H polymorphism in age-related macular degeneration. *Science* 308:385–389.

LaVail, M. M., Gorrin, G. M., and Repaci, M. A. (1987). Genetic regulation of light damage to photoreceptors. *Invest. Ophthalmol. Vis. Sci.* 28:1043–1048.

Mackay, D., Ionides, A., Kibar, Z., Rouleau, G., Berry, V., Moore, A., Shiels, A., and Bhattacharya, S. (1999). Connexin46 mutations in autosomal dominant congenital cataract. *Am. J. Hum. Genet.* 64:1357–1364.

Mandal, M. N., and Ayyagari, R. (2006). Complement factor H: Spatial and temporal expression and localization in the eye. *Invest. Ophthalmol. Vis. Sci.* 47:4091–4097.

Mata, N. L., Tzekov, R. T., Liu, X., Weng, J., Birch, D. G., and Travis, G. H. (2001). Delayed dark-adaptation and lipofuscin accumulation in abcr +/− mice: Implications for involvement of ABCR in age-related macular degeneration. *Invest. Ophthalmol. Vis. Sci.* 42:1685–1690.

Mata, N. L., Weng, J., and Travis, G. H. (2000). Biosynthesis of a major lipofuscin fluorophore in mice and humans with abcr-mediated retinal and macular degeneration. *Proc. Natl. Acad. Sci. U.S.A.* 97:7154–7159.

McLaughlin, M. E., Sandberg, M. A., Berson, E. L., and Dryja, T. P. (1993). Recessive mutations in the gene encoding the beta-subunit of rod phosphodiesterase in patients with retinitis pigmentosa. *Nat. Genet.* 4:130–134.

Nadeau, J. H., Davisson, M. T., Doolittle, D. P., Grant, P., Hillyard, A. L., Kosowsky, M. R., and Roderick, T. H. (1992). Comparative map for mice and human. *Mamm. Genome* 3:480–536.

Noben-Trauth, K., Naggert, J. K., North, M. A., and Nishina, P. M. (1996). A candidate gene for the mouse mutation tubby. *Nature* 380:534–538.

Quiring, R., Walldor, U., Kloter, U., and Gehring, W. J. (1994). Homology of the eyeless gene of *Drosophila* to the small eye gene in mice and aniridia in human. *Science* 265:765–769.

Radu, R. A., Mata, N. L., Bagla, A., and Travis, G. H. (2004). Light exposure stimulates formation of A2E oxiranes in a mouse model of Stargardt's macular degeneration. *Proc. Natl. Acad. Sci. U.S.A.* 101:5928–5933.

Rees, M. I., Watts, P., Fenton, I., Clarke, A., Snell, R. G., Owen, M. J., and Gray, J. (2000). Further evidence of autosomal dominant congenital zonular pulverulent cataracts linked to 13q11 (CZP3) and a novel mutation in connexin 46 (GJA-3). *Hum. Genet.* 106:206–209.

Rodriguez de Cordoba, S., Esparza-Gordillo, J., Goicoechea de Jorge, E., Lopez-Trascasa, M., and Sanchez-Corral, P. (2004). The human complement factor H: Functional roles, genetic variations and disease associations. *Mol. Immunol.* 41: 355–367.

Rome, C. E., Grimm, C., Hafezi, F., Marti, A., and Wenzel, A. (1998). Apoptotic cell death in retinal degenerations. *Prog. Retin Eye Res.* 17:443–464.

Sheils, A., Mackay, D., Ionides, A., Berry, V., Moore, A., and Bhattacharya, S. (1998). A missense mutation in the human connexin 50 gene underlies autosomal dominant "zonular pulverulent" cataract, on chromosome 1q. *Am. J. Hum. Genet.* 62:526–532.

Smith, R. S., Hawes, N. L., Chang, B., Roderick, T. H., Akeson, E. C., Heckenlively, J. R., Gong, X., Wang, X., and Davisson, M. T. (2000). Lop12, a new mouse mutation causing lens opacity similar to human Coppock cataract. *Genomics* 63:314–320.

Smith, R. S., Sundberg, J. P., and Linder, C. C. (1997). Mouse mutations as models for studying cataracts. *Pathobiology* 65: 146–154.

Travis, G. H., Brennan, M. B., Danielson, P. E., Kozak, C. A., and Sutcliffe, J. G. (1989). Identification of a photoreceptor-specific mRNA encoded by the gene responsible for retinal degeneration slow (rds). *Nature* 338:70–73.

Vasireddy, V., Jablonski, M. M., Mandal, M. N., Raz-Prag, D., Wang, X. F., Nizol, L., Iannaccone, A., Musch, D. C., et al. (2006). Elovl4 5-bp-deletion knock-in mice develop progressive photoreceptor degeneration. *Invest. Ophthalmol. Vis. Sci.* 47:4558–4568.

Weil, D., Blanchard, S., Kaplan, J., Guilford, P., Gibson, F., Walsh, J., Mburu, P., Varela, A., Levilliers, J., et al. (1995). Defective myosin VIIA gene responsible for Usher syndrome type 1B. *Nature* 374:60–61.

Weng, J., Mata, N. L., Azarian, S. M., Tzekov, R. T., Birch, D. G., and Travis, G. H. (1999). Insights into the function of rimprotein in photoreceptors and etilogy of Stargardt's disease from the phenotype in abcr knockout mice. *Cell* 98:13–23.

West, S. K., and Valmadrid, C. T. (1995). Epidemiology of risk factors for age-related cataract. *Surv. Ophthalmol.* 39:323–334.

Zareparsi, S., Branham, K. E., Li, M., Shah, S., Klein, R. J., Ott, J., Hoh, J., Abecasis, G. R., and Swaroop, A. (2005). Strong association of the Y402H variant in complement factor H at 1q32 with susceptibility to age-related macular degeneration. *Am. J. Hum. Genet.* 77:149–153.

Zhang, K., Kniazeva, M., Han, M., Li, W., Yu, Z., Yang, Z., Li, Y., Metzker, M. L., Allikmets, R., et al. (2001). A 5-bp deletion in ELOVL4 is associated with two related forms of autosomal dominant macular dystrophy. *Nat. Genet.* 27:89–93.

VII ADVANCED GENOMIC TECHNOLOGIES: APPLICATIONS TO THE MOUSE VISUAL SYSTEM

49 New Genetic Technologies for Studying the Morphology, Physiology, and Development of Mouse Retinal Neurons

TUDOR C. BADEA AND JEREMY NATHANS

Despite its comparatively reduced visual abilities, the mouse is becoming one of the most important organisms for investigating the physiology, organization, and development of the mammalian visual system. This trend reflects the ease with which genetic manipulations can be performed in the whole animal, including manipulation of defined subsets of neurons. Mouse studies have made significant contributions to the three main and interrelated areas of vision research: the molecular mechanisms of neuronal function and development, circuits and information coding, and pathological mechanisms of disease. In each of these areas, the modern mouse geneticist's approach consists largely in introducing or removing various genetic elements and asking how neuronal or glial structure, function, or development has been modified.

This chapter surveys current genetic approaches used to visualize subpopulations of cells or to alter their function or development. The emphasis is on retinal neurons, although the experimental approaches we discuss apply equally to glia and to visual pathways beyond the retina. Rather than providing an exhaustive summary, we highlight examples that illustrate general principles.

Gene transfer and gene targeting methods

In some situations, it is feasible to directly deliver DNA or RNA to target cells in the living animal, for example by injecting them into the eye as recombinant viruses or by using electroporation (Matsuda and Cepko, 2004; Kachi et al., 2005; Bi et al., 2006). With these approaches the researcher can achieve a decrement in gene expression by RNA interference (RNAi), or the ectopic production of reporters, light-activated channels, or other proteins. This is especially attractive for animals in which germ-line manipulation is difficult or impossible or in which the eye is particularly accessible to injection. In addition, ex vivo experiments, in which isolated retinas are maintained in culture, allow gene delivery by the aforementioned approaches, as well as by particle-mediated gene transfer (the "gene gun") (Wellmann et al., 1999; Gan et al., 2000; O'Brien and Lummis, 2004). Individual neurons can also be labeled using particle-mediated transfer of lipophilic dyes (Sun et al., 2002; Pignatelli and Strettoi, 2004). Applications of somatic cell gene transfer technologies include visualizing cell lineages and neuronal morphology by expressing histochemical reporters (Price et al., 1987; Turner et al., 1990), and modifying or monitoring function, for example, by RNAi or expression of a fluorescent calcium indicator. In some cases of somatic cell gene transfer, gene expression can be limited to a defined subset of neurons with a cell type–specific promoter. More commonly, the inefficient gene delivery process produces a sparse population of transduced cells, permitting the identities of individual cells to be determined later based on morphology and position, a strategy that was used in the retroviral marking of neuronal lineages (Turner et al., 1990). Because somatic cell gene transfer approaches are not specific to the mouse, they are not the focus of this review. However, they represent valuable alternatives to germ-line manipulation and can also be used in conjunction with the germ-line approaches discussed in this chapter.

Among techniques for altering the germ line, the insertion of transgenes (figure 49.1) is conceptually the simplest. Classically, this has involved the random insertion of relatively small constructs in which promoters with more or less restricted expression patterns control reporter genes (such as *E. coli* β-galactosidase; human placental alkaline phosphatase [PLAP], or fluorescent proteins such as green fluorescent protein [GFP]), genetic modulators (such as Cre recombinase or the ligand-controlled reverse tetracycline transactivator [rtTA]), or, more recently, modulators of physiological function (such as drug- or light-activated ion channels). Reporter genes are usually enzymes with

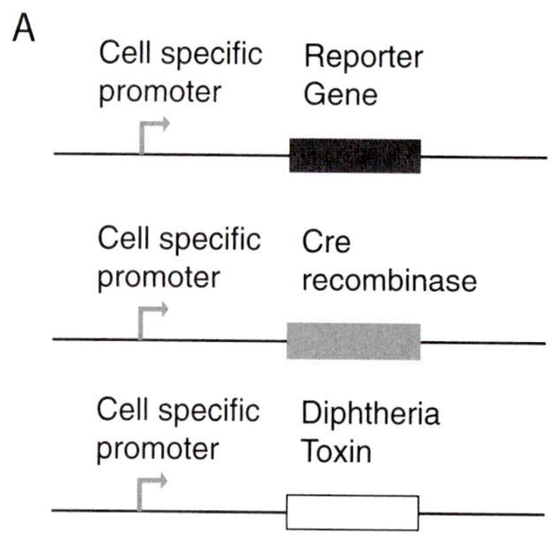

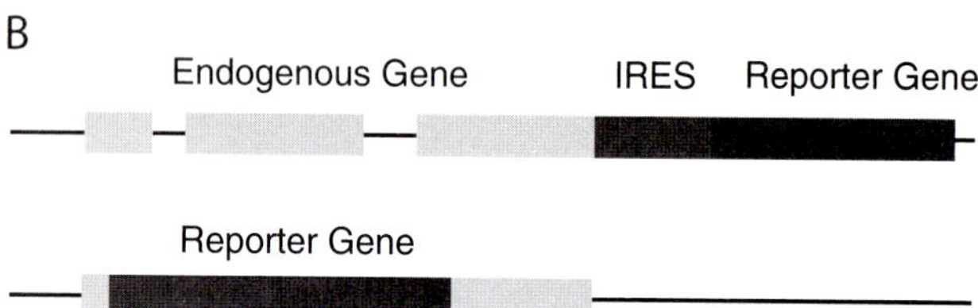

FIGURE 49.1 Transgenic approaches. Transgenic constructs are stably inherited genetic elements that integrate at random chromosomal locations and with a variable number of copies at the site of integration. *A*, Typical transgenes are composed of promoter elements that can direct transcription in more or less restricted cell populations and various cDNAs encoding reporter genes (such as PLAP or GFP), genetic regulators (represented here by the Cre recombinase), or other functional effectors (represented here by the α subunit of diphtheria toxin, which ablates the cell in which it is expressed). *B*, Bacterial artificial chromosome (BAC) transgenes are also randomly integrated in the genome; however, they carry larger segments of DNA and often reproduce more faithfully the expression pattern of the endogenous gene. The desired genetic elements can be placed under the control of the transgene by means of an internal ribosomal entry site (IRES) as a second translation unit (*top*), or they can replace the transgene coding region (*bottom*).

well-established histochemical stains, such as β-galactosidase or PLAP, or fluorescent proteins such as GFP. Transgene constructs are injected into the pronuclei of fertilized eggs and the resulting founders are screened by polymerase chain reaction (PCR) or Southern blotting for the presence of the transgene (Hogan et al., 1986). These founders will transmit the stably integrated transgene through the germ line to their offspring, which can then be analyzed to determine the pattern of transgene expression. In general, only a fraction of the lines express the injected transgene, and the expression pattern may vary substantially from line to line. In addition, transgene expression patterns are often variegated (i.e., expressed in only a subset of the expected cells), an effect that appears to reflect the chromatin structure at the site of integration. Finally, many transgenes are expressed in subsets of cells distinct from the ones in which the promoter segment used to drive expression is normally active (Xiang et al., 1996). In some situations, variegation or misexpression has proved useful, as described later in the chapter.

The utility of the classic transgenic approach depends on the availability of promoter segments that can drive expression in defined subsets of neurons. So far, this has been the case in only a few instances, most notably in primary sensory neurons that express receptor proteins in a cell type–specific manner. In the mouse retina, rhodopsin is produced in rod photoreceptors, short-wavelength-sensitive (S) photopigment is produced in S cones, middle-wavelength-sensitive (M) photopigment is produced in M cones, and melanopsin is produced in a special class of light-responsive retinal ganglion cells (RGCs). Even in this relatively simple system, however, there is an imperfect correlation between cell type and molecular marker: in mice and other rodents, some cones coexpress both S and M photopigment genes (Rohlich et al., 1994; Applebury et al., 2000). A second route to cell type–specific promoters for transgene expression in the retina is through the use of genes that are expressed by many neuronal populations elsewhere in the CNS but are restricted in the retina to one or a few cell types. Two examples are the genes encoding choline acetyltransferase and tyrosine hydroxylase, which are expressed in starburst and dopaminergic amacrine cells, respectively (Tauchi and Masland, 1984; Gustincich et al., 1997). Many other promoters are available for broad classes of neurons; for example, the Crx promoter is expressed in all photoreceptors (Furukawa et al., 2002).

Bacterial artificial chromosome (BAC) transgenesis (figure 49.1*B*) represents a variant strategy in which a large chromosomal fragment containing the gene of interest is typically engineered to direct the expression of a foreign protein (Heintz, 2001). The rationale for this strategy is that a large (100–200 kb) fragment, often containing the entire gene of interest, will more faithfully reproduce the endogenous expression pattern than a small promoter fragment, and will therefore direct reporter expression more precisely to that cell population. In some instances in which a transgene is normally expressed in multiple cell types or at multiple stages of development, it is desirable to activate the transgene in a subset of these cells or only during a limited temporal window. This can be achieved by using conditional expression systems, which are discussed at the end of the chapter.

The second major class of germ-line genetic manipulation involves targeted alterations using embryonic stem (ES) cells. This typically involves reporter insertion (knock-in), target gene deletion (knockout), or a combination of the two (figure 49.2). Briefly, in this approach, the construct of interest is introduced into ES cells, where it recombines with the target locus by homologous recombination. The potentially difficult steps are (1) construction of the targeting plasmid, (2) screening for the correct homologous recombination event among many ES clones, and (3) the subsequent generation

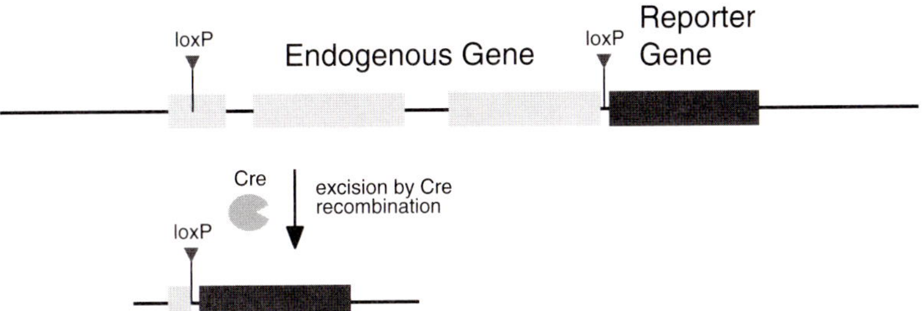

Figure 49.2 Knock-in and knockout strategies. In the example shown here, the endogenous exons of the target gene are flanked by loxP sites, and the endogenous transcription unit is followed by a reporter gene that is transcriptionally silent prior to Cre-mediated recombination. Recombination induced by Cre deletes the endogenous gene's exons and thereby allows the expression of the reporter gene under the same 5′ transcriptional regulatory elements as the endogenous gene. We note here that any regulatory elements located within introns would be deleted. This technique can be used to guide functional and morphological analyses of the cells that normally express the target gene. These cells can be studied in the heterozygous or homozygous mutant state, depending on whether the other allele of the gene is wild type or mutant (assuming that the gene is autosomal).

of the mutant mouse by injection of ES lines into early embryos. However, the advantages are substantial. Knock-in lines generally exhibit less variegation and more faithful patterns of reporter gene expression than transgenic lines, the dosage of the modified gene is well defined, and the line-to-line variability in expression that is seen in transgenic lines (reflecting the different locations and copy numbers of the transgene) is eliminated. As a result of this last characteristic, the number of lines to be screened is substantially reduced.

Targeted gene manipulations are increasingly being used in combination with site-specific DNA rearrangement catalyzed by sequence-specific Cre or Flp recombinases (Branda and Dymecki, 2004), which can be expressed (from a second locus) in defined subsets of cells and, in the case of the CreER(T) fusion protein, can also be controlled pharmacologically. This approach has been used to circumvent problems of lethality or other severe phenotypes associated with the ubiquitous loss of gene function that in many cases is observed with the standard knockout allele. With the availability of new mouse lines that express the recombinases under cell type–specific control, this approach is increasingly being used to produce changes in gene function in defined subsets of cells and to map the cell types and time windows in which a particular gene acts.

In the following sections we describe specific examples of these approaches as they have been applied to different retinal cell types. At the end of the chapter we discuss techniques for temporal control of gene expression.

Photoreceptors

Promoter sequences of bovine (Zack et al., 1991), human (Wang et al., 1992; Chen et al., 1994; Chiu and Nathans, 1994a), and murine (Chiu and Nathans, 1994b) photopigment genes have been used to drive expression of β-galactosidase or PLAP reporters in transgenic mice. These experiments showed that photopigment promoter transgenes from various mammals generally recapitulate the expression patterns of the corresponding endogenous genes. However, the expression of these transgenes exhibits substantial variegation, and, in the case of the human S cone photopigment promoter, misexpression was also observed in a subset of cone bipolar cells (Chen et al., 1994; Chiu and Nathans, 1994a). Interestingly, the human long-wavelength (L) pigment promoter and 5′ enhancer drives transgene expression in both M and S cones in the mouse (Wang et al., 1992). With larger photopigment promoter segments, expression is generally observed in a larger fraction of the expected target cells (Zack et al., 1991). For example, transgenic constructs carrying 11 kb of the mouse rhodopsin locus, including 4.5 kb of 5′ flanking sequences and all of the introns and exons, efficiently express rhodopsin in rod photoreceptors, which facilitated the study of a rhodopsin mutant responsible for retinitis pigmentosa (Sung et al., 1994).

One of the most informative genetic approaches is the targeted ablation of a specific cell type to assess its role in the circuitry of the system. Soucy et al. (1998) used this strategy to assess the role of cones in the scotopic (dim light) visual pathway. Prior studies had shown that rods transmit their signals via metabotropic glutamate receptors on rod bipolar cells, all of which are of the ON type; these bipolar cells then synapse onto AII amacrine cells in the innermost division of the inner plexiform layer (IPL). The AII amacrine cells in turn feed the rod signals into the cone pathway by means of gap junctions with ON cone bipolar cells and by sign-inverting glycinergic synapses with OFF cone bipolar cells. From this circuitry, it would be predicted that the glutamate analogue L-(+)-2-amino-4-phosphonobutyric acid (APB), which selectively activates metabotropic glutamate receptors, and therefore blocks both rod-to-rod bipolar and cone-to-ON-cone bipolar synaptic signals, should inhibit both ON and OFF responses of RGCs under scotopic conditions. However, Soucy and colleagues observed that applying APB to the retina ex vivo effectively abolished only ON responses under scotopic conditions; OFF responses remained largely intact. Soucy and colleagues also observed that strychnine, which blocks glycinergic signaling from AII amacrine cells to OFF cone bipolar cells, failed to inhibit the scotopic OFF RGC response. A second, APB-resistant pathway involving electrical coupling between rods and cones had previously been identified in the rabbit retina and could, in theory, have accounted for these data (DeVries and Baylor, 1995). To address this possibility, a human red pigment gene promoter was used to drive the expression of the α subunit of diphtheria toxin in cones, but not in rods or other cell types (Soucy et al., 1998). This transgene selectively eliminates nearly all cones, leaving only a few survivors in the inferior retina. Not surprisingly, retinas prepared from these animals failed to respond to light stimuli in the photopic (high light level) range. Under scotopic conditions, the RGC responses were nearly normal, as assayed by multielectrode array recordings. Interestingly, the scotopic APB-resistant OFF pathway responses were comparable to those in wild-type mice, indicating that, under these experimental conditions, cones are not required for the transmission of rod signals to OFF RGCs. These data implicated a third and previously unknown pathway leading from rod photoreceptors to OFF RGCs, which has since been characterized as a direct synaptic contact between rods and OFF cone bipolar cells (Hack et al., 1999; Tsukamoto et al., 2001; Fyk-Kolodziej et al., 2003; Li et al., 2004).

Bipolar cells

The role of gap junctions in the bipolar-AII amacrine cell circuit has been investigated with the use of transgenic and knockout/knock-in mice. Connexins are the building blocks of gap junctions, providing a direct electrical connection between neurons. In the mouse retina, connexin 36 and connexin 45 are expressed in distinct subsets of neurons. For example, an ON cone bipolar cell type specifically labeled by GFP in the BPGus-GFP transgenic mouse line expresses connexin 36 but not connexin 45 (Han and Massey, 2005; Lin and Masland, 2005). Replacing the open reading frame of the connexin 36 gene with a bicistronic gene encoding both PLAP and β-galactosidase revealed connexin 36 gene expression in photoreceptors, several classes of bipolar cells, and AII amacrine cells (Deans et al., 2001, 2002). In retinas from a connexin 36 knockout mouse, scotopic responses for both ON- and OFF-center RGCs were abolished, and there was a defect in gap junctional coupling between AII amacrine cells and cone bipolar cells. Although the RGC defect might well be a direct consequence of the AII amacrine-bipolar cell defect, connexin 36 is also expressed at other points within this circuit, such as the rod-to-cone gap junction, which might contribute to the phenotype (Deans et al., 2002; Völgyi et al., 2004). Conditionally knocking out connexin 36 in defined subsets of neurons should resolve this issue.

More recently, the role of connexin 45 has been investigated using a conditional knock-in strategy. Since a knockout of connexin 45 is embryonic lethal, a knock-in allele was constructed in which exon 3 (encompassing the entire open reading frame) was flanked by loxP sites and followed by the coding region for GFP (see figure 49.2 for an analogous knock-in strategy). After crossing in a Nestin-Cre transgene, which leads to Cre-mediated recombination principally in the CNS and is compatible with viability, several types of OFF and ON cone bipolar cells, but not rod bipolar cells, were seen to express this connexin gene, as judged by the localization of GFP. In addition, in the conditional mutant mouse, the electroretinogram (ERG) b-wave, which is thought to largely represent bipolar cell depolarization, was greatly reduced under scotopic but not photopic conditions, suggesting an involvement of connexin 45 in the pathway leading from rods to cone bipolar cells (Maxeiner et al., 2005; Schubert et al., 2005).

In the retina, expression of the metabotropic glutamate receptor mGluR6 is restricted to rod and ON cone bipolar cells. In mGluR6 knockout mice, the ERG b-wave is abolished, and visually evoked potentials in the superior colliculus are severely reduced. Nevertheless, the general architecture of the retina is preserved, and the mice can be trained to respond to light stimuli (Masu et al., 1995; Tagawa et al., 1999).

Signaling through mGluR6 appears to require the $G_{o\alpha}$ subunit of heterotrimeric G proteins, since the $G_{o\alpha}$ gene knockout phenocopies the mGluR6 phenotype in the retina (Dhingra et al., 2000, 2002). A 9.5 kb upstream region encompassing the promoter of the mGluR6 gene is sufficient to drive β-galactosidase expression in the correct cell types (Ueda et al., 1997). This information was used to construct the corresponding GFP line, and by imaging the GFP-expressing retinas ex vivo, Morgan et al. (2006) were able to observe the development of axonal and dendritic processes of bipolar cells and to show that they derive from basal and apical processes of the postmitotic precursor. This example nicely illustrates the utility of ex vivo imaging with a fluorescent reporter that is limited to one or a few cell types.

Several other useful genetic tools have been generated for the study of bipolar cells. A BAC transgenic line has been constructed in which the Pcp-2 gene (Purkinje cell protein-2, a protein/gene of unknown function, also known as L7) was modified to carry an internal ribosome entry site (IRES)-Cre coding region in the 3′ untranslated region, resulting in Cre expression specifically in rod bipolar cells (Zhang et al.,

2005). To trace synaptic connections and projection patterns, wheat germ agglutinin (WGA), a plant lectin known to be transported anterogradely along axons (Yoshihara et al., 1999), has been introduced as a transgene under the control of the L7 promoter, which drives expression in rod bipolar cells (Hanno et al., 2003). The level of WGA production is high enough to observe retrograde transsynaptic transport to photoreceptors, as well as anterograde transsynaptic transport of the protein to RGCs, revealing their axonal projections into the brain.

The intracellular concentrations of ions associated with signaling and membrane voltage changes can be visualized with subcellular spatial resolution using genetically encoded fluorescent reporters. Kuner and Augustine in 2000 reported that fluorescence resonance energy transfer (FRET) between cyan fluorescent protein (CFP) and yellow fluorescent protein (YFP) is dependent on chloride concentration. If a CFP-YFP fusion protein (Clomeleon) is excited with a wavelength suitable for CFP, the energy can be efficiently transferred to YFP, but the efficiency of energy transfer decreases with increasing chloride concentration. By expressing this construct in neurons one can monitor the opening of chloride channels such as GABA receptors. In one application of this technique, the Thy-1 promoter, which is discussed in detail in the next section, was used to drive the expression of transgenic Clomeleon in a diverse population of retinal neurons to study the ionic basis of ON versus OFF bipolar cell responses (Duebel et al., 2006). At the synapse between photoreceptors and bipolar cells, ON bipolar cells invert the polarity of the membrane potential (by using mGluRs) and OFF bipolar cells conserve the polarity (by using ionotropic glutamate receptors). It was previously inferred that ON and OFF bipolar cells have different dendrite:soma internal chloride (iCl) ratios. The YFP:CFP emission ratio of the transgenic Clomeleon showed that ON bipolar neurons have a high iCl in their dendrites, and therefore the opening of chloride channels (following GABA release from horizontal cells) leads to an outward chloride flux and membrane depolarization. By contrast, OFF bipolar cells have a low dendritic iCl concentration and respond to chloride channel opening with chloride influx and membrane hyperpolarization. By this simple mechanism, GABA release from horizontal cells produces receptive field antagonism in both the ON and OFF channels.

In cone bipolar cells, the transgenic Clomeleon was used to measure iCl in various cell compartments at resting membrane potential. Even though the iCl at the resting potential varies among different cells, the dendritic iCl was consistently higher and the axonal (i.e., output) arbor iCl was consistently lower than that of the soma. Moreover, two morphologically distinct bipolar cell types, type 7 and type 9, had distinct dendrite:soma iCl ratios, with type 9 having significantly higher dendritic iCl. Application of GABA to these two cell types had different effects, inducing chloride influx in type 7 and efflux in type 9 cells. Interestingly, one of the Thy-1–Clomeleon lines expresses the transgene in a bipolar cell subpopulation in which the dendritic arbors exclusively contact S cones (Haverkamp et al., 2005).

Amacrine cells

As noted earlier in this chapter, transgene expression patterns can vary considerably among different mouse lines carrying the same construct, depending on the location of transgene integration. Although this is not always a desirable characteristic, sometimes the "wrong" expression pattern turns out to be useful. As an example, expression of a β-galactosidase transgene driven by the vasoactive intestinal peptide (VIP) promoter was observed in a subpopulation of amacrine cells that do not normally express VIP (Nirenberg and Meister, 1997). Since these cells appeared quite uniform with respect to their distribution across the retina and dendritic arborization, they were considered to be members of one specific amacrine cell class, V-amacrine cells. The V-amacrine cells were photoablated with approximately 95% efficiency by incubating with the cell-permeant β-galactosidase substrate fluorescein-D-galactopyranoside, followed by intense illumination in the presence of aminoethyl carbazole (Nirenberg and Cepko, 1993). Multielectrode array recordings revealed a significant increase in response latency and response duration in ON-transient RGCs in the photoablated retinas (Nirenberg and Meister, 1997). Immunohistochemical characterization indicated that V-amacrine cells are GABA-ergic, consistent with the observation that picrotoxin, a GABA receptor antagonist, has effects on response latency and duration that resemble the effects of photoablation. These data suggest that V-amacrine cells shape RGC responses via GABA release, although their exact place in the inner retinal circuitry remains to be elucidated.

A second subpopulation of amacrine cells that have been labeled genetically consists of dopaminergic amacrine cells. Gustincich et al. (1997) isolated a transgenic mouse line that expresses PLAP under the control of the tyrosine hydroxylase (TH) promoter in dopaminergic amacrine cells. Interestingly, PLAP expression was also observed in a second class of wide-field amacrine cells, with dendritic arbors stratifying in the middle of the IPL; the dendritic arbors of dopaminergic amacrine cells stratify only in the outermost strata of the IPL. After enzymatic dissociation of the transgenic retina, live dopaminergic amacrine cells were identified by staining with fluorescent anti-PLAP antibody (PLAP is a glyosyl phosphatidyl inositol [GPI]-anchored protein that accumulates on the extracellular face of the plasma membrane) and studied electrophysiologically. With this approach, Gustincich et al. showed that these cells fire spontaneous action potentials that are repressed by GABA. Moreover, by immunopurifying the PLAP-expressing neurons, it was possible to analyze their mRNAs and identify additional genes that may be involved in dopaminergic amacrine cell function (Gustincich et al., 2004). A similar transgenic approach has recently been used to generate a mouse line expressing Cre recombinase in dopaminergic neurons in the retina and brain (Gelman et al., 2003).

Ever since the original descriptions of cholinergic amacrine cells (also called starburst amacrine cells), there has been debate as to the physiological function of these cells (Hayden et al., 1980; Masland et al., 1984). Starburst amacrine cells have radially symmetrical dendritic arbors that stratify in either of two narrow zones within the IPL, they release GABA as well as acetylcholine, and they have a retinal coverage factor estimated to be between 10 and 70, depending on the species. Because of the unusual distribution of inputs and outputs and their costratification with the two arbors of direction-selective (DS) RGCs, starburst amacrine cells have long been thought to be involved in DS responses to moving stimuli. A variety of approaches have been taken to test this hypothesis. In one approach, calcium imaging of DS responses in the dendritic arbors of starburst amacrine cells showed that these arbors have highly asymmetrical responses to stimuli moving across the retina in different directions (Euler et al., 2002). A second approach used a genetic tagging technique to ablate starburst amacrine cells from the mouse retina and then determined the effect of this ablation on DS RGC responses (Yoshida et al., 2001). A human interleukin-2 receptor α subunit (hIL-2Rα)–GFP fusion protein was expressed as a transgene under the control of the mGluR2 promoter. One of the transgenic lines expressed hIL-2Rα–GFP only in starburst amacrine cells, a subset of the cells that express mGluR2. A monoclonal anti-hIL-2Rα antibody conjugated to a bacterial toxin was injected intraocularly in this transgenic line, resulting in an almost complete ablation of starburst amacrine cells. Concomitant with this ablation, there was an almost complete loss of DS RGC responses and an increase in the spiking rate of presumptive DS RGCs regardless of the direction of the stimulus. In addition, the optokinetic reflex was abolished, while pupillary constriction was preserved. This study demonstrated an essential role for starburst amacrine cells in the DS circuitry, and of DS RGC responses in the optokinetic reflex.

Conditional gene deletion has been used to define the role of cholinergic signaling by starburst amacrine cells in the spontaneous waves of activity that characterize the developing retina. Cre-mediated recombination can be induced throughout much of the retina by using a transgene expressing Cre under the control of an intronic enhancer from the *Pax6* gene (Pax6αCre) (Marquardt et al., 2001). This transgene is active in proliferating retinal precursors beginning at embryonic day E9.5, prior to the differentiation of all retinal cell types. Interestingly, the expression pattern of this transgene excludes a wedge-shaped domain in the center of the retina. Using the Pax6αCre line, it is possible to ablate any loxP-flanked gene in the retina while largely avoiding the deleterious effects of gene deletion in the rest of the embryo. To eliminate cholinergic signaling in the retina, the gene encoding choline acetyltransferase (ChAT), an enzyme required for the synthesis of acetylcholine, was deleted using the Pax6αCre line (Stacy et al., 2005). ChAT is expressed in all cholinergic neurons in the body, but in the retina it is expressed only by starburst amacrine cells. This elimination of retinal cholinergic signaling had little or no effect on retinal morphology but delayed by several days the appearance of the spontaneous waves of activity. It would be interesting to investigate the long-term effects of this manipulation on DS RGCs.

In the context of new genetic tools for visualizing neurons, special mention should be made of mouse lines carrying fluorescent proteins under the control of the Thy-1 promoter (Feng et al., 2000). Thy-1 is a GPI-anchored cell-surface protein of uncertain function that was originally identified on thymocytes (T cells) in both mice and humans. It was subsequently found in the retina, where it decorates the surface of all or nearly all RGCs. Feng and colleagues made the extremely useful observation that transgenic lines in which any of a variety of fluorescent reporters—GFP, CFP, YFP, RFP—are driven by a Thy-1 promoter typically show reporter expression in relatively small numbers of neurons, with different lines expressing the reporter in different neuronal subtypes. Each of these lines generally carries multiple transgene copies integrated at a single site, and, perhaps because of this high copy number, several of the lines produce readily detectable fluorescence in both large and small arbors in those retinal neurons that express the transgene. The sparse expression that is a characteristic of the Thy-1 transgenic lines is also important for tracing the full extent and ramification of individual arbors. In one application of this system, the GFP-M line has been used to visualize a variety of wide-field amacrine cells that would have been difficult to completely fill by tracer injection (Lin and Masland, 2006).

Retinal ganglion cells

RGCs are the projection neurons of the vertebrate retina. They have been a focus of intense interest for over a century not only because they encode and transmit all of the information captured by the eye but also because they offer an excellent system for studying axonal pathfinding and target selection by projection neurons (Hartline, 1938; Kuffler, 1953; Attardi and Sperry, 1963; Schnitzer and Meister, 2003). At the time of this writing, a literature search with the key words "retinal ganglion cell" and "mouse" yielded 178 papers, of which 140 were published in the past 10 years.

Although a majority of these studies focus on RGC development, the ability to discriminate individual RGCs using genetic techniques will likely lure an increasing number of physiologists and systems neuroscientists to ask their favorite questions in this system. Several classification systems for RGC cell types derived by genetic and nongenetic approaches have been published (Sun et al., 2002; Badea and Nathans, 2004; Kong et al., 2005; Coombs et al., 2006). Here we describe several genetic approaches that have proved useful in the study of RGCs.

It has been known for some time that ipsilateral RGC projections are diminished in albino mice (Guillery et al., 1973). To more precisely assess the role of melanin (or lack of melanin) in RGC axonal pathfinding, Cronin et al. (2001, 2003) adapted the components of the lac repressor-lac operator system, one of the best-studied prokaryotic gene regulatory systems, to generate an inducible gene expression system in the mouse. In *E. coli*, the lac repressor protein (lacI) binds to and inhibits transcription from promoter elements containing the lac operator. This transcriptional repression can be abolished by addition of isopropyl-thiogalactoside (IPTG), a synthetic lactose analogue that binds the repressor protein and decreases its affinity for the operator. Cronin and colleagues synthesized a DNA segment encoding the lacI gene (the natural *E. coli* sequence is extensively methylated and transcriptionally silenced when introduced in mammalian cells) and then created transgenic mice in which the synthetic lacI DNA (synlacI) is under the control of the chicken β-actin promoter, leading to its expression in many tissues and cell types. These transgenic mice were crossed to a line carrying a tyrosinase transgene with three lac operators inserted near the promoter. In the absence of the synlacI transgene, the tyrosinase transgene produces tyrosinase, and therefore induces coat and retinal pigmented epithelium melanin production (i.e., pigmentation) in an albino genetic background. In the presence of the synlacI transgene, coat color and eye pigmentation revert to the albino phenotype. However, if IPTG is administered in the food, the tyrosinase transgene is derepressed, resulting in pigmentation. Using this system, the authors were able to demonstrate that tyrosinase activity is required during an early time window when RGC axons are growing (Cronin et al., 2003).

The Thy-1-GFP-H line, similar to the M line mentioned earlier in the context of amacrine cell analysis, has also proved useful in the study of RGC morphology. In one study, RGC dendritic morphologies were quantified during the period surrounding eyelid opening, and the effect of dark rearing on the stratification of RGC dendritic arbors within the IPL was measured (Tian and Copenhagen, 2003). It was found that in P10 retinas (just before eye opening), about 50% of labeled RGCs were bistratified, and that under normal light exposure conditions this number decreased to 30% by P30. However, when animals were reared in the dark, the fraction of labeled RGCs that were bistratified was still around 50% at P30, indicating that light exposure plays a role in RGC stratification or differentiation. These data were further supported by multielectrode array recordings which showed a decrease in the number of ON-OFF RGCs between P10 and P30 under normal rearing conditions and the persistence of ON-OFF RGCs in dark-reared animals.

By crossing the Thy-1-GFP alleles with other transgenes expressing fluorescent proteins, one can begin to ask questions about the wiring of various cell types, such as bipolar cells and RGCs (Lin and Masland, 2005). Moreover, crossing these transgenes into various gene knockout backgrounds can provide insights into the development of the labeled cell types (Lin et al., 2004). We note that one potential challenge with a strategy of this type is that the promoter that drives the transgenic reporter may be under the control of the gene that is knocked out, in which case a change in transgene expression may reflect this regulatory relationship rather than a change in the fate of the labeled cell.

An especially useful reporter for the study of projection neurons is the τ-β-galactosidase fusion protein (tau-lacZ). Tau is a microtubule-associated protein, and as a result, tau-lacZ nicely labels axonal microtubules. The tau-lacZ reporter has been knocked into the genes encoding several transcription factors expressed in RGCs (Pak et al., 2004; Pratt et al., 2004; Quina et al., 2005), as well as the gene encoding melanopsin, a photopigment expressed in a subset of RGCs (Hattar et al., 2002). In melanopsin tau-lacZ knock-in mice, β-galactosidase accumulation has been used to catalogue the central targets for these RGCs (Hattar et al., 2006).

Genetic cell-labeling techniques have also made contributions to our understanding of RGC physiology. For example, reporters of intracellular calcium have been expressed in RGCs using the tetracycline-inducible system (Hasan et al., 2004; described in the next section), allowing real-time measurements of intracellular calcium in conjunction with the electrical activity of the cells. These genetically encoded fluorescent reporters should facilitate optical measurements across large cell populations.

Genetic systems for site-specific recombination and drug-controlled gene expression

The Cre-lox recombinase system has been noted at several points in the preceding sections. An application of the Cre-lox technology that was not previously discussed involves using site-specific recombination as an indelible marker of lineage. In one version of this lineage analysis, the Cre coding region is inserted into a gene that is expressed in the progenitors of a particular lineage, for example a gene encoding one of the basic helix-loop-helix (bHLH) transcription factors that are transiently expressed during neural development. By crossing in a reporter that is expressed only following Cre-mediated deletion of a loxP-flanked transcription termination signal, one can visualize all the progeny of the cells in which the bHLH gene was previously active (Zirlinger et al., 2002; Yang et al., 2003; Ma and Wang, 2006).

A somewhat more flexible version of this approach uses a Cre-recombinase that is fused to the ligand-binding domain of a mutated estrogen receptor (ER(T)) that recognizes the synthetic ligand 4-hydroxytamoxifen (4-HT) instead of the endogenous ligand estrogen (Feil et al., 1996; Brocard et al., 1997). The Cre-ER(T) fusion protein is sequestered in the cytosol in the absence of 4-HT; systemic or local administration of 4-HT releases the fusion protein, which then migrates to the nucleus and catalyzes site-specific recombination (figure 49.3*B*). By using CreER(T), the timing of the site-specific recombination event can be controlled to within 1 day at any time in the life of the mouse simply by administering 4-HT; for prenatal exposure, 4-HT is administered to the mother. The efficiency of this process depends on several factors: (1) the abundance of the CreER(T) fusion protein, (2) the availability of the target locus for recombination, which appears to be determined by local chromatin environment, (3) the amount of 4-HT delivered, and (4) the differentiation state of the target cell.

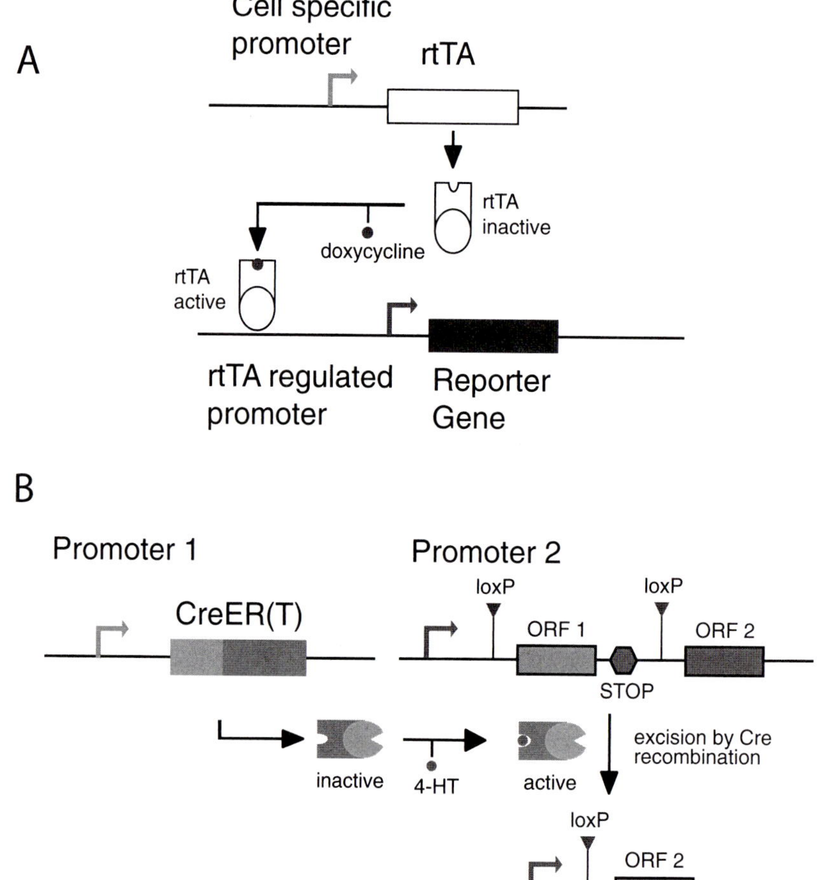

FIGURE 49.3 Pharmacological control of gene expression. Pharmacological approaches can be used to express genetic elements with improved spatial and temporal control or in a more restricted cell population. *A*, A transgene driven by a cell-specific promoter expresses rtTA, a doxycycline-sensitive transcriptional regulator. Unliganded rtTA is inactive but can be activated by the administration of doxycycline, causing it to bind to a specific DNA recognition site (tetO), and induce the transcription of a second genetic element. Thus, by generating one cell-specific transgene and crossing it to various rtTA-sensitive reporters, one can activate a reporter or a functional modulator of the target cells in a timed fashion, depending on doxycycline administration. *B*, A target locus (controlled by promoter 2) can be modified by the activity of a drug-sensitive Cre recombinase, CreER(T), expressed under the control of promoter 1. CreER(T) is produced in an inactive form and is activated by the administration of 4-HT (4-hydroxytamoxifen). The active recombinase then deletes open reading frame (ORF) 1, allowing ORF 2 to be transcribed under the control of promoter 2. This strategy can be used for conditional gene ablation, if the second locus is arranged as shown in figure 49.2, or for the conditional overexpression of reporter genes or other elements. Since the final pattern of ORF 2 expression is controlled by the spatial intersection of the expression patterns of promoters 1 and 2, as well as by 4-HT, this combinatorial strategy exhibits great flexibility for labeling and manipulating neuronal targets.

In an initial application of this method for lineage tracing, a CreER(T) line with ubiquitous expression was generated by knocking CreER(T) coding sequences into the ROSA26 locus (Zambrowicz et al., 1997; Badea et al., 2003). ROSA26 is a genetic locus identified by Soriano and colleagues during an insertional mutagenesis screen. The ROSA26 locus becomes transcriptionally active early in development, and transcription persists in all or nearly all cells in the body from that time on. Crossing the ROSA26-CreER(T) line to one that carries a ubiquitously expressed and Cre-activated PLAP (the Z/AP line constructed by Lobe et al., 1999) permits histochemical identification of those cells that have inherited a Cre-mediated recombination event (Badea et al., 2003). As expected, administering 4-HT at earlier or later developmental times generates, respectively, larger or smaller clones. Also as expected, the ROSA26-CreER(T);Z/AP combination generates labeled clones throughout the body at a density that depends on the 4-HT dose. Lineage tracing with ROSA26-CreER(T);Z/AP revealed the previously defined patterns of radial clones of retinal neurons (Price et al., 1987; Turner et al., 1990), and it also showed that retinal capillaries are composed of the intermingled progeny of a relatively small number of endothelial progenitors (Badea et al., 2003).

A second application of the CreER(T) technology is in the production of tissues with very low densities of genetically labeled neurons for morphological analysis. This approach has been used to generate a catalogue of all the major neuronal cell types in the retina by using ROSA26-CreER(T);Z/AP mice with both systemic and intraocular 4-HT injections (Badea and Nathans, 2004). The resulting set of labeled neurons has provided the raw material for a quantitative analysis of the patterns of stratification and dendritic arborization for all the major cell types. For example, in analyzing the arbors of polyaxonal amacrine cells, the data show that the lengths of individual dendrites can be comparable to the diameter of the retina, a finding also obtained with Thy-1 transgenic mice (Lin and Masland, 2006). The ROSA26-CreER(T);Z/AP labeling method has more recently been applied to the study of neuronal morphologies in various mutant retinas (Badea and Nathans, unpublished results).

Finally, we note that reversible drug control of gene expression, as described for synlacI/IPTG control of melanin production, is still a largely untapped technology for visual system studies. The rtTA is currently the system most widely used in both mammalian cell cultures and mice (Urlinger et al., 2000; Hasan et al., 2004; figure 49.3*A*). In this system, the tetracycline repressor (TetR), which in *E. coli* maintains the gene encoding the tetracycline efflux pump in a repressed state in the absence of tetracycline, has been engineered to bind rather than release its DNA target in the presence of tetracycline or related drugs, such as doxycycline (hence the adjective "reverse" in rtTA). The rtTA protein also carries a eukaryotic transcriptional activation domain, and therefore, when it binds to its DNA target (tetO), previously engineered into the gene of interest, transcription ensues. Coding sequences for rtTA, as well as for Cre, have recently been introduced into transgenic mice under the control of the Thy-1 promoter (Campsall et al., 2002; Kerrison et al., 2005).

Conclusion

We hope that the examples presented here make a convincing argument for using the mouse as a genetic model organism for the study of visual system function and development. However, the examples also illustrate the need to develop additional tools to target more refined subpopulations of neurons. We anticipate that combinations of gene expression cassettes with partially overlapping expression patterns—for example, one cell type–specific promoter controlling CreER(T) and a second cell type–specific promoter controlling a Cre-dependent reporter—will be developed in the near future to provide improved specificity by the intersection of their expression patterns. These and other advances should ultimately provide investigators with the ability to precisely control both cell type and temporal patterns of neuronal gene expression.

REFERENCES

Applebury, M. L., Antoch, M. P., Baxter, L. C., Chun, L. L., Falk, J. D., Farhangfar, F., Kage, K., Krzystolik, M. G., Lyass, L. A., et al. (2000). The murine cone photoreceptor: A single cone type expresses both S and M opsins with retinal spatial patterning. *Neuron* 27:513–523.

Attardi, D. G., and Sperry, R. W. (1963). Preferential selection of central pathways by regenerating optic fibers. *Exp. Neurol.* 7:46–64.

Badea, T. C., and Nathans, J. (2004). Quantitative analysis of neuronal morphologies in the mouse retina visualized by using a genetically directed reporter. *J. Comp. Neurol.* 480:331–351.

Badea, T. C., Wang, Y., and Nathans, J. (2003). A noninvasive genetic/pharmacologic strategy for visualizing cell morphology and clonal relationships in the mouse. *J. Neurosci.* 23:2314–2322.

Bi, A., Cui, J., Ma, Y. P., Olshevskaya, E., Pu, M., Dizhoor, A. M., and Pan, Z. H. (2006). Ectopic expression of a microbial-type rhodopsin restores visual responses in mice with photoreceptor degeneration. *Neuron* 50:23–33.

Branda, C. S., and Dymecki, S. M. (2004). Talking about a revolution: The impact of site-specific recombinases on genetic analyses in mice. *Dev. Cell* 6:7–28.

Brocard, J., Warot, X., Wendling, O., Messaddeq, N., Vonesch, J. L., Chambon, P., and Metzger, D. (1997). Spatio-temporally controlled site-specific somatic mutagenesis in the mouse. *Proc. Natl. Acad. Sci. U.S.A.* 94:14559–14563.

Campsall, K. D., Mazerolle, C. J., De Repentingy, Y., Kothary, R., and Wallace, V. A. (2002). Characterization of transgene expression and Cre recombinase activity in a panel of Thy-1 promoter-Cre transgenic mice. *Dev. Dyn.* 224:135–143.

Chen, J., Tucker, C. L., Woodford, B., Szel, A., Lem, J., Gianella-Borradori, A., Simon, M. I., and Bogenmann, E. (1994). The human blue opsin promoter directs transgene expression in short-wave cones and bipolar cells in the mouse retina. *Proc. Natl. Acad. Sci. U.S.A.* 91:2611–2615.

Chiu, M. I., and Nathans, J. (1994a). Blue cones and cone bipolar cells share transcriptional specificity as determined by expression of human blue visual pigment-derived transgenes. *J. Neurosci.* 14:3426–3436.

Chiu, M. I., and Nathans, J. (1994b). A sequence upstream of the mouse blue visual pigment gene directs blue cone-specific transgene expression in mouse retinas. *Vis. Neurosci.* 11:773–780.

Coombs, J., van der List, D., Wang, G. Y., and Chalupa, L. M. (2006). Morphological properties of mouse retinal ganglion cells. *Neuroscience* 140:123–136.

Cronin, C. A., Gluba, W., and Scrable, H. (2001). The lac operator-repressor system is functional in the mouse. *Genes Dev.* 15:1506–1517.

Cronin, C. A., Ryan, A. B., Talley, E. M., and Scrable, H. (2003). Tyrosinase expression during neuroblast divisions affects later pathfinding by retinal ganglion cells. *J. Neurosci.* 23: 11692–11697.

Deans, M. R., Gibson, J. R., Sellitto, C., Connors, B. W., and Paul, D. L. (2001). Synchronous activity of inhibitory networks in neocortex requires electrical synapses containing connexin 36. *Neuron* 31:477–485.

Deans, M. R., Volgyi, B., Goodenough, D. A., Bloomfield, S. A., and Paul, D. L. (2002). Connexin36 is essential for transmission of rod-mediated visual signals in the mammalian retina. *Neuron* 36:703–712.

DeVries, S. H., and Baylor, D. A. (1995). An alternative pathway for signal flow from rod photoreceptors to ganglion cells in mammalian retina. *Proc. Natl. Acad. Sci. U.S.A.* 92:10658–10662.

Dhingra, A., Jiang, M., Wang, T. L., Lyubarsky, A., Savchenko, A., Bar-Yehuda, T., Sterling, P., Birnbaumer, L., and Vardi, N. (2002). Light response of retinal ON bipolar cells requires a specific splice variant of $G\alpha_o$. *J. Neurosci.* 22:4878–4884.

Dhingra, A., Lyubarsky, A., Jiang, M., Pugh, E. N., Jr., Birnbaumer, L., Sterling, P., and Vardi, N. (2000). The light response of ON bipolar neurons requires $G\alpha_o$. *J. Neurosci.* 20:9053–9058.

Duebel, J., Haverkamp, S., Schleich, W., Feng, G., Augustine, G. J., Kuner, T., and Euler, T. (2006). Two-photon imaging reveals somatodendritic chloride gradient in retinal ON-type bipolar cells expressing the biosensor Clomeleon. *Neuron* 49: 81–94.

Euler, T., Detwiler, P. B., and Denk, W. (2002). Directionally selective calcium signals in dendrites of starburst amacrine cells. *Nature* 418:845–852.

Feil, R., Brocard, J., Mascrez, B., LeMeur, M., Metzger, D., and Chambon, P. (1996). Ligand-activated site-specific recombination in mice. *Proc. Natl. Acad. Sci. U.S.A.* 93:10887–10890.

Feng, G., Mellor, R. H., Bernstein, M., Keller-Peck, C., Nguyen, Q. T., Wallace, M., Nerbonne, J. M., Lichtman, J. W., and Sanes, J. R. (2000). Imaging neuronal subsets in transgenic mice expressing multiple spectral variants of GFP. *Neuron* 28:41–51.

Furukawa, A., Koike, C., Lippincott, P., Cepko, C. L., and Furukawa, T. (2002). The mouse Crx 5′-upstream transgene sequence directs cell-specific and developmentally regulated expression in retinal photoreceptor cells. *J. Neurosci.* 22: 1640–1647.

Fyk-Kolodziej, B., Qin, P., and Pourcho, R. G. (2003). Identification of a cone bipolar cell in cat retina which has input from both rod and cone photoreceptors. *J. Comp. Neurol.* 464: 104–113.

Gan, W. B., Grutzendler, J., Wong, W. T., Wong, R. O., and Lichtman, J. W. (2000). Multicolor "DiOlistic" labeling of the nervous system using lipophilic dye combinations. *Neuron* 27: 219–225.

Gelman, D. M., Noain, D., Avale, M. E., Otero, V., Low, M. J., and Rubinstein, M. (2003). Transgenic mice engineered to target Cre/loxP-mediated DNA recombination into catecholaminergic neurons. *Genesis* 36:196–202.

Guillery, R. W., Scott, G. L., Cattanach, B. M., and Deol, M. S. (1973). Genetic mechanisms determining the central visual pathways of mice. *Science* 179:1014–1016.

Gustincich, S., Contini, M., Gariboldi, M., Puopolo, M., Kadota, K., Bono, H., LeMieux, J., Walsh, P., Carninci, P., et al. (2004). Gene discovery in genetically labeled single dopaminergic neurons of the retina. *Proc. Natl. Acad. Sci. U.S.A.* 101:5069–5074.

Gustincich, S., Feigenspan, A., Wu, D. K., Koopman, L. J., and Raviola, E. (1997). Control of dopamine release in the retina: A transgenic approach to neural networks. *Neuron* 18:723–736.

Hack, I., Peichl, L., and Brandstatter, J. H. (1999). An alternative pathway for Rod signals in the rodent retina: rod photoreceptors, cone bipolar cells, and the localization of glutamate receptors. *Proc. Natl. Acad. Sci. U.S.A.* 96:14130–14135.

Han, Y., and Massey, S. C. (2005). Electrical synapses in retinal ON cone bipolar cells: Subtype-specific expression of connexins. *Proc. Natl. Acad. Sci. U.S.A.* 102:13313–13318.

Hanno, Y., Nakahira, M., Jishage, K., Noda, T., and Yoshihara, Y. (2003). Tracking mouse visual pathways with WGA transgene. *Eur. J. Neurosci.* 18:2910–2914.

Hartline, H. (1938). The response of single optic nerve fibers of the vertebrate eye to illumination of the retina. *Am. J. Physiol.* 121:400–415.

Hasan, M. T., Friedrich, R. W., Euler, T., Larkum, M. E., Giese, G., Both, M., Duebel, J., Waters, J., Bujard, H., et al. (2004). Functional fluorescent Ca2+ indicator proteins in transgenic mice under TET control. *PLoS Biol.* 2:e163.

Hattar, S., Kumar, M., Park, A., Tong, P., Tung, J., Yau, K. W., and Berson, D. M. (2006). Central projections of melanopsin-expressing retinal ganglion cells in the mouse. *J. Comp. Neurol.* 497:326–349.

Hattar, S., Liao, H. W., Takao, M., Berson, D. M., and Yau, K. W. (2002). Melanopsin-containing retinal ganglion cells: Architecture, projections, and intrinsic photosensitivity. *Science* 295:1065–1070.

Haverkamp, S., Wässle, H., Duebel, J., Kuner, T., Augustine, G. J., Feng, G., and Euler, T. (2005). The primordial, blue-cone color system of the mouse retina. *J. Neurosci.* 25:5438–5445.

Hayden, S. A., Mills, J. W., and Masland, R. M. (1980). Acetylcholine synthesis by displaced amacrine cells. *Science* 210: 435–437.

Heintz, N. (2001). BAC to the future: The use of bac transgenic mice for neuroscience research. *Nat. Rev. Neurosci.* 2:861–870.

Hogan, B., Costantini, F., and Lacy, E. (1986). *Manipulating the mouse embryo: A laboratory manual.* Cold Spring Harbor, NY: Cold Spring Harbor Laboratory.

KACHI, S., OSHIMA, Y., ESUMI, N., KACHI, M., ROGERS, B., ZACK, D. J., and CAMPOCHIARO, P. A. (2005). Nonviral ocular gene transfer. *Gene Ther.* 12:843–851.

KERRISON, J. B., DUH, E. J., YU, Y., OTTESON, D. C., and ZACK, D. J. (2005). A system for inducible gene expression in retinal ganglion cells. *Invest. Ophthalmol. Vis. Sci.* 46:2932–2939.

KONG, J. H., FISH, D. R., ROCKHILL, R. L., and MASLAND, R. H. (2005). Diversity of ganglion cells in the mouse retina: Unsupervised morphological classification and its limits. *J. Comp. Neurol.* 489:293–310.

KUFFLER, S. W. (1953). Discharge patterns and functional organization of mammalian retina. *J. Neurophysiol.* 16:37–68.

KUNER, T., and AUGUSTINE, G. J. (2000). A genetically encoded ratiometric indicator for chloride: Capturing chloride transients in cultured hippocampal neurons. *Neuron* 27:447–459.

LI, W., KEUNG, J. W., and MASSEY, S. C. (2004). Direct synaptic connections between rods and OFF cone bipolar cells in the rabbit retina. *J. Comp. Neurol.* 474:1–12.

LIN, B., and MASLAND, R. H. (2005). Synaptic contacts between an identified type of ON cone bipolar cell and ganglion cells in the mouse retina. *Eur. J. Neurosci.* 21:1257–1270.

LIN, B., and MASLAND, R. H. (2006). Populations of wide-field amacrine cells in the mouse retina. *J. Comp. Neurol.* 499:797–809.

LIN, B., WANG, S. W., and MASLAND, R. H. (2004). Retinal ganglion cell type, size, and spacing can be specified independent of homotypic dendritic contacts. *Neuron* 43:475–485.

LOBE, C. G., KOOP, K. E., KREPPNER, W., LOMELI, H., GERTSENSTEIN, M., and NAGY, A. (1999). Z/AP, a double reporter for Cre-mediated recombination. *Dev. Biol.* 208:281–292.

MA, W., and WANG, S. Z. (2006). The final fates of neurogenin2-expressing cells include all major neuron types in the mouse retina. *Mol. Cell Neurosci.* 31:463–469.

MARQUARDT, T., ASHERY-PADAN, R., ANDREJEWSKI, N., SCARDIGLI, R., GUILLEMOT, F., and GRUSS, P. (2001). Pax6 is required for the multipotent state of retinal progenitor cells. *Cell* 105:43–55.

MASLAND, R. H., MILLS, J. W., and CASSIDY, C. (1984). The functions of acetylcholine in the rabbit retina. *Proc. R. Soc. Lond. B. Biol. Sci.* 223:121–139.

MASU, M., IWAKABE, H., TAGAWA, Y., MIYOSHI, T., YAMASHITA, M., FUKUDA, Y., SASAKI, H., HIROI, K., NAKAMURA, Y., et al. (1995). Specific deficit of the ON response in visual transmission by targeted disruption of the mGluR6 gene. *Cell* 80:757–765.

MATSUDA, T., and CEPKO, C. L. (2004). Electroporation and RNA interference in the rodent retina in vivo and in vitro. *Proc. Natl. Acad. Sci. U.S.A.* 101:16–22.

MAXEINER, S., DEDEK, K., JANSSEN-BIENHOLD, U., AMMERMULLER, J., BRUNE, H., KIRSCH, T., PIEPER, M., DEGEN, J., KRUGER, O., et al. (2005). Deletion of connexin 45 in mouse retinal neurons disrupts the rod/cone signaling pathway between AII amacrine and ON cone bipolar cells and leads to impaired visual transmission. *J. Neurosci.* 25:566–576.

MORGAN, J. L., DHINGRA, A., VARDI, N., and WONG, R. O. (2006). Axons and dendrites originate from neuroepithelial-like processes of retinal bipolar cells. *Nat. Neurosci.* 9:85–92.

NIRENBERG, S., and CEPKO, C. (1993). Targeted ablation of diverse cell classes in the nervous system in vivo. *J. Neurosci.* 13: 3238–3251.

NIRENBERG, S., and MEISTER, M. (1997). The light response of retinal ganglion cells is truncated by a displaced amacrine circuit. *Neuron* 18:637–650.

O'BRIEN, J., and LUMMIS, S. C. (2004). Biolistic and diolistic transfection: Using the gene gun to deliver DNA and lipophilic dyes into mammalian cells. *Methods* 33:121–125.

PAK, W., HINDGES, R., LIM, Y. S., PFAFF, S. L., and O'LEARY, D. D. (2004). Magnitude of binocular vision controlled by islet-2 repression of a genetic program that specifies laterality of retinal axon pathfinding. *Cell* 119:567–578.

PIGNATELLI, V., and STRETTOI, E. (2004). Bipolar cells of the mouse retina: A gene gun, morphological study. *J. Comp. Neurol.* 476: 254–266.

PRATT, T., TIAN, N. M., SIMPSON, T. I., MASON, J. O., and PRICE, D. J. (2004). The winged helix transcription factor Foxg1 facilitates retinal ganglion cell axon crossing of the ventral midline in the mouse. *Development* 131:3773–3784.

PRICE, J., TURNER, D., and CEPKO, C. (1987). Lineage analysis in the vertebrate nervous system by retrovirus-mediated gene transfer. *Proc. Natl. Acad. Sci. U.S.A.* 84:156–160.

QUINA, L. A., PAK, W., LANIER, J., BANWAIT, P., GRATWICK, K., LIU, Y., VELASQUEZ, T., O'LEARY, D. D., GOULDING, M., and TURNER, E. E. (2005). Brn3a-expressing retinal ganglion cells project specifically to thalamocortical and collicular visual pathways. *J. Neurosci.* 25:11595–11604.

ROHLICH, P., VAN VEEN, T., and SZEL, A. (1994). Two different visual pigments in one retinal cone cell. *Neuron* 13:1159–1166.

SCHNITZER, M. J., and MEISTER, M. (2003). Multineuronal firing patterns in the signal from eye to brain. *Neuron* 37:499–511.

SCHUBERT, T., MAXEINER, S., KRUGER, O., WILLECKE, K., and WEILER, R. (2005). Connexin45 mediates gap junctional coupling of bistratified ganglion cells in the mouse retina. *J. Comp. Neurol.* 490:29–39.

SOUCY, E., WANG, Y., NIRENBERG, S., NATHANS, J., and MEISTER, M. (1998). A novel signaling pathway from rod photoreceptors to ganglion cells in mammalian retina. *Neuron* 21:481–493.

STACY, R. C., DEMAS, J., BURGESS, R. W., SANES, J. R., and WONG, R. O. (2005). Disruption and recovery of patterned retinal activity in the absence of acetylcholine. *J. Neurosci.* 25:9347–9357.

SUN, W., LI, N., and HE, S. (2002). Large-scale morphological survey of mouse retinal ganglion cells. *J. Comp. Neurol.* 451: 115–126.

SUNG, C. H., MAKINO, C., BAYLOR, D., and NATHANS, J. (1994). A rhodopsin gene mutation responsible for autosomal dominant retinitis pigmentosa results in a protein that is defective in localization to the photoreceptor outer segment. *J. Neurosci.* 14: 5818–5833.

TAGAWA, Y., SAWAI, H., UEDA, Y., TAUCHI, M., and NAKANISHI, S. (1999). Immunohistological studies of metabotropic glutamate receptor subtype 6-deficient mice show no abnormality of retinal cell organization and ganglion cell maturation. *J. Neurosci.* 19:2568–2579.

TAUCHI, M., and MASLAND, R. H. (1984). The shape and arrangement of the cholinergic neurons in the rabbit retina. *Proc. R. Soc. Lond. B. Biol. Sci.* 223:101–119.

TIAN, N., and COPENHAGEN, D. R. (2003). Visual stimulation is required for refinement of ON and OFF pathways in postnatal retina. *Neuron* 39:85–96.

TSUKAMOTO, Y., MORIGIWA, K., UEDA, M., and STERLING, P. (2001). Microcircuits for night vision in mouse retina. *J. Neurosci.* 21:8616–8623.

TURNER, D. L., SNYDER, E. Y., and CEPKO, C. L. (1990). Lineage-independent determination of cell type in the embryonic mouse retina. *Neuron* 4:833–845.

UEDA, Y., IWAKABE, H., MASU, M., SUZUKI, M., and NAKANISHI, S. (1997). The mGluR6 5′ upstream transgene sequence directs a cell-specific and developmentally regulated expression in retinal rod and ON-type cone bipolar cells. *J. Neurosci.* 17:3014–3023.

Urlinger, S., Baron, U., Thellmann, M., Hasan, M. T., Bujard, H., and Hillen, W. (2000). Exploring the sequence space for tetracycline-dependent transcriptional activators: Novel mutations yield expanded range and sensitivity. *Proc. Natl. Acad. Sci. U.S.A.* 97:7963–7968.

Völgyi, B., Deans, M. R., Paul, D. L., and Bloomfield, S. A. (2004). Convergence and segregation of the multiple rod pathways in mammalian retina. *J. Neurosci.* 24:11182–11192.

Wang, Y., Macke, J. P., Merbs, S. L., Zack, D. J., Klaunberg, B., Bennett, J., Gearhart, J., and Nathans, J. (1992). A locus control region adjacent to the human red and green visual pigment genes. *Neuron* 9:429–440.

Wellmann, H., Kaltschmidt, B., and Kaltschmidt, C. (1999). Optimized protocol for biolistic transfection of brain slices and dissociated cultured neurons with a hand-held gene gun. *J. Neurosci. Methods* 92:55–64.

Xiang, M., Zhou, L., and Nathans, J. (1996). Similarities and differences among inner retinal neurons revealed by the expression of reporter transgenes controlled by Brn-3a, Brn-3b, and Brn-3c promotor sequences. *Vis. Neurosci.* 13:955–962.

Yang, Z., Ding, K., Pan, L., Deng, M., and Gan, L. (2003). Math5 determines the competence state of retinal ganglion cell progenitors. *Dev. Biol.* 264:240–254.

Yoshida, K., Watanabe, D., Ishikane, H., Tachibana, M., Pastan, I., and Nakanishi, S. (2001). A key role of starburst amacrine cells in originating retinal directional selectivity and optokinetic eye movement. *Neuron* 30:771–780.

Yoshihara, Y., Mizuno, T., Nakahira, M., Kawasaki, M., Watanabe, Y., Kagamiyama, H., Jishage, K., Ueda, O., Suzuki, H., et al. (1999). A genetic approach to visualization of multisynaptic neural pathways using plant lectin transgene. *Neuron* 22:33–41.

Zack, D. J., Bennett, J., Wang, Y., Davenport, C., Klaunberg, B., Gearhart, J., and Nathans, J. (1991). Unusual topography of bovine rhodopsin promoter-lacZ fusion gene expression in transgenic mouse retinas. *Neuron* 6:187–199.

Zambrowicz, B. P., Imamoto, A., Fiering, S., Herzenberg, L. A., Kerr, W. G., and Soriano, P. (1997). Disruption of overlapping transcripts in the ROSA beta geo 26 gene trap strain leads to widespread expression of beta-galactosidase in mouse embryos and hematopoietic cells. *Proc. Natl. Acad. Sci. U.S.A.* 94:3789–3794.

Zhang, X. M., Chen, B. Y., Ng, A. H., Tanner, J. A., Tay, D., So, K. F., Rachel, R. A., Copeland, N. G., Jenkins, N. A., et al. (2005). Transgenic mice expressing Cre-recombinase specifically in retinal rod bipolar neurons. *Invest. Ophthalmol. Vis. Sci.* 46:3515–3520.

Zirlinger, M., Lo, L., McMahon, J., McMahon, A. P., and Anderson, D. J. (2002). Transient expression of the bHLH factor neurogenin-2 marks a subpopulation of neural crest cells biased for a sensory but not a neuronal fate. *Proc. Natl. Acad. Sci. U.S.A.* 99:8084–8089.

50 Adenoassociated Virus Gene Therapy in Mouse Models of Retinal Degeneration

SHANNON E. BOYE, SANFORD L. BOYE, AND WILLIAM W. HAUSWIRTH

A variety of therapeutic strategies aimed at combating inherited retinal diseases have recently been developed. In general, these strategies can be divided into three categories: gene therapy, pharmacological neuroprotection, and stem or precursor cell therapy. Of these approaches, only gene therapy is capable of curing a disease state. The others seek either to halt or slow the progression of an existing disorder or to replace key retinal cells once they are lost or become dysfunctional. Of course, if tissue replacement utilizes a sufficient number of normal cells, a cure may also be effected. This chapter focuses on gene-based therapeutic approaches for treating retinal degeneration (RD) in mouse models.

Gene therapy vectors

The history of gene therapy is best illustrated by the attempts to develop a lasting treatment for cystic fibrosis (CF). The earliest CF gene therapy trials utilized recombinant adeno-associated virus (AAV), which was found to be ineffective, owing to problems with delivery to the target cell and insufficient expression levels (Griesenbach et al., 2006; Flotte et al., 2007). In addition to AAV, two other candidate gene therapy vectors, adenovirus and lentivirus, were investigated for their therapeutic potential for treating CF. However, the occurrence of two high-profile adverse events in humans involving these vectors affected their utility in CF and other clinical studies. The systemic administration of an adenovirus vector for ornithine transcarbamylase (OCT) deficiency in which adenovirus vector was delivered to the liver resulted in a fatality (Raper et al., 2003). It was concluded that the high dose of vector (required because of poor expression from vector) given to this patient was immunogenic. Additionally, administration of a lentiviral vector to patients with X-linked severe combined immunodeficiency syndrome resulted in site-specific integration of the vector near a specific pro-oncogene, which resulted in three cases of leukemia, one of which was ultimately fatal (Williams, 2006). AAV's relatively nonimmunogenic properties and apparent lack of chromosomal integration indicated that it was inherently safer and more effective than the aforementioned viral vectors. Newer AAV vectors have been designed to address earlier shortcomings and are now in the process of being evaluated for the treatment of CF (Flotte et al., 2005). These same advances in AAV vector technology are being applied to the gene therapy of various other disorders, including disorders of the eye (Warrington and Herzog, 2006).

Adenoassociated virus vectors

Although there are a number of strategies for delivering genes to cells, the nature of the target tissue and the therapeutic requirements for the disease normally dictate which choice is optimal. Viruses of the Parvoviridae family have shown the most promise in gene therapy, particularly for retinal disease. A member of this family, human AAV has been widely exploited as a vector for gene delivery because of its advantages over other viral gene therapy vectors, namely, safety, long-term expression, the ability to transduce terminally differentiated cells, and selective (as well as broad) tropism through the use of the numerous AAV serotypes currently available. AAV is a nonpathogenic, replication-deficient dependovirus that contains a single-stranded genome of 4.7 kb flanked by inverted terminal repeats (ITRs), each 145 bases in length (Srivastava et al., 1983; Flotte and Berns, 2005). Specific sites within these ITRs control the conversion of single-stranded AAV genomes to their double-stranded DNA state necessary for subsequent transcription and translation (Qing et al., 1997, 1998; Mah et al., 1998).

Wild-type AAV is not associated with any pathological condition in humans. Recombinant AAV (rAAV) is produced by removing all native AAV coding sequences, leaving only the short ITRs flanking the promoter and cDNA of interest. This eliminates the virus's ability to integrate site specifically into the genome; the integration events that do occur are very infrequent and require chromosomal breakage (Miller et al., 2004). Thus, the overall risk of an AAV integration event activating an oncogene is considered low. AAV vectors do, however, promote long-term transgene expression by remaining in the transduced cell in a circular, double-stranded episomal form (Song et al., 2001, 2004; Duan et al., 2003). In other words, AAV-delivered DNA remains in the host cell nucleus as an independent genetic unit and not as part of the host cell's genome. In vivo expression has been documented to persist for more than 6 years in a dog model of Leber congenital amaurosis (Acland et al., 2005; G. Acland and G. Aguirre, pers. comm., 2007). Additionally, AAV vectors have been shown to efficiently transduce terminally differentiated, nondividing cells. This is clearly vital for treating retinal diseases, most of which involve malfunction of photoreceptors or other terminally differentiated retinal cells.

There are more than 100 different variants of AAV, categorized into serotypes and genomovars (Gao et al., 2004). Among these genomic variants is a broad diversity of AAV serotypes that utilize a range of different receptors (Flotte and Berns, 2005). The nine AAV serotypes currently in wide use, AAV serotypes 1, 2, 3, 4, 5, 6, 7, 8, and 9, differ from each other to varying degrees in their capsid protein sequence critical for serotype determination. Capsid variations confer distinct tissue and cell affinities and, as a result, define the speed of expression onset and the overall intensity of transgene expression by AAV vectors. AAV serotype 2 (AAV2) was the first used for gene transfer to the rodent retina via subretinal injection and was subsequently shown to promote broad transduction of photoreceptors and retinal pigmented epithelium (RPE) (Bennett et al., 1997; Flannery et al., 1997; Ali et al., 1998). Subsequently other serotypes have shown potential for targeting transgene expression to specific subsets of cells in the mouse retina. Typically, non-serotype 2 AAV vectors are made by packaging the vector DNA flanked by serotype 2 ITRs into the desired capsid serotype, a process termed pseudotyping. Almost all non-serotype 2 vectors to date have been made by this technique. AAV5, like AAV2, targets photoreceptors and RPE after subretinal injection, but does so with greater efficiency than AAV2 (Yang et al., 2002). AAV1 and AAV6, two closely related serotypes, have both been shown to transduce primarily RPE (Xiao et al., 1999). AAV4 is the only serotype to be expressed solely in RPE, based on results in rat, dog, and nonhuman primate, and would therefore be expected to do the same in mouse (Weber et al., 2003). AAV3 does not appear to transduce retinal cells at all after subretinal injection (Yang et al., 2002). Although AAV7 and AAV8 have not been as comprehensively evaluated in the mouse retina as other serotypes, there is some evidence that both transduce RPE and photoreceptors, with AAV8 being more efficient (Lauramore, 2004). The transduction characteristics of AAV9 in mouse retina have yet to be reported in the literature. The use of ITRs from serotypes other than AAV2 has been reported for an AAV5 capsid containing serotype 5 ITRs (Yang et al., 2002). This vector had a similar transduction pattern to that for AAV5 pseudotyped with serotype 2 ITRs, in that it was more efficient at targeting photoreceptors and RPE than standard AAV2.

When injected into the vitreous of mouse and rat, AAV2 has proven to be the most efficient serotype for targeting expression to the inner retina, primarily retinal ganglion cells (RGCs; Ali et al., 1998; Auricchio et al., 2001; Liang et al., 2001a; Martin et al., 2003). In addition to targeting expression to the inner retina, limited spread of expressed transgene to the optic nerve and brain has also been observed (Dudus et al., 1999). The transduction patterns of various AAV serotypes following subretinal or intravitreal delivery are summarized in table 50.1.

In addition to serotype selection, promoter choice aids significantly in defining the retinal cell specificity of transgene expression. For broad transgene expression in the retina, the cytomegalovirus (CMV) immediate early promoter has historically been used (Ali et al., 1998). More recently, the chimeric CMV-chicken β-actin promoter/CMV enhancer (CBA) has been used in applications where high-level, long-term expression of protein in a broad variety of cells is required (Raisler et al., 2002; Pang et al., 2006). In cases where a single cell type is the target of therapy, nonviral cell-specific promoters enhance the safety of AAV vectors by reducing possible toxicity associated with the transduction of nontarget cell types. AAV-mediated expression targeted to photoreceptors was first achieved in rat using 472 bps (−386/+85) of the proximal mouse rhodopsin promoter (Rho, also commonly referred to as mOP)

Table 50.1

Transduction characteristics of various AAV serotypes following subretinal or intravitreal administration to the mouse retina

AAV Serotype*	Injection Route	Transduction Pattern
AAV2/2	Subretinal	Photoreceptors, RPE
AAV2/2	Intravitreal	Ganglion cells
AAV2/5	Subretinal	Photoreceptors, RPE
AAV2/5	Intravitreal	None
AAV2/1	Subretinal	Primarily RPE
AAV2/1	Intravitreal	None
AAV2/6	Subretinal	Primarily RPE
AAV2/4	Subretinal	Solely RPE
AAV2/3	Subretinal	None
AAV2/7	Subretinal	Photoreceptors, RPE
AAV2/8	Subretinal	Photoreceptors, RPE
AAV5/5	Subretinal	Photoreceptors, RPE

*The first number indicates the serotype of the ITRs flanking vector DNA, and the second number represents the serotype of capsid protein.

in conjunction with AAV2 (Flannery et al., 1997). It has subsequently been shown to be the case for mouse as well (Min et al., 2005; Pawlyk et al., 2005). Some controversy exists as to whether mOP targets both rods and cones, but several recent studies have provided convincing evidence that cones are indeed transduced when using this promoter, particularly in conjunction with AAV5 (Glushakova et al., 2006a; Haire et al., 2006). A human blue cone opsin promoter originally shown to preferentially target cone photoreceptors in rat has also been shown to effectively target cones in mouse retina when used with AAV5 (Glushakova et al., 2006b). In addition, a human red cone opsin promoter fragment used in conjunction with AAV5 has also been shown to preferentially target cones in mouse retina (Alexander et al., 2005). Promoter analysis indicates that RPE-specific expression can be achieved using portions of the vitelliform macular dystrophy 2 (VMD2) promoter of the bestrophin gene (the gene responsible for Best disease) or the RPE65 promoter (Boulanger et al., 2000, 2002; Esumi et al., 2004, 2007). This has been confirmed in mouse when these promoters have been used in conjunction with AAV1 (Glushakova and Hauswirth, 2004).

Regulatable systems of gene expression are desirable in cases where continuous, high levels of expression of a therapeutic agent may be harmful to retina. Two have been used in conjunction with AAV vectors targeted in the retina: the tetracycline-inducible and the rapamycin-inducible transcriptional regulatory systems. Although both have been studied in rat (McGee-Sanftner et al., 2001; Auricchio, Rivera, et al., 2002; Smith et al., 2005), it is reasonable to expect that the results are equally applicable to mouse.

This chapter focuses on the application of AAV-mediated gene therapy in several different mouse models of inherited RD. In all studies mentioned, AAV-mediated somatic gene transfer resulted in significant functional improvement, as assessed by electroretinography (ERG) or behavior, or by regeneration or stabilization of retinal structure. In some cases, knowledge gained from initial work in mice has set the stage for the development of human clinical trials. A comprehensive list of these studies and the type of vector, promoter, and transgene used is given in table 50.2.

Antiangiogenic gene therapy

Although many clinical RDs are the result of mutations in genes expressed in the retina, some are secondary to systemic disease. The mammalian retina is one of the most metabolically active tissues in the body and therefore demands very high levels of oxygen via both the retinal and choroidal blood vessels. Systemic disease such as diabetes or retinopathy of prematurity (ROP) can result in retinal hypoxia that subsequently leads to retinal neovascularization. Age-related macular degeneration (AMD), the leading cause of blindness in developed countries, in its "wet form" is characterized by neovascularization originating in the choroidal vasculature. Normal retinal and choroidal vessel beds are maintained by a balance of several endogenous proteins, including positive growth factors such as vascular endothelial growth factor (VEGF) and antiangiogenic proteins such as pigmented epithelium–derived factor (SERPINF1, more commonly referred to as PEDF). Traditional treatments (laser, photodynamic therapy) seek to delay the progression of the disease by destroying new, pathogenic blood vessels. They do not, however, address the underlying cause, that being the recurring, inappropriate proliferation of the retinal or choroidal vasculature. The delivery of proteins with antiangiogenic properties has proved somewhat successful in patients with various neovascular or neovascular-associated diseases (O'Reilly et al., 1994, 1997; Stellmach et al., 2001). Two such therapies currently available to patients with neovascular AMD are Pfizer's Macugen (pegaptanib), a pegylated aptamer of VEGF, and Genentech's Lucentis (ranibizumab), an anti-VEGF antibody. However, both require repeated intraocular injections for extended periods of time, thus posing risk and compliance issues for patients. In animal models, AAV-mediated gene transfer of antiangiogenic proteins to various cells of the retina has been employed to combat both retinal and choroidal neovascularization, thus suggesting AAV-vectored genes may be an attractive, long-term alternative for the treatment of local neovascular disease.

Therapy for retinal neovascularization

The oxygen-induced retinopathy (OIR) mouse model, more commonly referred to as the ROP mouse, has been developed for the study of retinal neovascular disease (Smith et al., 1994). Newborn mice are placed in a hyperoxic (ca. 75% oxygen) chamber for 5 days. This high-oxygen environment induces retinal capillary ablation, which, when mice are returned to normoxic conditions, results in relative hypoxia and retinal ischemia. This in turn leads to VEGF-mediated retinal neovascularization like that seen in humans with neovascular retinal disease.

A variety of antiangiogenic treatments have been tested in the ROP mouse. In one study, AAV2 was used to deliver *PEDF*, under the control of the CBA promoter, to the intravitreal or subretinal space of a newborn mouse eye (Raisler et al., 2002). The contralateral control eye received an equivalent injection of PBS. Retinal neovascularization was quantified in both treated and untreated (contralateral) eyes by counting the number of vascular endothelial cell nuclei above the inner limiting membrane in P17 eyes. The number of neovascular nuclei observed in eyes treated with AAV2-*PEDF* was significantly reduced relative to that in control eyes. Similar results were obtained when AAV serotype 1

Table 50.2

Summary of mouse models treated with AAV gene therapy

Mouse Model	Description of Model	Related Disease or Disorder in Human	AAV Vector	Serotype	Function of Transgene Delivered	Reference
ROP	Oxygen-induced retinopathy	Retinopathy of prematurity and other vasculopathologies	CBA-*PEDF*	2	Angiogenic regulator	Raisler et al., 2002
ROP	Oxygen-induced retinopathy	Retinopathy of prematurity and other vasculopathologies	CMV-*PEDF*	1	Angiogenic regulator	Auricchio, Behling, et al., 2002
ROP	Oxygen-induced retinopathy	Retinopathy of prematurity and other vasculopathologies	CBA-*VEGF* (exon 6–7)	2	Angiogenic regulator	Deng et al., 2005
ROP	Oxygen-induced retinopathy	Retinopathy of prematurity and other vasculopathologies	CMV-s*Flt1*	2	Inhibitor of VEGF, antiangiogenic	Bainbridge et al., 2002
ROP	Oxygen-induced retinopathy	Retinopathy of prematurity and other vasculopathologies	CMV-*Timp3*	1	Regulates structure of basement membrane	Auricchio, Behling, et al., 2002
ROP	Oxygen-induced retinopathy	Retinopathy of prematurity and other vasculopathologies	CMV-*endostatin*	1	Antimitogenic factor	Auricchio, Behling, et al., 2002
ROP	Oxygen-induced retinopathy	Retinopathy of prematurity and other vasculopathologies	CBA-*K1K3* (angiostatin)	2	Angiogenic regulator	Raisler et al., 2002
CNV laser	Laser-induced choroidal neovascularization	Age-related macular degeneration	CBA-*PEDF*	2	Angiogenic regulator	Mori et al., 2002
$Prph2^{Rd2/Rd2}$*	Knockout of peripherin2	Autosomal dominant RP, macular dystrophies	Rho-*prph2*	2	Stabilization of discs in outer segments	Ali et al., 2000, and Sarra et al., 2001
$Rs1^{-/-}$	Knockout of retinoschisin	X-linked retinoschisis	CMV-*Rs1*	2	Structural and synaptic integrity of retinal neurons	Zeng et al., 2004
$Rs1^{-/-}$	Knockout of retinoschisin	X-linked retinoschisis	mOP-*RS1*	5	Structural and synaptic integrity of retinal neurons	Min et al., 2005
$GC1^{-/-}$	Knockout of guanylate cyclase-1	LCA 1	mOP-*bGC1*/ CBA-*bGC1*	5	cGMP production, phototransduction	Haire et al., 2006
$Rpe65^{-/-}$	Knockout of RPE65	LCA 2	CMV-*RPE65*	1	Retinal isomerohydrolase	Dejneka et al., 2003
rd12	Mutation in RPE65	LCA 2	CBA-*RPE65*	5	Retinal isomerohydrolase	Pang et al., 2006
$Rpgrip^{-/-}$	Knockout of RP GTPase Regulator (RPGR)–interacting protein	Leber congenital amaurosis (LCA)	mOP-*Rpgrip*	2	Protein trafficking through connecting cilia of rods and cones	Pawlyk et al., 2005

Table 50.2
Summary of mouse models treated with AAV gene therapy (continued)

Mouse Model	Description of Model	Related Disease or Disorder in Human	AAV Vector	Serotype	Function of Transgene Delivered	Reference
MPS VII	Mutation in β-glucuronidase (GUSB)	Mucopolysaccharidosis type VII	CBA-*GUSB*	2	Degradation of chondroitin, heparan, and dermatan sulfate proteoglycans	Hennig et al., 2004
Ppt1$^{-/-}$	Knockout of palmitoyl protein thioesterase1	Infantile neuronal ceroid lipofuscinosis (INCL)	CMV-*PPT1*	2	Lysosomal hydrolase	Griffey et al., 2005
Gnat2^{Cpfl3}	Mutation in α subunit of cone transducin	Achromatopsia	PR2.1-*Gnat2*	5	G protein involved in phototransduction	Hauswirth, unpublished data
Rho$^{-/-}$	Knockout of rhodopsin	Retinitis pigmentosa	CMV-*CNTF*-IRES-*GFP*	2	Neurotrophic factor	Liang, Dejneka, et al., 2001
Prph2$^{Rd2/Rd2}$	Mutation (insertional gene disruption) in peripherin2	Autosomal dominant RP, macular dystrophies	CBA-*GDNF* and Rho-*Prph2*	2	Neurotrophic factor and stabilization of discs in outer segments	Buch et al., 2006

*Also referred to as rds.
bOp, bovine rhodopsin promoter; CBA, chimeric CMV-chicken beta actin promoter; CMV, cytomegalovirus immediate early promoter; mOP, murine opsin promoter; PR2.1, human red cone opsin promoter.

was used to deliver *PEDF* under the control of the CMV promoter (Auricchio, Behling, et al., 2002). These were the first studies to show that intravitreal AAV conferred stable and effective expression of an antiangiogenic transgene.

VEGF has been demonstrated to be a key mediator of retinal neovascularization. VEGF isoforms bind two tyrosine kinase receptors expressed on the surface of endothelial cells, VEGF receptor 1 (FLT1) and VEGF receptor 2 (KDR) (De Vries et al., 1992; Gitay-Goren et al., 1992; Jakeman et al., 1992).

When activated by VEGF, these receptors stimulate endothelial cell proliferation and migration, vasopermeability, and vasculature organization and modeling. VEGF has been shown to be upregulated by hypoxia in various types of neovascular retinopathies (Adamis et al., 1994; Aiello et al., 1994), as well as in animal models of retinal ischemia (Miller et al., 1994; Pierce et al., 1995; Shima et al., 1996). Various anti-VEGF strategies have been developed that target either the expression of the protein or its interaction with its receptors. Antisense oligonucleotides, soluble VEGF receptors, receptor mimics, and small interfering RNAs targeting *VEGF* have all been shown to inhibit neovascularization in mouse models (Aiello et al., 1995; Robinson et al., 1996; Reich et al., 2003). However, the transient nature of all of these reagents may well hinder their therapeutic application.

In vitro studies have shown that VEGF peptides derived from exons 6 and 7 inhibit VEGF-mediated angiogenesis (Soker et al., 1997; Jia et al., 2001). These peptides were found to block the interaction of VEGF with the KDR receptor and coreceptor, neuropilin-1 (NPN1), thereby inhibiting VEGF-induced mitogenesis and migration of endothelial cells (Jia et al., 2001). Taking advantage of the antiangiogenic properties of these peptides by delivering both to the ROP mouse retina via an AAV serotype 2 vector under the control of a CBA promoter effectively inhibited retinal neovascularization (Deng et al., 2005). In this study, vector was administered to newborn pups prior to exposing them to the hyperoxic environment.

A related study sought to prevent ocular neovascularization by expressing a soluble version of the VEGF receptor 1, SFLT1, in the ROP mouse retina. AAV2 was used to deliver *SFlt1* under the control of the CMV promoter to the intravitreal space of ROP mouse eyes (Bainbridge et al., 2002). In this case, vector was delivered after the mouse was exposed to the hyperoxic environment. Utilizing a secretable gene product expressed by retinal cells not normally responsible for production of SFLT1 allowed vector injection into the vitreous rather than the subretinal space, a much less challenging technique. Treatment resulted in a 50% reduction of retinal neovascularization, with efficacy quantified as previously described.

Another vascular retinopathy characterized by early-onset ocular neovascularization is Sorsby's fundus dystrophy. Mutations in the gene for tissue inhibitor of matrix metalloproteinase-3 (*TIMP3*) have been identified in Sorsby's patients (Weber et al., 1994). The antiangiogenic properties of TIMP3 in vitro (Anand-Apte et al., 1997) prompted AAV1-mediated delivery of this transgene, under the control of the CMV promoter, to the subretinal space of newborn pups prior to placing them in the hyperoxic environment. The number of neovascular retinal endothelial cell nuclei in eyes treated with AAV1-*Timp3* was significantly less than in those injected with control vector (AAV1-*GFP* or AAV1-*lacZ*), proving that TIMP3 exerts angiostatic effects in vivo (Auricchio, Behling, et al., 2002).

The same study also addressed whether endostatin exhibited anti-angiogenic properties in the ROP mouse. Endostatin, encoded by a natural fragment of collagen XVIII (*Col18a1*), has been shown to inhibit ocular angiogenesis when secreted intravascularly from hepatocytes transduced by viral vectors (O'Reilly et al., 1997; Mori et al., 2001). Using the same protocol as in their TIMP3 experiment, it was shown that AAV1-mediated endostatin expression, driven by the CMV promoter, was also able to reduce angiogenesis in the ROP mouse (Auricchio, Behling, et al., 2002).

Another potent inhibitor of angiogenesis is angiostatin, a proteolytic fragment of plasminogen. Kringle domains 1 through 3 of angiostatin (K1K3), has been shown to have angiostatic effects in tumor bearing mice (O'Reilly et al., 1994, 1996; Wu et al., 1997). AAV2 was used to deliver *K1K3* under the control of a CBA promoter to either the subretinal or intravitreal space of newborn mouse pups with contralateral eyes receiving only PBS (Raisler et al., 2002). In ROP mice, the number of inner retinal vascular endothelial cells treated intravitreally or subretinally with AAV2-CBA-*K1K3* was again significantly less than in control eyes.

Therapy for choroidal neovascularization

The laser-induced choroidal neovascularization protocol was developed first in nonhuman primates (Ryan, 1982). Subsequently used in other mammalian species, including mouse (Miller et al., 1990), this model employs the use of a laser to rupture Bruch's membrane, which leads to recruitment of inflammatory and neovascular mediators promoting the proliferation of choroidal vessels into the retina proper. This pathology mimics that seen in the late stages of wet AMD. The extent of CNV is measured in the mouse 2–4 weeks post laser treatment in choroidal flat mounts prepared from animals that have been perfused with a fluorescent dye (Raisler et al., 2002). In a study using the laser CNV mouse model to test the effects of the antiangiogenic protein PEDF, mice were given intravitreal or subretinal injections of AAV2 containing a CBA promoter driving expression of either PEDF or GFP as a control (Mori et al., 2002). At 4–6 weeks post injection, the Bruch's membranes of these mice were ruptured by laser photocoagulation at three sites per eye. After 14 days, the area of CNV at the laser hole was measured by imaging choroidal flat mounts of mice that had been perfused with fluorescein-labeled dextran. Mice treated with AAV-CBA-*PEDF* before laser treatment, either subretinally or intravitreally, showed significantly smaller mean areas of CNV than mice injected with control vector. Thus, the principle of AAV-vectored antiangiogenic gene therapy utilizing soluble factors has been well established in mouse models for both retinal and choroidal neovascularization.

Gene replacement therapy

Gene replacement strategies are primarily designed for autosomal recessive diseases in which a defective gene is complemented, in trans, with a wild-type counterpart that will produce a normal functional protein, thereby preventing the pathology. It is usually important to express the desired transgene in the cell type in which it is normally expressed, and autosomal recessive retinal diseases are no exception. A number of successful retinal gene replacement studies have been performed in mice using genes that all play significant roles in the structural integrity or function of the retina. Several of these proof-of-principle mouse studies hold great promise for human application.

Therapy for Structural Defects in Retinal Disease

The oldest and most studied mouse model for structural disorders of the retina is the retinal degeneration slow (rds) or peripherin-2 ($Prph2^{Rd2/Rd2}$) mouse. The $Prph2^{Rd2/Rd2}$ mouse is homozygous for a null mutation (large DNA insertion) in the *Prph2* gene, encoding a photoreceptor-specific membrane glycoprotein (Travis et al., 1989) necessary for the stabilization of disc rims in photoreceptor outer segments. As a consequence of its absence, the $Prph2^{Rd2/Rd2}$ mouse is incapable of developing normal photoreceptor discs and outer segments (Sanyal and Jansen, 1981; Molday 1994). In addition to loss of photoreceptor function, rhodopsin is downregulated, and photoreceptors eventually suffer apoptotic cell death (Reuter and Sanyal, 1984; Nir et al., 1990; Chang et al., 1993). In humans, mutations in *PRPH2* cause autosomal dominant retinitis pigmentosa and macular dystrophy. As in the $Prph2^{Rd2/Rd2}$ mouse, these human diseases are characterized by progressive photoreceptor cell death and loss of visual function (Gregory-Evans and Bhattacharya, 1998). AAV2 carrying a normal mouse *Prph2* under the control of a bovine rhodopsin promoter was subretinally injected at P10 into $Prph2^{Rd2/Rd2}$ mice and resulted in preservation of vestigial rhodopsin-containing outer segments and improved photoreceptor function (Ali et al., 2000). However, subsequent experiments noted that ultrastructural improvements in photoreceptors depended on the age at which animals were treated (Sarra et al., 2001). Also, in all cases, there was no significant slowing of the rate of photoreceptor cell loss. Attempts at promoting photoreceptor cell survival in the *Prph2*$^{Rd2/Rd2}$ mouse via AAV delivered neurotrophic factors are discussed later.

X-linked juvenile retinoschisis (XLRS) is caused by mutations in the gene for retinioschisin-1 (*RS1*) (Sauer et al., 1997) that encodes a protein secreted from photoreceptor and bipolar cells as a multimeric complex of identical subunits linked by disulfide bonds (Molday et al., 2001; Reid et al., 2003; Wu and Molday, 2003). Each subunit contains a discoidin domain that has been implicated in cell adhesion and cell-cell interactions (Baumgartner et al., 1998). Patients with XLRS have intraretinal macular voids that form in a spoke-wheel-like pattern, peripheral retinal schisis, and functional changes classically illustrated by a depressed rod ERG b-wave and a fairly normal a-wave. The net effect is a single electronegative ERG waveform. The murine orthologue of the human retinoschisis gene, when knocked out in the mouse (*Rs1*$^{-/-}$), mimics some of the pathology seen in human patients, including disorganization of multiple retinal layers, duplication and mislocalization of ganglion cells, shortening of photoreceptor inner and outer segments, and mislocalization of photoreceptor nuclei (Weber et al., 2002). In one study, AAV2 was used to deliver RS1 under the control of a CMV promoter to the intravitreal space of 13-week-old *Rs1*$^{-/-}$ mice (Zeng et al., 2004). Contralateral eyes received an injection of PBS. Treatment resulted in retinoschisin protein distributed throughout the retina, as well as a reversal of the electronegative waveform through restoration of the normal, positive b-wave. However, treatment failed to improve retinal structure (Zeng et al., 2004). In another study, in order to target RS1 properly to photoreceptors, AAV5 containing human *RS1* under the control of the mOP promoter was delivered to the subretinal space of P15 *Rs1*$^{-/-}$ mice. Treatment led to a normal distribution of retinoschisin and progressive and significant improvement in both retinal function (ERG) and retinal morphology (Min et al., 2005). Photoreceptors were preserved and ERG signals improved for at least 5 months post treatment (Min et al., 2005). Thus, it appears that replacement of either the mouse or human form of RS1 conferred varying levels of synaptic integrity, depending on what AAV serotype, promoter, and delivery route was used. Taken together, these results provide hope that this type of therapy may be useful for XLRS patients.

Therapy for Functional Defects in the Retina

Leber congenital amaurosis. Leber congenital amaurosis (LCA) is an early-onset form of congenital blindness. Thus far, 10 genes associated with LCA have been identified or mapped. The first to be discovered, and therefore assigned to the LCA1 locus, was the retinal-specific guanylate cyclase gene (*GUCY2D*) (Perrault et al., 1996). Since its discovery nine others, including *RPE65* and *RP1GRIP1*, have been identified (Marlhens et al., 1998; Perrault et al., 1999; Dryja et al., 2001; Gerber et al., 2001). All LCA patient pedigrees are consistent with an autosomal recessive inheritance pattern, yet each gene has proved to be involved in strikingly different physiological pathways.

A mouse model of LCA1 was created by knocking out guanylate cyclase-1 (*GC1*) (Yang et al., 1999). Rods in *GC1*$^{-/-}$ mice do not degenerate, whereas cone loss progresses from central to peripheral retina and peaks between 9 and 16 weeks of age, with very few cones remaining at 6 months of age (Coleman et al., 2004). Cone-mediated ERGs are barely detectable at 1 month of age, while rods exhibit ERG amplitudes 30%–50% of those in congenic control mice but decrease until they plateau at 5 months of age (Yang et al., 1999). Additionally, cone arrestin and cone α-transducin fail to properly translocate between photoreceptor outer and inner segments in response to light. Recent studies have shown that subretinal AAV5-mediated delivery of bovine GC1 under control of either mOP or CBA promoters to P21 *GC1*$^{-/-}$ mice resulted in restoration of correct light-activated cone arrestin translocation (Haire et al., 2006). These results suggest that early therapeutic intervention may be required for the optimal treatment of LCA1.

A mouse model of LCA2, the *Rpe65* knockout mouse, was generated in 1998 (Redmond et al., 1998). RPE65 is a 61-kd protein that is primarily expressed in the microsomal membrane fraction of the retinal pigmented epithelium (RPE) and is the isomerohydrolase responsible for converting all-*trans*-retinyl ester to 11-*cis*-retinol in the visual cycle (Mata et al, 2004; Moiseyev et al., 2005). Rod outer segment discs in the *Rpe65*$^{-/-}$ mouse are disorganized and rod ERGs abolished, while an apparent cone signal remains. However, this ERG signal is not a true cone response but rather a highly desensitized rod response that is being detected under standard cone assay conditions (Seeliger et al., 2001). *Rpe65*$^{-/-}$ mice lack rhodopsin but maintain opsin apoprotein, and, owing to their inability to isomerize all-*trans*-retinal ester to its *cis*-form, all-*trans*-retinyl esters accumulate in the RPE (Redmond et al., 1998). AAV1 was used for in utero delivery of human *RPE65*, driven by a CMV promoter, to *Rpe65*$^{-/-}$ mice (Dejneka et al., 2004). Gene transfer into E14 fetuses resulted in efficient transduction of the RPE, restoration of ERG signals, and measurable rhodopsin after P6. Some animals responded with nearly normal ERG amplitudes and levels of rhodopsin. A naturally occurring model of LCA2, the rd12 mouse, contains a nonsense mutation in the *Rpe65* gene rendering the enzyme dysfunctional (Pang et al., 2005). As was noted in *Rpe65*$^{-/-}$ mice, rd12 mice have profoundly diminished rod ERGs, an absence of 11-*cis*-retinaldehyde and rhodopsin, massive accumulation of retinyl esters in the RPE, and slow photoreceptor degeneration (Pang et al., 2005). Subretinal treatment of P14 mice with a serotype 5 vector containing human *RPE65* cDNA, driven by the CBA promoter, resulted in RPE65 expression only in RPE cells, restoration of 11-*cis*-retinaldehyde, the presence of substantial levels of rhodopsin, and near normal rod and cone ERG amplitudes (Pang et al., 2006). Retinyl ester levels were also reduced to normal, and related to this, funduscopy and retinal morphology remained normal. All parameters of restored retinal health remained stable for at least 7 months. Perhaps most important, visually cued behavioral tests revealed that mice treated in only one eye performed as well as normal, wild-type mice. These results confirm that gene therapy can restore normal vision-dependent behavior in a congenitally blind animal. The promising results obtained in both LCA2 mouse models and the earlier Briard dog results (Acland et al., 2001), coupled with the preclinical safety studies done in rat, dog, and nonhuman primate, have laid the groundwork for upcoming clinical trials for LCA2, likely the first AAV human gene therapy trial in the eye (Jacobson et al., 2006a, 2006b).

A third mouse model of LCA is the retinitis pigmentosa GTPase regulator interacting protein (*Rpgrip*) knockout mouse (Hong et al., 2000). RPGRIP is a protein located in the ciliary axoneme of rod and cone photoreceptors (Hong et al., 2000, 2003) that serves to tether retinitis pigmentosa GTPase regulator (RPGR) to this structure (Zhao et al., 2003). In turn, RPGR is proposed to play a role in regulating protein transport through the connecting cilium of photoreceptors to outer segments (Hong et al., 2000). *Rpgrip*$^{-/-}$ mice display photoreceptor degeneration beginning at P15, as well as early-onset loss of ERG signals. AAV2-mediated delivery of RPGRIP driven by a 236 bp (−218/+17) mOP promoter and delivered to the subretinal space of P18–P20 *Rpgrip*$^{-/-}$ mice resulted in RPGRIP localized normally to the connecting cilium, photoreceptor preservation, and ERG recovery (Pawlyk et al., 2005).

Lysosomal storage disease. Lysosomes are responsible for the breakdown of intracellular macromolecules and are characterized by the nature of the material stored within. Defects in the enzymes that degrade lysosomal contents can lead to inability to turn over lysosomal material, resulting in a broad spectrum of more than 40 clinical disorders, two of which are mucopolysaccharidosis type VII (MPS VII) and infantile neuronal ceroid lipofuscinosis (INCL).

MPS VII is a member of a group of diseases caused by deficiencies in enzymes responsible for the breakdown of glycosaminoglycans (GAGs). MPS VII is caused by a deficiency in the enzyme β-glucuronidase (Sly et al., 1973) and leads to progressive RD and vision impairment. MPS VII mice lack β-glucuronidase activity due to a single base pair deletion in *Gusb* (Birkenmeier et al., 1989; Sands and Birkenmeier, 1993) and display progressive shortening of photoreceptor outer segments, apoptotic photoreceptor death, accumulation of lysosomal storage bodies in the RPE, and diminished ERG amplitudes (Birkenmeier et al., 1989; Lazarus et al., 1993; Ohlemiller et al., 2000; Birkenmeier et al., 1991; Stramm et al., 1990). AAV2 was used to deliver *GUSB*, driven by the CBA promoter, to the intravitreal space of 4-week-old MPS VII mice. At 16 weeks of age, vector-treated eyes had near normal levels of β-glucuronidase, preservation of cells in the outer nuclear layer, decreased RPE lysosomal storage, and significantly improved rod ERGs (Hennig et al., 2004). A similar vector administered systemically to newborn MPS VII mice prior to the initiation of disease resulted in almost complete ERG protection (Daly et al., 1999a, 1999b, 2001).

A second lysosomal storage disease having an ocular pathology is INCL, a neurodegenerative disorder described as the earliest onset form of Batten disease. INCL is caused by mutations in the palmitoyl protein thioesterase-1 gene (*PPT1*), a lysosomal hydrolase that is trafficked to the lysosome via the mannose-6-phosphate receptor (Vesa et al., 1995; Sleat et al., 1996). A *Ppt1* knockout mouse model of INCL displays significant rod and cone ERG deficits as early as 2 months of age, as well as progressive RD relative to congenic controls (Gupta et al., 2001; Griffey et al., 2005). Intravitreal delivery of AAV2 carrying human *PPT1* driven by the CMV promoter into P18–P21 PPT$^{-/-}$ mice resulted in increased PPT1 expression, significant improvements in rod and cone ERGs, and a slower rate of degeneration relative to that in untreated controls (Griffey et al., 2005). It is likely that use of an AAV5 vector or subretinal injection may increase the amount of PPT1 expression in photoreceptors and lead to improved histopathological protection.

Achromatopsia. Achromatopsia, also known as rod monochromatism, is an early-onset form of severe color blindness that results from defects in cone photoreceptors. A mouse model of recessive achromatopsia was found by ERG screening in the mouse strain collection at the Jackson Laboratory. The mutation, termed cpfl3, for cone photoreceptor function loss-3, was mapped to mouse chromosome 3, the same location as human *GNAT2* (Chang et al., 2006). *GNAT2* encodes the α subunit of cone transducin, the G protein involved in phototransduction, and, when mutated in the Cpfl3 mouse, renders the G protein nonfunctional. As a result, cone photoreceptors are unable to sustain the phototransduction cascade in response to light, leading to a very weak photopic cone response at 3 weeks of age that is lost by 9 weeks (Chang et al., 2006). Rod ERG responses are initially normal but also diminish somewhat with age. Cone transducin α immunolabeling was minimally detectable and was accompanied by some photoreceptor outer segment disorganization. Subretinal injection of AAV5 containing *Gnat2* cDNA driven by a cone-targeting PR2.1 promoter partially preserved retinal structure, completely restored photopic cone responses, and restored visual acuity to near normal (Alexander et al., 2007). These studies, which targeted transgene expression specifically to cones, hold promise for analogous cone therapy in other models of achromatopsia, as well as for other cone-targeted retinal diseases.

Neurotrophic factor gene therapy. Neurotrophic cell survival factors have shown promise in preserving photoreceptor cells from apoptosis, the common fate of photoreceptors in many RT diseases. In surveys of neurotrophic factors injected directly into the vitreous of various rodent models of photoreceptor degeneration, a number have been shown to promote photoreceptor survival (Faktorovich et al., 1990; LaVail et al., 1992, 1998). AAV-mediated delivery of cDNAs for such factors is an attractive option that would not require multiple injections and could supplement gene replacement therapies. AAV2-mediated delivery of ciliary neurotrophic factor (CNTF) has been evaluated in several mouse models of RD, including the rhodopsin knockout mouse ($Rho^{-/-}$), the peripherin knockout ($Prph^{Rd2/Rd2}$) mouse, and a heterozygous *Prph2* mouse with a transgenic copy of the P216L mutant *Prph2* allele ($rds^{+/-P216L}$) (Liang et al., 2001a, 2001b; Bok et al., 2002; Schlichenbrede et al., 2003; Buch et al., 2006). All studies showed that vectored CNTF expression promotes photoreceptor survival. Although not evaluated in the $Rho^{-/-}$ mouse (Liang et al., 2001a), in both $Prph2^{Rd2/Rd2}$ and $rds^{+/-P216L}$ mice, photoreceptor function, as evaluated by ERG, was either not improved or reduced in vector injected eyes relative to untreated controls (Bok et al., 2002; Schlichenbrede et al., 2003; Buch et al., 2006). This treatment-related loss in photoreceptor function also appeared to be dose dependent and occurred in normal eyes as well (Bok et al., 2002; Buch et al., 2006). Additionally, in the $Prph2^{Rd2/Rd2}$ mouse, when AAV-mediated CNTF expression was supplemented with either AAV2-*Prph2* or AAV2-*rhodopsin*, there was still no improvement relative to untreated control eyes. Taken together, these results suggest that CNTF dosing may be crucial to avoid any negative effects of the neurotrophin (Schlichenbrede et al., 2003). Indeed, in a recent study, AAV-mediated CNTF expression was found to be deleterious to photoreceptor function in wild-type, C57BL6, mice (Rhee et al., 2007). What remains to be determined is the dosage of CNTF delivered in vivo by AAV vectors relative to that expected in a clinical trial, and to what extent toxicity seen in one species, the mouse, can be carried over into the human.

In contrast, AAV-mediated glial cell line–derived neurotrophic factor (GDNF) expression driven by the CBA promoter in the $Prph2^{Rd2/Rd2}$ mouse slowed photoreceptor loss and, more importantly, did not have the adverse effects on photoreceptor function that were seen with CNTF. In addition, when used in combination with the appropriate gene replacement therapy, enhanced photoreceptor function was observed (Buch et al., 2006).

Conclusions and future directions for adenoassociated virus gene therapy in the mouse retina

A large body of evidence supports the use of AAV as an effective vector for gene delivery to the mouse retina. Optimization of gene therapy strategies, as well as the development of new mouse models of human retinal disease, suggests that appropriately designed AAV-mediated gene therapy may eventually be applied broadly to human subjects. Current research is focusing on mouse models that are more "human-like" and therefore may address the species differences between man and mouse. One such study is the development of the neural retina leucine zipper knockout ($Nrl^{-/-}$) mouse. As determined by structural and functional characteristics, the $Nrl^{-/-}$ mouse, in contrast to the normal rod-dominant mouse retina, contains an all cone-like retina (Daniele et al., 2005). This mouse may be a better rodent model of the cone-rich human macula, suggesting that subjecting the $Nrl^{-/-}$ mouse to ROP conditioning or laser-induced CNV, for example, may provide a better model for central field loss in neovascular disorders such as diabetic retinopathy and AMD. Additionally, crossing the $Nrl^{-/-}$ mouse with known cone degeneration models may aid in the development of more effective cone-targeted gene therapies.

Although this chapter has summarized gene replacement strategies in mouse models of RD that are predominantly inherited in an autosomal recessive fashion, progress has also been made toward addressing autosomal dominantly inherited RD. To date, most of this work has been carried out in the P23H rhodopsin rat, the primary current model for a common form of autosomal dominant retinitis pigmentosa (Dresner et al., 1998; Lewin et al., 1998; LaVail et al., 2000). A mouse model mimicking autosomal dominant macular dystrophy is the ELOVL4 mouse (Raz Praq et al., 2006; Vasireddy et al., 2006), which contains a heterozygous knock-in carrying the same 5 bp deletion in the *ELOVL4* gene associated with dominant Stargardtlike macular degeneration (STGD3) in humans. The ELOVL4 mouse has a retinal phenotype similar to STGD3 patients (Vasireddy et al., 2006), and attempts are currently under way to mediate the mouse disease using AAV vectors.

Another recent advance in the field of AAV gene delivery is the development of self-complementary AAV vectors (scAAV), which package double-stranded DNA in the viral capsid, in contrast to single-stranded DNA in standard AAV vectors. This modification overcomes the rate-limiting step for AAV-vectored transgene expression, the conversion of vector single-stranded DNA into double-stranded DNA by the host cell (McCarty et al., 2001, 2003). Studies have shown that scAAV mediates quicker and more efficient transgene expression than standard AAV vectors in mouse brain and retina (Fu et al., 2006; Hauswirth et al., 2006). scAAV-mediated gene therapy may therefore be of use in the treatment of disorders that require immediate, high-level intervention, particularly for some very rapidly degenerating mouse models of retinal disease.

In summary, based on a broad variety of successfully treated mouse models of retinal RD, the clinical future for AAV-vectored gene therapy seems bright.

REFERENCES

Acland, G. M., Aguirre, G. D., Bennett, J., Aleman, T. S., Cideciyan, A. V., Bennicelli, J., Dejneka, N. S., Pearce-Kelling, S. E., Maguire, A. M., et al. (2005). Long-term restoration of rod and cone vision by single dose rAAV-mediated gene transfer to the retina in a canine model of childhood blindness. *Mol. Ther.* 12:1072–1082.

Acland, G. M., Aguirre, G. D., Ray, J., Zhang, Q., Aleman, T. S., Cideciyan, A. V., Pearce-Kelling, S. E., Anand, V., Zeng, Y., et al. (2001). Gene therapy restores vision in a canine model of childhood blindness. *Nat. Genet.* 28:92–95.

Adamis, A. P., Miller, J. W., Bernal, M. T., D'Amico, D. J., Folkman, J., Yeo, T. K., and Yeo, K. T. (1994). Increased vascular endothelial growth factor levels in the vitreous of eyes with proliferative diabetic retinopathy. *Am. J. Ophthalmol.* 118:445–450.

Aiello, L. P., Avery, R. L., Arrigg, P. G., Keyt, B. A., Jampel, H. D., Shah, S. T., Pasquale, L. R., Thieme, H., Iwamoto, M. A., et al. (1994). Vascular endothelial growth factor in ocular fluid of patients with diabetic retinopathy and other retinal disorders. *N. Engl. J. Med.* 331:1480–1487.

Aiello, L. P., Pierce, E. A., Foley, E. D., Takagi, H., Chen, H., Riddle, L., Ferrara, N., King, G. L., and Smith, L. E. (1995). Suppression of retinal neovascularization in vivo by inhibition of vascular endothelial growth factor (VEGF) using soluble VEGF-receptor chimeric proteins. *Proc. Natl. Acad. Sci. U.S.A.* 92: 10457–10461.

Alexander, J. J., Li, Q., Timmers, A., Hawes, N., Chang, B., and Hauswirth, W. W. (2005). Restoration of cone function in a mouse model of achromatopsia by rAAV mediated promoter targeted expression of cone specific α-transducin. *Invest. Ophthalmol. Vis. Sci.* 46. ARVO E-Abstract 5207.

Alexander, J. J., Umino, Y., Everhart, D., Chang, B., Min, S. H., Li, Q., Timmers, A. M., Hawes, N. L., Pang, J. J., et al. (2007). Restoration of cone function in a mouse model of achromatopsia. *Nat. Med.* May 21 (Epub ahead of print).

Ali, R. R., Reichel, M. B., De Alwis, M., Kanuga, N., Kinnon, C., Levinsky, R. J., Hunt, D. M., Bhattacharya, S. S., and Thrasher, A. J. (1998). Adeno-associated virus gene transfer to mouse retina. *Hum. Gene Ther.* 9:81–86.

Ali, R. R., Sarra, G. M., Stephens, C., Alwis, M. D., Bainbridge, J. W., Munro, P. M., Fauser, S., Reichel, M. B., Kinnon, C., et al. (2000). Restoration of photoreceptor ultrastructure and function in retinal degeneration slow mice by gene therapy. *Nat. Genet.* 25:306–310.

Anand-Apte, B., Pepper, M. S., Voest, E., Montesano, R., Olsen, B., Murphy, G., Apte, S. S., and Zetter, B. (1997). Inhibition of angiogenesis by tissue inhibitor of metalloproteinase-3. *Invest. Ophthalmol. Vis. Sci.* 38:817–823.

Auricchio, A., Behling, K. C., Maguire, A. M., O'Connor, E. M., Bennett, J., Wilson, J. M., and Tolentino, M. J. (2002). Inhibition of retinal neovascularization by intraocular viral-mediated delivery of anti-angiogenic agents. *Mol. Ther.* 6:490–494.

Auricchio, A., Kobinger, G., Anand, V., Hildinger, M., O'Connor, E., Maguire, A. M., Wilson, J. M., and Bennett, J. (2001). Exchange of surface proteins impacts on viral vector cellular specificity and transduction characteristics: The retina as a model. *Hum. Mol. Genet.* 10:3075–3081.

Auricchio, A., Rivera, V. M., Clackson, T., O'Connor, E. E., Maguire, A. M., Tolentino, M. J., Bennett, J., and Wilson, J. M. (2002). Pharmacological regulation of protein expression from adeno-associated viral vectors in the eye. *Mol. Ther.* 6: 238–242.

Bainbridge, J. W., Mistry, A., De Alwis, M., Paleolog, E., Baker, A., Thrasher, A. J., and Ali, R. R. (2002). Inhibition of retinal neovascularisation by gene transfer of soluble VEGF receptor sFlt-1. *Gene Ther.* 9:320–326.

Baumgartner, S., Hofmann, K., Chiquet-Ehrismann, R., and Bucher, P. (1998). The discoidin domain family revisited: New members from prokaryotes and a homology-based fold prediction. *Protein Sci.* 7:1626–1631.

Bennett, J., Duan, D., Engelhardt, J. F., and Maguire, A. M. (1997). Real-time, noninvasive in vivo assessment of adeno-associated virus-mediated retinal transduction. *Invest. Ophthalmol. Vis. Sci.* 38:2857–2863.

Birkenmeier, E. H., Barker, J. E., Vogler, C. A., Kyle, J. W., Sly, W. S., Gwynn, B., Levy, B., and Pegors, C. (1991). Increased life span and correction of metabolic defects in murine mucopolysaccharidosis type VII after syngeneic bone marrow transplantation. *Blood* 78:3081–3092.

Birkenmeier, E. H., Davisson, M. T., Beamer, W. G., Ganschow, R. E., Vogler, C. A., Gwynn, B., Lyford, K. A., Maltais, L. M., and Wawrzyniak, C. J. (1989). Murine mucopolysaccharidosis type VII: Characterization of a mouse with beta-glucuronidase deficiency. *J. Clin. Invest.* 83:1258–1266.

Bok, D., Yasumura, D., Matthes, M. T., Ruiz, A., Duncan, J. L., Chappelow, A. V., Zolutukhin, S., Hauswirth, W., and LaVail, M. M. (2002). Effects of adeno-associated virus-vectored ciliary neurotrophic factor on retinal structure and function in mice with a P216L rds/peripherin mutation. *Exp. Eye Res.* 74:719–735.

Boulanger, A., Liu, S., Henningsgaard, A. A., Yu, S., and Redmond, T. M. (2000). The upstream region of the Rpe65 gene confers retinal pigment epithelium-specific expression in vivo and in vitro and contains critical octamer and E-box binding sites. *J. Biol. Chem.* 275:31274–31282.

Boulanger, A., and Redmond, T. M. (2002). Expression and promoter activation of the Rpe65 gene in retinal pigment epithelium cell lines. *Curr. Eye Res.* 24:368–375.

Buch, P. K., MacLaren, R. E., Duran, Y., Balaggan, K. S., MacNeil, A., Schlichtenbrede, F. C., Smith, A. J., and Ali, R. R. (2006). In contrast to AAV-mediated cntf expression, AAV-mediated Gdnf expression enhances gene replacement therapy in rodent models of retinal degeneration. *Mol. Ther.* 14:700–709.

Chang, B., Dacey, M. S., Hawes, N. L., Hitchcock, P. F., Milam, A. H., Atmaca-Sonmez, P., Nusinowitz, S., and Heckenlively,

J. R. (2006). Cone photoreceptor function loss-3, a novel mouse model of achromatopsia due to a mutation in Gnat2. *Invest. Ophthalmol. Vis. Sci.* 47:5017–5021.

Chang, G. Q., Hao, Y., and Wong, F. (1993). Apoptosis: Final common pathway of photoreceptor death in rd, rds, and rhodopsin mutant mice. *Neuron* 11:595–605.

Coleman, J. E., Zhang, Y., Brown, G. A., and Semple-Rowland, S. L. (2004). Cone cell survival and downregulation of GCAP1 protein in the retinas of GC1 knockout mice. *Invest. Ophthalmol. Vis. Sci.* 45:3397–3403.

Daly, T. M., Ohlemiller, K. K., Roberts, M. S., Vogler, C. A., and Sands, M. (2001). Prevention of systemic clinical disease in MPS VII mice following AAV-mediated neonatal gene transfer. *Gene Ther.* 8:1291–1298.

Daly, T. M., Okuyama, T., Vogler, C., Haskins, M. E., Muzyczka, N., and Sands, M. (1999a). Neonatal intramuscular injection with recombinant adeno-associated virus results in prolonged β-glucuronidase expression in situ and correction of liver pathology in mucopolysaccharidosis type VII mice. *Hum. Gene Ther.* 10:85–94.

Daly, T. M., Vogler, C., Levy, B., Haskina, M. E., and Sands, M. S. (1999b). Neonatal gene transfer leads to widespread correction of pathology in a murine model of lysosomal storage disease. *Proc. Natl. Acad. Sci. U.S.A.* 96:2296–2300.

Daniele, L. L., Lillo, C., Lyubarsky, A. L., Nikonov, S. S., Philp, N., Mears, A. J., Swaroop, A., Williams, D. S., and Pugh, E. N., Jr. (2005). Cone-like morphological, molecular, and electrophysiological features of the photoreceptors of the Nrl knockout mouse. *Invest. Ophthalmol. Vis. Sci.* 46:2156–2167.

Dejneka, N. S., Surace, E. M., Aleman, T. S., Cideciyan, A. V., Lyubarsky, A., Savchenko, A., Redmond, T. M., Tang, W., Wei, Z., et al. (2004). In utero gene therapy rescues vision in a murine model of congenital blindness. *Mol. Ther.* 9:182–188.

Deng, W. T., Yan, Z., Dinculescu, A., Pang, J., Teusner, J. T., Cortez, N. G., Berns, K. I., and Hauswirth, W. W. (2005). Adeno-associated virus-mediated expression of vascular endothelial growth factor peptides inhibits retinal neovascularization in a mouse model of oxygen-induced retinopathy. *Hum. Gene Ther.* 16:1247–1254.

De Vries, C., Escobedo, J. A., Ueno, H., Houck, K., Ferrara, N., and Williams, L. T. (1992). The fms-like tyrosine kinase, a receptor for vascular endothelial growth factor. *Science* 255: 989–991.

Drenser, K. A., Timmers, A. M., Hauswirth, W. W., and Lewin, A. S. (1998). Ribozyme-targeted destruction of RNA associated with autosomal-dominant retinitis pigmentosa. *Invest. Ophthalmol. Vis. Sci.* 39:681–689.

Dryja, T. P., Adams, S. M., Grimsby, J. L., McGee, T. L., Hong, D. H., Li, T., Andreasson, S., and Berson, E. L. (2001). Null RPGRIP1 alleles in patients with Leber congenital amaurosis. *Am. J. Hum. Genet.* 68:1295–1298.

Duan, D., Yue, Y., and Engelhardt, J. F. (2003). Consequences of DNA-dependent protein kinase catalytic subunit deficiency on recombinant adeno-associated virus genome circularization and heterodimerization in muscle tissue. *J. Virol.* 77:4751–4759.

Dudus, L., Anand, V., Acland, G. M., Chen, S. J., Wilson, J. M., Fisher, K. J., Maguire, A. M., and Bennett, J. (1999). Persistent transgene product in retina, optic nerve and brain after intraocular injection of rAAV. *Vision Res.* 39:2545–2553.

Esumi, N., Kachi, S., Campochiaro, P. A., and Zack, D. J. (2007). VMD2 promoter requires two proximal E-box sites for its activity in vivo and is regulated by the MITF-TFE family. *J. Biol. Chem.* 282:1838–1850.

Esumi, N., Oshima, Y., Li, Y., Campochiaro, P. A., and Zack, D. J. (2004). Analysis of the VMD2 promoter and implication of E-box binding factors in its regulation. *J. Biol. Chem.* 30: 19064–19073.

Faktorovich, E. G., Steinberg, R. H., Yasumura, D., Matthes, M. T., and LaVail, M. M. (1990). Photoreceptor degeneration in inherited retinal dystrophy delayed by basic fibroblast growth factor. *Nature* 347:83–86.

Flannery, J. G., Zolotukhin, S., Vaquero, M. I., LaVail, M. M., Muzyczka, N., and Hauswirth, W. W. (1997). Efficient photoreceptor-targeted gene expression in vivo by recombinant adeno-associated virus. *Proc. Natl. Acad. Sci. U.S.A.* 94:6916–6921.

Flotte, T. R. (2005). Recent developments in recombinant AAV-mediated gene therapy for lung diseases. *Curr. Gene Ther.* 5(3):361–366.

Flotte, T. R., and Berns, K. I. (2005). Adeno-associated virus: A ubiquitous commensal of mammals. *Hum. Gene Ther.* 16:401–407.

Flotte, T. R., Ng, P., Dylla, D. E., McCray, P. B., Jr, Wang, G., Kolls, J. K., and Hu, J. (2007). Viral vector-mediated and cell-based therapies for treatment of cystic fibrosis. *Mol. Ther.* 15(2):229–241.

Fu, H., Muenzer, J., Samulski, R. J., Breese, G., Sifford, J., Zeng, X., and McCarty, D. M. (2003). Self-complementary adeno-associated virus serotype 2 vector: Global distribution and broad dispersion of AAV-mediated transgene expression in mouse brain. *Mol. Ther.* 8:911–917.

Gao, G., Vandenberghe, L. H., Alvira, M. R., Lu, Y., Calcedo, R., Zhou, X., and Wilson, J. M. (2004). Clades of adeno-associated viruses are widely disseminated in human tissues. *J. Virol.* 78:6381–6388.

Gerber, S., Perrault, I., Hanein, S., Barbet, F., Ducroq, D., Ghazi, I., Martin-Coignard, D., Leowski, C., Homfray, T., et al. (2001). Complete exon-intron structure of the RPGR-interacting protein (RPGRIP1) gene allows the identification of mutations underlying Leber congenital amaurosis. *Eur. J. Hum. Genet.* 9:561–571.

Gitay-Goren, H., Soker, S., Vlodavsky, I., and Neufeld, G. (1992). The binding of vascular endothelial growth factor to its receptors is dependent on cell surface-associated heparin-like molecules. *J. Biol. Chem.* 267:6093–6098.

Glushakova, L. G., and Hauswirth, W. W. (2004). Unpublished results.

Glushakova, L. G., Timmers, A. M., Issa, T. M., Cortez, N. G., Pang, J., Teusner, J. T., and Hauswirth, W. W. (2006a). Does recombinant adeno-associated virus-vectored proximal region of mouse rhodopsin promoter support only rod-type specific expression in vivo? *Mol. Vis.* 12:298–309.

Glushakova, L. G., Timmers, A. M., Pang, J., Teusner, J. T., and Hauswirth, W. W. (2006b). Human blue-opsin promoter preferentially targets reporter gene expression to rat s-cone photoreceptors. *Invest. Ophthalmol. Vis. Sci.* 47:3505–3513.

Gregory-Evans, K., and Bhattacharya, S. S. (1998). Genetic blindness: Current concepts in the pathogenesis of human outer retinal dystrophies. *Trends Genet.* 14:103–108.

Griesenbach, U., Geddes, D. M., and Alton, E. W. (2006). Gene therapy progress and prospects: Cystic fibrosis. *Gene Ther.* 13 (14):1061–1067.

Griffey, M., Macauley, S. L., Ogilvie, J. M., and Sands, M. S. (2005). AAV2-mediated ocular gene therapy for infantile neuronal ceroid lipofuscinosis. *Mol. Ther.* 12:413–421.

Gupta, P., Soyombo, A. A., Atashband, A., Wisniewski, K. E., Shelton, J. M., Richardson, J. A., Hammer, R. E., and Hofmann, S. L. (2001). Disruption of PPT1 or PPT2 causes neuronal ceroid lipofuscinosis in knockout mice. *Proc. Natl. Acad. Sci. U.S.A.* 98:13566–13571.

Haire, S. E., Pang, J., Boye, S. L., Sokal, I., Craft, C. M., Palczewski, K., Hauswirth, W. W., and Semple-Rowland, S. L. (2006). Light-driven cone arrestin translocation in cones of postnatal guanylate cyclase-1 knockout mouse retina treated with AAV-GC1. *Invest. Ophthalmol. Vis. Sci.* 47:3745–3753.

Hauswirth, W. W., Petrs-Silva, H., Min, S-H., Liu, J. M., Mani, S., Chiodo, V. A., Ding, M., Linden, R., and Boye, S. L. (2006). Self-complementary AAV vectors promote fast and efficient transduction of mouse retina. *Invest. Ophthalmol. Vis. Sci.* 47. E-Abstract 838.

Hennig, A. K., Ogilvie, J. M., Ohlemiller, K. K., Timmers, A. M., Hauswirth, W. W., and Sands, M. S. (2004). AAV-mediated intravitreal gene therapy reduces lysosomal storage in the retinal pigmented epithelium and improves retinal function in adult MPS VII mice. *Mol. Ther.* 10:106–116.

Hong, D. H., Pawlyk, B., Shang, J., Sandberg, M. A., Berson, E. L., and Li, T. (2000). A retinitis pigmentosa GTPase regulator (RPGR)-deficient mouse model for X-linked retinitis pigmentosa (RP3). *Proc. Natl. Acad. Sci. U.S.A.* 97:3649–3654.

Hong, D. H., Pawlyk, B., Sokolov, M., Strissel, K. J., Yang, J., Tulloch, B., Wright, A. F., Arshavsky, V. Y., and Li, T. (2003). RPGR isoforms in photoreceptor connecting cilia and the transitional zone of motile cilia. *Invest. Ophthalmol. Vis. Sci.* 44:2413–2421.

Jacobson, S. G., Acland, G. M., Aguirre, G. D., Aleman, T. S., Schwartz, S. B., Cideciyan, A. V., Zeiss, C. J., Komaromy, A. M., Kaushal, S., et al. (2006a). Safety of recombinant adeno-associated virus type 2-RPE65 vector delivered by ocular subretinal injection. *Mol. Ther.* 13:1074–1084.

Jacobson, S. G., Boye, S. L., Aleman, T. S., Conlon, T. J., Zeiss, C. J., Roman, A. J., Cideciyan, A. V., Schwartz, S. B., Komaromy, A. M., et al. (2006b). Safety in nonhuman primates of ocular AAV2-RPE65, a candidate treatment for blindness in Leber congenital amaurosis. *Hum. Gene Ther.* 17:845–858.

Jakeman, L. B., Winer, J., Bennett, G. L., Altar, C. A., and Ferrara, N. (1992). Binding sites for vascular endothelial growth factor are localized on endothelial cells in adult rat tissues. *J. Clin. Invest.* 89:244–253.

Jia, H., Jezequel, S., Lohr, M., Shaikh, S., Davis, D., Soker, S., Selwood, D., and Zachary, I. (2001). Peptides encoded by exon 6 of VEGF inhibit endothelial cell biological responses and angiogenesis induced by VEGF. *Biochem. Biophys. Res. Commun.* 283:164–173.

Lauramore, M. (2004). Retinal cell tropism of adeno-associated viral (AAV) vector serotypes. Master's thesis, University of Florida, Gainesville. Available: http://etd.fcla.edu/UF/UFE0005301/lauramore_a.pdf.

LaVail, M. M., Unoki, K., Yasumura, D., Matthes, M. T., Yancopoulos, G. D., and Steinberg, R. H. (1992). Multiple growth factors, cytokines, and neurotrophins rescue photoreceptors from the damaging effects of constant light. *Proc. Natl. Acad. Sci. U.S.A.* 89:11249–11253.

LaVail, M. M., Yasumura, D., Matthes, M. T., Drenser, K. A., Flannery, J. G., Lewin, A. S., and Hauswirth, W. W. (2000). Ribozyme rescue of photoreceptor cells in P23H transgenic rats: Long-term survival and late-stage therapy. *Proc. Natl. Acad. Sci. U.S.A.* 97:11488–11493.

LaVail, M. M., Yasumura, D., Matthes, M. T., Lau-Villacorta, C., Unoki, K., Sung, C. H., and Steinberg, R. H. (1998). Protection of mouse photoreceptors by survival factors in retinal degenerations. *Invest. Ophthalmol. Vis. Sci.* 39:592–602.

Lazarus, H. S., Sly, W. S., Kyle, J. W., and Hageman, G. S. (1993). Photoreceptor degeneration and altered distribution of interphotoreceptor matrix proteoglycans in the mucopolysaccharidosis VII mouse. *Exp. Eye Res.* 56:531–541.

Lewin, A. S., Drenser, K. A., Hauswirth, W. W., Nishikawa, S., Yasumura, D., Flannery, J. G., and LaVail, M. M. (1998). Ribozyme rescue of photoreceptor cells in a transgenic rat model of autosomal dominant retinitis pigmentosa. *Nat. Med.* 4:967–971.

Liang, F. Q., Aleman, T. S., Dejneka, N. S., Dudus, L., Fisher, K. J., Maguire, A. M., Jacobson, S. G., and Bennett, J. (2001a). Long-term protection of retinal structure but not function using RAAV.CNTF in animal models of retinitis pigmentosa. *Mol. Ther.* 4:461–472.

Liang, F. Q., Dejneka, N. S., Cohen, D. R., Krasnoperova, N. V., Lem, J., Maguire, A. M., Dudus, L., Fisher, K. J., and Bennett, J. (2001b). AAV-mediated delivery of ciliary neurotrophic factor prolongs photoreceptor survival in the rhodopsin knockout mouse. *Mol. Ther.* 3:241–248.

Mah, C., Qing, K., Khuntirat, B., Ponnazhagan, S., Wang, X. S., Kube, D. M., Yoder, M. C., and Srivastava, A. (1998). Adeno-associated virus type 2–mediated gene transfer: Role of epidermal growth factor receptor protein tyrosine kinase in transgene expression. *J. Virol.* 72(12):9835–9843.

Marlhens, F., Griffoin, J. M., Bareil, C., Arnaud, B., Claustres, M., and Hamel, C. P. (1998). Autosomal recessive retinal dystrophy associated with two novel mutations in the RPE65 gene. *Eur. J. Hum. Genet.* 6:527–531.

Martin, K. R., Quigley, H. A., Zack, D. J., Levkovitch-Verbin, H., Kielczewski, J., Valenta, D., Baumrind, L., Pease, M. E., Klein, R. L., et al. (2003). Gene therapy with brain-derived neurotrophic factor as a protection: Retinal ganglion cells in a rat glaucoma model. *Invest. Ophthalmol. Vis. Sci.* 44:4357–4365.

Mata, N. L., Moghrabi, W. N., Lee, J. S., Bui, T. V., Radu, R. A., Horwitz, J., and Travis, G. H. (2004). Rpe65 is a retinyl ester binding protein that presents insoluble substrate to the isomerase in retinal pigment epithelial cells. *J. Biol. Chem.* 279(1):635–643.

McCarty, D. M., Fu, H., Monahan, P. E., Toulson, C. E., Naik, P., and Samulski, R. J. (2003). Adeno-associated virus terminal repeat (TR) mutant generates self-complementary vectors to overcome the rate-limiting step to transduction in vivo. *Gene Ther.* 10:2112–2118.

McCarty, D. M., Monahan, P. E., and Samulski, R. J. (2001). Self-complementary recombinant adeno-associated virus (scAAV) vectors promote efficient transduction independently of DNA synthesis. *Gene Ther.* 8:1248–1254.

McGee Sanftner, L. H., Rendahl, K. G., Quiroz, D., Coyne, M., Ladner, M., Manning, W. C., and Flannery, J. G. (2001). Recombinant AAV-mediated delivery of a tet-inducible reporter gene to the rat retina. *Mol. Ther.* 3:688–696.

Miller, J. W., Adamis, A. P., Shima, D. T., D'Amore, P. A., Moulton, R. S., O'Reilley, M. S., Folkman J., Dvorak, H. F., Brown, L. F., et al. (1994). Vascular endothelial growth factor/vascular permeability factor is temporally and spatially correlated with ocular angiogenesis in a primate model. *Am. J. Pathol.* 145:574–584.

Miller, D. G., Petek, L. M., and Russell, D. W. (2004). Adeno-associated virus vectors integrate at chromosome breakage sites. *Nat. Genet.* 36:767–773.

Miller, H., Miller, B., Ishibashi, T., and Ryan, S. J. (1990). Pathogenesis of laser-induced choroidal subretinal neovascularization. *Invest. Ophthalmol. Vis. Sci.* 31:899–908.

Min, S. H., Molday, L. L., Seeliger, M. W., Dinculescu, A., Timmers, A. M., Janssen, A., Tonagel, F., Tanimoto, N., Weber, B. H., et al. (2005). Prolonged recovery of retinal structure/function after gene therapy in an Rs1h-deficient mouse model of X-linked juvenile retinoschisis. *Mol. Ther.* 12:644–651.

Moiseyev, G., Chen, Y., Takahashi, Y., Wu, B. X., and Ma, J. X. (2005). RPE65 is the isomerohydrolase in the retinoid visual cycle. *Proc. Natl. Acad. Sci. U.S.A.* 102:12413–12418.

Molday, L. L., Hicks, D., Sauer, C. G., Weber, B. H., and Molday, R. S. (2001). Expression of X-linked retinoschisis protein RS1 in photoreceptor and bipolar cells. *Invest. Ophthalmol. Vis. Sci.* 42:816–825.

Molday, R. S. (1994). Peripherin/rds and rom-1: Molecular properties and role in photoreceptor cell degeneration. *Prog. Retin. Eye Res.* 271–299.

Mori, K., Ando, A., Gehlbach, P., Nesbitt, D., Takahashi, K., Goldsteen, D., Penn, M., Chen, C. T., Mori, K., et al. (2001). Inhibition of choroidal neovascularization by intravenous injection of adenoviral vectors expressing secretable endostatin. *Am. J. Pathol.* 159:313–320.

Mori, K., Gehlbach, P., Yamamoto, S., Duh, E., Zack, D. J., Li, Q., Berns, K. I., Raisler, B. J., Hauswirth, W. W., et al. (2002). AAV-mediated gene transfer of pigment epithelium–derived factor inhibits choroidal neovascularization. *Invest. Ophthalmol. Vis. Sci.* 43:1994–2000.

Nir, I., Agarwal, N., and Papermaster, D. S. (1990). Opsin gene expression during early and late phases of retinal degeneration in rds mice. *Exp. Eye Res.* 51:257–267.

Ohlemiller, K. K., Vogler, C. A., Roberts, M., Galvin, N., and Sands, M. S. (2000). Retinal function is improved in a murine model of a lysosomal storage disease following bone marrow transplantation. *Exp. Eye Res.* 71:469–481.

O'Reilly, M. S., Boehm, T., Shing, Y., Fukai, N., Vasios, G., Lane, W. S., Flynn, E., Birkhead, J. R., Olsen, B. R., et al. (1997). Endostatin: An endogenous inhibitor of angiogenesis and tumor growth. *Cell* 88:277–285.

O'Reilly, M. S., Holmgren, L., Chen, C., and Folkman, J. (1996). Angiostatin induces and sustains dormancy of human primary tumors in mice. *Nat. Med.* 2:689–692.

O'Reilly, M. S., Holmgren, L., Shing, Y., Chen, C., Rosenthal, R. A., Moses, M., Lane, W. S., Cao, Y., Sage, E. H., et al. (1994). Angiostatin: A novel angiogenesis inhibitor that mediates the suppression of metastases by a Lewis lung carcinoma. *Cell* 79:315–328.

Pang, J. J., Chang, B., Hawes, N. L., Hurd, R. E., Davisson, M. T., Li, J., Noorwez, S. M., Malhotra, R., McDowell, J. H., et al. (2005). Retinal degeneration 12 (rd12): A new, spontaneously arising mouse model for human Leber congenital amaurosis (LCA). *Mol. Vis.* 11:152–162.

Pang, J. J., Chang, B., Kumar, A., Nusinowitz, S., Noorwez, S. M., Li, J., Rani, A., Foster, T. C., Chiodo, V. A., et al. (2006). Gene therapy restores vision-dependent behavior as well as retinal structure and function in a mouse model of RPE65 Leber congenital amaurosis. *Mol. Ther.* 13:565–572.

Pawlyk, B. S., Smith, A. J., Buch, P. K., Adamian, M., Hong, D. H., Sandberg, M. A., Ali, R. R., and Li, T. (2005). Gene replacement therapy rescues photoreceptor degeneration in a murine model of Leber congenital amaurosis lacking RPGRIP. *Invest. Ophthalmol. Vis. Sci.* 46:3039–3045.

Perrault, I., Rozet, J. M., Calvas P., et al. (1996). Retinal-specific guanylate cyclase gene mutations in Leber's congenital amaurosis. *Nat. Genet.* 14:461–464.

Perrault, I., Rozet, J. M., Gerber, S., Ghazi, I., Leowski, C., Ducroq, D., Souied, E., Dufier, J. L., Munnich, A., et al. (1999). Leber congenital amaurosis. *Mol. Genet. Metab.* 68:200–208.

Pierce, E. A., Avery, R. L., Foley, E. D., Aiello, L. P., and Smith, L. E. (1995). Vascular endothelial growth factor/vascular permeability factor expression in a mouse model of retinal neovascularization. *Proc. Natl. Acad. Sci. U.S.A.* 92:905–909.

Qing, K., Khuntirat, B., Mah, C., Kube, D. M., Wang, X. S., Ponnazhagan, S., Zhou, S., Dwarki, V. J., Yoder, M. C., et al. (1998). Adeno-associated virus type 2–mediated gene transfer: Correlation of tyrosine phosphorylation of the cellular single-stranded D sequence-binding protein with transgene expression in human cells in vitro and murine tissues in vivo. *J. Virol.* 72(2):1593–1599.

Qing, K., Wang, X. S., Kube, D. M., Ponnazhagan, S., Bajpai, A., and Srivastava, A. (1997). Role of tyrosine phosphorylation of a cellular protein in adeno-associated virus 2–mediated transgene expression. *Proc. Natl. Acad. Sci. U.S.A.* 94(20):10879–10884.

Raisler, B. J., Berns, K. I., Grant, M. B., Beliaev, D., and Hauswirth, W. W. (2002). Adeno-associated virus type-2 expression of pigmented epithelium-derived factor or Kringles 1–3 of angiostatin reduce retinal neovascularization. *Proc. Natl. Acad. Sci. U.S.A.* 99:8909–8914.

Raper, S. E., Chirmule, N., Lee, F. S., Wivel, N. A., Bagg, A., Gao, G. P., Wilson, J. M., and Batshaw, M. L. (2003). Fatal systemic inflammatory response syndrome in a ornithine transcarbamylase deficient patient following adenoviral gene transfer. *Mol. Genet. Metab.* 80(1–2):148–158.

Raz-Prag, D., Ayyagari, R., Fariss, R. N., Mandal, M. N., Vasireddy, V., Majchrzak, S., Webber, A. L., Bush, R. A., Salem, N., Jr., et al. (2006). Haploinsufficiency is not the key mechanism of pathogenesis in a heterozygous Elovl4 knockout mouse model of STGD3 disease. *Invest. Ophthalmol. Vis. Sci.* 47:3603–3611.

Redmond, T. M., Yu, S., Lee, E., Bok, D., Hamasaki, D., Chen, N., Goletz, P., Ma, J. X., Crouch, R. K., et al. (1998). Rpe65 is necessary for production of 11-*cis*-vitamin A in the retinal visual cycle. *Nat. Genet.* 20:344–351.

Reich, S. J., Fosnot, J., Kuroki, A., Tang, W., Yang, X., Maguire, A. M., Bennett, J., and Tolentino, M. J. (2003). Small interfering RNA (siRNA) targeting VEGF effectively inhibits ocular neovascularization in a mouse model. *Mol. Vis.* 9:210–216.

Reid, S. N., Yamashita, C., and Farber, D. B. (2003). Retinoschisin, a photoreceptor-secreted protein, and its interaction with bipolar and muller cells. *J. Neurosci.* 23:6030–6040.

Reuter, J. H., and Sanyal, S. (1984). Development and degeneration of retina in rds mutant mice: The electroretinogram. *Neurosci. Lett.* 48:231–237.

Rhee, K. D., Ruiz, A., Duncan, J. L., Hauswirth, W. W., LaVail, M. M., Bok, D., and Yang, X. J. (2007). Molecular and cellular alterations induced by chronic expression of ciliary neurotrophic factor in a mouse model of retinitis pigmentosa. *Invest. Ophthalmol. Vis. Sci.* 48:1389–1400.

Robinson, G. S., Pierce, E. A., Rook, S. L., Foley, E., Webb, R., and Smith, L. E. (1996). Oligodeoxynucleotides inhibit retinal neovascularization in a murine model of proliferative retinopathy. *Proc. Natl. Acad. Sci. U.S.A.* 93:4851–4856.

Ryan, S. J. (1982). Subretinal neovascularization: Natural history of an experimental model. *Arch. Ophthalmol.* 100(11):1804–1809.

Sands, M. S., and Birkenmeier, E. H. (1993). A single-base-pair deletion in the beta-glucuronidase gene accounts for the phenotype of murine mucopolysaccharidosis type VII. *Proc. Natl. Acad. Sci. U.S.A.* 90:6567–6571.

Sanyal, S., and Jansen, H. G. (1981). Absence of receptor outer segments in the retina of rds mutant mice. *Neurosci. Lett.* 21:23–26.

Sarra, G. M., Stephens, C., de Alwis, M., Bainbridge, J. W., Smith, A. J., Thrasher, A. J., and Ali, R. R. (2001). Gene replacement therapy in the retinal degeneration slow (rds) mouse: The effect on retinal degeneration following partial transduction of the retina. *Hum. Mol. Genet.* 10:2353–2361.

Sauer, C. G., Gehrig, A., Warneke-Wittstock, R., Marquardt, A., Ewing, C. C., Gibson, A., Lorenz, B., Jurklies, B., and Weber, B. H. (1997). Positional cloning of the gene associated with X-linked juvenile retinoschisis. *Nat. Genet.* 17:164–170.

Schlichtenbrede, F. C., MacNeil, A., Bainbridge, J. W., Tschernutter, M., Thrasher, A. J., Smith, A. J., and Ali, R. R. (2003). Intraocular gene delivery of ciliary neurotrophic factor results in significant loss of retinal function in normal mice and in the Prph2Rd2/Rd2 model of retinal degeneration. *Gene Ther.* 10:523–527.

Seeliger, M. W., Grimm, C., Stahlberg, F., Friedburg, C., Jaissle, G., Zrenner, E., Guo, H., Reme, C. E., Humphries, P., et al. (2001). New views on RPE65 deficiency: The rod system is the source of vision in a mouse model of Leber congenital amaurosis. *Nat. Genet.* 29:70–74.

Shima, D. T., Gougos, A., Miller, J. W., Tolentino, M., Robinson, G., Adamis, A. P., and D'Amore, P. A. (1996). Cloning and mRNA expression of vascular endothelial growth factor in ischemic retinas of *Macaca fascicularis*. *Invest. Ophthalmol. Vis. Sci.* 37:1334–1340.

Sleat, D. E., Sohar, I., Lackland, H., Majercak, J., and Lobel, P. (1996). Rat brain contains high levels of mannose-6-phosphorylated glycoproteins including lysosomal enzymes and palmitoyl-protein thioesterase, an enzyme implicated in infantile neuronal lipofuscinosis. *J. Biol. Chem.* 271:19191–19198.

Sly, W. S., Quinton, B. A., McAlister, W. H., and Rimoin, D. L. (1973). Beta glucuronidase deficiency: Report of clinical, radiologic, and biochemical features of a new mucopolysaccharidosis. *J. Pediatr.* 82:249–257.

Smith, J. R., Verwaerde, C., Rolling, F., Naud, M. C., Delanoye, A., Thillaye-Goldenberg, B., Apparailly, F., and De Kozak, Y. (2005). Tetracycline-inducible viral interleukin-10 intraocular gene transfer, using adeno-associated virus in experimental autoimmune uveoretinitis. *Hum. Gene Ther.* 16(9):1037–1046.

Smith, L. E., Wesolowski, E., McLellan, A., Kostyk, S. K., D'Amato, R., Sullivan, R., and D'Amore, P. A. (1994). Oxygen-induced retinopathy in the mouse. *Invest. Ophthalmol. Vis. Sci.* 35:101–111.

Soker, S., Gollamudi-Payne, S., Fidder, H., Charmahelli, H., and Klagsbrun, M. (1997). Inhibition of vascular endothelial growth factor (VEGF)-induced endothelial cell proliferation by a peptide corresponding to the exon 7-encoded domain of VEGF165. *J. Biol. Chem.* 272:31582–31588.

Song, S., Laipis, P. J., Berns, K. I., and Flotte, T. R. (2001). Effect of DNA-dependent protein kinase on the molecular fate of the rAAV2 genome in skeletal muscle. *Proc. Natl. Acad. Sci. U.S.A.* 98:4084–4088.

Song, S., Lu, Y., Choi, Y. K., Han, Y., Tang, Q., Zhao, G., Berns, K. I., and Flotte, T. R. (2004). DNA-dependent PK inhibits adeno-associated virus DNA integration. *Proc. Natl. Acad. Sci. U.S.A.* 101:2112–2116.

Srivastava, A., Lusby, A. W., Berns, K. I. (1983). Nucleotide sequence and organization of the adenoassociated virus 2 genome. *J. Virol.* 45:555–564.

Stellmach, V., Crawford, S. E., Zhou, W., and Bouck, N. (2001). Prevention of ischemia-induced retinopathy by the natural ocular antiangiogenic agent pigment epithelium-derived factor. *Proc. Natl. Acad. Sci. U.S.A.* 98:2593–2597.

Stramm, L. E., Wolfe, J. H., Schuchman, E. H., Haskins, M. E., Patterson, D. F., and Aguirre, G. D. (1990). Beta-glucuronidase mediated pathway essential for retinal pigment epithelial degradation of glycosaminoglycans: Disease expression and in vitro disease correction using retroviral mediated cDNA transfer. *Exp. Eye Res.* 50:521–532.

Travis, G. H., Brennan, M. B., Danielson, P. E., Kozak, C. A., and Sutcliffe, J. G. (1989). Identification of a photoreceptor-specific mRNA encoded by the gene responsible for retinal degeneration slow (rds). *Nature* 338:70–73.

Vasireddy, V., Jablonski, M. M., Mandal, M. N., Raz-Prag, D., Wang, X. F., Nizol, L., Iannaccone, A., Musch, D. C., Bush, R. A., et al. (2006). Elovl4 5-bp-deletion knock-in mice develop progressive photoreceptor degeneration. *Invest. Ophthalmol. Vis. Sci.* 47:4558–4568.

Vesa, J., Hellsten, E., Verkruyse, L. A., Camp, L. A., Rapola, J., Santavuori, P., Hofmann, S. L., and Peltonen, L. (1995). Mutations in the palmitoyl protein thioesterase gene causing infantile neuronal ceroid lipofuscinosis. *Nature* 376:584–587.

Warrington, K. H., Jr., and Herzog, R. W. (2006). Treatment of human disease by adeno-associated viral gene transfer. *Hum. Genet.* 119(6):571–603.

Weber, B. H., Schrewe, H., Molday, L. L., Gehrig, A., White, K. L., Seeliger, M. W., Jaissle, G. B., Friedburg, C., Tamm, E., et al. (2002). Inactivation of the murine X-linked juvenile retinoschisis gene, Rs1h, suggests a role of retinoschisin in retinal cell layer organization and synaptic structure. *Proc. Natl. Acad. Sci. U.S.A.* 99(9):6222–6227.

Weber, B. H., Vogt, G., Wolz, W., Ives, E. J., and Ewing, C. C. (1994). Sorsby's fundus dystrophy is genetically linked to chromosome 22q13-qter. *Nat. Genet.* 7:158–161.

Weber, M., Rabinowitz, J., Provost, N., Conrath, H., Folliot, S., Briot, D., Cherel, Y., Chenuaud, P., Samulski, J., et al. (2003). Recombinant adeno-associated virus serotype 4 mediates unique and exclusive long-term transduction of retinal pigmented epithelium in rat, dog, and nonhuman primate after subretinal delivery. *Mol. Ther.* 7:774–781.

Williams, D. A. (2006). Vector insertion, mutagenesis and transgene toxicity. *Mol. Ther.* 14(4):457.

Wu, W. W., and Molday, R. S. (2003). Defective discoidin domain structure, subunit assembly, and endoplasmic reticulum processing of retinoschisin are primary mechanisms responsible for X-linked retinoschisis. *J. Biol. Chem.* 278:28139–28146.

Wu, Z., O'Reilly, M. S., Folkman, J., and Shing, Y. (1997). Suppression of tumor growth with recombinant murine angiostatin. *Biochem. Biophys. Res. Commun.* 236:651–654.

Xiao, W., Chirmule, N., Berta, S. C., McCullough, B., Gao, G., and Wilson, J. M. (1999). Gene therapy vectors based on adeno-associated virus type 1. *J. Virol.* 73:3994–4003.

Yang, G. S., Schmidt, M., Yan, Z., Lindbloom, J. D., Harding, T. C., Donahue, B. A., Engelhardt, J. F., Kotin, R., and Davidson, B. L. (2002). Virus-mediated transduction of murine retina with adeno-associated virus: Effects of viral capsid and genome size. *J. Virol.* 76:7651–7560.

Yang, R. B., Robinson, S. W., Xiong, W. H., Yau, K. W., Birch, D. G., and Garbers, D. L. (1999). Disruption of a retinal guanylyl cyclase gene leads to cone-specific dystrophy and paradoxical rod behavior. *J. Neurosci.* 19:5889–5897.

Zeng, Y., Takada, Y., Kjellstrom, S., Hiriyanna, K., Tanikawa, A., Wawrousek, E., Smaoui, N., Caruso, R., Bush, R. A., et al. (2004). RS-1 gene delivery to an adult Rs1h knockout mouse model restores ERG b-wave with reversal of the electronegative waveform of X-linked retinoschisis. *Invest. Ophthalmol. Vis. Sci.* 45:3279–3285.

Zhao, Y., Hong, D. H., Pawlyk, B., Yue, G., Adamian, M., Grynberg, M., Godzik, A., and Li, T. (2003). The retinitis pigmentosa GTPase regulator (RPGR)- interacting protein: Subserving RPGR function and participating in disk morphogenesis. *Proc. Natl. Acad. Sci. U.S.A.* 100:3965–3970.

51 Delivery of Plasmids into the Visual System Using Electroporation

TAKAHIKO MATSUDA AND CONSTANCE L. CEPKO

The ability to alter gene expression in vivo has opened a wide range of investigations into gene structure and function. In addition, it has provided a means to visualize specific cells, track cells with a particular history of gene expression, and alter cellular physiology, and it has allowed the production of models of disease. To facilitate the rapid introduction of gene constructs into the visual system, we used electroporation for delivery to the embryonic and early postnatal retina and brain. Plasmids that allow controlled expression of genes or short hairpin RNAs for RNA interference (RNAi) vectors have been developed. These methods open up the possibility of relatively rapid assessment of gene structure and function.

Comparison of gene transfer methods

Electroporation can be compared to other methods of gene delivery in vivo. Several types of viral vectors, including murine oncoretrovirus (Price et al., 1987; Turner and Cepko, 1987), lentivirus (Miyoshi et al., 1997), adenovirus (Bennett et al., 1994; Jomary et al., 1994; Li et al., 1994), and adeno-associated virus (Ali et al., 1996), are in use. There are advantages and disadvantages inherent in the use of viral vectors. The disadvantages are these: (1) It is time-consuming to prepare high-titer virus stocks to achieve efficient gene transfer. (2) Viral vectors have a size limitation for insert DNA. (3) In general, such vectors do not readily allow introduction of more than two genes into the same cells. (4) Biosafety is a concern for some viral vectors with broad host ranges. However, an advantage that cannot be overlooked for some applications (e.g., lineage analysis) is that integration of the oncoretroviral genome gives stable gene expression throughout all progeny of an infected cell. Electroporated DNA does not integrate efficiently. For some species, transgenic animals can be made by injecting DNA into fertilized eggs. However, producing such strains is invariably slow and often very expensive.

Electroporation bypasses many of the disadvantages cited earlier (Matsuda and Cepko, 2004). This method is faster and in some cases safer than viral gene transfer methods. The efficiency of electroporation into at least some areas of the developing visual system is quite good, and transgene expression persists for more than a month. There does not appear to be a limitation in terms of the species that can be targeted. Various types of DNA constructs, including RNAi vectors as well as conventional gene expression vectors, are readily introduced into the retina without DNA size limitation. We have even successfully electroporated bacterial artificial chromosome (BAC) constructs, although with more difficulty and low levels of expression (Cherry and Cepko, 2008). More than two different DNA constructs can be introduced at once. We found that at least five plasmids can be coelectroporated into the same cells without a significant reduction in coelectroporation frequency. We have also generated a series of cell type–specific promoter constructs that direct expression to specific retinal cell types and have achieved temporal control using recombinases.

When considering the options for gene transfer, one should carefully evaluate whether transient or stable, clonal or nonclonal gene expression is desirable, as well as the feasibility of applying the various methods to the species under study. In addition, it is important to recognize that electroporation, like most viral transduction methods, does not transduce 100% of cells in a targeted area. Transgenic animals can provide more uniform transduction, and if this is required, then electroporation and viral methods cannot be used.

Method of electroporation

Retina in Vivo The basic strategy for in vivo electroporation into the retinas of newborn mouse and rat pups is to inject DNA into the subretinal space between the retina and retinal pigment epithelium (RPE) (figure 51.1*A*). Electrodes are then placed on the heads of the pups and electric pulses are applied to the eyes (figure 51.2). The DNA constructs are transduced into the scleral side of the retina, where undiffentiated mitotic and newly postmitotic cells exist (figure 51.3). Because DNAs are preferentially transduced into undifferentiated progenitor/precursor cells, only late-born cell types (rod, bipolar, Müller glia, and a subset of amacrine cells) are labeled by electroporation at P0 (figures 51.4 and 51.5). It is not clear whether electroporation into progenitor/precursor cells is more effective than into mature neurons because of an inherent difference in cell types or whether this is simply due to the location of progenitor/precursor cells adjacent to the DNA injection site, the subretinal space. In addition to this strategy, it is also theoretically possible to transfect DNAs from the vitreous side of the retina by injecting DNAs into the vitreous chamber, and applying electric pulses in the direction opposite to that used for subretinal injections (see figure 51.1*B*). Indeed, other groups reported that DNA constructs could be transduced to ganglion cells, which line the surface of the retina facing the vitreous body, by in vivo electroporation using this strategy (Dezawa et al., 2002; Huberman et al., 2005; Kachi et al., 2005). However, our data show that the transfection efficiency of the vitreal side (ganglion cells) of the neonatal retina, as well as of the adult retina, is much lower than of the scleral side (progenitor/precursor cells) of the neonatal retina (see figure 51.8). Again, it is not clear why this injection site results in less successful transduction. It could result from physiological differences between ganglion cells/displaced amacrine cells and progenitor/precursor cells; for example, it could be the case that DNA plasmids may not be readily transcribed in these neurons. Alternatively, or in addition, it could result from such things as access of the electroporated plasmids to the nuclear

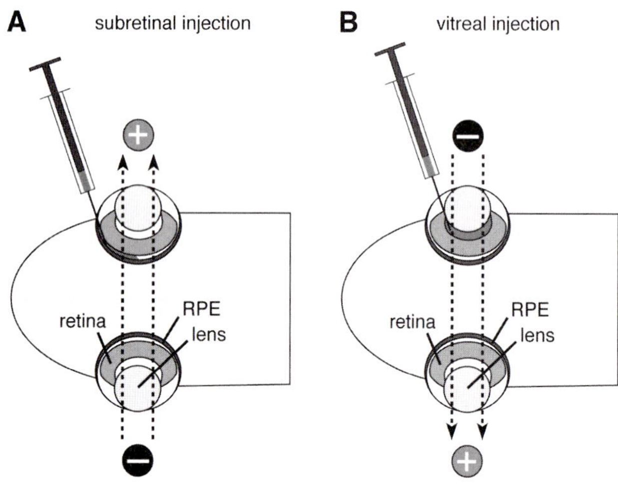

Figure 51.1 Strategy for in vivo electroporation *A*, Electroporation to the scleral (RPE) side of the retina. *B*, Electroporation to the vitreal side of the retina. See color plate 50.

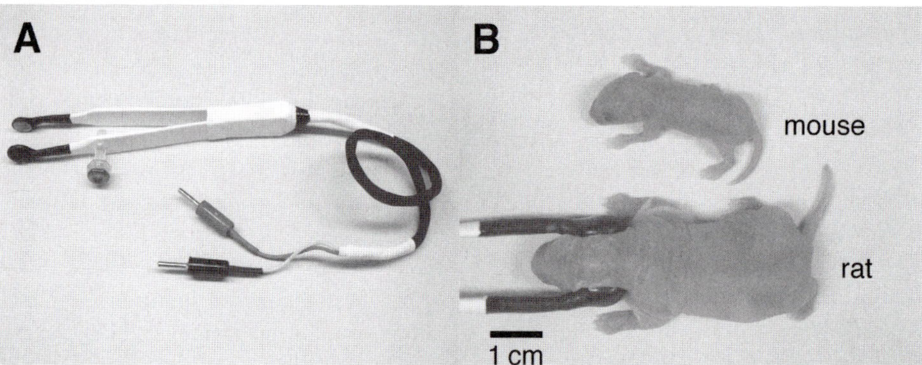

Figure 51.2 Electrodes and procedure for in vivo electroporation. Tweezer-type electrodes (*A*) are placed to hold the head of newborn (P0) rat or mouse (*B*). See color plate 51.

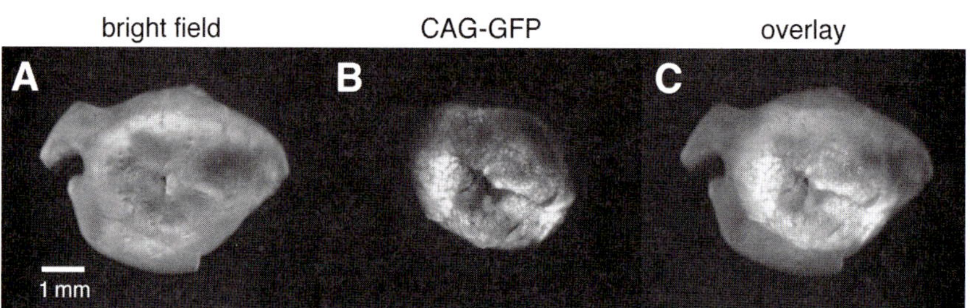

Figure 51.3 Whole-mount preparation of rat retina in vivo electroporated at P0 with CAG-GFP (Matsuda and Cepko, 2004), a GFP expression vector driven by the CAG (chicken β-actin promoter with cytomegalovirus enhancer) promoter and harvested at P21. Images are from the scleral side. Bright-field (*A*), GFP (*B*), and merged (*C*) images are shown. See color plate 52.

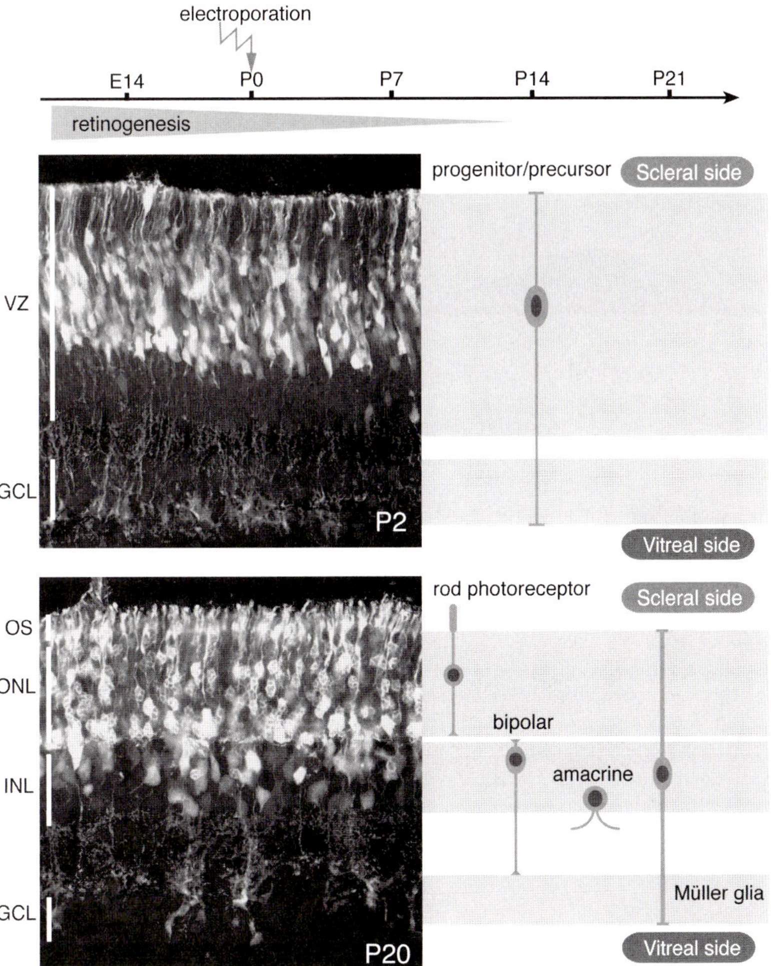

Figure 51.4 In vivo electroporated retina (P0 electroporation, section). Rat retinas were in vivo electroporated with CAG-GFP at P0 and harvested at P2 (*top panel*) or P20 (*bottom panel*). At P2, most of the GFP-positive cells have the morphology of progenitor/precursor cells, suggesting that DNAs are preferentially transfected to progenitor/precursor cells. Retinogenesis is completed within the first 2 weeks after birth. At P20, GFP is observed in four differentiated cell types: rod photoreceptors, bipolar cells, amacrine cells, and Müller glia. Early-born cell types (cone, horizontal, and ganglion cells) are not labeled by P0 electroporation. GCL, ganglion cell layer; INL, inner nuclear layer; ONL, outer nuclear layer; OS, outer segment; VZ, ventricular zone. See color plate 53.

compartment of the neurons. For example, electroporated plasmids may enter a cellular compartment, such as axons, Müller glial endfeet, or blood vessels, or even get trapped in basement membrane rather than go directly into the ganglion cell cytoplasm.

To deliver DNAs into early-born cell types (cone, horizontal, ganglion, and amacrine cells) whose progenitor/precursor cells exist primarily in the embryonic retina, one needs to electroporate DNAs into embryonic retinas (see figure 51.5). Two approaches are used for in vivo (in utero) electroporation into embryonic retinas. One utilizes ultrasound to guide delivery of the plasmid DNA to the subretinal space, or early optic vesicle, such as in murine embryos at E9.5. One can also deliver plasmid DNA to pups in utero without ultrasound, from about E13 for mouse or E14 for rat. This approach involves a learning period during which the practitioner becomes familiar with the landmarks of the embryonic structures as seen through the uterine wall (Turner et al., 1990). Delivery to the embryonic tissue again appears to result in uptake of the DNA primarily by cycling cells or newborn neurons. Because embryonic cells tend to undergo more rounds of cell division than postnatal progenitor cells, the DNA is diluted out more rapidly. Retention of the plasmid in the neurons that are generated soon after electroporation is apparent, because those are the cells that are most strongly marked; an example is the amacrine cells and cone photoreceptors following delivery at E14 in the mouse (figure 51.6).

Retina in Vitro In organ cultures of embryonic or neonatal retina, progenitor cells differentiate into neurons and glia and form three layers, mimicking normal development.

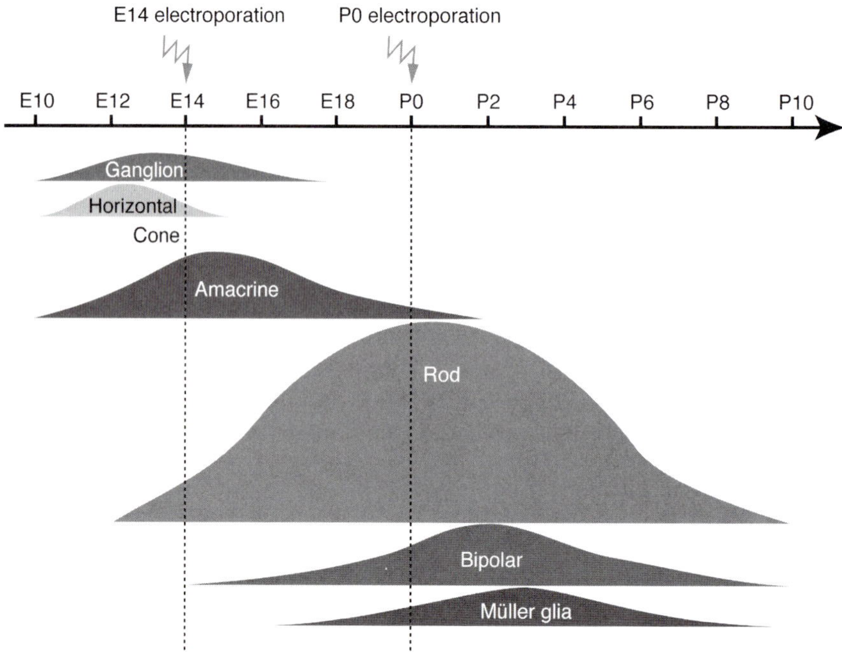

FIGURE 51.5 Timing of electroporation and labeled cell types. Birth order of retinal cells in the mouse retina is shown. As DNAs are preferentially transfected into undifferentiated progenitor/precursor cells by electroporation, electroporation at P0 labels only late-born cell types (rod, bipolar, Müller glia, and a subset of amacrine cells), which are generated from P0 retinal progenitors. On the other hand, electroporation at E14 can label early-born cell types (cone, horizontal, ganglion, and amacrine cells), which are generated from E14 retinal progenitors.

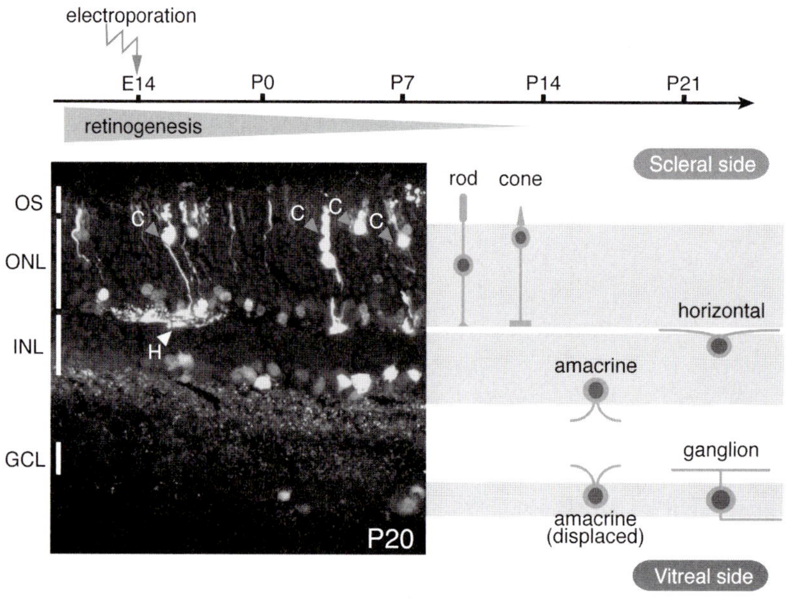

FIGURE 51.6 In vivo electroporated retina (E14 electroporation, section). Mouse embryonic retinas were electroporated with UB-GFP (Matsuda and Cepko, 2004), a GFP expression vector driven by the human ubiquitin promoter, at E14 in utero, and harvested at P20. Early-born cell types (cone, amacrine, horizontal, and ganglion cells) are clearly labeled with GFP, while late-born cell types (bipolar and Müller glial cells), which are generated from E14 RPCs after several rounds of cell division, are poorly labeled. This is probably due to dilution of introduced plasmids. *Red arrowheads* indicate the labeled cone photoreceptors. *Yellow arrowhead* indicates the labeled horizontal cell. GCL, ganglion cell layer; INL, inner nuclear layer; ONL, outer nuclear layer; OS, outer segment. See color plate 54.

Taking advantage of this propensity, we also developed a system to electroporate DNAs into isolated retinas (in vitro electroporation; see Matsuda and Cepko, 2004) using a micro-electroporation chamber (figures 51.7 and 51.8). Electroporated retinas are cultured for a few days to weeks.

Compared with in vivo electroporation, in vitro electroporation has several advantages. First, in vitro electroporation is easier and less skill dependent than in vivo electroporation. All retinas subjected to electroporation become GFP (RFP) positive when GFP (RFP) expression vectors are used. Second, it is relatively easy to handle a large number of retinas in a day. Third, in vitro electroporation can be easily applied not only to postnatal retinas, but also to embryonic retinas, to which in vivo electroporation (in utero electroporation) is more difficult to apply. Fourth, real-time monitoring of GFP (RFP)-transduced cells is possible under a fluorescent microscope. However, in vitro electroporation has several disadvantages inherent to organ culture. First, the morphology of cultured retina is frequently poor, and photoreceptor outer segments are poorly formed. Second, it is hard to culture retinas for a long period. In our

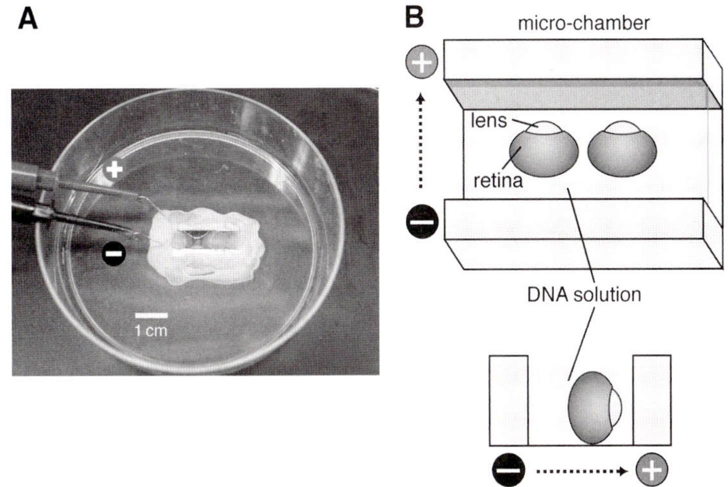

FIGURE 51.7 *A*, Microchamber for in vitro electroporation. *B*, Orientation of the retina in the chamber. Maximum transduction efficiency can be obtained when the scleral side is facing the minus electrode. See color plate 55.

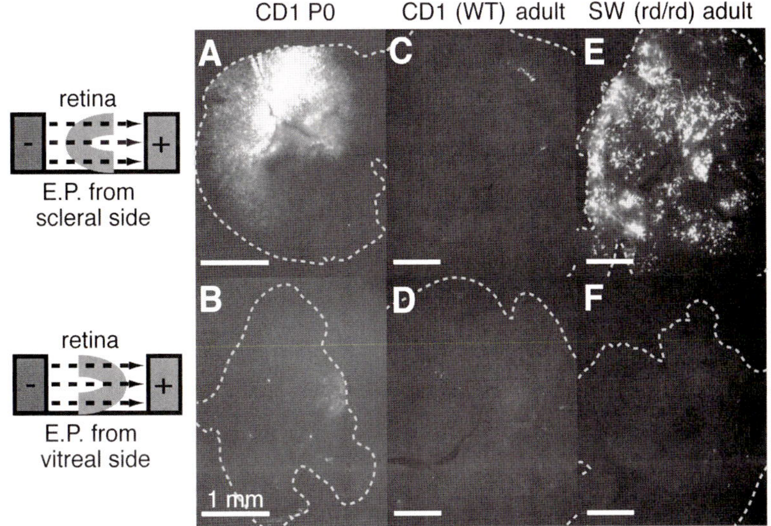

FIGURE 51.8 In vitro electroporated retinal explant (whole mount). Mouse retinas of P0 CD1 (*A* and *B*), adult CD1 (*C* and *D*), or adult Swiss Webster mice with a retinal degeneration mutation (*E* and *F*) were in vitro electroporated with CAG-GFP from the scleral side (*A*, *C*, and *E*) or from the vitreal side (*B*, *D*, and *F*) and cultured for 5 days. Images *A*, *C*, and *E* are from the scleral side and images *B*, *D*, and *F* are from the vitreal side. Note that only the scleral side of developing retina or of degenerated retina is highly transfectable. In *E*, most of the GFP-positive cells are Müller glial cells. See color plate 56.

experience, retinas tend to become unhealthy when cultured for more than 2 weeks.

Brain in Vivo The delivery of plasmid DNAs to the brain has been used by several groups previously (Fukuchi-Shimogori and Grove, 2001; Saito and Nakatsuji, 2001; Tabata and Nakajima, 2001). The same issues discussed earlier pertain here as well, such as dilution of DNA following early delivery (Shimogori et al., 2004). Marking of visual cortex has been achieved (Akaneya et al., 2005; Huberman et al., 2005). It is likely that most areas adjacent to a ventricle will allow successful plasmid uptake and expression following electroporation. Ventricular zones are adjacent to the ventricular lumina, into which DNA can be readily injected, and they are also the area where progenitor cells reside. As discussed earlier for the retina, it appears that these two criteria offer the ideal circumstances for successful electroporation. Injection into tissue rather than into a lumen does not result in effective electroporation, likely because only the DNA that remains in the needle track is available for uptake. In addition, it is unclear whether the neurons, which are more mature in developing tissue, will successfully take up and express such plasmids.

Controlling expression following electroporation

One advantage to using transgenic animals rather than viral vectors or even (often) electroporation is the ability to use regulatable promoters and recombinases to control gene expression. We have created a series of plasmids to realize these advantages for electroporated genes, or RNAi constructs (Matsuda and Cepko, 2007).

Temporal Regulation Conditionally active Cre recombinases are composed of Cre and the mutated ligand binding domains of the human estrogen receptor (ER^{T2}). They are activated by 4-hydroxytamoxifen (4-OHT) and have been used to temporally control gene expression in transgenic mice (Branda and Dymecki, 2004). We tested the 4-OHT-responsible Cre recombinases, $CreER^{T2}$ (single fusion; Feil et al., 1997) and $ER^{T2}CreER^{T2}$ (double fusion; Casanova et al., 2002), in vivo in the rat retina. These recombinases were expressed under control of the ubiquitous CAG promoter (Niwa et al., 1991) (figure 51.9*A*). A Cre-dependent expression vector (Kanegae et al., 1995) containing the CAG promoter, a floxed stop cassette, and a reporter gene (DsRed) was used as a recombination indicator (termed CALNL-DsRed; figure 51.9*B*). When P0 rat retinas were coelectroporated with CAG-$CreER^{T2}$, CALNL-DsRed (recombination indicator), and CAG-GFP (transfection control) and harvested at P21, very high background recombination (DsRed expression) was detected even without 4-OHT stimulation (figure 51.9*D*). $ER^{T2}Cre$ (N-terminal ER^{T2} fusion) also had very high background recombination activity. In contrast, $ER^{T2}CreER^{T2}$ double fusion had no detectable recombination activity without 4-OHT (figure 51.9*E*). When 4-OHT was injected intraperitoneally into the transfected rats at P20, an induction of DsRed expression was clearly detected 24 hours after 4-OHT administration (figure 51.9*F*). Similar results were observed when $CreER^{T2}$ and $ER^{T2}CreER^{T2}$ were transfected into 293 T cells or E14.5 mouse brain. These results indicate that at least for in vivo electroporation studies, $ER^{T2}CreER^{T2}$, but not $CreER^{T2}$ ($ER^{T2}Cre$), can lead to tight regulation of the onset of transgene expression.

It is not clear why the double ER^{T2} domain construct was required for tight regulation of recombinase activity. The heat shock protein 90 (Hsp90) interacts with the ER domain in the cytosol and thereby prevents the translocation of CreER fusion protein to the nucleus where DNA recombination occurs (Picard, 1994). The double fusion may have a higher affinity for Hsp90 to form a tighter complex. Alternatively, the $ER^{T2}CreER^{T2}$ fusion may have less activity due to the double fusion, and thus less background activity. It is also possible that degradation of $CreER^{T2}$ ($ER^{T2}Cre$) results in generation of "active Cre" lacking the regulatory domain, while $ER^{T2}CreER^{T2}$ is still inactive even after losing one regulatory domain.

Cell Type–Specific Regulation Using Specific Promoters To restrict transgene expression to specified cell types in the retina, several retinal cell type–specific promoters were obtained using the literature to guide construction or were developed in our laboratory. Regulatory sequences for rhodopsin (expressed in rods; Zack et al., 1991), Nrl (expressed in rods; Swaroop et al., 1992), Crx (expressed in photoreceptors and weakly in bipolars; Chen et al., 1997; Furukawa et al., 1997b), calcium-binding protein 5 (Cabp5, expressed in subsets of bipolar cells; Haeseleer et al., 2000), N-myc downstream-regulated gene 4 (Ndrg4, expressed in amacrines; Punzo and Cepko, 2008), cellular retinaldehyde-binding protein (Cralbp, expressed in Müller glia; Kennedy et al., 1998), clusterin (expressed in Müller glia; Blackshaw et al., 2004), Rax (expressed in progenitors and Müller glia; Furukawa et al., 1997a; Mathers et al., 1997), and Hes1 (expressed in progenitors and Müller glia; Tomita et al., 1996) were characterized for this purpose. When these promoters were used to express DsRed, DsRed was detected only in specific cell types in the retina (figure 51.10 and table 51.1). Using fluorescent protein variants (CFP, YFP, and DsRed) as reporters, we could visualize different cell types simultaneously (figure 51.11).

The cell type–specific promoters were also used to regulate expression of Cre recombinase (figure 51.12). This type of construct was coelectroporated with CALNL-DsRed, a recombination indicator. Following the action of Cre, DsRed

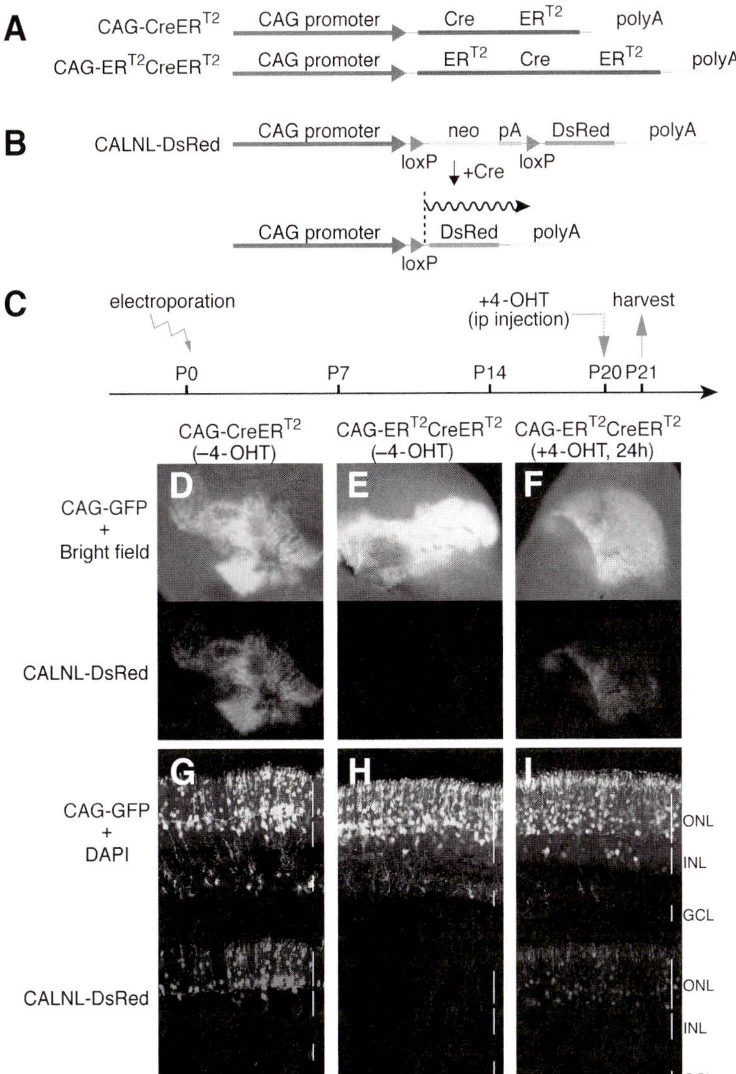

FIGURE 51.9 Temporal regulation of gene expression in the retina using inducible Cre recombinases. *A*, CAG-CreER^{T2}: Fusion protein (CreER^{T2}) between Cre recombinase and the mutated ligand-binding domain (ER^{T2}) of the human estrogen receptor is expressed under the control of the CAG promoter. CAG-ER^{T2}CreER^{T2}: Fusion protein (ER^{T2}CreER^{T2}) composed of Cre and two ER^{T2} domains is expressed under the control of the CAG promoter. CreER^{T2} and ER^{T2}CreER^{T2} are conditionally activated in response to 4-OHT. *B*, CALNL-DsRed: Cre/loxP-dependent inducible expression vector. DsRed is expressed only in the presence of Cre. *C*, A scheme of the experiment. *D–I*, P0 rat retinas were coelectroporated with three plasmids: CAG-GFP (transfection control), CALNL-DsRed (recombination indicator), and CAG-CreER^{T2} (*D*) or CAG-ER^{T2}CreER^{T2} (*E* and *F*). The retinas were stimulated without 4-OHT (*D* and *E*) or with 4-OHT (*F*) by IP injection at P20 and then harvested at P21. Whole-mount preparations of the harvested retinas are shown. *G–I*, Sections of the retinas shown in *D–F*. Cell nuclei were stained with DAPI. When CreER^{T2} was used, significant background recombination was observed even in the absence of 4-OHT. On the other hand, ER^{T2}CreER^{T2} had no detectable basal activity in the absence of 4-OHT. GCL, ganglion cell layer; INL, inner nuclear layer; ONL, outer nuclear layer. See color plate 57.

would be expressed from the ubiquitous CAG promoter. In all cases, DsRed expression levels in the retina were higher when DsRed was expressed from the CAG promoter rather than any of the cell type–specific promoters. The rhodopsin promoter-Cre construct specifically induced the expression of DsRed in rods. Similarly, the Nrl promoter-Cre construct led to the expression of DsRed only in rods, indicating that both promoters are restricted to rods and are not even transiently active in other cell types, including multipotent progenitors. Interestingly, when the Cabp5 promoter-Cre construct was used, a subset of rods, as well as bipolars, was labeled with DsRed. The ratio of the number of DsRed-positive rods to that of DsRed-positive bipolars was approximately 1 : 1. This might suggest that the Cabp5 promoter is active in the progenitors that produce rod and bipolar cells. The Ndrg4 promoter-Cre construct induced the expression

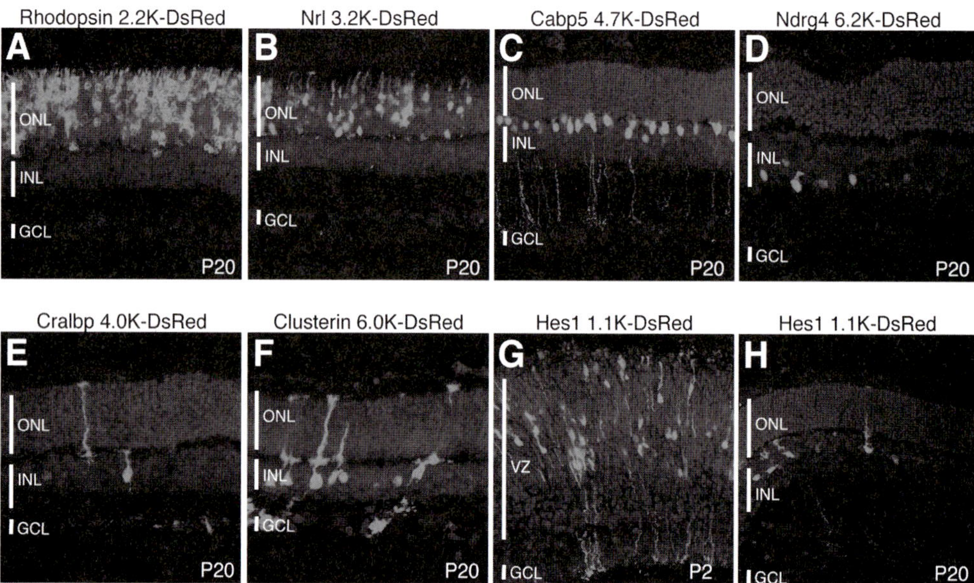

Figure 51.10 Spatial regulation of gene expression in the retina using cell type–specific promoters. Retinal cell type–specific promoters were fused to DsRed cDNA and electroporated into P0 rat retinas. The retinas were harvested at P20 (*A–F* and *H*) or P2 (*G*), sectioned, and stained with DAPI. Promoters of rhodopsin (*A*), Nrl (*B*), Cabp5 (*C*), Ndrg4 (*D*), Cralbp (*E*), clusterin (*F*), and Hes1 (*G* and *H*) were used to express DsRed. GCL, ganglion cell layer; INL, inner nuclear layer; ONL, outer nuclear layer. See color plate 58.

Table 51.1

Labeled cell types observed following electroporation with retinal cell type–specific promoters

Reporter Construct	Cell Types (Signal Intensity)
Rhodopsin promoter 2.2kb-DsRed	Rod (+++++)
Nrl promoter 3.2kb-DsRed	Rod (+++)
Crx promoter 5.0kb-DsRed	Rod (+) + Bip (+++)
Cabp5 promoter 4.7kb-DsRed	Bip (+++)
Ndrg4 promoter 6.2kb-DsRed	Ama (++++)
Cralbp promoter 4.0kb-DsRed	MG (+++)
Clusterin promoter 6.2kb-DsRed	MG (+++)
Rax promoter 7.2kb-DsRed (P2)	Prog (+)
Rax promoter 7.2kb-DsRed (P20)	Not detected
Hes1 promoter 1.1kb-DsRed (P2)	Prog (+++)
Hes1 promoter 1.1kb-DsRed (P20)	MG (++)
Rhodopsin promoter 2.2kb-Cre	Rod (++++++)
Nrl promoter 3.2kb-Cre	Rod (++++)
Crx promoter 5.0kb-Cre	Rod (++++) + Bip (++++)
Cabp5 promoter 4.7kb-Cre	Rod (+++) + Bip (++++)
Ndrg4 promoter 6.2kb-Cre	Rod (+++) + Ama (+++++)
Cralbp promoter 4.0kb-Cre	Rod (+++) Bip (+++) + MG (++++)
Clusterin promoter 6.2kb-Cre	Rod (+++) Bip (+++) + MG (++++)
Rax promoter 7.2kb-Cre	Rod (+++) Bip (+++) + Ama (+++) + MG (+++)
Hes1 promoter 1.1kb-Cre	Rod (+++) Bip (+++) + Ama (+++) + MG (+++)

Note: Results of figure 51.10 (expression patterns of DsRed directly driven by cell type–specific promoters) and figure 51.12 (expression patterns of DsRed induced by Cre recombinase driven by cell type–specific promoters) are summarized in the table. DNA constructs were transfected at P0, and P2 or P20 retinas were analyzed. Cell types were determined based on cell morphology and location. Relative expression levels of DsRed in each experiment are indicated.

Ama, amacrine cells; Bip, bipolar cells; MG, Müller glial cells; Prog, progenitor cells.

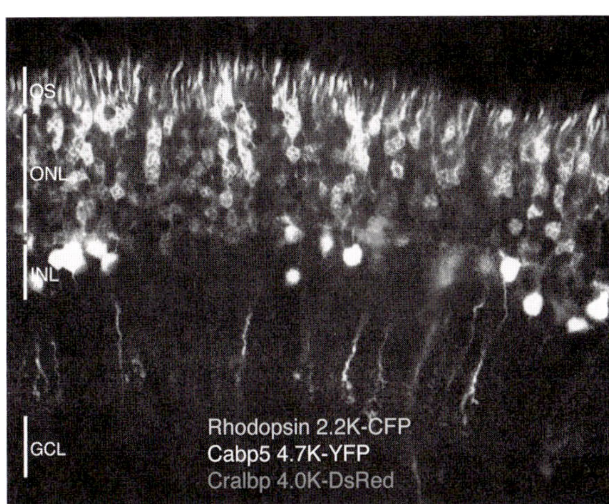

FIGURE 51.11 Multicolor labeling of the retina using cell type–specific promoters. P0 rat retina was electroporated with three reporter constructs: rhodopsin promoter 2.2K-CFP (specific for rods), Cabp5 promoter 4.7K-YFP (specific for a subset of bipolar cells), and Cralbp promoter 4.0K-DsRed (specific for Müller glia). The retina was harvested at P20, sectioned, and stained with DAPI. GCL, ganglion cell layer; INL, inner nuclear layer; ONL, outer nuclear layer; OS, outer segment. See color plate 59.

of DsRed in amacrines as well as in a subset of rods. The Cralbp promoter-Cre construct and the clusterin promoter-Cre construct induced the expression of DsRed in Müller glia and a small population of rod and bipolar cells. The Hes1 promoter-Cre construct and the Rax promoter-Cre construct induced the expression of DsRed in rod, bipolar, amacrine, and Müller glial cells. The expression patterns of DsRed were analyzed at P20, with the results summarized in table 51.1.

TEMPORAL AND CELL TYPE–SPECIFIC REGULATION By combining the temporal regulation afforded by ER^{T2}-$CreER^{T2}$ with the cell type–specific regulation provided by the promoters, we could inducibly express a reporter gene specifically in a desired cell type, such as "differentiated" Müller glia. As shown in figure 51.13, the clusterin promoter was cloned upstream of $ER^{T2}CreER^{T2}$, and the resulting plasmid was coelectroporated with CALNL-DsRed (recombination indicator) and CAG-GFP (transfection control) into P0 rat retinas. The retinas were stimulated with 4-OHT at P14, the time point when retinogenesis is complete (Young, 1985; Rapaport et al., 2004), and then analyzed at P16. Without 4-OHT stimulation, DsRed expression was not detected. When 4-OHT was injected into the rats, clear DsRed expression was detected in a subset of GFP-positive cells. The retinal sections showed that all the DsRed-positive cells examined were morphologically Müller glia. These results show that $ER^{T2}CreER^{T2}$ can be used with retinal cell type–specific promoters to achieve precise temporal and cell type–specific regulation in the retina.

CONDITIONAL RNAI To conditionally knock down gene expression in the retina, Cre-dependent inducible RNAi vectors utilizing the micro-RNA30 (mir30)-based shRNA expression system (Zeng et al., 2002; Paddison et al., 2004) were made. The mir30-based shRNA expression system has several advantages over conventional RNAi vectors expressing shRNAs directly from pol III promoters, such as the U6 promoter. First, shRNA can be expressed using pol II promoters (e.g., CAG promoter). Second, it is technically simple to put the regulatory elements (e.g., transcriptional stop cassette) into the expression vectors. Figure 51.14 shows the mir30-based vectors expressing shRNA under the control of the CAG promoter (CAG-mir30 and CALSL-mir30). CALSL-mir30 is a Cre-dependent inducible RNAi vector carrying a floxed transcriptional stop cassette immediately after the CAG promoter. CALSL-mir30 also was used with the rhodopsin promoter-Cre construct in the retina. P0 rat retinas were coelectroporated with four plasmids, CALSL-mir30(GFPshRNA) expressing an shRNA against GFP (GFPshRNA), CAG-GFP, CAG-DsRed, and the rhodopsin promoter-Cre, and analyzed at P20. Without the Cre construct, transfected retinal cells were clearly labeled by both GFP and DsRed. With the rhodopsin promoter-Cre construct, GFP expression in the ONL was specifically silenced while that in the INL cells was not affected, demonstrating that CALSL-mir30 can be used to conditionally knock down gene expression in the retina. These experiments showed there is a very high cotransfection efficiency. In order for cells to be both red and green, they must have been successfully electroporated with both CAG-GFP and CAG-DsRed. The coexpression rate of these two genes was nearly 100%, both in this case, where four plasmids were coelectroporated, and in many previous cases with two or three coelectroporated plasmids (Matsuda and Cepko, 2004).

The Cre/loxP recombination-dependent inducible vectors with the CAG promoter have several useful features. First, it is possible to inducibly express genes in specific cell types at specific time points. Second, after Cre/loxP-mediated recombination, strong "output signals" driven by the CAG promoter can be obtained. Expression of fluorescent reporter genes directly from cell type–specific promoters frequently results in such low levels of expression as to render the constructs unusable for some applications, such as the detection of live-labeled cells. We found there was a much greater sensitivity for the detection of expression when cell type–specific promoters were used with Cre plus CALNL-DsRed. Finally, these vectors can be used to trace the fate of progenitor and precursor cells labeled upon Cre/loxP-mediated recombination. Using these vectors, we showed that several cell type–specific promoters are weakly active in progenitors and/or other cell types. Two explanations for this observation, which are not mutually

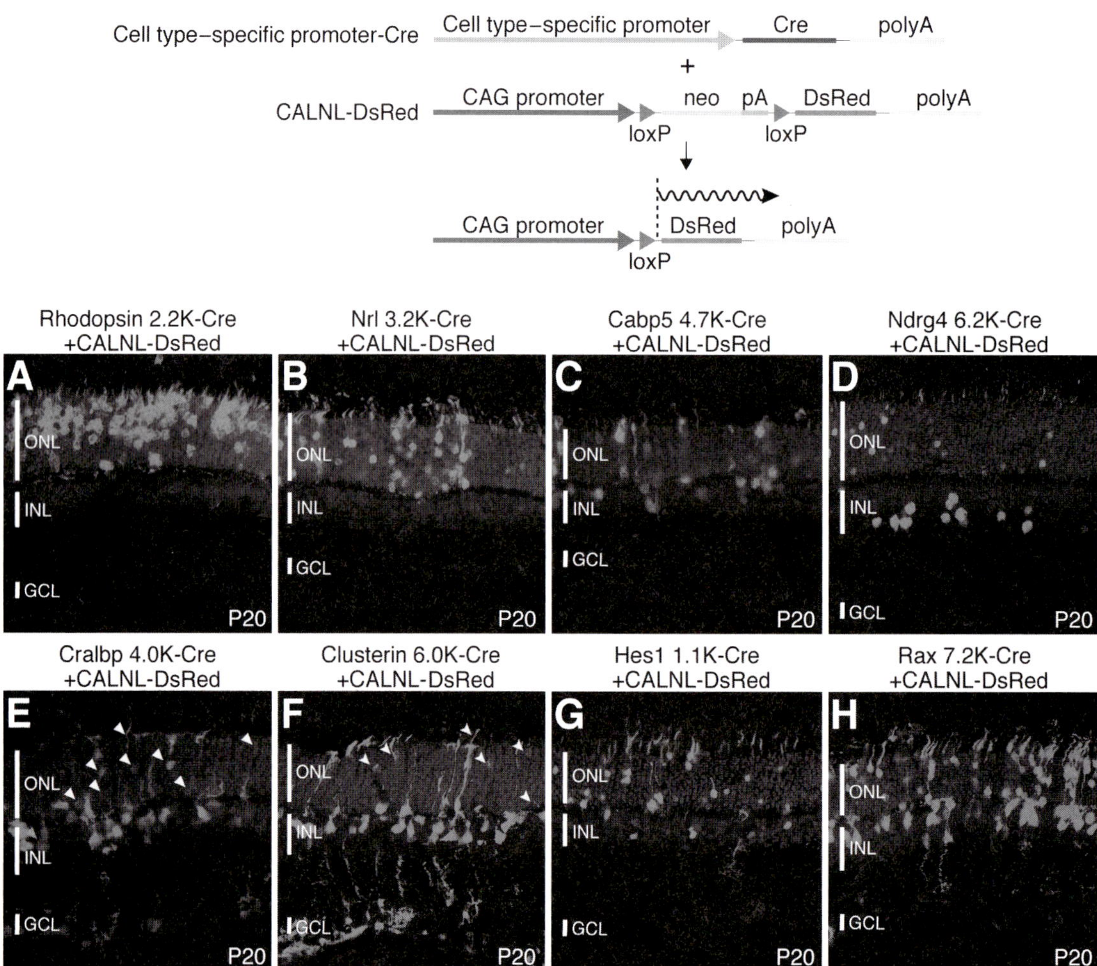

Figure 51.12 Lineage tracing experiments in the retina using the Cre/loxP system and cell type–specific promoters. P0 rat retinas were coelectroporated with retinal cell type–specific promoter Cre and CALNL-DsRed (recombination indicator). DsRed expression, induced by Cre/loxP-mediated recombination, was driven by the ubiquitous CAG promoter. The retinas were harvested at P20, sectioned, and stained with DAPI. Promoters of rhodopsin (*A*), Nrl (*B*), Cabp5 (*C*), Ndrg4 (*D*), Cralbp (*E*), clusterin (*F*), Hes1 (*G*), and Rax (*H*) were used to express Cre. *Yellow arrowheads* indicate the labeled rods. *Blue arrowhead* indicates the labeled bipolar cell. GCL, ganglion cell layer; INL, inner nuclear layer; ONL, outer nuclear layer. See color plate 60.

exclusive, can be considered. Lineage analyses using retroviral vectors have shown that clones with bipolar, Müller glia, or amacrine cells almost always also contain rods, even if the clone is of only two cells (Turner and Cepko, 1987). If these promoters are weakly active in progenitors that give rise to multiple cell types, then one might see labeling of rods, along with labeling of the cell type that normally is the only cell type to express a particular promoter. This idea is supported by two previous observations. Most of the known Müller glia–specific genes of the adult retina are also expressed in progenitors (Blackshaw et al., 2004), and two genes thought to be restricted to amacrine and horizontal cells could be observed in progenitors (Alexiades and Cepko, 1997). An additional explanation is that these promoters, transiently introduced into the retina by electroporation, are slightly "leaky," and such leakiness was detected by the more sensitive reporter (Cre plus CALNL-DsRed).

Future applications

There are many obvious applications for electroporation in studies of the visual system. Standard gain- and loss-of-function protocols are being employed in which a gene is over- or misexpressed or is targeted with RNAi. However, the flexibility offered by the high efficiency of coelectroporation enables many more types of experiments to be performed. For example, the best control for the specificity of an RNAi event is gene rescue; that is, one supplies a version of the endogenous gene that is targeted by RNAi but that

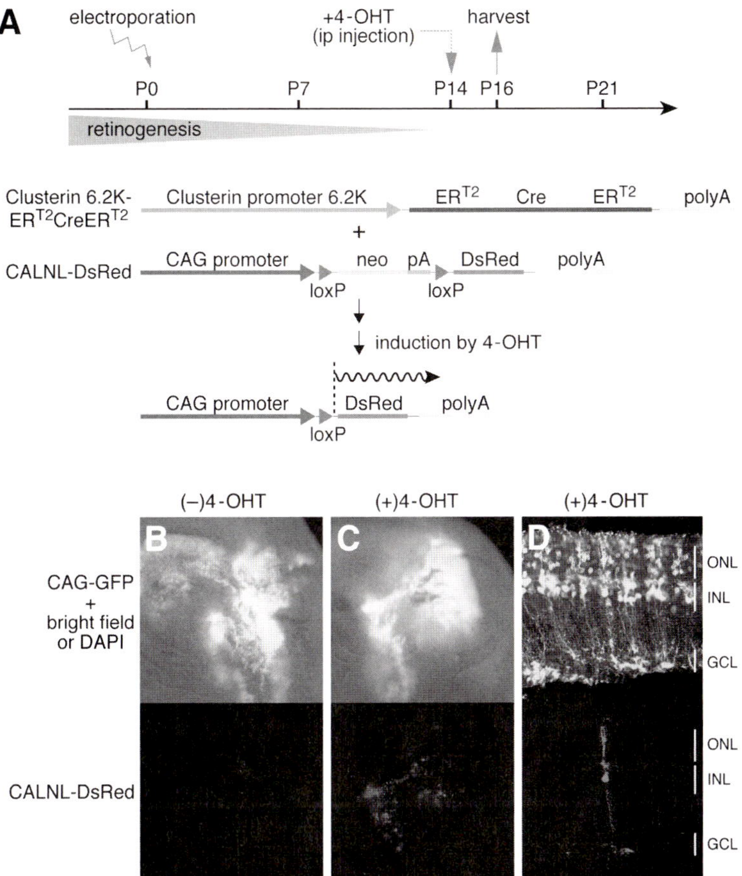

FIGURE 51.13 Inducible expression in the differentiated Müller glia (*A*). Clusterin promoter was fused to ER^{T2}CreER^{T2} cDNA and coelectroporated into P0 rat retinas with CALNL-DsRed (recombination indicator) and CAG-GFP (transfection control). Retinas were stimulated with or without 4-OHT at P14 by IP injection, then harvested at P16. *B*, Whole-mount preparation of the transfected retina harvested at P16 without 4-OHT stimulation. No DsRed expression was detected. *C*, Whole-mount preparation of the transfected retina stimulated with 4-OHT at P14 and harvested at P16. *D*, The retina shown in *C* was sectioned and stained with DAPI. Only Müller glial cells are labeled with DsRed. See color plate 61.

does not encode the targeted sequence. This is easily done by coelectroporating the plasmid encoding the RNAi and the resistant version of the targeted gene. One can also perform epistasis experiments. For example, one can target a transcription factor by RNAi and simultaneously supply a putative target of that transcription factor whose expression is controlled by a noncognate promoter to look for rescue. One can use the recombinases to turn on expression of either the RNAi or the rescue cassette to perform rescue or knockdown in specific cells or at specific times. Promoter constructs also allow one to mark subsets of cells and follow their migration, and so on. Their physiology can be controlled by the controlled expression of genes that might silence their neuronal activity.

Another application of interest to neuroscientists is to track the synaptic partners of an electroporated cell. Since the transient expression following electroporation can be relatively high level, one can provide enough of a transsynaptic tracer (e.g., WGA) to find the synaptically connected partners of an electroporated cell, which itself can be readily identified by labeling with an electroporation reporter, for example, GFP. In addition, electroporation of Cre plasmids, RNAi plasmids, and the like into mice in which engineering of the germ line has been carried out is being done. For example, rather than create a mouse strain that expresses Cre under control of a specific promoter, one can simply electroporate a Cre plasmid into a mouse that has a germ line with a floxed allele of a gene of interest. Many additional applications will be discovered through the creative use of these protocols and reagents as more neuroscientists discover the ease and flexibility of this system of gene transfer.

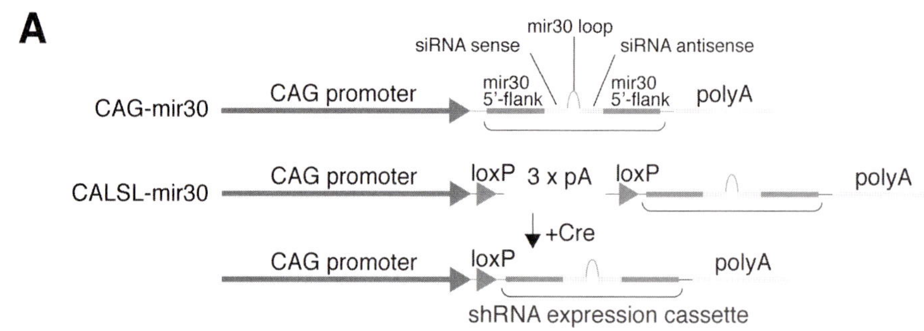

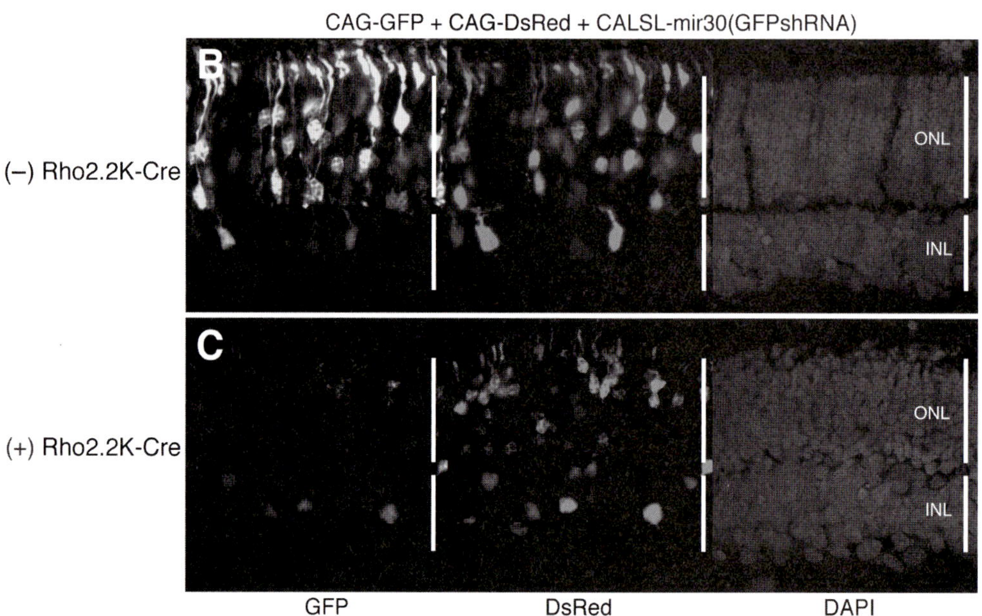

Figure 51.14 Inducible RNAi in the retina. *A*, CAG-mir30: The mir30 expression cassette is expressed under the control of the CAG promoter. The mir30 expression cassette has the hairpin stem composed of siRNA sense and antisense strands (22nt each), a loop derived from human mir30 (19nt), and 125nt mir30 flanking sequences on both sides of the hairpin. The mir30 primary transcript is processed to generate the mature shRNA. CALSL-mir30: Cre-dependent inducible shRNA expression vector carrying a floxed transcriptional stop cassette (3xpolyA signal sequences). Only in the presence of Cre, the mir30 expression cassette is expressed under the control of the CAG promoter. *B* and *C*, Conditional GFP knockdown in the retina. CAG-GFP and CAG-DsRed and CALSL-mir30(GFPshRNA) expressing an shRNA against GFP were coelectroporated without (*B*) or with (*C*) the rhodopsin promoter Cre into P0 rat retinas. The retinas were harvested at P20, sectioned, and stained with DAPI. Rod-specific GFP knockdown was observed in the presence of the rhodopsin promoter Cre. See color plate 62.

REFERENCES

Akaneya, Y., Jiang, B., and Tsumoto, T. (2005). RNAi-induced gene silencing by local electroporation in targeting brain region. *J. Neurophysiol.* 93:594–602.

Alexiades, M. R., and Cepko, C. L. (1997). Subsets of retinal progenitors display temporally regulated and distinct biases in the fates of their progeny. *Development* 124:1119–1131.

Ali, R. R., Reichel, M. B., Thrasher, A. J., Levinsky, R. J., Kinnon, C., Kanuga, N., Hunt, D. M., and Bhattacharya, S. S. (1996). Gene transfer into the mouse retina mediated by an adeno-associated viral vector. *Hum. Mol. Genet.* 5:591–594.

Bennett, J., Wilson, J., Sun, D., Forbes, B., and Maguire, A. (1994). Adenovirus vector-mediated in vivo gene transfer into adult murine retina. *Invest. Ophthalmol. Vis. Sci.* 35:2535–2542.

Blackshaw, S., Harpavat, S., Trimarchi, J., Cai, L., Huang, H., Kuo, W. P., Weber, G., Lee, K., Fraioli, R. E., et al. (2004). Genomic analysis of mouse retinal development. *PLoS Biol.* 2: E247.

Branda, C. S., and Dymecki, S. M. (2004). Talking about a revolution: The impact of site-specific recombinases on genetic analyses in mice. *Dev. Cell* 6:7–28.

Casanova, E., Fehsenfeld, S., Lemberger, T., Shimshek, D. R., Sprengel, R., and Mantamadiotis, T. (2002). ER-based double iCre fusion protein allows partial recombination in forebrain. *Genesis* 34:208–214.

Chen, S., Wang, Q. L., Nie, Z., Sun, H., Lennon, G., Copeland, N. G., Gilbert, D. J., Jenkins, N. A., and Zack, D. J. (1997). Crx, a novel Otx-like paired-homeodomain protein, binds to and transactivates photoreceptor cell-specific genes. *Neuron* 19: 1017–1030.

Cherry, T. J., and Cepko, C. L. (2008). Unpublished results.

Dezawa, M., Takano, M., Negishi, H., Mo, X., Oshitari, T., and Sawada, H. (2002). Gene transfer into retinal ganglion cells by in vivo electroporation: A new approach. *Micron* 33:1–6.

Feil, R., Wagner, J., Metzger, D., and Chambon, P. (1997). Regulation of Cre recombinase activity by mutated estrogen receptor ligand-binding domains. *Biochem. Biophys. Res. Commun.* 237:752–757.

Fukuchi-Shimogori, T., and Grove, E. A. (2001). Neocortex patterning by the secreted signaling molecule FGF8. *Science* 294:1071–1074.

Furukawa, T., Kozak, C. A., and Cepko, C. L. (1997a). Rax, a novel paired-type homeobox gene, shows expression in the anterior neural fold and developing retina. *Proc. Natl. Acad. Sci. U.S.A.* 94:3088–3093.

Furukawa, T., Morrow, E. M., and Cepko, C. L. (1997b). Crx, a novel otx-like homeobox gene, shows photoreceptor-specific expression and regulates photoreceptor differentiation. *Cell* 91: 531–541.

Haeseleer, F., Sokal, I., Verlinde, C. L., Erdjument-Bromage, H., Tempst, P., Pronin, A. N., Benovic, J. L., Fariss, R. N., and Palczewski, K. (2000). Five members of a novel Ca^{2+}-binding protein (CABP) subfamily with similarity to calmodulin. *J. Biol. Chem.* 275:1247–1260.

Huberman, A. D., Murray, K. D., Warland, D. K., Feldheim, D. A., and Chapman, B. (2005). Ephrin-As mediate targeting of eye-specific projections to the lateral geniculate nucleus. *Nat. Neurosci.* 8:1013–1021.

Jomary, C., Piper, T. A., Dickson, G., Couture, L. A., Smith, A. E., Neal, M. J., and Jones, S. E. (1994). Adenovirus-mediated gene transfer to murine retinal cells in vitro and in vivo. *FEBS Lett.* 347:117–122.

Kachi, S., Oshima, Y., Esumi, N., Kachi, M., Rogers, B., Zack, D. J., and Campochiaro, P. A. (2005). Nonviral ocular gene transfer. *Gene Ther.* 12:843–851.

Kanegae, Y., Lee, G., Sato, Y., Tanaka, M., Nakai, M., Sakaki, T., Sugano, S., and Saito, I. (1995). Efficient gene activation in mammalian cells by using recombinant adenovirus expressing site-specific Cre recombinase. *Nucleic Acids Res.* 23:3816–3821.

Kennedy, B. N., Huang, J., Saari, J. C., and Crabb, J. W. (1998). Molecular characterization of the mouse gene encoding cellular retinaldehyde-binding protein. *Mol. Vis.* 4:14–21.

Li, T., Adamian, M., Roof, D. J., Berson, E. L., Dryja, T. P., Roessler, B. J., and Davidson, B. L. (1994). In vivo transfer of a reporter gene to the retina mediated by an adenoviral vector. *Invest. Ophthalmol. Vis. Sci.* 35:2543–2549.

Mathers, P. H., Grinberg, A., Mahon, K. A., and Jamrich, M. (1997). The Rx homeobox gene is essential for vertebrate eye development. *Nature* 387:603–607.

Matsuda, T., and Cepko, C. L. (2004). Electroporation and RNA interference in the rodent retina in vivo and in vitro. *Proc. Natl. Acad. Sci. U.S.A.* 101:16–22.

Matsuda, T., and Cepko, C. L. (2007). Controlled expression of transgenes introduced by in vivo electroporation. *Proc. Natl. Acad. Sci. U.S.A.* 104:1027–1032.

Miyoshi, H., Takahashi, M., Gage, F. H., and Verma, I. M. (1997). Stable and efficient gene transfer into the retina using an HIV-based lentiviral vector. *Proc. Natl. Acad. Sci. U.S.A.* 94:10319–10323.

Niwa, H., Yamamura, K., and Miyazaki, J. (1991). Efficient selection for high-expression transfectants with a novel eukaryotic vector. *Gene* 108:193–199.

Paddison, P. J., Cleary, M., Silva, J. M., Chang, K., Sheth, N., Sachidanandam, R., and Hannon, G. J. (2004). Cloning of short hairpin RNAs for gene knockdown in mammalian cells. *Nat. Methods* 1:163–167.

Picard, D. (1994). Regulation of protein function through expression of chimaeric proteins. *Curr. Opin. Biotechnol.* 5:511–515.

Price, J., Turner, D., and Cepko, C. (1987). Lineage analysis in the vertebrate nervous system by retrovirus-mediated gene transfer. *Proc. Natl. Acad. Sci. U.S.A.* 84:156–160.

Punzo, C. and Cepko, C. L. (2008). Unpublished results.

Rapaport, D. H., Wong, L. L., Wood, E. D., Yasumura, D., and LaVail, M. M. (2004). Timing and topography of cell genesis in the rat retina. *J. Comp. Neurol.* 21:304–324.

Saito, T., and Nakatsuji, N. (2001). Efficient gene transfer into the embryonic mouse brain using in vivo electroporation. *Dev. Biol.* 240:237–246.

Shimogori, T., Banuchi, V., Ng, H. Y., Strauss, J. B., and Grove, E. A. (2004). Embryonic signaling centers expressing BMP, WNT and FGF proteins interact to pattern the cerebral cortex. *Development* 131:5639–5647.

Swaroop, A., Xu, J. Z., Pawar, H., Jackson, A., Skolnick, C., and Agarwal, N. (1992). A conserved retina-specific gene encodes a basic motif/leucine zipper domain. *Proc. Natl. Acad. Sci. U.S.A.* 89:266–270.

Tabata, H., and Nakajima, K. (2001). Efficient in utero gene transfer system to the developing mouse brain using electroporation: Visualization of neuronal migration in the developing cortex. *Neuroscience* 103:865–872.

Tomita, K., Ishibashi, M., Nakahara, K., Ang, S. L., Nakanishi, S., Guillemot, F., and Kageyama, R. (1996). Mammalian hairy and Enhancer of split homolog 1 regulates differentiation of retinal neurons and is essential for eye morphogenesis. *Neuron* 16:723–734.

Turner, D. L., and Cepko, C. L. (1987). A common progenitor for neurons and glia persists in rat retina late in development. *Nature* 28:131–136.

Turner, D. L., Snyder, E. Y., and Cepko, C. L. (1990). Lineage-independent determination of cell type in the embryonic mouse retina. *Neuron* 4:833–845.

Young, R. W. (1985). Cell differentiation in the retina of the mouse. *Anat. Rec.* 212:199–205.

Zack, D. J., Bennett, J., Wang, Y., Davenport, C., Klaunberg, B., Gearhart, J., and Nathans, J. (1991). Unusual topography of bovine rhodopsin promoter-lacZ fusion gene expression in transgenic mouse retinas. *Neuron* 6:187–199.

Zeng, Y., Wagner, E. J., and Cullen, B. R. (2002). Both natural and designed micro RNAs can inhibit the expression of cognate mRNAs when expressed in human cells. *Mol. Cell* 9: 1327–1333.

52 Genetic Knockouts in Ophthalmic Research and Drug Discovery

DENNIS S. RICE

The study of mouse genetics has had a tremendous impact on medical research over the last few decades. Ophthalmology is no exception and has benefited from the mouse, which exhibits significant homology with the human genome (Waterston et al., 2002). In fact, the first scientific publication of an inheritable defect in the central nervous system (CNS) in mice was *rodless* (subsequently shown to be a mutation in the β subunit of cGMP phosphodiesterase). Mutations in the human homologue result in retinitis pigmentosa and blindness. More recently, knockout strains have been used to predict drug actions in humans (Zambrowicz et al., 2003). Phenotypic screens are used to examine mouse knockouts for physiological parameters that are beneficial in the clinic. This chapter provides a general introduction to the importance of mouse genetics in understanding ocular development and the physiology of particular cell types and highlights several examples of significant contributions by mouse models to the discovery and development of new therapies in human ophthalmic disease.

Cell types in the retina

The neural retina and the retinal pigmented epithelium (RPE) are derived from neuroectodermal precursors in the optic vesicle, which emerges from the ventral diencephalon (Mann, 1964). The vesicle invaginates, forming the optic cup, in which the inner layer becomes the neural retina and the outer layer becomes the RPE. The neural retina in mice is organized into three cellular layers separated by plexiform layers that contain synaptic connections among retinal neurons. The laminar organization of the mouse retina was described in a monograph entitled *The Structure of the Retina*, first published in 1892 by the legendary anatomist, Santiago Ramón y Cajal (1972). Relying primarily on the Golgi method to label cellular elements in detail, Ramón y Cajal described the major cell types of the mouse retina. This description of retinal cytoarchitecture established the foundation for future studies aimed at understanding anatomical and physiological relationships in the vertebrate retina.

In routine histological sections, the mouse retina appears relatively simple and neatly organized into three cellular layers (figure 52.1*A*). Cells within these layers can be grouped into neuronal or glial cell types. Within a given general cell type, there are often multiple morphologies and neurochemical signatures that expand the list to 50–60 different cell types (Haverkamp and Wässle, 2000). The ganglion cell layer (GCL) in mice contains one or two rows of cells, depending on the central or peripheral location of the field in view (figure 52.1*B*). The GCL is populated by ganglion cells, the sole projection neurons of the retina that transmit signals through the optic nerve to the central visual nuclei. The GCL also contains retinal astrocytes, displaced amacrine cells, and cells that make up the superficial retinal vasculature, endothelial cells and mural cells. The inner nuclear layer (INL) is located in the neural retina and is five to seven cell layers thick, depending on the retinal locale in view (see figure 52.1*A*). The INL is home to a diverse population of retinal cells, such as amacrine cells, Müller glial cells, bipolar neurons, and horizontal cells (figure 52.1*B–D*).

The outer nuclear layer (ONL) contains rod and cone photoreceptors that detect illumination gradients (see figure 52.1*A*). Approximately 10–15 rows of nuclei populate the ONL, with rods far outnumbering cones in this nocturnal species (Carter-Dawson and LaVail, 1979). With few exceptions, cone cell nuclei are located at the periphery of the ONL (figure 52.2*A*). Photoreceptors are further specialized into outer and inner segments. These specializations are easily observed in routine sections. Inner segments enable the synthesis and transport of proteins destined for the outer segments. The outer segments contain stacked discs of membranes that capture photons and convert this energy to chemical messengers that travel back toward the INL to ultimately affect synaptic transmission of RGCs.

Cones account for approximately 2%–3% of the photoreceptor population in mice (Carter-Dawson and LaVail, 1979; Jeon et al., 1998). Figure 52.2*B* shows a reliable histological marker for cone photoreceptors, the lectin peanut agglutinin (PNA), which labels the interphotoreceptor matrix associated with cone but not rod photoreceptors (Johnson et al., 1986). Although mice lack a central specialization observed in other mammals, the density of cones (approximately 3,500 cones/mm^2) is comparable to the approximately 3,000 cones/mm^2 observed in the parafoveal primate retina (Curcio et al., 1990; Jeon et al., 1998). Rod

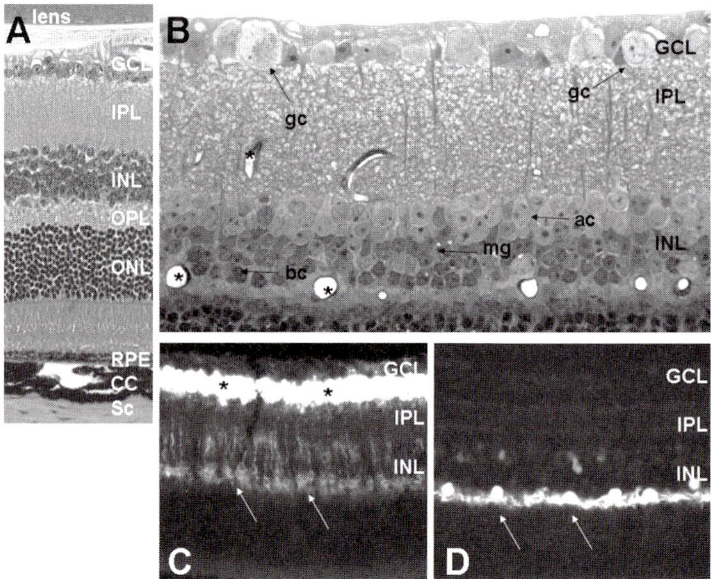

FIGURE 52.1 Anatomy and cell types in the adult mouse retina. *A*, The neural retina contains three cellular layers known as the ganglion cell layer (GCL), inner nuclear layer (INL), and outer nuclear layer (ONL). Two synaptic layers connect cells in the nuclear layers, the inner plexiform layer (IPL) and the outer plexiform layer (OPL). The retinal pigmented epithelium (RPE) contains melanin and protects and supports the photoreceptors in the ONL. The choriocapillaris (CC) is also pigmented and provides vascular supply to the RPE. The sclera (Sc) supports the outer eye. *B*, Higher magnification view of the inner retina. Ganglion cells (gc) are located in the GCL. Amacrine cells (ac) reside in the inner portion of the INL and stain much less intensely than the neighboring Müller glia (mg), located in the middle region of the INL. Bipolar cells (bc) are located on the outer portion of the INL (*asterisks* indicate capillaries). *C*, Many immunohistochemical markers can be used to identify individual cell types in the mouse retina. Anti-PKCα antibodies recognize the rod bipolar cell bodies (*arrows*) and their synaptic terminals (*asterisks*) in the IPL, near the GCL. *D*, Anticalbindin recognizes horizontal cells (*arrows*) in the outer portion of the INL. For a detailed list of molecular reagents to study individual cell types in the mouse retina, the reader should consult Haverkamp and Wässle (2000).

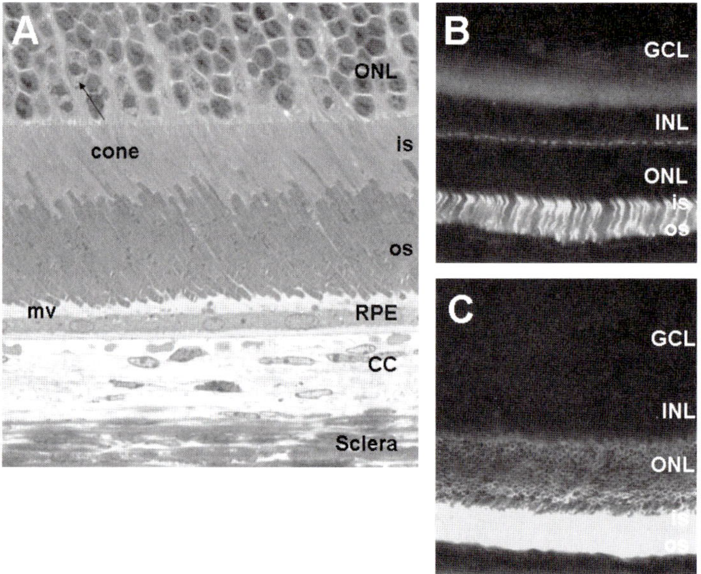

FIGURE 52.2 Anatomy of the outer retina. *A*, Phototransduction occurs in photoreceptors located in the outer nuclear layer (ONL). Cone photoreceptors are easily distinguished from the much more numerous rod photoreceptors by their heterochromatin (*arrow*) and location within the ONL, which is close to the inner segments (is). Outer segments (os) contain the light-sensitive pigments that capture photons. Their tips are engulfed by apical microvilli (mv) that extend from the retinal pigmented epithelium (RPE). The section in this image was obtained from an albino mouse that lacked pigmentation in the RPE or choriocapillaris (CC). *B*, The PNA-lectin conjugated to FITC is an excellent marker to visualize cone outer segments and inner segments in the mouse retina. *C*, Rods can be visualized with antirhodopsin antibodies.

photoreceptor density averages 437,000 cells/mm^2 and therefore represents approximately 97% of total photoreceptors. Rods can be identified with a variety of antibodies; antirhodopsin is one of the most commonly used (figure 52.2*C*).

The first synaptic relay in light sensation occurs at the level of the outer plexiform layer (OPL) and involves the transmission between rod photoreceptors and rod bipolar cells during low light or nocturnal conditions, and between cones and cone bipolar cells under photopic or bright-light conditions. Rod bipolar cells are routinely visualized with anti-PKCα antibodies (see figure 52.1*C*). These synaptic connections mark the interface between the ONL and the INL. Unlike other neuronal cell types in the INL, horizontal cells are defined by a single morphology, the axon-bearing horizontal cell. Calbindin immunoreactivity (see figure 52.1*D*) is an excellent marker for horizontal cells in the mouse retina (Haverkamp and Wässle, 2000). Rod photoreceptors establish contact at the axon terminal system and cone photoreceptors provide synaptic input to the horizontal cell dendrite. Horizontal cells provide reciprocal communication to photoreceptors and input to bipolar cells. Cone and rod bipolar cells relay visual stimuli from photoreceptors to a synaptic-rich region known as the inner plexiform layer (IPL), which contains connections formed among bipolar, amacrine, and ganglion cells (see figure 52.1*A* and *B*).

The retinal pigmented epithelium

Photoreceptors are intimately associated with an adjacent layer of cells in the outer retina known as the retinal pigmented epithelium. This epithelium is derived from neuroectoderm that also differentiates into the neural retina (Strauss, 2005). Thus, both neural retina and RPE are lateral extensions of the CNS. RPE cells appear cuboidal in cross section and hexagonal when viewed in whole-mount preparations. The RPE is one of the most intriguing cell types in the eye because of its location and functions within the retina proper. RPE cells are highly polarized, exhibiting a basal side that faces Bruch's membrane and an apical side that extends microvilli to surround the adjacent photoreceptor outer segments (see figure 52.2*A*). As the name implies, this epithelium contains numerous melanin granules, which give the cell a dark brown appearance in routine histological preparations (see figure 52.1*A*). The RPE is the first cell type in the body to express pigmentation, which is visible in the dorsal eye cup at approximately embryonic day 11.5 (E11.5; Strongin and Guillery, 1981). The basal side of the RPE is characterized by numerous infoldings that increase the surface area of the RPE membrane and facilitate transport and secretion (Strauss, 2005). These general characteristics of the RPE cell provide an adequate preamble to the important role this cell type serves in retinal development, physiology, and disease.

The RPE is positioned between the highly vascular choriocapillaris and the avascular photoreceptor layer of the neural retina (see figure 52.2*A*). Tight junctions that are present between apical surfaces of adjacent RPE cells establish the blood-retinal barrier at this location, while the endothelium is responsible for the barrier within the neural retina. Insofar as the RPE represents a barrier in the retina, one major function of this cell type is to transport water, electrolytes, and metabolic waste from the subretinal space to the choriocapillaris and import nutrients such as glucose and retinol from the systemic circulation (Strauss, 2005). Retinol (vitamin A) is important in visual sensation because it is a major source of 11-*cis*-retinaldehyde, the chromophore that binds opsins in photoreceptors. Light isomerizes 11-*cis*-retinal to all-*trans*-retinaldehyde, which initiates the signal transduction cascade and photoreceptor membrane hyperpolarization. The 11-*cis*-retinaldehyde–opsin receptor complex is restored in a process known as the retinoid visual cycle, and the RPE plays an important role in this process (Dowling, 1960).

A number of genes identified in humans and mice have been shown to encode critical components of the retinoid visual cycle, and mutations in these genes result in poor visual sensitivity and photoreceptor degeneration (Besch et al., 2003). Recent studies in mice have suggested that modulation of the retinoid cycle may be a new therapeutic strategy to treat RPE and retinal diseases. For example, the RPE65 gene encodes a protein of 533 amino acids that is required for conversion of all-*trans*-retinyl esters to 11-*cis*-retinol in the RPE (Redmond et al., 1998). Mutations that affect RPE65 activity result in Leber congenital amaurosis in humans, which is characterized by a severe, early-onset retinal dystrophy (Gu et al., 1997; Marlhens et al., 1997; Redmond et al., 2005).

The RPE65 protein is specifically expressed in RPE cells, and knockout of RPE65 in mice results in very low levels of 11-*cis*-retinal and its esters, while *trans*-retinyl esters accumulate in the RPE (Bavik et al., 1992; Redmond et al., 1998). Electroretinograms (ERGs) are severely attenuated, despite the presence of photoreceptors and outer segments (Redmond et al., 1998; Pang et al., 2005). The most obvious pathology is the shortening of outer segments in mice lacking RPE65, confirming that proteins that are intrinsic to RPE cells can often affect neighboring photoreceptors. Photoreceptor cell loss occurs in the absence of RPE65, but this event is likely secondary to biochemical changes in the visual cycle (Woodruff et al., 2003). Oral administration of 9-*cis*-retinal in mice lacking RPE65 led to recovery of light sensitivity and rod function (Van Hooser et al., 2000).

Administration of 9-*cis*-retinoid also restored visual pigment and retinal function in mice lacking the enzyme lecithin:retinol acyltransferase (LRAT), which is critical for the esterification of all-*trans*-retinol (Batten et al., 2005).

Mutations in LRAT result in early-onset retinal dystrophy in humans (Thompson et al., 2001). The product of LRAT activity is a substrate for RPE65, which produces 11-*cis*-retinol that is further oxidized to 11-*cis*-retinal in the RPE (Maeda et al., 2006a). Recently, functional recovery of photoreceptors was observed following 9-*cis*-retinal treatment in mice lacking the oxidative enzymes required for the final step in the reconversion of the bleached chromophore (Maeda et al., 2006b). These studies suggest that improvement in photoreceptor sensitivity is possible regardless of the primary genetic defect affecting the RPE biochemical synthetic pathway for 11-*cis*-retinal.

A major function of the RPE cells is to phagocytose photoreceptor outer segments, which are shed daily by the photoreceptors (Young and Bok, 1969). As a result, proteins that function in photoreceptors also affect neighboring RPE cells. ABCA4 is a member of the ATP-binding cassette transporter family and is localized in the outer segments of rod and cone photoreceptors (Cideciyan et al., 2004). Mutations in the ABCA4 gene are responsible for a number of photoreceptor degenerations in humans, such as Stargardt disease, atypical retinitis pigmentosa, and cone-rod dystrophy (Allikmets, 2000). Stargardt disease shares pathological features with AMD and is associated with accumulation of lipofuscin pigments in RPE cells and loss of central vision (Cideciyan et al., 2004). Mice lacking ABCA4, also known as rim protein (RmP), exhibit delayed dark adaptation with relatively normal retinal anatomy and photoreceptor sensitivity (Weng et al., 1999; Radu et al., 2003). Most important, these mice exhibit a dramatic accumulation of *N*-retinylidene-*N*-retinylethanolamine (A2E), the major fluorophore in lipofuscin that accumulates in RPE cells (Weng et al., 1999). Biophysical studies using recombinant protein and analysis of ABCA4 knockout mice suggest that ABCA4 functions as a flippase for *N*-retinylidene-phosphatidylethanolamine (*N*-ret-PE), the Schiff-base conjugate of all-*trans*-retinal and phosphatidylethanolamine. Hydrolysis of *N*-ret-PE in the photoreceptor cytoplasm releases all-*trans*-retinaldehyde, which is reduced to all-*trans*-retinol, which enters the RPE and is subsequently esterified by LRAT (Weng et al., 1999; McBee et al., 2001; Maeda et al., 2006b). In the absence of flippase activity, the *N*-ret-PE is thought to accumulate in the inner disc compartment. The models predict that following phagocytosis, outer segments containing high levels of the *N*-ret-PE adduct enter the phagolysosomal pathway in the RPE, which promotes the formation of A2E in lipofuscin upon light exposure. Accumulation of lipofuscin in the ABCA4 knockout is blocked when mice are reared in total darkness, confirming the light cycle dependency of this pathobiology (Mata et al., 2000).

Mutations in a different photoreceptor-specific protein known as elongation of very long chain fatty acids (ELOVL4) result in Stargardt disease in humans (Zhang et al., 2001). Knockout of ELOVL4 in mice results in a lethal phenotype, while heterozygous mice exhibit very mild morphological defects in the retina (Raz-Prag et al., 2006). Mice genetically engineered to overexpress the human mutation in ELOVL4 exhibit lipofuscin accumulation in the RPE and progressive photoreceptor degeneration (Karan et al., 2005; Vasireddy et al., 2006). Although more work needs to be done to establish the biochemical activity of this gene, this evidence suggests that factors involved in long chain polyunsaturated fatty acid content in photoreceptors could play a significant role in the propensity for lipofuscin accumulation and retinal degeneration.

Lipofuscin appears in the RPE during senescence as a by-product of the retinoid visual cycle and phagocytosis of the outer segments (Dorey et al., 1989). Studies in the ABCA4 and ELOVL4 genetic models implicate phospholipid biosynthesis and appropriate processing of retinoid cycle by-products as key cellular events that affect accumulation of lipofuscin in the RPE. High levels of lipofuscin and A2E in RPE cells are toxic to cells and may contribute to degenerations observed in retinal disease patients (Sparrow et al., 2000; Suter et al., 2000). Recently, the photo-oxidation products of A2E have been shown to activate the complement cascade in vitro (Zhou et al., 2006). Strong genetic associations with AMD have been described recently for complement factor alleles in humans (Edwards et al., 2005; Haines et al., 2005; Klein et al., 2005). The light dependency of lipofuscin accumulation, along with other environmental factors, suggests that modulation of the visual cycle and complement cascade are potential therapeutic strategies for macular degeneration.

Recent studies have shown that small molecule antagonists of the visual cycle protect against light-induced degeneration and lipofuscin accumulation in disease models (Maiti et al., 2006). This pharmacological approach recapitulated the phenotype in the RPE65 knockout mice, which exhibited a reduction in lipofuscin during senescence (Katz and Redmond, 2001). Moreover, mice lacking RPE65 are resistant to the light-induced degeneration challenge assay (Grimm et al., 2000). Importantly, inhibiting the visual cycle protects against light-induced degeneration and attenuates lipofuscin accumulation in the ABCR knockout mouse as well (Sieving et al., 2001; Radu et al., 2003, 2005; Maiti et al., 2006).

Most knockouts are maintained on a mixed genetic background between 129/SvJ and C57BL/6J. These two inbred strains are homozygous for RPE65 alleles that render mice either susceptible (Leu450) or resistant (Met450) to light-induced degeneration, most likely as a result of altered rhodopsin regeneration kinetics (Danciger et al., 2000; Kim et al., 2004). Indeed, the B6;129 F_2 hybrid background shows different sensitivity to light damage when the RPE65 alleles are compared (figure 52.3). The ability to combine different alleles of RPE65 in mice also harboring targeted mutations in other genes can reveal molecular modulators in the retinoid visual cycle. Collectively, these studies highlight the important interactions that occur between photoreceptors and RPE cells, and they identify new strategies to modulate human retinal diseases associated with lipofuscin accumulation and deficiencies in the visual cycle.

The intricate relationship that exists between the RPE and adjacent photoreceptors is critical to maintain normal visual function. The RPE is also important during retinal development (Strauss, 2005). Detailed studies of retinal development in hypopigmentation mutants have demonstrated that RGCs that normally project to ipsilateral central visual targets instead misroute at the optic chiasm and cross the midline, inappropriately reaching the contralateral central nuclei (LaVail et al., 1978; Dräger and Olsen, 1980; Jeffery, 1997). There is a delay in retinal development and rod number is decreased in albinos lacking functional tyrosinase, the key enzyme in the synthesis of melanin (Ilia and Jeffery, 1999). These studies implied that the enzymatic product of tyrosinase, which could be melanin, controls important aspects of retinal development.

Enzyme replacement therapy or product supplementation, as demonstrated in the retinoid cycle, is a viable strategy and mouse models have provided examples of proof of concept–type experiments. For example, during melanin synthesis, tyrosinase oxidizes L-tyrosine to L-dopaquinone, which is further converted to melanin. One product of this enzymatic reaction is L-3,4-dihydroxyphenylalanine (L-dopa). Transgenic mice that express tyrosine hydroxylase in the RPE rescue the retinal abnormalities in albino mice (Lavado et al., 2006). This result was attributed to direct action of L-dopa during retinal development as the transgene was expressed in mice lacking functional tyrosinase and, therefore, could not convert L-dopa to melanin. This clever genetic experiment demonstrates that either L-dopa or a metabolite is critical for normal retinal development and that supplementation could rescue defects that arise due to a deficiency in tyrosinase (Ilia and Jeffery, 1999).

Vascular cell types

Cells in the inner retina are nourished by three vascular beds that develop during the first 2 postnatal weeks in mice. Cellular regulation of vascular retinal development in mice remains one of the most intensely studied biological questions, owing to the accessibility of the developing vasculature in the postnatal eye. All aspects of angiogenesis occur in this organ, and the increasing availability of mouse genetic

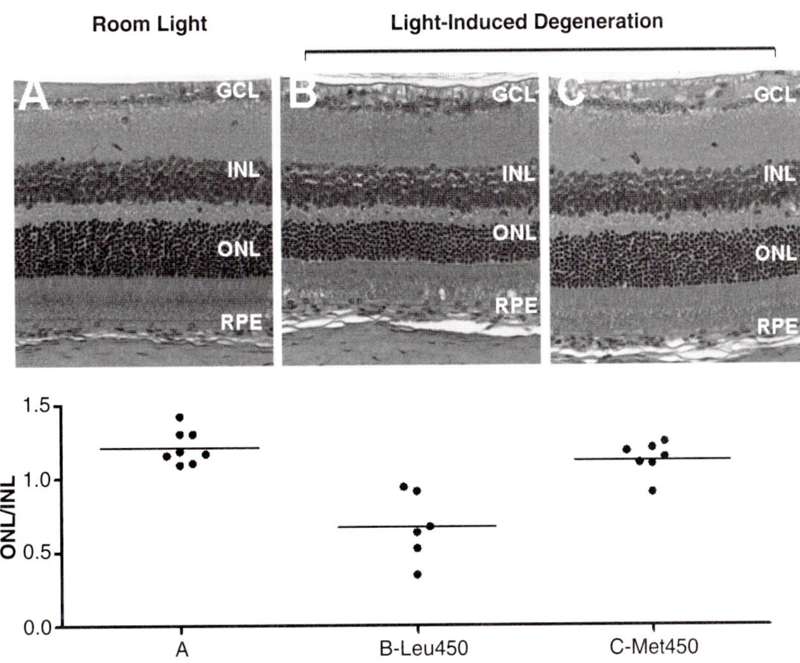

Figure 52.3 Light-induced degeneration in 129;B6 mice that are homozygous for either the Leu450 allele or Met450 allele of the RPE65 gene. Each dot represents the mean thickness of the ONL/INL from measurements obtained 400 μm on either side of the optic nerve head. *A*, Mice exposed to room light (40 lux) exhibit an ONL:INL ratio greater than 1.0 ($n = 8$). *B*, Mice homozygous for the Leu450 allele in the RPE65 gene are sensitive to 5 hours of light damage (5,000 lux) as shown in this histological section ($n = 6$). Sections were generated 7 days post light exposure. *C*, Mice ($n = 7$) homozygous for the Met450 allele in the RPE65 gene are resistant to light damage.

models and the ability to apply agents directly to the postnatal eye have enabled detailed studies of cell types and mechanisms involved in physiological angiogenesis. Pathological angiogenesis contributes to diseases in humans such as cancer and is a serious threat to vision in "wet" AMD and diabetic retinopathy (Folkman, 1995). Therefore, studies of the mouse intraocular vasculature have provided some of the most exciting insights into cellular regulation of blood vessel development, maintenance, and pathobiology.

The process of vascularization in the mouse eye is well described, and several excellent reviews are available (Fruttiger, 2002; Dorrell and Friedlander, 2006). Before birth, the developing neural retina is avascular, although the hyloid vasculature nourishes the developing lens and surrounding tissues. As neuronal differentiation proceeds, increasing metabolic activity of the inner retina results in physiological hypoxia that is thought to initiate formation of the retinal vasculature (Zhang et al., 1999, 2003). The first vascular bed arises during postnatal days P1–P10 and is known as the superficial vascular plexus, which supports ganglion cells (Connolly et al., 1988). During the second postnatal week, the superficial vessels branch to descend toward the outer retina, where they elaborate into a second vascular plexus, which nourishes cells located in the distal INL. During the second and third postnatal weeks, a third vascular plexus forms through angiogenic sprouting at the level of the innermost region of the INL (figure 52.4).

The orderly appearance of retinal vasculature during the first 3 postnatal weeks is orchestrated by specific cell types and guidance cues. Evidence obtained in a number of species, including mice, indicates that the initial vascular plexus arises through the directed migration of endothelial cells along a preassembled grid of astrocytes (Dorrell and Friedlander, 2006). These astrocytes originate from the optic stalk and migrate radially prior to the arrival of endothelial cells at the optic nerve head. Genetic models have been instrumental in elucidating molecular details of these complex cellular interactions. For example, mice lacking platelet-derived growth factor-A (PDGF-A) exhibit a decrease in the complexity of the astrocytic grid, and consequently the coverage of the superficial vascular plexus is also decreased (Gerhardt et al., 2003). PDGF-A is expressed by RGCs and interacts with its receptor, PDGFR-α, present on astrocytes (Mudhar et al., 1993). Transgenic mice that overexpress PDGF under the control of the neuron-specific enolase promoter exhibit overgrowth of retinal vasculature due to increased density of astrocytes. Conversely, blocking PDGF-A function attenuates retinal vascular development by perturbing the complexity of the astrocyte network (Fruttiger et al., 1996). The cell adhesion molecule R-cadherin also appears to be important for the astrocyte-mediated guidance of the superficial vascular plexus (Dorrell et al., 2002). Mice deficient in the nuclear hormone receptor Tlx exhibit impaired astrocyte development and loss of R-cadherin expression, with concomitant disruption in vascular development, further confirming the intimate association between astrocytes and the developing capillaries (Miyawaki et al., 2004). Astrocytes continue their important role in vascular biology in adult retina by enabling the formation of the blood-retina barrier (Janzer and Raff, 1987).

The relative hypoxia of the newborn retina is believed to stimulate expression of various pro-angiogenic factors that drive endothelial cell proliferation and migration (Stone et al., 1995; Gerhardt and Betsholtz, 2005; Dorrell and Friedlander, 2006). VEGF-A is among one of the best characterized of these pro-angiogenic factors, and alternative splicing of *Vegf* mRNA generates multiple isoforms that have different diffusion capabilities within the extracellular matrix (Ferrara et al., 2003). VEGF is produced by astrocytes prior to the arrival of endothelial cells (Stone et al., 1995; Gariano, 2003; Gerhardt et al., 2003). At the leading edge of the developing capillaries, specialized endothelial cells termed tip cells extend and retract actin-rich filopodia along the glial cell network and the surrounding matrix (Dorrell et al., 2002; Gerhardt et al., 2003). These endothelial tip cell pioneers are followed closely by endothelial cells in the stalk, which are proliferating to form a patent capillary network superimposed on the astrocytic grid (Gariano, 2003; Gerhardt and Betsholtz, 2005). Studies in mice designed to express individual isoforms of VEGF-A demonstrate that tip cell migration and normal vascular patterning in the developing retina and brain are dependent on the establishment of tightly regulated VEGF-A gradients (Ruhrberg et al., 2002; Stalmans et al., 2002; Gerhardt et al., 2003). Moreover, VEGF-A signaling through VEGF receptor 2 (VEGFR2) affects simultaneously tip cell migration and stalk cell proliferation, and the cellular mechanism for this effect remains an area of intense research (Gerhardt et al., 2003; Gerhardt and Betsholtz, 2005). VEGFR2 protein is highly expressed in tip cells, and antagonism of VEGFR2 signaling retracts tip cell filopodia, providing further support that VEGF-A is involved in the guided migration of tip cells.

Genetic knockout studies targeting a single allele of VEGF-A in mice result in lethality between E11 and E12. The heterozygous embryos displayed defective vascularization in several organs, confirming the essential role of VEGF in blood vessel formation (Carmeliet et al., 1996; Ferrara et al., 1996). Moreover, knockout of the VEGFR2 results in embryonic lethality around day 9 and is characterized by failed angiogenesis and hematopoiesis, along with disorganized blood vessels (Shalaby et al., 1995).

These studies established a clear role for VEGF-A signaling in physiological angiogenesis. The clinical utility of VEGF in pathological angiogenesis is evidenced as VEGF-

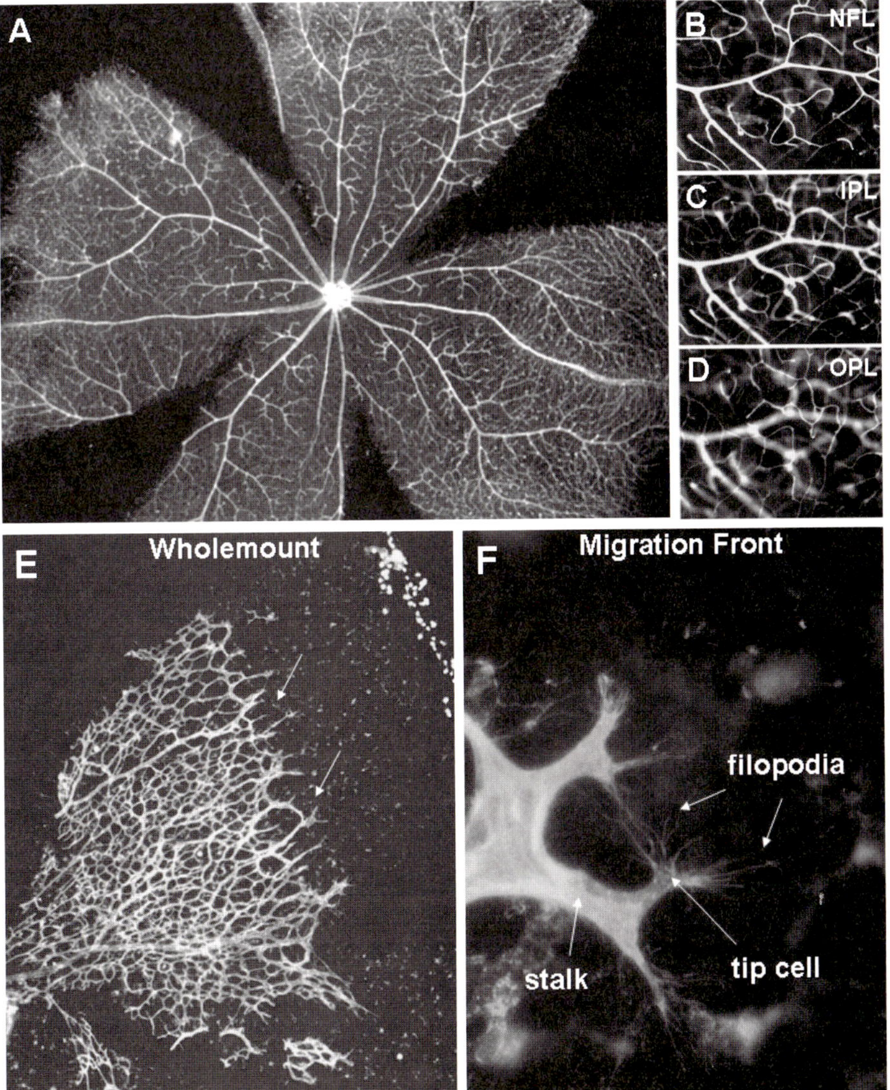

FIGURE 52.4 The retinal vasculature in mice contains three vessel beds. *A*, Whole-mount retinal preparation from a wild-type mouse stained with isolectin B4 conjugated to fluorescein. The retinal vasculature covers the entire retinal surface. *B–D*, Images taken at different depths through the retinal vasculature, starting at the most superficial layer, the nerve fiber layer (NFL [*B*]), which provides capillaries to the inner plexiform layer (IPL [*C*]), which are continuous with those capillaries in the outer plexiform layer (OPL [*D*]). *E*, Retinal whole mount obtained from a P6 mouse and stained with isolectin B4. The optic nerve head is at the *lower left* of the image, and the retinal periphery is in the *upper right*. The vasculature is developing toward the retinal periphery through the movement of the migration front (*arrows*). *F*, A higher magnification image of the migration front shows pioneer endothelial cells, termed tip cells, that direct the migration of the vasculature by extending actin-rich filipodia. Endothelial cells in the stalk form the nascent capillary bed.

blocking antibodies are now approved for wet AMD and colorectal cancer. Of note, the phenotypes observed in the heterozygous knockout of VEGF predicted the clinical efficacy of VEGF inhibition and provide a benchmark of the embryonic lethal phenotypes in mouse knockouts as a reliable indicator for potentially very potent modulators of vascular development and homeostasis.

The endothelial network, initially sculpted by astrocytes, is further remodeled into the mature vasculature that exhibits a stereotypical pattern. This process involves vascular pruning to establish a mature vessel density concurrent with the establishment of hemodynamic flow and increased oxygen levels in perfused tissue (Alon et al., 1995; Benjamin et al., 1998). Stabilization into a functional vessel requires intimate association with mural cells, such as pericytes and smooth muscle cells (Fischer et al., 2006). The dynamic interactions that occur between pericytes and endothelial cells are little understood at the molecular level, and studies using mouse genetic models are making inroads into this complex interaction among these cell types (Jain, 2003;

Armulik et al., 2005). The clinical significance of this question is great, as loss of pericytes and the appearance of microaneurysms are early hallmarks of retinopathy in diabetic patients (Speiser et al., 1968). Continued vessel occlusion results in increased vascular permeability, edema, and the formation of new vessels that proliferate into the vitreous.

Pericyte recruitment lags behind vessel formation (Benjamin et al., 1998). Pericyte coverage progresses from arterioles to venules, and the process does not reach completion before 3 weeks from birth. Remodeling of retinal vessels is complete before the establishment of pericyte coverage, indicating that mural cell investment marks the end of vascular remodeling capacity. Several gene knockout studies have shown that mural cells affect blood vessel branching, remodeling, and stabilization. For example, mice with a targeted deletion in either angiopoietin-1 or its receptor Tie2 exhibit defects in angiogenesis and vessel remodeling and maturation (Sato et al., 1995; Suri et al., 1996). Loss of pericytes and smooth muscle cells is evident in these animals. Most of the evidence suggests that these defects arise via an intrinsic block in signaling within endothelial cells, which specifically express Tie2, although alternative models have been suggested (Armulik et al., 2005). Endothelial tip cells secrete platelet-derived growth factor-B (PDGF-B), presumably in response to VEGF signaling (Lindahl et al., 1997; Dorrell and Friedlander, 2006). Mice deficient in PDGF-B are embryonic lethal and exhibit attenuation in pericyte proliferation and decreased vessel coverage. Vascular hemorrhaging, presumably as a result of vessels that are not fully invested by pericytes, is a common pathology observed in these mice. Pericyte loss, microvascular aneurysms, and lethality occur in mice lacking the PDGF-B receptor, which is expressed on mural cells (Benjamin et al., 1998; Hellstrom et al., 2001). In the absence of appropriate pericyte coverage, endothelial cells proliferate and become permeable, leading to impaired perfusion and hypoxia. These highlighted examples, and many others identified through mouse genetic studies, demonstrate a reciprocal cell-cell communication in which endothelial cells promote mural cell proliferation and migration and mural cells help support and stabilize endothelial cells (Hellstrom et al., 1999; Armulik et al., 2005).

Retinopathy of prematurity in premature infants is a pathogenesis of retinal blood vessels that arises as a result of high oxygen exposure to compensate for the underdeveloped lungs. Exposure of developing retinal vasculature to high oxygen decreases VEGF expression, leading to dropout of newly formed capillaries (Alon et al., 1995; Benjamin et al., 1998). Upon return to room air (normoxic conditions), VEGF is upregulated and neovascularization occurs. Pericyte investment is thought to be important for the ability of endothelial cells to respond to increasing oxygen tension. Fully invested capillaries, as is the case in mature vasculature, are largely refractory to the oxygen-induced vasobliteration (Alon et al., 1995; Benjamin et al., 1998). Novel strategies aimed at modulating cellular interactions between pericytes and endothelial cells are likely to emerge, given their important role in establishing and maintaining vascular integrity.

Additional guidance cues have been discovered through knockout mice that act to repel and keep tip cell endothelial pioneers on track toward formation of the complex vascular network. Using a knock-in reporter gene to monitor Unc5B expression, Lu and colleagues demonstrated high levels of Unc5B in endothelial tip cells in the retina and arteriole endothelial cells in more mature vessels (Lu et al., 2004). Unc5 proteins are membrane-bound receptors for axon guidance molecules known as netrins. Depending on the genetic background, homozygous Unc5B deficient mice were lethal by E12.5, exhibiting severe vascular phenotypes. Exuberant branching of vessels was observed in several organs, and endothelial tip cells demonstrated increased filopodial extensions in mice lacking Unc5B.

Vascular patterning arises through cellular interactions with both attractive and repulsive cues, which is reminiscent of guidance mechanisms that control the trajectories of neuronal projections during CNS development. Additional molecules involved in axon guidance have been shown to be involved in vascular patterning through gene knockout studies in mice. This list includes plexins, semaphorins, neuropilins, ephrins, and their receptors (Carmeliet and Tessier-Lavigne, 2005; Eichmann et al., 2005). The discovery of tip cells in endothelium that closely resemble growth cones of developing axons suggests that mechanisms acting during axonal guidance may directly apply to those controlling blood vessel patterning. Conversely, manipulations using cellular or molecular strategies in the relatively simple architecture of mouse retinal vasculature may yield insights into mechanisms that could be applied to promote reestablishment of neuronal connections in neurodegenerative conditions affecting the eye, such as glaucoma.

The availability of large numbers of genetic knockouts, combined with reliable markers to identify individual cell types, will continue to illustrate the power of mouse models to reveal additional cell types and molecules that affect both physiological and pathological angiogenesis (Jain, 2003). Many gene deletions in mice result in prenatal lethality or reduced viability as a consequence of blood vessel defects. In viable animals, genes affecting blood vessel formation and vascular integrity can be identified using noninvasive imaging techniques, such as angiography. For example, disruption of the endothelial cell–specific protein EGFL7 results in abnormal ocular blood vessel anatomy in some adult mice (figure 52.5*A*). EGFL7 is a secreted protein

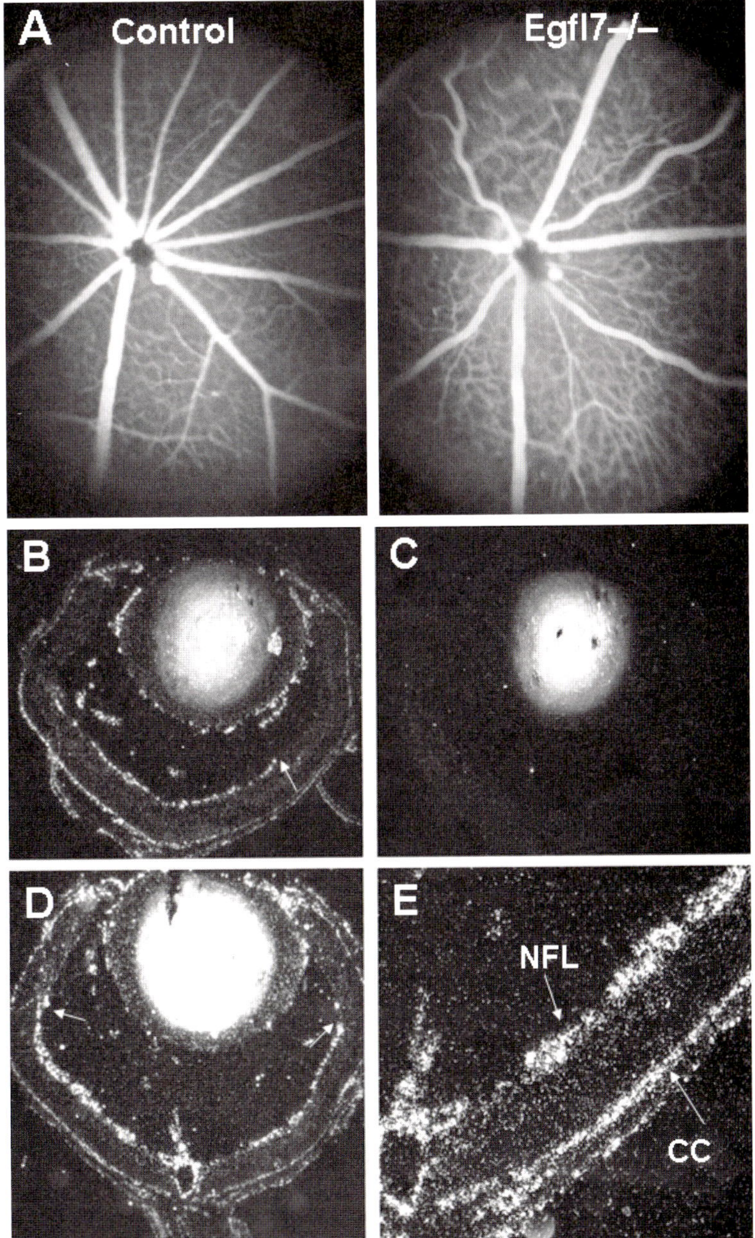

Figure 52.5 EGFL7 affects vascular anatomy. *A*, Angiography of wild-type mice (control) and mice lacking the secreted protein EGFL7 (−/−). In control eyes, blood vessels project directly toward the retinal periphery, while branches dive down toward the deeper levels of the retina to form the capillary beds. In the EGFL7−/− retina, vessels often meander on their way toward the retinal periphery. *B–E*, In situ hybridization of *Egfl7* in the postnatal mouse eye. *B*, At P3, Egfl7 expression in endothelial cells is present in the migrating front of the developing capillaries (*arrow*). Hyloid vessels and the choriocapillaris surround the eye, and iris vessels also express *Egfl7*. *C*, No signal in the P3 eye is observed when an *Egfl7* sense probe is used in the hybridization. *D*, At P6, the developing vasculature approaches the retinal periphery and *Eglf7* is present in these developing endothelial cells (*arrows*). *E*, Higher magnification of the P6 retina shown in *D*. *Egfl7* expression is present on the nerve fiber layer and the choriocapillaris (*arrows*), consistent with a developing retinal vasculature in the mouse eye.

that is highly expressed during embryonic and neonatal development (figure 52.5*B–E*). Expression levels decrease in mature vasculature, but Egfl7 expression is upregulated in vascular injury and in tumor models (Parker et al., 2004; Campagnolo et al., 2005). The abnormal vasculature observed in the eye of adult animals is due to a developmental defect in endothelial cell migration. Therefore, genetic screens in mice using embryonic lethality or noninvasive imaging in viable mice will lead to the identification of new targets for pathological angiogenesis.

Cell types in the anterior chamber

Glaucoma is a disease that affects RGCs, amacrine cells, and the optic nerve. This sight-threatening condition is often associated with increased ocular pressure, a major risk factor for glaucomatous disease. Regulation of intraocular pressure (IOP) is a balance between the production of aqueous humor at the ciliary body and drainage of aqueous humor at the iridocorneal angle (Civan and Macknight, 2004). Aqueous humor is produced by cells in the ciliary body that are nourished by a rich vascular supply. The humor travels through the pupil into the anterior chamber, where it encounters a series of cell types derived from the neural crest and mesoderm (Gould et al., 2004). These cells collectively form the drainage structures known as the conventional and uveoscleral (sometimes referred to as the nonconventional) outflow pathways. Traditionally, the conventional outflow pathway is thought to be dependent on pressure and involves cell types present in the trabecular meshwork, Schlemm's canal, and episcleral veins (Crowston and Weinreb, 2005). Aqueous humor is also drained through the uveoscleral pathway, which is a route through extracellular spaces in the iris, ciliary muscle, choroid, and sclera, where it ultimately collects in the lymphatics. The facility of the uveoscleral outflow remains an area of intense investigation (Crowston and Weinreb, 2005).

Although cell types involved in fluid dynamics have been well described, the molecular mechanisms involved in this process are only now being discovered. This exciting area of research is made possible by the development of several methods to measure IOP, determine the aqueous humor flow and episcleral venous pressure, and calculate total outflow facility in mice (John et al., 1998; Aihara et al., 2003a, 2003b; Crowston et al., 2004a). Mice have IOPs that are consistent with those in normotensive humans (Savinova et al., 2001). The dynamics of humor production and turnover are also comparable to those in humans (Aihara et al., 2003a), and mice respond to pharmacological agents that affect human aqueous humor production and outflow facility (Avila et al., 2001a, 2002; Aihara et al., 2002; Husain et al., 2006). These characteristics are leading to great interest in using mouse models to study processes associated with regulation of IOP and glaucoma.

Prostaglandin analogues are among the most widely prescribed drugs to manage ocular hypertension and glaucoma in the clinic. The mechanism by which these analogues lower IOP is still under investigation, but evidence suggests that IOP reductions occur by increasing outflow facility (Weinreb et al., 2002; Crowston and Weinreb, 2005). Prostaglandin analogues have been tested in a number of species, and a single topical application in mice lowers IOP within 6 hours (Aihara et al., 2002; Ota, Murata, et al., 2005; Husain et al., 2006). The intraocular metabolites of these analogues bind with high affinity to the FP receptor expressed primarily in cell types associated with aqueous production and flow (Anthony et al., 2001; Weinreb et al., 2002). Mice deficient in several of the prostanoid receptors have been studied to clarify the role of individual receptors involved in IOP effects of these hypotensive agents (Crowston et al., 2004b, 2005; Ota, Aihara, et al., 2005; Ota et al., 2006a, 2006b). A single application of latanoprost, travaprost, bimatoprost, or unoprostone to wild-type mice or mice deficient in the EP1 or EP2 receptors was effective at lowering IOP, indicating that EP receptors are not involved in the pharmacological actions of these analogues. In contrast, when these agents were applied to mice lacking the FP receptor, their ocular hypotensive action was no longer observed. These results clearly demonstrate that the FP receptor is required during the initial IOP-lowering effects of these clinical agents.

In the previous example, genetic knockouts provided the ability to determine the molecular target of clinically important compounds. Application of pharmacological agents to mice that lack specific genes also enables the direct test of on- versus off-target side effects (Zambrowicz et al., 2003). However, the phenotype of the knockout is also capable of predicting the potential utility of modulators for clinical applications. For example, several secreted and membrane proteins, such as type 1 collagen, aquaporin 1 and aquaporin 4 (AQP1 and AQP4, respectively), and the adenosine receptor 3 (AR3) have been shown to affect IOP in knockout mice. Mice deficient in type 1 collagen exhibited elevated IOP, while knockout of AQP1, AQP4, or AR3 resulted in lower IOP (Avila et al., 2001b; Zhang et al., 2002; Aihara et al., 2003c). The few studies that have focused on cellular mechanisms that control aqueous humor facility have concluded that mice appear to be excellent models in which to study the dynamics of pressure regulation (Lindsey and Weinreb, 2005). Combined with the increasing number of mouse genetic knockouts and new techniques amenable to the small mouse eye, the future looks very bright for new therapies aimed at specific cell types in the outflow pathway.

Ocular cell types are derived from the neural ectoderm, surface ectoderm, and mesenchymal and neural crest. Mouse genetics have played a leading role in elucidating cell migrations and communications that form and maintain the complexity and function of this organ. Therapeutic strategies under investigation or in clinical practice have established proof of concept in genetic models, and the predictive efficacy of the therapeutic was revealed through studies of gene knockouts. Mouse knockouts in challenge assays for pathological stresses, such as ischemia, ocular inflammation, and dry eye, can reveal individual genes with important functions in disease mechanisms (Da and Verkman, 2004; Pflugfelder et al., 2005; Liao et al., 2006). Mouse genetics will continue to be the core technology to study cell-cell interactions and physiological responses in mammalian biology and contribute to the next generation of therapeutics aimed at treating ocular disease.

ACKNOWLEDGMENTS The author thanks Kim Paes (Lexicon), Claire Gelfman (Lexicon), Weilan Ye (Genentech), and Maike Schmidt (Genentech) for scientific contributions to this chapter and Alex Turner for critical review of the manuscript.

REFERENCES

Aihara, M., Lindsey, J. D., and Weinreb, R. N. (2002). Reduction of intraocular pressure in mouse eyes treated with latanoprost. *Invest. Ophthalmol. Vis. Sci.* 43:146–150.

Aihara, M., Lindsey, J. D., and Weinreb, R. N. (2003a). Aqueous humor dynamics in mice. *Invest. Ophthalmol. Vis. Sci.* 44: 5168–5173.

Aihara, M., Lindsey, J. D., and Weinreb, R. N. (2003b). Episcleral venous pressure of mouse eye and effect of body position. *Curr. Eye. Res.* 27:355–362.

Aihara, M., Lindsey, J. D., and Weinreb, R. N. (2003c). Ocular hypertension in mice with a targeted type I collagen mutation. *Invest. Ophthalmol. Vis. Sci.* 44:1581–1585.

Allikmets, R. (2000). Simple and complex ABCR: Genetic predisposition to retinal disease. *Am. J. Hum. Genet.* 67:793–799.

Alon, T., Hemo, I., Itin, A., Pe'er, J., Stone, J., and Keshet, E. (1995). Vascular endothelial growth factor acts as a survival factor for newly formed retinal vessels and has implications for retinopathy of prematurity. *Nat. Med.* 1:1024–1028.

Anthony, T. L., Lindsey, J. D., Aihara, M., and Weinreb, R. N. (2001). Detection of prostaglandin EP(1), EP(2), and FP receptor subtypes in human sclera. *Invest. Ophthalmol. Vis. Sci.* 42: 3182–3186.

Armulik, A., Abramsson, A., and Betsholtz, C. (2005). Endothelial/pericyte interactions. *Circ. Res.* 97:512–523.

Avila, M. Y., Carre, D. A., Stone, R. A., and Civan, M. M. (2001a). Reliable measurement of mouse intraocular pressure by a servo-null micropipette system. *Invest. Ophthalmol. Vis. Sci.* 42: 1841–1846.

Avila, M. Y., Stone, R. A., and Civan, M. M. (2001b). A(1)-, A(2A)- and A(3)-subtype adenosine receptors modulate intraocular pressure in the mouse. *Br. J. Pharmacol.* 134:241–245.

Avila, M. Y., Stone, R. A., and Civan, M. M. (2002). Knockout of A3 adenosine receptors reduces mouse intraocular pressure. *Invest. Ophthalmol. Vis. Sci.* 43:3021–3026.

Batten, M. L., Imanishi, Y., Tu, D. C., Doan, T., Zhu, L., Pang, J., Glushakova, L., Moise, A. R., Baehr, W., et al. (2005). Pharmacological and rAAV gene therapy rescue of visual functions in a blind mouse model of Leber congenital amaurosis. *PLoS Med.* 2:e333.

Bavik, C. O., Busch, C., and Eriksson, U. (1992). Characterization of a plasma retinol-binding protein membrane receptor expressed in the retinal pigment epithelium. *J. Biol. Chem.* 267:23035–23042.

Benjamin, L. E., Hemo, I., and Keshet, E. (1998). A plasticity window for blood vessel remodelling is defined by pericyte coverage of the preformed endothelial network and is regulated by PDGF-B and VEGF. *Development* 125:1591–1598.

Besch, D., Jagle, H., Scholl, H. P., Seeliger, M. W., and Zrenner, E. (2003). Inherited multifocal RPE-diseases: Mechanisms for local dysfunction in global retinoid cycle gene defects. *Vision Res.* 43:3095–3108.

Campagnolo, L., Leahy, A., Chitnis, S., Koschnick, S., Fitch, M. J., Fallon, J. T., Loskutoff, D., Taubman, M. B., and Stuhlmann, H. (2005). EGFL7 is a chemoattractant for endothelial cells and is up-regulated in angiogenesis and arterial injury. *Am. J. Pathol.* 167:275–284.

Carmeliet, P., Ferreira, V., Breier, G., Pollefeyt, S., Kieckens, L., Gertsenstein, M., Fahrig, M., Vandenhoeck, A., Harpal, K., et al. (1996). Abnormal blood vessel development and lethality in embryos lacking a single VEGF allele. *Nature* 380: 435–439.

Carmeliet, P., and Tessier-Lavigne, M. (2005). Common mechanisms of nerve and blood vessel wiring. *Nature* 436:193–200.

Carter-Dawson, L. D., and LaVail, M. M. (1979). Rods and cones in the mouse retina. I. Structural analysis using light and electron microscopy. *J. Comp. Neurol.* 188:245–262.

Cideciyan, A. V., Aleman, T. S., Swider, M., Schwartz, S. B., Steinberg, J. D., Brucker, A. J., Maguire, A. M., Bennett, J., Stone, E. M., et al. (2004). Mutations in ABCA4 result in accumulation of lipofuscin before slowing of the retinoid cycle: A reappraisal of the human disease sequence. *Hum. Mol. Genet.* 13:525–534.

Civan, M. M., and Macknight, A. D. (2004). The ins and outs of aqueous humour secretion. *Exp. Eye Res.* 78:625–631.

Connolly, S. E., Hores, T. A., Smith, L. E., and D'Amore, P. A. (1988). Characterization of vascular development in the mouse retina. *Microvasc. Res.* 36:275–290.

Crowston, J. G., Aihara, M., Lindsey, J. D., and Weinreb, R. N. (2004a). Effect of latanoprost on outflow facility in the mouse. *Invest. Ophthalmol. Vis. Sci.* 45:2240–2245.

Crowston, J. G., Lindsey, J. D., Aihara, M., and Weinreb, R. N. (2004b). Effect of latanoprost on intraocular pressure in mice lacking the prostaglandin FP receptor. *Invest. Ophthalmol. Vis. Sci.* 45:3555–3559.

Crowston, J. G., Lindsey, J. D., Morris, C. A., Wheeler, L., Medeiros, F. A., and Weinreb, R. N. (2005). Effect of bimatoprost on intraocular pressure in prostaglandin FP receptor knockout mice. *Invest. Ophthalmol. Vis. Sci.* 46:4571–4577.

Crowston, J. G., and Weinreb, R. N. (2005). Glaucoma medication and aqueous humor dynamics. *Curr. Opin. Ophthalmol.* 16: 94–100.

Curcio, C. A., Sloan, K. R., Kalina, R. E., and Hendrickson, A. E. (1990). Human photoreceptor topography. *J. Comp. Neurol.* 292:497–523.

Da, T., and Verkman, A. S. (2004). Aquaporin-4 gene disruption in mice protects against impaired retinal function and cell death after ischemia. *Invest. Ophthalmol. Vis. Sci.* 45:4477–4483.

Danciger, M., Matthes, M. T., Yasamura, D., Akhmedov, N. B., Rickabaugh, T., Gentleman, S., Redmond, T. M., LaVail, M. M., and Farber, D. B. (2000). A QTL on distal chromosome 3 that influences the severity of light-induced damage to mouse photoreceptors. *Mamm. Genome* 11:422–427.

Dorey, C. K., Wu, G., Ebenstein, D., Garsd, A., and Weiter, J. J. (1989). Cell loss in the aging retina: Relationship to lipofuscin accumulation and macular degeneration. *Invest. Ophthalmol. Vis. Sci.* 30:1691–1699.

Dorrell, M. I., Aguilar, E.,and Friedlander, M. (2002). Retinal vascular development is mediated by endothelial filopodia, a preexisting astrocytic template and specific R-cadherin adhesion. *Invest. Ophthalmol. Vis. Sci.* 43:3500–3510.

Dorrell, M. I., and Friedlander, M. (2006). Mechanisms of endothelial cell guidance and vascular patterning in the developing mouse retina. *Prog. Retin. Eye Res.* 25:277–295.

Dowling, J. E. (1960). Chemistry of visual adaptation in the rat. *Nature* 188:114–118.

Dräger, U. C., and Olsen, J. F. (1980). Origins of crossed and uncrossed retinal projections in pigmented and albino mice. *J. Comp. Neurol.* 191:383–412.

Edwards, A. O., Ritter, R. III, Abel, K. J., Manning, A., Panhuysen, C., and Farrer, L. A. (2005). Complement factor H polymorphism and age-related macular degeneration. *Science* 308:421–424.

Eichmann, A., Le Noble, F., Autiero, M., and Carmeliet, P. (2005). Guidance of vascular and neural network formation. *Curr. Opin. Neurobiol.* 15:108–115.

Ferrara, N., Carver-Moore, K., Chen, H., Dowd, M., Lu, L., O'Shea, K. S., Powell-Braxton, L., Hillan, K. J., and Moore, M. W. (1996). Heterozygous embryonic lethality induced by targeted inactivation of the VEGF gene. *Nature* 380:439–442.

Ferrara, N., Gerber, H. P., and LeCouter, J. (2003). The biology of VEGF and its receptors. *Nat. Med.* 9:669–676.

Fischer, C., Schneider, M., and Carmeliet, P. (2006). Principles and therapeutic implications of angiogenesis, vasculogenesis and arteriogenesis. *Handb. Exp. Pharmacol.* 176(Pt 2):157–212.

Folkman, J. (1995). Angiogenesis in cancer, vascular, rheumatoid and other disease. *Nat. Med.* 1:27–31.

Fruttiger, M. (2002). Development of the mouse retinal vasculature: Angiogenesis versus vasculogenesis. *Invest. Ophthalmol. Vis. Sci.* 43:522–527.

Fruttiger, M., Calver, A. R., Kruger, W. H., Mudhar, H. S., Michalovich, D., Takakura, N., Nishikawa, S., and Richardson, W. D. (1996). PDGF mediates a neuron-astrocyte interaction in the developing retina. *Neuron* 17:1117–1131.

Gariano, R. F. (2003). Cellular mechanisms in retinal vascular development. *Prog. Retin. Eye Res.* 22:295–306.

Gerhardt, H., and Betsholtz, C. (2005). How do endothelial cells orientate? Exs:3–15.

Gerhardt, H., Golding, M., Fruttiger, M., Ruhrberg, C., Lundkvist, A., Abramsson, A., Jeltsch, M., Mitchell, C., Alitalo, K., et al. (2003). VEGF guides angiogenic sprouting utilizing endothelial tip cell filopodia. *J. Cell. Biol.* 161:1163–1177.

Gould, D. B., Smith, R. S., and John, S. W. (2004). Anterior segment development relevant to glaucoma. *Int. J. Dev. Biol.* 48:1015–1029.

Grimm, C., Wenzel, A., Hafezi, F., Yu, S., Redmond, T. M., and Reme, C. E. (2000). Protection of Rpe65-deficient mice identifies rhodopsin as a mediator of light-induced retinal degeneration. *Nat. Genet.* 25:63–66.

Gu, S. M., Thompson, D. A., Srikumari, C. R., Lorenz, B., Finckh, U., Nicoletti, A., Murthy, K. R., Rathmann, M., Kumaramanickavel, G., et al. (1997). Mutations in RPE65 cause autosomal recessive childhood-onset severe retinal dystrophy. *Nat. Genet.* 17:194–197.

Haines, J. L., Hauser, M. A., Schmidt, S., Scott, W. K., Olson, L. M., Gallins, P., Spencer, K. L., Kwan, S. Y., Noureddine, M., et al. (2005). Complement factor H variant increases the risk of age-related macular degeneration. *Science* 308:419–421.

Haverkamp, S., and Wässle, H. (2000). Immunocytochemical analysis of the mouse retina. *J. Comp. Neurol.* 424:1–23.

Hellstrom, M., Gerhardt, H., Kalen, M., Li, X., Eriksson, U., Wolburg, H., and Betsholtz, C. (2001). Lack of pericytes leads to endothelial hyperplasia and abnormal vascular morphogenesis. *J. Cell. Biol.* 153:543–553.

Hellstrom, M., Kalen, M., Lindahl, P., Abramsson, A., and Betsholtz, C. (1999). Role of PDGF-B and PDGFR-beta in recruitment of vascular smooth muscle cells and pericytes during embryonic blood vessel formation in the mouse. *Development* 126:3047–3055.

Husain, S., Andy Whitlock, N., Rice, D. S., and Crosson, C. E. (2006). Effects of latanoprost on rodent intraocular pressure. *Exp. Eye Res.* 83:1453–1458.

Ilia, M., and Jeffery, G. (1999). Retinal mitosis is regulated by dopa, a melanin precursor that may influence the time at which cells exit the cell cycle: Analysis of patterns of cell production in pigmented and albino retinae. *J. Comp. Neurol.* 405:394–405.

Jain, R. K. (2003). Molecular regulation of vessel maturation. *Nat. Med.* 9:685–693.

Janzer, R. C., and Raff, M. C. (1987). Astrocytes induce blood-brain barrier properties in endothelial cells. *Nature* 325:253–257.

Jeffery, G. (1997). The albino retina: An abnormality that provides insight into normal retinal development. *Trends Neurosci.* 20:165–169.

Jeon, C. J., Strettoi, E., and Masland, R. H. (1998). The major cell populations of the mouse retina. *J. Neurosci.* 18:8936–8946.

John, S. W., Smith, R. S., Savinova, O. V., Hawes, N. L., Chang, B., Turnbull, D., Davisson, M., Roderick, T. H., and Heckenlively, J. R. (1998). Essential iris atrophy, pigment dispersion, and glaucoma in DBA/2J mice. *Invest. Ophthalmol. Vis. Sci.* 39:951–962.

Johnson, L. V., Hageman, G. S., and Blanks, J. C. (1986). Interphotoreceptor matrix domains ensheath vertebrate cone photoreceptor cells. *Invest. Ophthalmol. Vis. Sci.* 27:129–135.

Karan, G., Lillo, C., Yang, Z., Cameron, D. J., Locke, K. G., Zhao, Y., Thirumalaichary, S., Li, C., Birch, D. G., et al. (2005). Lipofuscin accumulation, abnormal electrophysiology, and photoreceptor degeneration in mutant ELOVL4 transgenic mice: A model for macular degeneration. *Proc. Natl. Acad. Sci. U.S.A.* 102:4164–4169.

Katz, M. L., and Redmond, T. M. (2001). Effect of Rpe65 knockout on accumulation of lipofuscin fluorophores in the retinal pigment epithelium. *Invest. Ophthalmol. Vis. Sci.* 42:3023–3030.

Kim, S. R., Fishkin, N., Kong, J., Nakanishi, K., Allikmets, R., and Sparrow, J. R. (2004). Rpe65 Leu450Met variant is associated with reduced levels of the retinal pigment epithelium lipofuscin fluorophores A2E and iso-A2E. *Proc. Natl. Acad. Sci. U.S.A.* 101:11668–11672.

Klein, R. J., Zeiss, C., Chew, E. Y., Tsai, J. Y., Sackler, R. S., Haynes, C., Henning, A. K., SanGiovanni, J. P., Mane, S. M., et al. (2005). Complement factor H polymorphism in age-related macular degeneration. *Science* 308:385–389.

Lavado, A., Jeffery, G., Tovar, V., de la Villa, P., and Montoliu, L. (2006). Ectopic expression of tyrosine hydroxylase in the pigmented epithelium rescues the retinal abnormalities and visual function common in albinos in the absence of melanin. *J. Neurochem.* 96:1201–1211.

LaVail, J. H., Nixon, R. A., and Sidman, R. L. (1978). Genetic control of retinal ganglion cell projections. *J. Comp. Neurol.* 182:399–421.

Liao, T., Ke, Y., Shao, W. H., Haribabu, B., Kaplan, H. J., Sun, D., and Shao, H. (2006). Blockade of the interaction of leukotriene b4 with its receptor prevents development of autoimmune uveitis. *Invest. Ophthalmol. Vis. Sci.* 47:1543–1549.

Lindahl, P., Johansson, B. R., Leveen, P., and Betsholtz, C. (1997). Pericyte loss and microaneurysm formation in PDGF-B-deficient mice. *Science* 277:242–245.

Lindsey, J. D., and Weinreb, R. N. (2005). Elevated intraocular pressure and transgenic applications in the mouse. *J. Glaucoma* 14:318–320.

Lu, X., Le Noble, F., Yuan, L., Jiang, Q., De Lafarge, B., Sugiyama, D., Breant, C., Claes, F., De Smet, F., et al. (2004). The netrin receptor UNC5B mediates guidance events controlling morphogenesis of the vascular system. *Nature* 432:179–186.

Maeda, A., Maeda, T., Imanishi, Y., Golczak, M., Moise, A. R., and Palczewski, K. (2006a). Aberrant metabolites in mouse models of congenital blinding diseases: Formation and storage of retinyl esters. *Biochemistry* 45:4210–4219.

Maeda, A., Maeda, T., and Palczewski, K. (2006b). Improvement in rod and cone function in mouse model of fundus albipunctatus after pharmacologic treatment with 9-cis-retinal. *Invest. Ophthalmol. Vis. Sci.* 47:4540–4546.

Maiti, P., Kong, J., Kim, S. R., Sparrow, J. R., Allikmets, R., and Rando, R. R. (2006). Small molecule RPE65 antagonists limit the visual cycle and prevent lipofuscin formation. *Biochemistry* 45:852–860.

Mann, I. (1964). *Development of the human eye.* New York: Grune and Stratton.

Marlhens, F., Bareil, C., Griffoin, J. M., Zrenner, E., Amalric, P., Eliaou, C., Liu, S. Y., Harris, E., et al. (1997). Mutations in RPE65 cause Leber's congenital amaurosis. *Nat. Genet.* 17: 139–141.

Mata, N. L., Weng, J., and Travis, G. H. (2000). Biosynthesis of a major lipofuscin fluorophore in mice and humans with ABCR-mediated retinal and macular degeneration. *Proc. Natl. Acad. Sci. U.S.A.* 97:7154–7159.

McBee, J. K., Palczewski, K., Baehr, W., and Pepperberg, D. R. (2001). Confronting complexity: The interlink of phototransduction and retinoid metabolism in the vertebrate retina. *Prog. Retin. Eye Res.* 20:469–529.

Miyawaki, T., Uemura, A., Dezawa, M., Yu, R. T., Ide, C., Nishikawa, S., Honda, Y., Tanabe, Y., and Tanabe, T. (2004). Tlx, an orphan nuclear receptor, regulates cell numbers and astrocyte development in the developing retina. *J. Neurosci.* 24: 8124–8134.

Mudhar, H. S., Pollock, R. A., Wang, C., Stiles, C. D., and Richardson, W. D. (1993). PDGF and its receptors in the developing rodent retina and optic nerve. *Development* 118:539–552.

Ota, T., Aihara, M., Narumiya, S., and Araie, M. (2005). The effects of prostaglandin analogues on IOP in prostanoid FP-receptor-deficient mice. *Invest. Ophthalmol. Vis. Sci.* 46:4159–4163.

Ota, T., Aihara, M., Saeki, T., Narumiya, S., and Araie, M. (2006a). The effects of prostaglandin analogues on prostanoid EP1, EP2, and EP3 receptor-deficient mice. *Invest. Ophthalmol. Vis. Sci.* 47:3395–3399.

Ota, T., Aihara, M., Saeki, T., Narumiya, S., and Araie, M. (2006b). The IOP-lowering effects and mechanism of action of tafluprost in prostanoid receptor-deficient mice. *Br. J. Ophthalmol.* 91:673–676.

Ota, T., Murata, H., Sugimoto, E., Aihara, M., and Araie, M. (2005). Prostaglandin analogues and mouse intraocular pressure: Effects of tafluprost, latanoprost, travoprost, and unoprostone, considering 24-hour variation. *Invest. Ophthalmol. Vis. Sci.* 46:2006–2011.

Pang, J. J., Chang, B., Hawes, N. L., Hurd, R. E., Davisson, M. T., Li, J., Noorwez, S. M., Malhotra, R., et al. (2005). Retinal degeneration 12 (rd12): A new, spontaneously arising mouse model for human Leber congenital amaurosis (LCA). *Mol. Vis.* 11:152–162.

Parker, L. H., Schmidt, M., Jin, S. W., Gray, A. M., Beis, D., Pham, T., Frantz, G., Palmieri, S., Hillan, K., et al. (2004). The endothelial-cell-derived secreted factor Egfl7 regulates vascular tube formation. *Nature* 428:754–758.

Pflugfelder, S. C., Farley, W., Luo, L., Chen, L. Z., de Paiva, C. S., Olmos, L. C., Li, D. Q., and Fini, M. E. (2005). Matrix metalloproteinase-9 knockout confers resistance to corneal epithelial barrier disruption in experimental dry eye. *Am. J. Pathol.* 166:61–71.

Radu, R. A., Han, Y., Bui, T. V., Nusinowitz, S., Bok, D., Lichter, J., Widder, K., Travis, G. H., and Mata, N. L. (2005). Reductions in serum vitamin A arrest accumulation of toxic retinal fluorophores: A potential therapy for treatment of lipofuscin-based retinal diseases. *Invest. Ophthalmol. Vis. Sci.* 46: 4393–4401.

Radu, R. A., Mata, N. L., Nusinowitz, S., Liu, X., Sieving, P. A., and Travis, G. H. (2003). Treatment with isotretinoin inhibits lipofuscin accumulation in a mouse model of recessive Stargardt's macular degeneration. *Proc. Natl. Acad. Sci. U.S.A.* 100:4742–4747.

Ramón y Cajal, S. (1972). *The structure of the retina.* Springfield, IL: Charles C Thomas.

Raz-Prag, D., Ayyagari, R., Fariss, R. N., Mandal, M. N., Vasireddy, V., Majchrzak, S., Webber, A. L., Bush, R. A., Salem, N., Jr., et al. (2006). Haploinsufficiency is not the key mechanism of pathogenesis in a heterozygous Elovl4 knockout mouse model of STGD3 disease. *Invest. Ophthalmol. Vis. Sci.* 47: 3603–3611.

Redmond, T. M., Poliakov, E., Yu, S., Tsai, J. Y., Lu, Z., and Gentleman, S. (2005). Mutation of key residues of RPE65 abolishes its enzymatic role as isomerohydrolase in the visual cycle. *Proc. Natl. Acad. Sci. U.S.A.* 102:13658–13663.

Redmond, T. M., Yu, S., Lee, E., Bok, D., Hamasaki, D., Chen, N., Goletz, P., Ma, J. X., Crouch, R. K., et al. (1998). Rpe65 is necessary for production of 11-cis-vitamin A in the retinal visual cycle. *Nat. Genet.* 20:344–351.

Ruhrberg, C., Gerhardt, H., Golding, M., Watson, R., Ioannidou, S., Fujisawa, H., Betsholtz, C., and Shima, D. T. (2002). Spatially restricted patterning cues provided by heparin-binding VEGF-A control blood vessel branching morphogenesis. *Genes. Dev.* 16:2684–2698.

Sato, T. N., Tozawa, Y., Deutsch, U., Wolburg-Buchholz, K., Fujiwara, Y., Gendron-Maguire, M., Gridley, T., Wolburg, H., Risau, W., et al. (1995). Distinct roles of the receptor tyrosine kinases Tie-1 and Tie-2 in blood vessel formation. *Nature* 376: 70–74.

Savinova, O. V., Sugiyama, F., Martin, J. E., Tomarev, S. I., Paigen, B. J., Smith, R. S., and John, S. W. (2001). Intraocular pressure in genetically distinct mice: An update and strain survey. *BMC Genet.* 2:12.

Shalaby, F., Rossant, J., Yamaguchi, T. P., Gertsenstein, M., Wu, X. F., Breitman, M. L., and Schuh, A. C. (1995). Failure of blood-island formation and vasculogenesis in Flk-1-deficient mice. *Nature* 376:62–66.

Sieving, P. A., Chaudhry, P., Kondo, M., Provenzano, M., Wu, D., Carlson, T. J., Bush, R. A., and Thompson, D. A. (2001). Inhibition of the visual cycle in vivo by 13-cis retinoic acid protects from light damage and provides a mechanism for night blindness in isotretinoin therapy. *Proc. Natl. Acad. Sci. U.S.A.* 98:1835–1840.

Sparrow, J. R., Nakanishi, K., and Parish, C. A. (2000). The lipofuscin fluorophore A2E mediates blue light-induced damage to retinal pigmented epithelial cells. *Invest. Ophthalmol. Vis. Sci.* 41:1981–1989.

Speiser, P., Gittelsohn, A. M., and Patz, A. (1968). Studies on diabetic retinopathy. 3. Influence of diabetes on intramural pericytes. *Arch. Ophthalmol.* 80:332–337.

Stalmans, I., Ng, Y. S., Rohan, R., Fruttiger, M., Bouche, A., Yuce, A., Fujisawa, H., Hermans, B., Shani, M., et al. (2002). Arteriolar and venular patterning in retinas of mice selectively expressing VEGF isoforms. *J. Clin. Invest.* 109:327–336.

Stone, J., Itin, A., Alon, T., Pe'er, J., Gnessin, H., Chan-Ling, T., and Keshet, E. (1995). Development of retinal vasculature is mediated by hypoxia-induced vascular endothelial growth factor. (VEGF) expression by neuroglia. *J. Neurosci.* 15:4738–4747.

Strauss, O. (2005). The retinal pigment epithelium in visual function. *Physiol. Rev.* 85:845–881.

Strongin, A. C., and Guillery, R. W. (1981). The distribution of melanin in the developing optic cup and stalk and its relation to cellular degeneration. *J. Neurosci.* 1:1193–1204.

Suri, C., Jones, P. F., Patan, S., Bartunkova, S., Maisonpierre, P. C., Davis, S., Sato, T. N., and Yancopoulos, G. D. (1996). Requisite role of angiopoietin-1, a ligand for the TIE2 receptor, during embryonic angiogenesis. *Cell* 87:1171–1180.

Suter, M., Reme, C., Grimm, C., Wenzel, A., Jaattela, M., Esser, P., Kociok, N., Leist, M., and Richter, C. (2000). Age-related macular degeneration: The lipofusion component *N*-retinyl-*N*-retinylidene ethanolamine detaches proapoptotic proteins from mitochondria and induces apoptosis in mammalian retinal pigment epithelial cells. *J. Biol. Chem.* 275: 39625–39630.

Thompson, D. A., Li, Y., McHenry, C. L., Carlson, T. J., Ding, X., Sieving, P. A., Apfelstedt-Sylla, E., and Gal, A. (2001). Mutations in the gene encoding lecithin retinol acyltransferase are associated with early-onset severe retinal dystrophy. *Nat. Genet.* 28:123–124.

Van Hooser, J. P., Aleman, T. S., He, Y. G., Cideciyan, A. V., Kuksa, V., Pittler, S. J., Stone, E. M., Jacobson, S. G., and Palczewski, K. (2000). Rapid restoration of visual pigment and function with oral retinoid in a mouse model of childhood blindness. *Proc. Natl. Acad. Sci. U.S.A.* 97:8623–8628.

Vasireddy, V., Jablonski, M. M., Mandal, M. N., Raz-Prag, D., Wang, X. F., Nizol, L., Iannaccone, A., Musch, D. C., Bush, R. A., et al. (2006). Elovl4 5-bp-deletion knock-in mice develop progressive photoreceptor degeneration. *Invest. Ophthalmol. Vis. Sci.* 47:4558–4568.

Waterston, R. H., Lindblad-Toh, K., Birney, E., Rogers, J., Abril, J. F., Agarwal, P., Agarwala, R., Ainscough, R., Alexandersson, M., et al. (2002). Initial sequencing and comparative analysis of the mouse genome. *Nature* 420:520–562.

Weinreb, R. N., Toris, C. B., Gabelt, B. T., Lindsey, J. D., and Kaufman, P. L. (2002). Effects of prostaglandins on the aqueous humor outflow pathways. *Surv. Ophthalmol.* 47(Suppl. 1): S53–S64.

Weng, J., Mata, N. L., Azarian, S. M., Tzekov, R. T., Birch, D. G., and Travis, G. H. (1999). Insights into the function of Rim protein in photoreceptors and etiology of Stargardt's disease from the phenotype in abcr knockout mice. *Cell* 98:13–23.

Woodruff, M. L., Wang, Z., Chung, H. Y., Redmond, T. M., Fain, G. L., and Lem, J. (2003). Spontaneous activity of opsin apoprotein is a cause of Leber congenital amaurosis. *Nat. Genet.* 35:158–164.

Young, R. W., and Bok, D. (1969). Participation of the retinal pigment epithelium in the rod outer segment renewal process. *J. Cell. Biol.* 42:392–403.

Zambrowicz, B. P., Turner, C. A., and Sands, A. T. (2003). Predicting drug efficacy: Knockouts model pipeline drugs of the pharmaceutical industry. *Curr. Opin. Pharmacol.* 3:563–570.

Zhang, D., Vetrivel, L., and Verkman, A. S. (2002). Aquaporin deletion in mice reduces intraocular pressure and aqueous fluid production. *J. Gen. Physiol.* 119:561–569.

Zhang, K., Kniazeva, M., Han, M., Li, W., Yu, Z., Yang, Z., Li, Y., Metzker, M. L., Allikmets, R., et al. (2001). A 5-bp deletion in ELOVL4 is associated with two related forms of autosomal dominant macular dystrophy. *Nat. Genet.* 27:89–93.

Zhang, W., Ito, Y., Berlin, E., Roberts, R., and Berkowitz, B. A. (2003). Role of hypoxia during normal retinal vessel development and in experimental retinopathy of prematurity. *Invest. Ophthalmol. Vis. Sci.* 44:3119–3123.

Zhang, Y., Porat, R. M., Alon, T., Keshet, E., and Stone, J. (1999). Tissue oxygen levels control astrocyte movement and differentiation in developing retina. *Brain Res. Dev. Brain Res.* 118:135–145.

Zhou, J., Jang, Y. P., Kim, S. R., and Sparrow, J. R. (2006). Complement activation by photooxidation products of A2E, a lipofuscin constituent of the retinal pigment epithelium. *Proc. Natl. Acad. Sci. U.S.A.* 103:16182–16187.

53 Beyond Positional Cloning of Single Gene Mutations: Use of Mouse Models to Examine Allelic Variance and to Identify Genetic Modifiers

PATSY M. NISHINA AND JUERGEN K. NAGGERT

Mouse models have proven to be extremely useful in the study of heritable ocular diseases. They have provided candidate genes for similar human diseases and whole animal systems to test potential therapeutic interventions. Environmental factors influencing vision, such as light and diet, can be easily studied in mice. In addition, as a robust renewable resource, they have allowed the systematic exploration of disease etiology, progression, and pathologies, which in turn has led to the generation of hypotheses about the functions of particular molecules and mechanisms underlying disease. Finally, mouse models can be an important tool for examining allelic effects (e.g., variability in phenotypes attributable to different mutations within a single gene) and for identifying genetic background modifiers (e.g., variability in phenotypes attributable to nonallelic interactions). Both are discussed in this chapter.

Four key factors make mouse models particularly effective for dissecting allelic effects and identifying modifier loci. First, mice are inbred, that is, all animals from a given strain are genetically identical. Therefore, phenotypic variability observed when comparing different mutations within the same molecule in the same inbred strain background would suggest allelic effects, barring differences in animal husbandry, whereas phenotypic variability observed in two different, genetically defined strains carrying the same mutant allele would suggest the presence of genetic modifier loci. Second, methods have been developed to induce mutations through chemical mutagenesis or by germ-line manipulation through genetic engineering. These approaches, particularly the latter, allow researchers to affect spatial or temporal expression to examine the function or roles of particular domains within genes. Third, the reagents and resources in the form of genomic information are tremendous, and new data in the form of sequences and single nucleotide polymorphisms over multiple strains are forthcoming with ever increasing frequency (Pletcher et al., 2004; Rudd et al., 2005; Shifman et al., 2006; see also www.jax.org/phenome/snp.html). These advances in particular will assist in the actual identification of the modifying genes and the pathways through which these genes function. Finally, a large number of noninvasive clinical tools have been adapted to the small eyes of the mouse, allowing for monitoring of phenotypic variability. These tools include slit lamp biomicroscopy, indirect ophthalmoscopy, fluorescein angiography, fundus photography, and electroretinography (ERG). In addition, methods to assess visually evoked potentials (VEPs; Ridder and Nusinowitz, 2006) and behavioral parameters such as visual acuity and contrast sensitivity (Douglas et al., 2005) are available. Finally, new noninvasive methods to access the morphological features of the retina by optical coherence tomography in a living animal are currently being developed by a number of groups. These methods will also extend our ability to carry out repeated measures to study disease progression and treatment modalities in a single mouse over time.

Allelic effects as a cause of phenotypic variation

Particular alleles may define clinical outcome or disease progression. They may also reveal the functional importance of a particular domain of a gene or protein and the response to environmental stresses or treatment modalities. The availability of mouse models bearing different alleles of the same gene is likely to increase as more animals are generated through chemical mutagenesis and targeted transgenesis to introduce clinically relevant disease alleles from human patients into the mouse genome. These models will be instrumental in elucidating the function of molecules and will provide an in vivo system in which to identify subpopulations of patients who harbor different mutations in the same molecule, and to test genotype-specific therapeutic modalities.

Defining Disease Progression, Clinical Outcome, or Important Domains In general, loss-of-function alleles produce a different phenotype than do missense mutations effecting hypomorphic or gain-of-function alleles. It can be argued that insofar as most mutations identified in humans are generally not null mutations, to elucidate the role that molecules may play in vision an array of alleles for each protein should be studied.

The best example of an allelic series affecting disease progression was generated by chemical mutagenesis in the gene encoding phosphodiesterase 6b (Hart et al., 2005). Four of the seven mutations identified by the MRC Harwell ENU Mutagenesis program were phenotypically identical to the original *Pdeb6b*^{rd1} mutation, which is found in many standard inbred strains (e.g., C3H/HeJ, SJL/J, FVB/N) and leads to a rapid panretinal rod photoreceptor degeneration by 3 weeks of age (Bowes et al., 1990). Three of the four predicted loss-of-function alleles were nonsense mutations leading to the introduction of premature stop codons, the fourth was a splice site mutation that would severely disrupt normal splicing. Two of the three remaining alleles that led to a slower progressing phenotype were missense mutations and the third was a splice site mutation that still allowed a small percentage of normal transcript to be formed. Interestingly, mice with the *Pdeb6b*^{atrd3} allele, which carries an amino acid change from asparagine to serine in the highly conserved residue 606, near a putative catalytic domain, showed earlier impaired vision and a greater loss of rod photoreceptors than did *Pdeb6b*^{atrd1} mice, which carry a histidine-620-glutamine mutation that occurs in a relatively conserved residue within a putative catalytic domain. Further study of these alleles may provide additional insight into the functional significance of the domains in which these missense mutations occur.

Although mutations in *Pde6b* can lead to photoreceptor degeneration, they can also lead to congenital stationary night blindness (CSNB) in humans without apparent morphological changes. Recently, Tsang et al. (2007) introduced a CSNB allele, *Pde6b*^{H258N}, by transgenic means into the *Pdeb6b*^{rd1} background and rescued the photoreceptors. ERG abnormalities were observed; however, the actual amplitude of the waveforms appeared to depend on the genetic background.

Another recent example of alternative alleles providing insight into the potential function of a gene similarly arose from a chemical mutagenesis screen (http://nmf.jax.org/index.html). Through positional candidate cloning, *nmf247* was identified as a point mutation in the splice acceptor site in intron 6 of *Rpgrip1* that leads to a deletion of exon 7 and a premature stop codon in exon 9 (Won et al., 2007). Interestingly, the *Rpgrip1*^{nmf247} allele appeared to be more severe than the previously reported null allele (Zhao et al., 2003) in that outer segments were rarely observed and the rate of photoreceptor degeneration was extremely rapid, with most cell bodies gone by 3 weeks of age. In the rare case in which outer segments developed, they were enlarged and vertically oriented, as described in the null allele (Zhao et al., 2003). The recent report of a shorter murine splice variant of *Rpgrip1* (Lu and Ferreira, 2005) and closer inspection of the null allele, which was an insertional mutation into exon 14, indicated that the original null allele potentially affected only the full-length form of *Rpgrip1*, whereas both splice variants would have been missing in *Rpgrip1*^{nmf247} mice. This observation suggests that the short form of RPGRIP1 or an otherwise unidentified splice variant may be important in the initiation of normal outer segment development, a hypothesis that is testable with the availability of the *nmf247* mouse model.

Defining Responses to Environmental Influences It is perhaps not surprising that different alleles of the same gene produce different responses to environmental influences. Understanding these different responses to nongenetic factors such as light exposure may yield insights into clinical prognosis as well as the function of the molecules studied in relation to the environmental influence tested.

Four alleles of *Rpe65*, a molecule that is abundantly expressed in the retinal pigmented epithelium (RPE), have been described in mice (Hamel et al., 1993; Redmond et al., 1998; Pang et al., 2005). A targeted null mutation of the *Rpe65* gene demonstrated that in the absence of functional RPE65 protein, outer segments become disorganized and a slow photoreceptor degeneration ensues (Redmond et al., 1998). The findings that *Rpe65*$^{-/-}$ mice do not have 11-*cis*-retinyl esters in their RPE and accumulate all-*trans*-retinyl esters suggested a disruption of the isomerization of all-*trans*-retinyl esters to 11-*cis*-retinal (Redmond et al., 1998). Moiseyev et al. (2005) hypothesized and provided evidence that RPE65 acts as an isomerohydrolase in the retinoid visual cycle. Perhaps it is not surprising, then, that alterations in RPE65 might affect retinal responses to light exposure. Danciger et al. (2000) noted that of nine albino mouse strains, the C57BL/6J-c^{2J} (c2J) strain demonstrated marked resistance to light-induced photoreceptor damage. A genome-wide scan for the resistance/susceptibility alleles in progeny of a (c2J × BALB/c)F(1) × c2J backcross revealed a major locus (accounting for 50% of the protective effect) on chromosome 3 and three other weak but significant contributing regions on chromosomes 9, 12, and 14. The protective effect observed in the c2J background was determined to result from a single nucleotide polymorphism (SNP) in the *Rpe65* gene. The c2J strain has methionine at residue 450, while the other eight susceptible albino strains studied carried leucine at codon 450. BALB/cBy retinas, which were more susceptible to light damage, regenerate rhodopsin at a faster rate than retinas from c2J (Wenzel et al., 2001), indicating that the kinetics of regeneration, and not the absolute levels of rhodopsin, are important in light-induced degeneration. These observations are clinically relevant, as they suggest that naturally occurring variants that do not in themselves cause significant overt disease may influence visual outcome when challenged with environmental stresses.

Another example of allelic variants that affect different phenotypes on light exposure are those in the rhodopsin gene. Mutations in the rhodopsin gene, a G protein–coupled receptor, are responsible for 30% of autosomal dominant cases of retinitis pigmentosa (RP) in humans. Rhodopsin-deficient mice generated by homologous recombination showed that the presence of rhodopsin is necessary for proper outer segment development and photoreceptor survival (Humphries et al., 1997). Panretinal loss of photoreceptor cell bodies was observed in $Rho^{-/-}$ mice by 3 months of age. Mutational screening of the rhodopsin gene in a dog model of RP found an amino acid change from threonine to arginine at residue 4 (Kijas et al., 2002). The dogs showed a very slow recovery after exposure to bleaching light levels and local areas of degeneration. Of direct clinical relevance is the observation that moderate levels of light, such as those used in clinical examinations, increased the rate of retinal degeneration in these dogs (Cideciyan et al., 2005). We have recently identified two new rhodopsin alleles in our Models for Translational Vision Research (MTVR) program, Rho^{Mtvr1} and Rho^{Mtvr4}, which carry missense mutations induced by chemical mutagenesis that are phenotypically similar to the dog model (E. Budzynski, pers. comm., 2007). Degeneration of photoreceptors is focal and occurs only on direct light exposure. The observations from these models have important clinical implications, as individuals with this type of rhodopsin mutation may be more susceptible to light-induced damage, and early identification of these individuals may delay vision impairment if a reduction in light exposure is included in their treatment plan.

Defining Response to Treatment Because particular mutations at similar sites in the rhodopsin gene result in different clinical outcomes, the response to treatment may also be genotype dependent. RHO P23H is one of the most frequently occurring mutations associated with autosomal dominant RP in humans. A transgenic mouse, VPP, made with mutations in three amino acids, including P23H, exhibits a slow degeneration of both rods and cones, as assessed by ERG amplitudes and histology (Naash et al., 1993). Administration of recombinant human erythropoietin had no effect on the rate of photoreceptor degeneration in VPP mice but was able to protect mice from light-induced damage (Grimm et al., 2004). On the other hand, vitamin A supplementation slowed the rate of retinal degeneration in T17M transgenic mice but not in mice expressing the P347S allele of rhodopsin (Li et al., 1998).

Genetic modifiers as a cause of phenotypic variation

The phenotypic outcomes of a particular mutation may also be influenced by specific alleles of other genes in the genome, the so-called genetic modifiers. The phenomenon is also referred to as epistatic or nonlinear interaction between genes, so that the effects of variation in gene A are observed only in the presence of a particular variant of gene B. In mice, the existence of genetic modifiers was originally postulated from the variation in phenotype observed when spontaneous mutations were crossed onto different inbred backgrounds (Hummel et al., 1972). An early example of genetic modification in the visual system (LaVail et al., 1978) was demonstrated in mutants of the *c* locus in which differences in retinal ganglion cell projections could not be fully explained by allelic effects. Additionally, as large numbers of models with targeted mutations created on a 129Sv/J and C57BL/6 (B6) background have been generated, researchers have reported phenotypic variability, as the genetically engineered alleles were moved from the mixed 129/B6 background onto B6 (Ikeda et al., 1999; Humphries et al., 2001). In these cases, the effects of the modifier are observed only in the context of a primary mutation. The phenomenon of phenotypic modifications is currently recognized as a useful tool for identifying factors that interact with genes involved in known pathways or for providing entry points into the function of novel genes (Nadeau, 2003; Vincent, 2003; Linder, 2006). That is, they may provide additional information about genetic contributions to the phenotype for which treatment may already be available, or they may reveal additional steps in a biological pathway that may be more amenable to treatment. As more genes modifying the progression of ocular diseases caused by specific mutations are discovered, it is envisioned that these modifiers will unlock doors to new treatment modalities and help physicians make better diagnoses and treatment plans, perhaps by defining subgroups within a disease population. Examples of phenotypic variability in different genetic backgrounds where the primary mutation is the same are given in table 53.1. Examples of cases in which genetic modifier loci have been mapped or identified are less frequent; these are given in table 53.2. With the recent increase in available genomic information, the actual identification of genetic modifiers is expected to increase. Potential strategies for the identification of genetic modifiers are discussed later in the chapter.

Table 53.1

Genetic modification of ocular phenotypes observed in different strain backgrounds

Model	Effect of Genetic Modification	Strains Involved in Modification (Resistant → Susceptible)	References
Retinal degeneration 3 (*rd3*)	Variability in onset and progression of photoreceptor degeneration	RBF/Dn, Meta-In(1)Rk, Rb(11.13)4Bnr and In-30	Heckenlively, 1993
Rhodopsin$^{-/-}$	Variable rate of photoreceptor degeneration	C57BL/6 and 129/SvJ	Humphries et al., 2001
Nr2e3^{rd7}	Suppression of retinal spotting and photoreceptor degeneration	B6.Cg-*rd7/rd7* and CAST/EiJ	Akhmedov et al., 2000
Trp53	Attenuation of vitreal opacity, retinal folds and retrolental fibroplasia in the 129/SvJ background	129/SvJ and C57BL/6	Ikeda et al., 1999
Bmp4	Anterior segment dysgenesis with elevated intraocular pressure	C57BL/6J, BliA CAST/Ei, C3H/HeJ AKR/J, BALB/C 129/SvEvTac	Chang et al., 2001
isa, iris stromal atrophy, DBA/2J	Increased cell death	AKXD-28/Ty	Anderson et al., 2001
ipd, iris pigment dispersion	Milder phenotype	AKXD-28/Ty	Anderson et al., 2001
Nr2e1^{frc}	Thinning of optic layers, differences in ERG responses, and retinal vascular development	B6129F1, 129P3/JEms, and C57BL/6	Young et al., 2002
Crb1^{rd8}	Retinal dysplasia and photoreceptor degeneration	C57BL/6 and C3H/HeJ	Mehalow et al., 2003

Table 53.2

Genetic modifier loci that have been mapped and/or cloned

Model	Effect of Genetic Modification	Strains Involved in Modification (Resistant → Susceptible)	Map Location and/or Modifier Identity	References
tubby (*tub* or *rd5*)	Delay of photoreceptor degeneration	AKR/J and C57BL/6	Chrs 11 (*motr1*), 2, and 8	Ikeda et al., 2002a
Light-induced photoreceptor damage model	Resistance to light damage	BALB/c2J and albino strains	*Rpe65*^{Leu450Met}	Danciger et al., 2000; Wenzel et al., 2001
isa, iris stromal atrophy, DBA/2J	Increased cell death	AKXD-28/Ty		Anderson et al., 2001
ipd, iris pigment dispersion	Milder phenotype	AKXD-28/Ty		Anderson et al., 2001
Chx10^{orJ}	Partial recovery of visual function	CASA/Rk and 129/SvJ	Chrs 6 and 14	Wong, et al., 2006
VPP and *Rpe65*^{Leu450Met}	Reduced photoreceptor degeneration		*Rpe65*^{Leu450Met}	Naash et al., 1993; Samardzija et al., 2006

Examples of Genetic Modification of Retinal Degenerative Disease in Mice Recent figures indicate the existence of at least 181 cloned or mapped genes that, when mutated, lead to retinal disease in humans (Retnet: www.sph.uth.tmc.edu/Retnet/disease.htm). Although modifiers have been reported for a small percentage of these genes, because genes do not act in isolation, one would expect that most mutations are modified to some extent by interaction with other genes. In mice, an example of variable expressivity in photoreceptor degeneration as a result of genetic background was reported in 1993 for retinal degeneration 3 (*rd3*) mutant mice (Heckenlively, 1993). The onset and progression of degeneration differed among strains RBF/Dn, Meta-In(1)Rk, Rb(11.13)4Bnr, and In-30, all carrying the same *rd3* allele. Scotopic ERGs were extinguished in the first two strains by 6 weeks of age, and outer nuclear layer (ONL) degeneration was observed as early as 14 days of age and progressed through 8 weeks. In contrast, mice homozygous for the *rd3* mutation on strain In-30 manifested milder retinal dysfunction in which scotopic ERGs were not extinguished until 16 weeks of age, and ONL degeneration began at 3 weeks and progressed through 16 weeks of age (Heckenlively, 1993; Linberg et al., 2005). Since this first report of genetic modification, genetic background modification of photoreceptor degenerations has been reported for a number of models. Mice deficient in rhodopsin (*Rho*$^{-/-}$ mice) were protected by modifiers from the B6 genetic background when compared with the 129Sv background (Humphries et al., 2001). In the B6 background, *Rho*$^{-/-}$ mice were reported to have greater cone photoreceptor function and a greater number of photoreceptor nuclei. However, modification is specific for the mutant gene. Unlike the genetic modification observed for *Rho*$^{-/-}$ mice, in tubby mice (Ikeda et al., 2002a), the B6 background is more susceptible to photoreceptor degeneration and the AKR and CAST strain backgrounds afford some protection.

Modifier genes may also completely suppress a mutant phenotype (Ikeda et al., 1999; Akhmedov et al., 2000). In an intercross between strains B6.Cg-*Nr2e3*$^{rd7/rd7}$ and CAST/Ei, some F_2 mice homozygous for the *Nr2e3*^{rd7} mutation were free of the characteristic retinal spotting phenotype (Akhmedov et al., 2000). Subsequent studies have shown that suppression of retinal spotting and subsequent photoreceptor degeneration correlates with suppression of the excess blue cone production that underlies the retinal whorls and folds (Haider et al., 2006). A similar suppression of the disease phenotype was observed in some F_2 *Nr2e3*^{rd7} mice from intercrosses with the AKR/J and NON.NODn2b/J strains. Interestingly, none of the modifier regions identified from intercrosses between B6.Cg-*Nr2e3*^{rd7}/*Nr2e3*^{rd7} and any of these strains overlapped (Haider et al., in press). Therefore, not only are genetic modifiers specific to mutations, as described with *Rho*$^{-/-}$ and tubby mice, they may also be different in different strain combinations.

Some modifiers have also demonstrated new phenotypes (Mehalow et al., 2003). The retinal degeneration 8 (*rd8*) mutation in crumbs1 (*Crb1*), originally identified in a mixed background between strains C57BL/6 and C3H/HeJ, exhibited large spots in the inferior nasal quadrant of the retina. These spots corresponded to areas of retinal dysplasia as shown by histological analysis. When the *Crb1*^{rd8} mutation was moved onto the C57BL/6 background by 10 backcross generations, the dysplastic phenotype disappeared, suggesting that unlinked C3H/HeJ alleles were lost during the process of introgressing the mutation onto the B6 background. Subsequent intercrosses with the B6.C3H-*Crb1*^{rd8}/*Crb1*^{rd8} mice and C3H/HeJ mice restored the dysplastic phenotype, indicating that the genetic modification is likely conferred by C3H/HeJ (M. M. Edwards, pers. comm., 2007).

In studies with mice where both environmental factors and allelic variability of primary mutations can be controlled, genetic modification may be more evident and tractable. However, genetic modification can still be complex, and for a given disorder, a combination of modifier genes may act together to create a cumulative effect on the expression of a phenotype. For example, in F_2 *tub/tub* progeny of an intercross between B6.Cg-*tub/tub* and the AKR/J strain, a significant range of photoreceptor cell survival was observed. Several chromosomal regions were identified to cosegregate with the thickness of the ONL (Ikeda et al., 2002a). At 20 weeks of age, B6.Cg-*tub/tub* mice normally have 5%–10% of residual ONL thickness remaining, whereas ONL thickness in F_2 mice from the intercross ranged from 5% to 80%. One modifier on chromosome 11, modifier of tubby retinal degeneration 1 (*motr1*), was detected with high statistical significance in a genome-wide scan, and two additional loci on chromosomes 2 and 8 showed suggestive linkage. Protective alleles came from both the AKR (*motr1* and the chromosome 2 locus) and B6 backgrounds (the chromosome 8 locus). Interestingly, Williams et al. (1998) were able to map the natural variation in ganglion cell number in two recombinant inbred strain sets, BXD and BXH, to the same genomic regions containing the tubby modifiers. Identification of these and other modifier loci should offer insight into the particular pathways through which the primary mutant gene functions and into the pathways involved in degeneration.

Strategies for cloning genetic modifiers

As mentioned in the previous section, some genetic modifiers have been identified. The number is small when compared with the number of disease genes known to cause ocular disease, however. Therefore, it seems probable that many modifiers await discovery. Identifying these genes could help improve treatment for individuals affected by ocular diseases by defining pathways through which disease-causing genes function. At this juncture, it seems appropriate to consider methods that are evolving to identify variants that modify phenotypes or that have been used in other systems to identify modifier genes. An integrated approach using a combination of strategies is likely to provide the best opportunity for efficiently identifying genetic modifiers (Cervino et al., 2006).

Chromosomal Localization of Modified Traits The first step in identifying a genetic modifier is to establish a robust, reproducible method for phenotyping the modification, either qualitative (e.g., the presence or absence of a particular phenotype) or quantitative (e.g., the onset, rate, or severity of a particular phenotype). Because severity is characterized as a continuous distribution rather than in discrete subsets, it is grouped with the quantitative traits.

In the next step, the source of modification is chromosomally localized in progeny from backcrosses or intercrosses of mice that carry the primary mutation with another strain whose genetic makeup is able to modify the phenotype. Phenotypic modification that is observed only in mice carrying the primary mutation is mapped by comparing phenotypic variation to sequence variation throughout the genome (e.g., genome-wide scan). Once a region is found in which there is significant skewing of a genotype that correlates with the phenotypic modification, the region can be narrowed by further recombinational linkage analysis and testing for sequence differences among biologically relevant genes contained within the chromosomal area that might explain the modifying effects. If multiple regions are identified, candidate regions can be investigated individually for their ability to modify a given phenotype by construction of congenic strains in which the modifier region and the primary mutation are placed in the same genetic background by successive backcrossing. If the primary mutation is in the C57BL/6 background and modification is observed with strains A/J or PWD/Ph, then the congenic process may be hastened by intercrossing the primary mutation to the consomic or chromosomal substitution strain (Silver, 1995) bearing the chromosome on which the modification is observed. In addition, existing congenic lines that cover the modifier region in question can be used as a resource to verify or to identify the modifier (Ikeda et al., 2002a).

Segregating Crosses with Multiple Strains Although quantitative trait loci (QTL) mapping and recombinational linkage analysis are powerful tools, these traditional methods require large numbers of animals. It is important, therefore, that these methods be made more efficient. One way in which the efficiency of QTL mapping can be improved is by performing multiple crosses with different strains in which the primary mutation is segregating. Detecting the same modifier in multiple strains suggests that it may be derived from a common ancestral allele. Although recombinations were previously thought of as random events, hot spots for recombination have been shown in various strain combinations (Kelmenson et al., 2005); the use of multiple crosses narrows the confidence interval significantly by increasing the number of recombinations, both ancestral and new, within the region (Wang et al., 2004).

Haplotype Analysis A modifier region identified through multiple cross-mappings can be further narrowed by comparing the genomic sequences of the parental strains (reviewed in DiPetrillo et al., 2005; Flint et al., 2005). Haplotype analysis is one method used for such a comparison. This method utilizes the fact that inbred mouse strains are derived from a limited set of ancestors, so that alleles of genes are shared between several inbred strains. These alleles are part of an ancestral haplotype surrounding that gene, and haplotype blocks can be identified by the identity of marker alleles within the haplotype between inbred strains. Since these haplotype blocks are on the order of 40 kb to 1.5 Mb long, the genomic area in which the modifier locus resides can be narrowed by identifying the shared ancestral haplotype block in the strains that modify the phenotype. Conversely, areas where no haplotype sharing is observed can be excluded as candidate regions for the modifier. Practically, a dense SNP map is compiled across the map position from the multiple strain cross and is compared between the strains that modify the phenotype and those that do not. Regions where all the modifying strains share the same SNP alleles and are different from the alleles of the nonmodifying strains can be considered candidate regions. The attraction of this technique is that it can reduce the necessity to generate large numbers of mice to narrow a region considerably, and in many cases the SNP information may already be available through the mouse resequencing project (www.informatics.jax.org/menus/strain_menu.shtml; http://genome.perlegen.com/browser/index.html). This technique has been used in mice to narrow modifier regions in studies investigating cancer (Wang and You, 2005) and cardiomyopathy (Wheeler et al., 2005). The power of haplotype analysis was shown in a study of hypertension, in which a QTL region was narrowed from 18 cM to 2.3 cM using haplotype analysis (DiPetrillo et al., 2004). Not all modifiers, however, are captured by ancestral haplotypes. Genetic variation is continually acquired, and at least some modifier alleles are due to mutations that occurred after the common inbred strains were established and are private to one or a few inbred strains (Ikeda et al., 2002b).

Gene Expression Profiling or Microarray Analysis A growing body of literature supports the usefulness of combining the mapping of modifier loci with expression profiling, especially in the identification of complex traits (Wayne and McIntyre, 2002; Tabakoff et al., 2003). In an elegant study, Dyck et al. (2003) combined these two techniques to understand the development of gallstones in C57L/J mice that carry the *Lith1* gallstone-susceptibility locus. This study used expression profiling, through microarray analysis, to identify differences in gene expression between the C57L/J mice and gallstone-resistant AKR/J mice. Numerous genes involved in fatty acid metabolism were identified. Through literature searches of common regulatory elements within antioxidant systems, the nuclear transcription factor *Nrf2*, which maps to the *Lith1* locus, was identified. Thus, the combination of modifier mapping and expression profiling in conjunction with pathway analysis is a powerful tool. Locus mapping identifies chromosomal regions that are associated with a known phenotype but may contain many genes. Expression profiling identifies genes whose expression levels differ between two populations (i.e., modified and unmodified) but whose association with the observed phenotype is unknown. By combining these two techniques, it is possible to use data acquired in the mapping phase to filter data acquired in the expression profiling phase, either by identifying a misregulated gene within the modifier region or by identifying a misregulated pathway, a component of which resides in the modifier region, suggesting it as a candidate gene.

Modifier Screens Using Mutagenesis Although mutagenesis screens have been used for years to identify modifiers in lower organisms (Carrera et al., 1998; Therrien et al., 2000; Mutsuddi et al., 2004), it has only recently been used for this purpose in mice. Mice with mutations in a gene that is believed to interact with genetic modifiers can be mutated using *N*-ethylnitrosurea (ENU), a chemical mutagen, and the resulting offspring screened for an altered phenotype. For example, an ENU modifier screen was used to identify genes that suppress thrombocytopenia (lack of blood platelets) in a mouse model $Mpl^{-/-}$ (Carpinelli et al., 2004). In this study, mutant males were treated with ENU and mated to untreated females. Blood collected from G_1 progeny were assessed for platelet levels. Mice that showed improved platelet levels were backcrossed to $Mpl^{-/-}$ mice to verify heritability of suppression. DNA from males with heritable suppression was then used to map candidate modifiers. This study produced two candidate modifier alleles of the *c-Myb* gene. These alleles were shown to reduce c-MYB activity, subsequently suppressing the thrombocytopenia phenotype (Carpinelli et al., 2004). More recently, a sensitized screen to identify alterations in dopaminergic homeostasis was carried out in mice with a disrupted dopamine transporter (Speca et al., 2006). Seven phenodeviant lines with abnormal locomotor activity were identified, two of which were dependent on the presence of the DAT mutation and two others that affected dopamine neurotransmission. Hence, sensitized mutagenesis-driven modifier screens in mice could also be a powerful adjunct for identification of genetic modifiers for retinal disease genes.

Summary

The variability in onset, progression, severity, phenotypic expression, or response to treatment, which is a common observation for many diseases, may be due to interactions of mutant alleles with genetic modifiers, or alternatively to environmental or allelic effects. The heterogeneity within the human population makes it difficult to assess the underlying cause of the phenotypic disease variability. However, understanding the nature of the variability may be important in effecting optimum treatment modalities. Model organisms, such as the mouse, can play an important and necessary role in elucidating the cause of variation in phenotype and in response to treatment.

REFERENCES

Akhmedov, N. B., Piriev, N. I., Chang, B., Rapoport, A. L., Hawes, N. L., Nishina, P. M., Nusinowitz, S., Heckenlively, J. R., Roderick, T. H., et al. (2000). A deletion in a photoreceptor-specific nuclear receptor mRNA causes retinal degeneration in the rd7 mouse. *Proc. Natl. Acad. Sci. U.S.A.* 97(10): 5551–5556.

Bowes, C., Li, T., Danciger, M., Baxter, L. C., Applebury, M. L., and Farber, D. B. (1990). Retinal degeneration in the rd mouse is caused by a defect in the beta subunit of rod cGMP-phosphodiesterase. *Nature* 347(6294):677–680.

Carpinelli, M. R., Hilton, D. J., Metcalf, D., Antonchuk, J. L., Hyland, C. D., Mifsud, S. L., Di Rago, L., Hilton, A. A., Willson, T. A., et al. (2004). Suppressor screen in Mpl−/− mice: c-Myb mutation causes supraphysiological production of platelets in the absence of thrombopoietin signaling. *Proc. Natl. Acad. Sci. U.S.A.* 101(17):6553–6558.

Carrera, P., Abrell, S., Kerber, B., Walldorf, U., Preiss, A., Hoch, M., and Jackle, H. (1998). A modifier screen in the eye reveals control genes for Kruppel activity in the *Drosophila* embryo. *Proc. Natl. Acad. Sci. U.S.A.* 95(18):10779–10784.

Cervino, A. C., Darvasi, A., Fallahi, M., Mader, C. C., and Tsinoremas, N. F. (2006). An integrated in-silico gene mapping strategy in inbred mice. *Genetics*, ePub ahead of print.

Cideciyan, A. V., Jacobson, S. G., Aleman, T. S., Gu, D., Pearce-Kelling, S. E., Sumaroka, A., Acland, G. M., and Aguirre, G. D. (2005). In vivo dynamics of retinal injury and repair in the rhodopsin mutant dog model of human retinitis pigmentosa. *Proc. Natl. Acad. Sci. U.S.A.* 102(14):5233–5238.

Danciger, M., Matthes, M. T., Yasamura, D., Akhmedov, N. B., Rickabaugh, T., Gentleman, S., Redmond, T. M., LaVail, M. M., and Farber, D. B. (2000). A QTL on distal chromosome 3 that influences the severity of light-induced damage to mouse photoreceptors. *Mamm. Genome* 11(6):422–427.

DiPetrillo, K., Tsaih, S. W., Sheehan, S., Johns, C., Kelmenson, P., Gavras, H., Churchill, G. A., and Paigen, B. (2004). Genetic analysis of blood pressure in C3H/HeJ and SWR/J mice. *Physiol. Genomics* 17(2):215–220.

DiPetrillo, K., Wang, X., Stylianou, I. M., and Paigen, B. (2005). Bioinformatics toolbox for narrowing rodent quantitative trait loci. *Trends Genet.* 21(12):683–692.

Douglas, R. M., Alam, N. M., Silver, B. D., McGill, T. J., Tschetter, W. W., and Prusky, G. T. (2005). Independent visual threshold measurements in the two eyes of freely moving rats and mice using a virtual-reality optokinetic system. *Vis. Neurosci.* 22(5):677–684.

Dyck, P. A., Hoda, F., Osmer, E. S., and Green, R. M. (2003). Microarray analysis of hepatic gene expression in gallstone-susceptible and gallstone-resistant mice. *Mamm. Genome* 14(9): 601–610.

Flint, J., Valdar, W., Shifman, S., and Mott, R. (2005). Strategies for mapping and cloning quantitative trait genes in rodents. *Nat. Rev. Genet.* 6(4):271–286.

Grimm, C., Wenzel, A., Stanescu, D., Samardzija, M., Hotop, S., Groszer, M., Naash, M., Gassmann, M., and Reme, C.

(2004). Constitutive overexpression of human erythropoietin protects the mouse retina against induced but not inherited retinal degeneration. *J. Neurosci.* 24(25):5651–5658.

Haider, N. B., DeMarco, P., Nystuen, A. M., Huang, X., Smith, R. S., McCall, M. A., Naggert, J. K., and Nishina, P. M. (2006). The transcription factor, *Nr2e3*, functions in retinal progenitors to suppress cone cell generation. *Vision Neurosci.* 23(6): 917–929.

Haider, N. B., Zhang, W., Hurd, R., Ikeda, A., Nystuen, A. M., Naggert, J. K., and Nishina, P. M. (in press). Mapping of genetic modifiers of $Nr2e3^{rd7/rd7}$ that suppress retinal degeneration and restore blue cone cells to normal quantity. *Mamm. Genome.*

Hamel, C. P., Tsilou, E., Pfeffer, B. A., Hooks, J. J., Detrick, B., and Redmond, T. M. (1993). Molecular cloning and expression of RPE65, a novel retinal pigment epithelium–specific microsomal protein that is post-transcriptionally regulated in vitro. *J. Biol. Chem.* 268(21):15751–15757.

Hart, A. W., McKie, L., Morgan, J. E., Gautier, P., West, K., Jackson, I. J., and Cross, S. H. (2005). Genotype-phenotype correlation of mouse Pde6b mutations. *Invest. Ophthalmol. Vis. Sci.* 46(9):3443–3450.

Heckenlively, J. R., Chang, B. Peng, C., Hawes, N. L., and Roderick, T. H. (1993). Variable expressivity of rd-3 retinal degeneration dependent on background strain. In J. G. Hollyfield, R. E. Anderson, and M. M. LaVail (Eds.), *Retinal degeneration.* New York: Plenum Press.

Hummel, K. P., Coleman, D. L., and Lane, P. W. (1972). The influence of genetic background on expression of mutations at the diabetes locus in the mouse. I. C57BL-KsJ and C57BL-6J strains. *Biochem. Genet.* 7(1):1–13.

Humphries, M. M., Kiang, S., McNally, N., Donovan, M. A., Sieving, P. A., Bush, R. A., Machida, S., Cotter, T., Hobson, A., et al. (2001). Comparative structural and functional analysis of photoreceptor neurons of Rho−/− mice reveal increased survival on C57BL/6J in comparison to 129Sv genetic background. *Vision Neurosci.* 18(3):437–443.

Humphries, M. M., Rancourt, D., Farrar, G. J., Kenna, P., Hazel, M., Bush, R. A., Sieving, P. A., Sheils, D. M., McNally, N., et al. (1997). Retinopathy induced in mice by targeted disruption of the rhodopsin gene. *Nat. Genet.* 15(2): 216–219.

Ikeda, A., Naggert, J. K., and Nishina, P. M. (2002a). Genetic modification of retinal degeneration in tubby mice. *Exp. Eye Res.* 74(4):455–461.

Ikeda, A., Zheng, Q. Y., Zuberi, A. R., Johnson, K. R., Naggert, J. K., and Nishina, P. M. (2002b). Microtubule-associated protein 1A is a modifier of tubby hearing (moth1). *Nat. Genet.* 30 (4):401–405.

Ikeda, S., Hawes, N. L., Chang, B., Avery, C. S., Smith, R. S., and Nishina, P. M. (1999). Severe ocular abnormalities in C57BL/6 but not in 129/Sv p53-deficient mice. *Invest. Ophthalmol. Vis. Sci.* 40(8):1874–1878.

Kelmenson, P. M., Petkov, P., Wang, X., Higgins, D. C., Paigen, B. J., and Paigen, K. (2005). A torrid zone on mouse chromosome 1 containing a cluster of recombinational hotspots. *Genetics* 169(2):833–841.

Kijas, J. W., Cideciyan, A. V., Aleman, T. S., Pianta, M. J., Pearce-Kelling, S. E., Miller, B. J., Jacobson, S. G., Aguirre, G. D., and Acland, G. M. (2002). Naturally occurring rhodopsin mutation in the dog causes retinal dysfunction and degeneration mimicking human dominant retinitis pigmentosa. *Proc. Natl. Acad. Sci. U.S.A.* 99(9):6328–6333.

LaVail, J. H., Nixon, R. A., and Sidman, R. L. (1978). Genetic control of retinal ganglion cell projections. *J. Comp. Neurol.* 182 (3):399–421.

Li, T., Sandberg, M. A., Pawlyk, B. S., Rosner, B., Hayes, K. C., Dryja, T. P., and Berson, E. L. (1998). Effect of vitamin A supplementation on rhodopsin mutants threonine-17 → methionine and proline-347 → serine in transgenic mice and in cell cultures. *Proc. Natl. Acad. Sci. U.S.A.* 95(20):11933–11938.

Linberg, K. A., Fariss, R. N., Heckenlively, J. R., Farber, D. B., and Fisher, S. K. (2005). Morphological characterization of the retinal degeneration in three strains of mice carrying the rd-3 mutation. *Vision Neurosci.* 22(6):721–734.

Linder, C. C. (2006). Genetic variables that influence phenotype. *ILAR J.* 47(2):132–140.

Lu, X., and Ferreira, P. A. (2005). Identification of novel murine- and human-specific RPGRIP1 splice variants with distinct expression profiles and subcellular localization. *Invest. Ophthalmol. Vis. Sci.* 46(6):1882–1890.

Mehalow, A. K., Kameya, S., Smith, R. S., Hawes, N. L., Denegre, J. M., Young, J. A., Bechtold, L., Haider, N. B., Tepass, U., et al. (2003). CRB1 is essential for external limiting membrane integrity and photoreceptor morphogenesis in the mammalian retina. *Hum. Mol. Genet.* 12(17):2179–2189.

Moiseyev, G., Chen, Y., Takahashi, Y., Wu, B. X., and Ma, J. X. (2005). RPE65 is the isomerohydrolase in the retinoid visual cycle. *Proc. Natl. Acad. Sci. U.S.A.* 102(35):12413–12418.

Mutsuddi, M., Marshall, C. M., Benzow, K. A., Koob, M. D., and Rebay, I., (2004). The spinocerebellar ataxia 8 noncoding RNA causes neurodegeneration and associates with staufen in *Drosophila. Curr. Biol.* 14(4):302–308.

Naash, M. I., Hollyfield, J. G., al-Ubaidi, M. R., and Baehr, W.. (1993). Simulation of human autosomal dominant retinitis pigmentosa in transgenic mice expressing a mutated murine opsin gene. *Proc. Natl. Acad. Sci. U.S.A.* 90(12):5499–5503.

Nadeau, J. H. (2003). Modifier genes and protective alleles in humans and mice. *Curr. Opin. Genet. Dev.* 13(3):290–295.

Pang, J. J., Chang, B., Hawes, N. L., Hurd, R. E., Davisson, M. T., Li, J., Noorwez, S. M., Malhotra, R., McDowell, J. H., et al. (2005). Retinal degeneration 12 (rd12): A new, spontaneously arising mouse model for human Leber congenital amaurosis (LCA). *Mol. Vis.* 11:152–162.

Pletcher, M. T., McClurg, P., Batalov, S., Su, A. I., Barnes, S. W., Lagler, E., Korstanje, R., Wang, X., Nusskern, D., et al. (2004). Use of a dense single nucleotide polymorphism map for in silico mapping in the mouse. *PLoS Biol.* 2(12):e393.

Redmond, T. M., Yu, S., Lee, E., Bok, D., Hamasaki, D., Chen, N., Goletz, P., Ma, J. X., Crouch, R. K., et al. (1998). Rpe65 is necessary for production of 11-*cis*-vitamin A in the retinal visual cycle. *Nat. Genet.* 20(4):344–351.

Ridder, W. H., III, and Nusinowitz, S. (2006). The visual evoked potential in the mouse: Origins and response characteristics. *Vision. Res.* 46(6–7):902–913.

Rudd, M. F., Williams, R. D., Webb, E. L., Schmidt, S., Sellick, G. S., and Houlston, R. S. (2005). The predicted impact of coding single nucleotide polymorphisms database. *Cancer Epidemiol. Biomarkers Prev.* 14(11 Pt. 1):2598–2604.

Shifman, S., Bell, J. T., Copley, R. R., Taylor, M. S., Williams, R. W., Mott, R., and Flint, J.. (2006). A high-resolution single nucleotide polymorphism genetic map of the mouse genome. *PLoS Biol.* 4(12):e395.

Silver, L. (1995). *Mouse genetics.* Oxford: Oxford University Press.

Speca, D. J., Rabbee, N., Chihara, D., Speed, T. P., and Peterson, A. S. (2006). A genetic screen for behavioral mutations that perturb dopaminergic homeostasis in mice. *Genes Brain Behav.* 5(1):19–28.

Tabakoff, B., Bhave, S. V., and Hoffman, P. L. (2003). Selective breeding, quantitative trait locus analysis, and gene arrays identify candidate genes for complex drug-related behaviors. *J. Neurosci.* 23(11):4491–4498.

Therrien, M., Morrison, D. K., Wong, A. M., and Rubin, G. M. (2000). A genetic screen for modifiers of a kinase suppressor of Ras-dependent rough eye phenotype in *Drosophila. Genetics* 156(3):1231–1242.

Tsang, S. H., Woodruff, M., Jun, L., Mahajan, V., Yamashita, C. K., Pedersen, R., Lin, C. S., Goff, S. P., Rosenberg, T., et al. (2007). Transgenic mice carrying the H258N mutation in the gene encoding the beta-subunit of phosphodiesterase-6 (PDE6B) provide a model for human congenital stationary night blindness. *Hum. Mutat.* 28(3):243–254.

Vincent, A. L. (2003). Searching for modifier genes. *Clin. Exp. Ophthalmol.* 31(5):374–375.

Wang, D., and You, M. (2005). Five loci, SLT1 to SLT5, controlling the susceptibility to spontaneously occurring lung cancer in mice. *Cancer Res.* 65(18):8158–8165.

Wang, X., Korstanje, R. Higgins, D., and Paigen, B. (2004). Haplotype analysis in multiple crosses to identify a QTL gene. *Genome Res.* 14(9):1767–1772.

Wayne, M. L., and McIntyre, L. M. (2002). Combining mapping and arraying: An approach to candidate gene identification. *Proc. Natl. Acad. Sci. U.S.A.* 99(23):14903–14906.

Wenzel, A., Reme, C. E., Williams, T. P., Hafezi, F., and Grimm, C. (2001). The Rpe65 Leu450Met variation increases retinal resistance against light-induced degeneration by slowing rhodopsin regeneration. *J. Neurosci.* 21(1):53–58.

Wheeler, F. C., Fernandez, L., Carlson, K. M., Wolf, M. J., Rockman, H. A., and Marchuk, D. A. (2005). QTL mapping in a mouse model of cardiomyopathy reveals an ancestral modifier allele affecting heart function and survival. *Mamm. Genome* 16(6):414–423.

Williams, R. W., Strom, R. C., and Goldowitz, D. (1998). Natural variation in neuron number in mice is linked to a major quantitative trait locus on Chr 11. *J. Neurosci.* 18(1):138–146.

Won, J., Gifford, E. J., Smith, R. S., Hicks, W. L., Naggert, J. K., and Nishina, P. M. (2007). Allelic variation suggests *Rpgrip1* is important for outersegment development. *Invest. Ophthalmol. Vis. Sci.* 48. E-abstract, 4490.

Zhao, Y. D., Hong, H., Pawlyk, B., Yue, G., Adamian, M., Grynberg, M., Godzik, A., and Li, T. (2003). The retinitis pigmentosa GTPase regulator (RPGR)-interacting protein: Subserving RPGR function and participating in disk morphogenesis. *Proc. Natl. Acad. Sci. U.S.A.* 100(7):3965–3970.

54 The Mouse Eye Transcriptome: Cellular Signatures, Molecular Networks, and Candidate Genes for Human Disease

ELDON E. GEISERT AND ROBERT W. WILLIAMS

The laboratory mouse occupies a unique position at the intersection of basic vision science and clinical medicine. The advantages of this species include its small size and rapid rate of reproduction, its extremely well-characterized genome, and the many well-honed techniques used to engineer gene variants, knockouts, and knock-ins. Temporal and spatial patterns of gene expression can be controlled with impressive precision in eye, retina, brain, and many other tissues of mice (see chapter 39, this volume). Human gene variants, usually those that cause disease, can be inserted into the mouse genome to study mechanisms of normal function, disease progression, and drug efficacy (Pennesi et al., 2003). In a dramatic recent example, Jacobs et al. (2007) inserted the human red opsin gene (*OPN1LW*) into mice, thereby converting this normally color-blind species into a functional trichromat able to discriminate between red and green. Even more radical engineering is practical. For example, it is now possible to produce so-called humanized mice in which the proteins in an organ such as the liver (Kondo et al., 2002) or the immune system (Shultz et al., 2007) are replaced through genetic engineering by human equivalents. One can only speculate that comparable work humanizing the mouse eye and retina is not far behind. The future holds the potential for having mouse models that will exactly recapitulate human disease affecting vision, allowing us the opportunity to define the fundamental defect in disease states and to develop and test new therapies to prevent the loss of sight.

There are also more subtle and perhaps equally important ways in which mice are having an impact on biomedical research and clinical medicine. Populations of diverse strains of mice can be used to model human genetic diversity. Although most biologists use mice to model actions of specific genes—each in isolation on a fixed genetic background (usually C57BL/6J)—a growing number of geneticists are using groups of different strains of mice, particularly offspring of the 16 strains that have been sequenced (Frazer et al., 2007), to model the complexity of human populations. Diverse strains of mice and their progeny can be used to test the utility and predictability of personalized medicine. Approximately 10 million common sequence variants, including single nucleotide polymorphisms (SNPs), insertions, deletions, duplications, and even retrotransposons, contribute to much of human biological diversity. Roughly the same types and numbers of genomic sequence variants account for phenotypic differences among common inbred strains of mice, which, unlike humans, can be raised in nearly identical environments. For example, the two oldest strains of mice, the glaucoma-prone DBA/2J and the comparatively normal C57BL/6J, differ at roughly 1.5 million SNPs, as well as an additional large number of microsatellites and copy number variants. It is now practical to use a relatively modest number of strains, from 10 to 100, to model the response diversity and wide spectrum of disease burden of complex human populations rather than just to model that action of a single gene in a single inbred strain. It is finally practical to exploit variation among strains as if it were a "natural" genomic manipulation (Williams et al., 1996). Variation of this type can provide insight into interactions among genes, transcripts, and proteins expressed in the eye, retina, and brain. This more holistic approach tends to scale better to the whole genome than do studies of single alleles on single genetic backgrounds.

In the first half of this chapter, we discuss the current state of mouse genomics with special reference to the expression of genes in the mouse eye. How many genes are expressed in different parts of the eye? What online resources are now available to track progress in eye genomics in mouse and human? How well are researchers able to use online resources to computationally annotate or infer gene function in the same way that protein function is often inferred by common structural motifs? In the second half of this chapter, we return to the topic of the population genetics of the mouse eye and review a powerful new data set, the Hamilton Eye Institute Mouse Eye Database, which includes many analytical tools to study associations between variation in gene expression and functional differences in the eye, retina, and brain of a large number of highly diverse strains of mice.

Mouse and human genomes

Early in 2001, initial draft sequences of the human genome were published nearly simultaneously by the International Human Genome Sequencing Consortium (McPherson et al., 2001) and Celera Genomics (Venter et al., 2001). A few months after release of the human sequence, Celera assembled a commercial draft of the mouse genome that combined public and private sequence data from five strains of mice (A/J, C57BL/6J, DBA/2J, 129X1/SvJ, and 129S1/SvImJ). The first public assembly of the genome of strain C57BL/6J was released late in 2002 (Waterston et al., 2002). The strong position of C57BL/6J as the most important and widely used inbred strain was reinforced by this public release. This accounts for the now almost obligatory step of transferring (or introgressing, to use the geneticist's term) all interesting mutations into the C57BL/6 (B6 or "black-six") genome.

The revelation of human and mouse genomes has catalyzed a large and unanticipated revolution in the production and use of online genomic databases. Use was initially confined mainly to molecular biologists and bioinformaticists. At present, however, a significant proportion of the biomedical research community has come to take these resources for granted as a vital research infrastructure on par with PubMed. Over the last few years, dynamic Web editions of human, mouse, rat, chimpanzee, dog, yeast, *Drosophila*, and *C. elegans* genomes at NCBI, UCSC, and Ensemble have had an enormous impact on the way biomedical research is conducted. These Web portals or knowledgebases represent dynamic encyclopedias that form a framework for most genetic, genomic, molecular, cellular, systems, and clinical research. Learning how to use and evaluate these resources is becoming as important as learning how to read and critique the literature.

Initial comparative analysis of mammalian genomes found that the mouse genome is slightly shorter than the human genome (2.6 billion nucleotides vs. 3.0 billion nucleotides), probably due to "trivial" differences in noncoding sequence and repetitive DNA. As expected, the mouse and human genomes contain very close to the same number of classic protein-coding genes, now estimated at 27,000 ± 3,000 in mammals. A large part of the mouse genome can be partitioned into chromosome strands that are roughly equivalent to homologous strands of human chromosomes, a feature that is referred to as conserved synteny (similar strings). Like many interesting research efforts, our improved understanding of genome sequence and the process of transcription has revealed how much we now do not understand. While the genome is often referred to metaphorically as an encyclopedia, or even as a simple string of letters, it is actually a deviously clever and an incomplete patchwork of code. This code cannot be understood except in the context of a whole organism and its environmental history. Having sequence and global transcriptome data in hand has taught molecular biologists and bioinformaticists to be humble in their claims of having seen a path to a brave new postgenomic world. To give one example, we now have a much greater appreciation of the complex role of noncoding RNAs, micro-RNAs, guide RNAs, and antisense RNA sequences in regulating transcription and translation. There is now good evidence that more of the genome (perhaps as much as 30%), including intergenic "junk DNA," is transcribed, and that only a fraction of transcripts are destined to be translated into mature protein. There is also strong evidence of far more alternative transcript use, with estimates that up to 80%–90% of genes have two or more variants. The supposedly bland world of DNA and RNA has suddenly become much more of a jungle and may even rival the proteome in its intricacy and complexity (Kampa et al., 2004; Kapranov et al., 2007).

Sequence Differences Among Mice: A Great New Resource With genomic sequence data from five different inbred strains, Celera was able to systematically extract close to 3 million SNPs (Waterston et al., 2002; Lindblad-Toh et al., 2005). This resource introduced a new approach to genomics in which missense mutations and premature stop codons can be hunted down directly in databases. For example, among the 1.5 million SNPs that distinguish between the two oldest inbred strains of mice, C57BL/6J and DBA/2J, a subset of 42 is located in the tyrosine-related protein 1 (*Tyrp1*, also known as the brown locus), including two missense mutations that alter protein sequence (figure 54.1). This first wave of SNP variants for five strains was followed three years later (Frazer et al., 2007) by a massive amount of array-based sequence data generated by Perlegen Sciences for the National Institute for Environment Health Sciences (table 54.1). Perlegen used massive wafers covered with 25-nucleotide DNA strands (68 wafers per genome) to sequence precisely the same gene-rich 1.5 billion base pairs of DNA across a panel of 15 highly diverse strains, including four wild subspecies from which virtually all common strains trace their descent—WSB/EiJ (*Mus musculus domesticus*), PWD/PhJ (*M. m. musculus*), MOLF/EiJ (*M. m. molossinus*), and CAST/EiJ (*M. m. castaneus*).

The result of this massive effort is an open database that provides access to about 10 million high-quality SNPs that can be downloaded and sorted at several sites, including the SNP browser at GeneNetwork, www.genenetwork.org/webqtl/snpBrowser (see figure 54.1). Although these new SNPs have not garnered the attention of the original sequencing efforts, they are extremely powerful resources. The millions of SNPs that are now a fixed resource for inbred strains neatly match the 8–10 million common SNPs segregating in human populations (www.hapmap.org). In both mouse and human these SNPs are collectively responsible for much of the phenotypic diversity and differences in health and disease. For example, the first missense mutations in *Tyrp1* (figure 54.1, *top*) change the wild-type TGT cysteine codon at position 86 in exon 2 (note the Gs and As in the *top row*) present in virtually all mammals to a TAT codon in DBA/2J that codes for a mutant tyrosine residue. This SNP is responsible for the brown locus phenotype. The second missense SNP in exon 5 (rs28091461, the less severe b-"light" allele) results in an arginine (R) to histidine (H) replacement at amino acid position 326. These mutations in a key melanocyte catalase disturb melanin production and lead to oculocutaneous albinism type 3 (OCA3) in humans. In mice, these mutations also contribute significantly to glaucoma susceptibility (see chapter 39, this volume).

To ensure a low error rate, both Celera and Perlegen used stringent criteria to define SNPs. This conservative approach and the focus on gene-rich regions have led to the prediction that there are actually in excess of 40 million common SNPs fixed in the genomes of these 16 common strains (Frazer et al., 2007). There are also many other types of genetic polymorphism variants, including insertions, deletions, polymorphic transposons, duplications, and inversions. In sum, just a small cohort of inbred strains provides direct access to roughly four times the level of common variation segregating in humans. Before the genome projects, this genetic variation remained undiscovered, but after sequencing several

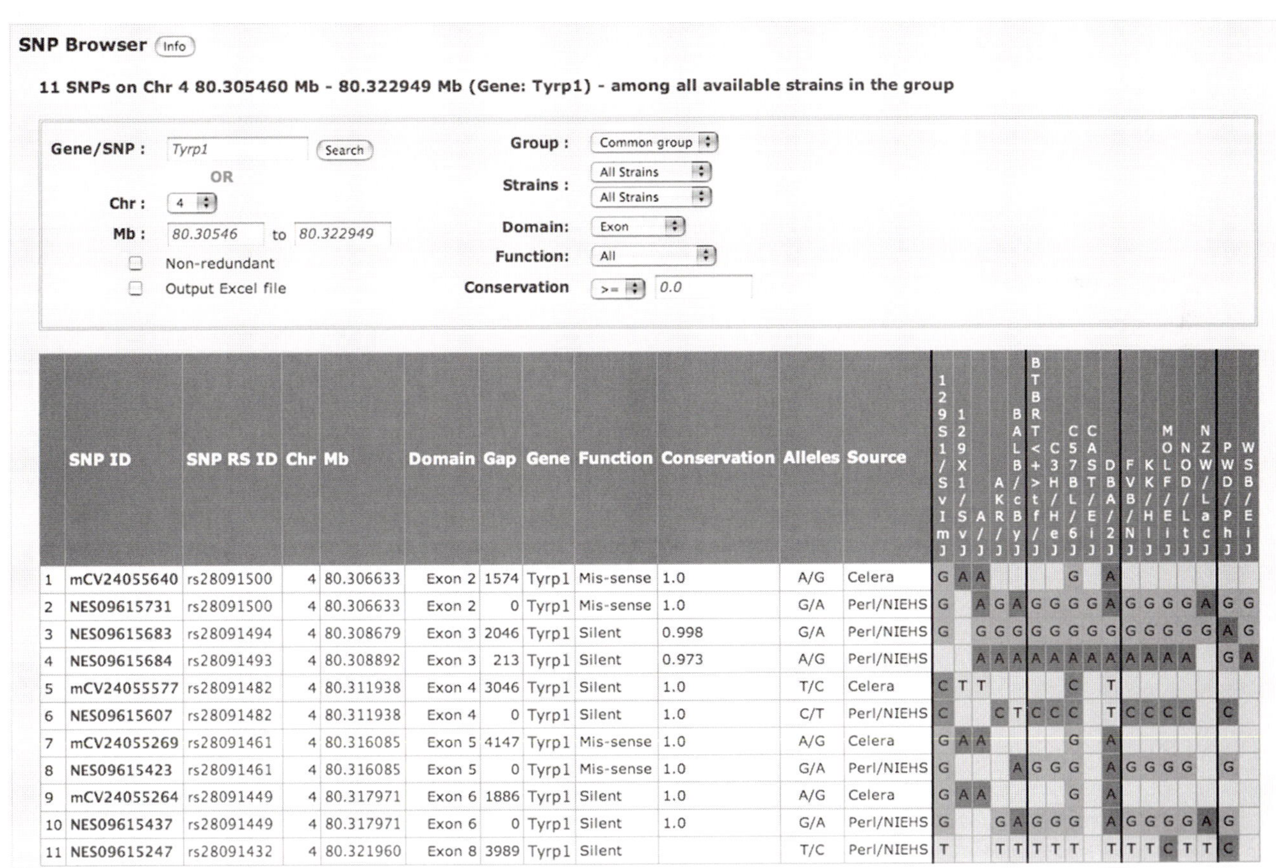
SNP Browser (Info)

11 SNPs on Chr 4 80.305460 Mb - 80.322949 Mb (Gene: Tyrp1) - among all available strains in the group

Gene/SNP : Tyrp1 (Search)
OR
Chr : 4
Mb : 80.30546 to 80.322949
Non-redundant
Output Excel file
Group : Common group
Strains : All Strains / All Strains
Domain: Exon
Function: All
Conservation >= 0.0

	SNP ID	SNP RS ID	Chr	Mb	Domain	Gap	Gene	Function	Conservation	Alleles	Source	129S1/SvImJ	129X1/SvJ	A/J	AKR/J	BALB/cByJ	BTBR T<+>tf/J	C3H/HeJ	C57BL/6J	CAST/EiJ	DBA/2J	FVB/NJ	KK/HlJ	MOLF/EiJ	NOD/LtJ	NZW/LacJ	PWD/PhJ	WSB/EiJ
1	mCV24055640	rs28091500	4	80.306633	Exon 2	1574	Tyrp1	Mis-sense	1.0	A/G	Celera	G	A	A					G		A							
2	NES09615731	rs28091500	4	80.306633	Exon 2	0	Tyrp1	Mis-sense	1.0	G/A	Perl/NIEHS	G		A	G	A	G	G	G	G	A	G	G	G	G	A	G	G
3	NES09615683	rs28091494	4	80.308679	Exon 3	2046	Tyrp1	Silent	0.998	G/A	Perl/NIEHS	G		G	G	G	G	G	G	G	G	G	G	G	G	G	A	G
4	NES09615684	rs28091493	4	80.308892	Exon 3	213	Tyrp1	Silent	0.973	A/G	Perl/NIEHS			A	A	A	A	A	A	A	A	A	A	A	A		G	A
5	mCV24055577	rs28091482	4	80.311938	Exon 4	3046	Tyrp1	Silent	1.0	T/C	Celera	C	T	T					C		T							
6	NES09615607	rs28091482	4	80.311938	Exon 4	0	Tyrp1	Silent	1.0	C/T	Perl/NIEHS	C			C	T	C	C	C		T	C	C	C	C		C	
7	mCV24055269	rs28091461	4	80.316085	Exon 5	4147	Tyrp1	Mis-sense	1.0	A/G	Celera	G	A	A					G		A							
8	NES09615423	rs28091461	4	80.316085	Exon 5	0	Tyrp1	Mis-sense	1.0	G/A	Perl/NIEHS	G				A	G	G	G		A	G	G	G	G		G	
9	mCV24055264	rs28091449	4	80.317971	Exon 6	1886	Tyrp1	Silent	1.0	A/G	Celera	G	A	A					G		A							
10	NES09615437	rs28091449	4	80.317971	Exon 6	0	Tyrp1	Silent	1.0	G/A	Perl/NIEHS	G			G	A	G	G	G		A	G	G	G	G	A	G	
11	NES09615247	rs28091432	4	80.321960	Exon 8	3989	Tyrp1	Silent		T/C	Perl/NIEHS	T			T	T	T	T	T		T	T	T	C	T	T	C	

FIGURE 54.1 The SNPs within the exons of the tyrosine-related protein 1 (*Tyrp1*) are shown from the SNP browser page of GeneNetwork. This is a list limited to the 11 SNPs found in the exons of *Tyrp1* (total of 126 SNPs in the gene) within the 17 strains of mice examined. At the top of the page the critical information can be selected. For this analysis we examined *Tyrp1*. The chromosomal location is listed. We also selected all strains in the database, exons only, and all functions of the SNPs. The listing at the bottom of the page is self-explanatory, with SNP ID, SNP RS ID, chromosome (Chr), megabase pair (Mb), domain, gap, gene, function of the SNP (Function), conservation, alleles, source, and the specific SNPs in the strains examined. Notice that four of the SNPs create missense mutations, and the remainder of those found in exons are silent.

Table 54.1

Top strains of mice currently sequenced, along with several pertinent ocular phenotypes

Strain	Sequencing Status	Ocular Trait
C57BL/6J	8X shotgun	Pigmented appearance: black; related genotype: a/a. C57BL/6J was the DNA source for the international collaboration that generated the first high-quality draft sequence of the mouse genome.
DBA/2J	1.3X + Perlegen	Dilute brown. Glaucoma model, large eye; interacting loci cause severe iris atrophy and glaucoma in DBA/2J mice. Retinal histopathology reveals a loss of RGCs, as well as GABAergic and cholinergic amacrine cells (Moon et al., 2005).
A/J	1.3X + Perlegen	*Tyr*-negative albino
129S1/SvImJ	1.3X + Perlegen	*Tyr*-negative albino white-bellied agouti
129X1/SvJ	Celera	*Tyr* chinchilla pink eye ocular albino
CAST/EiJ	Perlegen	Agouti
BTBR T^+ tf/J	Perlegen	Black and tan, tufted
MOLF/EiJ	Perlegen	White-bellied agouti; related genotype: A^w/A^w. Homozygous for the retinal degeneration allele *Pde6b*^{rd1}.
KK/HlJ	Perlegen	*Tyr*-negative albino KK/HlJ male mice exhibit diabetic symptoms that include hyperglycemia, hyperinsulinemia, and insulin resistance.
AKR/J	Perlegen	*Tyr*-negative albino
PWD/PhJ	Perlegen	Agouti
NZW/LacJ	Perlegen	*Tyrp1b/Tyrp1b p Tyrc/p Tyrc* albino; *Pde6b*^{rd1}
BALB/cByJ	Perlegen	*Tyr*-negative albino
WSB/EiJ		White-bellied agouti
C3H/HeJ	Perlegen	Agouti carries *Pde6b*^{rd1}, resulting in retinal degeneration by weaning age
FVB/NJ	Perlegen	*Tyr*-negative albino carries *Pde6b*^{rd1}, resulting in retinal degeneration
NOD/LtJ	Perlegen	*Tyr*-negative albino

Note: The level of coverage and quality produced by Perlegen Sciences' array-based resequencing technology is equivalent to that of 1.5 × whole-genome shotgun sequencing. For mouse strains and phenotypes, see www.informatics.jax.org/external/festing/mouse/STRAINS.shtml.

different genomes we are finding that the genome contains a surprising number of variations. With the online genomic resources available to investigators, scientists are able to mine these data sources, producing a rapidly evolving understanding of the structure of the genome.

Gene expression in the mouse eye: Results and resources

Recent advances in genomic technologies have facilitated the large-scale examination of tissues, defining transcript abundance for tens of thousands of genes simultaneously in single experiments. There are two basic technological approaches. In the first, mRNA is isolated, processed, and directly sequenced (expressed sequence tags [ESTs] or serial analysis of gene expression [SAGE]). In the second approach, mRNA or its cDNA derivative is hybridized to a complementary probe (microarray methods), and rather than counting mRNA molecules, one measures the binding affinity as an indirect measure of mRNA concentration. In both of these applications mRNA is isolated using oligo-dT to hybridize the poly-A tail of the message. This approach selectively isolates RNA that will be translated into protein (approximately 3% of the total RNA in the cell), eliminating the highly abundant ribosomal RNA and transfer RNA. The advantage to these methods is the rapid interrogation of all mRNAs. The disadvantage is that untranslated RNAs are not interrogated by these methods and we are not examining the full complexity of transcriptional activity. The EST analysis and the SAGE analysis directly sequence copies of mRNA and can accurately measure the levels of abundant messages. Furthermore, the quality of the database and detection of rare messages can be increased by increasing the number of sequenced clones or cDNA fragments. Microarray has the advantage of examining a large number of transcripts in a single hybridization step. However, microarray methods have two significant disadvantages. For abundant transcripts, the probe can be saturated and will not reflect the true level of message, and for rare transcripts the hybridization may be below the level of detection.

Expressed sequence tag and serial analysis of gene expression analysis

Many different genes are expressed in the diverse tissue types that make up the eye. Early estimates based on the short sequences (300–500 base pairs long) derived from mRNAs

(ESTs) indicated that retina alone produced around 15,000 unique transcripts (Williams, Strom, Zhou, et al., 1998). The UniGene EST collection binds together a set of ESTs that trace back to the same genome location, and often to a single well-known gene. This puts the UniGene collection at a halfway point between the modest number of canonical protein-coding genes and the high number of transcript variants. In the mouse there are a total of around 86,000 UniGene EST clusters (build 163), of which 24,000 are derived from mouse eye tissues. This is roughly twice the number found in organs such as liver (12,000) and heart (11,000), but somewhat less than that found in whole brain (30,000). Unfortunately, differences among tissue and organs have as much to do with ascertainment biases and database coverage as they do with inherent differences in mRNA and cellular diversity. This point is driven home by the fact that the number of UniGene clusters in humans is 50% greater than that in mice (124,000), a difference that is almost certainly technical. However, as in the mouse, the number of human UniGene clusters associated with ocular tissues is close to 24,000.

The National Eye Institute's NEIBank is an excellent resource to explore the fine details of EST sets extracted from different ocular tissues in several species (http://neibank.nei.nih.gov). NEIBank includes EST/UniGene collection libraries from whole eye and several discrete ocular tissue types, including the ciliary body (human only), the choroid/retinal pigmented epithelium (human, mouse, other), cornea (mouse, human, other), iris (human, rat, zebrafish), lacrimal gland (human and mouse), lens (human, mouse, rat, kangaroo, dog, zebrafish, rabbit, guinea pig, cow, rhesus monkey), optic nerve (human only), trabecular meshwork (human and rat), and retina (human, mouse, rat, dog, zebrafish, rabbit, guinea pig). The NEIBank retinal mRNA library for adult mouse (NbLib0027) consists of approximately 35,000 UniGene clusters and ESTs. Only one-third (12,224) are represented by multiple hits or clones. Not surprisingly, at the top of the list is rhodopsin, represented by 1,050 counts. In other words, rhodopsin sequence was identified in 1,050 independently sequenced clones. If we sum the unique transcripts in NEIBank across all mouse eye libraries, the total reaches about 28,000 (table 54.2). This sum does not include those genes, ESTs, and UniGene clusters that are only active during development. What we can conclude is that a significant proportion of the genome, certainly well over half of all coding genes, is expressed in the eye, with an exceedingly high level of expression in the retina.

SAGE analysis, like EST analysis, directly sequences short segments of cDNA, offering the ability to improve the quality of the data set by increasing the number of cDNAs sequenced. For the eye, the SAGE database of the Cepko group (http://itstgp01.med.harvard.edu/retina) examines the expression patterns in the developing mouse eye. In the case of the Cepko database, SAGE tags are 14 bases in length and are used to identify specific transcripts in the developing C57BL/6 retina (Blackshaw et al., 2004). This high-quality database identifies transcripts expressed at very high levels and low levels. The data are presented in an easy-to-use, highly interactive format presenting SAGE data for different tissues of the eye and at different developmental stages ranging from embryonic day 12.5 to adult. Using this resource one can examine the level of expression of individual transcripts to uncover developmental expression patterns. In addition to the SAGE database, in situ hybridizations of retinal sections are included for many of the mouse transcripts. The data presented at the Cepko site are a starting point for functional analysis of the role of genes in retinal development. For example, Blackshaw et al. (2004) identified genes expressed in the adult retina that formed a photoreceptor-enriched catalogue of transcripts within the inner retina. This group of genes has a correlated developmental expression pattern with rhodopsin and may offer prime candidate genes for human disease.

Table 54.2

Numbers of clones in different EST libraries in the NEIBank

Mouse Eye	Human Eye	Mouse Retina	Number of Clones
28,300	14,342	34,885	1 or more
8,347	5,277	12,224	2 or more
5,240	3,193	8,413	3 or more
3,619	2,058	6,207	4 or more
2,644	1,442	4,757	5 or more
1,997	1,040	3,697	6 or more
1,494	801	2,955	7 or more
1,175	628	2,374	8 or more
956	516	1,920	9 or more
782	433	1,576	10 or more
673	374	1,330	11 or more
570	326	1,110	12 or more
370	241	712	15 or more
221	143	397	20 or more
133	97	230	25 or more
99	68	178	30 or more

Note: Shown are the EST copy number in the mouse eye (NbLib0032 353 highest copy number for *Cryg*), the human (NbLib0079 NEI site 339 highest copy number for *Cryg*), and the mouse retina (NbLib0027 1050 max, for *Rho*). Data were extracted from the NEIBank (http://neibank.nei.nih.gov).

Microarray analysis

The advent of microarray technology in the 1990s led to a revolution in the way data are collected and analyzed. With a single chip, one can interrogate tens of thousands of transcripts. This created the need for massive databases and the skilled management of bioinformatic resources. These databases contain significant amounts of data for transcript levels within the eye, retina, and other ocular tissues. In the case of the eye and retina, the data are confounded by the fact that the structures are composed of many different tissue types formed by unique cells. From these data one can extract some unique cellular signatures; however, the results may not accurately reflect each of the cell types and may include lack of cell-level specificity. Furthermore, the data do not provide the investigator with any information concerning translational regulation (protein expression) or post-translational modifications important in protein regulation. Nonetheless, several microarray databases offer unique opportunities for vision researchers to investigate the regulation of the gene expression during eye development and in different strains of the mouse.

For the development of the eye there is a wonderful microarray-based Web site maintained by the Friedlander group at Scripps Institute. This site is a source of information for the postnatal developmental expression pattern of transcripts in mouse retina. The Friedlander group used Affymetrix microarrays to identify the relative levels of gene expression during the postnatal development of the mouse eye (Dorrell et al., 2004). (The data are presented at www.scripps.edu/cb/friedlander/gene_expression.) The developmental expression patterns of groups of genes are illustrated in a format that allows the investigator to query the developmental expression patterns of a specific gene or groups of genes. These Web sites can serve as references to define the molecular signatures of different tissues in the eye, along with the developmental regulation of gene expression. They also provide an excellent resource with which to follow the developmental expression patterns of genes expressed in the eye or retina. Their analysis provides the investigator with developmental expression patterns of groups of genes. These clusters of genes are specifically related to the developmental patterns of cell birth and maturation. For example, the last group of genes to be upregulated is related to phototransduction and the maturation of rods. The Friedlander database, like many vision-related mouse databases, is based on information generated from only one strain of mouse, the C57BL/6 mouse.

One important goal of genomic research is to combine expression data with variation in phenotype. In the mouse, this can be accomplished by examining strain differences as related to differential susceptibility to disease or naturally occurring differences in phenotype. For the mouse there are several resources that define phenotypic variability. Two examples are the Jackson Laboratory mouse phenotype database (http://phenome.jax.org/pub-cgi/phenome/mpdcgi?rtn=docs/home) and GeneNetwork Phenotypes (www.genenetwork.org). The mouse strains also serve as a rich genomic resource, with expression genetics allowing us to correlate phenotype variation with genomic locus. Quantifying mRNA levels with microarray-based systems has allowed for a rapid interrogation or transcript expression in the mouse. Expression genetics allows for a conceptually unique approach of using this transcript expression data to locate genomic loci controlling disease or phenotype. Furthermore, by using mouse genetic panels such as the BXD strain set, we can provide insights into the genetic networks controlling differences in gene expression and phenotypic variation.

The Hamilton Eye Institute Mouse Eye Database We have created the Hamilton Eye Institute Mouse Eye Database (HEIMED, available at www.genenetwork.org) to bring expression genetics to the vision research community. By examining variations at the transcript level we can define correlations in gene expression to genomic loci revealing higher-order transcriptional networks, as well as loci capable of modulating morphological features in the eye, for example, retinal ganglion cell (RGC) number. This approach can lead to dissection of entire networks of genes controlling transcriptional networks within the eye that dictate specific ocular phenotypes. To bring this power of expression genetics and the mouse strain set to the study of the eye, we developed a highly interactive database, HEIMED. This database estimates mRNA expression in whole eyes of young adult mice of many lines generated using the Affymetrix M430 2.0 array, which contains more than 45,000 probe sets representing more than 39,000 transcripts. Within the HEIMED, data from a total of 98 mouse strains is presented, including 67 BXD strains; the two parental strains (C57BL/6J and DBA/2J), along with their reciprocal F1s; and 27 strains from the mouse diversity panel (plus B6 and D2 for a total of 29 common strains) were generated by crossing C57BL/6J with DBA/2J. The BXDs are particularly useful for systems genetics because all of the BXDs are fully mapped and both parental strains are fully sequenced.

The BXD Genetic Reference Panel of Mice The BXD strain set is an integral part of HEIMED and our eye databases. This unique strain set was originally developed in the laboratory of Benjamin Taylor and was transferred to the Jackson Laboratory from Dr. Taylor's research colony at his retirement (Taylor et al., 1999). The two parental mouse strains, C57BL/6J and DBA/2J, were inbred strains developed relatively early. These strains have contrasting characteristics. The C57BL/6J is a very widely used inbred strain that was originally developed to be refractory to tumors; in contrast, the DBA/2J strain was developed to be susceptible to tumors. These inbred genetic differences have produced one strain (C57BL/6J) that is resistant to CNS damage and another (DBA/2J) that is susceptible to injury (Inman et al., 2002). The DBA/2J mice used in the traditional set of BXD strains carried a mutation in the *Tyrp1* gene that contributed to iris stromal atrophy. In 1997, a second mutation in *Gpnmb* resulted in a significant increase in iris diseases, causing pigment dispersion in the DBA/2J strain (Chang et al., 1999). In the advanced BXD RI strain set, which was developed from DBA/2J mice carrying both mutations (Peirce et al., 2004), 15 strains carry both the *Tyrp1* and *Gpnmb* mutations and should develop iris disease similar to that observed in the DBA/2J strain. Since the BXD RI strain set is fully mapped and since each strain can be sampled an unlimited number of times, these mice are ideal for use as a mapping panel to identify genomic loci controlling specific phenotypes such as ganglion cell number (Williams et al., 1996) or controlling genetic networks (Vazquez-Chona et al., 2005).

The BXD RI strain set is at the core of our novel analytical of tool set and QTL mapping algorithms (www.genenetwork.org). This includes an SNP database for sequenced mouse strains, along with unique sequence analysis software developed by the Williams group. The collective purpose of these tools and techniques is to extract and test molecular networks that affect gene expression in the eye and the retina. Examples of the innovative use of this approach are described in articles published in *Science* (Brem et al., 2002) and *Nature* (Schadt et al., 2003) that have highlighted the power of treating expression data as a quantitative trait and using QTL mapping methods to systematically identify upstream controllers that are responsible for individual differences in transcript abundance (Jansen and Nap, 2001). Our group has been using QTL mapping methods of this type for more than 6 years (Williams et al., 1996; Hittalmani et al., 2003; Wang et al., 2003; Chesler et al., 2004; Vazquez-Chona et al., 2005), and we welcome the opportunity to bring these approaches to the vision research community, specifically for study of the retina (Vazquez-Chona et al., 2005) (see www.genenetwork.org and the HEIMED). The precision with which we can map QTLs that modulate retina transcript networks is determined by the quality of genetic maps that we assemble for RI strains. With the sequence data, we can now completely define all breakpoints in the set of 80 BXD RI strains. These strains incorporate approximately 7,000 recombinations. Ideally, we would know the precise location of each of these breakpoints within 100,000 base pairs. This would have been almost unthinkable a few years ago. Now it is simply a matter of finding polymorphic loci that distinguish the parental strains.

Using HEIMED, we can extract the molecular signatures of specific tissues or cell types by looking for genes that correlate across the entire genome and are coexpressed with tissue-specific or cell-specific marker genes. If we examine these molecular signatures in the HEIMED database, we can begin to unravel the unique genetic networks that regulate tissue-specific expression patterns. An example of this type of analysis is genes that covary with rhodopsin (*Rho*). Unlike other approaches that identify all of the genes expressed in a cell type (in the case of rhodopsin it is rods), HEIMED generates a list of genes that are uniquely expressed in rods, forming a unique signature for this cell type. If we examine the top 100 transcripts that correlate with *Rho*, we can observe a unique molecular signature for photoreceptors with genes expressed in rods (e.g., *Pde6b*, *Gnat1*, *Guca1b*, *Nrl*, *Pde6g*, *Pdc*, *Vtn*, *Rp1*, and *Cabp4*) with similar expression patterns across the reference panel of mice. The genetic covariance with the rod-specific transcripts not only defines a unique rod signature; it can also be used to define genes associated with human retinal diseases. Pearson and Spearman correlations were used to rank candidates with expression tightly coupled ($r > 0.9$ for the first 100 probe sets) with rhodopsin across all strains. Thirty of the top 100 covariates with rhodopsin are genes currently associated with retinal disease in humans. For example, *Rdh12* ($r = 0.98$ with rhodopsin) has a well-characterized association with Leber's congenital amaurosis (LCA3). Examples of other known disease genes that covary with rhodopsin are listed in table 54.3. The genomic locations of other genes that covary with rhodopsin suggest that they are candidate genes for human disease. Their genomic locations in the mouse were converted to human chromosome locations using mouse/human synteny maps.

We examined the location of human diseases with human disease loci with unidentified disease-causing genes in the RetNet database (www.sph.uth.tmc.edu/Retnet/disease.htm). This analysis allowed us to generate strong biological candidates for uncloned human disease loci, using HEIMED in combination with GeneNetwork. The eight candidate genes for human retinal diseases are listed in table 54.4. These results are one example of the power and potential of mouse genomics for understanding retinal disease in the human.

An example of a tissue-specific molecular signature is the cornea. If we use *Aldh3a1*, the gene for aldehyde dehydrogenase family 3, subfamily A1, as a marker for the cornea and run this on the trait correlation function of GeneNetwork, we then retrieve a set of transcripts that appears to be a molecular signature of the cornea. The transcripts in the list include *Aldh3a1*, keratin 12, members of the KLF transcription factor family, and the corneal crystalline Tkt. If we examine the list of genes from HEIMED, we find they represent a series of genes that are expressed in the cornea, with some genes being unique to the cornea. By comparing these genes with the total gene expression in the cornea as represented in the NEIBank (NbLib0116, adult mouse cornea; http://neibank.nei.nih.gov/index.shtml), we find that 9 of the top 10 genes on the HEIMED corneal list are highly represented in the NEIBank list. These include aldehyde dehydrogenase family 3, subfamily A1 (*Aldh3a1*, 32 independent

Table 54.3

Cloned human disease genes found in our correlative analysis of rhodopsin expression in the mouse, with 23 cloned human disease genes and references for the original and cloning of the gene

Gene	Disease*	Human Locus	Mapping Reference	Cloning Reference
Crb1	Leber congenital amaurosis, AR Retinitis pigmentosa, AR Other AD retinopathies	1q31.3	den Hollander et al., 1999b	den Hollander et al. 1999a
Sag	Retinitis pigmentosa, AR CSNB, AR	2q37.1	Ngo et al., 1990	Ngo et al., 1990
Rho	CSNB, AD Retinitis pigmentosa, AR, AD	3q22.1	Nathans et al., 1986	Nathans and Hogness, 1984
Gnat1	CSNB, AD	3p21.31	Sparkes et al., 1987	Lerman and Minna, 2000
Pde6b	CSNB, AD Retinitis pigmentosa, AR	4p16.3	Bateman et al., 1992	Pittler et al., 1993
Cnga1	Retinitis pigmentosa, AR	4p12	Dhallan et al., 1991	Kaupp et al., 1989
Pde6a	Retinitis pigmentosa, AR	5q33.1	Ovchinnikov et al., 1987	Pittler et al., 1990
Guca1b	Macular degeneration, AD	6p21.1	Surguchov et al., 1997	Payne et al., 1999
Guca1a	Cone or cone-rod dystrophy, AD	6p21.1	Subbaraya et al., 1994	Subbaraya et al., 1994
Tulp1	Leber congenital amaurosis, AR Retinitis pigmentosa, AR	6p21.3	North et al., 1997	North et al., 1997
Rp1	Retinitis pigmentosa, AR, AD	8q12.1	Pierce et al., 1999	Pierce et al., 1999
Kcnv2	Cone or cone-rod dystrophy, AR	9q24.2	Ottschytsch et al., 2002	Ottschytsch et al., 2002
Cabp4	CSNB, AR	11q13.1	Haeseleer et al., 2004	Haeseleer et al., 2000
Rom1	Retinitis pigmentosa, AD	11q12.3	Bascom et al., 1990	Bascom et al., 1989
Nrl	Retinitis pigmentosa, AD, AR	14q11.2	Yang-Feng and Swaroop, 1992	Swaroop et al., 1991
Rdh12	Leber congenital amaurosis, AR	14q24.1	Haeseleer et al., 2002	Haeseleer et al., 2002
Nr2e3	Retinitis pigmentosa, AR Other AR retinopathy	15q23	Kobayashi et al., 1999	Kobayashi et al., 1999
Cngb1	Retinitis pigmentosa, AR	16q13	γ subunit: Ardell et al., 1995 β subunit: Ardell et al., 1996	γ subunit: Ardell et al., 1995 β subunit: Ardell et al., 1996
Aipl1	Cone or cone-rod dystrophy, AD	17p13.2	Sohocki et al., 1999	Sohocki et al., 1999
Unc119	Cone or cone-rod dystrophy, AD	17q11	Swanson et al., 1998	Higashide et al., 1996
Fscn2	Macular degeneration, AD	17q25.3	Tubb et al., 2000	Saishin et al., 1997
Crx	Retinitis pigmentosa, AD Cone or cone-rod dystrophy, AD	19q13.32	Freund et al., 1997	Freund et al., 1997
Rs1	XL retinoschisis	Xp22.13	Dahl et al., 1987	Sauer et al., 1997

AD, autosomal dominant; AR, autosomal recessive; CSNB, congenital stationary night blindness; XL, x-linked.

Table 54.4

Eight candidate genes for mapped human disease

Gene	Disease	Human Locus	Mouse Locus	Mapping Reference
RP32	Severe AR RP	1p34.3–p13.3	4 at 154.132529 Mb	Zhang et al., 2005
AXPC1	AR ataxia	1q31.1–1q32.3	1 at 134.282002 Mb	Higgins et al., 1997
RP29	AR RP	4q32.1–4q34.3	8 at 26.0 cM	Hameed et al., 2001
MCDR3	AD macular dystrophy	5pter–5p13.1	15 at 6.994909 Mb	Michaelides et al., 2003
LOC387715	ARMD, complex etiology	10q26.13	Chr 7 F_3	Jakobsdottir et al., 2005
USH1A, USH1	AR Usher syndrome, French	14q32.11–14qter	4 at 150.799494 Mb	Kaplan et al., 1991
RP22	AR RP	16p12.3–16p12.1	7 at 60.0 cM	Finckh et al., 1998
CACD	AD central areolar choroidal dystrophy	17pter–17p13.1	11 at 68.798082	Lotery et al., 1996

Note: Most of the data came from the website RetNet. The eye signal is the average expression level across all strains of the specific transcript in the eye expressed on a log scale. The clones are expressed at a level of 2 log units less in BXD24, which has acquired a mutation that causes photoreceptor degeneration.

AR, autosomal recessive; RP, retinitis pigmentosa.

clones); keratin complex 1; acidic gene 12 (*Krt1-12*, 44 independent clones); transketolase (*Tkt*, five independent clones); and uroplakin 1B (*Upk1b*, three independent clones). Furthermore, many of the genes in the list are key features of the corneal proteome (see chapter 57, this volume). These include the corneal crystallins, *Aldh3A1* and *Tkt*, which are highly expressed in the cornea (Piatigorsky, 2000; Estey et al., 2007). The list also includes genes of unknown function in the cornea, such as *Upk1b*. Uroplakin1b is thought of as a bladder protein expressed in the transitional epithelium as part of a complex with the other two known uroplakin proteins (Min et al., 2006; Sun, 2006). The ability to extract this corneal transcriptome signature from the whole eye database illustrates the power of HEIMED. The minor but consistent variations in corneal gene expression across the strains of mice in the data set allow the software to extract a group of genes uniquely expressed in the cornea from a data set consisting of the transcriptome of the whole eye.

Genetic networks in the mouse eye

In addition to providing molecular signatures of different cell types and tissues of the eye, HEIMED can reveal genetic networks that underlie phenotypic differences in the mouse eye. The genetic heterogeneity in inbred mice results in significant variation in phenotypes. These genetic heterogeneities can result in differences in behavior, neural structure, number of neurons, protein expression, and relative abundance of mRNA species. The simplest example is a Mendelian trait with a specific phenotype such as albinism. With the number of inbred strains available, the expression levels of specific transcripts can easily be examined. For example we can look at the levels of tyrosinase (*Tyr*) across a number of strains (figure 54.2). The lack of tyrosinase function is directly related to a common mouse phenotype, albinism. In figure 54.2, the level of *Tyr* is illustrated for 21 inbred strains (the data are from HEIMED). The pigmented strains are represented by *solid bars* and the albino strains by *white bars*. In general, strains with lower levels of *Tyr* are animals that are albino and not all albino mice have low levels of *Tyr* transcript. This points out the simple nature of most mutations. The lack of pigment is related not to the level of the *Tyr* transcript but to the normal functioning of the tyrosinase protein. This example of *Tyr* serves as a simple caution always to relate the analysis of data to the biology of the system, especially when examining levels of transcripts. This serves as a word of caution as we begin to examine the differences in the genomes of inbred strains and specific transcriptome profiles within the eye. These genomic or genetic differences may or may not be fully reflected in

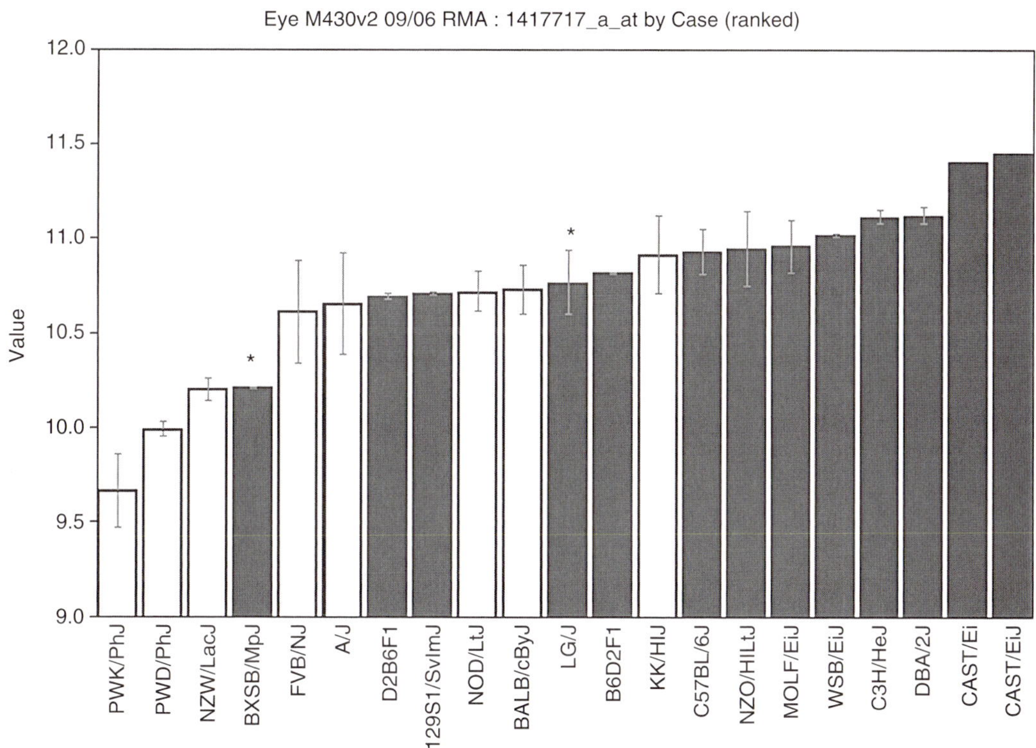

Figure 54.2 Expression levels of tyrosinase (*Tyr*) are shown for many of the inbred strains from the mouse diversity panel (see names along the ordinate). The scale to the left is a log scale of transcript level expressed as a mean and standard deviation as defined by the Affymetrix chip. Note the low levels of *Tyr* in most of the albino mice (*white bars*). The strains that have not been sequenced are indicated by an *asterisk* above the histogram bar.

protein expression levels or alterations in functional interactions of the protein. In most cases, the ultimate predictor of phenotype is the protein, not the transcript.

Unlike the simple Mendelian trait of albinism, where a single base mutation can cause a complete lack of protein function, most physical traits are regulated by complex genetic interactions that result in modest variation in different transcripts. The genomic loci regulating these complex traits can be difficult to extract from a genetically diverse outbred population. The genetic variability in inbred strains and recombinant inbred strains (such as the BXD strain set) offers unique opportunities to define genomic loci regulating complex traits. The study of these complex traits is facilitated by the availability of many different inbred strains of mice and specific Web-based genomic tools, many of which can be found at GeneNetwork. In this highly interactive database, numerous phenotypes are presented from sets of inbred panels of mice, including CNS phenotypes for cerebellum (Neumann et al., 1993), hippocampus (Lu et al., 2001; Kempermann et al., 2006), striatum (Rosen and Williams, 2001), and amygdala (Mozhui et al., 2007). Of specific interest to the vision community are data sets related to the eye, the retina, and the central visual system.

At the University of Tennessee, the Williams group has used these genetically variable populations of mouse strains to define regulatory loci controlling specific phenotypes. These phenotypic characterizations include variability in retinal ganglion cell (RGC) number, eye weight, and cell number in the lateral geniculate nucleus (Williams, Strom, and Goldowitz, 1998; Seecharan et al., 2003). For example, the population of RGCs in the mouse has a bimodal distribution, from a low of approximately 45,000–50,000 in CAST/Ei and BXD27 to a high of 75,000 in BXD5 and BXD32 (Williams et al., 1996; Williams, Strom, and Goldowitz, 1998; Seecharan et al., 2003). A major QTL on chromosome 11 that modulates RGC population size, *Nnc1*, has been mapped to a 4 Mb interval (peak at 98 Mb, 1.5 LOD confidence interval 97–101 Mb). Within this locus are genomic elements (potential candidate genes) that are involved in regulation of the number of RGCs in the mouse retina (Williams et al., 1996). In addition, Williams, Strom, and Goldowitz (1998) mapped two other contributing loci on chromosome 2 and chromosome 8 by simply quantifying the number of RGCs in 38 recombinant inbred strains and using composite interval-mapping techniques. This type of quantitative method was also used to map genomic loci controlling eye weight (Zhou and Williams, 1999) and cell number in the lateral geniculate nucleus (Seecharan et al., 2003). The traditional QTL mapping strategy defines loci that regulate a physical trait. This approach allows a systematic approach to defining a major genomic loci regulating a complex trait, such as RGC number in the mouse. Furthermore, we can use the QTL mapping methods as the basis for defining genetic networks controlling gene expression and phenotypes.

The power of inbred strains extends beyond their use as a tool to map genomic loci controlling physical traits. These reference panels of mice can also be used to unravel genetic networks controlling the structure of the eye, its development, and its response to diseases. By treating the changes in mRNA levels as a physical phenotype, differences in transcriptional control can be evaluated using traditional QTL mapping methods to define groups of transcripts with similar patterns of expression. These similar patterns of expression reveal commonality in regulatory networks that are correlated to specific genomic loci. By combining gene expression profiling with genetic linkage analysis, the location of genetic elements that modulate expression levels of specific groups of genes can be identified (Darvasi, 1998; Broman, 2005). This type of expression genetics has been used to identify genes underlying complex traits, diseases, and behavioral phenotypes (Morley et al., 2004; Bystrykh et al., 2005). Examples of this type of integrated gene expression profiling and linkage analysis are studies that have identified genes predisposing individuals to hypertension (*Cd36*) and atherosclerosis (*ABCG5* and *ABCG8*) (Aitman et al., 1999; Berge et al., 2000). These studies illustrate the power of combining gene expression profiling with linkage analysis to study gene expression.

Quantitative trait locus mapping in the Hamilton Eye Institute Mouse Eye Database

The QTL mapping functions in GeneNetwork can be used as a tool to understand the genetic networks controlling changes observed in traditional micoarray studies. As stated earlier, the genetic variability in inbred strains and mouse diversity (BXD) strain sets can be used to define groups of transcripts with similar patterns of expression. These similar patterns reveal commonality in regulatory networks that are correlated with specific genomic loci. By combining gene expression profiling with genetic linkage analysis, the location of genetic elements that modulate expression levels of specific groups of genes can be identified (Darvasi, 1998; Broman, 2005). The high levels of heritable variation in gene expression allow researchers to correlate the expression variability with one or more regions of the genome. Some of these loci modulate genes within the interval where they are located (*cis*-acting), although most loci modulate genes from a distance, at a different genomic location (*trans*-acting). HEIMED allows exploration of the genetic variability in the BXD RI strains and selected inbred strains. To examine regulatory networks, the BXD RI strain set plays a preeminent role in identifying QTLs controlling the level of gene expression. This analysis can be used to define *cis*-acting and *trans*-acting QTLs.

Three transcripts (*Tyrp1*, *Gpnmb*, and *Tyr*) were selected. The *Tyrp1* gene and the *Gpnmb* gene show strong *cis*-QTLs (figure 54.3*A* and *C*); *Tyr* demonstrates a strong *trans*-QTL. The *Tyr* gene is quite variable across mouse strains; there is a twofold difference in gene expression across the BXD RI strains and other inbred strains. Running a genome-wide scan by selecting the interval mapping function reveals a linkage of expression variability of *Tyr* with a locus on chromosome 4 (see figure 54.3*A*). Note that the peak linkage on chromosome 4 likelihood ratio statistic (LRS) is more than 40 megabases and is at the same locus as the *Tyrp1* gene itself. The strong *cis*-QTL of *Tyrp1* at the same genomic locus as the *trans*-QTL for *Tyr* makes *Tyrp1* a potential candidate gene controlling the gene expression variability of *Tyr*.

Defining genetic networks in traditional microarray experiments

Like many groups, we have used microarray methods to profile global changes following specific experimental manipulations. In this process, changes in gene expression are identified and analyzed to define functional patterns of expression. For most microarray studies, this is the end of the process. However, with the bioinformatics tools offered on GeneNetwork, the analysis of microarray gene clusters can be extended to define genetic networks regulating these changes in gene expression. To illustrate this process, we take an example from our research group.

We have used microarray techniques to obtain a picture of the global changes occurring in the retina following injury (Vazquez-Chona et al., 2004). The transcriptome-wide analysis was designed to look at the temporal regulation of transcripts controlling retinal wound healing. This gene expression profiling identified clusters of genes that are regulated in specific temporal patterns (Vazquez-Chona et al., 2004). From all these data, the response of the retina to injury could be subdivided into three temporal phases of gene expression: early acute, delayed subacute, and late chronic. Transcripts in each phase appear to be functionally related and reflect known cellular changes. The global changes occurring after injury are similar across different injury models, including mechanical trauma, ischemia, and increased intraocular pressure. The similarities in these profiles suggest that the changes in gene expression are part of common biochemical and cellular processes involved in the response of the retina to injury. As with many microarray experiments, this description of changes in the transcriptome leaves one with clusters of genes and little understanding of the basic mechanisms involved in regulating gene expression. To take the analysis to the next level, we used the databases and bioinformatics tools on GeneNetwork to examine the common regulatory elements controlling the clusters of genes in the temporal response to injury.

The basic approach to extract the underlying genetic networks involves, in sequence, identifying robust changes in gene expression following injury; defining regulatory loci (*trans*-QTLs), using genetic analysis of transcript data at GeneNetwork; and predicting candidate regulators, using bioinformatic resources that are available online. We defined a set of acute phase genes that are commonly expressed in the retina, brain, and spinal cord after traumatic injury (Vazquez-Chona et al., 2005). We then used the expression QTL analysis combined transcriptome profiling with linkage analysis to reveal variability in the chromosomal loci modulating gene expression. The analysis was made using the BXD RI strain sets and the bioinformatics tools available at genenetwork.org. Expression of acute phase genes in BXD RI mouse forebrains is modulated by a major QTL on chromosome 12 between 15 and 32 Mb. With the loci identified, the next step was to identify the candidate genes.

The identification of candidate genes within specific intervals of the BXD strain set is simplified by the nature of the strain set and the expression data set. For a gene to have a QTL that can be mapped, there must be significant variability in gene expression across the BXD strain set. In HEIMED, 10,000 probe sets have significant variability and have a significant LRS score. The second feature that identifies a potential candidate gene is that it must either be within the locus or have a *cis*-QTL. Within HEIMED, 5,000 probe sets have significant *cis*-QTLs. Within the chromosome 12 interval, there are three good candidate genes, *Id2*, *Lpin1*, and *Sox11*. All these transcripts have strong *cis*-QTLs and are known either to be transcription factors (Yokota and Mori, 2002; Jankowski et al., 2006) or to have the potential to localize to the cell's nucleus (Peterfy et al., 2005). Thus, these three genes are ideal candidates to be upstream regulators of the injury network.

The novel combination of microarray analysis, expression genetics, and bioinformatics provides a new and powerful approach to defining regulatory elements in the genome. Using this approach, we were able to generate specific, testable hypotheses to define the pathways that regulate proliferative and reactive responses in the retina and elsewhere in the CNS. As more diverse gene expression data sets become available, a comparison of gene expression and regulation in different biological contexts should help identify the regulatory elements controlling the reactive response in the retina.

Conclusion

The preceding analysis provides a glimpse into the revolution in genomics and genetics that is allowing us to examine and compare gene expression in different tissues. By defining the genetic variability among strains, we can now account

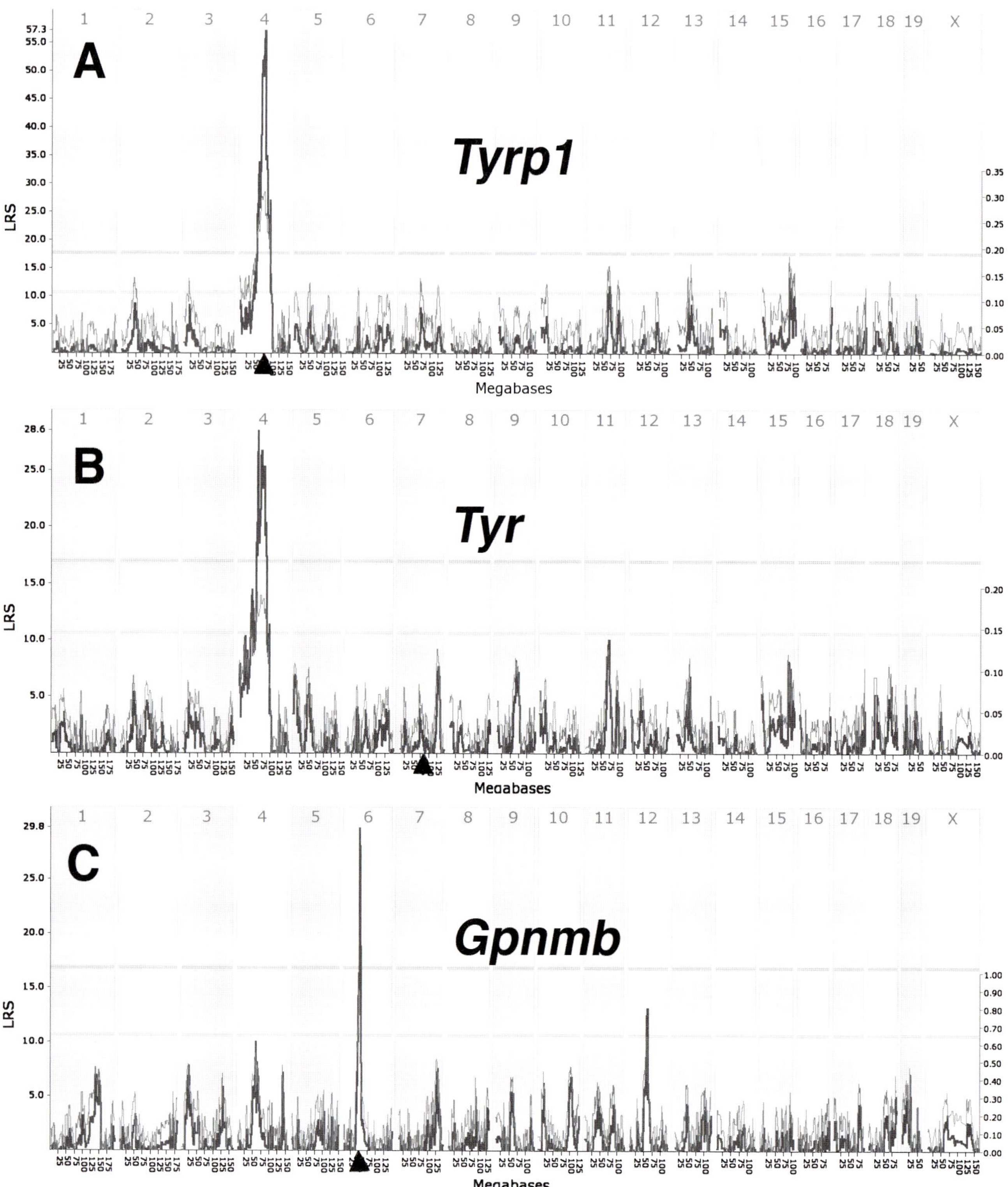

FIGURE 54.3 Interval mapping computes linkage maps for the entire genome. The numbers across the top of the three panels indicate mouse chromosomes, from Chr 1 to Chr X. We used the genetic analysis of transcript expression at GeneNetwork to define genomic loci that control transcript abundance variability in mouse eye. The variability in transcript abundance in the segregating population of BXD RI strains makes it possible to map transcript abundance to a specific chromosomal locus. Genetic linkage maps (*A–C*) show genes with significant LRS scores (the significance level is indicated by the upper line). *A*, Individual genome-wide maps for *Tyrp1* demonstrating a strong *cis*-QTL (the location of the gene is indicated by the *black triangle*). *B*, Genome-wide scan for *Tyr*, a gene with a strong *trans*-QTL. *C*, Genome-wide scan for *Gpnmb*, an additional gene with a strong *cis*-QTL. Maps were generated by linking transcript variability against 8,222. The linkage between transcript variation and genetic differences at a particular genetic locus is measured in terms of likelihood ratio statistic (LRS, *solid line*). *Dashed horizontal lines* mark transcript-specific significance thresholds for genome-wide $P < 0.05$ (*upper band*) and genome-wide $P < 0.63$ (*lower band*). The *triangle* indicates gene location. Linkage maps were generated using the interval mapping tool at GeneNetwork.

for many phenotypic differences in the mouse eye. The mouse eye is genetically unique in that findings in the mouse can directly apply to understanding gene expression in human conditions leading to the loss of sight. Defining the genetic variability and differences in gene expression across strains of mice that are fully mapped and sequenced allows a direct correlation between eye phenotypes and disease states with genomic loci and candidate genes. Transcriptome-wide analysis of the eye allows us to define genetic variability between strains not only to specific cellular phenotypes, but also to the response of cells to changes in the state of the eye. Using HEIMED allows the vision research community to define molecular signatures within the tissues of the eye, identify candidate genes for human disease, begin to understand genetic networks regulating tissue-specific gene expression, and identify the complex interactions of genomic loci that underlie the complex structures of the eye. As technology progresses, it should be possible to use cell type–specific analysis of mRNA and protein expression across large genetically defined and manipulated panels of mice. The use of these methods in large genetic reference panels of mice and the multiscale integration of the resultant data should allow for the definition of genes responsible for complex genetic diseases. We are currently using this approach to define genomic loci and candidate genes associated with susceptibility and resistance retinal ganglion to cell death in human diseases.

ACKNOWLEDGMENTS Support for the acquisition of microarray data sets was generously provided by Dr. Barrrett Haik, chair of the Department of Ophthalmology and director of the Hamilton Eye Institute. This work is supported by the National Eye Institute (RO1EY17841), the Integrative Neuroscience Initiative on Alcoholism (U01AA13499, U24AA13513), the Human Brain Project (P20-DA21131), NCI (U01CA105417), and the Biomedical Informatics Research Network, NCRR (U24RR021760). All arrays were processed at the VA Medical Center, Memphis, by Dr. Yan Jiao and Dr. Weikuan Gu. We thank Dr. Lu Lu for his contributions to every aspect of the HEIMED project, Bill Orr for his assistance, and Dr. Mohamed Nassr for his assistance in data analysis.

REFERENCES

Aitman, T. J., Glazier, A. M., Wallace, C. A., Cooper, L. D., Norsworthy, P. J., Wahid, F. N., Al-Majali, K. M., Trembling, P. M., Mann, C. J., et al. (1999). Identification of Cd36 (Fat) as an insulin-resistance gene causing defective fatty acid and glucose metabolism in hypertensive rats. *Nat. Genet.* 21(1):76–83.

Ardell, M. D., Aragon, I., Oliveira, L., Porche, G. E., Burke, E., and Pittler, S. J. (1996). The beta subunit of human rod photoreceptor cGMP-gated cation channel is generated from a complex transcription unit. *FEBS Lett.* 389(2):213–218.

Ardell, M. D., Makhija, A. K., Oliveira, L., Miniou, P., Viegas-Pequignot, E., and Pittler, S. J. (1995). cDNA, gene structure, and chromosomal localization of human GAR1 (CNCG3L), a homolog of the third subunit of bovine photoreceptor cGMP-gated channel. *Genomics* 28(1):32–38.

Bascom, R. A., Connell, G., Garcia-Heras, J., Collins, L., Ledbetter, D., Molday, R. S., Kalnins, V., and McInnes, R. R. (1990). Molecular and ultrastructural characterization of the products of the human retinopathy candidate genes ROM1 and RDS (abstr.). *Am. J. Hum. Genet.* 47(Suppl.):A101.

Bascom, R., Manara, S., Gallie, B., Willard, H., Kalnins, V., and McInnes, R. R. (1989). Identification of a new mammalian photoreceptor-specific gene family (abstr.). *Am. J. Hum. Genet.* 45: A172.

Bateman, J. B., Klisak, I., Kojis, T., Mohandas, T., Sparkes, R. S., Li, T. S., Applebury, M. L., Bowes, C., and Farber, D. B. (1992). Assignment of the beta-subunit of rod photoreceptor cGMP phosphodiesterase gene PDEB (homolog of the mouse rd gene) to human chromosome 4p16. *Genomics* 12(3): 601–603.

Berge, K. E., Tian, H., Graf, G. A., Yu, L., Grishin, N. V., Schultz, J., Kwiterovich, P., Shan, B., Barnes, R., et al. (2000). Accumulation of dietary cholesterol in sitosterolemia caused by mutations in adjacent ABC transporters. *Science* 290(5497):1771–1775.

Blackshaw, S., Harpavat, S., Trimarchi, J., Cai, L., Huang, H., Kuo, W. P., Weber, G., Lee, K., Fraioli, R. E., et al. (2004). Genomic analysis of mouse retinal development. *PLoS Biol.* 2(9): E247.

Brem, R. B., Yvert, G., Clinton, R., and Kruglyak, L. (2002). Genetic dissection of transcriptional regulation in budding yeast. *Science* 296(5568):752–755.

Broman, K. W. (2005). The genomes of recombinant inbred lines. *Genetics* 169(2):1133–1146.

Bystrykh, L., Weersing, E., Dontje, B., Sutton, S., Pletcher, M. T., Wiltshire, T., Su, A. I., Vellenga, E., Wang, J., et al. (2005). Uncovering regulatory pathways that affect hematopoietic stem cell function using "genetical genomics". *Nat. Genet.* 37(3):225–232.

Chang, B., Smith, R. S., Hawes, N. L., Anderson, M. G., Zabaleta, A., Savinova, O., Roderick, T. H., Heckenlively, J. R., Davisson, M. T., et al. (1999). Interacting loci cause severe iris atrophy and glaucoma in DBA/2J mice. *Nat. Genet.* 21(4): 405–409.

Chesler, E. J., Lu, L., Wang, J., Williams, R. W., and Manly, K. F. (2004). WebQTL: Rapid exploratory analysis of gene expression and genetic networks for brain and behavior. *Nat. Neurosci.* 7(5):485–486.

Dahl, N., Goonewardena, P., Chotai, J., Wadelius, C., Lindsten, J., and Pettersson, U. (1987). DNA linkage analysis of X-chromosome linked retinoschisis (abstr.). *Cytogenet. Cell Genet.* 46:602.

Darvasi, A. (1998). Experimental strategies for the genetic dissection of complex traits in animal models. *Nat. Genet.* 18(1):19–24.

den Hollander, A. I., ten Brink, J. B., de Kok, Y. J., van Soest, S., van den Born, L. I., van Driel, M. A., van de Pol, D. J., Payne, A. M., Bhattacharya, S. S., et al. (1999a). Mutations in a human homologue of *Drosophila* crumbs cause retinitis pigmentosa (RP12). *Nat. Genet.* 23(2):217–221.

den Hollander, A. I., van Driel, M. A., de Kok, Y. J., van de Pol, D. J., Hoyng, C. B., Brunner, H. G., Deutman, A. F., and Cremers, F. P. (1999b). Isolation and mapping of novel candidate genes for retinal disorders using suppression subtractive hybridization. *Genomics* 58(3):240–249.

Dhallan, R. S., Macke, J., Eddy, R. L., Shows, T. B., Reed, R. R., Yau, K.-W., and Nathans, J. (1991). The human rod photoreceptor cyclic GMP gated channel gene maps to chromosome 4 (abstr.). *Cytogenet. Cell Genet.* 58:1886.

Dorrell, M. I., Aguilar, E., Weber, C., and Friedlander, M. (2004). Global gene expression analysis of the developing postnatal mouse retina. *Invest. Ophthalmol. Vis. Sci.* 45(3):1009–1019.

Estey, T., Piatigorsky, J., Lassen, N., and Vasiliou, V. (2007). ALDH3A1: A corneal crystallin with diverse functions. *Exp. Eye Res.* 84(1):3–12.

Finckh, U., Xu, S., Kumaramanickavel, G., Schurmann, M., Mukkadan, J. K., Fernandez, S. T., John, S., Weber, J. L., Denton, M. J., et al. (1998). Homozygosity mapping of autosomal recessive retinitis pigmentosa locus (RP22) on chromosome 16p12.1–p12.3. *Genomics* 48(3):341–345.

Frazer, K. A., Eskin, E., Kang, H. M., Bogue, M. A., Hinds, D. A., Beilharz, E. J., Gupta, R. V., Montgomery, J., Morenzoni, M. M., et al. (2007). A sequence-based variation map of 8.27 million SNPs in inbred mouse strains. *Nature* 448(7157): 1050–1053.

Freund, C. L., Gregory-Evans, C. Y., Furukawa, T., Papaioannou, M., Looser, J., Ploder, L., Bellingham, J., Ng, D., Herbrick, J. A., et al. (1997). Cone-rod dystrophy due to mutations in a novel photoreceptor-specific homeobox gene (CRX) essential for maintenance of the photoreceptor. *Cell* 91(4):543–553.

Haeseleer, F., Imanishi, Y., Maeda, T., Possin, D. E., Maeda, A., Lee, A., Rieke, F., and Palczewski, K. (2004). Essential role of Ca^{2+}-binding protein 4, a Cav1.4 channel regulator, in photoreceptor synaptic function. *Nat. Neurosci.* 7(10):1079–1087.

Haeseleer, F., Jang, G. F., Imanishi, Y., Driessen, C. A., Matsumura, M., Nelson, P. S., and Palczewski, K. (2002). Dual-substrate specificity short chain retinol dehydrogenases from the vertebrate retina. *J. Biol. Chem.* 277(47):45537–45546.

Haeseleer, F., Sokal, I., Verlinde, C. L., Erdjument-Bromage, H., Tempst, P., Pronin, A. N., Benovic, J. L., Fariss, R. N., and Palczewski, K. (2000). Five members of a novel Ca(2+)-binding protein (CABP) subfamily with similarity to calmodulin. *J. Biol. Chem.* 275(2):1247–1260.

Hameed, A., Khaliq, S., Ismail, M., Anwar, K., Mehdi, S. Q., Bessant, D., Payne, A. M., and Bhattacharya, S. S. (2001). A new locus for autosomal recessive RP (RP29) mapping to chromosome 4q32–q34 in a Pakistani family. *Invest. Ophthalmol. Vis. Sci.* 42(7):1436–1438.

Higashide, T., Murakami, A., McLaren, M. J., and Inana, G. (1996). Cloning of the cDNA for a novel photoreceptor protein. *J. Biol. Chem.* 271(3):1797–1804.

Higgins, J. J., Morton, D. H., Patronas, N., and Nee, L. E. (1997). An autosomal recessive disorder with posterior column ataxia and retinitis pigmentosa. *Neurology* 49(6):1717–1720.

Hittalmani, S., Huang, N., Courtois, B., Venuprasad, R., Shashidhar, H. E., Zhuang, J. Y., Zheng, K. L., Liu, G. F., Wang, G. C., et al. (2003). Identification of QTL for growth- and grain yield-related traits in rice across nine locations of Asia. *TAG Theoretical Appl. Genet.* 107(4):679–690.

Inman, D., Guth, L., and Steward, O. (2002). Genetic influences on secondary degeneration and wound healing following spinal cord injury in various strains of mice. *J. Comp. Neurol.* 451(3): 225–235.

International HapMap Consortium. (2005). A haplotype map of the human genome. *Nature* 437(7063):1299–1320.

Jacobs, G. H., Williams, G. A., Cahill, H., and Nathans, J. (2007). Emergence of novel color vision in mice engineered to express a human cone photopigment. *Science* 315(5819): 1723–1725.

Jakobsdottir, J., Conley, Y. P., Weeks, D. E., Mah, T. S., Ferrell, R. E., and Gorin, M. B. (2005). Susceptibility genes for age-related maculopathy on chromosome 10q26. *Am. J. Hum. Genet.* 77(3):389–407.

Jankowski, M. P., Cornuet, P. K., McIlwrath, S., Koerber, H. R., and Albers, K. M. (2006). SRY-box containing gene 11 (Sox11) transcription factor is required for neuron survival and neurite growth. *Neuroscience* 143(2):501–514.

Jansen, R. C., and Nap, J. P. (2001). Genetical genomics: The added value from segregation. *Trends Genet.* 17(7):388–391.

Kampa, D., Cheng, J., Kapranov, P., Yamanaka, M., Brubaker, S., Cawley, S., Drenkow, J., Piccolboni, A., Bekiranov, S., et al. (2004). Novel RNAs identified from an in-depth analysis of the transcriptome of human chromosomes 21 and 22. *Genome Res.* 14(3):331–342.

Kaplan, J., Gerber, S., Bonneau, D., Rozet, J., Briard, M., Dufier, J., Munnich, A., and Frézal, J. (1991). Probable location of Usher type I gene on chromosome 14q by linkage with D14S13 (MLJ14 probe). *Cytogenet. Cell Genet.* 58:1988.

Kapranov, P., Cheng, J., Dike, S., Nix, D. A., Duttagupta, R., Willingham, A. T., Stadler, P. F., Hertel, J., Hackermuller, J., et al. (2007). RNA maps reveal new RNA classes and a possible function for pervasive transcription. *Science* 316(5830): 1484–1488.

Kaupp, U. B., Niidome, T., Tanabe, T., Terada, S., Bonigk, W., Stuhmer, W., Cook, N. J., Kangawa, K., Matsuo, H., et al. (1989). Primary structure and functional expression from complementary DNA of the rod photoreceptor cyclic GMP-gated channel. *Nature* 342(6251):762–766.

Kempermann, G., Chesler, E. J., Lu, L., Williams, R. W., and Gage, F. H. (2006). Natural variation and genetic covariance in adult hippocampal neurogenesis. *Proc. Natl. Acad. Sci. U.S.A.* 103 (3):780–785.

Kobayashi, M., Takezawa, S., Hara, K., Yu, R. T., Umesono, Y., Agata, K., Taniwaki, M., Yasuda, K., and Umesono, K. (1999). Identification of a photoreceptor cell-specific nuclear receptor. *Proc. Natl. Acad. Sci. U.S.A.* 96(9):4814–4819.

Kondo, S., Schutte, B. C., Richardson, R. J., Bjork, B. C., Knight, A. S., Watanabe, Y., Howard, E., de Lima, R. L., Daack-Hirsch, S., et al. (2002). Mutations in IRF6 cause Van der Woude and popliteal pterygium syndromes. *Nat. Genet.* 32 (2):285–289.

Lerman, M. I., and Minna, J. D. (2000). The 630-kb lung cancer homozygous deletion region on human chromosome 3p21.3: Identification and evaluation of the resident candidate tumor suppressor genes. The International Lung Cancer Chromosome 3p21.3 Tumor Suppressor Gene Consortium. *Cancer Res.* 60 (21):6116–6133.

Lindblad-Toh, K., Wade, C. M., Mikkelsen, T. S., Karlsson, E. K., Jaffe, D. B., Kamal, M., Clamp, M., Chang, J. L., Kulbokas, E. J., III, et al. (2005). Genome sequence, comparative analysis and haplotype structure of the domestic dog. *Nature* 438(7069):803–819.

Lotery, A. J., Ennis, K. T., Silvestri, G., Nicholl, S., McGibbon, D., Collins, A. D., and Hughes, A. E. (1996). Localisation of a gene for central areolar choroidal dystrophy to chromosome 17p. *Hum. Mol. Genet.* 5(5):705–708.

Lu, L., Airey, D. C., and Williams, R. W. (2001). Complex trait analysis of the hippocampus: Mapping and biometric analysis of two novel gene loci with specific effects on hippocampal structure in mice. *J. Neurosci.* 21(10):3503–3514.

McPherson, J. D., Marra, M., Hillier, L., Waterston, R. H., Chinwalla, A., Wallis, J., Sekhon, M., Wylie, K., Mardis, E. R., et al. (2001). A physical map of the human genome. *Nature* 409(6822):934–941.

Michaelides, M., Johnson, S., Tekriwal, A. K., Holder, G. E., Bellmann, C., Kinning, E., Woodruff, G., Trembath, R. C., Hunt, D. M., et al. (2003). An early-onset autosomal dominant macular dystrophy (MCDR3) resembling North Carolina macular dystrophy maps to chromosome 5. *Invest. Ophthalmol. Vis. Sci.* 44(5):2178–2183.

Min, G., Wang, H., Sun, T. T., and Kong, X. P. (2006). Structural basis for tetraspanin functions as revealed by the cryo-EM structure of uroplakin complexes at 6-A resolution. *J. Cell Biol.* 173 (6):975–983.

Morley, M., Molony, C. M., Weber, T. M., Devlin, J. L., Ewens, K. G., Spielman, R. S., and Cheung, V. G. (2004). Genetic analysis of genome-wide variation in human gene expression. *Nature* 430(7001):743–747.

Mozhui, K., Hamre, K. M., Holmes, A., Lu, L., and Williams, R. W. (2007). Genetic and structural analysis of the basolateral amygdala complex in BXD recombinant inbred mice. *Behav. Genet.* 37(1):223–243.

Nathans, J., and Hogness, D. S. (1984). Isolation and nucleotide sequence of the gene encoding human rhodopsin. *Proc. Natl. Acad. Sci. U.S.A.* 81(15):4851–4855.

Nathans, J., Thomas, D., and Hogness, D. S. (1986). Molecular genetics of human color vision: The genes encoding blue, green, and red pigments. *Science* 232(4747):193–202.

Neumann, P. E., Garretson, J. D., Skabardonis, G. P., and Mueller, G. G. (1993). Genetic analysis of cerebellar folial pattern in crosses of C57BL/6J and DBA/2J inbred mice. *Brain Res.* 619(1–2):81–88.

Ngo, J. T., Klisak, I., Sparkes, R. S., Mohandas, T., Yamaki, K., Shinohara, T., and Bateman, J. B. (1990). Assignment of the S-antigen gene (SAG) to human chromosome 2q24–q37. *Genomics* 7(1):84–87.

North, M. A., Naggert, J. K., Yan, Y., Noben-Trauth, K., and Nishina, P. M. (1997). Molecular characterization of TUB, TULP1, and TULP2, members of the novel tubby gene family and their possible relation to ocular diseases. *Proc. Natl. Acad. Sci. U.S.A.* 94(7):3128–3133.

Ottschytsch, N., Raes, A., Van Hoorick, D., and Snyders, D. J. (2002). Obligatory heterotetramerization of three previously uncharacterized Kv channel alpha-subunits identified in the human genome. *Proc. Natl. Acad. Sci. U.S.A.* 99(12):7986–7991.

Ovchinnikov, YuA., Gubanov, V. V., Khramtsov, N. V., Ischenko, K. A., Zagranichny, V. E., Muradov, K. G., Shuvaeva, T. M., and Lipkin, V. M. (1987). Cyclic GMP phosphodiesterase from bovine retina: Amino acid sequence of the alpha-subunit and nucleotide sequence of the corresponding cDNA. *FEBS Lett.* 223(1):169–173.

Payne, A. M., Downes, S. M., Bessant, D. A., Plant, C., Moore, T., Bird, A. C., and Bhattacharya, S. S. (1999). Genetic analysis of the guanylate cyclase activator 1B (GUCA1B) gene in patients with autosomal dominant retinal dystrophies. *J. Med. Genet.* 36(9):691–693.

Peirce, J. L., Lu, L., Gu, J., Silver, L. M., and Williams, R. W. (2004). A new set of BXD recombinant inbred lines from advanced intercross populations in mice. *BMC Genet.* 5:7.

Pennesi, G., Mattapallil, M. J., Sun, S. H., Avichezer, D., Silver, P. B., Karabekian, Z., David, C. S., Hargrave, P. A., McDowell, J. H., et al. (2003). A humanized model of experimental autoimmune uveitis in HLA class II transgenic mice. *J. Clin. Invest.* 111(8):1171–1180.

Peterfy, M., Phan, J., and Reue, K. (2005). Alternatively spliced lipin isoforms exhibit distinct expression pattern, subcellular localization, and role in adipogenesis. *J. Biol. Chem.* 280(38): 32883–32889.

Piatigorsky, J. (2000). Review: A case for corneal crystallins. *J. Ocul. Pharmacol. Ther.* 16(2):173–180.

Pierce, E. A., Quinn, T., Meehan, T., McGee, T. L., Berson, E. L., and Dryja, T. P. (1999). Mutations in a gene encoding a new oxygen-regulated photoreceptor protein cause dominant retinitis pigmentosa. *Nat. Genet.* 22(3):248–254.

Pittler, S. J., Baehr, W., Wasmuth, J. J., McConnell, D. G., Champagne, M. S., vanTuinen, P., Ledbetter, D., and Davis, R. L. (1990). Molecular characterization of human and bovine rod photoreceptor cGMP phosphodiesterase alpha-subunit and chromosomal localization of the human gene. *Genomics* 6(2): 272–283.

Pittler, S. J., Keeler, C. E., Sidman, R. L., and Baehr, W. (1993). PCR analysis of DNA from 70-year-old sections of rodless retina demonstrates identity with the mouse rd defect. *Proc. Natl. Acad. Sci. U.S.A.* 90(20):9616–9619.

Rosen, G. D., and Williams, R. W. (2001). Complex trait analysis of the mouse striatum: Independent QTLs modulate volume and neuron number. *BMC Neurosci.* 2:5.

Saishin, Y., Shimada, S., Morimura, H., Sato, K., Ishimoto, I., Tano, Y., and Tohyama, M. (1997). Isolation of a cDNA encoding a photoreceptor cell-specific actin-bundling protein: retinal fascin. *FEBS Lett.* 414(2):381–386.

Sauer, C. G., Gehrig, A., Warneke-Wittstock, R., Marquardt, A., Ewing, C. C., Gibson, A., Lorenz, B., Jurklies, B., and Weber, B. H. (1997). Positional cloning of the gene associated with X-linked juvenile retinoschisis. *Nat. Genet.* 17(2):164–170.

Schadt, E. E., Monks, S. A., Drake, T. A., Lusis, A. J., Che, N., Colinayo, V., Ruff, T. G., Milligan, S. B., Lamb, J. R., et al. (2003). Genetics of gene expression surveyed in maize, mouse and man. *Nature* 422(6929):297–302.

Seecharan, D. J., Kulkarni, A. L., Lu, L., Rosen, G. D., and Williams, R. W. (2003). Genetic control of interconnected neuronal populations in the mouse primary visual system. *J. Neurosci.* 23(35):11178–11188.

Shultz, L. D., Pearson, T., King, M., Giassi, L., Carney, L., Gott, B., Lyons, B., Rossini, A. A., and Greiner, D. L. (2007). Humanized NOD/LtSz-scid IL2 receptor common gamma chain knockout mice in diabetes research. *Ann. N.Y. Acde. Sci.* 1103:77–89.

Sohocki, M. M., Malone, K. A., Sullivan, L. S., and Daiger, S. P. (1999). Localization of retina/pineal-expressed sequences: Identification of novel candidate genes for inherited retinal disorders. *Genomics* 58(1):29–33.

Sparkes, R. S., Cohn, V. H., Mohandas, T., Zollman, S., Cire-Eversole, P., Amatruda, T. T., Reed, R. R., Lochrie, M. A., and Simon, M. I. (1987). Mapping of genes encoding the subunits of guanine nucleotide-binding protein (G-proteins) in humans (abstr.). *Cytogenet. Cell Genet.* 46:696.

Subbaraya, I., Ruiz, C. C., Helekar, B. S., Zhao, X., Gorczyca, W. A., Pettenati, M. J., Rao, P. N., Palczewski, K., and Baehr, W. (1994). Molecular characterization of human and mouse photoreceptor guanylate cyclase-activating protein (GCAP) and chromosomal localization of the human gene. *J. Biol. Chem.* 269(49):31080–31089.

Sun, T. T. (2006). Altered phenotype of cultured urothelial and other stratified epithelial cells: Implications for wound healing. *Am. J. Physiol.* 291(1):F9–F21.

Surguchov, A., Bronson, J. D., Banerjee, P., Knowles, J. A., Ruiz, C., Subbaraya, I., Palczewski, K., and Baehr, W. (1997). The human GCAP1 and GCAP2 genes are arranged in a tail-to-tail array on the short arm of chromosome 6 (p21.1). *Genomics* 39(3):312–322.

Swanson, D. A., Chang, J. T., Campochiaro, P. A., Zack, D. J., and Valle, D. (1998). Mammalian orthologs of *C. elegans* unc-119 highly expressed in photoreceptors. *Invest. Ophthalmol. Vis. Sci.* 39(11):2085–2094.

Swaroop, A., Xu, J. Z., Agarwal, N., and Weissman, S. M. (1991). A simple and efficient cDNA library subtraction procedure: Isolation of human retina-specific cDNA clones. *Nucl. Acids Res.* 19(8):1954.

Taylor, B. A., Wnek, C., Kotlus, B. S., Roemer, N., MacTaggart, T., and Phillips, S. J. (1999). Genotyping new BXD recombinant inbred mouse strains and comparison of BXD and consensus maps. *Mamm. Genome* 10(4):335–348.

Tubb, B. E., Bardien-Kruger, S., Kashork, C. D., Shaffer, L. G., Ramagli, L. S., Xu, J., Siciliano, M. J., and Bryan, J. (2000). Characterization of human retinal fascin gene (FSCN2) at 17q25: Close physical linkage of fascin and cytoplasmic actin genes. *Genomics* 65(2):146–156.

Vazquez-Chona, F., Khan, A. N., Chan, C. K., Moore, A. N., Dash, P. K., Hernandez, M. R., Lu, L., Chesler, E. J., Manly, K. F., et al. (2005). Genetic networks controlling retinal injury. *Mol. Vision* 11:958–970.

Vazquez-Chona, F., Song, B. K., and Geisert, E. E., Jr. (2004). Temporal changes in gene expression after injury in the rat retina. *Invest. Ophthalmol. Vis. Sci.* 45(8):2737–2746.

Venter, J. C., Adams, M. D., Myers, E. W., Li, P. W., Mural, R. J., Sutton, G. G., Smith, H. O., Yandell, M., Evans, C. A., et al. (2001). The sequence of the human genome. *Science* 291 (5507):1304–1351.

Wang, X., Le Roy, I., Nicodeme, E., Li, R., Wagner, R., Petros, C., Churchill, G. A., Harris, S., Darvasi, A., et al. (2003). Using advanced intercross lines for high-resolution mapping of HDL cholesterol quantitative trait loci. *Genome Res.* 13(7): 1654–1664.

Waterston, R. H., Lindblad-Toh, K., Birney, E., Rogers, J., Abril, J. F., Agarwal, P., Agarwala, R., Ainscough, R., Alexandersson, M., et al. (2002). Initial sequencing and comparative analysis of the mouse genome. *Nature* 420(6915):520–562.

Williams, R. W., Strom, R. C., and Goldowitz, D. (1998). Natural variation in neuron number in mice is linked to a major quantitative trait locus on Chr 11. *J. Neurosci.* 18(1):138–146.

Williams, R. W., Strom, R. C., Rice, D. S., and Goldowitz, D. (1996). Genetic and environmental control of variation in retinal ganglion cell number in mice. *J. Neurosci.* 16(22):7193–7205.

Williams, R. W., Strom, R. C., Zhou, G., and Yan, Z. (1998). Genetic dissection of retinal development. *Semin. Cell Development. Biol.* 9(3):249–255.

Yang-Feng, T. L., and Swaroop, A. (1992). Neural retina-specific leucine zipper gene NRL (D14S46E) maps to human chromosome 14q11.1–q11.2. *Genomics* 14(2):491–492.

Yokota, Y., and Mori, S. (2002). Role of Id family proteins in growth control. *J. Cell. Physiol.* 190(1):21–28.

Zhang, Q., Zulfiqar, F., Xiao, X., Riazuddin, S. A., Ayyagari, R., Sabar, F., Caruso, R., Sieving, P. A., Riazuddin, S., et al. (2005). Severe autosomal recessive retinitis pigmentosa maps to chromosome 1p13.3–p21.2 between D1S2896 and D1S457 but outside ABCA4. *Hum. Genet.* 118(3–4):356–365.

Zhou, G., and Williams, R. W. (1999). Eye1 and Eye2: Gene loci that modulate eye size, lens weight, and retinal area in the mouse. *Invest. Ophthalmol. Vis. Sci.* 40(5):817–825.

55 Mouse Models, Microarrays, and Genetic Networks in Retinal Development and Degenerative Disease

SUNIL K. PARAPURAM AND ANAND SWAROOP

Retinal degenerative diseases (RDs) are a major cause of untreatable blindness in the Western world (Bressler et al., 2003; Hartong et al., 2006). A vast majority of RDs are categorized as orphan diseases, affecting fewer than 200,000 individuals in the population; nevertheless, these diseases collectively represent an important health problem (Weleber, 2005). Of almost 200 mapped RD loci, as many as 130 genes have been identified (www.sph.uth.tmc.edu/Retnet/sum-dis.htm). These studies have assisted in better clinical diagnosis and management (Kalloniatis and Fletcher, 2004; Hartong et al., 2006). However, the precise molecular events and cellular pathways of disease pathogenesis are relatively less well understood, and effective treatment paradigms are still not available for most retinopathies. A major challenge has been the heterogeneity of mutations resulting in photoreceptor degeneration, making it economically impractical for pharmaceutical companies to invest in therapies that may alleviate the pathology in small subsets of populations. Mutational heterogeneity is illustrated most noticeably in the case of rhodopsin, where at least 88 mutations can cause the autosomal dominant type of retinitis pigmentosa (RP) yet two alleles lead to RP only in a homozygous state (Gal et al., 1997). Another impediment is that the affected individuals exhibit extensive variations in disease phenotype even though the same gene may be involved. Thus, the design of therapeutic strategies must take into account the complexity of retinal phenotypes and the heterogeneity of gene defects.

Gene therapy, a paradigm for individualized treatment, has been used extensively to deliver a functional gene to counter the effect of a nonfunctional gene or to eliminate a mutant allele in animal models of RD (Acland et al., 2001; Hauswirth and Lewin, 2000; Mori et al., 2002; Dinculescu et al., 2005). A number of generalized approaches are also being developed to surmount the complex diversity of RDs; these include the surgical implantation of optoelectronic retinal prostheses (Zrenner, 2002; Humayun et al., 2003; Rizzo et al., 2004), transplantation of cells (Gouras et al., 1994; Lund et al., 2001; MacLaren et al., 2006), and treatment with growth or survival factors (Faktorovich et al., 1990; Frasson et al., 1999; Delyfer et al., 2004). All of these therapeutic strategies suffer from certain limitations. Gene therapy protocols need to address extensive heterogeneity in gene mutations, apart from safety and efficacy problems associated with viral vectors. For electronic chips, limited field of vision and resolution are among some of the difficulties. Transplantation of cells faces different kinds of hurdles, including functional integration into the retina, biocompatibility, long-term survival of cell transplants, and ethical issues. In the case of treatments involving growth and survival factors, the delivery of optimal amounts and their usefulness or side effects over the long term constitute primary concerns. We therefore need to incorporate additional paradigms for effective design of therapies for RDs.

Comprehensive studies have established that dysfunction or death of rod and cone photoreceptors are the primary cause of blindness in the vast majority of RDs (Rattner et al., 1999; Pacione et al., 2003). A better understanding of photoreceptor development, function, and survival would greatly assist in effective design of treatments for blinding retinal diseases. This chapter first discusses gene profiling using microarrays and the construction of regulatory networks underlying photoreceptor differentiation. We then describe a systematic approach to delineating molecular pathways of photoreceptor cell death caused by inherited gene defects, with a goal of developing novel treatment paradigms.

Expression profiling using microarrays

Microarrays of oligonucleotides or DNA fragments derived from expressed sequence regions allow simultaneous measurement of expression changes in thousands of genes under a given condition (Duggan et al., 1999; Zareparsi et al.,

2004). Temporal gene profiles of a specific tissue or cell type can provide valuable information for constructing networks or pathways involved in a complex biological process, such as differentiation or disease pathogenesis. The choice of a specific microarray platform (e.g., cDNA array, short vs. long oligonucleotide arrays) for expression profiling depends on the purpose of the experiments. Because our goal is to compare gene profiles from multiple different experiments (i.e., profiles from the retina or photoreceptors of multiple mutant mice at different stages of disease progression), it is highly desirable to employ stringent quality control and minimize intersample experimental variations. Therefore, we have optimized conditions for microarray analysis using mouse GeneChips MOE430.2.0 (www.affymetrix.com); these microarrays include 45,101 probe sets corresponding to about 39,000 transcripts of 34,000 annotated genes. Discussions of microarrays and associated methods can be found in several recent publications (Duggan et al., 1999; Livesey et al., 2000; Mu et al., 2001; Farjo et al., 2002; Yoshida et al., 2002; Diaz et al. 2003; Hackam et al., 2004; Zareparsi et al., 2004).

A major challenge in gene profiling experiments is the extraction of useful information from enormous data sets. The mammalian retina consists of six major types of neurons and one type of glia; however, many distinct subtypes can be identified based on morphology and function (Masland, 2001). Global profiling of the retina would reveal average changes in expression of genes in many different cell types; several of these would reflect manifestations secondary to RD. Notably, a number of photoreceptor-specific genes are mutated in RDs, and even when the mutant gene is widely expressed, photoreceptors are considered the primary site of disease in a majority of patients with RD. In patients with RP and in most *rd* mouse mutants, rods appear to be the first retinal cell type that is affected. Even in age-related macular degeneration (AMD), increased loss of rods is observed in the central visual field during early stages (Curcio et al., 1996). It is therefore likely that gene profiling of purified rod (and cone) photoreceptors rather than the whole retina will yield more useful data for network or pathway construction to fully comprehend differentiation or degenerative disease.

NRL and gene profiling of purified rod (and cone) photoreceptors

The basic motif-leucine zipper transcription factor (TF), NRL (Swaroop et al., 1992), is essential for rod photoreceptor differentiation; loss of NRL in mice (*Nrl*$^{-/-}$) results in transformation of postmitotic rod precursors to cones (Mears et al., 2001; Daniele et al., 2005; Akimoto et al., 2006), whereas ectopic expression of NRL converts cones to rods (Oh et al., 2007). NRL is expressed preferentially in rods and the pineal gland (Swain et al., 2001; Akimoto et al., 2006). We recently used *Nrl* promoter to direct the expression of GFP (Nrlp-EGFP transgene) in mice (*wt-Gfp*) and successfully marked the rod photoreceptors with GFP at the time of birth (Akimoto et al., 2006). GFP tagging allowed us to identify and purify rod photoreceptors at different stages of development using flow cytometry (FACS analysis) (figure 55.1). Evaluation of retinas from the *Nrl*$^{-/-}$-*Gfp* mice (generated by breeding *wt-Gfp* mice with the *Nrl*$^{-/-}$ mice) provided a direct demonstration of the transformation of rods to cones in the absence of NRL, and this also led to efficient enrichment of cone photoreceptors by FACS (Akimoto et al., 2006). To produce gene signatures of developing and mature rods or cones, we used total RNA from 1–5 × 10^5 FACS-purified cells for linear amplification. Biotin-labeled fragmented cDNAs derived from the amplification were then hybridized to mouse GeneChips (Affymetrix). Profiling of rods (from *wt-Gfp* retina) and cones (from *Nrl*$^{-/-}$-*Gfp* retina) at five distinct stages of development revealed comprehensive sets of differentially expressed genes that distinguish photoreceptors from other cell types (Akimoto et al., 2006). This expression analysis also uncovered the advantages of profiling purified cells, as many changes were missed when profiles of the entire retina were studied. Differential gene expression patterns at specific developmental stages provide basic data sets for higher-order analysis, such as clustering, to identify genes that behave similarly and those unique to a particular cell. However, construction of regulatory networks or pathways is a major challenge, requiring sophisticated statistical tools to bring out features such as key regulators (nodes or hubs), the hierarchies they sustain, and the genes they regulate.

Characteristics of biological networks and relevance to photoreceptors

The rationale for generating regulatory networks is to explain the spatial and temporal execution of specific cellular functions (Davidson et al., 2003). Networks consist of nodes representing molecules (such as protein, DNA, RNA and metabolites) and edges that explain the association between nodes. Networks offer a quantifiable description based on factors such as degree or connectivity between hubs, degree distribution, path length, and clustering coefficient between the various elements (Barabasi and Oltvai, 2004; Blais and Dynlacht, 2005). A majority of biological networks are scale-free and, unlike random networks, are nonuniform, having few highly connected hubs and many nodes that have only a few links (Barabasi and Albert, 1999). Many networks also display the "small world" property with high clustering but small characteristic path lengths between two nodes (Watts and Strogatz, 1998). Transcriptional and posttranscription regulatory networks can describe many of the cellular

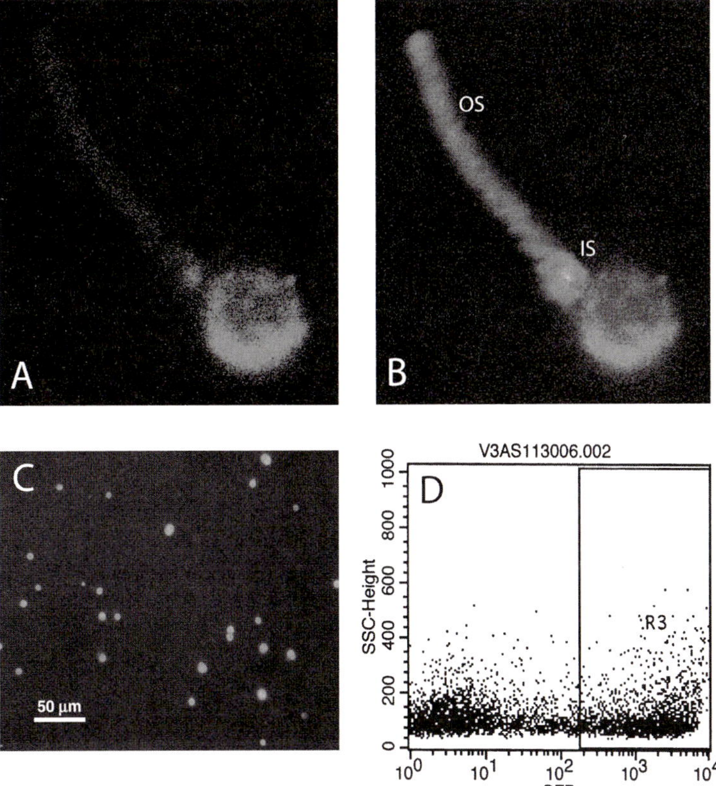

FIGURE 55.1 *A*, A single rod photoreceptor isolated from adult *wt-Gfp* mice shows the expression of GFP. *B*, The same cell shows staining for rhodpsin (red) in the outer segment (OS) and inner segment (IS) regions and bis-benzimide staining (blue) for the nucleus. *C*, Samples of dissociated cells are viewed under the microscope before (shown) and after flow sorting. *D*, Flow cytometry allows the GFP-positive population of cells to be gated (R3) and sorted separately. See color plate 63.

activities and are subdivided into physical and functional networks. Although physical networks are represented by interactions such as protein-protein/DNA/RNA or RNA-RNA, the functional networks represent the outcome of these interactions, such as regulation of gene expression or signaling pathways (Walhout, 2006). Analysis of high-throughput yeast two-hybrid data has revealed about 2,800 interactions among 8,100 human proteins tested, discovering more than 300 new connections to more than 100 disease-associated proteins (Rual et al., 2005). Alterations in transcriptome and proteomic signatures in metastatic and clinically localized prostate cancer, along with the concordance between the protein and transcript levels, were able to predict clinical outcomes in prostate cancer and other solid tumors (Varambally et al., 2005). Though biological network assemblies are still in their infancy, numerous recent studies represent important steps toward understanding complex physiological processes.

At this stage, it is not conceivable to decipher the single master network that would describe all the transcribed genes, expressed proteins, and protein-protein interactions in the entire retina (or even in rod and cone photoreceptors) at a single specific developmental stage. Hence, our goal is to establish gene regulatory networks in rod photoreceptors under normal and disease conditions. This information can then be integrated into protein expression and interaction networks. These subnetworks are not independent; instead, they link with each other to form more complex patterns. Hence, the biological process can be visualized as the highly regulated and progressive generation of subnetworks that combine together to describe the unique properties of a specific cell type during differentiation or disease (Blais and Dynlacht, 2005; Fraser and Marcotte, 2004).

Hierarchy in regulatory networks underlying photoreceptor development

A key question pertaining to photoreceptor development is how NRL expression in postmitotic photoreceptor precursors initiates the cascade of molecular events that suppress the cone-specific differentiation pathway and establish rod lineage and function. In many cases TFs form key hubs of a regulatory network and display a hierarchical organization because they regulate the expression of one or more genes. Extensive pyramid-shaped hierarchical structures have been described in the regulatory networks of *E. coli* and *S. cerevisiae*, with most of the transcription factors occupying the lower stratum and only a few master transcription factors occupying the top echelon (Yu and Gerstein, 2006). A similar hierarchical structure was identified in *C. elegans*, where three or more layers of transcriptional control existed (Deplancke et al., 2006). Establishing such hierarchies in the regulatory network of rod development would require integration of large gene expression data sets, obtained from as many stages of differentiation as possible (from birth to maturation). It would also be necessary to perform comprehensive gene profiling of purified rods after altering the function (e.g., by RNAi, transgenics, or knockout) of one or more key NRL-interacting proteins (such as CRX) and of NRL's downstream targets (such as NR2E3). This can be easily accomplished by breeding the *wt-Gfp* mice with various mutant strains (figure 55.2).

To dissect the role of NRL and other transcriptional regulators (such as NR2E3 and CRX) in photoreceptor differentiation, we have also generated a number of transgenic mouse lines on wild-type (wt) or *Nrl*$^{-/-}$ background (Yoshida et al., 2004; Cheng et al., 2006; Oh et al., 2007). We are now producing gene profiles of FACS-purified rods with specific genetic mutation or transgenes and have begun constructing cluster networks. We have developed methods using transitive coexpression analysis to tightly cluster functionally related genes by simultaneously including their biological and statistical importance, even when their expression profiles are dissimilar (Zhu et al., 2005). These clusters would form initial components in constructing networks that could explain the role of transcription factors and signaling molecules in controlling rod differentiation.

Mouse models of retinal degenerative disease and pathways of photoreceptor cell death

Mouse models of RDs provide candidate genes for human retinopathies, insights into the mechanisms of disease pathogenesis, and comprehensive evaluation of treatment techniques. Careful ocular phenotyping of naturally occurring inbred strains of mice have already identified at least 35 mutants that exhibit different types of RD (Rattner and Nathans, 1999; Frederick et al., 2000; Bessant et al., 2001; Chang et al., 2002; Pacione et al., 2003). Several of the *rd* strains (e.g., *rd1*, *rd2* [*rds*], *rd3*, *rd7*, *rd16*) have led to the discovery of *Pde6b*, *Prph2*, *Rd3*, *Nr2e3*, and *Cep290/Nphp6*, respectively, as genes involved in photoreceptor biology (Travis et al., 1989; Bowes et al., 1990; Akhmedov et al., 2000; Chang et al., 2006; Friedman et al., 2006); their corresponding homologues in humans have similar biological functions and are mutated in retinopathies (McLaughlin et al., 1993; Travis and Hepler, 1993; Haider et al., 2000; Wright et al., 2004; den Hollander et al., 2006; Friedman et al., 2006; Sayer et al., 2006). Numerous transgenic and knockout mouse models have also been generated in various laboratories to investigate the physiological function of respective genes and associated disease mechanisms (Humphries et al., 1997; Redmond et al., 1998; Furukawa et al. 1999; Hong et al., 2000; Mears et al., 2001; Zhao et al., 2003; Cheng et al., 2006; Lee et al., 2006).

With a goal of developing knowledge-based treatments and therapies, we proposed a comprehensive approach to

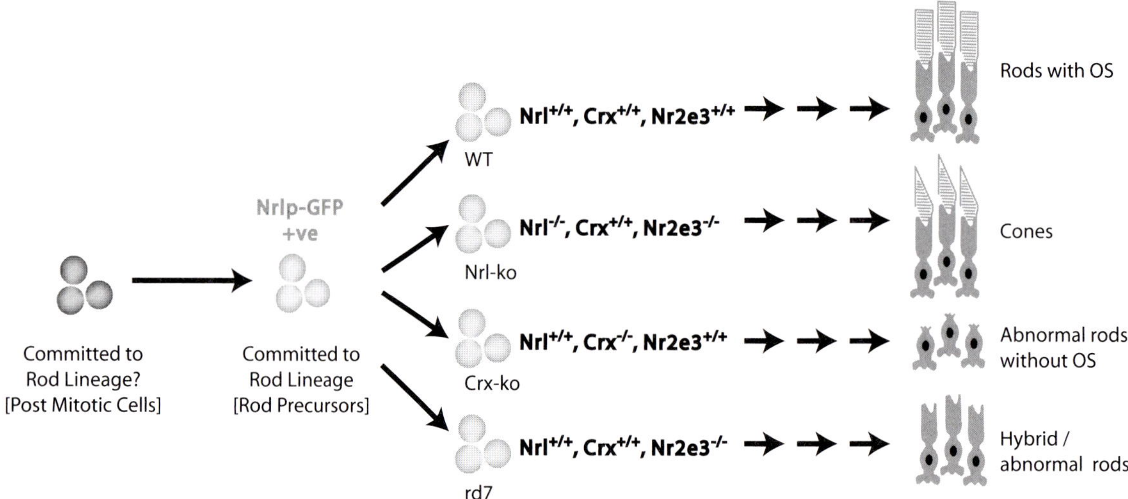

FIGURE 55.2 Role of regulatory genes (NRL, CRX, and NR2E3) in the network(s) leading to rod and/or cone differentiation can be studied by loss of their function in mice. Breeding mutant mice with the *wt-Gfp* mice can provide GFP-tagged rods that can be isolated for gene profiling.

examine commonalities in pathways of photoreceptor cell death caused by mutations in different mutant genes (Yu et al., 2004) (figure 55.3). Though multiple, distinct mutations in more than 100 genes result in RD, it is believed that apoptosis is the final step in photoreceptor cell death (Portera-Cailliau et al., 1994; Wong, 1995; Travis, 1998). Thus, it is intuitive to hypothesize that diverse genetic defects eventually converge at a few specific signaling pathways that finally induce apoptosis. The failure to prevent degeneration by inhibition of certain apoptotic pathways (Doonan et al., 2005) indicates that it might either be too late to rescue a cell if apoptotic pathways are set in motion or all apoptotic pathways may need to be simultaneously blocked. We reasoned that delineation of early steps in the cell death pathway induced by distinct genetic mutations would identify common pre-apoptotic signaling (PAS) molecules (see figure 55.3). These molecules can serve as better targets for drug discovery, as photoreceptors may not yet be committed to apoptosis. In addition, PAS-targeted drugs may benefit a larger group of affected RD individuals.

Given that photoreceptor degeneration in most *rd* mutant mice (akin to affected individuals) manifests over a relatively long time frame, an adaptive cellular response should result in altered gene expression profiles as disease progresses. We therefore propose that the temporal profiling of gene expression during disease progression would reveal how a specific genetic mutation causes the death of photoreceptors. Meta-analysis of temporal gene profiles from multiple mouse mutants should then uncover common PAS molecules.

Degeneration network(s) by expression profiling of photoreceptors from rd *mice*

The key question is how inherited mutation(s) in a large number of genes cause rod (or cone) dysfunction, eventually leading to cell death. We can analyze this in the context of networks. A scale-free network has the ability to withstand errors because of the redundancy of the wiring and the robustness of various modules that function in a cell (Hartwell et al., 1999; Albert et al., 2000). However, the capacity for error tolerance also means that the system is prone to attacks (Albert et al., 2000). It is not difficult to imagine the breakdown of cellular functions due to a deleterious mutation in a critical component. Usually, the more connected a gene or protein is in a regulatory network, the more essential it is for the survival and function of the cell (Jeong et al., 2001; Deplancke et al., 2006). Thus, if and when regulatory networks of a cell, such as a rod photoreceptor, are delineated, one might be able to trace the problem and the effects that a mutation has on the module or the hub or the entire network, leading to RD. We need not simulate the mutation leading to the network breakdown, as numerous RD mouse models are already available. Our goals are therefore to produce gene profiles of rod photoreceptors isolated from various mouse models of RD and to compare these with the gene patterns or networks of normal rods. To accomplish this, we are breeding *rd* mouse strains with *wt-Gfp* mice to obtain homozygous *rd* mutants that have the GFP transgene, permitting FACS purification of mutant rod

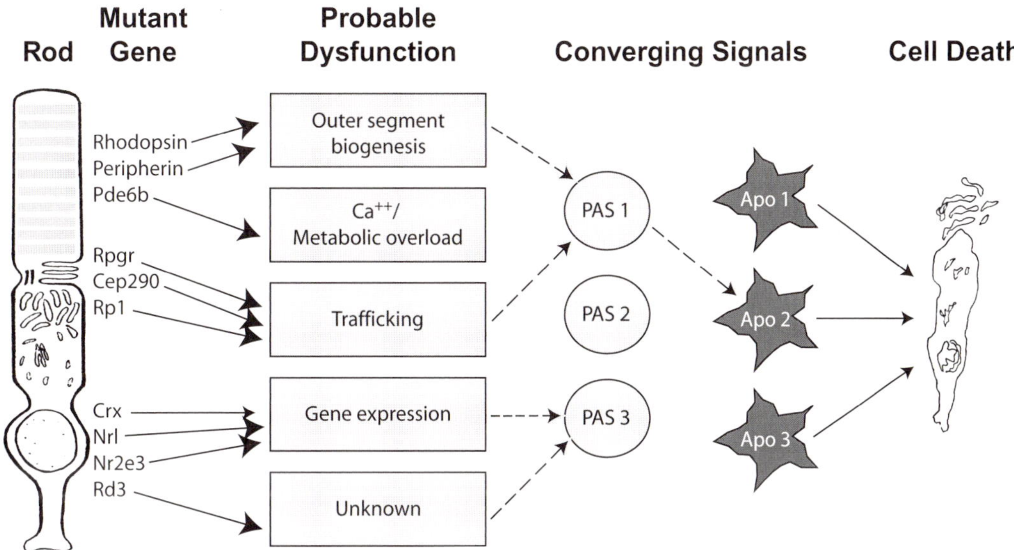

Figure 55.3 Apoptosis is the final step in photoreceptor cell death, even though RDs are caused by defects in different genes. We hypothesize that signaling pathways generated by different gene mutations (as indicated) will eventually converge on a few pre-apoptotic signals (PAS 1, 2, 3, . . .), which then induce apoptotic (Apo 1, 2, 3, . . .) pathways, resulting in photoreceptor cell death. Genetic mutations that affect similar pathways may induce the same PAS, which can be targeted for drug therapy (Modified from Yu et al., 2004.)

photoreceptors. In the case of autosomal recessive mutations, a relevant mouse strain that is homozygous for both the Nrlp-EGFP transgene and the *rd* mutant gene can be obtained by the F_3 generation. In fact, a single copy of a GFP transgene is sufficient for rod enrichment by FACS.

Gene profiling of rods carrying a specific gene mutation during various stages of disease progression will generate extensive data sets that can be used for constructing the pathways or networks leading to photoreceptor cell death. As indicated in figure 55.3, we compare temporal rod gene expression profiles from various *rd* mutants, with a goal of elucidating commonalities in cell death pathways or cross-talk in signaling networks. One can speculate that pathways from mutant genes that have similar functions may share more commonalities. Likewise, mice with early-onset RD may share more common signaling molecules than *rd* mice exhibiting slower photoreceptor disease. Identification of PAS molecules can lead to novel discovery targets, which could be modulated by drugs to prevent network errors and to alter the course of photoreceptor dysfunction or death. In most RDs, it is the rods that degenerate first, and the degeneration of cones is due to a by-stander effect (Ripps, 2002); thus, many laboratories have attempted to preserve cone function (Mohand et al., 2000; Leveillard et al., 2004). PAS-targeted drugs, therefore, may contribute to cone survival and vision.

Future considerations

In the field of ocular development and pathology, numerous investigators have amassed impressive data on gene expression patterns under normal and disease (mutant) conditions (Blackshaw et al., 2001; Sharon et al., 2002; Yoshida et al., 2002, 2004; Chowers et al., 2003; Farkas et al., 2004; Hackam et al., 2004; Akimoto et al., 2006; Cheng et al., 2006). However, progress in network construction has been relatively slow. A major problem is the lack of coordinated efforts with standard criteria and uniform gene profiling platforms that allow meta-analysis of large data sets obtained by different investigators. Even though we have focused on generating gene networks for rod differentiation and degeneration by exploiting our research on NRL, this approach can be applied to other cell types and tissues and to other disease paradigms. Studies of retinal proteome (Ethen et al., 2006) and protein interactions will undoubtedly complement the gene profiling data sets. It is our hope that collaborative studies will be undertaken by different laboratories using uniform standard profiling platforms to create integrative networks for better understanding of retinal (or photoreceptor) development, function, and disease.

ACKNOWLEDGMENTS Work was supported by grants from the National Institutes of Health (EY011115, EY007961, and EY007003), the Foundation for Fighting Blindness, Research to Prevent Blindness, and the Elmer and Sylvia Sramek Foundation. We thank Andy Goldberg and the members of the Swaroop laboratory, particularly Matthew Brooks, Hong Cheng, Radu Cojocaru, James Friedman, Hemant Khanna, Ritu Khanna, and Edwin Oh, for comments and discussions.

REFERENCES

Acland, G. M., Aguirre, G. D., Ray, J., Zhang, Q., Aleman, T. S., Cideciyan, A. V., Pearce-Kelling, S. E., Anand, V., Zeng, Y., et al. (2001). Gene therapy restores vision in a canine model of childhood blindness. *Nat. Genet.* 28:92–95.

Akhmedov, N. B., Piriev, N. I., Chang, B., Rapoport, A. L., Hawes, N. L., Nishina, P. M., Nusinowitz, S., Heckenlively, J. R., Roderick, T. H., et al. (2000). A deletion in a photoreceptor-specific nuclear receptor mRNA causes retinal degeneration in the rd7 mouse. *Proc. Natl. Acad. Sci. U.S.A.* 97:5551–5556.

Akimoto, M., Cheng, H., Zhu, D., Brzezinski, J. A., Khanna, R., Filippova, E., Oh, E. C., Jing, Y., Linares, J. L., et al. (2006). Targeting of GFP to newborn rods by Nrl promoter and temporal expression profiling of flow-sorted photoreceptors. *Proc. Natl. Acad. Sci. U.S.A.* 103:3890–3895.

Albert, R., Jeong, H., and Barabasi, A. L. (2000). Error and attack tolerance of complex networks. *Nature* 406:378–382.

Barabasi, A. L., and Albert, R. (1999). Emergence of scaling in random networks. *Science* 286:509–512.

Barabasi, A. L., and Oltvai, Z. N. (2004). Network biology: Understanding the cell's functional organization. *Nat. Rev. Genet.* 5:101–113.

Bessant, D. A., Ali, R. R., and Bhattacharya, S. S. (2001). Molecular genetics and prospects for therapy of the inherited retinal dystrophies. *Curr. Opin. Genet. Dev.* 11:307–316.

Blackshaw, S., Fraioli, R. E., Furukawa, T., and Cepko, C. L. (2001). Comprehensive analysis of photoreceptor gene expression and the identification of candidate retinal disease genes. *Cell* 107:579–589.

Blais, A., and Dynlacht, B. D. (2005). Constructing transcriptional regulatory networks. *Genes Dev.* 19:1499–1511.

Bowes, C., Li, T., Danciger, M., Baxter, L. C., Applebury, M. L., and Farber, D. B. (1990). Retinal degeneration in the rd mouse is caused by a defect in the beta subunit of rod cGMP-phosphodiesterase. *Nature* 347:677–680.

Bressler, N. M., Bressler, S. B., Congdon, N. G., Ferris, F. L., III, Friedman, D. S., Klein, R., Lindblad, A. S., Milton, R. C. and Seddon, J. M. (2003). Potential public health impact of Age-Related Eye Disease Study results: AREDS Report No. 11. *Arch. Ophthalmol.* 121:1621–1624.

Chang, B., Hawes, N. L., Hurd, R. E., Davisson, M. T., Nusinowitz, S., and Heckenlively, J. R. (2002). Retinal degeneration mutants in the mouse. *Vision Res.* 42:517–525.

Chang, B., Khanna, H., Hawes, N., Jimeno, D., He, S., Lillo, C., Parapuram, S. K., Cheng, H., Scott, A., et al. (2006). In-frame deletion in a novel centrosomal/ciliary protein CEP290/NPHP6 perturbs its interaction with RPGR and results in early-onset retinal degeneration in the rd16 mouse. *Hum. Mol. Genet.* 15: 1847–1857.

Cheng, H., Aleman, T. S., Cideciyan, A. V., Khanna, R., Jacobson, S. G., and Swaroop, A. (2006). In vivo function of the orphan nuclear receptor NR2E3 in establishing photoreceptor identity during mammalian retinal development. *Hum. Mol. Genet.* 15:2588–2602.

Chowers, I., Liu, D., Farkas, R. H., Gunatilaka, T. L., Hackam, A. S., Bernstein, S. L., Campochiaro, P. A., Parmigiani, G., and Zack, D. J. (2003). Gene expression variation in the adult human retina. *Hum. Mol. Genet.* 12:2881–2893.

Curcio, C. A., Medeiros, N. E., and Millican, C. L. (1996). Photoreceptor loss in age-related macular degeneration. *Invest. Ophthalmol. Vis. Sci.* 37:1236–1249.

Daniele, L. L., Lillo, C., Lyubarsky, A. L., Nikonov, S. S., Philp, N., Mears, A. J., Swaroop, A., Williams, D. S., and Pugh, E. N., Jr. (2005). Cone-like morphological, molecular, and electrophysiological features of the photoreceptors of the Nrl knockout mouse. *Invest. Ophthalmol. Vis. Sci.* 46:2156–2167.

Davidson, E. H., McClay, D. R., and Hood, L. (2003). Regulatory gene networks and the properties of the developmental process. *Proc. Natl. Acad. Sci. U.S.A.* 100:1475–1480.

Delyfer, M. N., Leveillard, T., Mohand-Said, S., Hicks, D., Picaud, S., and Sahel, J. A. (2004). Inherited retinal degenerations: Therapeutic prospects. *Biol. Cell* 96:261–269.

den Hollander, A. I., Koenekoop, R. K., Yzer, S., Lopez, I., Arends, M. L., Voesenek, K. E., Zonneveld, M. N., Strom, T. M., Meitinger, T., et al. (2006). Mutations in the CEP290 (NPHP6) gene are a frequent cause of Leber congenital amaurosis. *Am. J. Hum. Genet.* 79:556–561.

Deplancke, B., Mukhopadhyay, A., Ao, W., Elewa, A. M., Grove, C. A., Martinez, N. J., Sequerra, R., Doucette-Stamm, L., Reece-Hoyes, J. S., et al. (2006). A gene-centered *C. elegans* protein-DNA interaction network. *Cell* 125:1193–1205.

Diaz, E., Yang, Y. H., Ferreira, T., Loh, K. C., Okazaki, Y., Hayashizaki, Y., Tessier-Lavigne, M., Speed, T. P., and Ngai, J. (2003). Analysis of gene expression in the developing mouse retina. *Proc. Natl. Acad. Sci. U.S.A.* 100:5491–5496.

Dinculescu, A., Glushakova, L., Min, S. H., and Hauswirth, W. W. (2005). Adeno-associated virus-vectored gene therapy for retinal disease. *Hum. Gene Ther.* 16:649–663.

Doonan, F., Donovan, M., and Cotter, T. G. (2005). Activation of multiple pathways during photoreceptor apoptosis in the rd mouse. *Invest. Ophthalmol. Vis. Sci.* 46:3530–3538.

Duggan, D. J., Bittner, M., Chen, Y., Meltzer, P., and Trent, J. M. (1999). Expression profiling using cDNA microarrays. *Nat. Genet.* 21:10–14.

Ethen, C. M., Reilly, C., Feng, X., Olsen, T. W., and Ferrington, D. A. (2006). The proteome of central and peripheral retina with progression of age-related macular degeneration. *Invest. Ophthalmol. Vis. Sci.* 47:2280–2890.

Faktorovich, E. G., Steinberg, R. H., Yasumura, D., Matthes, M. T., and LaVail, M. M. (1990). Photoreceptor degeneration in inherited retinal dystrophy delayed by basic fibroblast growth factor. *Nature* 347:83–86.

Farjo, R., Yu, J., Othman, M. I., Yoshida, S., Sheth, S., Glaser, T., Baehr, W., and Swaroop, A. (2002). Mouse eye gene microarrays for investigating ocular development and disease. *Vision Res.* 42:463–470.

Farkas, R. H., Qian, J., Goldberg, J. L., Quigley, H. A., and Zack, D. J. (2004). Gene expression profiling of purified rat retinal ganglion cells. *Invest. Ophthalmol. Vis. Sci.* 45:2503–2513.

Fraser, A. G., and Marcotte, E. M. (2004). Development through the eyes of functional genomics. *Curr. Opin. Genet. Dev.* 14:336–342.

Frasson, M., Picaud, S., Leveillard, T., Simonutti, M., Mohand-Said, S., Dreyfus, H., Hicks, D., and Sabel, J. (1999). Glial cell line-derived neurotrophic factor induces histologic and functional protection of rod photoreceptors in the rd/rd mouse. *Invest. Ophthalmol. Vis. Sci.* 40:2724–2734.

Frederick, J., Bronson, J. D., and Baehr, W. (2000). Animal models of inherited retinal diseases. *Methods Enzymol.* 316: 515–526.

Friedman, J. S., Chang, B., Kannabiran, C., Chakarova, C., Singh, H. P., Jalali, S., Hawes, N. L., Branham, K., Othman, M., et al. (2006). Premature truncation of a novel protein, RD3, exhibiting subnuclear localization is associated with retinal degeneration. *Am. J. Hum. Genet.* 79:1059–1070.

Furukawa, T., Morrow, E. M., Li, T., Davis, F. C., and Cepko, C. L. (1999). Retinopathy and attenuated circadian entrainment in Crx-deficient mice. *Nat. Genet.* 23:466–470.

Gal, A., Apfelstedt-Sylla, E., Janecke, A. R., and Zrenner, E. (1997). Rhodopsin mutations in inherited retinal dystrophies and dysfunctions. *Prog. Ret. Eye Res.* 16:51–79.

Gouras, P., Du, J., Kjeldbye, H., Yamamoto, S., and Zack, D. J. (1994). Long-term photoreceptor transplants in dystrophic and normal mouse retina. *Invest. Ophthalmol. Vis. Sci.* 35:3145–3153.

Hackam, A. S., Strom, R., Liu, D., Qian, J., Wang, C., Otteson, D., Gunatilaka, T., Farkas, R. H., Chowers, I., et al. (2004). Identification of gene expression changes associated with the progression of retinal degeneration in the rd1 mouse. *Invest. Ophthalmol. Vis. Sci.* 45:2929–2942.

Haider, N. B., Jacobson, S. G., Cideciyan, A. V., Swiderski, R., Streb, L. M., Searby, C., Beck, G., Hockey, R., Hanna, D. B., et al. (2000). Mutation of a nuclear receptor gene, NR2E3, causes enhanced S cone syndrome, a disorder of retinal cell fate. *Nat. Genet.* 24:127–131.

Hartong, D. T., Berson, E. L., and Dryja, T. P. (2006). Retinitis pigmentosa. *Lancet* 368:1795–1809.

Hartwell, L. H., Hopfield, J. J., Leibler, S., and Murray, A. W. (1999). From molecular to modular cell biology. *Nature* 402: C47–C52.

Hauswirth, W. W., and Lewin, A. S. (2000). Ribozyme uses in retinal gene therapy. *Prog. Retin. Eye Res.* 19:689–6710.

Hong, D. H., Pawlyk, B. S., Shang, J., Sandberg, M. A., Berson, E. L., and Li, T. (2000). A retinitis pigmentosa GTPase regulator (RPGR)-deficient mouse model for X-linked retinitis pigmentosa (RP3). *Proc. Natl. Acad. Sci. U.S.A.* 97:3649–3954.

Humayun, M. S., Weiland, J. D., Fujii, G. Y., Greenberg, R., Williamson, R., Little, J., Mech, B., Cimmarusti, V., Van Boemel, G., et al. (2003). Visual perception in a blind subject with a chronic microelectronic retinal prosthesis. *Vision Res.* 43:2573–2581.

Humphries, M. M., Rancourt, D., Farrar, G. J., Kenna, P., Hazel, M., Bush, R. A., Sieving, P. A., Sheils, D. M., McNally, N., et al. (1997). Retinopathy induced in mice by targeted disruption of the rhodopsin gene. *Nat. Genet.* 15:216–219.

Jeong, H., Mason, S. P., Barabasi, A. L., and Oltvai, Z. N. (2001). Lethality and centrality in protein networks. *Nature* 411: 41–42.

Kalloniatis, M., and Fletcher, E. L. (2004). Retinitis pigmentosa: Understanding the clinical presentation, mechanisms and treatment options. *Clin. Exp. Optom.* 87:65–80.

Lee, E. S., Burnside, B., and Flannery, J. G. (2006). Characterization of peripherin/rds and rom-1 transport in rod photoreceptors of transgenic and knockout animals. *Invest. Ophthalmol. Vis. Sci.* 47:2150–2160.

Leveillard, T., Mohand-Said, S., Lorentz, O., Hicks, D., Fintz, A. C., Clerin, E., Simonutti, M., Forster, V., Cavusoglu, N., et al. (2004). Identification and characterization of rod-derived cone viability factor. *Nat. Genet.* 36:755–759.

Livesey, F. J., Furukawa, T., Steffen, M. A., Church, G. M., and Cepko, C. L. (2000). Microarray analysis of the transcriptional network controlled by the photoreceptor homeobox gene Crx. *Curr. Biol.* 10:301–310.

Lund, R. D., Kwan, A. S., Keegan, D. J., Sauve, Y., Coffey, P. J., and Lawrence, J. M. (2001). Cell transplantation as a treatment for retinal disease. *Prog. Retin. Eye Res.* 20:415–449.

MacLaren, R. E., Pearson, R. A., MacNeil, A., Douglas, R. H., Salt, T. E., Akimoto, M., Swaroop, A., Sowden, J. C., and Ali, R. R. (2006). Retinal repair by transplantation of photoreceptor precursors. *Nature* 444:203–207.

Masland, R. H. (2001). The fundamental plan of the retina. *Nat. Neurosci.* 4:877–886.

McLaughlin, M. E., Sandberg, M. A., Berson, E. L., and Dryja, T. P. (1993). Recessive mutations in the gene encoding the beta-subunit of rod phosphodiesterase in patients with retinitis pigmentosa. *Nat. Genet.* 4:130–134.

Mears, A. J., Kondo, M., Swain, P. K., Takada, Y., Bush, R. A., Saunders, T. L., Sieving, P. A., and Swaroop, A. (2001). Nrl is required for rod photoreceptor development. *Nat. Genet.* 29: 447–452.

Mohand-Said, S., Hicks, D., Dreyfus, H., and Sahel, J. A. (2000). Selective transplantation of rods delays cone loss in a retinitis pigmentosa model. *Arch. Ophthalmol.* 118:807–811.

Mori, K., Gehlbach, P., Yamamoto, S., Duh, E., Zack, D. J., Li, Q., Berns, K. I., Raisler, B. J., Hauswirth, W. W., et al. (2002). AAV-mediated gene transfer of pigment epithelium-derived factor inhibits choroidal neovascularization. *Invest. Ophthalmol. Vis. Sci.* 43:1994–2000.

Mu, X., Zhao, S., Pershad, R., Hsieh, T. F., Scarpa, A., Wang, S. W., White, R. A., Beremand, P. D., Thomas, T. L., et al. (2001). Gene expression in the developing mouse retina by EST sequencing and microarray analysis. *Nucleic Acids Res.* 29: 4983–4993.

Oh, E.C.T., Khan, N., Novelli, E., Khanna, H., Strettoi, E., and Swaroop, A. (2007). Transformation of cone precursors to functional rod photoreceptors by bZIP transcription factor NRL. *Proc. Natl. Acad. Sci. U.S.A.* 104:1679–1684.

Pacione, L. R., Szego, M. J., Ikeda, S., Nishina, P. M., and McInnes, R. R. (2003). Progress toward understanding the genetic and biochemical mechanisms of inherited photoreceptor degenerations. *Annu. Rev. Neurosci.* 26:657–700.

Portera-Cailliau, C., Sung, C. H., Nathans, J., and Adler, R. (1994). Apoptotic photoreceptor cell death in mouse models of retinitis pigmentosa. *Proc. Natl. Acad. Sci. U.S.A.* 91:974–978.

Rattner, A., Sun, H., and Nathans, J. (1999). Molecular genetics of human retinal disease. *Annu. Rev. Genet.* 33:89–131.

Redmond, T. M., Yu, S., Lee, E., Bok, D., Hamasaki, D., Chen, N., Goletz, P., Ma, J. X., Crouch, R. K., et al. (1998). Rpe65 is necessary for production of 11-cis-vitamin A in the retinal visual cycle. *Nat. Genet.* 20:344–351.

Ripps, H. (2002). Cell death in retinitis pigmentosa: Gap junctions and the "bystander" effect. *Exp. Eye Res.* 74:327–336.

Rizzo, J. F., III, Goldbaum, S., Shahin, M., Denison, T. J., and Wyatt, J. (2004). In vivo electrical stimulation of rabbit retina with a microfabricated array: Strategies to maximize responses for prospective assessment of stimulus efficacy and biocompatibility. *Restor. Neurol. Neurosci.* 22:429–443.

Rual, J. F., Venkatesan, K., Hao, T., Hirozane-Kishikawa, T., Dricot, A., Li, N., Berriz, G. F., Gibbons, F. D., Dreze, M., et al. (2005). Towards a proteome-scale map of the human protein-protein interaction network. *Nature* 437:1173–1178.

Sayer, J. A., Otto, E. A., O'Toole, J. F., Nurnberg, G., Kennedy, M. A., Becker, C., Hennies, H. C., Helou, J., Attanasio, M., et al. (2006). The centrosomal protein nephrocystin-6 is mutated in Joubert syndrome and activates transcription factor ATF4. *Nat. Genet.* 38:674–681.

Sharon, D., Blackshaw, S., Cepko, C. L., and Dryja, T. P. (2002). Profile of the genes expressed in the human peripheral retina, macula, and retinal pigment epithelium determined through serial analysis of gene expression (SAGE). *Proc. Natl. Acad. Sci. U.S.A.* 99:315–320.

Swain, P. K., Hicks, D., Mears, A. J., Apel, I. J., Smith, J. E., John, S. K., Hendrickson, A., Milam, A. H., and Swaroop, A. (2001). Multiple phosphorylated isoforms of NRL are expressed in rod photoreceptors. *J. Biol. Chem.* 276:36824–36830.

Swaroop, A., Xu, J. Z., Pawar, H., Jackson, A., Skolnick, C., and Agarwal, N. (1992). A conserved retina-specific gene encodes a basic motif/leucine zipper domain. *Proc. Natl. Acad. Sci. U.S.A.* 89:266–270.

Travis, G. H. (1998). Mechanisms of cell death in the inherited retinal degenerations. *Am. J. Hum. Genet.* 62:503–508.

Travis, G. H., Brennan, M. B., Danielson, P. E., Kozak, C. A., and Sutcliffe, J. G. (1989). Identification of a photoreceptor-specific mRNA encoded by the gene responsible for retinal degeneration slow (rds). *Nature* 338:70–73.

Travis, G. H., and Hepler, J. E. (1993). A medley of retinal dystrophies. *Nat. Genet.* 3:191–192.

Varambally, S., Yu, J., Laxman, B., Rhodes, D. R., Mehra, R., Tomlins, S. A., Shah, R. B., Chandran, U., Monzon, F. A., et al. (2005). Integrative genomic and proteomic analysis of prostate cancer reveals signatures of metastatic progression. *Cancer Cell* 8:393–406.

Walhout, A. J. (2006). Unraveling transcription regulatory networks by protein-DNA and protein-protein interaction mapping. *Genome Res.* 16:1445–1454.

Watts, D. J., and Strogatz, S. H. (1998). Collective dynamics of "small-world" networks. *Nature* 393:440–442.

Weleber, R. G. (2005). Inherited and orphan retinal diseases: Phenotypes, genotypes, and probable treatment groups. *Retina* 25:S4–S7.

Wong, F. (1995). Photoreceptor apoptosis in animal models: Implications for retinitis pigmentosa research. *Arch. Ophthalmol.* 113: 1245–1247.

Wright, A. F., Reddick, A. C., Schwartz, S. B., Ferguson, J. S., Aleman, T. S., Kellner, U., Jurklies, B., Schuster, A., Zrenner, E., et al. (2004). Mutation analysis of NR2E3 and NRL genes in enhanced S cone syndrome. *Hum. Mutat.* 24: 439.

Yoshida, S., Mears, A. J., Friedman, J. S., Carter, T., He, S., Oh, E., Jing, Y., Farjo, R., Fleury, G. A., et al. (2004). Expression profiling of the developing and mature $Nrl^{-/-}$ mouse retina: Identification of retinal disease candidates and transcriptional regulatory targets of Nrl. *Hum. Mol. Genet.* 13:1487–1503.

Yoshida, S., Yashar, B. M., Hiriyanna, S., and Swaroop, A. (2002). Microarray analysis of gene expression in the aging human retina. *Invest. Ophthalmol. Vis. Sci.* 43:2554–2560.

Yu, H., and Gerstein, M. (2006). Genomic analysis of the hierarchical structure of regulatory networks. *Proc. Natl. Acad. Sci. U.S.A.* 103:14724–14731.

Yu, J., Mears, A. J., Yoshida, S., Farjo, R., Carter, T. A., Ghosh, D., Hero, A., Barlow, C., and Swaroop, A. (2004). From disease genes to cellular pathways: A progress report. *Novartis Found. Symp.* 255:147–160 [discussion 160–164, 177–178].

Zareparsi, S., Hero, A., Zack, D. J., Williams, R. W., and Swaroop, A. (2004). Seeing the unseen: Microarray-based gene expression profiling in vision. *Invest. Ophthalmol. Vis. Sci.* 45:2457–2562.

Zhao, Y., Hong, D. H., Pawlyk, B., Yue, G., Adamian, M., Grynberg, M., Godzik, A., and Li, T. (2003). The retinitis pigmentosa GTPase regulator (RPGR)-interacting protein: Subserving RPGR function and participating in disk morphogenesis. *Proc. Natl. Acad. Sci. U.S.A.* 100:3965–3970.

Zhu, D., Hero, A. O., Cheng, H., Khanna, R., and Swaroop, A. (2005). Network constrained clustering for gene microarray data. *Bioinformatics* 21:4014–4020.

Zrenner, E. (2002). Will retinal implants restore vision? *Science* 295:1022–1025.

56 Retinal Vascular and Retinal Pigment Epithelium Gene Expression

MICHAEL I. DORRELL AND MARTIN FRIEDLANDER

The highly ordered, compact structure of the mammalian retina is well suited for the unimpeded transmission of light and its subsequent transduction into electrical signals that will be transformed into images in the visual cortex of the brain. The processing and orderly transmission of these signals from the posteriorly located photoreceptors through multiple intraretinal synapses with a variety of other neuronal cell types is critically dependent on maintenance of this highly ordered retinal structure. For reviews of neural retinal structure and synaptic formations, see Lukasiewicz (2005) and Mumm et al. (2005). This orderly development of the retinal structure is dependent on early cell guidance mechanisms to mediate appropriate cell-cell relationships, followed by long-term mechanisms that maintain retinal homeostasis and ensure that the striated retinal plexuses and neuronal synapses are not disrupted. Both the retinal pigment epithelium (RPE) and the retinal vasculature play important roles in maintaining retinal homeostasis and ultimately retinal function. Anatomical or physiological abnormalities of either system can lead to retinal dysfunction and loss of vision.

To better understand how structural and functional homeostasis is established and maintained by various cellular components of the retina, numerous studies have focused on the RPE and retinal vasculature. A discussion of all the experiments defining individual gene expression and function in the RPE or retinal vasculature is well beyond the scope of this chapter. Thus, we mainly discuss large-scale gene expression analyses, focusing specifically on challenges faced in obtaining interpretable RPE and retinal vascular gene expression data, strategies to overcome these challenges, and future applications of RPE and retinal vascular gene expression studies.

The RPE is a pigmented monolayer of polarized cells located just posterior to the photoreceptors, with many important retinal functions (figure 56.1). The RPE basolateral surface lies on Bruch's membrane and mediates selective transport of nutrients from the blood vessels of the choriocapillaris to the outer neural retina, as well as removal of water and waste products from the subretinal space to the blood. Tight junctions between the RPE cells allow the photoreceptor environment to remain separate from the fenestrated choriocapillaris while facilitating selective molecular transport between the two tissue beds, thus maintaining the outer blood-retinal barrier. The apical membranes of RPE cells form numerous long processes that partially envelop photoreceptor outer segments. This close interaction allows RPE cells to play a central supporting role for photoreceptor function by (1) regulating retinal (vitamin A) metabolism and distribution, a process required for the visual cycle and maintenance of photoreceptor excitability, and (2) phagocytosis of the photoreceptor outer segments that are shed daily, a process essential for photoreceptor survival (Futter, 2006). (For good reviews of RPE and visual function, see de Jong, 2006, and Strauss, 2005.) When RPE function is lost, retina function is affected dramatically. For example, mutations in RPE-specific genes are linked to numerous forms of retinal degeneration (Chong and Bird, 1999), and abnormalities in the RPE are associated with age-related macular degeneration (AMD; de Jong, 2006; Zarbin, 2004).

Appropriate development and function of the retinal vasculature are also critical for maintaining proper visual function. The very high metabolic activity of the retina demands a substantial blood supply to provide oxygen, nutritional elements, and removal of metabolic waste products. Equally important, it is now believed that paracrine support functions are provided by vascular endothelial cells (ECs) for retinal neuronal elements (Otani and Friedlander, 2005). During development, retinal vessels in the mouse retina form three vascular plexuses in a highly reproducible manner, leading to the formation of distinct vascular and avascular zones within the inner neural retina (see figure 56.1). This process is similar to retinal vascular development in humans during the third trimester in utero. The choriocapillaris forms posterior to the RPE monolayer and Bruch's membrane and supplies the vast majority of oxygen and nutrients to the retinal photoreceptors in the outer nuclear layer. Mechanisms of vascular guidance in the mouse retina

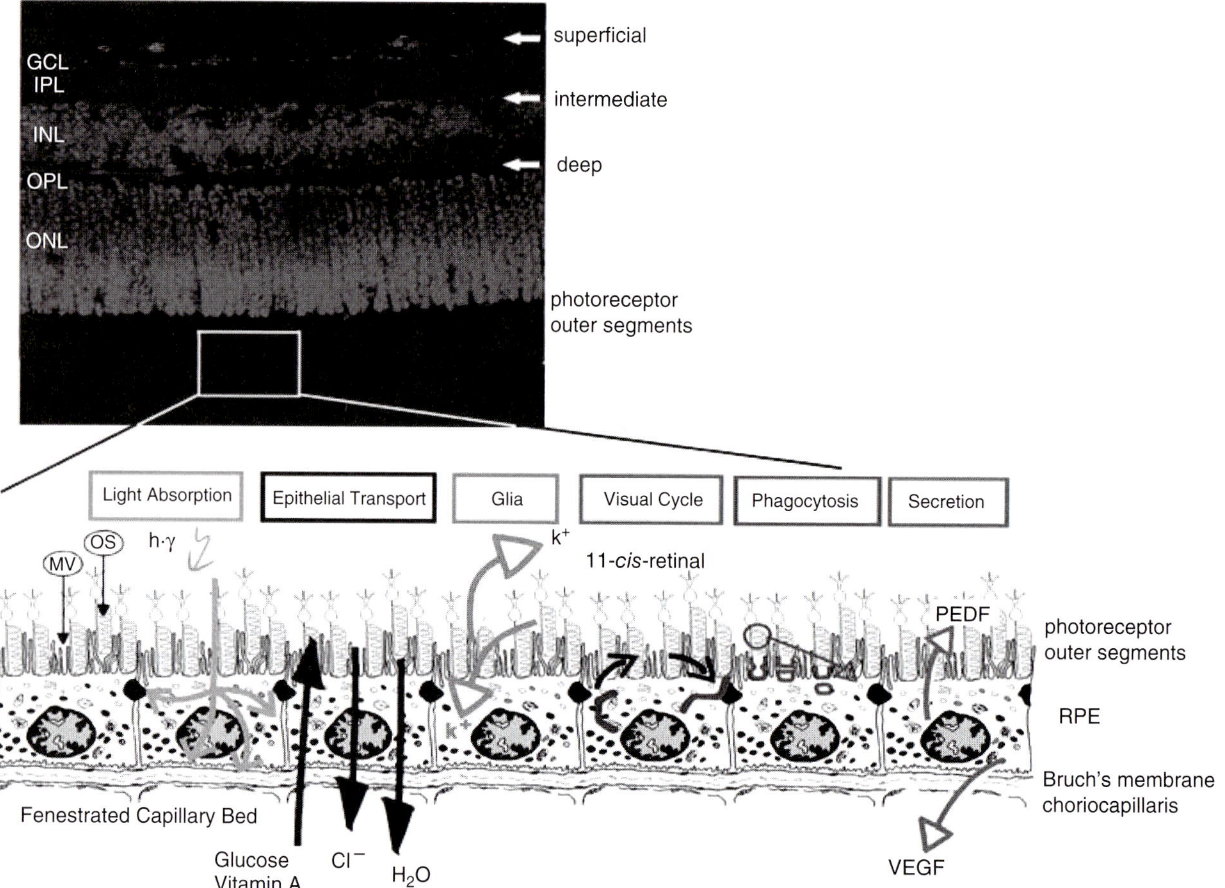

FIGURE 56.1 *Top*, The retina is a complex, striated tissue with highly organized neuronal layers. The inner retinal vasculature forms three distinct plexuses: The superficial plexus forms within the ganglion cell layer (GCL), the intermediate plexus forms at the inner edge of the inner nuclear layer (INL), and the deep plexus forms at the outer edge of the INL. *Bottom*, Posterior to the retina are the RPE, Bruch's membrane, and the choriocapillaris. The RPE performs many functions that are critical to retinal function. See color plate 64. (*Top*, From Dorrell and Friedlander, 2006. *Bottom*, From Strauss, 2005.)

have been extensively reviewed elsewhere (Dorrell and Friedlander, 2006). If any of the retinal or choroidal vascular layers fail to develop, the retina will lack adequate oxygen and nutrients, leading to cellular death and vision loss. Improper vascular organization or excessive neovascularization can also be quite detrimental to retinal function. For proof of the importance of maintaining a normal, appropriate retinal vasculature, one need only consider the vast majority of diseases that can cause a catastrophic loss of vision. Most of these diseases, which include AMD, diabetic retinopathy, retinopathy of prematurity, and others, have vascular components that contribute directly to pathological manifestation of the disease (Adamis et al., 1999; Eichler et al., 2004). Proper functioning of the RPE and vascular endothelium are critical to maintaining normal retinal function. Thus, analysis of gene expression in these cells should provide insight into how they facilitate normal retinal function and contribute to disease when they malfunction.

Methods of testing gene expression in the retina

Methods to study gene expression have improved vastly in the past decade, particularly with the advent of and subsequent improvements in microarray and SAGE technologies. Microarray gene chips now allow researchers to study the expression of thousands of different genes simultaneously. Commercial products such as Affymetrix gene arrays now offer comprehensive analysis of genome-wide expression in human and mouse, as well as many other species often used for experimental purposes (for more information on Affymetrix chips, see www.affymetrix.com). These arrays mediate non-hypothesis-driven analysis of the expression levels of multiple, if not all, genes rather than a specific subset of predescribed genes. However, both technical and biological variability need to be considered when analyzing microarray data. Technical variation is caused by differences arising from nonbiological, technical aspects of the experiment, such as differences in RNA preparation, RNA degradation, array labeling, irregularities in individual arrays, hybridization, washing, and image analysis. Biological variation results from natural variability within the biological system itself. These variables can arise from individual differences, litter effects, or other variables such as pathogen load or diet. Replication is essential to overcome these variables and to increase the likelihood of identifying true positives and reduce the incidence of false positives. In an optimal situation, technical and biological variability are tested separately by (1) testing the same RNA sample or RNA prepared from the same source, and applying to separate arrays (testing technical variability), and (2) testing RNA samples from separate individuals or sources (testing biological variability). Because of the cost of microarray experiments and limited sample availability, particularly when analyzing retinal material, extensive replicates may not be practical. In these instances, biological replications often suffice, since technical variability is innately accounted for within biological replicates; RNA must be prepared separately from each source and ultimately hybridized to separate chips. However, important information regarding the source of variability (i.e., is the variability due to technical problems or natural biological variability?) will be lost. It is also important to validate microarray results using more traditional techniques such as RT-PCR, in situ hybridization, and in vivo analysis of transgenic and knockout mice. In evaluating published reports on gene expression using large-scale array analysis, these major issues should be considered: (1) Were adequate numbers and controls used? (2) Were conclusions validated using other techniques of gene expression analysis? For further details on the use of microarrays for ocular gene expression analysis and important discussions about analyzing and validating results obtained using microarray analysis, see the review by Zareparsi et al. (2004) and chapter 55, this volume.

Another form of nonbiased, large-scale gene expression analysis known as serial analysis of gene expression (SAGE) was described in 1995 (Velculescu et al., 1995). SAGE is a sequencing-based method for gene expression profiling that facilitates the global and quantitative characterization of a transcriptome by specifically targeting the 3′ region of expressed gene transcripts. Standard protocols utilize predetermined restriction enzymes (most utilize the *Nla*III site CATG) to release 14 base-pair sequences, referred to as SAGE tags, located after the last defined restriction site in the 3′ part of the detected transcript. The 14 bp tags are then ligated together into longer concatemers, which are cloned for DNA sequencing. The sequence of each tag is detected and compared with a preconstructed reference database that predicts SAGE tags for each known gene. In this way, most individual SAGE tags can be assigned to specific genes using available NCBI sequences (SAGEmap). Each tag detected in a sample represents a single parent transcript (expressed gene), and the frequency of detection of each transcript is directly related to the gene expression level. Thus, SAGE data give both qualitative (identification of expressed genes) and quantitative data (absolute measures of gene expression levels are possible). When a specific SAGE tag does not map to a sequence in the reference database, it suggests that the SAGE tag has detected a novel transcript. For a comprehensive review of SAGE data, see Wang (2006).

Unlike microarray analysis, which relies on specific gene sequences immobilized to each chip, SAGE does not rely on previous knowledge of the gene sequence. Thus, SAGE can be useful to detect any expressed gene and historically has been very successful for detecting novel genes that are expressed in the retina (Blackshaw et al., 2004) or various other tissues. However, SAGE is generally more expensive than microarray analysis, and as more and more genomes have been sequenced and as our understanding of individual genes within those genomes has increased, microarrays are becoming all-inclusive for many different species. SAGE can detect alternatively spliced variants and antisense transcripts, which is generally not possible using standard microarray analysis, although specific arrays can be made to detect both of these products for specific genes. The sensitivity of SAGE is better than that of microarrays, but microarrays generally provide better specificity for each gene; SAGE analysis can misidentify a sequence because of sequence redundancy in multiple genes or sequencing errors. Controls for both technical and biological variability, similar to those previously described for microarray analysis, are also required for the effective use of SAGE analysis.

SAGE analysis has been used effectively to determine gene expression during early retinal development in the mouse (Blackshaw et al., 2004). Based on the temporal onset of specific gene expression in relation to neuronal cell differentiation, this study was able to define subsets of retinal progenitor cells and provided useful methods for predicting genes whose function might be related to retinal neuronal cell differentiation (Blackshaw et al., 2004). In another study, SAGE was used to specifically profile genes expressed in RPE isolated from human retinas (Sharon et al., 2002). This study demonstrated that the gene expression profile of RPE was significantly different from the rest of the human retina. Interestingly, relatively high percentages (ca. 9.5%) of the identified RPE genes with known functions were involved in phagocytosis and protein degradation. In contrast, the neural retina devotes less than 3% of its transcripts to these processes, demonstrating a strong commitment of the RPE to the critical function of rod outer segment phagocytosis (Sharon et al., 2002). This study also identified 22 previously unknown elements that appear to be exclusively expressed by the RPE. Ongoing studies and new SAGE data will continue to increase our understanding of the role of specific gene expression in RPE and retinal vascular function.

Isolation of retinal pigment epithelium or vasculature from retinas

Recent advances in analytical techniques have greatly enhanced gene expression research, and it is now possible to obtain large amounts of data from single experiments. However, separating the retinal vascular cells or RPE cells from other more prominent neuronal and glial components remains one of the main difficulties in the specific analysis of RPE or vascular gene expression in the retina. This is particularly true when using large-scale, "unbiased" techniques such as array or SAGE analysis. Although RPE and vascular components of the retina are absolutely critical to normal retinal function, the relative percentage of these cell types in the retina is low. The RPE is a monolayer, and the retinal vasculature exists as three small vascular plexuses in the inner neural retina and the single-layer choriocapillaris. Because the RPE and vascular beds constitute only a small percentage of the retinal cells, important information about gene expression in the RPE or retinal vasculature can easily be lost among genes expressed in more abundant retinal neuronal and glial cells when analyzing gene expression using RNA isolated from whole retinas.

One such study used microarray analysis to analyze gene expression during various stages of retinal vascular development by isolating mRNA from dissected whole retinas at various stages during postnatal development (Dorrell et al., 2004). Multiple genes involved in neuronal development and the transfer of visual signals also change dramatically during these developmental stages, and these genes are generally expressed at higher abundance. Thus, it is likely that many important vascular-related or RPE-specific genes remained "hidden" within background levels. Deciphering which observed changes in gene expression correlated with important roles during various stages of vascular development rather than roles in other, nonvascular retina developmental processes was difficult. Specific patterns of gene expression changes in relation to developmental progression were eventually linked to various functions such as neuronal differentiation, visual signal transfer, or vascular development (figure 56.2*A*) (Dorrell, Aguilar, et al., 2004). By correlating the expression profiles with potential function, an important function for R-cadherin in endothelial cell guidance during retinal vascular development emerged from this gene expression analysis study (figure 56.2*B–D*) (Dorrell et al., 2002). Using the large-scale gene expression analysis, R-cadherin expression was found to be correlated with major events during retinal vascular development. R-cadherin expression is high at birth and throughout the first week, when the superficial vascular plexus is actively forming. R-cadherin expression also peaks just prior to and during formation of the deep and intermediate vascular plexuses. Subsequent immunohistochemical and functional analyses demonstrated that R-cadherin expression is localized to sites of vascular development and is required for normal vascular guidance to the characteristic retinal plexuses (see figure 56.2*B–D*). Many other factors are likely to be involved in retinal vascular guidance during development and maintenance of vascular homeostasis, and future gene expression studies may help further characterize these mechanisms. However, specific isolation of retinal vascular components or RPE cells would greatly enhance the use of large-scale gene expression analysis in these particular fields.

Retinal Pigment Epithelium Isolation and Gene Expression Studies Multiple strategies are currently being used to isolate RPE or vascular components from the retina for subsequent gene expression analysis. Techniques for specifically isolating RPE cells free of other contaminating retinal cells have been described. Most of these techniques use various proteolytic enzymes to dissociate the extracellular matrix, allowing the RPE to be mechanically dissected free of the choroid and underlying neural retina (Castillo et al., 1995; Mayerson et al., 1985). Because pure RPE cells can be isolated, these techniques have been valuable for specifically studying RPE gene expression in vivo, particularly gene expression in RPE isolated from diseased human retinas. In 2002, cDNA libraries from native human RPE were used to profile RPE gene expression (Buraczynska et al., 2002). This study identified several RPE-specific genes, along with multiple genes expressed in RPE as well as in other ocular and nonocular tissues. As expected, a majority of the RPE-expressed, classifiable genes included genes involved in the metabolic pathway (21%) or gene regulation and protein expression (23%). A surprisingly large percentage of expressed genes were identified as growth factors and cell signaling molecules (13%), membrane transport molecules (5%), and molecules involved in protein trafficking (7%). This is consistent with a role for RPE in maintaining retinal homeostasis through controlled cytokine expression, transport of nutrients and ions, and maintenance of the interphotoreceptor matrix (Buraczynska et al., 2002).

RPE isolation protocols have also facilitated studies that assess changes in gene expression associated with various in vivo mouse models of disease. Using large-scale microarray analysis, RPE gene expression was compared between young (2-month-old) and older (2-year-old) mice to analyze changes in RPE gene expression associated with aging (Ida et al., 2003). A number of genes, mainly involving inflammation, stress response to oxidative stress, DNA damage, and heat shock, were found to be upregulated in isolated RPE cells from older mice. Interestingly, genes involved in stimulating neovascularization were also upregulated, supporting the hypothesis that changes in RPE function related to aging may contribute to the pathogenesis of "wet" AMD (Ida et al., 2003). Few genes were found to be downregulated in

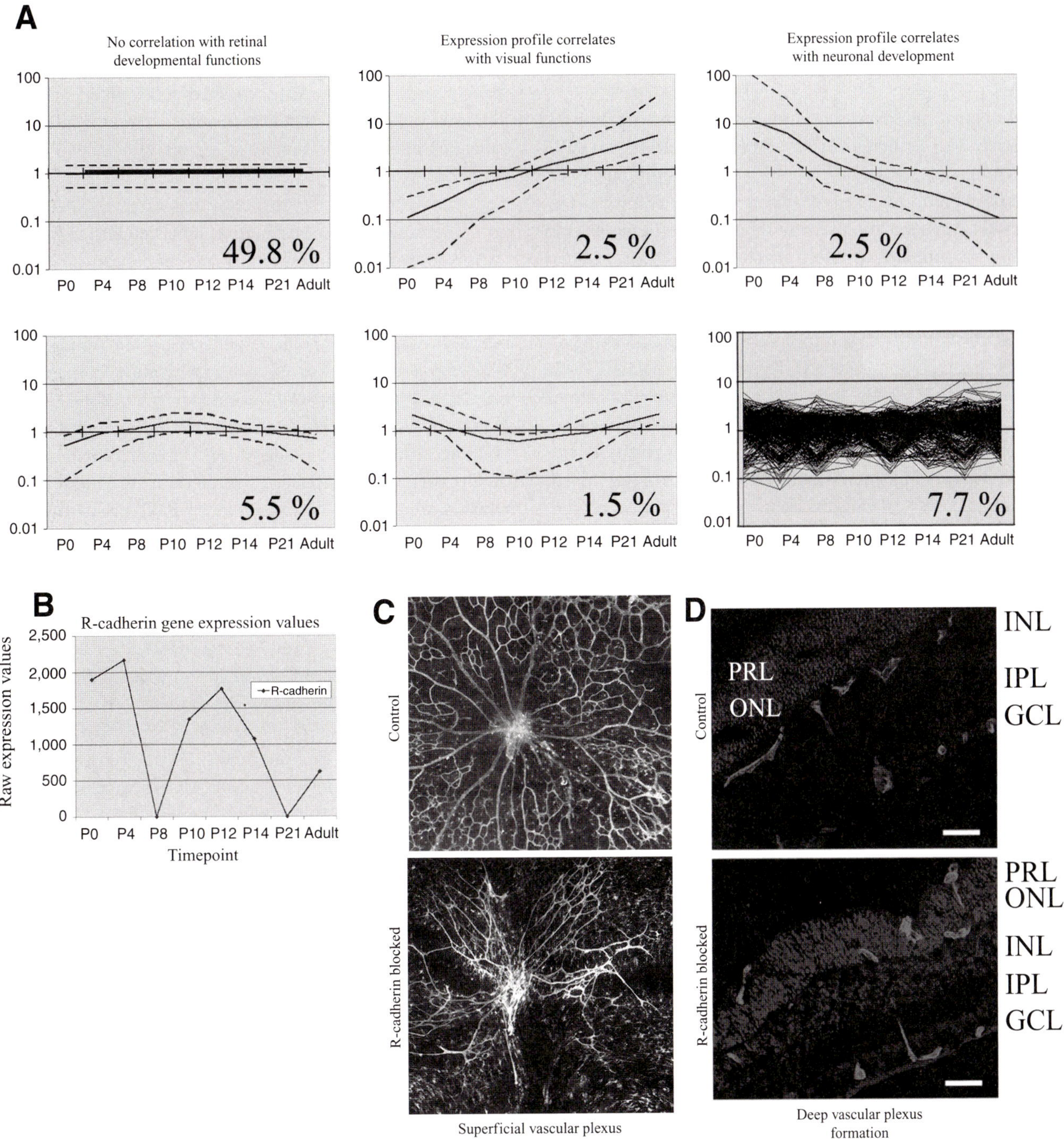

FIGURE 56.2 *A*, Gene expression profile clustering of mRNA from whole mouse retinas at different postnatal developmental stages. Based on expression profile, gene function could be classified as having probable involvement in the onset of vision (mouse retinal development nears completion and vision begins around P14), neuronal development and differentiation (nears completion around P14), or potential involvement in postnatal retinal vascular development (a process that undergoes multiple changes during these times, and thus gene expression would vary throughout). *B*, The expression profile of R-cadherin was determined to have a potential relationship to retinal vascular development. When R-cadherin function was blocked, the retinal vasculature failed to form normally in the superficial plexus (*C*), and guidance to the normal deep vascular plexuses was disrupted (*D*). Vessels migrated through the photoreceptor layer and into the subretinal space. See color plate 65. (Adapted from Dorrell et al., 2002, 2004.)

this study, although the study was not comprehensive, and important downregulation of certain genes may have been missed by the stringent constraints applied during the data analysis.

Although retina dissociation and subsequent isolation of RPE cells has facilitated many important studies on RPE gene expression, one must consider the possible effects of using proteolytic enzymes to dissociate the retina. Gene expression can change rapidly on removal of cells from their native environment, an effect that occurs as extracellular matrix components are broken down or as the cells' own membrane proteins are cleaved by enzymatic digestion. Thus, care should be taken to dissociate the retina using as gentle a proteolytic process as possible, and isolated RPE cells should be placed into RNA preservatives such as RNALater (Ambion) or Trizol (Invitrogen) quickly to minimize changes in gene expression that occur due to isolation techniques. In addition, it is critical that RPE isolation from all control and test samples is stringently performed in exactly the same manner so as not to increase the levels of technical variability discussed earlier.

Although RPE isolation is valuable for studying gene expression changes in vivo, the limited life span of normal, primary RPE cells in culture represents a substantial obstacle for cell and molecular analysis in vitro. However, the analysis of gene expression changes due to specific, controlled variables often requires in vitro studies. Several RPE cell lines have been developed that maintain many of the behavioral and physiological characteristics of primary RPE and express similar markers, such as RPE-65, cellular retinaldehyde–binding protein (CRALBP), and pigmented epithelium–derived factor (PEDF) (Kanuga et al., 2002; Lund et al., 2001). These cell lines, such as the commonly used ARPE-19 cell line, which is currently available from ATCC (catalogue no. CRL-2302), have been used in many in vitro studies to identify important RPE-related genes. Using the ARPE-19 cell line, researchers found correlative changes in gene expression following injury of the cultured monolayer. Not surprisingly, genes involved in wound repair, including DNA synthesis, DNA repair, cellular adhesion, cytokine expression, and signal transduction, were greatly upregulated during repair of the RPE monolayer. Also highly upregulated were interesting inflammatory associated genes such as mitogen-activated kinase, CD44, monocyte chemotactic protein (MCP-1), thymosin β-10, and hepatoma-derived growth factor (Singh et al., 2001). Upregulation of these genes suggests that the RPE may play a significant role during the early inflammatory response that accompanies many ocular diseases, such as proliferative vitreoretinopathy. In another study using ARPE-19 cells, various cellular adhesion molecules, growth factors, and chemokines generally involved in inflammation and repair, including MCP-1, were also greatly upregulated on vitreous treatment of the RPE cells, a process used to mimic the repair response observed in vivo due to proliferative vitreoretinopathy (Fan et al., 2002). Time-dependent changes in gene expression on phagocytosis of rod outer segments (Chowers et al., 2004), the response of RPE to oxidative stress (Alizadeh et al., 2001; Weigel et al., 2002), RPE cell differentiation (Alizadeh et al., 2000), and many other gene expression studies have also been performed using the ARPE-19 spontaneously transformed human RPE cell line.

As with any cell line, immortalization of the RPE cells, whether spontaneous or directed, can alter function and gene expression when compared to native RPE. Using microarray analysis, significant differences were found in the gene expression profiles of cultured primary human RPE cells from four separate donors compared to ARPE-19 cells. Hierarchical clustering demonstrated that despite being obtained from a wide range of ages (48–82 years), each of the primary RPE cell groups clustered together, and no significant overlap was observed with the ARPE-19 cell lines (figure 56.3) (Cai and Del Priore, 2006). Thus, despite the definite utility of these cell lines for determining alterations in gene expression due to specific controlled changes, actual gene expression changes to similar effects may differ in vivo, and caution should be used when generalizing results from ARPE-19 cells. It should be noted, however, that no clear differences were observed in the normal (nonstimulated) expression level of genes with functions related to angiogenesis, phagocytosis, or apoptosis (Cai and Del Priore, 2006), the major RPE functions for which ARPE-19 cells are often used. Thus, ARPE-19 cells might be useful for many important studies regarding RPE gene expression, but, as with most in vitro studies, the results ultimately need to be confirmed in vivo.

The differentiation state of RPE cells, and ultimately gene expression and cellular function, can be altered by different culture conditions, particularly when grown with different

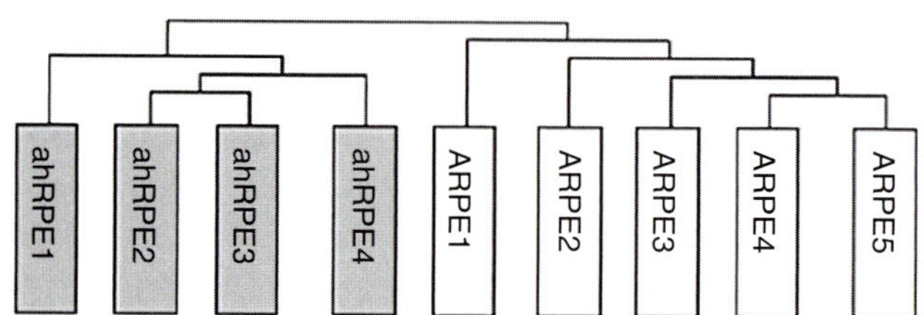

FIGURE 56.3 Hierarchic clustering analysis of human adult RPE from four different samples (ages ranging from 48 to 82 years) and five ARPE-19 cultures. The gene expression profiles from the four primary human samples and the five ARPE-19 samples cluster into two distinct groups with no discernable overlap, demonstrating significant differences between primary RPE and ARPE-19 cells. Thus, caution should be exercised when making conclusions of RPE gene expression from cultured, immortalized RPE cells. (Adapted from Cai and Del Priore, 2006.)

extracellular matrix components (Turowski et al., 2004). This should also be considered when using cell lines, since different levels of gene expression may be caused simply by differences in culture conditions. Another consideration is the use of specific culture conditions to help maximize similarities to RPE in vivo. For example, culture on porcine lens capsule membranes has been shown to maintain an in vivo-like differentiated state in ARPE-19 cells; apical microvilli formation is induced, and rod outer segment phagocytosis properties are maintained (Turowski et al., 2004). These factors should all be considered when using cultured RPE cells for gene expression studies.

Isolation of Retinal Vasculature and Subsequent Gene Expression Studies Isolating retinal ECs can be very difficult because much of the retinal vasculature is intricately associated with nonvascular tissue within the neural retinal layers (see figure 56.1*B*). Numerous EC lines are available, and isolation of primary ECs, such as human umbilical vein ECs (HUVECs), is common. However, analysis of cultured ECs is problematic because these cells, in culture, are significantly different from such cells in vivo, where the tissue microenvironment has a significant impact on the expression and downregulation of various genes. In addition, microvascular ECs from different organs, and even from different blood vessels within these organs (arterial, venous, microvascular capillaries, etc.), behave differently in response to certain stimuli such as cytokines or growth factors (Gumkowski et al., 1987). Thus, for obtaining useful retinal vascular gene expression data, the specific use of retinal microvascular ECs may be important. Several protocols for isolating retinal ECs have been published (Antonetti and Wolpert, 2003), although the isolation of retinal microvascular ECs from mice is quite difficult. In general, isolation protocols utilize proteolytic digestion of the retina, usually with solutions containing collagenase mixed with various other combinations of extracellular matrix digestion enzymes or trypsin, followed by purification of the ECs using immunoprecipitation with vascular-specific markers such as platelet-derived endothelial cellular adhesion molecule (PECAM; CD31). Few studies have been published that specifically address gene expression from retinal ECs in mouse models of disease, including no known large-scale gene expression studies to date, probably owing to the difficulty of obtaining pure primary ECs from mouse retinas. Certain retinal microvascular EC lines have been created, such as rat JG2/1 cells. These maintain many of the characteristics of primary ECs, such as expression of GLUT-1, the transferrin receptor, von Willebrand factor, and the RECA-1 antigen, high-affinity uptake of acetylated LDL, and isolectin *Griffonia simplicifolia* binding (Greenwood et al., 1996). However, a similar retinal EC line from mice has yet to be developed.

Many nonendothelial cells, such as astrocytes, pericytes, microglia, and perivascular macrophages, also play critical roles in both developmental and pathological neovascularization (Provis et al., 1997). Thus, studies analyzing gene expression related to changes in the retinal vasculature should also consider the role of these cells, since changes in their gene expression profiles may significantly affect retinal neovascularization. One of the main problems with isolating mouse vasculature from retinas is that the strong enzymes required to completely remove retinal ECs from the neural retina often result in EC death. Newer isolation techniques take advantage of gentle retinal dissociation techniques with lower concentrations of dissociation enzymes in an attempt to isolate small fragments of intact vessels (J. Greenwood, pers. comm.). Although complete purification of ECs or even vessel fragments may not be achieved, the substantial enhancement of vascular-associated cells and thus vascular-related RNA would represent an important step for retinal vascular gene expression studies. In addition, the co-isolation of closely associated astrocytes, pericytes, and microglia, which remain attached to ECs during the gentle dissociation and purification methods, may actually be advantageous. This allows culture and subsequent analysis of vascular fragments rather than ECs alone, and thus is likely to more closely recapitulate the in vivo retinal microvascular environment by including multiple vascular-related cells.

Another method of isolating retinal vasculature for subsequent gene expression analysis uses laser capture microdissection technology. Using microdissection, desired cells or tissue can be isolated from frozen sections. Generally, retinal sections are fixed and the vessels are stained using an endothelial marker such as PECAM or von Willebrand factor. Prior to laser capture, the slides are dehydrated in graded ethanol solutions and dried using acetone and xylene. For most laser capture microdissection techniques, the slide must be completely dry for efficient laser-induced capture of the desired cells. Moisture results in inefficient capture of the cells and lower resolution capture, causing nearby, undesired cells to be captured as well. Because gene expression analysis requires intact mRNA, extreme caution should be used throughout dissection, sectioning of the tissue, and laser capture, and all solutions and materials should be RNase free to ensure that the RNA is not degraded. If the RNA has been protected appropriately, RNA can be subsequently extrapolated from the isolated cells using any of a number of commercial micro-RNA isolation kits (e.g., Ambion, Qiagen). Advances in technique have made RNA amplification and subsequent gene array analysis a feasible method of evaluating gene expression from limited tissue (Luzzi et al., 2003), although certain variables are inevitably added when RNA is amplified, such as incomplete amplification of mRNA ends. Laser capture microdissection and subsequent microarray gene expression analysis has already been applied to brain microvascular studies (Liu et al., 2006), and similar studies are likely to be valuable in the retina.

Use of transgenics in gene expression analysis

The use of transgenic mice and genetic knockouts has also substantially enhanced our knowledge of gene function in the retina. As genes are identified whose expression patterns indicate a role in retinal function, the results of altering gene expression can be very informative. Analysis of mutants with altered gene expression levels, such as those that overexpress or underexpress a specific gene, or that have altered expression localization, can give important insights into a gene's function. For example, a particular role for VEGF isoforms during retinal vascular development and pathological neovascularization was demonstrated using mice engineered to express specific VEGF isoforms. These studies demonstrated that a combination of diffusible and relatively immobile isoforms of VEGF was required for normal vascular development. Either the combined expression of $VEGF_{120}$ (readily diffusible) and $VEGF_{188}$ (largely immobile) (Ishida et al., 2003) or the single-factor expression of $VEGF_{165}$ (Stalmans et al., 2002), which is partially diffusible through the retina, was required for normal retinal vascular development. Mice that solely expressed either $VEGF_{120}$ or $VEGF_{188}$ developed severely abnormal retinal vasculature characterized by abnormal vessel organization and size and inappropriate arterial and venous differentiation (Stalmans et al., 2002). Mice engineered to overexpress VEGF in the photoreceptors (by placing the VEGF gene behind a rhodopsin promoter) also developed abnormal retinal vascularization characterized by the formation of vascular sprouts that grew from the inner retinal vasculature toward the outer photoreceptor segments (Tobe et al., 1998). These studies demonstrate the utility of altered gene expression in determining functional roles for genes in retinal neovascularization.

Many genes expressed in the eye, particularly developmental genes, also have fundamental roles elsewhere that can lead to early lethality in mutants. Unfortunately, in many cases this has rendered conventional gene knockouts uninformative for analysis of specific gene functions in later stages of eye development. In addition, it is often difficult to analyze specific vascular- or RPE-related roles of genes in mice with global gene deficiencies. For these reasons, conditional knockouts have become necessary to elucidate the specific role of retinal vascular- or RPE-related genes. The advent of Cre/Lox technology has provided an important tool for manipulating gene expression in mice by allowing cell-specific activation or inactivation of genes. Conditional knockouts have now been created for vascular-associated cells, including ECs (Bjarnegard et al., 2004), astrocytes (Hirrlinger et al., 2006), myeloid cells (Cramer et al., 2003), and smooth muscle actin-expressing cells, such as arterial pericytes (Regan et al., 2000). Studies using these mice have already been instrumental in advancing our understanding of the critical roles for different genes and vascular-associated cell types in general neovascularization. As cell-specific Cre mice are combined with more Lox gene knockouts, and as these mice are further exploited for retinal research, we will continue to learn more about the importance of specific gene expression in relation to retinal vascular development and disease. Cre recombinase has also recently been linked to the tyrosinase related protein-1 (Trp-1) promoter, making future RPE specific knockouts possible (Marneros et al., 2005). Although the absolute specificity of this gene promoter for RPE cells remains somewhat controversial, it should suffice for eye-specific studies, and these and future RPE specific knockouts should quickly advance the studies of RPE specific gene expression and function as well.

Correlation of retinal pigment epithelium gene expression and retinal vascularization

A strong relationship between the RPE and retinal vasculature, both during retinal development and throughout adulthood, is becoming evident. The RPE clearly induces development of the choroidal vessels. $VEGF_{120}$ and $VEGF_{165}$ are both expressed by mouse RPE cells, and when VEGF expression was specifically eliminated in the RPE, the choroid became absent throughout development and adulthood; scleral tissue was observed just posterior to the RPE where the choroidal vascular plexus would normally be found (Marneros et al., 2005). Although multiple retinal abnormalities were observed in these mice, including microphthalmia and an absence of Bruch's membrane, the RPE seemed to differentiate normally, indicating that the vascular abnormalities were due to a lack of VEGF-mediated pro-angiogenic signaling by the RPE. Other growth factors, such as basic fibroblast growth factor (FGF-2), are also expressed by the RPE and have been suggested to play a critical role during normal retinal vascular development (Rousseau et al., 2000).

RPE abnormalities have also been correlated with the onset of age-related macular degeneration (AMD) (Campochiaro et al., 1999). VEGF overexpression in the RPE has been correlated with AMD progression in excised human diseased retinal tissue (Kliffen et al., 1997) as well as mouse models (Schwesinger et al., 2001; Spilsbury et al., 2000). In addition to the expression of pro-angiogenic factors that may promote choroidal neovascularization when expressed at abnormal levels, the lack of normal RPE expression of certain antiangiogenic factors may also contribute to abnormal retinal neovascularization. The RPE is known to express factors such as pigmented epithelium–derived factor (PEDF), which may help to maintain the normally quiescent retinal vasculature. PEDF expression is upregulated as retinal vascular development is completed (Behling et al., 2002), and retinas from patients with AMD have demonstrated a lack of normal PEDF expression in the RPE compared with age-matched donors without AMD (Bhutto et al., 2006).

In addition to the definite role of the RPE during normal and pathological choroidal neovascularization, new evidence suggests that the RPE may also play an underappreciated role during development of the vascular plexuses in the inner retina. In the postnatal Balb/c mouse, vessels branch from the superficial plexus around P8 and form the deep plexus at the outer edge of the inner nuclear layer (INL). Although the precise factors that initiate this process are not known, hypoxia in the deeper retina, caused by retinal thickening, photoreceptor maturation, and the concomitant increase in neuronal activity, is likely to be a main driving force (Zhang et al., 2003). As a result, the production of growth factors in the neural retina is increased, subsequently initiating the formation of the deep vascular plexuses. As the vessels migrate toward the deep retina, the ECs must be guided to the appropriate plexuses at the outer and inner edges of the INL. Filopodial processes, which can contact and respond to preexisting guidance cues, have been observed at the tips of ECs migrating toward the deep vascular plexus (Dorrell, et al., 2002). R-cadherin expression at the outer and inner edges of the INL correlates with vascularization of the deep and intermediate plexuses, and when R-cadherin mediated adhesion is disrupted, retinal vessels migrate directly past the deep plexus, into the normally avascular photoreceptor layer and subretinal space (Dorrell, et al., 2002; Dorrell, Otani, et al., 2004) (see figure 56.2*D*). A similar phenotype whereby vessels invade the ONL was also observed in transgenic mice with photoreceptor-induced overexpression of VEGF (Tobe et al., 1998). This indicates that normal guidance cues can be overcome either by overexpression of growth factors beyond the normal deep vascular plexus or by masking specific adhesion molecules critical for EC guidance. Abnormal vascular sprouts invading the outer retina and the subretinal space are also observed in mice lacking the very-low-density lipoprotein receptor (VLDLR) (Heckenlively et al., 2003). Unlike the subretinal vessels that form when R-cadherin mediated adhesion is blocked, which directly bypass the deep layers, these subretinal vessels develop a few days later as sprouts from the normal deep and intermediate retinal plexuses. VLDLR is known to mediate neuronal guidance during development of the neocortex in a mechanism involving R-cadherin (Rice et al., 2001; Trommsdorff et al., 1999) and these results suggest that VLDLR expression in the retina could potentially be functioning in a similar fashion during retinal vascular guidance.

In each of these situations, retinal vessels migrate through the photoreceptor layer and into the subretinal space alongside the RPE. Although many of the growth factors that initiate formation of the deep vascular plexuses definitely come from retinal glial and neuronal cells, these observations suggest that deep vascular sprouting may be promoted by the RPE as well. The pro-angiogenic cytokine gradient that induces development of the choroid may also participate in the development of inner retinal vascular plexuses, particularly the formation of the deep vascular plexuses. According to this hypothesis, ECs may be attracted toward the cytokine gradient formed by growth factor expression in the RPE, but normally they are guided to the deep and intermediate plexuses as they migrate. However, when these guidance cues are lost, such as the effects observed when normal R-cadherin or VLDLR function is lost, the vessels migrate past the normal deep and intermediate plexuses, through the photoreceptors, and into the subretinal space by default. More experimental evidence is certainly required to confirm or reject this hypothesis. The continued study of gene expression in both the RPE and the retinal vasculature should help answer this particular question and will continue to advance our understanding of the normal role of the RPE during normal and pathological retinal neovascularization.

Conclusion and future directions

Large-scale genomic analyses are very useful for identifying genes whose expression may be critical to various biological processes. However, gene expression analysis of the RPE and retinal vasculature is only a first step toward understanding the role these genes play in regulating normal and pathological retinal processes. As discussed in this chapter, the results of large-scale gene expression analyses need to be confirmed using other techniques, and protein expression levels must be tested before firm conclusions about the relevance of gene expression to biological function can be made. In addition, the biological effects of a particular gene's expression, and the effects of differing expression levels in varying circumstances, must be considered. For example, many housekeeping genes, which are generally expressed at high levels, can demonstrate differential gene expression levels. However, even statistically significant differences in the expression of these genes usually have low biological relevance. Because of high expression levels and constitutive functions, even relatively substantial changes in expression may not dramatically affect retinal vascular or RPE functions. By contrast, the function of many genes critical to normal RPE and retinal vascular function, such as cytokines and growth factors, can be significantly altered by marginal differences in expression levels. Small changes in the expression of these genes may have dramatic effects leading to the onset or progression of various diseases. Thus, the biological effects of differential gene expression need to be addressed.

Finally, many genes are regulated beyond the transcriptional level. For example, HIF1-α is a critical cellular oxygen sensor. It mediates a cell's response to hypoxia by turning on various stress response pathways and by initiating the expression of VEGF and other pro-angiogenic factors to initiate vessel growth and ultimately alleviate hypoxia. However, HIF1-α is constitutively expressed and is regulated by posttranslational degradation. Under normal oxygen conditions, HIF1-α is rapidly degraded, but in hypoxic conditions it becomes stabilized. Gene expression analysis alone would not detect the important changes in HIF1-α protein levels in cells exposed to different oxygen levels. Thus, whereas gene expression analysis is very useful, it is the amount of functional protein produced by cells that ultimately makes a difference. As techniques for detecting protein expression, such as large-scale proteomic analysis, continue to improve they will become more and more useful for the analysis of RPE and retinal vascular functions.

Since the early 1990s, gene expression analysis has seen a massive boom, largely helped by the advent of large-scale analysis techniques. As microarray technologies evolve to provide more sensitive temporal expression information, and as other techniques continue to provide information about spatial expression at the cellular level (i.e., microarray of laser-captured specimens), our understanding of normal and abnormal biological processes in the retina should be greatly enhanced. These large-scale techniques, such as microarray or SAGE, along with other more conventional techniques, such as RT-PCR and in situ hybridization, have already been instrumental in studying retinal gene expression. With the use of isolation techniques such as microdissection, specific RPE and retinal vascular gene expression analyses will continue to be possible. These studies will advance our understanding of the roles that RPE and the retinal vasculature play in normal retinal homeostasis, as well as help determine what effects alterations in normal gene expression levels might have on the progression of various ocular diseases.

ACKNOWLEDGMENTS Work was supported by the National Eye Institute (grant no. EY11254), the MacTel Foundation, Scripps Fonseca/Mericos Fund, the Robert Mealey Program for the Study of Macular Degenerations, the V. Kann Rasmussen Foundation, and the Horner Family Fund. MID was supported by a California Institute for Regenerative Medicine fellowship. We thank the entire Friedlander laboratory staff for their helpful contributions to the preparation of this chapter.

REFERENCES

ADAMIS, A. P., AIELLO, L. P., and D'AMATO, R. A. (1999). Angiogenesis and ophthalmic disease. *Angiogenesis* 3:9–14.

ALIZADEH, M., GELFMAN, C. M., BENCH, S. R., and HJELMELAND, L. M. (2000). Expression and splicing of FGF receptor mRNAs during APRE-19 cell differentiation in vitro. *Invest. Ophthalmol. Vis. Sci.* 41:2357–2362.

ALIZADEH, M., WADA, M., GELFMAN, C. M., HANDA, J. T., and HJELMELAND, L. M. (2001). Downregulation of differentiation specific gene expression by oxidative stress in ARPE-19 cells. *Invest. Ophthalmol. Vis. Sci.* 42:2706–2713.

ANTONETTI, D. A., and WOLPERT, E. B. (2003). Isolation and characterization of retinal endothelial cells. *Methods Mol. Med.* 89: 365–374.

BEHLING, K. C., SURACE, E. M., and BENNETT, J. (2002). Pigment epithelium-derived factor expression in the developing mouse eye. *Mol. Vis.* 8:449–454.

BHUTTO, I. A., MCLEOD, D. S., HASEGAWA, T., KIM, S. Y., MERGES, C., TONG, P., and LUTTY, G. A. (2006). Pigment epithelium-derived factor (PEDF) and vascular endothelial growth factor (VEGF) in aged human choroid and eyes with age-related macular degeneration. *Exp. Eye Res.* 82:99–110.

BJARNEGARD, M., ENGE, M., NORLIN, J., GUSTAFSDOTTIR, S., FREDRIKSSON, S., ABRAMSSON, A., TAKEMOTO, M., GUSTAFSSON, E., FASSLER, R., et al. (2004). Endothelium-specific ablation of PDGFB leads to pericyte loss and glomerular, cardiac and placental abnormalities. *Development* 131:1847–1857.

BLACKSHAW, S., HARPAVAT, S., TRIMARCHI, J., CAI, L., HUANG, H., KUO, W. P., WEBER, G., LEE, K., FRAIOLI, R. E., et al. (2004). Genomic analysis of mouse retinal development. *PLoS Biol.* 2: E247.

BURACZYNSKA, M., MEARS, A. J., ZAREPARSI, S., FARJO, R., FILIPPOVA, E., YUAN, Y., MACNEE, S. P., HUGHES, B., and SWAROOP, A. (2002). Gene expression profile of native human retinal pigment epithelium. *Invest. Ophthalmol. Vis. Sci.* 43:603–607.

CAI, H., and DEL PRIORE, L. V. (2006). Gene expression profile of cultured adult compared to immortalized human RPE. *Mol. Vis.* 12:1–14.

CAMPOCHIARO, P. A., SOLOWAY, P., RYAN, S. J., and MILLER, J. W. (1999). The pathogenesis of choroidal neovascularization in patients with age-related macular degeneration. *Mol. Vis.* 5:34.

CASTILLO, B. V., JR., LITTLE, C. W., DEL CERRO, C., and DEL CERRO, M. (1995). An improved method of isolating fetal human retinal pigment epithelium. *Curr. Eye Res.* 14:677–683.

CHONG, N. H., and BIRD, A. C. (1999). Management of inherited outer retinal dystrophies: Present and future. *Br. J. Ophthalmol.* 83:120–122.

CHOWERS, I., KIM, Y., FARKAS, R. H., GUNATILAKA, T. L., HACKAM, A. S., CAMPOCHIARO, P. A., FINNEMANN, S. C., and ZACK, D. J. (2004). Changes in retinal pigment epithelial gene expression induced by rod outer segment uptake. *Invest. Ophthalmol. Vis. Sci.* 45:2098–2106.

CRAMER, T., YAMANISHI, Y., CLAUSEN, B. E., FORSTER, I., PAWLINSKI, R., MACKMAN, N., HAASE, V. H., JAENISCH, R., et al. (2003). HIF-1alpha is essential for myeloid cell-mediated inflammation. *Cell* 112:645–657.

DE JONG, P. T (2006). Age-related macular degeneration. *N. Engl. J. Med.* 355:1474–1485.

DORRELL, M. I., AGUILAR, E., and FRIEDLANDER, M. (2002). Retinal vascular development is mediated by endothelial filopodia, a preexisting astrocytic template and specific R-cadherin adhesion. *Invest. Ophthalmol. Vis. Sci.* 43:3500–3510.

DORRELL, M. I., AGUILAR, E., WEBER, C., and FRIEDLANDER, M. (2004). Global gene expression analysis of the developing postnatal mouse retina. *Invest. Ophthalmol. Vis. Sci.* 45:1009–1019.

DORRELL, M. I., and FRIEDLANDER, M. (2006). Mechanisms of endothelial cell guidance and vascular patterning in the developing mouse retina. *Prog. Retin. Eye Res.* 25:277–295.

DORRELL, M. I., OTANI, A., AGUILAR, E., MORENO, S. K., and FRIEDLANDER, M. (2004). Adult bone marrow–derived stem cells use R-cadherin to target sites of neovascularization in the developing retina. *Blood* 103(9):3420–3427.

EICHLER, W., YAFAI, Y., WIEDEMANN, P., and REICHENBACH, A. (2004). Angiogenesis-related factors derived from retinal glial (Müller) cells in hypoxia. *Neuroreport* 15:1633–1637.

FAN, W., ZHENG, J. J., PEIPER, S. C., and MCLAUGHLIN, B. J. (2002). Changes in gene expression of ARPE-19 cells in response to vitreous treatment. *Ophthalmic. Res.* 34:357–365.

FUTTER, C. E. (2006). The molecular regulation of organelle transport in mammalian retinal pigment epithelial cells. *Pigment Cell Res.* 19:104–111.

GREENWOOD, J., PRYCE, G., DEVINE, L., MALE, D. K., DOS SANTOS, W. L., CALDER, V. L., and ADAMSON, P. (1996). SV40 large T immortalised cell lines of the rat blood-brain and blood-retinal barriers retain their phenotypic and immunological characteristics. *J. Neuroimmunol.* 71:51–63.

GUMKOWSKI, F., KAMINSKA, G., KAMINSKI, M., MORRISSEY, L. W., and AUERBACH, R. (1987). Heterogeneity of mouse vascular endothelium: In vitro studies of lymphatic, large blood vessel and microvascular endothelial cells. *Blood Vessels* 24:11–23.

HECKENLIVELY, J. R., HAWES, N. L., FRIEDLANDER, M., NUSINOWITZ, S., HURD, R., DAVISSON, M., and CHANG, B. (2003). Mouse model of subretinal neovascularization with choroidal anastomosis. *Retina* 23:518–522.

HIRRLINGER, P. G., SCHELLER, A., BRAUN, C., HIRRLINGER, J., and KIRCHHOFF, F. (2006). Temporal control of gene recombination in astrocytes by transgenic expression of the tamoxifen-inducible DNA recombinase variant CreERT2. *Glia* 54:11–20.

IDA, H., BOYLAN, S. A., WEIGEL, A. L., and HJELMELAND, L. M. (2003). Age-related changes in the transcriptional profile of mouse RPE/choroid. *Physiol. Genomics* 15:258–262.

ISHIDA, S., USUI, T., YAMASHIRO, K., KAJI, Y., AMANO, S., OGURA, Y., HIDA, T., OGUCHI, Y., AMBATI, J., et al. (2003). $VEGF_{164}$-mediated inflammation is required for pathological, but not physiological, ischemia-induced retinal neovascularization. *J. Exp. Med.* 198:483–489.

KANUGA, N., WINTON, H. L., BEAUCHENE, L., KOMAN, A., ZERBIB, A., HALFORD, S., COURAUD, P. O., KEEGAN, D., COFFEY, P., et al. (2002). Characterization of genetically modified human retinal pigment epithelial cells developed for in vitro and transplantation studies. *Invest. Ophthalmol. Vis. Sci.* 43:546–555.

KLIFFEN, M., SHARMA, H. S., MOOY, C. M., KERKVLIET, S., and DE JONG, P. T. (1997). Increased expression of angiogenic growth factors in age-related maculopathy. *Br. J. Ophthalmol.* 81:154–162.

LIU, X. S., ZHANG, Z. G., ZHANG, L., MORRIS, D. C., KAPKE, A., LU, M., and CHOPP, M. (2006). Atorvastatin downregulates tissue plasminogen activator-aggravated genes mediating coagulation and vascular permeability in single cerebral endothelial cells captured by laser microdissection. *J. Cereb. Blood Flow Metab.* 26:787–796.

LUKASIEWICZ, P. D. (2005). Synaptic mechanisms that shape visual signaling at the inner retina. *Prog. Brain Res.* 147:205–218.

LUND, R. D., ADAMSON, P., SAUVE, Y., KEEGAN, D. J., GIRMAN, S. V., WANG, S., WINTON, H., KANUGA, N., KWAN, A. S., et al. (2001). Subretinal transplantation of genetically modified human cell lines attenuates loss of visual function in dystrophic rats. *Proc. Natl. Acad. Sci. U.S.A.* 98:9942–9947.

LUZZI, V., MAHADEVAPPA, M., RAJA, R., WARRINGTON, J. A., and WATSON, M. A. (2003). Accurate and reproducible gene expression profiles from laser capture microdissection, transcript amplification, and high density oligonucleotide microarray analysis. *J. Mol. Diagn.* 5:9–14.

MARNEROS, A. G., FAN, J., YOKOYAMA, Y., GERBER, H. P., FERRARA, N., CROUCH, R. K., and OLSEN, B. R. (2005). Vascular endothelial growth factor expression in the retinal pigment epithelium is essential for choriocapillaris development and visual function. *Am. J. Pathol.* 167:1451–1459.

MAYERSON, P. L., HALL, M. O., CLARK, V., and ABRAMS, T. (1985). An improved method for isolation and culture of rat retinal pigment epithelial cells. *Invest. Ophthalmol. Vis. Sci.* 26:1599–1609.

MUMM, J. S., GODINHO, L., MORGAN, J. L., OAKLEY, D. M., SCHROETER, E. H., and WONG, R. O. (2005). Laminar circuit formation in the vertebrate retina. *Prog. Brain Res.* 147:155–169.

OTANI, A., and FRIEDLANDER, M. (2005). Retinal vascular regeneration. *Semin. Ophthalmol.* 20:43–50.

PROVIS, J. M., LEECH, J., DIAZ, C. M., PENFOLD, P. L., STONE, J., and KESHET, E. (1997). Development of the human retinal vasculature: Cellular relations and VEGF expression. *Exp. Eye Res.* 65:555–568.

REGAN, C. P., MANABE, I., and OWENS, G. K. (2000). Development of a smooth muscle-targeted Cre recombinase mouse reveals novel insights regarding smooth muscle myosin heavy chain promoter regulation. *Circ. Res.* 87:363–369.

RICE, D. S., NUSINOWITZ, S., AZIMI, A. M., MARTINEZ, A., SORIANO, E., and CURRAN, T. (2001). The reelin pathway modulates the structure and function of retinal synaptic circuitry. *Neuron* 31: 929–941.

ROUSSEAU, B., DUBAYLE, D., SENNLAUB, F., JEANNY, J. C., COSTET, P., BIKFALVI, A., and JAVERZAT, S. (2000). Neural and angiogenic defects in eyes of transgenic mice expressing a dominant-negative FGF receptor in the pigmented cells. *Exp. Eye Res.* 71: 395–404.

SCHWESINGER, C., YEE, C., ROHAN, R. M., JOUSSEN, A. M., FERNANDEZ, A., MEYER, T. N., POULAKI, V., MA, J. J., REDMOND, T. M., et al. (2001). Intrachoroidal neovascularization in transgenic mice overexpressing vascular endothelial growth factor in the retinal pigment epithelium. *Am. J. Pathol.* 158:1161–1172.

SHARON, D., BLACKSHAW, S., CEPKO, C. L., and DRYJA, T. P. (2002). Profile of the genes expressed in the human peripheral retina, macula, and retinal pigment epithelium determined through serial analysis of gene expression (SAGE). *Proc. Natl. Acad. Sci. U.S.A.* 99:315–320.

SINGH, S., ZHENG, J. J., PEIPER, S. C., and MCLAUGHLIN, B. J. (2001). Gene expression profile of ARPE-19 during repair of the monolayer. *Graefes Arch. Clin. Exp. Ophthalmol.* 239:946–951.

SPILSBURY, K., GARRETT, K. L., SHEN, W. Y., CONSTABLE, I. J., and RAKOCZY, P. E. (2000). Overexpression of vascular endothelial growth factor (VEGF) in the retinal pigment epithelium leads to the development of choroidal neovascularization. *Am. J. Pathol.* 157:135–144.

STALMANS, I., NG, Y. S., ROHAN, R., FRUTTIGER, M., BOUCHE, A., YUCE, A., FUJISAWA, H., HERMANS, B., SHANI, M., et al. (2002). Arteriolar and venular patterning in retinas of mice selectively expressing VEGF isoforms. *J. Clin. Invest.* 109:327–336.

STRAUSS, O. (2005). The retinal pigment epithelium in visual function. *Physiol. Rev.* 85:845–881.

TOBE, T., OKAMOTO, N., VINORES, M. A., DEREVJANIK, N. L., VINORES, S. A., ZACK, D. J., and CAMPOCHIARO, P. A. (1998). Evolution of neovascularization in mice with overexpression of vascular endothelial growth factor in photoreceptors. *Invest. Ophthalmol. Vis. Sci.* 39:180–188.

Trommsdorff, M., Gotthardt, M., Hiesberger, T., Shelton, J., Stockinger, W., Nimpf, J., Hammer, R. E., Richardson, J. A., and Herz, J. (1999). Reeler/Disabled-like disruption of neuronal migration in knockout mice lacking the VLDL receptor and ApoE receptor 2. *Cell* 97:689–701.

Turowski, P., Adamson, P., Sathia, J., Zhang, J. J., Moss, S. E., Aylward, G. W., Hayes, M. J., Kanuga, N., and Greenwood, J. (2004). Basement membrane-dependent modification of phenotype and gene expression in human retinal pigment epithelial ARPE-19 cells. *Invest. Ophthalmol. Vis. Sci.* 45:2786–2794.

Velculescu, V. E., Zhang, L., Vogelstein, B., and Kinzler, K. W. (1995). Serial analysis of gene expression. *Science* 270:484–487.

Wang, S. M. (2006). Understanding SAGE data. *Trends Genet.* doi:10.1016/j.tig.2006.11.001.

Weigel, A. L., Handa, J. T., and Hjelmeland, L. M. (2002). Microarray analysis of H_2O_2-, HNE-, or tBH-treated ARPE-19 cells. *Free Radic. Biol. Med.* 33:1419–1432.

Zarbin, M. A. (2004). Current concepts in the pathogenesis of age-related macular degeneration. *Arch. Ophthalmol.* 122:598–614.

Zareparsi, S., Hero, A., Zack, D. J., Williams, R. W., and Swaroop, A. (2004). Seeing the unseen: Microarray-based gene expression profiling in vision. *Invest. Ophthalmol. Vis. Sci.* 45: 2457–2462.

Zhang, W., Ito, Y., Berlin, E., Roberts, R., and Berkowitz, B. A. (2003). Role of hypoxia during normal retinal vessel development and in experimental retinopathy of prematurity. *Invest. Ophthalmol. Vis. Sci.* 44:3119–3123.

57 Gene Expression in Cornea and Lens

SHIVALINGAPPA K. SWAMYNATHAN AND JORAM PIATIGORSKY

Optimal vision depends on the transparence and refractive abilities of both cornea and lens, through which light traverses before reaching the retina. Embryonic induction, development, and postnatal maturation of the mouse lens and cornea involve a series of well-coordinated interactions between the neuroectoderm that forms the retina and the surface ectoderm that forms the lens and cornea (Chow and Lang, 2001; Cvekl and Tamm, 2004). One of the currently emerging unifying themes in developmental ophthalmology is that the transcription factors required for embryonic development of cornea and lens are also used for expression of crystallins, the specialized proteins characteristic of the differentiated states of lens and cornea, in the adult tissues. This chapter summarizes current knowledge and recent developments related to the regulation of gene expression in the mouse lens and cornea during embryonic and adult stages, with appropriate references to the human congenital eye defects associated with mutations in genes regulating eye development.

Development of lens and cornea

The lens arises by invagination of the thickened lens placode on the surface ectoderm in response to signals from the underlying optic vesicle (future retina) around embryonic day 11 (E11) in mice (figure 57.1). The anterior cells of the lens vesicle divide and remain cuboidal, while the posterior cells elongate, lose organelles, and differentiate into nondividing primary fiber cells, ultimately losing their nuclei. As development proceeds, proliferation of the anterior epithelial cells becomes progressively confined to the lens equator, where they continue to divide slowly throughout life and give rise to the cortical fiber cells. The lens cells accumulate high proportions of a few water-soluble proteins called crystallins. The transparent primary and secondary cortical fiber cells form the bulk of the lens and are responsible for its optical properties. Three major groups of crystallin gene families, α, β, and γ, each including several members, account for 90% of the water-soluble proteins in the mouse lens (Bloemendal and de Jong, 1991). It is of interest that different species often accumulate different proteins as lens crystallins, which are known as taxon-specific crystallins (Piatigorsky and Wistow, 1991; Wistow and Piatigorsky, 1988).

The cornea has a more complex cellular composition than the lens. The surface ectoderm anterior to the lens vesicle gives rise to the corneal epithelium. Underneath the epithelium, the cornea develops a thick extracellular collagen-filled stroma littered with keratocytes and a posterior monolayer of endothelial cells derived from the neural crest (Hay, 1979; Zieske, 2004). A significant number of corneal basal epithelial cells derived from the embryonic surface ectoderm remain undifferentiated in neonatal mice and serve as corneal epithelial progenitor cells. Following eye opening, around postnatal (PN) day 15, the progenitor cells divide and stratify to form the mature cornea by about 6 weeks of age (Hay, 1979; Zieske, 2004). This proliferation and differentiation continue in the adult mouse, allowing steady replacement of the sloughed off superficial epithelial cells by the slow division of basal cells; basal cells are replenished by stem cells originating from the limbal epithelium at the periphery of the cornea (Collinson et al., 2002; Cotsarelis et al., 1989; Nagasaki and Zhao, 2003). The corneal epithelial cells and keratocytes, like the lens fiber cells, accumulate a high proportion of a few intracellular proteins, called corneal crystallins, and these often differ in different species (Jester et al., 1999, 2005; Piatigorsky, 1998). In the mouse, the corneal crystallins aldehyde dehydrogenase 3A1 (Aldh3a1) and transketolase (Tkt) account for 50% and 10% of water-soluble proteins, respectively. In addition, the corneal epithelial cells accumulate high concentrations of cytokeratins (Krt12 in the case of mice) (Tanifuji-Terai et al., 2006).

The abundance of crystallins indicates that they serve specific optical roles (known for lens, hypothesized for cornea), yet they are also expressed in lower amounts in many tissues where they have strictly enzymatic or other cellular functions. In other words, the widely expressed lens and corneal crystallins gain optical functions by virtue of their high tissue-specific expression, a situation that has been called gene sharing (Piatigorsky and Wistow, 1989; Piatigorsky et al., 1988). The gene sharing relationship between tissue-specific expression and function of a gene and its encoded protein adds an intriguing general aspect to gene expression in lens and cornea (Piatigorsky, 2007).

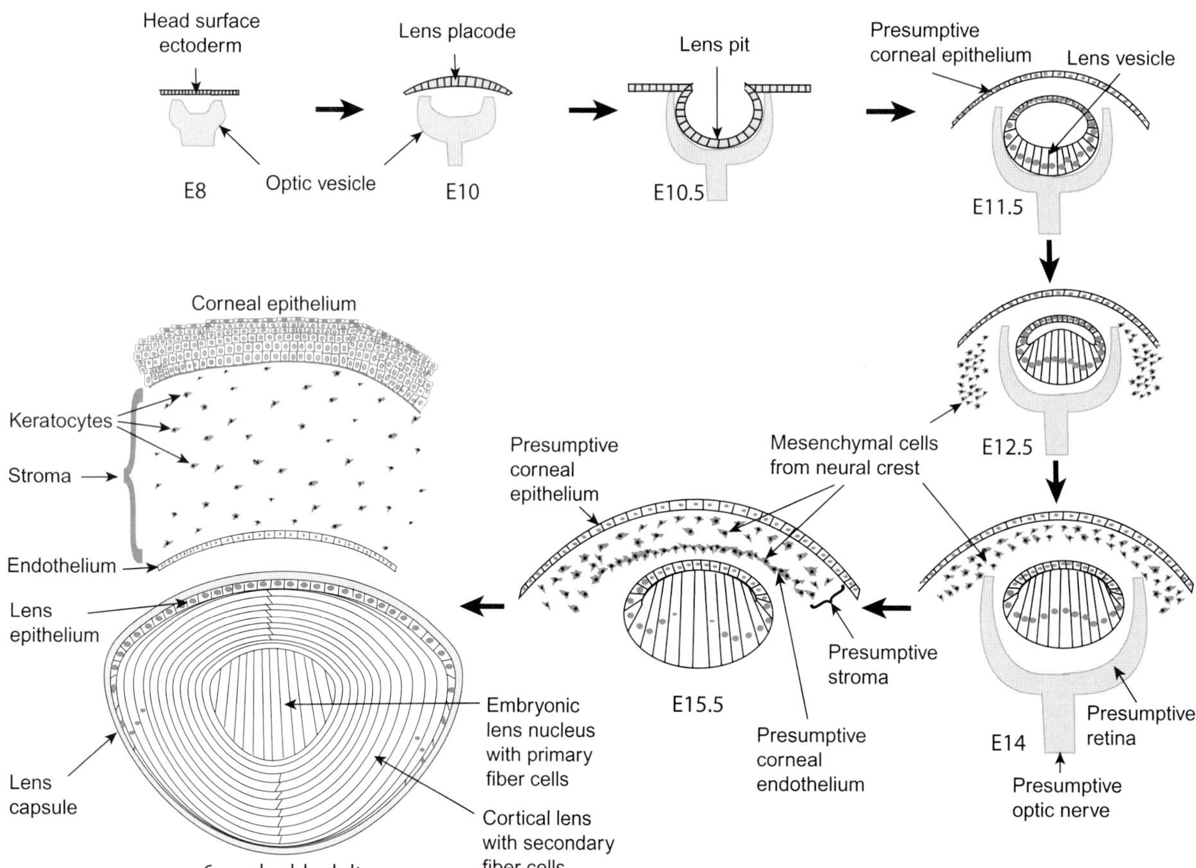

FIGURE 57.1 Schematic overview of the developing mouse eye. Progressive steps in the development of mouse eye at different embryonic days (E8, E10, . . .) and the 6-week-old adult lens and cornea are illustrated. Illustrations are not drawn to scale.

Large-scale analyses of gene expression in the cornea and lens

The basal layer of limbal epithelium between the cornea and the conjunctiva is enriched in stem cells that give rise to transient amplifying cells that migrate to the central corneal epithelium and become the basal epithelial cells. Laser capture microdissection followed by microarray analysis identified about 100 differentially expressed genes in limbal compared to corneal epithelial basal cells (Zhou et al., 2006). In another study, comparison of the rat limbal and central corneal transcripts by serial analysis of gene expression (SAGE) identified 759 transcripts specific for the limbus and 844 transcripts specific for the central cornea, with 2,292 transcripts present in both (Adachi et al., 2006). Comparison of PN9 and 6-week-old adult mouse corneas by SAGE demonstrated dynamic changes in gene expression during postnatal corneal maturation (Norman et al., 2004). Roughly one-third of the transcripts expressed in the cornea are present exclusively in the PN9 or mature corneas, and the remaining one-third are expressed at both stages. Abundantly expressed transcripts in the cornea are associated with diverse functions such as metabolism, redox activities, and barrier integrity (Norman et al., 2004).

In the lens, younger and transcriptionally active differentiating cells envelop a core of mature fiber cells lacking nuclei and cytoplasmic organelles. Microarray comparison of gene expression profiles of young elongating and mature fiber cells captured by laser microdissection identified 65 differentially expressed genes important for lens cell differentiation (Ivanov et al., 2005). In humans, the expression of as many as 1,196 transcripts is elevated and the expression of 1,278 transcripts is decreased by twofold or more in lens epithelial cells compared to cortical fiber cells (Hawse et al., 2005). These gene expression changes correspond to distinct pathways and functions important for the formation of lens fiber cells.

Endogenous noncoding microRNAs (miRNAs) inhibit the translation and affect the stability of target mRNAs, and thus have a role in the regulation of development and differentiation (Kloosterman and Plasterk, 2006). Studies of miRNAs in the eye are just beginning. So far, several miRNAs expressed in a distinct tissue- and cell-type-specific manner in different tissues of the eye have been detected using miRNA microarrays (Ryan et al., 2006). MiRNA (mir)-184, one of the abundant miRNAs in cornea and lens, is expressed in the corneal epithelium and in the lens germinative zone epithelial cells. Mir-205 is widely expressed in the anterior segment epithelia and epidermis (Ryan et al., 2006). Specific functions of these miRNAs are not known yet.

Transcription factors involved in the development of cornea and lens

Studies employing transgenic mice and targeted deletion of genes helped accumulate useful information about the network of transcription factors influencing the development of cornea and lens (figure 57.2). Here we briefly review the contribution of different transcription factors to the development of cornea and lens.

Homeobox Transcription Factors Homeobox-containing transcription factors have received preferential attention in studies on gene regulation during eye development, in view of their critical contribution. As indicated in the following discussion, in addition to their developmental roles, the homeobox transcription factors are also important regulators of crystallin gene expression.

Pax6. Pax6, a paired domain-homeobox transcription factor, is essential for the inductive interactions between the neuroectoderm and the surface ectoderm during early embryonic eye development (see figure 57.2) (Simpson and Price, 2002). Of historical interest, the importance of *Pax6* for eye development was first noted in *Drosophila*, where its homologue is known as *eyeless* (Gehring, 2004). In humans, mutations in PAX6 result in severe eye defects (Graw, 2003; Hanson, 2003; Hanson et al., 1994). Homozygous *Pax6* mutant mice develop only rudiments of the optic vesicle and die in the neonatal stage (Hogan et al., 1988). In heterozygotes, lens placode formation is delayed, resulting in a smaller lens with vacuolated fiber cells, frequently fused to

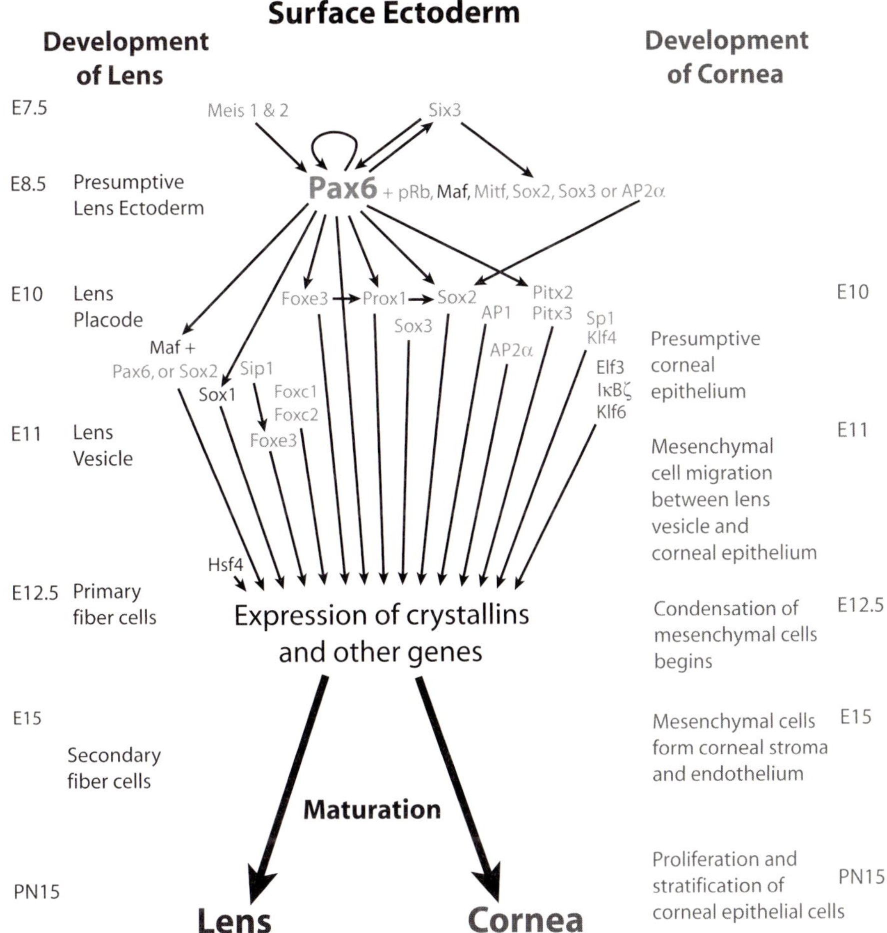

Figure 57.2 Transcription factors regulating the development of mouse lens and cornea. The network of transcription factors regulating the development of lens (red), or cornea (blue), or both (green) is shown, along with the embryonic age and the developmental stages of lens and cornea. Many of these transcription factors remain active in the mature lens and cornea. See color plate 66.

the cornea, resembling Peter's anomaly (Collinson et al., 2001). In the mouse, *Pax6* expression, first detected at E8 at the optic pit, head surface ectoderm, and neural ectoderm, is restricted to the lens placode, optic vesicle, and stalk at E9.5. After E13.5, *Pax6* is expressed in the proliferating anterior epithelial cells of the lens vesicle and the surface ectoderm, which gives rise to cornea, conjunctiva, and eyelids. In the adult mouse, *Pax6* is expressed in the lens epithelial cells, cornea, conjunctiva, iris, ciliary body, and retina (Koroma et al., 1997). Homeobox transcription factors Meis1 and Meis2, expressed in a pattern similar to Pax6, directly regulate *Pax6* expression in presumptive lens ectoderm by binding the *Pax6* lens placode enhancer (see figure 57.2) (Zhang et al., 2002).

Pax6 upregulates its own expression and influences eye development both directly, by controlling different genes encoding structural proteins required for eye formation, and indirectly, by controlling a number of genes encoding developmental transcription factors, including Six3, c-Maf, MafA/L-Maf, Prox1, Sox2, and FoxE3 (see figure 57.2) (Aota et al., 2003; Ashery-Padan et al., 2000; Brownell et al., 2000; Chauhan et al., 2002; Cvekl and Tamm, 2004; Cvekl et al., 2004; Duncan et al., 2000; Furuta and Hogan, 1998; Marquardt et al., 2001). Pax6 is autonomously required for formation of corneal epithelium, stroma, and endothelium between E10.5 and E16.5 (Collinson et al., 2003; Davis et al., 2003). The corneal epithelium in the heterozygous *Pax6* (*Small eye, Sey*) mouse is thinner, with a reduced number of cell layers, despite increased cell proliferation. The levels of desmoglein, β-catenin, γ-catenin, and the intermediate filament keratin-12 are reduced in the *Sey* cornea, suggesting defective intercellular adhesion (Davis et al., 2003), an idea supported by a recent report showing that *Pax6* heterozygote corneal epithelial cells have multiple glycoconjugate defects on the cell surface that restrict their ability to initiate migration in response to wound healing (Kucerova et al., 2006). Corneal epithelial cell proliferation is inhibited on overexpression of *Pax6* (Ouyang et al., 2006). The distribution of neural crest–derived cells is abnormal in *Sey* mouse from early developmental stages to the adult, indicating that normal distribution and integration of neural crest–derived cells depend on a proper dosage of Pax6 (Kanakubo et al., 2006).

Pax6 is actively involved in the repair and maintenance of the adult corneal surface. During corneal wound healing, the amount of Pax6 increases at the migrating front of the resurfacing corneal epithelium, where it upregulates matrix metalloproteinase gelatinase B (gelB; MMP-9). Two Pax6-binding sites exist within the gelB −522/+19 bp promoter fragment, which contains the necessary *cis*- elements for appropriate expression (Sivak et al., 2000). Pax6 paired domain controls the gelB promoter activity by interacting directly with one of these sites, and indirectly with the other site, through cooperative interactions with AP2α. A reduced Pax6 dosage in heterozygous *Sey* mice results in a loss of *gelB* expression at the migrating epithelial front, which correlates with an increase in inflammation (Sivak et al., 2004).

Pax6 influences target gene expression both independently and in association with other transcription factors such as pRb, MafA, MitF, Sox2, and Sox3 in a cooperative manner (see figure 57.2). Sox2 and Sox3 interact with Pax6, leading to synergistic transcriptional activation (Aota et al., 2003). In the lens, both *αA*- and *αB-crystallin* genes are upregulated (Cvekl and Piatigorsky, 1996; Cvekl et al., 1994, 1995; Gopal-Srivastava et al., 1996; Haynes et al., 1996), and *βB1-crystallin* (Duncan et al., 1998) and *γ-crystallin* (Yang et al., 2004) genes are downregulated by Pax6. Unlike the synergistic activation of *αB-crystallin* by Pax6 and c-Maf, Pax6 has no effect on c-Maf-mediated αA-crystallin promoter activation (Yang et al., 2004). Compound heterozygous mice with mutations in both *Pax6* and *Gli3*, a zinc finger transcription factor gene expressed in the embryonic eye, develop more extensive abnormalities in the retina, iris, lens, and cornea than do single *Gli3+/−* or *Pax6+/−* mutants (Zaki et al., 2006). The requirement for a normal *Gli3* gene dosage is greater in the absence of normal *Pax6* gene dosage, suggesting that these two transcription factors cooperate during eye morphogenesis.

Six3. Six3, a Six domain containing homeobox transcription factor, is expressed in the anterior neural ectoderm at E7, developing retinal field at E8, and head ectoderm that forms the lens placode at E9 in the mouse (Lagutin et al., 2001; Oliver et al., 1995). After E9, Pax6 and Six3, expressed in an overlapping manner, regulate the expression of each other (see figure 57.2) (Goudreau et al., 2002). Conditional deletion of mouse *Six3* in the presumptive lens ectoderm disrupts lens induction, resulting in the absence of the lens placode and lens in severe cases. Six3 influences eye development directly, by regulating the expression of structural and metabolic genes required for eye formation, and indirectly, by activating the expression of Pax6 in the lens preplacodal ectoderm (see figure 57.2) (Liu et al., 2006).

Prox1. Another well-conserved homeobox transcription factor influencing lens fiber cell elongation in the lens vesicle is Prox1 (see figure 57.2). Prox1 is expressed in the mouse at E9.5 in the lens placode, at E10.5 in the lens vesicle, and at E12.5 onward in the anterior epithelium, lens fiber cells, and surface ectoderm (Tomarev et al., 1998). Homozygous *Prox1* null mice, which die around E14.5, show defective fiber cell elongation, abnormal cellular proliferation, downregulated expression of the cell cycle inhibitors Cdkn1b (p27KIP1) and Cdkn1c (p57KIP2), misexpression of E-cadherin, inappropriate apoptosis, and absence of *γD*- and *γB-crystallin* expression (Wigle and Oliver, 1999). As the mutant lens cells fail to polarize and elongate properly, a hollow lens is formed. Prox1 binds and activates the mouse γD-crystallin promoter in vitro (Lengler et al., 2001).

POU homeodomain transcription factors. Bicoid-related POU homeodomain transcription factors Pitx2 and Pitx3 also regulate eye development (see figure 57.2). Deletion of *Pitx2*, normally expressed in the neural crest– and the mesoderm-derived precursors of the periocular mesenchyme, results in severe disruption of periocular mesenchyme structures and extrinsic defects in early optic nerve development. Studies with neural crest–specific *Pitx2* null mice (*Pitx2*-ncko) indicate that *Pitx2* is required in neural crest for specification of the corneal endothelium and stroma and the sclera (Evans and Gage, 2005). Central corneal thickness is reduced in heterozygous *Pitx2* mutant mice (Asai-Coakwell et al., 2006). Overexpression of Pitx2a isoform in the mouse corneal mesenchyme and iris lead to corneal opacification, corneal hypertrophy, irido-corneal adhesions, and severely degenerated retina resembling glaucoma and Axenfeld-Rieger syndrome (Homberg et al., 2004). In humans, PITX2 or FOXC1 mutations account for up to 50% of the Axenfeld-Rieger malformations of the anterior segment (Graw, 2003).

Mutations in *Pitx3*, normally expressed from E10 in the thickening lens placode and later in the lens vesicle, are responsible for the *aphakia* mutant mice in which lens differentiation is affected after E11 (Semina et al., 1997, 2000). In humans, PITX3 mutations lead to posterior polar cataract and variable anterior segment mesenchymal dysgenesis (Addison et al., 2005; Semina et al., 1998).

Sip1. Sip1, a Smad-interacting zinc-finger homeodomain transcription factor, is expressed after lens placode induction in the lens epithelium and immature lens fibers of the bow region (Yoshimoto et al., 2005). Conditional deletion of *Sip1* in the lens results in a small hollow lens connected to the surface ectoderm (Yoshimoto et al., 2005). Sip1 is required for lens fiber cell maturation, and γ-crystallin, a marker for mature fiber cells, is absent in the *Sip1* null lenses (Yoshimoto et al., 2005). Sip1 activates *Foxe3* expression in a Smad-binding domain–dependent manner in the lens (Yoshimoto et al., 2005).

Non-homeobox Transcription Factors Regulating the Development of Lens and Cornea

High mobility group transcription factors Sox1 and Sox2. Sox transcription factors belonging to the high mobility group (HMG) family of DNA-binding proteins are involved in the regulation of diverse developmental processes. The targeted deletion of *Sox1* in mice causes microphthalmia and cataract (Nishiguchi et al., 1998). Mutant lens fiber cells fail to elongate and lack expression of γ-crystallins, as direct interaction of Sox1 protein with γ-crystallin promoters is required for their expression. Both Sox1 and Sox2 bind upstream lens enhancer elements in the mouse *αB-crystallin* gene (Ijichi et al., 2004). Transcription factors AP2, Pax6, and Prox1 upregulate *Sox2* gene expression (see figure 57.2) (Lengler et al., 2001).

Hmgn1. The nucleosome-binding HMG protein Hmgn1, capable of altering the structure and activity of chromatin, affects the development of the corneal epithelium in mice (Birger et al., 2006). *Hmgn1* null mice develop a thin, poorly stratified corneal epithelium depleted of suprabasal wing cells and a disorganized basement membrane. Epithelial cell–specific markers glutathione-S-transferase (GST)-α4 and -ω1 are reduced in *Hmgn1* null corneas, while the components of adherens junctions—E-cadherin and α-, β- and γ-catenin—are upregulated (Birger et al., 2006).

Winged helix-forkhead transcription factors. Human congenital primary aphakia, a rare developmental disorder characterized by microphthalmia, anterior segment dysgenesis, and in severe cases the complete absence of lens, is caused by null mutations in FOXE3, a winged helix-forkhead transcription factor (Valleix et al., 2006). In the mouse, mutations in *Foxe3* result in the dysgenetic lens (dyl) mutant strain that has several defects in lens development and altered patterns of crystallin expression (Blixt et al., 2007; Brownell et al., 2000; Medina-Martinez et al., 2005). Foxe3 is initially expressed in the developing brain and the lens placode and later restricted to the anterior lens epithelium in a Pax6- and Sip1-dependent manner, and is turned off on fiber cell differentiation (Yoshimoto et al., 2005). Targeted disruption of mouse *Foxe3* results in an abnormal eye with a small, vacuolated lens. The anterior lens epithelium and the cornea do not separate, forming an unusual, multilayered tissue. These defects in lens development are accompanied by changes in the expression of DNase II-like acid DNase, Prox1, p57, and PDGF-α receptor (Blixt et al., 2007; Medina-Martinez et al., 2005).

Two other forkhead transcription factors, Foxc1 (Mf1) and Foxc2 (Mfh1), have nearly identical DNA binding domains, and largely overlapping expression patterns and functions in the developing eye (Hiemisch et al., 1998; Smith et al., 2000). *Foxc1*, expressed in the mesenchymal cells in the eye (Kidson et al., 1999; Kume et al., 1998), is restricted to the future trabecular meshwork by E16.5 (Kidson et al., 1999). *Foxc1* null mice die at birth with multiple abnormalities, including severe anterior segment developmental defects, such as fused lens and cornea, a thickened corneal epithelium, disorganized stroma, and missing endothelium (Hong et al., 1999; Kidson et al., 1999; Kume et al., 1998). *Foxc1* heterozygous mice are viable, with milder anterior segment defects (Hong et al., 1999; Smith et al., 2000). *Foxc1* and *Foxc2* double heterozygous mice have malformations of the ciliary body not seen in either heterozygous mouse alone (Smith et al., 2000). In humans, FOXC1 mutations cause anterior segment dysgenesis and glaucoma (Honkanen et al., 2003; Mears et al., 1998; Mirzayans et al., 2000; Nishimura et al., 1998).

Heat shock factor 4. The heat shock factors (HSFs) belonging to the basic domain/leucine zipper family of transcription factors consist of three members in mammals (Hsf1, 2, and 4). HSFs upregulate the stress-inducible promoters by interacting with the heat shock responsive elements. In the embryonic mouse lens, Hsf1 and Hsf2 are expressed at high levels. Their levels decrease in the adult lens, where Hsf4 takes over (Somasundaram and Bhat, 2004). αB-Crystallin promoter is upregulated by Hsf4, but not by Hsf1 or Hsf2 (Somasundaram and Bhat, 2004). *Hsf4* null mice show increased proliferation, premature, defective differentiation of the lens epithelial cells, and increased expression of growth factors FGF-1, FGF-4, and FGF-7, and develop early postnatal cataract with abnormal lens fiber cells containing inclusion-like structures (Fujimoto et al., 2004; Min et al., 2004). The human HSF4 locus is associated with autosomal recessive cataract (Smaoui et al., 2004) and autosomal dominant lamellar and Marner cataract (Bu et al., 2002).

Maf. Maf transcription factors belong to the basic domain/leucine zipper family whose consensus target site, T-MARE, is an extended version of an AP1 site. Three members of the large Maf family, c-Maf, MafB, and Nrl, are expressed in the mouse lens (Kawauchi et al., 1999). The expression of c-Maf is earliest and most prominent in lens fiber cells and persists throughout lens development (see figure 57.2) (Kawauchi et al., 1999; Ring et al., 2000). Homozygous *Maf* mutant embryos and newborns show defective lens fiber cell differentiation, with severely impaired expression of crystallin genes. Posterior lens cells in *Maf(lacZ)* mutant mice do not elongate, do not express *αA*- and any of the *β-crystallin* genes, and display inappropriately high levels of DNA synthesis at E11.5 (Kawauchi et al., 1999; Kim et al., 1999; Ring et al., 2000). Maf interacts with Pax6 and Sox to synergistically upregulate the mouse αB-crystallin and γF-crystallin promoter activities, respectively (see figure 57.2) (Rajaram and Kerppola, 2004; Yang et al., 2004). Synergistic activation of these promoters by Maf and Sox and their subnuclear localization are disrupted by a mutation in Maf that causes cataract (Rajaram and Kerppola, 2004).

Sp1/Krüppel-like transcription factors. Many Sp1/Krüppel-like transcription factors, members of the zinc finger family of DNA binding proteins, are expressed in the ocular surface and lens (see figure 57.2) (Chiambaretta et al., 2004; Norman et al., 2004). Expression of Sp1 in the ectoderm and lens vesicle at E11 is much lower than that in the cornea from E15.5 to late stages (Nakamura et al., 2005). Sp1 levels in the cornea decline gradually following eyelid opening. Evidence for the involvement of Sp1 in the regulation of corneal gene expression comes from the finding that Sp1 activates *involucrin* gene expression in the differentiating corneal epithelium (Adhikary et al., 2005b).

Expression of Krüppel-like transcription factor Klf4, one of the most highly expressed transcription factors in the mouse cornea (Norman et al., 2004), is detectable in the ocular surface from around E10 and is sustained in the adult cornea (see figure 57.2). Conditional deletion of *Klf4* in the surface ectoderm-derived structures of the eye leads to fragile corneal epithelium, swollen, vacuolated basal epithelial and endothelial cells, vacuolated lens, edematous stroma, and loss of conjunctival goblet cells (Swamynathan et al., 2007). Klf4 binds and activates keratin-12 and aquaporin-5 promoters in the corneal epithelium (Swamynathan et al., 2007). Klf4 cooperates with Oct3/4 and Sox2 and acts as a mediating factor that specifically binds to the proximal element to activate the Lefty1 core promoter in embryonic stem cells (Nakatake et al., 2006). Pluripotent stem cells could be derived from mouse embryonic or adult fibroblasts by introducing four factors, Oct3/4, Sox2, c-Myc, and Klf4, under embryonic stem cell culture conditions (Takahashi and Yamanaka, 2006). As each of these factors is present in the corneal limbus, it is likely that they are involved in the maintenance of limbal stem cells, the source of epithelial cells in the mature cornea.

Another Krüppel-like factor, Klf6, is expressed in the lens pit at E10.5, in the ectoderm, mesenchyme, and the lens epithelium at E12.5, and in the lens and corneal epithelium and corneal stroma at E15.5 (Nakamura et al., 2004). Later on, the expression of Klf6 remains high in the cornea but decreases in the lens. In humans, expression of KLF6 is elevated in keratoconus, a progressive disease associated with thinning and scarring of the cornea (Chiambaretta et al., 2006). KLF6 binds and downregulates the *α1-proteinase inhibitor* (*α1-PI*) gene in corneal epithelial cells and may thereby be involved in keratoconus (Chiambaretta et al., 2006). Human KLF6 binds and activates keratin-12 promoter in cultured cells (Chiambaretta et al., 2002).

I-κB-ζ. I-κB-ζ, a regulator of the transcription factor NF-κB, is expressed in the ocular surface epithelium, a part of the mucosal defense system (see figure 57.2) (Ueta et al., 2005). I-κB-ζ negatively regulates the pathological progression of ocular surface inflammation (Ueta et al., 2005). *I-κB-ζ* null mouse ocular surface shows chronic inflammation accompanied by loss of conjunctival goblet cells, indicating that I-κB-ζ is an integral part of the network of transcription factors required for ocular surface development (Ueta et al., 2005).

AP1. AP1, a group of dimeric complexes formed by the various Jun, Fos, Fra, and ATF proteins that regulate cell proliferation in response to various stimuli, is expressed in the lens and cornea (see figure 57.2) (Adhikary et al., 2005a; Ilagan et al., 1999; Norman et al., 2004; Okada et al., 2003; Shirai et al., 2004). AP1 activates mouse *αA-crystallin* expression through the conserved +25/+32 bp AP1 binding site (Ilagan et al., 1999). AP1 is necessary for expression of involucrin, a structural protein that is selectively expressed in differentiating corneal epithelial cells (Adhikary et al., 2005a, 2005b). In transgenic mice, removal of the AP1 site by truncation or point mutation results in a loss of *involucrin* expression, confirming the importance of AP1 for involucrin promoter activity during corneal epithelial cell differentiation.

AP2. The activating protein-2 (AP2) family of transcription factors, consisting of five different members, AP2α, AP2β, AP2γ, AP2δ, and AP2ε, stimulates proliferation and suppresses terminal differentiation in a cell-type-specific manner during embryonic development (Eckert et al., 2005). AP2α is expressed in the lens and corneal epithelium (see figure 57.2) (Ohtaka-Maruyama et al., 1998; West-Mays et al., 1999, 2003). *Ap2α* null embryos exhibit a range of phenotypes from a complete lack of eyes to defective lens attached to the overlying surface ectoderm (West-Mays et al., 1999). Conditional deletion of *Ap2α* in lens placode derivatives, including the corneal epithelium, results in a decrease in the expression of the cell-cell adhesion molecule E-cadherin, misexpression of laminin, entactin, and type IV collagen, and disruption of stromal collagen fibril organization, showing that AP2α is required for proper formation of the mouse cornea (Dwivedi et al., 2005; West-Mays et al., 2003). Pax6 and AP2α interact with each other and coordinate the expression of gelatinase-B (matrix metalloproteinase 9) and corneal epithelial repair (Sivak et al., 2004).

Elf3. Ese-1/Elf3, an epithelium-specific transcription factor, is upregulated in differentiating mouse corneal epithelium and in immortalized human corneal epithelial cells (HCEs), and transactivates *keratin-12* through Ets binding sites (Yoshida et al., 2000). Suppression of Ese-1/Elf3 by antisense RNA in HCE cells affects their differentiation, suggesting the involvement of Ese-1/Elf3 in differentiation of corneal epithelial cells (see figure 57.2).

Regulation of expression of specific genes in the lens and cornea

Crystallin Gene Expression in the Lens Differentiation of the lens is characterized by lens-preferred expression and accumulation of water-soluble crystallins, essential lens structural proteins required for light refraction and transparency (Piatigorsky, 1998; Piatigorsky and Wistow, 1989). Much effort in the last two decades shows that the lens-preferred expression of crystallins is an outcome of synergistic interactions between developmentally regulated transcription factors such as Pax6, c-Maf, MafA/L-Maf, MafB, Nrl, Sox1, Sox2, Rarβ/Rxrβ, Prox1, Six3, and Hsf4, ubiquitously expressed factors such as AP1, Creb, pRb, and Usf, and chromatin remodeling proteins such as Asc-2 and Cbp/p300 (figure 57.3) (Cvekl and Piatigorsky, 1996; Cvekl and Tamm, 2004; Cvekl et al., 2004).

αA-Crystallin. Mouse αA-crystallin, a marker of lens fiber cell differentiation and one of the most abundant mouse lens crystallins, is expressed at high levels in the developing lens, beginning around E10.5, and continuing in the adult lens (Robinson and Overbeek, 1996; Wawrousek et al., 1990). The mouse αA-crystallin promoter contains a Maf responsive element (MARE) at −110/−98 bp position, and overlapping binding sites for αACryBP1/PrdII/Mbp-1 (Brady et al., 1995; Kantorow et al., 1993; Nakamura et al., 1990), Maf (Wawrousek et al., 1990; Yang and Cvekl, 2005), and Pax6 (Cvekl et al., 1995) at −88 to +46 bp position (see figure 57.3). Pax6 and c-Maf activate *αA-crystallin* moderately and strongly, respectively, in a nonsynergistic manner (Yang and Cvekl, 2005; Yang et al., 2004, 2006).

Three conserved distal control regions (DCR1, −7706/−7492 bp; DCR2, −1900/−1670 bp; DCR3, +3650/+3856 bp) regulate mouse αA-crystallin promoter activity (see figure 57.3) (Yang et al., 2004). DCR1, bound by Pax6, stimulates αA-crystallin promoter activity in primary lens explants. DCR1/DCR2/αA-crystallin promoter activity resembles the native αA-crystallin promoter activity in lens epithelium and fiber cells. In contrast, the DCR3/αA-crystallin promoter activity is restricted to late lens fibers (Yang et al., 2004, 2006). Pax6, c-Maf, and CREB recruit chromatin-remodeling enzymes such as Brg1, Snf2h, CBP, and/or p300, thereby leading to localized histone acetylation and upregulation of *αA-crystallin* gene expression (Chen et al., 2002; Yang et al., 2006).

αB-Crystallin. Expression of αB-crystallin, a member of the small heat shock protein (sHSP) family, begins in the lens placode at E10 and continues at high levels in the lens epithelium and the lens fibers, and in moderate levels in many tissues (Haynes et al., 1996; Iwaki et al., 1989). A skeletal muscle–preferred, orientation-dependent enhancer containing five distinct *cis*-acting regulatory elements (αBE-1, αBE-4 αBE-2, αBE-3, and MRF, an E box) is present at −427/−259 bp position (see figure 57.3) (Gopal-Srivastava and Piatigorsky, 1993; Gopal-Srivastava et al., 1995; Swamynathan and Piatigorsky, 2002). The −426/+44 bp, −339/+44 bp, and −164/+44 bp promoter fragments retain activity in the lens as well as corneal epithelium, indicating

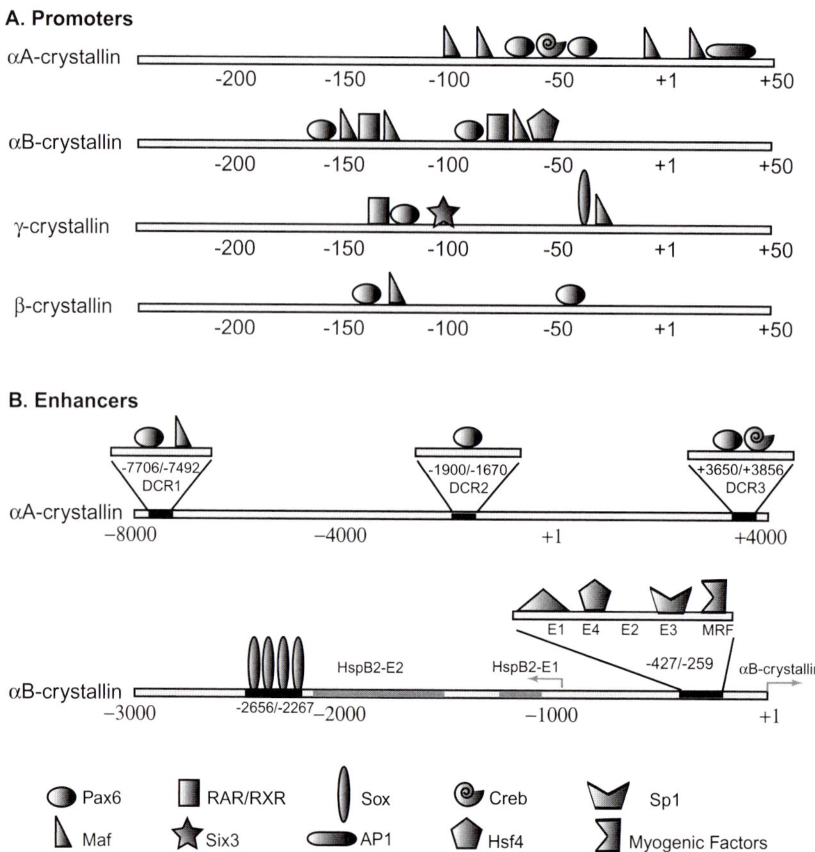

FIGURE 57.3 Organization of different transcription factor binding sites on crystallin promoters (*A*) and enhancers (*B*). Note the use of similar transcription factor binding sites on diverse crystallin promoters. DCR, distal control region. DNA fragments are not drawn to scale.

that the αB-crystallin enhancer is not required for basal promoter activity in the lens and cornea (Gopal-Srivastava et al., 2000). Another well-conserved lens-specific enhancer (−2656/−2267 bp) containing four putative Sox1- and Sox2-binding sites activates the αB-crystallin promoter, even though the *HspB2* gene is located in between this enhancer and the αB-crystallin promoter (see figure 57.3) (Ijichi et al., 2004).

Two well-conserved lens-specificity regions, LSR1 (−147/−118 bp) and LSR2 (−78/−46 bp), are bound by Pax6, Maf, and RARs and are required for the lens activity of the mouse αB-crystallin promoter (see figure 57.3) (Gopal-Srivastava et al., 1996; Yang et al., 2004). The −164/+44 bp and −115/+44 bp mouse αB-crystallin promoter activities are lens specific in transgenic mice, although the average activity is 30 times lower for the shorter fragment lacking LSR1. Site-specific mutation of LSR1 eliminates both Pax6 binding and the −164/+44 bp promoter activity in transgenic mice (Gopal-Srivastava et al., 1996). Pax6-mediated activation of the αB-crystallin −162/+45 bp promoter is more robust in association with any of the Mafs and RARβ/RXRβ (Yang et al., 2004).

β- and γ-Crystallins. β- and γ-crystallins are expressed in a lens fiber cell–specific manner. Several *cis*-elements required for lens-specific expression of the βB1-crystallin promoter have been identified by phylogenetic footprinting of the 5′ flanking sequence of the mouse, rat, human, and chicken *βB1-crystallin* genes (see figure 57.3) (Chen et al., 2001). The mouse *βB1-crystallin −1493/+44 CAT* transgene is expressed in the lens fiber cells (Chen et al., 2001). Transcription factor c-Maf directly activates many *β-crystallin* genes (see figure 57.3) (Ring et al., 2000).

Mutations in γ-crystallins lead to many dominant inherited cataracts in humans and mice (Garber et al., 1985; Graw, 1999). Sox1 binds a conserved element in the γ-crystallin promoter, and targeted deletion of *Sox1* causes reduced *γ-crystallin* expression, impaired fiber cell elongation, microphthalmia, and cataract (Nishiguchi et al., 1998). The heat shock factor HSF4 supports *γF-crystallin* expression in the lens fiber cells (Fujimoto et al., 2004). Pax6 represses the activation of the γF-crystallin promoter by large Mafs, Sox, and RARβ/RXRβ proteins in transiently transfected lens cells (Yang et al., 2004).

GENE EXPRESSION IN THE CORNEA Unlike the lens, where a large body of work has focused on understanding the regulation of a handful of crystallin genes, in the cornea there is a limited amount of work, spread among different genes.

Keratocan. Keratocan (Ktcn), a keratan sulfate proteoglycan of the extracellular matrix, is first expressed at E13.5 in the periocular mesenchymal cells and after E14.5 is restricted to the stromal keratocytes (Liu et al., 1998). In adult transgenic mice with *β-geo* transgene driven by 3.2 kb 5′ flanking sequence, exon 1 and 0.4 kb of intron 1 of *Ktcn*, β-Gal activity is detected only in cornea. Spatiotemporal expression patterns of the −3.2 kb fragment transgene recapitulate that of endogenous *Ktcn*, suggesting that the 3.2 kb *Ktcn* upstream sequence contains the necessary *cis*-elements to regulate *keratocan* gene expression (Liu et al., 2000).

Keratins. Keratin-12 (Krt12), one of the more than 30 different keratins (intermediate filament components), each with a specific expression pattern in different epithelial cells, is expressed specifically in the stratified corneal epithelium (Tanifuji-Terai et al., 2006). Heterozygous mutations in KRT12 cause Meesmann corneal dystrophy, an autosomal dominant disorder affecting the human corneal epithelium. *Krt12* null mice develop fragile corneal epithelium resembling Meesmann corneal dystrophy (Kao et al., 1996). During embryonic development, Krt12 expression is restricted to the suprabasal and/or superficial cells of the corneal epithelium from E15.5 to P10 in mice. After PN30, *Krt12* expression is detected sporadically in the basal corneal epithelium, and the number of Krt12-positive basal cells increases as the mice grow older (Tanifuji-Terai et al., 2006). Pax6, KLF4, and KLF6 stimulate Krt12 promoter activity (Liu et al., 1999). Expression of *Krt12* is delayed and down-regulated in the *Pax6+/−* corneal epithelium, implying abnormal differentiation (Ramaesh et al., 2005).

Corneal crystallins. An underlying assumption in many gene regulation–related studies is that gene expression is controlled mainly at the level of transcription. However, post-transcriptional regulation may play a significant role in the expression of abundant corneal crystallins aldehyde dehydrogenase IIIA1 (Aldh3a1) and transketolase (Tkt), which constitute roughly 50% and 10% of the water-soluble protein, respectively, and only about 1% each of the total mRNA in the adult cornea (Norman et al., 2004). *Aldh3a1* expression in the mouse is at least 500-fold higher in the corneal epithelial cells than in other tissues (Kays and Piatigorsky, 1997). In transgenic mice, a 13 kb mouse Aldh3a1 promoter fragment is active selectively in tissues that express the endogenous *Aldh3a1* gene; however, unlike the promoter activity of the endogenous wild-type gene, the promoter activity of the 13 kb fragment in the transgene is higher in the stomach and bladder than in the cornea. By contrast, a 4.4 kb mouse Aldh3a1 promoter fragment drives transgene expression in transgenic mice specifically in the corneal epithelial cells and not in other tissues, indicating that *cis*-control elements for corneal promoter activity reside within this smaller DNA fragment (Kays and Piatigorsky, 1997). Current experiments indicate that Aldh3a1 promoter activity is controlled by transcription factors that also control lens crystallin genes (Pax6, Oct1) as well as additional transcription factors expressed highly in the cornea (KLF4, KLF5). In addition, a suppressor sequence resides in the first intron of the mouse *Aldh3a1* gene, although it is not known at present how it might function in regulating endogenous gene expression (Davis et al., in press).

Another mouse corneal crystallin is Tkt, which is expressed at 30–50 times higher levels in the mature mouse cornea than in other tissues (Sax et al., 1996). Tkt mRNA levels increase six-fold in the mouse cornea in vivo within 1–2 days of eye opening. Both exposure to light and oxidative stresses appear to play a role in the up-regulation of *Tkt* gene expression after eye opening and during corneal maturation (Sax et al., 2000). The *Tkt* gene contains two transcription initiation sites separated by 630 bp, with a common initiator ATG codon (West-Mays et al., 1999). The distal transcription initiation site is used weakly in liver and the proximal GC-rich transcription initiation site (within intron 1) lacking a TATA box is used in the liver and for high corneal expression. There is little knowledge yet of the molecular basis for the high expression of *Tkt* in the mouse cornea.

Concluding remarks

The studies summarized in this chapter indicate that the mouse lens and cornea utilize many similar transcription factors for their development and maintenance. One of the striking similarities in gene expression in these two tissues is that many (not all) of these developmental transcription factors are also employed to express their highly specific multifunctional proteins, the crystallins. In view of the similarities between lens and cornea in their (1) origin from ectodermal cells during embryogenesis, (2) utilization of common transcription factors during embryonic development and postnatal maturation, (3) accumulation of crystallins, and (4) optical function, it has been proposed that the cornea and lens be considered as a single unit called the refracton (Piatigorsky, 2001). The refracton concept is not meant to equate the needs for and extents of refraction served by the lens and/or cornea of different species, both of which may differ considerably among species (especially aquatic versus terrestrial species) or even within the same species at different developmental times (such as an aquatic larva and terrestrial vertebrate, i.e., a toad) or at different behavioral times (such as an amphibious species in water or land, i.e., a frog or penguin). Rather, unifying the lens and cornea as the refracton underlines the numerous developmental and functional similarities of these two transparent eye structures, including especially the accumulation of taxon-specific, soluble proteins called collectively the lens or corneal crystallins, respectively. It is our hope that the refracton concept will stimulate cross-fertilization of ideas and knowledge concerning these refractive tissues of the eye by increasing dialogue and information exchange between basic scientists and clinicians presently specializing in the lens or the cornea.

We have witnessed substantial progress in our understanding of gene expression and its consequences for the development of the cornea and lens in the recent past. Many studies have utilized germ-line deletions or conditional inactivation of specific genes in the surface ectoderm–derived tissues of the eye. Improvements in our ability to delete or mutate specific genes in a spatiotemporally controlled manner will further aid this effort. We can look forward to the identification of additional roles for the transcription factors currently known to influence eye development, as well as to the discovery of novel transcription factors and new interactions among the transcription factors, in our quest to unravel the molecular basis, biological consequences, and medical implications of gene expression in the lens and cornea.

ACKNOWLEDGMENTS Work was supported by the intramural research program of the National Eye Institute, NIH. We are grateful to Dr. Janine Davis for a critical reading of the manuscript.

REFERENCES

Adachi, W., Ulanovsky, H., Li, Y., Norman, B., Davis, J., and Piatigorsky, J. (2006). Serial analysis of gene expression (SAGE) in the rat limbal and central corneal epithelium. *Invest. Ophthalmol. Vis. Sci.* 47:3801–3810.

Addison, P. K., Berry, V., Ionides, A. C., Francis, P. J., Bhattacharya, S. S., and Moore, A. T. (2005). Posterior polar cataract is the predominant consequence of a recurrent mutation in the PITX3 gene. *Br. J. Ophthalmol.* 89:138–141.

Adhikary, G., Crish, J. F., Bone, F., Gopalakrishnan, R., Lass, J., and Eckert, R. L. (2005a). An involucrin promoter AP1 transcription factor binding site is required for expression of involucrin in the corneal epithelium in vivo. *Invest. Ophthalmol. Vis. Sci.* 46:1219–1227.

Adhikary, G., Crish, J. F., Gopalakrishnan, R., Bone, F., and Eckert, R. L. (2005b). Involucrin expression in the corneal epithelium: An essential role for Sp1 transcription factors. *Invest. Ophthalmol. Vis. Sci.* 46:3109–3120.

Aota, S., Nakajima, N., Sakamoto, R., Watanabe, S., Ibaraki, N., and Okazaki, K. (2003). Pax6 autoregulation mediated by direct interaction of Pax6 protein with the head surface ectoderm-specific enhancer of the mouse Pax6 gene. *Dev. Biol.* 257:1–13.

Asai-Coakwell, M., Backhouse, C., Casey, R. J., Gage, P. J., and Lehmann, O. J. (2006). Reduced human and murine corneal thickness in an Axenfeld-Rieger syndrome subtype. *Invest. Ophthalmol. Vis. Sci.* 47:4905–4909.

Ashery-Padan, R., Marquardt, T., Zhou, X., and Gruss, P. (2000). Pax6 activity in the lens primordium is required for lens formation and for correct placement of a single retina in the eye. *Genes Dev.* 14:2701–2711.

Birger, Y., Davis, J., Furusawa, T., Rand, E., Piatigorsky, J., and Bustin, M. (2006). A role for chromosomal protein HMGN1 in corneal maturation. *Differentiation* 74:19–29.

Blixt, A., Landgren, H., Johansson, B. R., and Carlsson, P. (2007). Foxe3 is required for morphogenesis and differentiation of the anterior segment of the eye and is sensitive to Pax6 gene dosage. *Dev. Biol.* 302:218–229.

Bloemendal, H., and de Jong, W. W. (1991). Lens proteins and their genes. *Prog. Nucleic Acid Res. Mol. Biol.* 41:259–281.

Brady, J. P., Kantorow, M., Sax, C. M., Donovan, D. M., and Piatigorsky, J. (1995). Murine transcription factor alpha A-crystallin binding protein I. Complete sequence, gene structure, expression, and functional inhibition via antisense RNA. *J. Biol. Chem.* 270:1221–1229.

Brownell, I., Dirksen, M., and Jamrich, M. (2000). Forkhead Foxe3 maps to the dysgenetic lens locus and is critical in lens development and differentiation. *Genesis* 27:81–93.

Bu, L., Jin, Y., Shi, Y., Chu, R., Ban, A., Eiberg, H., Andres, L., Jiang, H., Zheng, G., et al. (2002). Mutant DNA-binding domain of HSF4 is associated with autosomal dominant lamellar and Marner cataract. *Nat. Genet.* 31:276–278.

Chauhan, B. K., Reed, N. A., Yang, Y., Cermak, L., Reneker, L., Duncan, M. K., and Cvekl, A. (2002). A comparative cDNA microarray analysis reveals a spectrum of genes regulated by Pax6 in mouse lens. *Genes Cells* 7:1267–1283.

Chen, Q., Dowhan, D. H., Liang, D., Moore, D. D., and Overbeek, P. A. (2002). CREB-binding protein/p300 co-activation of crystallin gene expression. *J. Biol. Chem.* 277: 24081–24089.

Chen, W. V., Fielding Hejtmancik, J., Piatigorsky, J., and Duncan, M. K. (2001). The mouse beta B1-crystallin promoter: Strict regulation of lens fiber cell specificity. *Biochim. Biophys. Acta.* 1519:30–38.

Chiambaretta, F., Blanchon, L., Rabier, B., Kao, W. W., Liu, J. J., Dastugue, B., Rigal, D., and Sapin, V. (2002). Regulation of corneal keratin-12 gene expression by the human Kruppel-like transcription factor 6. *Invest. Ophthalmol. Vis. Sci.* 43:3422–3429.

Chiambaretta, F., De Graeve, F., Turet, G., Marceau, G., Gain, P., Dastugue, B., Rigal, D., and Sapin, V. (2004). Cell and tissue specific expression of human Kruppel-like transcription factors in human ocular surface. *Mol. Vis.* 10:901–909.

Chiambaretta, F., Nakamura, H., De Graeve, F., Sakai, H., Marceau, G., Maruyama, Y., Rigal, D., Dastugue, B., Sugar, J., et al. (2006). Kruppel-like factor 6 (KLF6) affects the promoter activity of the alpha1-proteinase inhibitor gene. *Invest. Ophthalmol. Vis. Sci.* 47:582–590.

Chow, R. L., and Lang, R. A. (2001). Early eye development in vertebrates. *Annu. Rev. Cell. Dev. Biol.* 17:255–296.

Collinson, J. M., Morris, L., Reid, A. I., Ramaesh, T., Keighren, M. A., Flockhart, J. H., Hill, R. E., Tan, S. S., Ramaesh, K., et al. (2002). Clonal analysis of patterns of growth, stem cell activity, and cell movement during the development and maintenance of the murine corneal epithelium. *Dev. Dyn.* 224:432–440.

Collinson, J. M., Quinn, J. C., Buchanan, M. A., Kaufman, M. H., Wedden, S. E., West, J. D., and Hill, R. E. (2001). Primary defects in the lens underlie complex anterior segment abnormalities of the Pax6 heterozygous eye. *Proc. Natl. Acad. Sci. U.S.A.* 98:9688–9693.

Collinson, J. M., Quinn, J. C., Hill, R. E., and West, J. D. (2003). The roles of Pax6 in the cornea, retina, and olfactory epithelium of the developing mouse embryo. *Dev. Biol.* 255:303–312.

Cotsarelis, G., Cheng, S. Z., Dong, G., Sun, T. T., and Lavker, R. M. (1989). Existence of slow-cycling limbal epithelial basal cells that can be preferentially stimulated to proliferate: Implications on epithelial stem cells. *Cell* 57:201–209.

Cvekl, A., Kashanchi, F., Sax, C. M., Brady, J. N., and Piatigorsky, J. (1995). Transcriptional regulation of the mouse alpha A-crystallin gene: Activation dependent on a cyclic AMP-responsive element (DE1/CRE) and a Pax-6-binding site. *Mol. Cell. Biol.* 15:653–660.

Cvekl, A., and Piatigorsky, J. (1996). Lens development and crystallin gene expression: Many roles for Pax-6. *Bioessays* 18: 621–630.

Cvekl, A., Sax, C. M., Bresnick, E. H., and Piatigorsky, J. (1994). A complex array of positive and negative elements regulates the chicken alpha A-crystallin gene: Involvement of Pax-6, USF, CREB and/or CREM, and AP1 proteins. *Mol. Cell. Biol.* 14:7363–7376.

Cvekl, A., and Tamm, E. R. (2004). Anterior eye development and ocular mesenchyme: New insights from mouse models and human diseases. *Bioessays* 26:374–386.

Cvekl, A., Yang, Y., Chauhan, B. K., and Cveklova, K. (2004). Regulation of gene expression by Pax6 in ocular cells: A case of tissue-preferred expression of crystallins in lens. *Int. J. Dev. Biol.* 48:829–844.

Davis, J., Davis, D., Norman, B., and Piatigorsky, J. (in press). Synergistic activation of the corneal crystallin Aldh3a1 gene by Pax6, Oct-1, and p300: Shared transcriptional pathways in cornea and lens. *Invest. Ophthalmol. Vis. Sci.*

Davis, J., Duncan, M. K., Robison, W. G., Jr., and Piatigorsky, J. (2003). Requirement for Pax6 in corneal morphogenesis: A role in adhesion. *J. Cell. Sci.* 116:2157–2167.

Duncan, M. K., Cvekl, A., Li, X., and Piatigorsky, J. (2000). Truncated forms of Pax-6 disrupt lens morphology in transgenic mice. *Invest. Ophthalmol. Vis. Sci.* 41:464–473.

Duncan, M. K., Haynes, J. I., 2nd, Cvekl, A., and Piatigorsky, J. (1998). Dual roles for Pax-6: A transcriptional repressor of lens fiber cell-specific beta-crystallin genes. *Mol. Cell. Biol.* 18:5579–5586.

Dwivedi, D. J., Pontoriero, G. F., Ashery-Padan, R., Sullivan, S., Williams, T., and West-Mays, J. A. (2005). Targeted deletion of AP2alpha leads to disruption in corneal epithelial cell integrity and defects in the corneal stroma. *Invest. Ophthalmol. Vis. Sci.* 46:3623–3630.

Eckert, D., Buhl, S., Weber, S., Jager, R., and Schorle, H. (2005). The AP2 family of transcription factors. *Genome Biol.* 6:246.

Evans, A. L., and Gage, P. J. (2005). Expression of the homeobox gene Pitx2 in neural crest is required for optic stalk and ocular anterior segment development. *Hum. Mol. Genet.* 14:3347–3359.

Fujimoto, M., Izu, H., Seki, K., Fukuda, K., Nishida, T., Yamada, S., Kato, K., Yonemura, S., Inouye, S., et al. (2004). HSF4 is required for normal cell growth and differentiation during mouse lens development. *EMBO J.* 23:4297–4306.

Furuta, Y., and Hogan, B. L. (1998). BMP4 is essential for lens induction in the mouse embryo. *Genes Dev.* 12:3764–3775.

Garber, A. T., Winkler, C., Shinohara, T., King, C. R., Inana, G., Piatigorsky, J., and Gold, R. J. (1985). Selective loss of a family of gene transcripts in a hereditary murine cataract. *Science* 227:74–77.

Gehring, W. J. (2004). Historical perspective on the development and evolution of eyes and photoreceptors. *Int. J. Dev. Biol.* 48:707–717.

Gopal-Srivastava, R., Cvekl, A., and Piatigorsky, J. (1996). Pax-6 and alphaB-crystallin/small heat shock protein gene regulation in the murine lens. Interaction with the lens-specific regions, LSR1 and LSR2. *J. Biol. Chem.* 271:23029–23036.

Gopal-Srivastava, R., Haynes, J. I., 2nd, and Piatigorsky, J. (1995). Regulation of the murine alpha B-crystallin/small heat shock protein gene in cardiac muscle. *Mol. Cell. Biol.* 15: 7081–7090.

Gopal-Srivastava, R., Kays, W. T., and Piatigorsky, J. (2000). Enhancer-independent promoter activity of the mouse alphaB-crystallin/small heat shock protein gene in the lens and cornea of transgenic mice. *Mech. Dev.* 92:125–134.

Gopal-Srivastava, R., and Piatigorsky, J. (1993). The murine alpha B-crystallin/small heat shock protein enhancer: Identification of alpha BE-1, alpha BE-2, alpha BE-3, and MRF control elements. *Mol. Cell. Biol.* 13:7144–7152.

Goudreau, G., Petrou, P., Reneker, L. W., Graw, J., Loster, J., and Gruss, P. (2002). Mutually regulated expression of Pax6 and Six3 and its implications for the Pax6 haploinsufficient lens phenotype. *Proc. Natl. Acad. Sci. U.S.A.* 99:8719–8724.

Graw, J. (1999). Cataract mutations and lens development. *Prog. Retin. Eye. Res.* 18:235–267.

Graw, J. (2003). The genetic and molecular basis of congenital eye defects. *Nat. Rev. Genet.* 4:876–888.

Hanson, I. M. (2003). PAX6 and congenital eye malformations. *Pediatr. Res.* 54:791–796.

Hanson, I. M., Fletcher, J. M., Jordan, T., Brown, A., Taylor, D., Adams, R. J., Punnett, H. H., and van Heyningen, V. (1994). Mutations at the PAX6 locus are found in heterogeneous anterior segment malformations including Peters' anomaly. *Nat. Genet.* 6:168–173.

Hawse, J. R., DeAmicis-Tress, C., Cowell, T. L., and Kantorow, M. (2005). Identification of global gene expression differences between human lens epithelial and cortical fiber cells reveals specific genes and their associated pathways important for specialized lens cell functions. *Mol. Vis.* 11:274–283.

Hay, E. D. (1979). Development of the vertebrate cornea. *Int. Rev. Cytol.* 63:263–322.

Haynes, J. I., 2nd, Duncan, M. K., and Piatigorsky, J. (1996). Spatial and temporal activity of the alpha B-crystallin/small heat shock protein gene promoter in transgenic mice. *Dev. Dyn.* 207:75–88.

Hiemisch, H., Schutz, G., and Kaestner, K. H. (1998). The mouse Fkh1/Mf1 gene: cDNA sequence, chromosomal localization and expression in adult tissues. *Gene* 220:77–82.

Hogan, B. L., Hirst, E. M., Horsburgh, G., and Hetherington, C. M. (1988). Small eye (Sey): A mouse model for the genetic analysis of craniofacial abnormalities. *Development* 103(Suppl.): 115–119.

Holmberg, J., Liu, C. Y., and Hjalt, T. A. (2004). PITX2 gain-of-function in Rieger syndrome eye model. *Am. J. Pathol.* 165:1633–1641.

Hong, H. K., Lass, J. H., and Chakravarti, A. (1999). Pleiotropic skeletal and ocular phenotypes of the mouse mutation congenital hydrocephalus (ch/Mf1) arise from a winged helix/forkhead transcriptionfactor gene. *Hum. Mol. Genet.* 8:625–637.

Honkanen, R. A., Nishimura, D. Y., Swiderski, R. E., Bennett, S. R., Hong, S., Kwon, Y. H., Stone, E. M., Sheffield, V. C., and Alward, W. L. (2003). A family with Axenfeld-Rieger syndrome and Peters anomaly caused by a point mutation (Phe-112Ser) in the FOXC1 gene. *Am. J. Ophthalmol.* 135:368–375.

Ijichi, N., Tsujimoto, N., Iwaki, T., Fukumaki, Y., and Iwaki, A. (2004). Distal Sox binding elements of the alphaB-crystallin gene show lens enhancer activity in transgenic mouse embryos. *J. Biochem. (Tokyo)* 135:413–420.

Ilagan, J. G., Cvekl, A., Kantorow, M., Piatigorsky, J., and Sax, C. M. (1999). Regulation of alphaA-crystallin gene expression: Lens specificity achieved through the differential placement of similar transcriptional control elements in mouse and chicken. *J. Biol. Chem.* 274:19973–19978.

Ivanov, D., Dvoriantchikova, G., Pestova, A., Nathanson, L., and Shestopalov, V. I. (2005). Microarray analysis of fiber cell maturation in the lens. *FEBS Lett.* 579:1213–1219.

Iwaki, T., Kume-Iwaki, A., Liem, R. K., and Goldman, J. E. (1989). Alpha B-crystallin is expressed in non-lenticular tissues and accumulates in Alexander's disease brain. *Cell* 57:71–78.

Jester, J. V., Budge, A., Fisher, S., and Huang, J. (2005). Corneal keratocytes: Phenotypic and species differences in abundant protein expression and in vitro light-scattering. *Invest. Ophthalmol. Vis. Sci.* 46:2369–2378.

Jester, J. V., Moller-Pedersen, T., Huang, J., Sax, C. M., Kays, W. T., Cavangh, H. D., Petroll, W. M., and Piatigorsky, J. (1999). The cellular basis of corneal transparency: Evidence for "corneal crystallins". *J. Cell. Sci.* 112(Pt. 5):613–622.

Jordan, T., Hanson, I., Zaletayev, D., Hodgson, S., Prosser, J., Seawright, A., Hastie, N., and van Heyningen, V. (1992). The human PAX6 gene is mutated in two patients with aniridia. *Nat. Genet.* 1:328–332.

Kanakubo, S., Nomura, T., Yamamura, K., Miyazaki, J., Tamai, M., and Osumi, N. (2006). Abnormal migration and distribution of neural crest cells in Pax6 heterozygous mutant eye, a model for human eye diseases. *Genes Cells* 11:919–933.

Kantorow, M., Becker, K., Sax, C. M., Ozato, K., and Piatigorsky, J. (1993). Binding of tissue-specific forms of alpha A-CRYBP1 to their regulatory sequence in the mouse alpha A-crystallin-encoding gene: Double-label immunoblotting of UV-crosslinked complexes. *Gene* 131:159–165.

Kao, W. W., Liu, C. Y., Converse, R. L., Shiraishi, A., Kao, C. W., Ishizaki, M., Doetschman, T., and Duffy, J. (1996). Keratin 12–deficient mice have fragile corneal epithelia. *Invest. Ophthalmol. Vis. Sci.* 37:2572–2584.

Kawauchi, S., Takahashi, S., Nakajima, O., Ogino, H., Morita, M., Nishizawa, M., Yasuda, K., and Yamamoto, M. (1999). Regulation of lens fiber cell differentiation by transcription factor c-Maf. *J. Biol. Chem.* 274:19254–19260.

Kays, W. T., and Piatigorsky, J. (1997). Aldehyde dehydrogenase class 3 expression: Identification of a cornea-preferred gene promoter in transgenic mice. *Proc. Natl. Acad. Sci. U.S.A.* 94:13594–13599.

Kidson, S. H., Kume, T., Deng, K., Winfrey, V., and Hogan, B. L. (1999). The forkhead/winged-helix gene, Mf1, is necessary for the normal development of the cornea and formation of the anterior chamber in the mouse eye. *Dev. Biol.* 211:306–322.

Kim, J. I., Li, T., Ho, I. C., Grusby, M. J., and Glimcher, L. H. (1999). Requirement for the c-Maf transcription factor in crystallin gene regulation and lens development. *Proc. Natl. Acad. Sci. U.S.A.* 96:3781–3785.

Kloosterman, W. P., and Plasterk, R. H. (2006). The diverse functions of microRNAs in animal development and disease. *Dev. Cell* 11:441–450.

Koroma, B. M., Yang, J. M., and Sundin, O. H. (1997). The Pax-6 homeobox gene is expressed throughout the corneal and conjunctival epithelia. *Invest. Ophthalmol. Vis. Sci.* 38:108–120.

Kucerova, R., Ou, J., Lawson, D., Leiper, L. J., and Collinson, J. M. (2006). Cell surface glycoconjugate abnormalities and corneal epithelial wound healing in the Pax6+/− mouse model of aniridia-related keratopathy. *Invest. Ophthalmol. Vis. Sci.* 47:5276–5282.

Kume, T., Deng, K. Y., Winfrey, V., Gould, D. B., Walter, M. A., and Hogan, B. L. (1998). The forkhead/winged helix gene Mf1 is disrupted in the pleiotropic mouse mutation congenital hydrocephalus. *Cell* 93:985–996.

Lagutin, O., Zhu, C. C., Furuta, Y., Rowitch, D. H., McMahon, A. P., and Oliver, G. (2001). Six3 promotes the formation of ectopic optic vesicle-like structures in mouse embryos. *Dev. Dyn.* 221:342–349.

Lengler, J., Bittner, T., Munster, D., Gawad Ael, D., and Graw, J. (2005). Agonistic and antagonistic action of AP2, Msx2, Pax6, Prox1 and Six3 in the regulation of Sox2 expression. *Ophthalmic Res.* 37:301–309.

Lengler, J., Krausz, E., Tomarev, S., Prescott, A., Quinlan, R. A., and Graw, J. (2001). Antagonistic action of Six3 and Prox1 at the gamma-crystallin promoter. *Nucleic Acids Res.* 29:515–526.

Liu, C., Arar, H., Kao, C., and Kao, W. W. (2000). Identification of a 3.2 kb 5′-flanking region of the murine keratocan gene that directs beta-galactosidase expression in the adult corneal stroma of transgenic mice. *Gene* 250:85–96.

Liu, C. Y., Shiraishi, A., Kao, C. W., Converse, R. L., Funderburgh, J. L., Corpuz, L. M., Conrad, G. W., and Kao, W. W. (1998). The cloning of mouse keratocan cDNA and genomic DNA and the characterization of its expression during eye development. *J. Biol. Chem.* 273:22584–22588.

Liu, J. J., Kao, W. W., and Wilson, S. E. (1999). Corneal epithelium-specific mouse keratin K12 promoter. *Exp. Eye Res.* 68:295–301.

Liu, W., Lagutin, O. V., Mende, M., Streit, A., and Oliver, G. (2006). Six3 activation of Pax6 expression is essential for mammalian lens induction and specification. *EMBO J.* 25:5383–5395.

Marquardt, T., Ashery-Padan, R., Andrejewski, N., Scardigli, R., Guillemot, F., and Gruss, P. (2001). Pax6 is required for the multipotent state of retinal progenitor cells. *Cell* 105:43–55.

Mears, A. J., Jordan, T., Mirzayans, F., Dubois, S., Kume, T., Parlee, M., Ritch, R., Koop, B., Kuo, W. L., et al. (1998). Mutations of the forkhead/winged-helix gene, FKHL7, in patients with Axenfeld-Rieger anomaly. *Am. J. Hum. Genet.* 63:1316–1328.

Medina-Martinez, O., Brownell, I., Amaya-Manzanares, F., Hu, Q., Behringer, R. R., and Jamrich, M. (2005). Severe defects in proliferation and differentiation of lens cells in Foxe3 null mice. *Mol. Cell Biol.* 25:8854–8863.

Min, J. N., Zhang, Y., Moskophidis, D., and Mivechi, N. F. (2004). Unique contribution of heat shock transcription factor 4 in ocular lens development and fiber cell differentiation. *Genesis* 40:205–217.

Mirzayans, F., Gould, D. B., Heon, E., Billingsley, G. D., Cheung, J. C., Mears, A. J., and Walter, M. A. (2000). Axenfeld-Rieger syndrome resulting from mutation of the FKHL7 gene on chromosome 6p25. *Eur. J. Hum. Genet.* 8:71–74.

Nagasaki, T., and Zhao, J. (2003). Centripetal movement of corneal epithelial cells in the normal adult mouse. *Invest. Ophthalmol. Vis. Sci.* 44:558–566.

Nakamura, H., Chiambaretta, F., Sugar, J., Sapin, V., and Yue, B. Y. (2004). Developmentally regulated expression of KLF6 in the mouse cornea and lens. *Invest. Ophthalmol. Vis. Sci.* 45:4327–4332.

Nakamura, H., Ueda, J., Sugar, J., and Yue, B. Y. (2005). Developmentally regulated expression of Sp1 in the mouse cornea. *Invest. Ophthalmol. Vis. Sci.* 46:4092–4096.

Nakamura, T., Donovan, D. M., Hamada, K., Sax, C. M., Norman, B., Flanagan, J. R., Ozato, K., Westphal, H., and Piatigorsky, J. (1990). Regulation of the mouse alpha A-crystallin gene: Isolation of a cDNA encoding a protein that binds to a cis sequence motif shared with the major histocompatibility complex class I gene and other genes. *Mol. Cell Biol.* 10: 3700–3708.

Nakatake, Y., Fukui, N., Iwamatsu, Y., Masui, S., Takahashi, K., Yagi, R., Yagi, K., Miyazaki, J., Matoba, R., et al. (2006). Klf4 cooperates with Oct3/4 and Sox2 to activate the Lefty1 core promoter in embryonic stem cells. *Mol. Cell Biol.* 26: 7772–7782.

Nishiguchi, S., Wood, H., Kondoh, H., Lovell-Badge, R., and Episkopou, V. (1998). Sox1 directly regulates the gamma-crystallin genes and is essential for lens development in mice. *Genes Dev.* 12:776–781.

Nishimura, D. Y., Swiderski, R. E., Alward, W. L., Searby, C. C., Patil, S. R., Bennet, S. R., Kanis, A. B., Gastier, J. M., Stone, E. M., et al. (1998). The forkhead transcription factor gene FKHL7 is responsible for glaucoma phenotypes which map to 6p25. *Nat. Genet.* 19:140–147.

Norman, B., Davis, J., and Piatigorsky, J. (2004). Postnatal gene expression in the normal mouse cornea by SAGE. *Invest. Ophthalmol. Vis. Sci.* 45:429–440.

Ohtaka-Maruyama, C., Hanaoka, F., and Chepelinsky, A. B. (1998). A novel alternative spliced variant of the transcription factor AP2alpha is expressed in the murine ocular lens. *Dev. Biol.* 202:125–135.

Okada, Y., Saika, S., Shirai, K., Ohnishi, Y., and Senba, E. (2003). Expression of AP1 (c-Fos/c-Jun) in developing mouse corneal epithelium. *Graefes Arch. Clin. Exp. Ophthalmol.* 241: 330–333.

Oliver, G., Mailhos, A., Wehr, R., Copeland, N. G., Jenkins, N. A., and Gruss, P. (1995). Six3, a murine homologue of the sine oculis gene, demarcates the most anterior border of the developing neural plate and is expressed during eye development. *Development* 121:4045–4055.

Ouyang, J., Shen, Y. C., Yeh, L. K., Li, W., Coyle, B. M., Liu, C. Y., and Fini, M. E. (2006). Pax6 overexpression suppresses cell proliferation and retards the cell cycle in corneal epithelial cells. *Invest. Ophthalmol. Vis. Sci.* 47:2397–2407.

Piatigorsky, J. (1998). Gene sharing in lens and cornea: Facts and implications. *Prog. Retin. Eye Res.* 17:145–174.

Piatigorsky, J. (2001). Enigma of the abundant water-soluble cytoplasmic proteins of the cornea: The "refracton" hypothesis. *Cornea* 20:853–858.

Piatigorsky, J. (2007). *Gene sharing and evolution: Diversity of protein functions.* Cambridge, MA: Harvard University Press.

Piatigorsky, J., O'Brien, W. E., Norman, B. L., Kalumuck, K., Wistow, G. J., Borras, T., Nickerson, J. M., and Wawrousek, E. F. (1988). Gene sharing by delta-crystallin and argin-inosuccinate lyase. *Proc. Natl. Acad. Sci. U.S.A.* 85:3479–3483.

Piatigorsky, J., and Wistow, G. J. (1989). Enzyme/crystallins: Gene sharing as an evolutionary strategy. *Cell* 57:197–199.

Piatigorsky, J., and Wistow, G. (1991). The recruitment of crystallins: New functions precede gene duplication. *Science* 252: 1078–1079.

Rajaram, N., and Kerppola, T. K. (2004). Synergistic transcription activation by Maf and Sox and their subnuclear localization are disrupted by a mutation in Maf that causes cataract. *Mol. Cell. Biol.* 24:5694–5709.

Ramaesh, T., Ramaesh, K., Martin Collinson, J., Chanas, S. A., Dhillon, B., and West, J. D. (2005). Developmental and cellular factors underlying corneal epithelial dysgenesis in the Pax6+/− mouse model of aniridia. *Exp. Eye Res.* 81:224–235.

Ring, B. Z., Cordes, S. P., Overbeek, P. A., and Barsh, G. S. (2000). Regulation of mouse lens fiber cell development and differentiation by the Maf gene. *Development* 127:307–317.

Robinson, M. L., and Overbeek, P. A. (1996). Differential expression of alpha A- and alpha B-crystallin during murine ocular development. *Invest. Ophthalmol. Vis. Sci.* 37:2276–2284.

Ryan, D. G., Oliveira-Fernandes, M., and Lavker, R. M. (2006). MicroRNAs of the mammalian eye display distinct and overlapping tissue specificity. *Mol. Vis.* 12:1175–1184.

Sax, C. M., Kays, W. T., Salamon, C., Chervenak, M. M., Xu, Y. S., and Piatigorsky, J. (2000). Transketolase gene expression in the cornea is influenced by environmental factors and developmentally controlled events. *Cornea* 19:833–841.

Sax, C. M., Salamon, C., Kays, W. T., Guo, J., Yu, F. X., Cuthbertson, R. A., and Piatigorsky, J. (1996). Transketolase is a major protein in the mouse cornea. *J. Biol. Chem.* 271: 33568–33574.

Semina, E. V., Ferrell, R. E., Mintz-Hittner, H. A., Bitoun, P., Alward, W. L., Reiter, R. S., Funkhauser, C., Daack-Hirsch, S., and Murray, J. C. (1998). A novel homeobox gene PITX3 is mutated in families with autosomal-dominant cataracts and ASMD. *Nat. Genet.* 19:167–170.

Semina, E. V., Murray, J. C., Reiter, R., Hrstka, R. F., and Graw, J. (2000). Deletion in the promoter region and altered expression of Pitx3 homeobox gene in aphakia mice. *Hum. Mol. Genet.* 9:1575–1585.

Semina, E. V., Reiter, R. S., and Murray, J. C. (1997). Isolation of a new homeobox gene belonging to the Pitx/Rieg family: Expression during lens development and mapping to the aphakia region on mouse chromosome 19. *Hum. Mol. Genet.* 6:2109–2116.

Shirai, K., Saika, S., Okada, Y., Senba, E., and Ohnishi, Y. (2004). Expression of c-Fos and c-Jun in developing mouse lens. *Ophthalmic Res.* 36:226–230.

Simpson, T. I., and Price, D. J. (2002). Pax6: A pleiotropic player in development. *Bioessays* 24:1041–1051.

Sivak, J. M., Mohan, R., Rinehart, W. B., Xu, P. X., Maas, R. L., and Fini, M. E. (2000). Pax-6 expression and activity are induced in the reepithelializing cornea and control activity of the transcriptional promoter for matrix metalloproteinase gelatinase B. *Dev. Biol.* 222:41–54.

Sivak, J. M., West-Mays, J. A., Yee, A., Williams, T., and Fini, M. E. (2004). Transcription factors Pax6 and AP2alpha interact to coordinate corneal epithelial repair by controlling expression of matrix metalloproteinase gelatinase B. *Mol. Cell Biol.* 24:245–257.

Smaoui, N., Beltaief, O., BenHamed, S., M'Rad, R., Maazoul, F., Ouertani, A., Chaabouni, H., and Hejtmancik, J. F. (2004). A homozygous splice mutation in the HSF4 gene is associated with an autosomal recessive congenital cataract. *Invest. Ophthalmol. Vis. Sci.* 45:2716–2721.

Smith, R. S., Zabaleta, A., Kume, T., Savinova, O. V., Kidson, S. H., Martin, J. E., Nishimura, D. Y., Alward, W. L., Hogan, B. L., et al. (2000). Haploinsufficiency of the transcription factors FOXC1 and FOXC2 results in aberrant ocular development. *Hum. Mol. Genet.* 9:1021–1032.

Somasundaram, T., and Bhat, S. P. (2004). Developmentally dictated expression of heat shock factors: Exclusive expression of HSF4 in the postnatal lens and its specific interaction with alphaB-crystallin heat shock promoter. *J. Biol. Chem.* 279: 44497–44503.

Swamynathan, S. K., Katz, J. P., Kaestner, K. H., Ashery-Padan, R., Crawford, M. A., and Piatigorsky, J. (2007). Conditional deletion of mouse Klf4 gene results in corneal epithelial fragility, stromal edema and loss of conjunctival goblet cells. *Mol. Cell Biol.* 27:182–194.

Swamynathan, S. K., and Piatigorsky, J. (2002). Orientation-dependent influence of an intergenic enhancer on the promoter activity of the divergently transcribed mouse Shsp/alpha B-crystallin and Mkbp/HspB2 genes. *J. Biol. Chem.* 277:49700–49706.

Takahashi, K., and Yamanaka, S. (2006). Induction of pluripotent stem cells from mouse embryonic and adult fibroblast cultures by defined factors. *Cell* 126:663–676.

Tanifuji-Terai, N., Terai, K., Hayashi, Y., Chikama, T., and Kao, W. W. (2006). Expression of keratin 12 and maturation of corneal epithelium during development and postnatal growth. *Invest. Ophthalmol. Vis. Sci.* 47:545–551.

Tomarev, S. I., Zinovieva, R. D., Chang, B., and Hawes, N. L. (1998). Characterization of the mouse Prox1 gene. *Biochem. Biophys. Res. Commun.* 248:684–689.

Ueta, M., Hamuro, J., Yamamoto, M., Kaseda, K., Akira, S., and Kinoshita, S. (2005). Spontaneous ocular surface inflammation and goblet cell disappearance in I kappa B zeta gene-disrupted mice. *Invest. Ophthalmol. Vis. Sci.* 46:579–588.

Valleix, S., Niel, F., Nedelec, B., Algros, M. P., Schwartz, C., Delbosc, B., Delpech, M., and Kantelip, B. (2006). Homozygous nonsense mutation in the FOXE3 gene as a cause of congenital primary aphakia in humans. *Am. J. Hum. Genet.* 79: 358–364.

Wawrousek, E. F., Chepelinsky, A. B., McDermott, J. B., and Piatigorsky, J. (1990). Regulation of the murine alpha A-crystallin promoter in transgenic mice. *Dev. Biol.* 137:68–76.

West-Mays, J. A., Sivak, J. M., Papagiotas, S. S., Kim, J., Nottoli, T., Williams, T., and Fini, M. E. (2003). Positive influence of AP2alpha transcription factor on cadherin gene expression and differentiation of the ocular surface. *Differentiation* 71:206–216.

West-Mays, J. A., Zhang, J., Nottoli, T., Hagopian-Donaldson, S., Libby, D., Strissel, K. J., and Williams, T. (1999). AP2alpha transcription factor is required for early morphogenesis of the lens vesicle. *Dev. Biol.* 206:46–62.

Wigle, J. T., and Oliver, G. (1999). Prox1 function is required for the development of the murine lymphatic system. *Cell* 98: 769–778.

Wistow, G. J., and Piatigorsky, J. (1988). Lens crystallins: The evolution and expression of proteins for a highly specialized tissue. *Annu. Rev. Biochem.* 57:479–504.

Yang, Y., Chauhan, B. K., Cveklova, K., and Cvekl, A. (2004). Transcriptional regulation of mouse alphaB- and gammaF-crystallin genes in lens: Opposite promoter-specific interactions between Pax6 and large Maf transcription factors. *J. Mol. Biol.* 344:351–368.

Yang, Y., and Cvekl, A. (2005). Tissue-specific regulation of the mouse alphaA-crystallin gene in lens via recruitment of Pax6 and c-Maf to its promoter. *J. Mol. Biol.* 351:453–469.

Yang, Y., Stopka, T., Golestaneh, N., Wang, Y., Wu, K., Li, A., Chauhan, B. K., Gao, C. Y., Cveklova, K., et al. (2006). Regulation of alphaA-crystallin via Pax6, c-Maf, CREB and a broad domain of lens-specific chromatin. *EMBO J.* 25:2107–2118.

Yoshida, N., Yoshida, S., Araie, M., Handa, H., and Nabeshima, Y. (2000). Ets family transcription factor ESE-1 is expressed in corneal epithelial cells and is involved in their differentiation. *Mech. Dev.* 97:27–34.

Yoshimoto, A., Saigou, Y., Higashi, Y., and Kondoh, H. (2005). Regulation of ocular lens development by Smad-interacting protein 1 involving Foxe3 activation. *Development* 132:4437–4448.

Zaki, P. A., Collinson, J. M., Toraiwa, J., Simpson, T. I., Price, D. J., and Quinn, J. C. (2006). Penetrance of eye defects in mice heterozygous for mutation of Gli3 is enhanced by heterozygous mutation of Pax6. *BMC Dev. Biol.* 6:46.

Zhang, X., Friedman, A., Heaney, S., Purcell, P., and Maas, R. L. (2002). Meis homeoproteins directly regulate Pax6 during vertebrate lens morphogenesis. *Genes Dev.* 16:2097–2107.

Zhou, M., Li, X. M., and Lavker, R. M. (2006). Transcriptional profiling of enriched populations of stem cells versus transient amplifying cells: A comparison of limbal and corneal epithelial basal cells. *J. Biol. Chem.* 281:19600–19609.

Zieske, J. D. (2004). Corneal development associated with eyelid opening. *Int. J. Dev. Biol.* 48:903–911.

58 Proteomics of the Mouse Lens

WOLFGANG HOEHENWARTER AND PETER R. JUNGBLUT

Proteomics, the science surrounding all of a sample's protein constituents, and the eye lens have a long mutual history (Hoehenwarter et al., 2006b). The lens is a tissue whose function is to concentrate light and help produce a sharp visual image. It is completely avascular and consists mostly of the proteins of one superfamily, the crystallins (Wistow and Piatigorsky, 1988). Their short-range order and precise molecular arrangement in solution establish the refractive index and ultimately its function (Delaye and Tardieu, 1983).

Proteomics has extensively characterized these proteins in many species. A high-definition separation of all the urea-soluble protein constituents of the mouse lens was produced using large-scale carrier ampholyte-based two-dimensional gel electrophoresis (2DE) (Jungblut et al., 1998). This work produced 1,940 distinct dye-stained protein spots, many of which were excised from the gel and analyzed with matrix-assisted laser desorption ionization time-of-flight mass spectrometry. It became clear that most of the polypeptides of the eye lens of the mouse are indeed different modified crystallin proteins, or more appropriately crystallin protein species. In-depth studies have been completed in several wild-type and naturally occurring and induced mutant mouse strains and have identified numerous posttranslational modifications in the healthy lens and in the lens affected by cataract, and have elucidated some of the factors implicated in this disease. Future studies should establish the totality of the protein species, resolve proteins specifically involved in the onset and progression of cataract, and give an in-depth understanding of the tissue as a whole.

Major structural proteins of the lens: The crystallins

The proteins of the crystallin superfamily make up 80%–90% of the entire mass of lens proteins. They were originally classified according to their native size, and the first three letters of the Greek alphabet were assigned to them in descending order of their molecular weight (Mörner, 1893). α-Crystallin is the largest native crystallin, with a molecular weight of 300–>1,000 kd; β-crystallin is the next largest, with a molecular weight of between 40 and 200 kd; and γ-crystallins are the smallest crystallins, with a molecular weight of around 20 kd. Native α- and β-crystallins are multimers composed of several types of monomeric subunits; native γ-crystallins do not polymerize. More recent size exclusion chromatography has separated the native water-soluble crystallins of the adult lens more precisely into a large high-molecular-weight (HMW) fraction containing mostly α-crystallin and other proteins on the verge of insolubilization, a fraction containing α-crystallin, a higher and a lower molecular weight fraction of β-crystallin, β high (βH) and β low (βL), and a small fraction containing the γS-crystallin monomer, followed by the larger and lowest molecular weight γ-crystallin fraction.

The native crystallin proteins are in various stages of solution and can be thought of as bulk material that fills the otherwise empty lens cells. This material is transparent due to the supramolecular arrangement and short-range order of the proteins. This order is not random but is precisely defined at a molecular level. A disturbance of this homeostasis can lead to unfolding, improper folding, insolubilization, and aggregation of proteins. The insoluble aggregates diffract incident light, resulting in opacification of the lens and visual impairment. This is what is known as cataract (Harding, 1972; Carrell and Lomas, 1997).

The peculiarities of the lens, namely, the little protein biosynthesis and reduced metabolism and the exposure to light and its effects, have imparted a high degree of stability to the crystallins. They are also connected to the stress response (de Jong et al., 1989) next to their function as transparent structure. The protein concentration and the stochiometry of the crystallins in the regions of the lens vary, so a refractive index gradient is created. In most species the refractive index declines from center to periphery, which increases the convexity of the lens and can eliminate spherical and chromatic aberration (Fernald and Wright, 1983). This is especially so in the mouse, which has a lens nucleus with a very high protein content and little water.

The α-crystallins are clearly distinct from the β- and γ-crystallins in molecular evolution. In contrast, the β- and γ-crystallin proteins seem to have a common ancestor. This leads to the assumption of an initial α-crystallin and β-/γ-crystallin gene in an early archetype lens that differentiated into the multiple genes of the current crystallin protein families. The 16 major proteins of the α-, β-, and γ-crystallin protein families are highly conserved and ubiquitous in the lens of mammals (Lubsen et al., 1988), and are also present in many other species. Two in an evolutionary context, more distant members of the γ-crystallin protein family, are also known in the mouse, γN- and γS-crystallin (van Rens et al.,

1989; Wistow et al., 2005). In addition, a number of less abundant crystallin proteins with specific functions related to enzymes have been detected in the lens of various species (Wistow, 1993).

α-Crystallin Protein Family α-Crystallin is the most abundant protein in the lens. It constitutes between 30% and 50% of the total mass of lens proteins and is evenly distributed throughout the organ in most species. In the mouse, there are three unmodified α-crystallin polypeptides, αA-crystallin, αB-crystallin, and αA-insert crystallin. αA- and αB-crystallin are 57% identical in primary structure. αA-insert crystallin is unique to mammals and common in rodents and is also a product of the αA-crystallin gene. It is produced by alternative splicing of an insert exon in the first intron of the gene (Cohen et al., 1978).

α-Crystallin has never been crystallized, so its three-dimensional (3D) structure could not yet be determined by X-ray diffraction. The native proteins' large size also precludes nuclear magnetic resonance (NMR) measurements. However, the secondary and tertiary structure of the individual α-crystallin gene products are known. Circular dichroism and infrared measurements have determined that they are composed primarily of β strands with little α helix structure (Thomson and Augusteyn, 1989; Farnsworth et al., 1997). They are subdivided into a hydrophobic, globular N-terminal domain, a hydrophilic C-terminal domain in β sheet conformation, and a C-terminal extension. The amino acid composition and tertiary structure of the N-terminal domain are relatively varied in the polypeptides and between species but include three structure-function regions in α-helical conformation (Smith et al., 1996; Pasta et al., 2003). A large part of the C-terminal domain is known as the α-crystallin domain (Caspers et al., 1995) and is conserved in the protein family. The C-terminal extension is variable. We have constructed a tertiary structure model of αA-crystallin of the mouse using ab initio protein structure prediction algorithms (figure 58.1; Hoehenwarter et al., 2006a).

α-Crystallins undergo extensive posttranslational modification beginning at the earliest stages of lens development. These are mainly deamidation, phosphorylation, and N- and C-terminal truncation. The unmodified and modified α-crystallin monomers are the minimal subunits that assemble the functional native protein. Several models have been proposed that agree that they exchange dynamically (van den Oetelaar et al., 1990; Gesierich and Pfeil, 1996) and form small multimers as the building blocks of higher molecular order (Bova et al., 2000). Posttranslational modification of the monomers affects subunit multi- and oligomerization (Merck et al., 1992; Bova et al., 2000, Pasta et al., 2003; Thampi and Abraham 2003), quaternary structure dynamics (Bova et al., 2000; Pasta et al., 2003), and protein function (Takemoto et al., 1993; Pasta et al., 2003). The small heat shock protein HSP27 can also coassemble with the α-crystallin monomers. Thus, α-crystallin is a polydisperse and highly dynamic protein whose size, structure, and function vary according to the composition of its subunits.

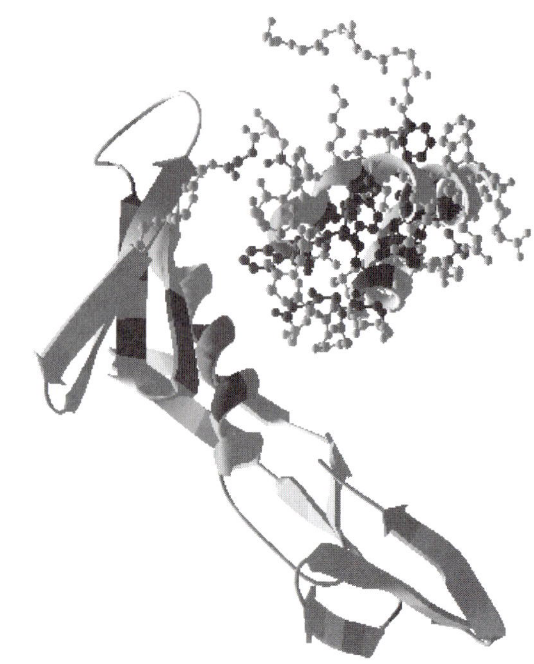

Figure 58.1 Model of αA-crystallin secondary and tertiary structure, colored according to the hydrophobicity of its amino acid residues. The most hydrophobic residues are colored dark blue; the least hydrophobic residues are colored red, as shown in color plate 67. The Rosetta algorithm on the HMMSTR server (www.bioinfo.rpi.edu/~bystrc/hmmstr/server.php) (Bystroff and Shao, 2002) available on the ExPASY (http://au.expasy.org/) home page was used for molecular modeling. Full-length αA-crystallin secondary structure was calculated at 29.5% α helix and 32% β sheet content. The N-terminal globular domain is organized into three helices, displayed as ribbons with hydrophobic side chains buried. Structure-function regions identified earlier (Smith et al., 1996; Pasta et al., 2003) make up the first two of these N-terminal α helices. The highly conserved residues 102–117 of the "α crystallin domain" (Caspers et al., 1995), containing the substantial first part of a DNA-binding motif (Singh et al., 1998), as well as an arginine residue 116 shown to be critical for molecular integrity (Bera et al., 2002), are predicted to have α-helical conformation and are displayed as ribbons. This is consistent with an older 3D model (Farnsworth et al., 1998) and makes the α-helical prediction that is somewhat higher than previous calculations (Farnsworth et al., 1997; Horwitz et al., 1998; Bova et al., 2000) seem plausible. However, it is inconsistent with site-directed spin label studies that demonstrate β sheet conformation for residues 109–120 (Berengian et al., 1997). The model confirms the β sheet secondary structure of residues 67–101, determined to be an alcohol dehydrogenase (ADH) and 1,1′-bi (4-anilino) naphtalene-5,5′-disulfonic acid (bis-ANS) binding site and to exhibit extensive chaperone activity (Farnsworth and Singh, 2004). See color plate 67.

α-Crystallin is a molecular chaperone (Horwitz, 1992; Jakob et al., 1993). The "α-crystallin domain" is implicit in all small heat shock proteins, and it was shown that αB-crystallin is indeed a member of this protein family (Klemenz et al., 1991). The small heat shock proteins interact with denatured proteins, keeping them in solution and in a refoldable conformation independently of ATP. The substrates of α-crystallin in the lens are the β- and γ-crystallins (Wang and Spector, 1994; Bloemendal et al., 2004), some enzymes, and elements of the cytoskeleton, such as the intermediate filament protein vimentin and the beaded filament. It is reasonable to assume that next to its role as transparent structural material, α-crystallin induces proper cytoskeleton architecture and prevents protein insolubilization, and that it is a major factor in upholding the clarity and function of the lens over years.

β- AND γ-CRYSTALLIN PROTEIN FAMILIES The β- and γ-crystallins are the other abundant major proteins in the lens. The families have very similar protein and gene structure and thus presumably have a common ancestor. In the lens of the mouse and most other mammals, there are seven unmodified β-crystallin polypeptides, four relatively acidic, termed βA1 through A4, and three more basic, termed βB1 through βB3. βA1- and βA3-crystallin are the products of the same gene and are the result of alternate translation initiation starting points. In the mouse, βA1-crystallin lacks the first 17 N-terminal amino acid residues of βA3-crystallin. There are six highly conserved, unmodified γ-crystallin polypeptides, γA–γF, whose genes are linked in one gene cluster, and two more distantly related polypeptides, γN- and γS-crystallin. The primary function of both the β- and γ-crystallins is as transparent material.

Data on the protein structure for both families are abundant. β- and γ-crystallins have similar secondary and tertiary structure. The monomers are composed mostly of β strands organized into four motifs of four antiparallel β strands each. The motifs are of the Greek key type, with the β strands 1, 2, and 4 forming a β sheet and strand 3 in a proximal position. This motif structure leaves many hydrophobic amino acid residue side chains exposed. The isolated β strand 3 interacts with β strand 4 of the β sheet of the neighboring motif, and the two motifs assemble into a complete globular domain with hydrophobic side chains buried. The monomers are subdivided into two globular domains separated by an unorganized stretch of primary structure, the connecting peptide. Also, primary structure can extend beyond the domains, which are then known as either the N- or C-terminal extensions.

The β-crystallin monomers are subunits that assemble the native higher molecular weight β-crystallin protein. The protein can be homo- or heteromeric (Bax et al., 1990; Slingsby and Bateman, 1990; Bateman et al., 2003) and is mostly a dimer (Slingsby and Bateman, 1990) or tetramer; however, further oligomerization is also known (Bateman et al., 2003). The connecting peptide is extended, which mediates the interaction of two globular domains from individual molecules in pseudo-twofold symmetry. The βB-crystallins have long unstructured N- and C- terminal extensions, the βA-crystallins have only N-terminal extensions. Their function is not clear, but there is evidence that the extensions are involved in promoting higher-order assembly of β-crystallin tetra- and oligomers, and that they may act as "spacers" in the supramolecular arrangement of the proteins (Nalini et al., 1994; Bateman et al., 2003).

The native protein is found throughout the fiber cells of the lens; however, the distribution of the individual β-crystallin monomers varies. βB2-crystallin is the major β-crystallin monomer in mammals, and synthesis of the β-crystallins is increased postnatally, so that the native protein is more abundant in the cortex than in the nucleus of the lens.

The γ-crystallin proteins are strictly monomers. The connecting peptide is bent, which brings the two globular domains of one molecule into close proximity and promotes intermolecular domain interaction around a pseudo-twofold axis (Blundell et al., 1981). The two motifs that constitute a domain have adopted a slight asymmetry that allows rows of hydrophobic residues to interdigitate much as in a zipper and creates an extra degree of close packing. The γ-crystallins lack N-terminal extensions, and their C-terminal extensions are very short, so the molecules as a whole are very compact, with only limited regions exposed for proteolysis. This guarantees maximum protein stability and allows a very close association, to a high degree excluding water (Mayr et al., 1994). Indeed, the γ-crystallins achieve the highest protein density and are particularly suited for the dehydrated conditions in the nucleus of the lens, where they are most abundant and create the highest refractive index. In this context, the proteins can only conditionally be considered monomeric; it seems more plausible that they have entered a state of macromolecular crowding in an almost completely dehydrated environment (Stevens et al., 1995). The γ-crystallins also have an unusually high content of cysteine residues, which may be involved in molecular bonds with other molecules in this tightly packed arrangement.

Proteomics and eye lens proteomics: An introduction

The high abundance and easy accessibility of the proteins of the lens have made the tissue a frequent subject of proteomics studies. Proteomics is a science dedicated to the comprehensive understanding of the totality and the dynamics of all of the protein constituents of a sample. Arbitrarily it began in 1975, when O'Farrell developed the 2DE technique combining isoelectric focusing (IEF) and sodium dodecyl sulfate polyacrylamide gel electrophoresis (SDS-PAGE) for large-scale separation of the proteins of biological samples (O'Farrell, 1975). With this technique, denatured proteins migrate to positions termed protein spots on the 2DE gel, as dictated by the relation of their chemical parameters to the applied 2DE parameters (Jungblut et al., 1997). High quality 2DE has a remarkable resolution capacity, being able to separate up to 10,000 sample constituents distinguished by a single amino acid or posttranslational modification (Klose and Kobalz, 1995). The separated proteins in the gel are visualized by staining them with a dye or by blotting them onto membranes and then staining them, resulting in a 2DE protein spot pattern.

The other premier technique employed for large-scale protein and peptide separation in proteomics is liquid chromatography (LC). LC is one of the oldest and best techniques for molecular separation in biochemical analysis, earning Archer Martin and Richard Synge the Nobel Prize for Chemistry in 1952. It is based on the individual behavior of soluble analytes in a mobile phase passed over and interacting differentially with a solid phase or matrix. Various combinations of liquid and solid phases featuring distinct molecular interaction and separation properties have been developed and tried over the years, leading to several popular LC approaches, among them affinity chromatography, ion exchange chromatography, reverse phase chromatography, and size exclusion chromatography. The combination of two or more of these techniques, in conjunction with relatively long durations (several hours) and low flow rates (nano-LC), has remarkable resolution power.

Following separation, it is desirable to identify as many proteins as completely as possible. Originally, purified or separated proteins were mostly analyzed by Edman degradation, a procedure that realizes protein primary structure beginning with a polypeptide's N-terminus (Edman, 1949). Primary structure information is the most basic and meaningful form of polypeptide characterization and presents the least degree of ambiguities.

A major breakthrough was reached in the late 1980s, when mass spectrometry became available for polypeptide analysis. Originally developed late in the nineteenth century, it is a technique that measures an ionized molecule's mass and charge. Ionized molecules from an ion source are manipulated by electric fields in an analyzer, where their recorded behavior prior to detection by an ion detector allows calculation of their physical parameters. So-called soft ionization techniques convert polypeptides to gas phase ions without damaging the molecules. The principal soft ionization techniques employed in proteomics are matrix-assisted laser desorption/ionization (MALDI) (Karas and Hillenkamp, 1988; Tanaka et al., 1988) and electrospray ionization (ESI) (Fenn et al., 1989). It is common to digest proteins either with enzymes or with chemicals and to analyze the resulting peptides with mass spectrometry, because mass accuracy, resolution, and charge minimization are all improved in the low mass range, under 3 kd.

The data acquired by mass spectrometry must be converted into meaningful information. A polypeptide's mass and charge allow the calculation of its primary structure; however, in light of the 20 proteinogenic amino acids and modifications, the possibilities for large peptides and proteins are considerable. In theory, the sequenced genomes of organisms contain the primary structures of all of an organism's primary translation products. This is an enormous asset for protein identification. Polypeptide masses recorded in mass spectra are used to search databases of conceptually translated genomics data according to primary structure segment masses, in many cases resulting in matches of the mass spectrometric data to amino acid sequences, producing peptide sequence suggestions and conclusive protein identification. This is termed peptide mass fingerprinting or peptide mass mapping (Henzel et al., 1993, Jungblut et al., 1997; Thiede et al., 2005). Modifications can be assessed from mass shifts using the identification as a reference. A number of software suites available commercially or free of charge on the Web expedite this process.

Today's generation of mass spectrometers deliver compositional and conformational information by fragmenting or promoting dissociation of the analyzed ions and applying a second round of mass spectrometry to the fragment ions. This is termed tandem mass spectrometry, or MS/MS (Senn et al., 1966; Biemann et al., 1966). Metastable dissociation of polypeptides occurs mainly at the peptide bond. If a peptide ion's charge is retained at the N-terminus following dissociation, the resulting fragment ion is termed b ion, while if the charge is retained at the C-terminus, the fragment ion is termed y ion. These ions allow the additive calculation of mass differences between fragment ion masses and the correlation of the mass differences with amino acid residues. A combination of mass, charge, and MS/MS data—or exclusively MS/MS data, if sufficiently available—can be used to determine protein primary structure, including modifications and modification sites.

Two-dimensional electrophoresis and lens proteomics go together from the outset. Already in 1975 Kibbelaar and Bloemendal applied the water-soluble and water-insoluble proteins of the whole lens, the size exclusion chromatography α, β_H, β_L, and γ fractions, and the urea-soluble proteins from the calf lens to urea PAGE combined with SDS-PAGE. They produced a first rudimentary protein spot pattern of the major lens proteins, the unmodified crystallins, and suggested α-crystallin interaction with membrane components (Kibbelaar and Bloemendal, 1975). With improvement in 2DE techniques, a definitive protein spot pattern or reference map for the crystallins and other components was achieved in 1982 for the water-soluble proteins of the bovine lens cortex, with a final definitive nomenclature for β-crystallins added in 1984 (Berbers et al., 1982, 1984). Similar investigations in chicken, mouse, rat, and human yielded comparable crystallin reference patterns and α-crystallin characterization with nomenclature and demonstrated the presence of the cytoskeleton proteins vimentin and actin in the urea-soluble fraction, presumably from the anterior epithelial cell layer and outer cortex (Garadi et al., 1983; Garber et al., 1984; Datiles et al., 1992).

Newer investigations have become increasingly comprehensive, often further characterizing crystallin proteins, confirming amino acid sequences predicted from cDNA or detecting discrepancies and annotating sequences and creating higher-quality reference maps, as well as detecting numerous noncrystallin lens proteins (Shih et al., 1998; Lampi et al., 2002; Hoehenwarter et al., 2005). A detailed reference map of the entire adult mouse lens proteome using high-resolution large-scale 2DE separated the urea-soluble proteins into 1,940 spots (Jungblut et al., 1998) and was ultimately followed by an in-depth analysis of the water-soluble and water-insoluble proteins at different ages (Ueda et al., 2002). A 2DE protein spot pattern of the young urea-soluble mouse lens proteome with the characteristic crystallin pattern produced in our laboratory is shown in figure 58.2. An accessible repository for mouse lens and other proteomics data is under preparation in the form of our 2DE database (www.mpiib-berlin.mpg.de/2D-PAGE).

Major LC investigations have characterized the infant to adult water-soluble and the adult water-insoluble human lens proteomes. Following size exclusion chromatography, water-soluble α, β_H, β_L, and γ fractions were applied to reverse phase chromatography on C4 columns for further fractionation. Whole proteins were then analyzed offline with ESI mass spectrometry. The crystallin proteins αA and αB, βB1, βB2, and βB3, A1, A3, and A4, and γC, γD, and γS were detected and changes in their abundance as well as posttranslational modifications with age were characterized (Ma et al., 1998). Another investigation subjected the water-insoluble monomeric α-crystallins to cation exchange chromatography before reverse phase chromatography and offline ESI mass spectrometry. A high degree of separation was achieved, and it was shown that α-crystallin is the major component of the water-insoluble lens proteins in humans, constituting about half of protein abundance. In addition, numerous α-crystallin protein species were identified and distinguished from the water-soluble fraction (Lund et al., 1996). Large-scale LC-based proteomic investigations of the mouse lens proteome have not been published.

In summary, the investigations described in this section and others not mentioned have proven invaluable for characterizing the proteins of the healthy lens as well as of morphological sections (Garland et al., 1996), and in elucidating some of the complex factors involved in cataract development (Garber et al., 1984; David et al., 1994; Calvin et al., 1996; Li et al., 2002) in the mouse and various other species.

Proteomics beyond genomics

The proteins in an organism are not limited to the primary translation products of its genes. Many proteins undergo posttranslational modification. Posttranslational modifications are covalent modifications to a protein's primary structure that can alter the function of the original unmodified protein. This introduces an additional vast level of functional activity that goes completely beyond the genome and cannot be assayed by genomics- or transciptomics-based research. The taxonomic term *protein species* was introduced in 1996 (Jungblut et al., 1996) to express this context. A protein species is defined as a polypeptide and possibly one or more other chemical groups that are covalently bonded. As such, it is the most basic term in protein taxonomy. It distinguishes proteins, posttranslationally modified forms of a protein, protein isoforms, different allelic forms of a protein, and any other primary structure variants as mature distinct molecules.

The proteome-wide identification of protein species is one of the major challenges facing proteomics today. A protein species is considered identified only when the entirety of its primary structure is known, so that it can be distinguished from another protein species that differs in only one primary structure element, such as one amino acid or chemical group or, ultimately, one atom. Current techniques, particularly 2DE and mass spectrometry, can achieve this on a small scale (Okkels et al., 2004).

LC procedures are also able to separate the protein species of a proteome but stop short of making them as readily accessible as 2DE. Their primary advantage is the relative speed at which complex protein mixtures can be assayed, thanks to the development of the electrospray ionization technique. Together with a connecting apparatus, it allows polypeptides to be eluted online or semi-online from chromatography into a mass spectrometer (Yates, 1998). To maximize separation performance, multiple steps of different types of chromatography can be combined. This is known as multidimensional protein identification technology, or MudPIT (Washburn et al., 2001). Strategies of this type that analyze peptides from protein digestion or internal cleavage generate between 10,000 and 100,000 distinct mass spectra, making comprehensive evaluation equally as laborious as the complete analysis of spots from 2DE (Swanson and Washburn, 2005; Hoehenwarter et al., 2006a). Although rapid detection of modifications is possible, the assignment of the identified peptides and modifications to individual molecules and thus the identification of the protein species are not.

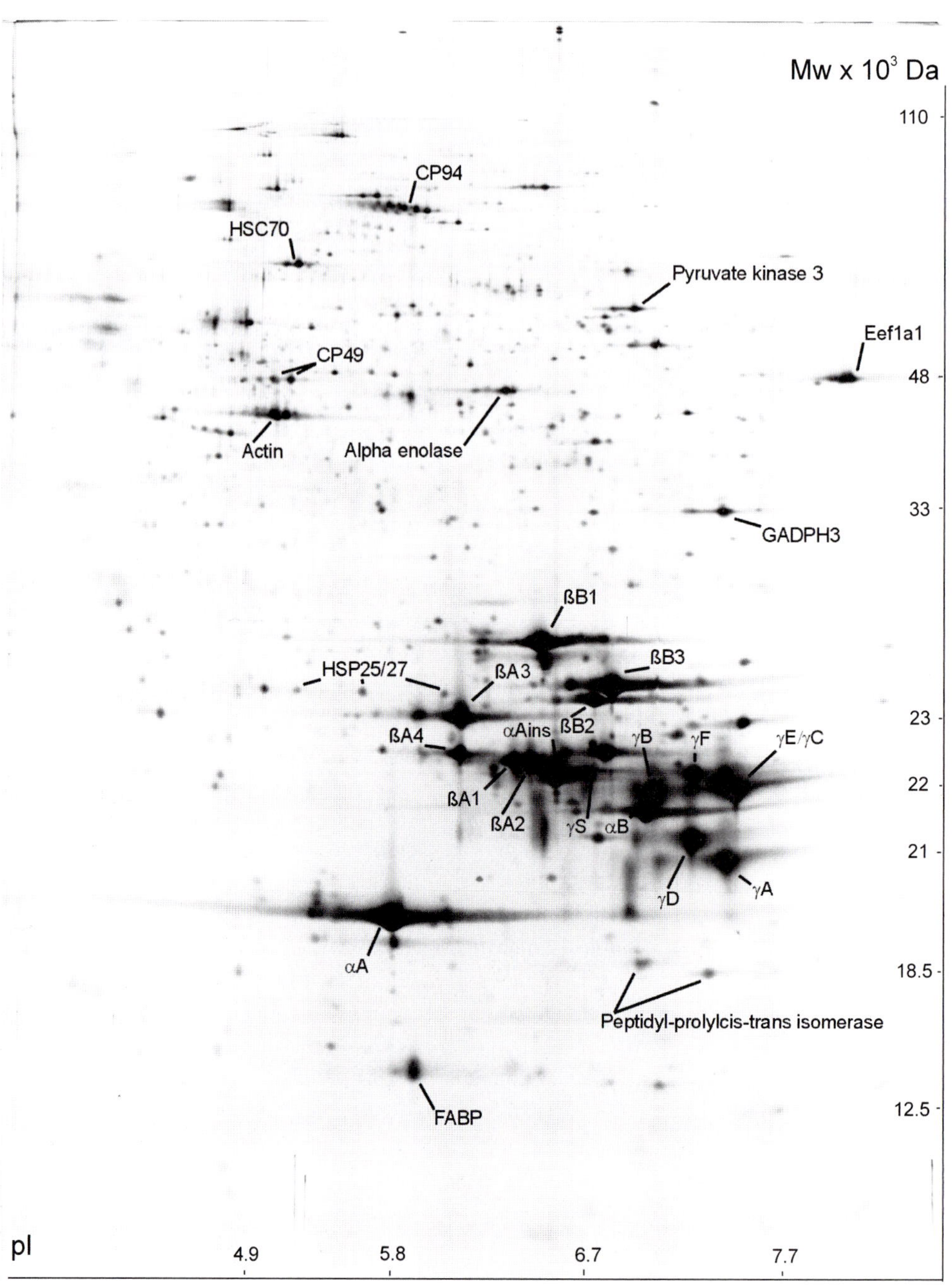

FIGURE 58.2 Protein spot pattern of the urea-soluble proteins of the 10-day-old mouse lens separated with large-scale 2DE and visualized with silver staining. Some identified proteins are indicated; the crystallin proteins are named as a token only.

The lens proteins of the crystallin superfamily undergo extensive posttranslational modification in all species. This process begins before birth and increases as the organism ages, with early-onset modifications becoming more abundant and additional modification types appearing. Indeed, the water-soluble proteins of the nucleus and cortex of the adult human lens were analyzed separately with 2DE, which revealed a nuclear protein spot pattern that is quite distinct from the previously described cortical or whole-lens pattern (Garland et al., 1996). This is evidence of a high degree of posttranslational modification in the very young lens, as the development of the nucleus is essentially prenatal, and so the nuclear protein species must be derived from posttranslational modification of the primary crystallin proteins. As this report and numerous others have made clear, many types of posttranslationally modified crystallins exist and are abundant in the healthy lens.

The fact that the protein species are mature molecules with individual primary structures implies that they have defined and possibly distinct functions in the supramolecular order of the transparent mass of proteins in the lens. This is illustrated for some αA-crystallin protein species separated with 2DE (figure 58.3). The protein species were analyzed with mass spectrometry; it was ascertained that they were products of the αA-crystallin gene, and a nomenclature was introduced (Hoehenwarter et al., 2008). One of the protein species, α-A_B, was analyzed in detail (Hoehenwarter et al., 2006a). The protein species's N-terminus is serine residue 42 of the full-length αA-crystallin protein and very probably the result of truncation by the calcium-dependent calpastatin protease Lp82. Its position on calibrated 2DE gels is in accordance with its theoretical molecular weight and pI. Nevertheless, the protein species was not identified, as only 50% sequence coverage was achieved with mass spectrometry. A model of its secondary and tertiary structure was produced with ab initio structure prediction algorithms (Bystroff and Shao, 2002). The insights gained from the model allowed the formulation of a hypothesis for the function of the protein species in the healthy lens. It is involved in the regulation of the size and function of the native protein. Together with other evidence, this discovery suggests that the protein species related to the primary translation products of the α-crystallin genes are also α-crystallin subunits, and that many more subunits than previously suspected influence the properties of the native HMW α-crystallin oligomer.

In contrast to the number of protein species apparently necessary for the development of the healthy lens, some crystallin protein species are known to induce cataract. Their conformation is incompatible with their environment, so they become insoluble, leading to opacities in the lens and visual impairment. Tryptophan oxidation to kynurenine was observed in γB- and γC-crystallins of adult mice (Jungblut et al., 1998), but a clear connection of this modification to cataract is missing. Certain protein species such as truncated βB1- or γ-cystallin (David et al., 1994; Gong et al., 1997; Descamps et al., 2005; Hoehenwarter et al., 2008) are specifically connected to the onset and development of cataract, their appearance in the lens unequivocally leading to the disease. Other protein species may be involved in cataractogenesis; however, they are also found in the healthy tissue. This duality is not fully understood, but it is conceivable that the protein species are deleterious only when their abundance is perpetuated beyond a certain threshold. Also, it has been shown that modifying factors are present in the lens of the mouse, and that the interactions of the crystallin protein species with these protein species affect the onset and development of cataract as well as healthy lens development (Hoehenwarter et al., 2008).

The concept of protein species with individual functions introduces a new level of complexity that is not unrealistic. These functions must be elucidated for a true understanding of the biological processes in the lens and other tissues, organs, and organisms. The first big step will be the complete identification of the proteome at the protein species level, meaning an exact description of native components. One of the techniques that could achieve this in the near future is the combination of multidimensional LC for protein species separation and MS/MS mass spectrometry of whole proteins for protein species identification. This approach,

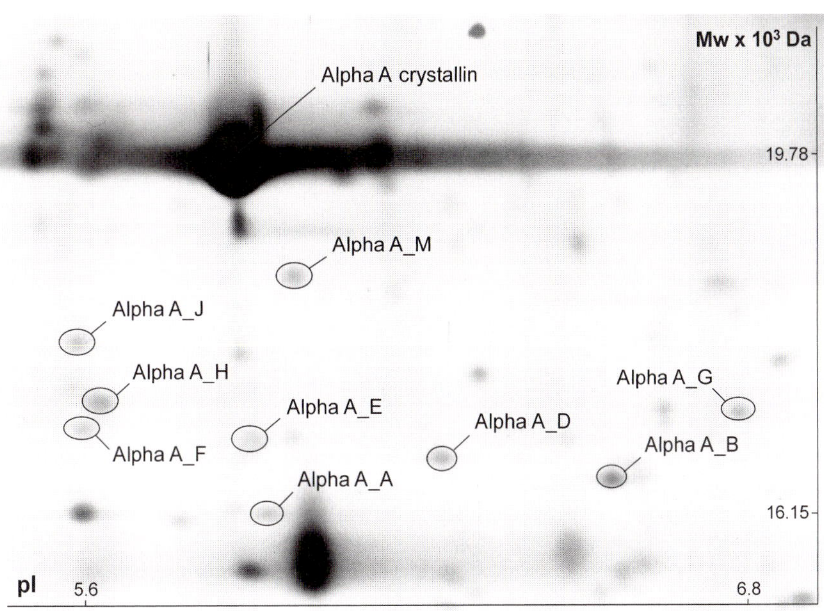

FIGURE 58.3 Section of a protein spot pattern of the urea-soluble proteins of the 10-day-old mouse lens separated with large-scale 2DE and visualized with silver staining that shows the full length αA-crystallin protein and some other αA-crystallin protein species.

known as top-down proteomics, has delivered encouraging results (Sze et al., 2002; Ge et al., 2002). Just recently the strategy's main limitation, that it could not be applied to proteins larger than 50 kd, was alleviated (Han et al., 2006), bringing routine proteome characterization within reach. Other modern mass spectrometry techniques have been used to determine the seminative quaternary structure of α-crystallin and could be applied to other protein species as well (Aquilina et al., 2003). A technique known as imaging mass spectrometry can be used to determine the distribution of proteins and protein species in tissues or organs (Crecelius et al., 2005). The combination of these and other technologies with an established proteome should allow the functional analysis of the totality of the protein species and make a true, in-depth understanding of the native situation conceivable in the eye lens and other tissues.

REFERENCES

Aquilina, J. A., Benesch, J. L., Bateman, O. A., Slingsby, C., and Robinson, C. V. (2003). Polydispersity of a mammalian chaperone: Mass spectrometry reveals the population of oligomers in alphaB-crystallin. *Proc. Natl. Acad. Sci. U.S.A.* 100:10611–10616.

Bateman, O. A., Sarra, R., Van Genesen, S. T., Kappe, G., Lubsen, N. H., and Slingsby, C. (2003). The stability of human acidic beta-crystallin oligomers and hetero-oligomers. *Exp. Eye Res.* 77:409–422.

Bax, B., Lapatto, R., Nalini, V., Driessen, H., Lindley, P. F., Mahadevan, D., Blundell, T. L., and Slingsby, C. (1990). X-ray analysis of beta B2-crystallin and evolution of oligomeric lens proteins. *Nature* 347:776–780.

Bera, S., Thampi, P., Cho, W. J., and Abraham, E. C. (2002). A positive charge preservation at position 116 of alpha A-crystallin is critical for its structural and functional integrity. *Biochemistry* 41:12421–12426.

Berbers, G. A., Boerman, O. C., Bloemendal, H., and de Jong, W. W. (1982). Primary gene products of bovine beta-crystallin and reassociation behavior of its aggregates. *Eur. J. Biochem.* 128:495–502.

Berbers, G. A., Hoekman, W. A., Bloemendal, H., de Jong, W. W., Kleinschmidt, T., and Braunitzer, G. (1984). Homology between the primary structures of the major bovine beta-crystallin chains. *Eur. J. Biochem.* 139:467–479.

Berengian, A. R., Bova, M. P., and Mchaourab, H. S. (1997). Structure and function of the conserved domain in alphaA-crystallin: Site-directed spin labeling identifies a beta-strand located near a subunit interface. *Biochemistry* 36:9951–9957.

Biemann, K., Cone, C., Webster, B. R., and Arsenault, G. P. (1966). Determination of the amino acid sequence in oligopeptides by computer interpretation of their high-resolution mass spectra. *J. Am. Chem. Soc.* 88:5598–5606.

Bloemendal, H., de Jong, W., Jaenicke, R., Lubsen, N. H., Slingsby, C., and Tardieu, A. (2004). Ageing and vision: Structure, stability and function of lens crystallins. *Prog. Biophys. Mol. Biol.* 86:407–485.

Blundell, T., Lindley, P., Miller, L., Moss, D., Slingsby, C., Tickle, I., Turnell, B., and Wistow, G. (1981). The molecular structure and stability of the eye lens: X-ray analysis of gamma-crystallin II. *Nature* 289:771–777.

Bova, M. P., McHaourab, H. S., Han, Y., and Fung, B. K. (2000). Subunit exchange of small heat shock proteins: Analysis of oligomer formation of alphaA-crystallin and Hsp27 by fluorescence resonance energy transfer and site-directed truncations. *J. Biol. Chem.* 275:1035–1042.

Bystroff, C., and Shao, Y. (2002). Fully automated ab initio protein structure prediction using I-SITES, HMMSTR and ROSETTA. *Bioinformatics* 18(Suppl. 1):S54–S61.

Calvin, H. I., Wu, J. X., Viswanadhan, K., and Fu, S. C. (1996). Modifications in lens protein biosynthesis signal the initiation of cataracts induced by buthionine sulfoximine in mice. *Exp. Eye Res.* 63:357–368.

Carrell, R. W., and Lomas, D. A. (1997). Conformational disease. *Lancet* 350:134–138.

Caspers, G. J., Leunissen, J. A., and de Jong, W. W. (1995). The expanding small heat-shock protein family, and structure predictions of the conserved "alpha-crystallin domain." *J. Mol. Evol.* 40:238–248.

Cohen, L. H., Westerhuis, L. W., de Jong, W. W., and Bloemendal, H. (1978). Rat alpha-crystallin A chain with an insertion of 22 residues. *Eur. J. Biochem.* 89:259–266.

Crecelius, A. C., Cornett, D. S., Caprioli, R. M., Williams, B., Dawant, B. M., and Bodenheimer, B. (2005). Three-dimensional visualization of protein expression in mouse brain structures using imaging mass spectrometry. *J. Am. Soc. Mass Spectrom.* 16:1093–1099.

Datiles, M. B., Schumer, D. J., Zigler J. S., Jr., Russell, P., Anderson, and L., Garland, D. (1992). Two-dimensional gel electrophoretic analysis of human lens proteins. *Curr. Eye Res.* 11:669–677.

David, L. L., Calvin, H. I., and Fu, S. C. (1994). Buthionine sulfoximine induced cataracts in mice contain insolubilized crystallins with calpain II cleavage sites. *Exp. Eye Res.* 59:501–504.

de Jong, W. W., Hendriks, W., Mulders, L. W., and Bloemendal, H. (1989). Evolution of eye lens crystallins: The stress connection. *Trends Biochem. Sci.* 14:354–368.

Delaye, M., and Tardieu, A. (1983). Short-range order of crystallin proteins accounts for eye lens transparency. *Nature* 302: 415–417.

Descamps, F. J., Martens, E., Proost, P., Starckx, S., Van den Steen, P. E., Van Damme, J., and Opdenakker, G. (2005). Gelatinase B/matrix metalloproteinase-9 provokes cataract by cleaving lens betaB1 crystallin. *FASEB J.* 19:29–35.

Edman, P. (1949). A method for the determination of the amino acid sequence in peptides. *Arch. Biochem.* 22:475–476.

Farnsworth, P., Frauwirth, H., Groth-Vasselli, B., and Singh, K. (1998). Refinement of 3D structure of bovine lens alpha A-crystallin. *Int. J. Biol. Macromol.* 22:175–185.

Farnsworth, P., Groth-Vasselli, B., Greenfield, N. J., and Singh, K. (1997). Effects of temperature and concentration on bovine lens alpha-crystallin secondary structure: A circular dichroism spectroscopic study. *Int. J. Biol. Macromol.* 20:283–291.

Farnsworth, P., and Singh, K. (2004). Structure function relationship among alpha-crystallin related small heat shock proteins. *Exp. Eye Res.* 79:787–794.

Fenn, J. B., Mann, M., Meng, C. K., Wong, S. F., and Whitehouse, C. M. (1989). Electrospray ionization for mass spectrometry of large biomolecules. *Science* 246:64–71.

Fernald, R. D., and Wright, S. E. (1983). Maintenance of optical quality during crystalline lens growth. *Nature* 301:618–620.

Garadi, R., Katar, M., and Maisel, H. (1983). Two-dimensional gel analysis of chick lens proteins. *Exp. Eye Res.* 36:859–869.

Garber, A. T., Goring, D., and Gold, R. J. (1984). Characterization of abnormal proteins in the soluble lens proteins of CatFraser mice. *J. Biol. Chem.* 259:10376–10379.

Garland, D. L., Duglas-Tabor, Y., Yimenez-Asensio, J., Datiles, M. B., and Magno, B. (1996). The nucleus of the human lens: Demonstration of a highly characteristic protein pattern by two-dimensional electrophoresis and introduction of a new method of lens dissection. *Exp. Eye Res.* 62:285–291.

Ge, Y., Lawhorn, B. G., ElNaggar, M., Strauss, E., Park, J. H., Begley, T. P., and McLafferty, F. W. (2002). Top down characterization of larger proteins (45 kDa) by electron capture dissociation mass spectrometry. *J. Am. Chem. Soc.* 124:672–678.

Gesierich, U., and Pfeil, W. (1996). The conformational stability of alpha-crystallin is rather low: Calorimetric results. *FEBS Lett.* 393:151–154.

Gong, X., Li, E., Klier, G., Huang, Q., Wu, Y., Lei, H., Kumar, N. M., Horwitz, J., and Gilula, N. B. (1997). Disruption of alpha3 connexin gene leads to proteolysis and cataractogenesis in mice. *Cell* 91:833–843.

Han, X., Jin, M., Breuker, K., and McLafferty, F. W. (2006). Extending top-down mass spectrometry to proteins with masses greater than 200 kilodaltons. *Science* 314:109–112.

Harding, J. J. (1972). Conformational changes in human lens proteins in cataract. *Biochem. J.* 129:97–100.

Henzel, W. J., Billeci, T. M., Stults, J. T., Wong, S. C., Grimley, C., and Watanabe, C. (1993). Identifying proteins from two-dimensional gels by molecular mass searching of peptide fragments in protein sequence databases. *Proc. Natl. Acad. Sci. U.S.A.* 90:5011–5015.

Hoehenwarter, W., Ackermann, R., Pleissner, K. P., Schmid, M., Stein, R., Zimny-Arndt, U., Kumar, N. M., and Jungblut, P. R. (2008). Modifying factors of the cataract pathology of the nucleus of the mouse eye lens. Unpublished manuscript.

Hoehenwarter, W., Ackermann, R., Zimny-Arndt, U., Kumar, N. M., and Jungblut, P. R. (2006a). The necessity of functional proteomics: Protein species and molecular function elucidation exemplified by in vivo alpha A crystallin N-terminal truncation. *Amino Acids* 31:317–323.

Hoehenwarter, W., Klose, J., and Jungblut, P. R. (2006b). Eye lens proteomics. *Amino Acids* 30:369–389.

Hoehenwarter, W., Kumar, N. M., Wacker, M., Zimny-Arndt, U., Klose, J., and Jungblut, P. R. (2005). Eye lens proteomics: From global approach to detailed information about phakinin and gamma E and F crystallin genes. *Proteomics* 5:245–257.

Horwitz, J. (1992). Alpha-crystallin can function as a molecular chaperone. *Proc. Natl. Acad. Sci. U.S.A.* 89:10449–10453.

Horwitz, J., Huang, Q. L., Ding, L., and Bova, M. P. (1998). Lens alpha-crystallin: Chaperone like properties. *Methods Enzymol.* 290:365–383.

Jakob, U., Gaestel, M., Engel, K., and Buchner, J. (1993). Small heat shock proteins are molecular chaperones. *J. Biol. Chem.* 268:1517–1520.

Jungblut, P., Otto, A., Favor, J., Lowe, M., Muller, E. C., Kastnetr, M., Sperling, K., and Klose, J. (1998). Identification of mouse crystallins in 2D protein patterns by sequencing and mass spectrometry: Application to cataract mutants. *FEBS Lett.* 435:131–137.

Jungblut, P., and Thiede, B. (1997). Protein identification from 2-DE gels by MALDI mass spectrometry. *Mass Spectrom. Rev.* 16:145–162.

Jungblut, P., Thiede, B., Zimny-Arndt, U., Muller, E. C., Scheler, C., Wittmann-Liebold, B., and Otto, A. (1996). Resolution power of two-dimensional electrophoresis and identification of proteins from gels. *Electrophoresis* 17:839–847.

Karas, M., and Hillenkamp, F. (1988). Laser desorption ionization of proteins with molecular masses exceeding 10,000 daltons. *Anal. Chem.* 60:2299–2301.

Kibbelaar, M., and Bloemendal, H. (1975). The topography of lens proteins based on chromatography and two-dimensional gel electrophoresis. *Exp. Eye Res.* 21:25–36.

Klemenz, R., Frohli, E., Steiger, R. H., Schafer, R., and Aoyama, A. (1991). Alpha B-crystallin is a small heat shock protein. *Proc. Natl. Acad. Sci. U.S.A.* 88:3652–3655.

Klose, J., and Kobalz, U. (1995). Two-dimensional electrophoresis of proteins: An updated protocol and implications for a functional analysis of the genome. *Electrophoresis* 16:1034–1059.

Lampi, K., Shih, M., Ueda, Y., Shearer, T. R., and David, L. L. (2002). Lens proteomics: Analysis of rat crystallin sequences and two-dimensional electrophoresis map. *Invest. Ophthalmol. Vis. Sci.* 43:216–224.

Li, W., Calvin, H. I., David, L. L., Wu, K., McCormack, A. L., Zhu, G. P., and Fu, S. C. (2002). Altered patterns of phosphorylation in cultured mouse lenses during development of buthionine sulfoximine cataracts. *Exp. Eye Res.* 75:335–346.

Lubsen, N. H., Aarts, H. J., and Schoenmakers, J. G. (1988). The evolution of lenticular proteins: The beta- and gamma-crystallin super gene family. *Prog. Biophys. Mol. Biol.* 51:47–76.

Lund, A. L., Smith, J. B., and Smith, D. L. (1996). Modifications of the water-insoluble human lens alpha-crystallins. *Exp. Eye Res.* 63:661–672.

Ma, H., Fukiage, C., Azuma, M., and Shearer, T. R. (1998). Cloning and expression of mRNA for calpain Lp82 from rat lens: Splice variant of p94. *Invest. Ophthalmol. Vis. Sci.* 39:454–461.

Mayr, E. M., Jaenicke, R., and Glockshuber, R. (1994). Domain interaction and connecting peptides in lens crystallins. *J. Mol. Biol.* 235:84–88.

Merck, K. B., De Haard-Hoekman, W. A., Oude Essink, B. B., Bloemendal, H., and De Jong, W. W. (1992). Expression and aggregation of recombinant alpha A-crystallin and its two domains. *Biochim. Biophys. Acta* 1130:267–276.

Mörner, C. T. (1893). Untersuchung der Proteinsubstanzen in den leichtbrechenden Medien des Auges. *Z. Physiol. Chem.* 18: 61–106.

Nalini, V., Bax, B., Driessen, H., Moss, D. S., Lindley, P. F., and Slingsby, C. (1994). Close packing of an oligomeric eye lens beta-crystallin induces loss of symmetry and ordering of sequence extensions. *J. Mol. Biol.* 236:1250–1258.

O'Farrell, P. H. (1975). High resolution two-dimensional electrophoresis of proteins. *J. Biol. Chem.* 250:4007–4021.

Okkels, L. M., Muller, E. C., Schmid, M., Rosenkrands, I., Kaufman, S. H., Andersen, P., and Jungblut, P. R. (2004). CFP10 discriminates between nonacetylated and acetylated ESAT-6 of *Mycobacterium tuberculosis* by differential interaction. *Proteomics* 4:2954–2960.

Pasta, S. Y., Raman, B., Ramakrishna, T., and Rao, C. M. (2003). Role of the conserved SRLFDQFFG region of alpha-crystallin, a small heat shock protein: Effect on oligomeric size, subunit exchange and chaperone-like activity. *J. Biol. Chem.* 278: 51159–51166.

Senn, M., Venkataraghavan, R., and McLafferty, F. W. (1966). Mass spectrometric studies of peptides. 3. Automated determination of amino acid sequences. *J. Am. Chem. Soc.* 88:5593–5597.

Shih, M., Lampi, K. J., Shearer, T. R., and David, L. L. (1998). Cleavage of beta crystallins during maturation of bovine lens. *Mol. Vis.* 4:4–11.

Singh, K., Groth-Vasselli, B., and Farnsworth, P. N. (1998). Interaction of DNA with bovine lens alpha-crystallin: Its functional implications. *Int. J. Biol. Macromol.* 22:315–320.

Slingsby, C., and Bateman, O. A. (1990). Quaternary interactions in eye lens beta-crystallins: Basic and acidic subunits of beta-crystallins favor heterologous association. *Biochemistry* 29:6592–6599.

Smith, J. B., Liu, Y., and Smith, D. L. (1996). Identification of possible regions of chaperone activity in lens alpha-crystallin. *Exp. Eye Res.* 63:125–128.

Stevens, A., Wang, S. X., Caines, G. H., and Schleich, T. (1995). 13C-NMR off resonance rotating frame spin-lattice relaxation studies of bovine lens gamma-crystallin self association: Effect of "macromolecular crowding." *Biochim. Biophys. Acta* 1246:82–90.

Swanson, S. K., and Washburn, M. P. (2005). The continuing evolution of shotgun proteomics. *Drug Discov. Today* 10:719–725.

Sze, S. K., Ge, Y., Oh, H., and McLafferty, F. W. (2002). Top-down mass spectrometry of a 29-kDa protein for characterization of any posttranslational modification to within one residue. *Proc. Natl. Acad. Sci. U.S.A.* 99:1774–1779.

Takemoto, L., Emmons, T., and Horwitz, J. (1993). The C-terminal region of alpha-crystallin: Involvement in protection against heat-induced denaturation. 294:435–438.

Tanaka, K., Waki, H., Ido, Y., Akita, S., Yoshida, Y., and Yoshida, T. (1988). Protein an polymer analysis up to m/z 100,000 by laser ionization time of flight mass spectrometry. *Rapid Commun. Mass Spectrom.* 2:151–153.

Thampi, P., and Abraham, E. C. (2003). Influence of the C-terminal residues on oligomerization of alpha A-crystallin. *Biochemistry* 42:11857–11863.

Thiede, B., Höhenwarter, W., Krah, A., Mattow, J., Schmid, M., Schmidt, F., and Jungblut, P. R. (2005). Peptide mass fingerprinting. *Methods* 35:237–247.

Thomson, J. A., and Augusteyn, R. C. (1989). On the structure of alpha-crystallin: Construction of hybrid molecules and homopolymers. *Biochim. Biophys. Acta* 994:246–252.

Ueda, Y., Duncan, M. K., and David, L. L. (2002). Lens proteomics: The accumulation of crystallin modifications in the mouse lens with age. *Invest. Ophthalmol. Vis. Sci.* 43:205–215.

van den Oetelaar, P. J., van Someren, P. F., Thomson, J. A., Siezen, R. J., and Hoenders, H. J. (1990). A dynamic quaternary structure of bovine alpha-crystallin as indicated from intermolecular exchange of subunits. *Biochemistry* 29:3488–3493.

van Rens, G. L., Raats, J. M., Driessen, H. P., Oldenburg, M., Wijnen, J. T., Khan, P. M., de Jong, W. W., and Bloemendal, H. (1989). Structure of the bovine eye lens gamma S-crystallin gene (formerly beta S). *Gene* 78:225–233.

Wang, K., and Spector, A. (1994). The chaperone activity of bovine alpha crystallin. Interaction with other lens crystallins in native and denatured states. *J. Biol. Chem.* 269:13601–13608.

Washburn, M. P., Wolters, D., and Yates, J. R., III (2001). Large-scale analysis of the yeast proteome by multidimensional protein identification technology. *Nat. Biotechnol.* 19:242–247.

Wistow, G. (1993). Possible tetramer-based quaternary structure for alpha-crystallins and small heat shock proteins. *Exp. Eye Res.* 56:729–732.

Wistow, G., and Piatigorsky, J. (1988). Lens crystallins: The evolution and expression of proteins for a highly specialized tissue. *Annu. Rev. Biochem.* 57:479–504.

Wistow, G., Watt, K., David, L., Gao, C., Bateman, O., Bernstein, S., Tomarev, S., Segovia, L., Slingsby, C., et al. (2005). GammaN-crystallin and the evolution of the beta-gamma-crystallin superfamily in vertebrates. *FEBS J.* 272:2276–2291.

Yates, J. R., III (1998). Mass spectrometry and the age of the proteome. *J. Mass Spectrom.* 33:1–19.

59 Genetic and Proteomic Analyses of the Mouse Visual Cycle

JOHN C. SAARI AND JOHN W. CRABB

The vertebrate eye paints upon the retina with bleached photopigments a picture of the luminous world outside.
—W. A. H. Rushton

Our retinas have evolved to provide useful detection of light over an extraordinary range of illumination intensities by using two sets of photoreceptors, rods and cones, which complement each other in sensitivity and in the speed and dynamic range of response. With this system, differentiation of the horizon from the moonless night sky is possible even though each rod photoreceptor of the human retina absorbs a photon on average once every 85 minutes. At the other end of the scale, a white ptarmigan can still be seen on a snowy slope in bright daylight, when the average cone photoreceptor absorbs more than 10^6 photons per second (Rodieck, 1998).

Despite enormous differences in physiological responses, the chemistry of light detection involved in both rods and cones of all vertebrate species is the same and involves photoisomerization of 11-*cis*-retinal, or a closely related derivative, to all-*trans*-retinal. Enzymatic regeneration of 11-*cis*-retinal takes place in all vertebrates in cells adjacent to the photoreceptor cells in a process originally called the visual cycle and more recently the retinoid cycle. Great advances have been made in the past decade in our understanding of the molecular events responsible for the regeneration of rod visual pigments. Detailed knowledge of a cone visual cycle remains elusive, although the evidence for involvement of Müller cells continues to accumulate.

This chapter considers advances in our understanding of the visual cycle that critically depended on the use of mouse genetics, alteration of the mouse genome, and proteomics. The rich history associated with many visual cycle components is mentioned only in passing, with relevant reviews cited. Throughout this chapter, we use standard conventions for denoting genes and gene products (examples: human gene, *RPE65*; mouse gene, *Rpe65*; protein, RPE65).

A variety of techniques have been employed over the years to study molecular aspects of the rod visual cycle. Early investigators made use of the color changes that accompanied photoisomerization of 11-*cis*-retinal, bound to opsin, to all-*trans*-retinal (purple to yellow) and reduction of all-*trans*-retinal to all-*trans*-retinol (yellow to colorless). Later, classic enzymology provided valuable information about the various reactions that make up the cycle, primarily relying on bovine tissue extracts. Molecular cloning of cDNAs and ectopic cDNA expression allowed the assignment of enzymatic activities to molecular entities. The sequencing of complete genomes identified orthologues of key enzymes and opened up comparative sequence analysis for mechanistic studies. Assignment of an in vivo activity to a molecular entity was not a trivial matter and required techniques for generating transgenic and knockout mice. For one enzyme of the cycle (lecithin:retinol acyltransferase, LRAT), the enzymatic activity in vitro clearly pointed to an in vivo function, as proven by the phenotype of mice with targeted disruption of the gene. In other cases, disruption of the genes had either little effect (*Rdh5*, *Rdh11*, *prRDH*, *Rdh12*, *Irbp*) or a partial effect (*Rlbp1*) on the rate of rhodopsin regeneration, suggesting functional redundancy at these steps. Analysis of disease-causing mutations in humans was not always helpful, presumably because of differences between the human and mouse visual systems.

Additional information regarding the visual cycle resulted from the identification and characterization of proteins using mass spectrometry, methodology referred to as proteomics. Indeed, the sensitivity and accuracy of these techniques have revolutionized structural component analysis, and future utilization promises to open up our understanding of the cell biology of retinoid processing.

Genetic analysis of the mouse visual cycle

The rod visual cycle is made up of a mixture of well-established and novel reactions occurring in two adjacent cell types. Diffusion of retinoids between the two cell types links the reactions into a cycle. Decades of research have established the reaction sequence in rod photoreceptors and retinal pigmented epithelium (RPE), and many of the enzymes that carry out these reactions in vivo have been identified. Nonetheless, details regarding the mechanisms of the reactions and possible reaction controls are lacking, and detailed information about the cell biology of retinoid processing in RPE is almost nonexistent. Furthermore, the nature of the diffusion of retinoids between the cell types is poorly understood.

The phototransduction cascade is activated by the absorption of a photon by 11-*cis*-retinal, the chromophore attached to rod opsin (figure 59.1). The photoisomerization product, all-*trans*-retinal, dissociates from opsin and is reduced to all-*trans*-retinol by NADPH, catalyzed by one or more retinol dehydrogenases (RDHs) of the rod outer segment. All-*trans*-retinol diffuses from the rod cell through the interphotoreceptor matrix and enters the RPE, where LRAT catalyzes its esterification with a long chain fatty acid. Isomerohydrolase (RPE65) simultaneously hydrolyzes the ester bond of all-*trans*-retinyl ester and isomerizes the double bond at position 11–12 to yield 11-*cis*-retinol and a fatty acid. Oxidation of 11-*cis*-retinol to 11-*cis*-retinal by NAD is catalyzed by one or more *cis*-specific RDHs (*cis*-RDHs) and returned to the rod outer segment for conjugation with opsin and regeneration of the visual pigment. Cellular retinol-binding protein type I (CRBPI) and cellular retinaldehyde-binding protein (CRALBP) are present in RPE and facilitate esterification and isomerization/oxidation of retinoids, respectively. Interphotoreceptor retinoid-binding protein (IRBP) is present in the interphotoreceptor matrix (IPM) and may protect retinoids during diffusion between cells and reduce their toxic effects. A brief description of our current understanding of the reactions of the rod visual cycle follows.

All-*trans*-Retinol Dehydrogenase Following photoisomerization of 11-*cis*-retinal, all-*trans*-retinal is released from opsin and reduced to all-*trans*-retinol by NADPH in the outer segments of photoreceptor cells. This reaction is accompanied by a change in color from yellow (all-*trans*-retinal) to colorless (all-*trans*-retinol) and was the first enzymatic visual cycle reaction to be studied in detail (Wald and Hubbard, 1949).

Based on their kinetic properties and substrate specificities, several short chain dehydrogenases/reductases (SDRs) have been proposed to catalyze the reduction of all-*trans*-retinal in vivo. However, studies of knockout mice have failed to identify a single enzyme whose absence has a major effect on the rate of visual pigment regeneration in vivo. This example points to the importance of mouse genetics in assigning in vivo functions to in vitro activities.

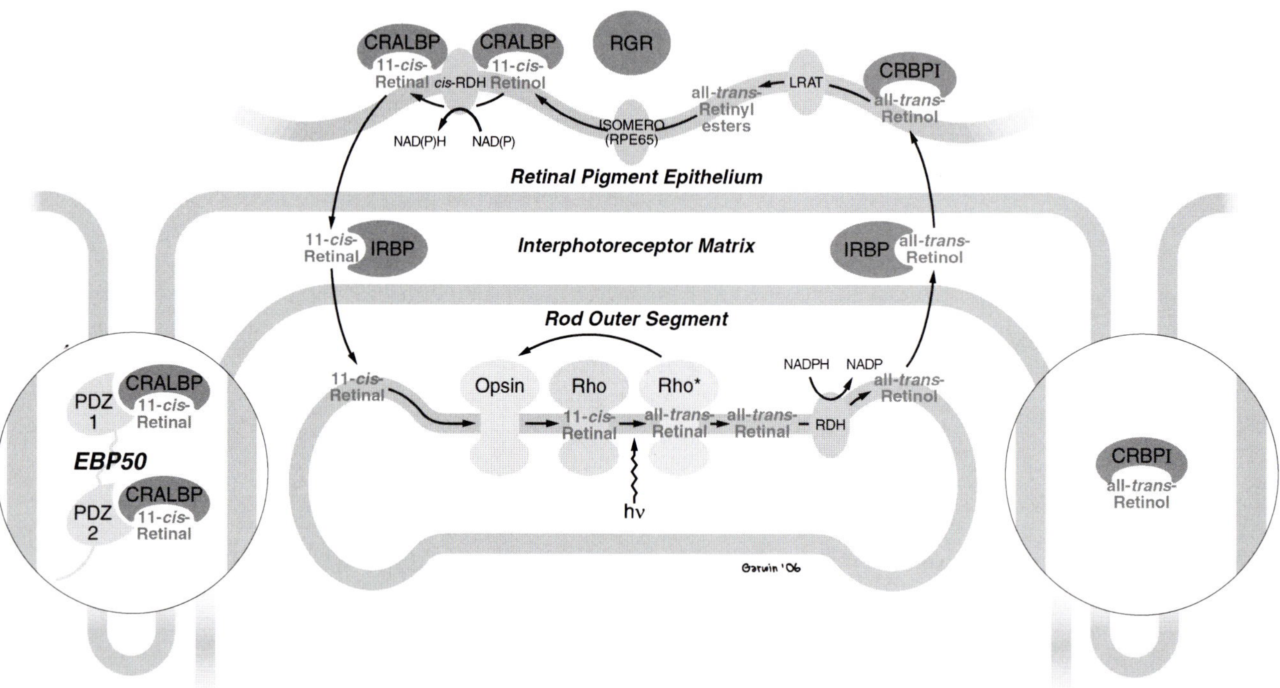

Figure 59.1 Hypothetical schematic of the rod photoreceptor visual cycle. Transcellular diffusion and intracellular enzymatic processing of visual cycle retinoids are shown. A retinal pigmented epithelial (RPE) cell is depicted with apical process extending toward a rod outer segment, with one disc membrane. Reactions and processes are as discussed in the text. *Circular insets* depict putative roles of components in RPE apical processes. *cis*-RDH, 11-*cis*-retinal dehydrogenase; CRALBP, cellular retinaldehyde-binding protein; CRBPI, cellular retinol-binding protein type I; EBP50, ERM-binding phosphoprotein of 50 kd, also known as NHERF-1 (sodium hydrogen exchanger regulatory factor type 1); IRBP, interphotoreceptor retinoid-binding protein; ISOMERO, isomerohydrolase, recently identified as RPE65; LRAT, lecithin:retinol acyltransferase; PDZ, a scaffold domain protein; RGR, retinal G protein–coupled receptor; RDH, all-*trans*-retinol dehydrogenase; Rho, rhodopsin; Rho*, activated rhodopsin (metarhodopsin II); RPE65, retinal pigmented epithelial protein of 65 kd. See color plate 68.

A cDNA encoding RetSDR1 was cloned during a search of a retinal cDNA library for SDR homologues (Haeseleer et al., 1998). In situ hybridization and immunocytochemistry revealed the gene to be highly expressed in cone outer segments; however, expression was also noted in cells of the inner retina. The expressed enzyme catalyzed the reduction of all-*trans*- but not 11-*cis*-retinal and required NADPH. Several hydroxysteroids were also substrates for the enzyme, and transcripts were noted in several other tissues (Cerignoli et al., 2002). At present, the function of this enzyme in cone outer segments is not known.

A cDNA-encoding prRDH (RDH8) was cloned during a screen of retina-specific genes (Rattner et al., 2000). Antibodies revealed that the enzyme was expressed in rod and cone photoreceptor outer segments. The expressed enzyme was specific for all-*trans*-retinal and NADPH, similar to the activity in rod outer segments. *prRdh*$^{-/-}$ mice developed normally, and their retinal morphology was normal (Maeda et al., 2005). As predicted, the rate of reduction of all-*trans*-retinal was reduced in *prRdh*$^{-/-}$ mouse extracts following a flash; however, the rate of rhodopsin regeneration was normal. This result is an indication that the overall rate of the visual cycle is controlled by a step downstream of RDH, presumably the isomerohydrolase step, and that another dehydrogenase remained to be identified.

Mutations in the *RDH12* gene in humans resulted in a severe form of retinal degeneration beginning in early childhood (Janecke et al., 2004). However, the enzyme is found in rod inner segments and not in outer segments, and disruption of the *Rdh12* gene in mice did not affect the rate of visual pigment regeneration or ERG responses (Kurth et al., 2007). *Rdh12*$^{-/-}$ mice also exhibited accelerated 11-*cis*-retinal production and increased susceptibility to light-induced photoreceptor degeneration (Maeda et al., 2006). The cause of the severe form of retinal dystrophy in humans with mutations in this gene remains unexplained but may be related to light damage.

ATP-Binding Cassette A4 The disc membrane of the rod photoreceptor cell is equipped with a transporter of the ATP-binding cassette (ABC)-transporter family that retrieves all-*trans*-retinal from the luminal side of the disc membrane. Topologically, the compartment within the discs is equivalent to the outside of the cell, removed from the cytosolic site of production of NADPH and presumably from the active site of all-*trans*-RDH. The transporter, originally known as ABCR and now called ABCA4, utilizes ATP to "flip" all-*trans*-retinal from the luminal side of the disc to the cytosolic side, where it can be reduced to all-*trans*-retinol. The actual substrate for the translocation may be all-*trans*-retinal linked to phosphatidylethanolamine as a Schiff base. Characterization of the phenotype of *Abca4*$^{-/-}$ mice (Weng et al., 1999) revealed that the rate of rhodopsin regeneration was normal, indicating that most of the all-*trans*-retinal must be released on the cytosolic side of the disc membrane. However, *Abca4*$^{-/-}$ mice accumulated all-*trans*-retinal and A2E, a novel pyridinium *bis*-retinoid characterized earlier as a component of lipofuscin. Mutations in the human *ABCA4* gene cause autosomal recessive Stargardt disease (Allikmets et al., 1997), a form of macular dystrophy with large accumulations of lipofuscin in RPE. Based on these observations, it seems likely that the main physiological role of ABCR is to retrieve the small (in comparison to the total flux of the visual cycle) amount of all-*trans*-retinal that is released on the lumenal side of the discs and thus to minimize accumulation of its toxic condensation products.

Lecithin:Retinol Acyltransferase In RPE, retinyl esters are primarily synthesized by LRAT via transfer of a fatty acyl group from the *sn-1* position of phosphatidylcholine to the hydroxyl of retinol (Berry et al., 1989; Saari and Bredberg, 1989). Molecular characterization of LRAT from retina revealed a small hydrophobic protein (25.3 kd) (Ruiz et al., 1999) encoded by a single gene in mouse and humans (Ruiz et al., 2001).

Lrat$^{-/-}$ mice were normal in appearance and grossly unremarkable; however, reduced fertility was noted in males. Development of the retina in *Lrat*$^{-/-}$ mice appeared normal; however, rod outer segments were shorter than normal in 4.5-month-old animals. Rhodopsin and retinoids, except for small amounts of all-*trans*-retinol, were virtually absent from retinas. ERG responses were grossly diminished, and the scotopic threshold was elevated by 5–6 log units (Batten et al., 2004).

The virtual absence of retinyl esters and 11-*cis*-retinal in retinas of *Lrat*$^{-/-}$ mice is consistent with the proposed role of LRAT in esterification of all-*trans*-retinol and of all-*trans*-retinyl ester as the substrate for the isomerohydrolase in the visual cycle (Deigner et al., 1989). Thus, in the absence of LRAT, the visual cycle would be blocked at the isomerohydrolase step by the absence of substrate. Other studies ruled out impaired uptake of blood-borne retinoids by RPE because oral gravage of 9-*cis*-retinyl acetate or succinate esters resulted in formation of isorhodopsin in the retina (Batten et al., 2005).

Isomerohydrolase The search for an isomerase is a fascinating story in which investigators followed two different paths for years, a search for a protein associated with the isomerase activity, and a search for a function for isomerohydrolase (RPE65), before realizing the two paths intersected.

The isomerase activity, which regenerates the 11-*cis*-retinoid configuration, is the signature enzyme of the visual cycle. Although many investigators assumed that all-*trans*-retinal would be isomerized directly to 11-*cis*-retinal, Rando's laboratory determined that the isomerization took place at the oxidation level of all-*trans*-retinol and discovered an enzymatic activity that converted all-*trans*-retinyl esters to 11-*cis*-retinol and a free fatty acid, a reaction termed an isomerohydrolase (Bernstein and Rando, 1986; Bernstein et al., 1987). Hydrolysis of the ester bond was proposed to provide the energy needed for generation of the hindered 11-*cis*-retinoid (Deigner et al., 1989). Attempts to purify the enzyme or to isolate a cDNA encoding the enzyme were unsuccessful for nearly two decades following the discovery of its activity.

Meanwhile, attempts to identify a retinol-binding protein (RBP) receptor led to the characterization of a major protein of RPE microsomes called p63 (Båvik et al., 1991). Subsequent studies demonstrated that its localization was not consistent with its proposed function. Other investigators, interested in proteins exclusively expressed by RPE cells, characterized a major protein of RPE microsomes, RPE65, which was identical to p63 (Hamel et al., 1993). *Rpe65*$^{-/-}$ mice were unable to synthesize 11-*cis*-retinoids and accumulated large amounts of all-*trans*-retinyl esters in their RPE (Redmond et al., 1998). Both rod and cone functions were affected, indicating that RPE65 was involved in rod and cone visual cycles (Seeliger et al., 2001). Although this phenotype would be expected if RPE65 were the isomerohydrolase, attempts to provide direct evidence for this contention were unsuccessful until 2005, when three laboratories, using different approaches, demonstrated that RPE65 was responsible for isomerohydrolase activity (Jin et al., 2005; Redmond et al., 2005; Moiseyev et al., 2006).

Differences in susceptibility to light damage observed in several strains of mice were traced to a L450M sequence variation in the *Rpe65* gene (Danciger et al., 2000). Subsequent studies revealed that this sequence variation also correlated with differences in the rate of rhodopsin regeneration. Strains of mice with L450 regenerated their visual pigment approximately four times faster and were more susceptible to light damage than strains of mice with M450 (Wenzel et al., 2001). The RPE65 content of M450 strains of mice was significantly lower than that of L450 strains, suggesting that the sequence variation affected the stability of RPE65. The rate of the isomerase reaction is the slow step in the mouse visual cycle (see discussion of retinoid flow). Thus, a decrease in the amount of RPE65 would be expected to reduce the flux of retinoid through this reaction, allow retinoid to accumulate as relatively innocuous all-*trans*-retinyl esters, and reduce the amount of visual pigment available for photoisomerization. (See also the discussion of CRALBP and light damage.)

The isomerohydrolase reaction also requires a lipid-binding protein for activity. Apo-cellular retinaldehyde-binding protein (CRALBP) performs this function most efficiently in vitro (Winston and Rando, 1998), but other proteins are effective at much higher concentrations. Presumably, the retinoid-binding protein relieves inhibition of the enzyme by binding the product of the reaction, 11-*cis*-retinol (Winston and Rando, 1998). This explanation is in keeping with the visual phenotype of *Rlbp1*$^{-/-}$ (*Cralbp*$^{-/-}$) mice, which show a delay in the visual cycle at the isomerohydrolase step (Saari et al., 2001). However, the requirement for CRALBP is not absolute because the visual cycle functions in its absence, although very slowly (see later discussion of CRALBP).

Detailed examination of RPE65 structure has provided considerable insight into molecular aspects of the catalytic activity (Moiseyev et al., 2006). RPE65 is a member of the carotenoid-cleavage oxygenase family of enzymes, which includes β-carotene 15,15′-monooxygenase (carotene cleavage enzyme). These enzymes coordinate an active site Fe^{2+} via four histidines, which are conserved in RPE65 and other members of the family. The crystal structure of an apocarotenoid 15,15′-oxygenase suggests that all-*trans*-apocarotenoids are transiently isomerized during catalysis of cleavage (Kloer et al., 2005). Mutation of the corresponding histidine residues in RPE65 abolished the isomerohydolase activity of the protein (Redmond et al., 2005). The addition of chelating agents to native RPE65 enzyme reduced the activity of the enzyme and the addition of Fe(II) restored the activity. Finally, native RPE65 bound Fe(II) with a nearly 1 to 1 stoichiometry. These studies suggest, in an evolutionary sense, that an ancestral Fe-binding protein gave rise to a branch with isomerase and carotenoid cleavage activity (e.g., carotene cleavage enzyme) and a branch with just isomerase activity (e.g., RPE65) and demonstrate a role for iron in the regeneration of visual pigments.

Retinal G Protein–Coupled Receptor Retinal G protein–coupled receptor (RGR) was first detected during a screen for RPE-specific proteins (Jiang et al., 1993). It was later found to be present in Müller cells also. The importance of RGR for retinal function and health was emphasized by the observation that mutations in the *RGR* gene in humans resulted in degeneration of the retina (Morimura et al., 1999). Sequence analysis revealed it to be a member of the G protein–coupled receptor family and to bind all-*trans*-retinal. Illumination of an RGR·all-*trans*-retinal complex resulted in photoisomerization of the retinoid to 11-*cis*-retinal, similar to the photoisomerization of all-*trans*-retinal bound to squid retinochrome. This striking result immediately suggested that a function of the protein might be to provide 11-*cis*-retinal during illumination via a photoisomerization reaction. Initially, characterization of *Rgr*$^{-/-}$ mice provided conflicting results regarding the effect of the absence of RGR on the rate of regeneration in the dark. More recently, careful attention to the sequence variation of the *Rpe65* gene at position 450 (see discussion of *RPE65*) in control and experimental groups of animals clearly revealed that the rate of regeneration of rhodopsin was three times slower in *Rgr*$^{-/-}$ mice (Wenzel et al., 2005). Surprisingly, the absence of RGR in mice affected regeneration both during light exposure and in the dark, indicating that RGR was not a photoisomerase. Molecular details about the role of RGR remain to be determined.

11-*cis*-Retinol Dehydrogenase In RPE, 11-*cis*-retinol, produced by the isomerohydrolase, is oxidized to 11-*cis*-retinal by an SDR. As with the SDRs in the outer segment, there is functional redundancy at this step. Two SDRs have been identified in extracts of RPE. Surprisingly, neither enzyme alone or in combination accounts completely for 11-*cis*-retinol oxidizing activity in vivo in the mouse.

Shortly after its discovery, RPE65, then known as p63, was noted to interact with another protein in RPE microsomes (Simon et al., 1995). Cloning and studies of the expressed protein revealed it to be a member of the SDR family of proteins (RDH5) and to catalyze the oxidation of 11-*cis*-retinol by NAD. Humans with mutations in the RDH5 gene have a condition called fundus albipunctatus, which is a slowly progressing form of retinitis pigmentosa characterized by delayed dark adaptation and, in some cases, late-onset cone dystrophy (Yamamoto et al., 1999; Nakamura et al., 2000). Thus, it was a surprise when the rate of rhodopsin regeneration was found to be normal in *Rdh5*$^{-/-}$ mice (Driessen et al., 2000). The only abnormality noted in these animals was an accumulation of 13-*cis*-retinyl esters in RPE. These results suggested that another SDR catalyzed the oxidation of 11-*cis*-retinol in mice.

RDH11 is expressed in prostate and also in RPE cells of the retina (Haeseleer et al., 2002). *Rdh11*$^{-/-}$ mice showed a phenotype similar to that of *Rdh5*$^{-/-}$ mice (Kim et al., 2005). The phenotype of *Rdh5*$^{-/-}$/*Rdh11*$^{-/-}$ (double knockout) mice was similar to that of *Rdh5*$^{-/-}$ mice but also displayed an abnormality in cone function. However, the flow of retinoids in the visual cycle was normal when moderate amounts of visual pigment were bleached (Kim et al., 2005), suggesting the existence of yet additional 11-*cis*-RDHs. No disease-causing mutations in the *RDH11* gene in humans have been reported. RDH10 is expressed in RPE and Müller cells but appears to be specific for all-*trans*-retinols (B. X. Wu et al., 2004).

Several lines of evidence suggest that oxidation of 11-*cis*-retinol by *cis*-RDHs of RPE microsomes is facilitated by CRALBP. When bound to CRALBP, the aldehyde group of 11-*cis*-retinal is sequestered from water-soluble carbonyl reagents yet is readily reduced by NADH and RPE microsomes (Saari and Bredberg, 1982). 11-*cis*-retinol bound to CRALBP is oxidized to 11-*cis*-retinal by the *cis*-retinol dehydrogenase(s) of RPE microsomes more rapidly than free retinol (Saari et al., 1994) and has a lower K_m (higher affinity) than free retinol for purified recombinant RDH5 (Golovleva et al., 2003).

Retinol-Binding Protein and the RBP Receptor RBP is a small protein (21 kd) secreted into the blood conjugated with all-*trans*-retinol, where it circulates associated with transthyretin. RBP is synthesized primarily in the liver and in lesser amounts in several tissues, including adipose tissue and RPE. In *Rbp*$^{-/-}$ mice, which are unable to mobilize hepatic vitamin A but develop normally, dietary vitamin A reaches peripheral tissues as retinyl esters carried by plasma lipoproteins. Retinal function is markedly diminished for the first few months after birth (Quadro et al., 1999), but *Rbp*$^{-/-}$ mice attain full visual function thereafter if maintained on a vitamin A-sufficient diet. Thus, it appears that for developmental purposes, most tissues are able to obtain vitamin A via circulating dietary retinyl esters, but the eye requires an RBP-dependent mechanism for the amount of vitamin A required for vision (Vogel et al., 2002).

Uptake of vitamin A from RBP was suggested to involve a receptor-mediated process in the 1970s (Bok and Heller, 1976), and decades later an RBP-receptor, STRA6, was identified (Kawaguchi et al., 2007). STRA6 was originally discovered as a gene responsive to retinoic acid. Homozygous mutations in *STRA6* in humans result in severe developmental malformations and mental retardation (Passuto et al., 2007). Based on the patterns of STRA6 expression in embryo and adult, it appears that STRA6 may play an important role in delivering vitamin A to many tissues in the embryo and a more restricted role in the adult, where it is primarily expressed in tissues making up blood-brain or blood-organ barriers (e.g., RPE, choroid plexus).

Cellular Retinol-Binding Protein Type I CRBPI is a small, water-soluble retinoid-binding protein with high affinity for all-*trans*-retinol and all-*trans*-retinal (Napoli, 1999). CRBPI is expressed in many tissues, including RPE and Müller cells of the eye (Bok et al., 1984; Saari et al., 1984). Evidence obtained in vitro suggested that the protein could be involved in promoting esterification and oxidation of retinol and hydrolysis of retinyl esters (Herr and Ong, 1992; Napoli, 1999). However, its physiological role in vivo was not clear until analysis of *CrbpI*$^{-/-}$ mice. Normal development, reproduction, and behavior of these animals ruled out a major role for CRBPI in retinoic acid production because retinoic acid signaling is required for all these processes. A reduced content and six times faster turnover of hepatic retinyl esters was in keeping with a role for the protein in delivery of all-*trans*-retinol for esterification by LRAT (Ghyselinck et al., 1999). Stores of retinyl esters in RPE were also reduced relative to wild type, and all-*trans*-retinol accumulated transiently during recovery from a flash (Saari et al., 2002). Overall, the results were in accord with a role for CRBPI in delivery of all-*trans*-retinol to LRAT for esterification in RPE and liver.

Interphotoreceptor Retinoid-Binding Protein Interphotoreceptor retinoid-binding protein (IRBP) is a water-soluble protein synthesized by photoreceptor cells and secreted into the interphotoreceptor matrix (IPM) (reviewed in Gonzalez-Fernandez, 2003). Localization of the protein in the extracellular compartment between photoreceptor and RPE cells (Bunt-Milam and Saari, 1983) and its ability to load with all-*trans*-retinol following bleaches of visual pigment suggested that the protein would be involved in transcellular diffusion of retinoids (reviewed in Pepperberg et al., 1993).

The retinas of $Irbp^{-/-}$ mice showed a loss of photoreceptor nuclei and changes in the structural integrity of photoreceptor outer segments from P11 to P30. However, the rate of progression of the condition was quite slow, and was unaffected by raising the animals in the dark (Ripps et al., 2000). Even after 6 months, the number of photoreceptor nuclei was reduced to only about 50% of the number in wild-type mice (Liou et al., 1998; Ripps et al., 2000). Surprisingly, the rate of visual pigment regeneration was unaffected (Palczewski et al., 1999) or was even modestly faster (Ripps et al., 2000) in the absence of IRBP. Attempts to detect other retinoid-binding proteins in IPM that might have substituted for IRBP have been unsuccessful.

IRBP appears to be necessary for release of 11-*cis*-retinal from cultured RPE cells (Carlson and Bok, 1992). One explanation for this finding is that a receptor mechanism is involved. However, the rate of visual pigment regeneration in $Irbp^{-/-}$ mice was nomal, and molecular information regarding this receptor has not yet appeared in the literature.

The role of IRBP in visual physiology remains enigmatic. The small enhancement of the rate of rhodopsin regeneration in the absence of IRBP and the slow progression of the associated retinal degeneration are consistent with a role for the protein in buffering the concentration of free (unbound) all-*trans*-retinal or 11-*cis*-retinal in the IPM during retinoid diffusion between RPE and photoreceptor cells. However, the absence of protection from retinal degeneration in dark-reared animals does not fully accommodate such a function. IRBP binds several hydrophobic substances in addition to retinoids, including docosahexaenoic acid and other fatty acids (Bazan et al., 1985), and may be involved in intercellular diffusion of these substances, including scavenging of oxidatively damaged retinoids and fatty acids.

Cellular Retinaldehyde-Binding Protein CRALBP is a water-soluble protein with high affinity for 11-*cis*-retinol or 11-*cis*-retinal, found in abundance in RPE and Müller cells (Saari and Crabb, 2005). These features and the protein's pronounced effects on enzymatic reactions of the visual cycle in vitro (Saari et al., 1994; Golovleva et al., 2003; Winston and Rando, 1998), suggested that it was involved in the regeneration of visual pigments.

No differences were detected in the gross retinal morphologies of control and $Rlbp1^{-/-}$ mice raised in the dark (Saari et al., 2001). However, the rate of visual pigment regeneration following flash illumination was slower by about 15 times in the $Rlbp1^{-/-}$ animals. PCR analysis of the *Rpe65* gene indicated that differences in the rate of regeneration of control and knockout mice could not be accounted for by the L450M sequence variation in the *Rpe65* gene (see section on RPE65). Analysis of visual cycle retinoids revealed that retinyl ester accumulated during the delay, suggesting that the isomerohydrolase step in the visual cycle was affected by the absence of CRALBP. Dark adaptation was delayed in both cone and rod visual pathways in $Rlbp1^{-/-}$ animals as measured by ERG. These results are consistent with studies in humans with mutations in the *RLBP1* gene demonstrating dramatic delays in both rod and cone branches of dark adaptation curves (Bursedt et al., 2001).

The results of these studies for the rod system are most readily understood if apo-CRALBP accepts 11-*cis*-retinol from the isomerohydrolase, a role for the protein that is well established in vitro (Winston and Rando, 1998). However, it is important to note that the absence of CRALBP in mice resulted only in a delay in visual pigment regeneration, not a complete block. Some other molecule may be present or induced in the knockout that can fulfill the role of CRALBP, if less efficiently.

Albino $Rlbp1^{-/-}$ mice were protected from light damage (Saari et al., 2001). Other laboratories also observed that delays in the visual cycle resulted in protection from light damage (Sieving et al., 2001; Grimm et al., 2000). Retinoid analysis of $Rlbp1^{-/-}$ mice established that a diminished regeneration rate caused photoreceptor retinoids to accumulate as the relatively innocuous retinyl esters in RPE during constant illumination (Garwin and Saari, 2008). This and the resulting diminished amount of potentially toxic all-*trans*-retinaldehyde in flux are likely to account for this protective effect. It is interesting to note that pharmacological inhibition of the visual cycle has been proposed as a potential means of delaying the onset of some inherited retinal diseases (reviewed in Travis et al., 2006).

Retinoid Flow in the Visual Cycle The kinetics of appearance and disappearance of visual cycle retinoids during recovery from a flash or from constant illumination has been followed over the years using methods with increasing resolving power and sensitivity. Initial studies reported the flow of retinoids between neural retina and RPE long before sophisticated methods of retinoid separation were available (Dowling, 1960). More recent studies employing high-performance liquid chromatography (HPLC) analysis have identified slow steps based on the accumulation and decay of visual cycle intermediates. Early HPLC studies (Saari et al., 1998) were done in mice of mixed genetic backgrounds, before the effect of *Rpe65* sequence variations on regeneration rates was understood (Wenzel et al., 2001). Nonetheless, these and other studies clearly demonstrated the accumulation and slow decay of all-*trans*-retinal during recovery in the dark following a flash (Dowling, 1960; Saari et al., 1998; Palczewski et al., 1999; Qtaishat et al., 1999). Later studies with inbred strains of mice corroborated the slow decay of all-*trans*-retinal and also noted the accumulation and slow decay of all-*trans*-retinyl esters during recovery in the dark (Saari et al., 2001). Thus, there appeared to be two slow steps in the flow of retinoids leading to regeneration of rhodopsin following a flash, one related to the reduction of all-*trans*-retinal and the other related to the isomerohydrolase step. Based on the apparent decay rates for the two intermediates, processing of all-*trans*-retinyl ester, presumably by isomerohydrolase, appeared to be the slowest step. A similar conclusion was reached via mathematical analysis of flash-recovery data (Lamb and Pugh, 2004).

Other studies had demonstrated that the rate of visual pigment regeneration characteristic of various strains of mice was proportional to the amount of RPE65 (isomerohydrolase) in their retinas (Grimm et al., 2000). Retinoid analysis of mice during steady illumination provided additional information (Garwin and Saari, 2008). All-*trans*-retinal rose to a maximum and decayed to low levels during the illumination period, whereas all-*trans*-retinyl esters accumulated to a plateau and remained elevated until the light was extinguished. These results demonstrate the two slow steps but indicate that decay of all-*trans*-retinyl esters (isomerohydrolase reaction) is the slower of the two.

Thus, retinoid analyses identified visual cycle intermediates that accumulated during recovery from either flash or steady illumination. Because both reactions that process these intermediates are complicated, we do not know what limits the rates. For instance, the rate of reduction of all-*trans*-retinal by NADPH could be controlled by several processes, including the intrinsic turnover rate and amount of the enzyme, the rate of production of NADPH, the rate of release of all-*trans*-retinal from opsin, or an active control process. Similarly, the rate of isomerization and cleavage of all-*trans*-retinyl ester could be limited by processes including the rate of the isomerohydrolase reaction itself, removal of product by apo-CRALBP, substrate delivery of all-*trans*-retinyl ester to the enzyme, or active control of the reaction rate.

Cone visual cycle

The cone visual cycle has been more difficult to approach experimentally because of the relatively few cones in most retinas used in the laboratory for biochemical studies. Circumstantial evidence has implicated Müller cells in cone visual pigment regeneration for decades. Recently, considerable progress has been made in characterizing reactions that may be involved in a cone visual cycle. It will be of great interest to learn whether novel reactions occur in Müller cells. Our understanding of this putative pathway lags behind that of the rod regeneration pathway.

It is not surprising that many aspects of visual pigment regeneration in rod and cone photoreceptor cells are dramatically different. Rod and cone visual pigments were designed to function in totally different illumination environments. In addition, rods outnumber cones in mammalian retinas by about 30 to one, setting up the possibility of competition for 11-*cis*-retinal. Bleached salamander cone photoreceptors in vitro will regenerate their visual pigment with exogenous 11-*cis*-retinol, whereas rods require 11-*cis*-retinal (Jones et al., 1989). It is possible that this specificity reduces the competition between rods and cones for 11-*cis*-retinoids. In salamander retina, isolated cones regenerate when 11-*cis*-retinal is applied to either their inner or outer segments, whereas rods regenerate only when 11-*cis*-retinal is applied to the outer segments (Jin et al., 1994). This implies that cones could utilize a source of 11-*cis*-retinoid near their inner segments, possibly Müller cells. Bleached cone photoreceptors in neural retina, separated from RPE, resensitize in the dark, whereas bleached rod photoreceptors require the apposition of RPE (Goldstein and Wolf, 1973), again implying that a source of 11-*cis*-retinol must exist within cells of the neural retina. Müller cells contain both CRBPI and CRALBP (Saari and Crabb, 2005), and cultured chicken Müller cells synthesize 11-*cis*-retinol from all-*trans*-retinol (Das et al., 1992; Muniz et al., 2006). Recently, enzyme activities of a putative cone visual cycle have been identified in retinal extracts of ground squirrels and chickens (Arshavsky, 2002; Mata et al., 2002). Thus, considerable indirect evidence exists for a distinct cone visual cycle in Müller cells. However, much of the evidence comes from studies of amphibian or avian retina, and it is not certain that the same features apply to mammalian retina. The cone visual cycle depicted in figure 59.2 is based on that proposed by Travis and co-workers (Mata et al., 2002).

Proteomic analysis of the visual cycle

Proteomics, within the context of this article, refers to the identification of the proteins within a tissue, organ, organelle, or tissue fraction using mass spectrometric analysis. Few studies have directly addressed questions related to the visual cycle with this approach. However, the information obtained from studies with other primary goals has often provided useful insight regarding visual cycle components.

Analysis of Interacting Components As discussed elsewhere in this chapter, apo-CRALBP is likely to bind 11-*cis*-

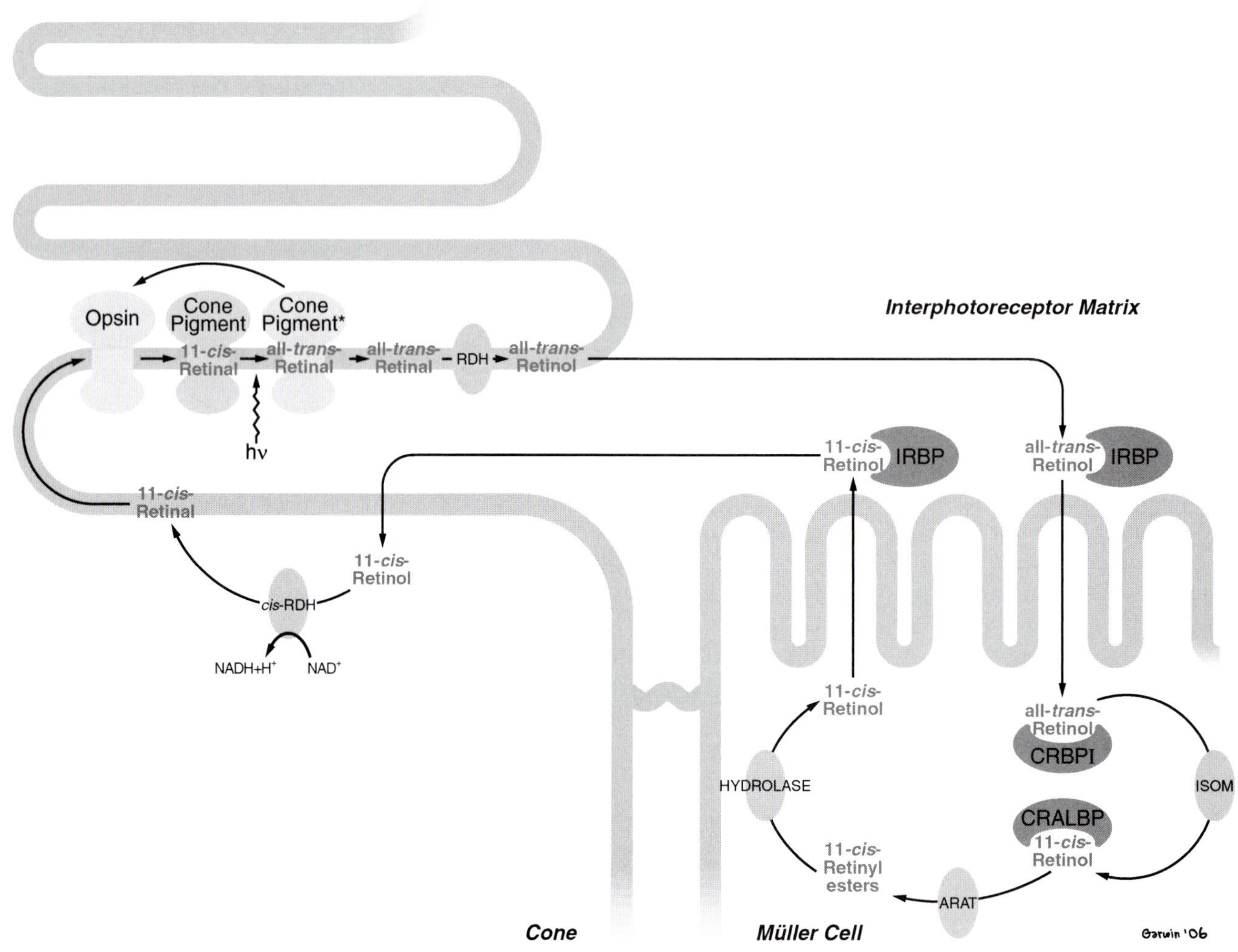

Figure 59.2 Hypothetical schematic of the cone photoreceptor visual cycle. Transcellular diffusion and intracellular enzymatic processing of cone visual cycle retinoids are shown. Structure at *left* depicts a portion of the inner and outer segments of a cone photoreceptor cell. Structure at *right* depicts the apical end of a Müller cell. The cells are joined by structures of the external limiting membrane (*short wavy line*). ARAT, acylCoA:retinol acyltransferase; HYDROLASE, 11-*cis*-retinyl ester hydrolase; ISOM, isomerase. See also the abbreviation key for figure 59.1. See color plate 69. (After Mata et al., 2002.)

retinol, the product of the isomerohydrolase reaction, and relieve product inhibition of the enzyme. Proteomic analyses have been used to analyze protein components interacting with CRALBP. In one approach, a component with high affinity for CRALBP was detected with a gel overlay assay and identified as EBP50/NHERF-1 (ERM-binding phosphoprotein50/sodium-hydrogen exchanger regulatory factor 1) by mass spectrometric analysis of the corresponding component from a two-dimensional (2D) gel (Nawrot et al., 2004). EBP50/NHERF-1 is a multivalent organizer that can link various proteins with affinity for its two PDZ domains to the cytoskeleton via a C-terminal domain that binds ezrin, radixin, or moesin, proteins with affinity for actin (Bretscher et al., 2002). CRALBP, EBP50/NHERF-1, ezrin, and actin are all found in the apical processes of RPE cells, indicating the potential for interaction in vivo (Nawrot et al., 2004). EBP50/NHERF-1 may organize a retinoid-processing complex in the apical processes of RPE (Nawrot et al., 2006).

In a second proteomic approach, a preparation enriched in mouse RPE apical processes was isolated using wheat germ agglutinin-affinity chromatography, and protein components within it were identified using mass spectrometry (Bonilha et al., 2004a). Several visual cycle components were identified, including IRBP, CRALBP, EBP50/NHERF-1, CRBPI, 11-RDH, and ezrin. Furthermore, this approach, in combination with immunohistochemistry, allowed identification of more than 200 proteins from preparations of mouse RPE apical microvilli that may participate in the maintenance, support, and biochemical processes occurring at this critical interface with photoreceptors (Bonilha et al., 2004b). These results support other studies providing evidence for a retinoid-processing complex in apical RPE.

In a third and ongoing approach, immunoprecipitation (IP) with or without iTRAQ quantitative mass spectrometric methods has been used to probe for visual cycle protein interactions in bovine RPE microsomes. IP experiments with the purified recombinant proteins RDH5 and CRALBP support a structural interaction in a C-terminal region of CRALBP (Wu et al., 2005). As noted earlier in the discussion of 11-*cis*-retinol dehydrogenase, several lines of evidence support a functional interaction between CRALBP and RDH5 (Saari and Bredberg, 1982; Saari et al., 1994; Golovleva et al., 2003). iTRAQ technology utilizes amine-specific tags and yields diagnostic reporter ions during MS/MS analysis of the labeled peptides, the intensity of which provides relative protein quantification. iTRAQ quantitative analysis of anti-CRALBP IP products from RPE microsomes supports a possible retinoid-processing protein complex composed of CRALBP, RPE65, LRAT, RDH5, and RGR (Gu et al., 2006). Comparative quantification of visual cycle reciprocal IP products is being used to further evaluate the composition of this putative RPE protein complex.

In other studies, proteomics has been instrumental in identifying posttranslational modifications and functional domains within visual cycle proteins. Two noteworthy examples include RPE65 and CRALBP. MALDI TOF mass spectrometric analyses of affinity purified RPE65 provided the first compelling evidence that RPE65 was posttranslationally modified and supported the presence in RPE of both a cytosolic, lower-mass isoform and a membrane-associated, higher-mass isoform (Ma et al., 2001). More recently, Rando and co-workers used mass spectrometry to characterize tryptic peptides from RPE65 and reported the presence of three palmitoylated cysteine residues in the membrane-associated isoform. They suggested that palmitoylation may serve as a switching mechanism controlling RPE65 ligand-binding selectivity (Xue et al., 2004). However, others have reported that mutating these three cysteine residues has little effect on isomerase activity, so the role of posttranslational modifications in RPE65 functions remains to be determined (Redmond et al., 2005; Takahashi et al., 2006).

Photoaffinity labeling and proteomic high-resolution topological analyses have been particularly useful in understanding the functional domains of CRALBP involved in ligand and protein interactions (Z. Wu et al., 2004). Eight photoaffinity-modified residues in human CRALBP were identified by liquid chromatography tandem mass spectrometry, several of which had been independently identified using other protein chemical methods and site-directed mutagenesis. Topological analysis of apo- and holo-CRALBP by hydrogen-deuterium exchange and mass spectrometry demonstrated that residues 198–255 incorporated significantly less deuterium when the retinoid-binding pocket was occupied with 11-*cis*-retinal. This hydrophobic region encompasses all but one of the photolabeled residues. In a structural model of CRALBP based on the crystal structures of three CRAL_TRIO family members, all of the photolabeled residues lined the ligand-binding cavity except one, which appears to reside in a flexible loop at the entrance/exit of the ligand cavity. The topological analyses also supported the solvent accessibility of CRALBP residues 147–157 and 262–275 and are consistent with a positively charged groove in the structural model that may be involved in protein interactions as proposed for other CRAL_TRIO family members (Z. Wu et al., 2004).

Conclusion

The past decade has produced an astounding amount of information on the pathway for regeneration of rod visual pigments, thanks to advances in mouse genetics, genetic manipulation, and proteomics. The pathway for regeneration of cones has been more difficult to approach experimentally because of the relatively small proportion of cones in mouse and bovine retinas. Despite these great advances, much remains to be learned about rod visual pigment regeneration. For example, the molecular entities responsible for the dehydrogenase activities of the visual cycle remain to be assigned, and the cone pathway remains poorly understood. In addition, the cell biology of retinoid processing and transfer remains to be worked out. We expect many of these problems to be solved as increasingly clever ways of utilizing mouse genomics and proteomics evolve.

ACKNOWLEDGMENTS Work was supported by NIH grant nos. EY02317, EY06603, EY014239, and EY015638 and by Research to Prevent Blindness, Inc., Foundation Fighting Blindness, the Cleveland Clinic Foundation, and the Milton and Ruth Steinbach fund. The authors thank Gregory G. Garwin for help with the illustrations.

REFERENCES

ALLIKMETS, R., SINGH, N., SUN, H., SHROYER, N. F., HUTCHINSON, A., CHIDAMBARAM, A., GERRARD, B., BAIRD, L., STAUFFER, D., et al. (1997). A photoreceptor cell-specific ATP-binding transporter gene (*ABCR*) is mutated in recessive Stargardt macular dystrophy. *Nat. Genet.* 15:236–246.

ARSHAVSKY, V. Y. (2002). Like night and day: Rods and cones have different pigment regeneration pathways. *Neuron* 36:1–4.

BATTEN, M. L., IMANISHI, Y., MAEDA, T., TU, D. C., MOISE, A. R., BRONSON, D., POSSIN, D., VAN GELDER, R. N., BAEHR, W., et al. (2004). Lecithin-retinol acyltransferase is essential for accumulation of all-*trans*-retinyl esters in the eye and in the liver. *J. Biol. Chem.* 279:10422–10432.

Batten, M. L., Imanishi, Y., Tu, D. C., Doan, T., Zhu, L., Pang, J., Glushakova, L., Moise, A. R., Baehr, W., et al. (2005). Pharmacological and rAAV gene therapy rescue of visual functions in a blind mouse model of Leber congenital amaurosis. *PLoS* 2:1177–1189.

Båvik, C. O., Eriksson, U., Allen, R. A., and Peterson, P. A. (1991). Identification and partial characterization of a retinal pigment epithelial membrane receptor for plasma retinol-binding protein. *J. Biol. Chem.* 266:14978–14985.

Bazan, N. G., Reddy, T. S., Redmond, T. M., Wiggert, B., and Chader, G. J. (1985). Endogenous fatty acids are covalently and noncovalently bound to interphotoreceptor retinoid-binding protein in the monkey retina. *J. Biol. Chem.* 260:13677–13680.

Bernstein, P. S., Law, W. C., and Rando, R. R. (1987). Isomerization of all-*trans*-retinoids to 11-*cis*-retinoids in vitro. *Proc. Natl. Acad. Sci. U.S.A.*, 84:1849–1853.

Bernstein, P., and Rando, R. R. (1986). *In vivo* isomerization of all-*trans*- to 11-*cis*-retinoids in the eye occurs at the alcohol oxidation state. *Biochemistry* 25:6473–6578.

Berry, R. J., Cañada, F. J., and Rando, R. R. (1989). Solubilization and partial purification of retinyl esters synthetase and retinoid isomerase from bovine ocular pigment epithelium. *J. Biol. Chem.* 264:9231–9238.

Bok, D., and Heller, J. (1967). Transport of retinol from the blood to the retina: An autoradiographic study of the pigment epithelial cell surface receptor for plasma retinol-binding protein. *Exp. Eye Res.* 22:395–402.

Bok, D., Ong, D. E., and Chytil, F. (1984). Immunocytochemical localization of cellular retinol binding protein in the rat retina. *Invest. Ophthalmol. Vis. Sci.* 25:877–883.

Bonilha, V. L., Bhattacharya, S. K., West, K. A., Crabb, J. S., Sun, J., Rayborn, M. E., Nawrot, M., Saari, J. C., and Crabb, J. W. (2004a). Support for a proposed retinoid-processing protein complex in apical retinal pigment epithelium. *Exp. Eye Res.* 79:419–422.

Bonilha, V. L., Bhattacharya, S. K., West, K. A., Sun, J., Crabb, J. W., Rayborn, M. E., and Hollyfield, J. G. (2004b). Proteomic characterization of isolated retinal pigment epithelium microvilli. *Mol. Cell. Proteomics* 3:1119–1127.

Bretscher, A., Edwards, K., and Fehon, R. G. (2002). ERM proteins and merlin: Integrators at the cell cortex. *Nat. Rev. Molec. Cell Biol.* 3:586–599.

Bunt-Milam, A. H., and Saari, J. C. (1983). Immunocytochemical localization of two retinoid-binding proteins in vertebrate retina. *J. Cell Biol.* 97:703–712.

Burstedt, M. S. I., Forsman-Semb, K., Golovleva, I., Janunger, T., Wachtmeister, L., and Sandgren, O. (2001). Ocular phenotype of Bothnia dystrophy, an autosomal recessive retinitis pigmentosa associated with an R234W mutation in the RLBP1 gene. *Arch. Ophthalmol.* 119:260–267.

Carlson, A., and Bok, D. (1992). Promotion of the release of 11-*cis*-retinal from cultured retinal pigment epithelium by interphotoreceptor retinoid-binding protein. *Biochemistry* 31:9056–9062.

Cerignoli, F., Guo, X., Cardinali, B., Rinaldi, C., Casaletto, J., Frati, L., Screpanti, I., Gudas, L. J., Gulino, A., et al. (2002). retSDR1, a short-chain retinol dehydrogenase/reductase, is retinoic acid-inducible and frequently deleted in human neuroblastoma cell lines. *Cancer Res.* 62:1196–1204.

Danciger, M., Matthes, M. T., Yasamura, D., Akhmedov, N. B., Rickabaugh, T., Gentleman, S., Redmond, T. M., LaVail, M. M., and Farber, D. B. (2000). A QTL on distal chromosome 3 that influences the severity of light-induced damage to mouse photoreceptors. *Mamm. Genome* 11:422–427.

Das, S. R., Bhardwaj, N., Kjeldbye, H., and Gouras, P. (1992). Müller cells of chicken retina synthesize 11-*cis*-retinol. *Biochem. J.* 285:907–913.

Deigner, P. S., Law, W. C., Canada, F. J., and Rando, R. R. (1989). Membranes as the energy source in the endergonic transformation of vitamin A to 11-*cis*-retinol. *Science* 244:968–971.

Dowling, J. (1960). Chemistry of visual adaptation in the rat. *Nature* 188:114–118.

Driessen, C. C. G. G., Winkens, J. J., Hoffmann, K., Kuhlmann, L. D., Janssen, B.P.M., Van Vugt, A. H. M., Van Hooser, J. P., Wieringa, B. E., Deutman, A. F., et al. (2000). Disruption of the 11-*cis*-retinol dehydrogenase gene leads to accumulation of *cis*-retinols and *cis*-retinyl esters. *Mol. Cell. Biol.* 20:4275–4287.

Garwin and Saari (2008). Unpublished results.

Ghyselinck, N. B., Bavik, C., Sapin, V., Mark, M., Bonnier, D., Hindelang, C., Dierich, A., Nilsson, C. B., Hakansson, H., et al. (1999). Cellular retinol-binding protein I is essential for vitamin A homeostasis. *EMBO J.* 18:4903–4914.

Goldstein, E. B., and Wolf, B. M. (1973). Regeneration of the green-rod pigment in the isolated frog retina. *Vision Res.* 13: 527–534.

Golovleva, I., Bhattacharya, S., Wu, Z., Shaw, N., Yang, Y., Andrabi, K., West, K. A., Burstedt, S. I., Forsman, K., et al. (2003). Disease-causing mutations in the cellular retinaldehyde-binding protein tighten and abolish ligand interactions. *J. Biol. Chem.* 278:12397–12402.

Gonzalez-Fernandez, F. (2003). Interphotoreceptor retinoid-binding protein: An old gene for new eyes. *Vision Res.* 43: 3021–3036.

Grimm, C., Wenzel, A., Hafezi, F., Yu, S., Redmond, T. M., and Reme, C. E. (2000). Protection of Rpe65-deficient mice identifies rhodopsin as a mediator of light-induced retinal degeneration. *Nat. Genet.* 25:63–66.

Gu, X., Crabb, J. S., Nawrot, M., Saari, J. C., and Crabb, J. W. (2006). Quantitative mass spectrometric analysis of visual cycle protein interactions. In *Proceedings of the 54th ASMS Conference on Mass Spectrometry and Allied Topics*, Seattle, Washington, May 28–June 1, 2006. Citation no. A063296.

Haeseleer, F., Huang, J., Lebioda, L., Saari, J. C., and Palczewski, K. (1998). Molecular characterization of a novel short-chain dehydrogenase/reductase that reduces all-*trans*-retinal. *J. Biol. Chem.* 273:21790–21799.

Haeseleer, F., Jang, G.-F., Imanishi, Y., Driessen, C. A. G. G., Matsumura, M., Nelson, P. S., and Palczewski, K. (2002). Dual substrate specficity short chain retinol dehydrogenases from the vertebrate retina. *J. Biol. Chem.* 277:45537–45546.

Hamel, C. P., Tsilou, E., Pfeffer, B. A., Hooks, J. J., Detrick, B., and Redmond, T. M. (1993). Molecular cloning and expression of RPE65, a novel retinal pigment epithelium-specific microsomal protein that is post-transcriptionally regulated in vitro. *J. Biol. Chem.* 268:15751–15757.

Herr, F. M., and Ong, D. E. (1992). Differential interaction of lecithin-retinol acyltransferase with cellular retinol binding proteins. *Biochemistry* 31:6748–6755.

Janecke, A. R., Thompson, E. A., Utermann, G., Becker, C., Hübner, C. A., Schmid, E., McHenry, C. L., Nair, A. R., Ruschendorf, F., et al. (2004). Mutations in *RDH12* encoding a photoreceptor cell retinol dehydrogenase cause childhood-onset severe retinal dystrophy. *Nat. Genet.* 36:850–854.

Jiang, M., Pandey, S., and Fong, H. K. W. (1993). An opsin homologue in the retina and pigment epithelium. *Invest. Ophthalmol. Vis. Sci.* 34:3669–3678.

Jin, J., Jones, G. J., and Cornwall, M. C. (1994). Movement of retinal along cone and rod photoreceptors. *Vis. Neurosci.* 11: 389–399.

Jin, M., Li, S., Moghrabi, W. N., Sun, H., and Travis, G. H. (2005). Rpe65 is the retinoid isomerase in bovine retinal pigment epithelium. *Cell* 122:449–459.

Jones, G. J., Crouch, R. K., Wiggert, B., Cornwall, M. C., and Chader, G. J. (1989). Retinoid requirements for recovery of sensitivity after visual-pigment bleaching in isolated photoreceptors. *Proc. Natl. Acad. Sci. U.S.A.* 86:9606–9610.

Kawaguchi, R., Yu, J., Honda, J., Whitelegge, J., Ping, P., Wiita, P., Bok, D., and Sun, H. (2007). A membrane receptor for retinol binding protein mediates cellular uptake of vitamin A. *Science* 315:820–825.

Kim, T. S., Maeda, A., Maeda, T., Heinlein, C., Kedishvili, N., Palczewski, K., and Nelson, P. S. (2005). Delayed dark adaptation in 11-*cis*-retinol dehydrogenase-deficient mice. *J. Biol. Chem.* 280:8694–8704.

Kloer, D. P., Ruch, S., Al-Babili, S., Beyer, P., and Schulz, G. E. (2005). The structure of a retinal-forming carotenoid oxygenase. *Science* 308:267–269.

Kurth, I., Thompson, D. A., Rüther, K., Feathers, K., Chrispell, J., Schroth, J., McHenry, C., Schweizer, M., Skosyrski, S., et al. (2007). Targeted disruption of the murine retinal dehydrogenase gene *Rdh12* does not inhibit visual cycle function. *Mol. Cell Biol.* 27:1370–1379.

Lamb, T. D., and Pugh E. N., Jr. (2004). Dark adaptation and the retinoid cycle of vision. *Prog. Retin. Eye Res.* 23:307–380.

Liou, G. I., Fei, Y., Peachey, N. S., Matragoon, S., Wei, S., Blaner, W. S., Wang, Y., Liu, C., Gottesman, M. E., et al. (1998). Early onset photoreceptor abnormalities induced by targeted disruption of the interphotoreceptor retinoid-binding protein gene. *J. Neurosci.* 18:4511–4520.

Ma, J., Zhang, J., Othersen, K. L., Moiseyev, G., Ablonczy, Z., Redmond, T. M., Chen, Y., and Crouch, R. K. (2001). Expression, purification, and MALDI analysis of RPE65. *Invest. Ophthalmol. Vis. Sci.* 42:1429–1435.

Maeda, A., Maeda, T., Imanishi, Y., Kuksa, V., Alexseev, A., Bronson, J. D., Zhang, H., Sun, W., Saperstein, D. A., et al. (2005). Role of photoreceptor-specific retinol dehydrogenase in the retinoid cycle *in vivo*. *J. Biol. Chem.* 280:18822–18832.

Maeda, A., Maeda, T., Imanishi, Y., Sun, W., Jastrzebska, B., Hatala, D. A., Winkens, H. J., Hofmann, K. P., Janssen, J. J., et al. (2006). Retinol dehydrogenase (RDH12) protects photoreceptors from light-induced degeneration in mice. *J Biol Chem.* 281:37697–37704.

Mata, N. L., Radu, R. A., Clemmons, R. S., and Travis, G. H. (2002). Isomerization and oxidation of vitamin A in cone-dominant retinas: A novel pathway for visual pigment regeneration in daylight. *Neuron* 36:69–80.

Moiseyev, G., Takahashi, Y., Chen, Y., Gentleman, S., Redmond, T. M., Crouch, R. K., and Ma, J.-X. (2006). RPE65 is an iron(II)-dependent isomerohydrolase in the retinoid visual cycle. *J. Biol. Chem.* 281:2835–2840.

Morimura, H., Saindelle-Ribeaudeau, F., Berson, E. L., and Dryja, T. P. (1999). Mutations in RGR, encoding a light-sensitive opsin homologue, in patients with retinitis pigmentosa. *Nat. Genet.* 23:393–394.

Muniz, A., Vilazana-Espinoza, E. T., Thackeray, B., and Tsin, A.T.C. (2006). 11-*cis*-acyl-CoA:retinol *O*-acyltransferase activity in the primary culture of chicken Müller cells. *Biochemistry* 45: 12265–12273.

Nakamura, M., Hotta, Y., Tanikawa, A., Terasake, H., and Miyake, Y. (2000). A high association with cone dystrophy in fundus albipunctatus by mutations of the *RHD5* gene. *Invest. Ophthalmol. Vis. Sci.* 41:3925–3932.

Napoli, J. L. (1999). Interactions of retinoid binding proteins and enzymes in retinoid metabolism. *Biochim. Biophys. Acta* 1440: 139–162.

Nawrot, M., Liu, T., Garwin, G. G., Crabb, J. W., and Saari, J. C. (2006). Scaffold proteins and the regeneration of visual pigments. *Photochem. Photobiol.* 82:1482–1488.

Nawrot, M., West, K., Huang, J., Possin, D. E., Bretscher, A., Crabb, J. W., and Saari, J. C. (2004). Cellular retinaldehyde-binding protein interacts with ERM-binding phosphoprotein 50 in retinal pigment epithelium. *Invest. Ophthalmol. Vis. Sci.* 45: 393–401.

Palczewski, K., Van Hooser, J. P., Garwin, G. G., Chen, J., Liou, G. I., and Saari, J. C. (1999). Kinetics of visual pigment regeneration in excised mouse eyes and in mice with a targeted disruption of the gene encoding interphotoreceptor retinoid-binding protein or arrestin. *Biochemistry* 38:12012–12019.

Pasutto, F., Sticht, H., Hammersen, G., Gillessen-Kaesbach, G., FitPatrick, D. R., Nürnberg, G., Brasch, F., Schirmer-Zimmermann, H., Tolmie, J. L., et al. (2007). Mutations in *STRA6* cause a broad spectrum of malformations including anophthalmia, congenital heart defects, diaphragmatic hernia, alveolar capillary dysplasia, lung hypoplasia, and mental retardation. *Am. J. Hum. Genet.* 80:550–560.

Pepperberg, D. R., Okajima, T.-I. L., Wiggert, B., Ripps, H., Crouch, R. K., and Chader, G. J. (1993). Interphotoreceptor retinoid-binding binding protein. *Mol. Neurobiol.* 7:61–84.

Quadro, L., Blaner, W. S., Salchow, D. J., Vogel, S., Piantedosi, R., Gouras, P., Freeman, S., Cosma, M. P., Colantuoni, V., et al. (1999). Impaired retinal function and vitamin A availability in mice lacking retinol-binding protein. *EMBO J.* 18:4633–4644.

Qtaishat, N. M., Okajima, T.-I. L., Li, S., Naash, M. I., and Pepperberg, D. R. (1999). Retinoid kinetics in eye tissues of VPP transgenic mice and their normal littermates. *Invest. Ophthalmol. Vis. Sci.* 40:1040–1049.

Rattner, A., Smallwood, P. M., and Nathans, J. (2000). Identification and characterization of all-*trans*-retinol dehydrogenase from photoreceptor outer segments, the visual cycle enzyme that reduces all-*trans*-retinal to all-*trans*-retinol. *J. Biol. Chem.* 275: 11034–11043.

Redmond, T. M., Poliakov, E., Yu, S., Tsai, J.-Y., and Gentleman, S. (2005). Mutation of key residues of RPE65 abolishes its enzymatic role as isomerohydrolase in the visual cycle. *Proc. Natl. Acad. Sci. U.S.A.* 102:13658–13663.

Redmond, T. M., Yu, S., Lee, E., Bok, D., Hamasaki, D., Chen, N., Goletz, P., Ma, J.-X., Crouch, R. K., et al. (1998). *Rpe65* is necessary for production of 11-cis-vitamin A in the retinal visual cycle. *Nat. Genet.* 20:344–351.

Ripps, H., Peachey, N. S., Xu, X., Nozell, S. E., Smith, S. B., and Liou, G. I. (2000). The rhodopsin cycle is preserved in IRBP "knockout" mice despite abnormalities in retinal structure and function. *Vis. Neurosci.* 17:97–105.

Rodieck, R. W. (1998). *The first steps in seeing.* Sunderland, MA: Sinauer.

Ruiz, A., Kuehn, M. H., Andorf, J. L., Stone, E., Hageman, G. S., and Bok, D. (2001). Genomic organization and mutation analysis of the gene encoding lecithin retinol acyltransferase in human retinal pigment epithelium. *Invest. Ophthalmol. Vis. Sci.* 42:31–37.

Ruiz, A., Winston, A., Lim, Y.-H. Gilbert, B. A., Rando, R. R., and Bok, D. (1999). Molecular and biochemical characterization of lecithin retinol acyltransferase. *J. Biol. Chem.* 274: 3834–3841.

Rushton, W. A. H. (1977). Visual adaptation. *Biophys. Struct. Mechanism* 3:159–162.

Saari, J. C., and Bredberg, L. (1982). Enzymatic reduction of 11-*cis*-retinal bound to cellular retinal-binding protein. *Biochim. Biophys. Acta* 716:266–272.

Saari, J. C., and Bredberg, D. L. (1989). Lecithin:retinol acyltransferase in retinal pigment epithelial microsomes. *J. Biol. Chem.* 264:8638–8640.

Saari, J. C., Bredberg, D. L., and Noy, N. (1994). Control of substrate flow at a branch in the visual cycle. *Biochemistry* 33: 3106–3112.

Saari, J. C., Bunt-Milam, A. H., Bredberg, D. L., and Garwin, G. G. (1984). Properties and immunocytochemical localization of three retinoid-binding proteins from bovine retina. *Vision Res.* 24:1595–1603.

Saari, J. C., and Crabb, J. W. (2005). Focus on molecules: Cellular retinaldehyde-binding protein (CRALBP). *Exp. Eye Res.* 81: 245–246.

Saari, J. C., Garwin, G. G., van Hooser, J. P., and Palczewski, K. (1998). Reduction of all-*trans*-retinal limits regeneration of visual pigment in mice. *Vision Res.* 38:1325–1333.

Saari, J. C., Nawrot, M., Garwin, G. G., Kennedy, M. J., Hurley, J. B., Ghyselinck, N. B., and Chambon, P. (2002). Analysis of the visual cycle in cellular retinol-binding protein type I (CRBPI) knockout mice. *Invest. Ophthalmol. Vis. Sci.* 43: 1730–1735.

Saari, J. C., Nawrot, M., Kennedy, B. N., Garwin, G. G., Hurley, J. B., Huang, J., Possin, D. E., and Crabb, J. W. (2001). Visual cycle impairment in cellular retinaldehyde binding protein (CRALBP) knockout mice results in delayed dark adaptation. *Neuron* 29:739–748.

Seeliger, M. W., Grimm, C., Stahlberg, F., Friedburg, C., Jaissle, G., Zrenner, E., Guo, H., Reme, C. E., Humphries, P., et al. (2001). New views on RPE65 deficiency: The rod system is the source of vision in a mouse model of Leber congenital amaurosis. *Nat. Genet.* 29:70–74.

Sieving, P. A., Chaudhry, P., Kondo, M., Provenzano, M., Wu, D., Carlson, T. J., Bush, R. A., and Thompson, D. A. (2001). Inhibition of the visual cycle in vivo by 13-*cis*-retinoic acid protects from light damage and provides a mechanism for night blindness in isotretinoid therapy. *Proc. Natl. Acad. Sci. U.S.A.* 98:1835–1840.

Simon, A., Hellman, U., Wernstedt, C., and Eriksson, U. (1995). The retinal pigment epithelial-specific 11-*cis* retinol dehydrogenase belongs to the family of short chain alcohol dehydrogenases. *J. Biol. Chem.* 270:1107–1112.

Takahashi, Y., Moiseyev, G., Chen, Y., and Ma, J.-X. (2006). The roles of three palmitoylation sites of RPE65 in its membrane association and isomerohydrolase activity. *Invest. Ophthalmol. Vis. Sci.* 47:5191–5196.

Travis, G. H., Golczak, M., Moise, A. R., and Palczewski, K. (2006). Diseases caused by defects in the visual cycle: Retinoids as potential therapeutic agents. *Annu. Rev. Pharmacol. Toxicol.* 47:469–512.

Vogel S., Piantedosi, R., O'Byrne, S. M., Kako, Y., Quadro, L., Gottesman, M. E., Goldberg, I. J., and Blaner, W. S. (2002). Retinol-binding protein-deficient mice: Biochemical basis for impaired vision. *Biochemistry* 41:15360–15368.

Wald, G., and Hubbard, R. (1949). The reduction of retinene$_1$ to vitamin A1 in vitro. *J. Gen. Physiol.* 32:367–389.

Weng, J., Mata, N. L., Azarian, S. M., Tzekov, R. T., Birch, D. G., and Travis, G. H. (1999). Insights into the function of rim protein in photoreceptors and etiology of Stargardt's disease from the phenotype in *abcr* knockout mice. *Cell* 98:13–23.

Wenzel, A., Oberhauser, V., Pugh, E. N., Jr., Lamb, T. D., Grimm, C., Samardzija, M., Fahl, E., Selliger, M. W., Reme, C. E., et al. (2005). The retinal G protein-coupled receptor (RGR) enhances isomerohydrolase activity independent of light. *J. Biol. Chem.* 280:29874–29884.

Wenzel, A., Remé, C. E., Williams, T. P., Hafezi, F., and Grimm, C. (2001). The *Rpe65* leu450met variation increases retinal resistance against light-induced degeneration by slowing rhodopsin regeneration. *J. Neurosci.* 21:53–58.

Winston, A., and Rando, R. R. (1998). Regulation of isomerohydrolase activity in the visual cycle. *Biochemistry* 37:2044–2050.

Wu, B. X., Moiseyev, G., Chen, Y., Rohrer, B., Crouch, R. K., and Ma, J.-X. (2004). Identification of RDH10, an all-*trans*-retinol dehydrogenase, in retinal Müller cells. *Invest. Ophthalmol. Vis. Sci.* 45:3857–3862.

Wu, Z., Bhattacharya, S. K., Jin, Z., Bonhila, V. L., Liu, T., Nawrot, M., Teller, D. C., Saari, J. C., and Crabb, J. W. (2005). CRALBP ligand and protein interactions. In J. G. Hollyfield, R. E. Anderson, and M. M. LaVail (Eds.), Retinal degenerative diseases. *Adv. Exp. Med. Biol.* 572:477–484.

Wu, Z., Hasan, A., Liu, T., Teller, D. C., and Crabb, J. W. (2004). Identification of the CRALBP ligand interactions by photoaffinity labeling, hydrogen/deuterium exchange and structural modeling. *J. Biol. Chem.* 279:27357–27364.

Xue, L., Gollapalli, D. R., Maiti, P., Jahng, W. J., and Rando, R. R. (2004). A palmitoylation switch mechanism in the regulation of the visual cycle. *Cell* 117:761–771.

Yamamoto, H., Simon, A., Eriksson, U., Harris, E., Berson, E. L., and Dryja, T. P. (1999). Mutations in the gene encoding 11-*cis*-retinol dehydrogenase cause delayed dark adaptation and fundus albipunctatus. *Nat. Genet.* 22:188–191.

CONTRIBUTORS

Badea, Tudor C. Johns Hopkins University Medical School, Baltimore, Maryland
Bear, Mark F. Picower Institute for Learning and Memory, Massachusetts Institute of Technology, Cambridge, Massachusetts
Berardi, Nicoletta Università di Firenze del Consiglio Nazionale delle Ricerche, Pisa, Italy
Berger, Wolfgang Division of Medical Molecular Genetics and Gene Diagnostics, Institute of Medical Genetics, University of Zurich, Zurich, Switzerland
Blankenship, Aaron G. Neurobiology Section, Division of Biological Sciences, University of California, La Jolla, California
Bloomfield, Stewart A. Department of Ophthalmology, New York University School of Medicine, New York, New York
Boye, Sanford L. Department of Ophthalmology and Molecular Genetics, University of Florida, Gainesville, Florida
Boye, Shannon E. Department of Ophthalmology and Molecular Genetics, University of Florida, Gainesville, Florida
Brown, Richard E. Department of Psychology, Dalhousie University, Nova Scotia, Canada
Burkhalter, Andreas Department of Anatomy and Neurobiology, Washington University School of Medicine, St. Louis, Missouri
Caspi, Rachel R. Laboratory of Immunology, National Eye Institute, National Institutes of Health, Bethesda, Maryland
Cenni, Maria Cristina Istituto di Neuroscienze del Consiglio Nazionale delle Ricerche, Pisa, Italy
Cepko, Constance L. Department of Genetics, Howard Hughes Medical Institute, Harvard Medical School, Boston, Massachusetts
Chalupa, Leo M. Section of Neurobiology, Physiology, and Behavior, University of California, Davis, California
Chang, Bo The Jackson Laboratory, Bar Harbor, Maine
Chen, Chinfei Division of Neuroscience and Neurobiology Program, Children's Hospital, Harvard Medical School, Boston, Massachusetts
Clancy, Barbara Department of Biology, University of Central Arkansas, Conway, Arkansas
Coombs, Julie L. Section of Neurobiology, Physiology, and Behavior, University of California, Davis, California
Crabb, John W. Department of Ophthalmic Research, Cole Eye Institute, Cleveland, Ohio
Danciger, Michael Department of Biology, Loyola Marymount University, Los Angeles, California
Daniele, Lauren L. Department of Ophthalmology, F. M. Kirby Center for Molecular Ophthalmology, University of Pennsylvania School of Medicine, Philadelphia, Pennsylvania
Dorrell, Michael I. Department of Cell Biology, Scripps Research Institute, La Jolla, California
Douglas, Robert M. Department of Ophthalmology and Vision Sciences, University of British Columbia, Vancouver, Canada
Dräger, Ursula C. Eunice Kennedy Shriver Center for Mental Retardation, University of Massachusetts Medical School, Waltham, Massachusetts
Dreher, Bogdan School of Medical Sciences and Bosch Institute, University of Sydney, Sydney, Australia
Dyer, Michael A. Department of Developmental Neurobiology, St. Jude Children's Research Hospital, Memphis, Tennessee
Erskine, Lynda School of Medical Sciences, Institute of Medical Sciences, University of Aberdeen, Aberdeen, Scotland
Feller, Marla B. Neurobiology Section, Division of Biological Sciences, University of California, Berkeley, California
Finlay, Barbara L. Department of Psychology, Cornell University, Ithaca, New York
Frenkel, Mikhail Y. Picower Institute for Learning and Memory, Massachusetts Institute of Technology, Cambridge, Massachusetts
Friedlander, Martin Department of Cell Biology, Scripps Research Institute, La Jolla, California
Galli-Resta, Lucia Istituto di Neuroscienze del Consiglio Nazionale delle Ricerche, Pisa, Italy
Geisert, Eldon E. Department of Ophthalmology, University of Tennessee Health Science Center, Memphis, Tennessee
Goldberg, Jeffrey L. Bascom Palmer Eye Institute, University of Miami, Miami, Florida
Graw, Jochen Institute of Developmental Genetics, German Research Center for Environmental Health, Helmholtz Center Munich, Neuherberg, Germany
Gregg, Ronald G. Departments of Ophthalmology and Visual Sciences and Biochemistry and Molecular Biology, University of Louisville, Louisville, Kentucky
Grubb, Matthew S. Medical Research Council Centre for Developmental Neurobiology, King's College London, London, England
Gubitosi-Klug, Rose A. Departments of Medicine and Ophthalmology, Case Western Reserve University, Cleveland, Ohio
Guido, William Department of Anatomy and Neurobiology, Virginia Commonweath University School of Medicine, Richmond, Virginia
Hauswirth, William W. Departments of Ophthalmology and Molecular Genetics, University of Florida, Gainesville, Florida
Hazlett, Linda D. Department of Anatomy/Cell Biology, Wayne State University School of Medicine, Detroit, Michigan
Hoehenwarter, Wolfgang Max Planck Institute for Infection Biology, Berlin, Germany
Hofer, Sonja B. Max Planck Institute of Neurobiology, Martinsried, Germany
Howell, Gareth R. The Jackson Laboratory, Bar Harbor, Maine
Hübener, Mark Max Planck Institute of Neurobiology, Martinsried, Germany
Isa, Tadashi Department of Developmental Physiology, National Institute for Physiological Sciences, Okazaki, Japan

Jang, Young P. Department of Ophthalmology, Columbia University, New York, New York

John, Simon W. M. The Jackson Laboratory, Bar Harbor, Maine

Jungblut, Peter R. Max Planck Institute for Infection Biology, Berlin, Germany

Karl, Mike O. University of Washington, School of Medicine, Seattle, Washington

Kellenberger, Antonia Institute of Human Anatomy and Embryology, University of Regensburg, Regensburg, Germany

Kern, Timothy S. Medicine and Ophthalmology, Case Western Reserve University, Cleveland, Ohio

Kim, So R. Department of Ophthalmology, Columbia University, New York, New York

Klein, William H. Department of Biochemistry and Molecular Biology, University of Texas, Houston, Texas

Lamba, Deepak University of Washington, School of Medicine, Seattle, Washington

Leamey, Catherine A. School of Medical Sciences and Bosch Institute, University of Sydney, Sydney, Australia

Luo, Tuanlian Eunice Kennedy Shriver Center for Mental Retardation, University of Massachusetts Medical School, Waltham, Massachusetts

Lyubarsky, Arkady Department of Ophthalmology, F. M. Kirby Center for Molecular Ophthalmology, University of Pennsylvania School of Medicine, Philadelphia, Pennsylvania

Maffei, Lamberto Istituto di Neuroscienze del Consiglio Nazionale delle Ricerche, Pisa, Italy

Marchant, Jeffrey K. Department of Anatomy and Cell Biology, Tufts University School of Medicine, Boston, Massachusetts

Mason, Carol A. Department of Pathology and Cell Biology, Center for Neurobiology and Behavior, Columbia University, New York, New York

Matsuda, Takahiko Department of Genetics and Howard Hughes Medical Institute, Harvard Medical School, Boston, Massachusetts

May, Christian-Albrecht Institut für Anatomie, Technological University of Dresden, Dresden, Germany

McCall, Maureen A. Department of Psychological and Brain Sciences, University of Louisville, Louisville, Kentucky

Mrsic-Flogel, Thomas D. Max Planck Institute of Neurobiology, Martinsried, Germany

Mu, Xiuqian Department of Biochemistry and Molecular Biology, University of Texas, Houston, Texas

Naggert, Juergen K. The Jackson Laboratory, Bar Harbor, Maine

Nathans, Jeremy Department of Molecular Biology and Genetics, Johns Hopkins University Medical School, Baltimore, Maryland

Nelson, Branden University of Washington, School of Medicine, Seattle, Washington

Nikonov, Sergei S. Department of Ophthalmology, F. M. Kirby Center for Molecular Ophthalmology, School of Medicine, University of Pennsylvania, Philadelphia, Pennsylvania

Nishina, Patsy M. The Jackson Laboratory, Bar Harbor, Maine

Panda, Satchidananda Regulatory Biology Laboratory, Salk Institute for Biological Studies, La Jolla, California

Parapuram, Sunil K. W. K. Kellogg Eye Center, University of Michigan, Ann Arbor, Michigan

Peachey, Neal S. Cleveland Veterans Affairs Medical Center, Cleveland Clinic Foundation, Cleveland, Ohio

Petros, Timothy J. Department of Pathology and Cell Biology, Center for Neurobiology and Behavior, Columbia University, New York, New York

Piatigorsky, Joram Laboratory of Molecular and Developmental Biology, National Eye Institute, National Institutes of Health, Bethesda, Maryland

Pinto, Lawrence H. Department of Neurobiology and Physiology and Center for Functional Genomics, Northwestern University, Evanston, Illinois

Porciatti, Vittorio Bascom Palmer Eye Institute, University of Miami Miller School of Medicine, Miami, Florida

Powers, Michael R. Oregon Health and Science University, Portland, Oregon; Bascom Palmer Eye Institute, University of Miami Miller School of Medicine, Miami, Florida

Protti, Dario A. School of Medical Sciences and Bosch Institute, University of Sydney, Sydney, Australia

Prusky, Glen T. Department of Neuroscience, Canadian Centre for Behavioural Neuroscience, University of Lethbridge, Alberta, Canada

Pugh, Edward N., Jr. Department of Ophthalmology, F. M. Kirby Center for Molecular Ophthalmology, University of Pennsylvania School of Medicine, Philadelphia, Pennsylvania

Reese, Benjamin E. Neuroscience Research Institute, University of California, Santa Barbara, California

Reh, Thomas A. Health Sciences Center, University of Washington, School of Medicine, Seattle, Washington

Rice, Dennis S. Lexicon Pharmaceuticals, The Woodlands, Texas

Robinson, Michael L. Zoology Department, Miami University, Oxford, Ohio

Saari, John C. Department of Ophthalmology, University of Washington, Seattle, Washington

Sakatani, Tomoya Department of Developmental Physiology, National Institute for Physiological Sciences, Okazaki, Japan

Sale, Alessandro Scuola Normale Superiore, Laboratory of Neurobiology, Pisa, Italy

Schaeffel, Frank Section of Neurobiology of the Eye, University Eye Hospital Tübingen, Tübingen, Germany

Sparrow, Janet R. Department of Ophthalmology, Columbia University, New York, New York

Stahl, John S. Department of Neurology, Case Western Reserve University, Cleveland, Ohio

Stone, Jonathan Research School of Biological Sciences, Australian National University, Canberra City, Australia

Strettoi, Enrica Istituto di Neuroscienze del Consiglio Nazionale delle Ricerche, Laboratorio di Neurofisiologia, Pisa, Italy

Swamynathan, Shivalingappa K. Laboratory of Molecular and Developmental Biology, National Eye Institute, National Institutes of Health, Bethesda, Maryland

Swaroop, Anand Neurobiology Neurodegeneration and Repair Laboratory, National Eye Institute, National Institutes of Health, Bethesda, Maryland; W. K. Kellogg Eye Center, University of Michigan, Ann Arbor, Michigan

Tamm, Ernst R. Institute of Human Anatomy and Embryology, University of Regensburg, Regensburg, Germany

Thompson, Hannah Institute of Ophthalmology, University College London, London, England

Tian, Ning Departments of Ophthalmology and Visual Science and Neurobiology, Yale University School of Medicine, New Haven, Connecticut

Troy, John B. Department of Biomedical Engineering, Northwestern University, Evanston, Illinois

Tucker, Priscilla K. Museum of Zoology, University of Michigan, Ann Arbor, Michigan

Valter, Krisztina Research School of Biological Sciences, Australian National University, Canberra City, Australia

Völgyi, Béla Department of Ophthalmology, New York University School of Medicine, New York, New York

Wagner, Elisabeth Eunice Kennedy Shriver Center for Mental Retardation, University of Massachusetts Medical School, Waltham, Massachusetts

Wang, Quanxin Department of Anatomy and Neurobiology, Washington University School of Medicine, St. Louis, Missouri

Williams, Robert W. Departments of Anatomy and Neurobiology and Pediatrics, University of Tennessee Health Science Center, Memphis, Tennessee

Wong, Aimée A. Department of Psychology, Dalhousie University, Nova Scotia, Canada

Zhou, Jilin Department of Ophthalmology, Columbia University, New York, New York

INDEX

Note: Page numbers followed by *f* indicate figures; page numbers followed by *t* indicate tables.

E

H

I

O